Rudolph's Fundamentals of

PEDIATRICS

Third Edition

Editors

Abraham M. Rudolph, MD
Emeritus Professor of Pediatrics and Senior Staff Member
Cardiovascular Research Institute
University of California, San Francisco
San Francisco, California

Robert K. Kamei, MD
Associate Professor of Clinical Pediatrics
Director, Residency Training Program
Department of Pediatrics
University of California, San Francisco
San Francisco, California

Kim J. Overby, MD
Pediatric Medical Care Coordinator
Child Welfare Division
Elwyn, Inc.
Elwyn, Pennsylvania

McGRAW-HILL
Medical Publishing Division

New York   Chicago   San Francisco   Lisbon   London   Madrid   Mexico City
Milan   New Delhi   San Juan   Seoul   Singapore   Sydney   Toronto

McGraw-Hill

A Division of The McGraw·Hill Companies

Rudolph's Fundamentals of Pediatrics, Third Edition

Copyright © 2002 by The **McGraw-Hill Companies**, Inc. Copyright © 1998 by Appleton & Lange, a Simon & Schuster Company; Copyright © 1994 by Appleton & Lange. All rights reserved. Printed in the United States of America. Except as permitted under the United States Copyright Act of 1976, no part of this publication may be reproduced or distributed in any form or by any means, or stored in a data base or retrieval system, without the prior written permission of the publisher.

1 2 3 4 5 6 7 8 9 0 DOC DOC 0 9 8 7 6 5 4 3 2
ISBN 0-8385-8450-0

Notice

Medicine is an ever-changing science. As new research and clinical experience broaden our knowledge, changes in treatment and drug therapy are required. The authors and the publisher of this work have checked with sources believed to be reliable in their efforts to provide information that is complete and generally in accord with the standards accepted at the time of publication. However, in view of the possibility of human error or changes in medical sciences, neither the authors nor the publisher nor any other party who has been involved in the preparation or publication of this work warrants that the information contained herein is in every respect accurate or complete, and they disclaim all responsibility for any errors or omissions or for the results obtained from use of such information contained in this work. Readers are encouraged to confirm the information contained herein with other sources. For example and in particular, readers are advised to check the product information sheet included in the package of each drug they plan to administer to be certain that the information contained in this work is accurate and that changes have not been made in the recommended dose or in the contraindications for administration. This recommendation is of particular importance in connection with new or infrequently used drugs.

This book was set in Adobe Garamond at Circle Graphics.
The editors were Shelley Reinhardt and Nicky Panton.
The production supervisor was Catherine H. Saggese.
The cover designer was Aimee Nordin.
The index was prepared by Jerry Ralya.

R.R. Donnelley and Sons Company was printer and binder.

This book is printed on acid-free paper.

Library of Congress Cataloging-in-Publication Data

Rudolph's fundamentals of pediatrics / editors, Abraham M. Rudolph, Robert K. Kamei,
Kim J. Overby.—3rd ed.
    p. ; cm.
  Includes bibliographical references and index.
  ISBN 0-8385-8450-0 (softcover : alk. paper)
  1. Pediatrics. I. Title: Fundamentals of pediatrics. II. Rudolph, Abraham M., 1924– III.
Kamei, Robert K. IV. Overby, Kim J.
  [DNLM: 1. Pediatrics. WS 200 R9165 2002]
RJ45 .R868 2002
618.92—dc21   2001054631

International Edition ISBN: 0-07-112442-X
Copyright © 2002. Exclusive rights by The McGraw-Hill Companies, Inc., for manufacture and export. This book cannot be re-exported from the country to which it is consigned by McGraw-Hill. The International Edition is not available in North America.

Contents

Authors

William Adelman, MD
Assistant Professor of Pediatrics
Uniformed Services University of the Health Sciences
Bethesda, Maryland;
Chief of Adolescent Medicine
Darnall Army Community Hospital
Fort Hood, Texas
Internet: William.adelman@amedd.army.mil
Adolescence

Ann Alpers, JD
Assistant Professor of Medicine
University of California, San Francisco
San Francisco, California
Internet: Anna@medicine.ucsf.edu
Ethical Issues in Pediatrics

Michael M. Brook, MD
Associate Professor
Department of Pediatrics
University of California, San Francisco
San Francisco, California
Internet: Mmbrook@pedcard.ucsf.edu
Circulation

Barbara A. Chini, MD
Assistant Professor of Pediatrics
University of Cincinnati School of Medicine;
Pediatric Pulmonologist
Children's Hospital Medical Center
Cincinnati, Ohio
Internet: barb.chini@chmcc.org
Respiratory Diseases

John Christodoulou, MB, BS, PhD, FRACP, CGHGSA
Associate Professor
Department of Paediatrics & Child Heath
University of Sydney;
Director, Western Sydney Genetics Program
Royal Alexandra Hospital for Children
Sydney, Australia
Internet: johnc@chw.edu.au
A Clinical Approach to Inborn Errors of Metabolism

Daniel L. Coury, MD
Professor of Clinical Pediatrics
The Ohio State University College of Medicine;
Chief, Section of Behavioral-Developmental Pediatrics
The Children's Hospital
Columbus, Ohio
Internet: dcoury@chi.osu.edu
Developmental & Behavioral Pediatrics

Cynthia R. Curry, MD
Director, Genetic Medicine
Valley Children's Hospital
Madera, California;
Professor of Pediatrics
University of California, San Francisco
San Francisco, California
Internet: Ccurry@valleychildrens.org
An Approach to Clinical Genetics

Mark E. Dato, MD, PhD
Section Head
Procter & Gamble Pharmaceuticals;
Adjunct Pediatric Pulmonologist
Children's Hospital Medical Center
Cincinnati, Ohio
Internet: Dato.me@pg.com
Respiratory Diseases

Francis J. DiMario, Jr., MD
Professor of Pediatrics and Neurology
The University of Connecticut School of Medicine
Farmington;
Associate Chair for Academic Affairs
Department of Pediatrics
and
Chief, Division of Pediatric Neurology
Connecticut Children's Medical Center
Hartford, Connecticut
Internet: Fdimari@ccmckids.org
The Nervous System

Dennis R. Durbin, MD
Assistant Professor of Pediatrics and Epidemiology
University of Pennsylvania School of Medicine;
Attending Physician
Division of Emergency Medicine
The Children's Hospital of Philadelphia
Philadelphia, Pennsylvania
Internet: Ddurbin@cceb.med.upenn.edu
Injuries & Emergencies

Lawrence F. Eichenfield, MD
Associate Clinical Professor of Pediatrics and
    Medicine (Dermatology)
University of California
San Diego School of Medicine;
Chief
Division of Pediatric and Adolescent Dermatology
Children's Hospital
San Diego, California
Internet: Leichenfield@chsd.org
Skin

Jonathan Ellen, MD
Associate Professor of Pediatrics, Epidemiology, and
 Family & Population Health Sciences
Division of General Pediatrics and Adolescent
  Medicine
Department of Pediatrics
Johns Hopkins University School of Medicine
Baltimore, Maryland
Internet: Jellen@jhmi.edu
Adolescence

Joel A. Fein, MD
Assistant Professor of Pediatrics
The University of Pennsylvania School of Medicine;
Attending Physician
Division of Emergency Medicine
The Children's Hospital of Philadelphia
Philadelphia, Pennsylvania
Internet: Fein@email.chop.edu
Injuries & Emergencies

Sheila Fallon Friedlander, MD
Associate Clinical Professor of Pediatrics and Medicine
  (Dermatology)
Division of Pediatric Dermatology
University of California, San Diego
  School of Medicine;
Staff Physician
Children's Hospital
San Diego, California
Internet: Sfriedlander@chsd.org
Skin

Stephen E. Gitelman, MD
Associate Professor of Clinical Pediatrics
Division of Pediatric Endocrinology;
and Director
Pediatric Diabetes Program
University of California, San Francisco
San Francisco, California
Internet: sgitelma@peds.ucsf.edu
Endocrinology

Caroline A. Hastings, MD
Pediatric Hematologist/Oncologist
Children's Hospital
Oakland, California;
Associate Clinical Professor
Department of Pediatrics
University of California, San Francisco
San Francisco, California
Internet: Chastings@mail.cho.org
Blood

Anna Huttenlocher, MD
Assistant Professor
Departments of Pediatrics and Pharmacology
University of Wisconsin Medical School;
Attending Physician
University of Wisconsin Hospital
Madison, Wisconsin
Internet: Huttenlocher@facstaff.wisc.edu
Immunologic Disorders

Ronald V. Keech, MD
Professor
Department of Ophthalmology
University of Iowa Hospitals and Clinics
Iowa City, Iowa
Internet: Ronald-keech@uiowa.edu
Ophthalmology

Donald Wayne Laney, Jr., MD
Assistant Professor of Pediatrics and Nutrition Sciences
University of Alabama School of Medicine,
   Birmingham;
Medical Director
North Alabama Children's Specialists
Huntsville, Alabama
Internet: Wlaney@pol.net
The Gastrointestinal Tract & Liver

Allan S. Lau, MD, FRCP(C)
Honorary Consultant
Department of Pediatrics
Queen Mary Hospital
Hong Kong
Internet: asylau@hkucc.hku.hk
Infectious Diseases

Deborah Lehman, MD
Associate Director of Pediatric Infectious Diseases and
Director, Pediatric HIV Center
Cedars Sinai Medical Center
Los Angeles, California;
Assistant Clinical Professor of Pediatrics
University of California
Los Angeles School of Medicine
Los Angeles, California
Internet: deborah.lehman@cshs.org
Infectious Diseases

Bernard Lo, MD
Professor of Medicine and Director
Program in Medical Ethics
University of California, San Francisco
San Francisco, California
Internet: Bernie@medicine.ucsf.edu
Ethical Issues in Pediatrics

Bertram H. Lubin, MD
Director of Medical Research
Children's Hospital Oakland Research Institute
Oakland, California
Internet: blubin@chori.org
Blood

Robert S. Mathias, MD
Associate Clinical Professor of Pediatrics
Division of Pediatric Nephrology
University of California, San Francisco
San Francisco, California
Internet: Rmathias@peds.ucsf.edu
Kidneys & Electrolytes

Mary Denise Moore, MD
Associate Professor of Clinical Pediatrics
University of Illinois College of Medicine at Rockford;
Staff Physician
Rockford Health System
Rockford, Illinois
Internet: Marymoore81@earthlink.net
Rheumatic Diseases

Phillip Moore, MD
Associate Professor
Department of Pediatrics, and
Director, Congenital Cardiac Catheterization Program
University of California, San Francisco
San Francisco, California
Internet: Pmoore@pedcard.ucsf.edu
Circulation

Kim J. Overby, MD
Pediatric Medical Care Coordinator
Child Welfare Division
Elwyn, Inc.
Elwyn, Pennsylvania
Internet: k.j.overby@worldnet.att.net
Pediatric Health Supervision

John Colin Partridge, MD, MPH
Clinical Professor
Department of Pediatrics
San Francisco General Hospital
San Francisco, California
Internet: cpartridge@sfghpeds.ucsf.edu
The Perinatal Period

Anthony A. Portale, MD
Professor of Pediatrics and Medicine;
Chief, Division of Pediatric Nephrology
University of California, San Francisco
San Francisco, California
Internet: Aportale@peds.ucsf.edu
Kidneys & Electrolytes

Donald E. Potter, MD
Clinical Professor of Pediatrics
Division of Pediatric Nephrology
University of California, San Francisco
San Francisco, California
Internet: Dpotter@peds.ucsf.edu
Kidneys & Electrolytes

Marta R. Rogido, MD
Assistant Professor of Pediatrics
Division of Neonatology
Emory University School of Medicine
Atlanta, Georgia
Internet: marta_rogido@oz.ped.emory.edu
The Perinatal Period

Stephen M. Rosenthal, MD
Professor of Pediatrics
Division of Pediatric Endocrinology
Department of Pediatrics
University of California San Francisco
San Francisco, California
Internet: Smr@itsa.ucsf.edu
Endocrinology

David R. Rozansky, MD, PhD
Assistant Professor
Division of Pediatric Nephrology
Department of Pediatrics
Oregon Health & Science University
Portland, Oregon
Internet: Rozansky@medicine.ucsf.edu
Kidneys & Electrolytes

Steven M. Selbst, MD
Professor of Pediatrics
Jefferson Medical College of Thomas Jefferson
    University
Philadelphia, Pennsylvania;
Vice Chairman and Residency Program Director
Department of Pediatrics;
Attending Physician
Division of Emergency Medicine
A.I. duPont Hospital for Children
Wilmington, Delaware
Internet: Sselbst@nemours.org
Injuries & Emergencies

Richard S. Shames, MD
Assistant Clinical Professor of Pediatrics
Stanford University School of Medicine
Stanford, California
Internet: Rshames@pdl.com
Allergy: Mechanisms & Disease Processes

John T. Smith, MD
Associate Clinical Professor
Department of Orthopedic Surgery
University of Utah School of Medicine
Salt Lake City, Utah
Internet: John.smith@hsc.utah.edu
Orthopedic Problems in Children

Augusto Sola, MD
Professor of Pediatrics
and Director, Division of Neonatology
Emory University School of Medicine
Atlanta, Georgia
Internet: augusto_sola@oz.ped.emory.edu
The Perinatal Period

Alan Uba, MD
Assistant Clinical Professor
Department of Pediatrics
University of California, San Francisco
San Francisco, California
Internet: auba@itsa.ucsf.edu
Infectious Diseases

George F. Van Hare, MD
Associate Professor
Department of Pediatrics
Stanford University School of Medicine
Stanford, California;
Associate Clinical Professor
Department of Pediatrics
University of California, San Francisco
San Francisco, California
Internet: Vanhare@leland.Stanford.EDU
Circulation

Diane Wara, MD
Professor of Pediatrics;
Chief, Division of Pediatric Immunology/Rheumatology;
Director, Pediatric Clinical Research Center
and Associate Dean for Women and Minority Affairs
University of California, San Francisco
San Francisco, California
Internet: warad@peds.ucsf.edu
Immunologic Disorders

Daniel C. West, MD
Assistant Professor of Pediatrics;
Director, Residency Training Program
University of California, Davis
Sacramento, California
Internet: Dcwest@ucdavis.edu
Cancer in Children

Judith V. Williams, MD
Assistant Professor of Clinical Internal Medicine
and Pediatrics
Eastern Virginia Medical School
Norfolk, Virginia
Skin

Robert W. Wilmott, MD
Professor and Chairman
Department of Pediatrics
St. Louis University School of Medicine
St. Louis, Missouri
Internet: wilmottr@slu.edu
Respiratory Diseases

Preface

In the first two editions, we attempted to create a text that provided a broad base of pediatric information using a problem-oriented clinical approach. From our experiences teaching medical students and residents in the clinical setting, we recognize that, while traditional textbooks provide an important source of information, they often do not present this material in a way that encourages the understanding of clinical problems from the clinician's perspective. Our book addresses what is most needed by students of pediatrics: an approach which provides not only a discussion of relevant normal and abnormal function, but also a framework for analyzing and integrating information around common symptom complexes. Learning pediatrics by focusing on presenting symptom complexes assists the student's ability to remember, process, and apply information in diagnosis and treatment.

We have been pleased and encouraged with the positive reception of the book by both students and faculty. For the third edition, we were fortunate to include Dr. Kim Overby as an editor. All chapters have been updated and more algorithms and tables have been added to help summarize information and facilitate the assimilation and application of material to the clinical setting. Sections have been rewritten and expanded for clarity and comprehensiveness. As with the first two editions, we made particular effort to indicate what is important because it is common, because it is treatable, or because it is harmful if overlooked. We have continued to limit the number of reference citations to include those which are of historical interest and those which provide a more extensive review.

As before, we remain grateful for our contributors' efforts in writing the chapters and responding to our comments and suggestions.

Abraham M. Rudolph, MD
Robert K. Kamei, MD
Kim J. Overby, MD

San Francisco, CA
February 2002

Pediatric Health Supervision

Kim J. Overby, MD

The goal of primary care pediatrics is to facilitate optimal health and well-being for children and their families. This is accomplished through a variety of interrelated activities, including problem surveillance and management, problem prevention, health promotion, and the coordination of care for special-needs children. The traditional focus on problem diagnosis and management has been broadened to include screening for disease and its precursors in asymptomatic populations. Pediatric providers have long recognized the value of preventive programs such as mass immunization and continue to lead the way in this area through an emphasis on regular health supervision, anticipatory guidance, and involvement in community-based prevention strategies. Recent emphasis also has been placed on the related concept of health promotion, whereby optimal health and well-being can be positively encouraged rather than focusing on avoiding problems. A by-product of the successes of modern medicine has been an increasing population of children with chronic illnesses, disabilities, and other special needs. The primary care provider is in a unique position to coordinate the often complex care of these children and facilitate communication among the individuals involved in their cases. These areas form the foundation for current recommendations regarding routine child health supervision (Tables 1–1 and 1–2), which are based largely on common sense and expert consensus. Much more research is needed to help providers determine the optimal schedule and content of the well-child visit.

Caring for children provides unique rewards and challenges. The interplay between environmental influences and factors intrinsic to the child becomes evident in many aspects of pediatric health and development. Continuity of care is based on a developmental framework that recognizes the constancy of growth and change throughout childhood. At each visit, the child's developmental level dictates the approach to the patient and much of the visit's content. Flexibility is essential in performing the physical examination. A focus on examining the least threatening areas first and using age-appropriate methods to minimize the child's anxiety is important. In pediatrics, the therapeutic alliance must necessarily include children and their families; therefore, the importance of establishing a trusting, long-term relationship cannot be overemphasized.

This chapter is divided into five main sections—Physical Growth, Motor and Psychological Development,

Counseling and Anticipatory Guidance, Screening, and Immunizations—and is intended to provide a functional overview of the major components of pediatric health supervision as well as some issues and problems frequently encountered in each of these areas. Issues with specific relevance to adolescents are covered in more depth in Chapter 2.

■ PHYSICAL GROWTH

Changes in physical size and appearance are visible manifestations of the complex morphologic, biochemical, and physiologic changes taking place during childhood. Pediatric health care providers routinely monitor weight, length, head circumference, dental development, and the appearance of secondary sexual characteristics to assess the overall adequacy of a child's growth. Common rules of thumb regarding physical growth patterns are presented in Tables 1–3 and 1–4. The normal progression of secondary sexual characteristics is discussed in Chapter 2.

In the absence of an absolute definition of normality, the adequacy of a child's growth is determined by comparison with others of similar age and sex and by the presence or absence of concordance between growth parameters and the consistency of growth patterns over time. Plotting a child's height, weight, and head circumference on a standard National Center for Health Statistics (NCHS) cross-sectional growth chart provides a statistical definition of normality by comparing that individual with others of similar age and.sex. The further a child's growth parameters are from population norms (traditionally defined as 2 SD above and below the mean), the greater the likelihood of a growth problem, but making assumptions about the adequacy of a child's growth on the basis of a single set of growth parameters can be misleading. By definition, approximately 5% of the population will be above and below the range of growth parameters statistically defined as normal. The standard NCHS growth curves were generated by measuring different groups of primarily white, middle-class children at each age, so extrapolating those data to children of different ethnic or racial backgrounds can erroneously label their growth as abnormal.

Table 1-1. Recommendations for Preventive Pediatric Health Care (RE9535) by the Committee on Practice and Ambulatory Medicine*

Age[5]	Prenatal[1]	Infancy[4]								Early Childhood[4]				
		Newborn[2]	2–4d[3]	By 1 mo	2 mo	4 mo	6 mo	9 mo	12 mo	15 mo	18 mo	24 mo	3 y	4 y
History														
Initial interval	•	•	•	•	•	•	•	•	•	•	•	•	•	•
Measurements														
Height and weight		•	•	•	•	•	•	•	•	•	•	•	•	•
Head circumference		•	•	•	•	•	•	•	•	•	•	•		
Blood pressure													•	•
Sensory screening														
Vision		S	S	S	S	S	S	S	S	S	S	S	O[6]	O
Hearing		O[7]	S	S	S	S	S	S	S	S	S	S	S	O
Developmental/ behavioral assessment[8]		•	•	•	•	•	•	•	•		•	•	•	•
Physical examination[9]		•	•	•	•	•	•	•	•	•	•	•	•	•
Procedures—general[10]														
Hereditary/Metabolic screening[11]		•←——→	•											
Immunization[12]		•		•	•	•		• ←→	•	←		•		→
Hematocrit or hemoglobin[13]								• ←→	•			•		•
Urinalysis														
Procedures—patients at risk														
Lead screening[16]								× ←→	•			★		
Tuberculin test[17]									★	★	★	★	★	★
Cholesterol screening[18]												★	★	★
STD screening[19]														
Pelvic exam[20]														
Anticipatory guidance[21]	•	•	•	•	•	•	•	•	•	•	•	•	•	•
Injury prevention[22]	•	•	•	•	•	•	•	•	•	•	•	•	•	•
Violence prevention[23]	•	•	•	•	•	•	•	•	•	•	•	•	•	•
Sleep positioning counseling[24]	•	•	•	•	•	•	•							
Nutrition counseling[25]	•	•	•	•	•	•	•	•	•	•	•	•	•	•
Dental Referral[26]									←				→	

Age⁵	Middle Childhood[4]				Adolescence[4]										
	5y	6y	8y	10y	11y	12y	13y	14y	15y	16y	17y	18y	19y	20y	21y
History															
Initial interval	•	•	•	•	•	•	•	•	•	•	•	•	•	•	•
Measurements															
Height and weight	•	•	•	•	•	•	•	•	•	•	•	•	•	•	•
Head circumference															
Blood pressure	•	•	•	•	•	•	•	•	•	•	•	•	•	•	•
Sensory screening															
Vision	O	O	O	O	S	O	S	S	O	S	S	O	S	S	S
Hearing	O	O	O	O	S	O	S	S	O	S	S	O	S	S	S
Developmental/ behavioral assessment[8]	•	•	•	•	•	•	•	•	•	•	•	•	•	•	•
Physical examination[9]	•	•	•	•	•	•	•	•	•	•	•	•	•	•	•
Procedures—general[10]															
Hereditary/Metabolic screening[11]	•→														
Immunization[12]	•	•	•	•	•	•	•	•	•	•	•	•	•	•	•
Hematocrit or hemoglobin[13]	•				←——[14]——→		•								•
Urinalysis															
Procedures—patients at risk															
Lead screening[16]	⋆	⋆	⋆	⋆	⋆	⋆	⋆	⋆	⋆	⋆	⋆	⋆	⋆	⋆	⋆
Tuberculin test[17]	⋆	⋆	⋆	⋆	⋆	⋆	⋆	⋆	⋆	⋆	⋆	⋆	⋆	⋆	⋆
Cholesterol screening[18]					⋆	⋆	⋆	⋆	⋆	⋆	⋆	⋆	⋆	⋆	⋆
STD screening[19]					⋆	⋆	⋆	⋆	⋆	⋆	⋆	⋆	⋆	⋆	⋆
Pelvic exam[20]					⋆	⋆	⋆	⋆	⋆	⋆	⋆	⋆	←——[20]——→		⋆
Anticipatory guidance[21]	•	•	•	•	•	•	•	•	•	•	•	•	•	•	•
Injury prevention[22]	•	•	•	•	•	•	•	•	•	•	•	•	•	•	•
Violence prevention[23]	•	•	•	•	•	•	•	•	•	•	•	•	•	•	•
Sleep positioning counseling[24]															
Nutrition counseling[25]	•	•	•	•	•	•	•	•	•	•	•	•	•	•	•
Dental Referral[26]	•	•	•	•	•	•	•	•	•	•	•	•	•	•	•

* Each child and family is unique; therefore, these **Recommendations for Preventive Pediatric Health Care** are designed for the care of children who are receiving competent parenting, have no manifestations of any important health problems, and are growing and developing in satisfactory fashion. **Additional visits may become necessary** if circumstances suggest variations from normal. These guidelines represent a consensus by the Committee on Practice and Ambulatory Medicine in consultation with national committees and sections of the American Academy of Pediatrics (AAP). The Committee emphasizes the great importance of continuity of care in comprehensive health supervision and the need to avoid **fragmentation of care.**

Special chemical, immunologic, and endocrine testing is usually carried out with specific indications. Testing other than newborn (e.g., inborn errors of metabolism, sickle disease, etc.) is discretionary with the physician.

• = to be performed; ⋆ = to be performed for patients at risk; S = subjective, by history; O = objective, by a standard testing method; ●——● = the range during which a service may be provided, with the dot indicating the preferred age.

(continued)

3

Table 1-1. *(Continued)*

1 A prenatal visit is recommended for parents who are at high risk, for first-time parents, and for those who request a conference. The prenatal visit should include anticipatory guidance, pertinent medical history, and a discussion of benefits of breast feeding and planned method of feeding per AAP statement "The Prenatal Visit" (1996).

2 Every infant should have a newborn evaluation after birth. Breast feeding should be encouraged and instruction and support offered. Every breast feeding infant should have an evaluation 48–72 h after discharge from the hospital to include weight, formal breast feeding evaluation, encouragement, and instruction as recommended in the AAP statement "Breastfeeding and the Use of Human Milk" (1997).

3 For newborns discharged in less than 48 h after delivery per AAP statement "Hospital Stay for Healthy Term Newborns" (1995).

4 Developmental, psychosocial, and chronic disease issues for children and adolescents may require frequent counseling and treatment visits separate from preventive care visits.

5 If a child comes under care for the first time at any point on the schedule, or if any items are not accomplished at the suggested age, the schedule should be brought up to date at the earliest possible time.

6 If the patient is uncooperative, rescreen within 6 mo.

7 All newborns should be screened per the AAP Task Force on Newborn and Infant Hearing statement, "Newborn and Infant Hearing Loss: Detection and Intervention" (1999).

8 By history and appropriate physical examination if suspicious, by specific objective developmental testing. Parenting skills should be fostered at every visit.

9 At each visit, a complete physical examination is essential, with infant totally unclothed, older child undressed and suitably draped.

10 These may be modified, depending on entry point into schedule and individual need.

11 Metabolic screening (e.g., thyroid, hemoglobinopathies, phenylketonuria, galactosemia) should be done according to state law.

12 Schedule(s) per the Committee on Infectious Diseases, published annually in the January edition of *Pediatrics.* Every visit should be an opportunity to update and complete a child's immunizations.

13 See AAP *Pediatric Nutrition Handbook* (1998) for a discussion of universal and selective screening options. Consider earlier screening for high-risk infants (e.g., premature infants and low birth weight infants). See also "Recommendations to Prevent and Control Iron Deficiency in the United States, *MMWR* 1998;47(RR-3):1–29.

14 All menstruating adolescents should be screened annually.

15 Conduct dipstick urinalysis for leukocytes annually for sexually active male and female adolescents.

16 For children at risk of lead exposure consult the AAP statement "Screening for Elevated Blood Levels" (1998). Additionally, screening should be done in accordance with state law where applicable.

17 TB testing per recommendations of the Committee on Infectious Diseases, published in the current edition of *Red Book: Report of the Committee on Infectious Diseases.* Testing should be done upon recognition of high-risk factors.

18 Cholesterol screening for high-risk patients per AAP statement "Cholesterol in Childhood" (1998). If family history cannot be ascertained and other risk factors are present, screening should be at the discretion of the physician.

19 All sexually active patients should be screened for sexually transmitted diseases (STDs).

20 All sexually active females should have a pelvic examination. A pelvic examination and routine Pap smear should be offered as part of preventive health maintenance between the ages of 18 and 21 y.

21 Age-appropriate discussion and counseling should be an integral part of each visit for care per the AAP *Guidelines for Health Supervision III* (1998).

22 From birth to age 12, refer to the AAP Injury prevention program (TIPP*) as described in *A Guide to Safety Counseling in Office Practice* (1994).

23 Violence prevention and management for all patients per AAP Statement "The Role of the Pediatrician in Youth Violence Prevention in Clinical Practice and at the Community Level" (1999).

24 Parents and caregivers should be advised to place healthy infants on their backs when putting them to sleep. Side positioning is a reasonable alternative but carries a slightly higher risk of sudden infant death syndrome. Consult the AAP statement "Changing Concepts of Sudden Infant Death Syndrome: Implications for Infant Sleeping Environment and Sleep Position" (2000).

25 Age appropriate nutrition counseling may be appropriate for some children. Subsequent examinations as prescribed by dentist.

26 Earlier initial dental examinations may be appropriate for some children. Subsequent examinations as prescribed by dentist.

Table 1–2. Recommended Frequency of GAPS Preventive Services

	Stage of Adolescence		
	Early (11–14 y)	*Middle (15–17 y)*	*Late (18–21 y)*
Health guidance			
Parenting	●	●	◗
Adolescent development	■	■	■
Safety practices	■	■	■
Diet and fitness	■	■	■
Healthy life-styles (sexual behavior, smoking, alcohol & drug use)	■	■	■
Screening			
Hypertension[1]	■	■	■
Hyperlipidemia[2]	HR-1		●
Eating disorders	■	■	■
Obesity	■	■	■
Tobacco use	■	■	■
Alcohol and drug use	■	■	■
Sexual behavior	■	■	■
Sexually transmissible diseases			
Gonorrhea	■[4]	■[4]	■[4]
Chlamydia	■[4]	■[4]	■[4]
Genital warts	■[4]	■[4]	■[4]
Syphilis	HR-2	HR-2	HR-2
HIV infection	HR-2	HR-2	HR-2
Cervical cancer	■[4]	■[4]	■[5]
Depression/suicide risk	■	■	■
Physical, sexual or emotional abuse	■	■	■
Learning problems	■	■	■
Tuberculosis	HR-3	HR-3	HR-3
Immunizations[3]			
Measles, mumps, and rubella	HR-4	HR-4	HR-4
Diphtheria and tetanus		HR-5	
Hepatitis B	HR-6	HR-6	HR-6

[1] Recommendation developed by the National Heart, Lung, and Blood Institute Second Task Force on Blood Pressure in Children.
[2] Recommendation developed by the National Cholesterol Education Program: Report of the Expert Panel on Blood Cholesterol Levels in Children and Adolescents (1991).
[3] Recommendation developed by the Advisory Committee for Immunization Practices.
[4] Screening should be performed if the adolescent is currently sexually active.
[5] Screening should be performed if the adolescent female is sexually active or 18 y of age or older.
● = once per time period; ■ = yearly; ◗ = optional; HIV = human immunodeficiency virus; HR = high-risk category.
HR-1: Test should be performed if there is a family history of cardiovascular disease before age 55 or parental history of high cholesterol. Physician may choose to perform the test if family history is unknown or if the adolescent has multiple risk factors for future cardiovascular disease.
HR-2: Syphilis test should be performed on and HIV test offered to adolescents who are at high risk for infection. This includes having had more than one sexual partner in past 6 mo, having exchanged sex for drugs, being a male who has engaged in sex with other males, having used intravenous drugs (HIV), having had other sexually transmitted diseases, having lived in an area endemic for infection, and having had a sexual partner who is at risk for infection.
HR-3: Test should be performed on adolescents who have been exposed to active tuberculosis, have lived in a homeless shelter, have been incarcerated, have lived in an area endemic for tuberculosis, or currently work in a health care setting.
HR-4: Vaccination should be provided to adolescents who have had only one previous vaccination for measles, mumps, and rubella.
HR-5: Vaccination should be given 10 y after previous diphtheria toxoid booster.
HR-6: Hepatitis B virus vaccination should be given to susceptible adolescents at high risk for infection (see HR-2).

Reproduced with permission from Elster AB, Kuznets NJ: *Guidelines for Adolescent Preventive Services (GAPS).* Baltimore: Williams & Wilkins, 1993.

Table 1–3. Typical Patterns of Physical Growth

Weight	Birth weight is regained by 10th–14th d
	Average weight gain/d: 0–6 mo = 20 g; 6–12 mo = 15 g
	Birth weight doubles at ~4 mo, triples at ~12 mo, quadruples at ~24 mo
	During second year, average weight gain/mo = ~0.25 kg.
	After age 2 y, average annual gain until adolescence = ~2.3 kg (5 lb)
Length/height	By end of first year, birth length increases by 50%
	Birth length doubles by 4 y, triples by 13 y
	Average height gain during second year = ~12 cm (5 in)
	After age 2 y, average annual growth until adolescence ≥5 cm (2 in)
Head circumference	Average head growth/week: 0–2 mo = ~0.5 cm, 2–6 mo = ~0.25 cm
	Average total head growth from 0–3 mo = ~5 cm, 3–6 mo = ~4 cm, 6–9 mo = ~2 cm, 9 mo–1 y = ~1 cm

Of even greater importance to the overall assessment of a child's growth is the observation of growth curves over time. Serial measurements provide the most accurate indication of whether physical growth is progressing normally for a given individual. Because most children track along a genetically determined percentile, significant deviations from a previously stable growth curve should provoke concern. However, downward crossing of percentiles during the first 2 years of life also can result from several normal growth variants (see section on Failure to Thrive).

Another aspect of growth assessment involves observing the relation between growth parameters in a given child. For most individuals, general concordance is observed between percentiles for height, weight, and head circumference. Major discrepancies between or disproportionate fall-off in growth parameters suggest a variety of specific growth problems (see section on Failure to Thrive).

Routine surveillance of a child's growth provides a framework for periodic discussions regarding normal growth patterns, nutritional needs, and developmental feeding behaviors of infants and children. The primary care provider is also in a unique position to detect and orchestrate subsequent evaluation and management of a variety of growth problems. Knowledge of normal and pathologic growth patterns is essential to this process. The following section focuses on several of the most common

Table 1–4. Chronology of Tooth Eruption and Exfoliation

	Eruption	
	Maxillary	**Mandible**
Primary[1]		
Central incisor	10 (8–12)	8 (6–10)
Lateral incisor	11 (9–13)	13 (10–16)
Canine	19 (16–22)	20 (17–23)
First molar	16 (13–19 boys) (14–19 girls)	16 (14–18)
Second molar	29 (25–33)	27 (23–31 boys) (24–30 girls)
Permanent[2]		
Central incisor	7–7.5	6–6.5
Lateral incisor	8–8.5	7.2–7.7
Canine	11–11.6	9.7–10.2
First premolar	10–10.3	10–10.7
Second premolar	10.7–11.2	10.7–11.5
First molar	6–6.3	6–6.2
Second molar	12.2–12.7	11.7–12
Third molar	20.5	20–20.5

	Exfoliation[3]			
			Mean age (y/mo)	
Rank	**Mandibular arch**	**Maxillary arch**	**Boys**	**Girls**
First	Central incisors		8.0	5.7
Second		Central incisors	6.10	6.7
Third	Lateral incisors		7.2	6.10
Fourth		Lateral incisors	7.10	7.5
Fifth	Canines		10.5	9.7
Sixth	First molars		10.8	10.2
Seventh		First molars	10.11	10.6
Eighth		Canines	11.3	10.7
Ninth	Second molars	Second molars	11.9	11.5

[1] **Mean age in months ±1 SD.** Adapted and reproduced, with permission, from Lunt RC, Law DB: *J Am Dent Assoc* 1974; 89:878.

[2] **Mean age in years.** Adapted and reproduced, with permission, from Burdi AR: The development and eruption of the human dentitions. In: *Pediatric Dental Medicine.* Forrester DJ, Fleming J (editors). Lea & Febiger, 1981.

[3] Adapted and reproduced, with permission, from Rica LW et al: Chronology and sequence of exfoliation of primary teeth. *J Am Dent Assoc* 1982;105:641.

growth concerns pediatricians must confront, including failure to thrive, obesity, and variations in head size and shape. Short stature and variations in pubertal development are discussed in Chapter 19.

Common Growth Concerns

FAILURE TO THRIVE

The term *failure to thrive*, first used to describe the malnourished and depressed condition of many institutionalized infants in the early 1900s, remains a descriptive rather than a diagnostic label. It is applied generally to children whose attained weights or rates of weight gain are significantly below those of other children of similar age and sex. Depending on the length and severity of malnourishment, linear growth and head circumference can be affected. Although the adverse acute and long-term consequences of childhood malnutrition are well established, the point at which deviations from age-related norms exceed normal growth variation and place the child at risk is less certain. Lack of consensus regarding specific anthropomorphic criteria for identifying the child who is failing to thrive is reflected in the number of commonly used definitions (Table 1–5).

Growth failure in infancy and childhood can result from a wide range of factors, including serious medical disease, behavioral and neurologic feeding problems, parental misinformation, poverty, and dysfunctional and/or abusive child–caregiver interactions (Table 1–6). On the one hand, in most cases, an underlying organic etiology is not found; when one is identified, it rarely presents with growth failure as its only manifestation. On the other hand, psychosocial and behavioral feeding problems resulting in growth failure are common and should no longer be perceived as diagnoses of exclusion. Whether primarily organic or psychosocial in origin, all children who fail to thrive suffer the physical and psychological consequences of malnutrition and are at significant risk for long-term physical and psychodevelopmental sequelae. In recognition of this fact and because biologic, psychosocial, and behavioral problems frequently coexist, the approach to the child with apparent growth failure has shifted from attempts to define a purely organic or nonorganic etiology to assessing physical and psychosocial risk factors, the degree of malnourishment, and the resultant physiologic and psychodevelopmental consequences for that child. Key aspects of the evaluation are a review of past and present growth data, a thorough history and physical examination, developmental and behavioral assessments, observation of a feeding, assessment of situation-specific and global child–parent interactions, and selected laboratory studies based on concerns raised by the evaluation (Table 1–7). By performing each aspect of the evaluation, the provider should attempt to answer several questions that are key to arriving at the correct diagnosis and an appropriate treatment plan (Table 1–8).

Because many parents occasionally worry about their children's growth and several normal variants can be confused with growth failure, the first issue that must be addressed is whether the child is truly failing to thrive. This question can be answered best by reviewing the child's past and present growth data for deviations from population norms, consistency over time, and concordance between growth parameters. Care must be taken when applying NCHS growth norms, which were derived primarily from a white, middle-class population, to children of different ethnic or racial backgrounds. Children who are genetically short or small tend to be small at birth, and their growth parameters are consistent with those of their parents. They have normal weight for height (both equally below the 3rd percentile), growth curves that fall below but parallel to NCHS curves, normal skinfold thickness, and bone age consistent with chronologic age.

The shape and placement of growth curves over time provide important information (Figure 1–1). Children who are growing normally parallel their genetically determined percentiles on the standard NCHS growth curves. Children who are genetically small parallel the standard curves at the low end of, or just below, the statistically defined normal range of heights and weights in the population. Children who have suffered a significant prenatal event leading to growth failure typically are proportionately small for gestational age at birth and, with time, continue to fall further away from population means on all parameters. The postnatal onset of a growth problem is manifest by a downward trend in a previously stable growth curve. Although the downward crossing of percentiles always should provoke concern, during the first 2 years of life this pattern also can result from two normal growth variants that might be difficult to differentiate

Table 1–5. Definitions of Failure to Thrive

Attained growth
  Weight <3rd percentile on NCHS growth chart
  Weight for height <5th percentile on NCHS growth chart
  Weight 20% or more below ideal weight for height
  Triceps skin fold thickness ≤5 mm

Rate of growth
  Depressed rate of weight gain
    <20 g/d from 0–3 mo of age
    <15 g/d from 3–6 mo of age
  Falloff from previously established growth curve: downward
    crossing of ≥2 major percentiles on NCHS growth charts
  Documented weight loss

NCHS = National Center for Health Statistics.

Table 1–6. Causes of Inadequate Weight Gain

Inadequate intake
  Lack of appetite
    Chronic disease (e.g., CNS pathology, gastrointestinal
      disorders, chronic infections)
    Anemia (e.g., iron deficiency)
    Psychosocial problems (e.g., apathy)
  Difficulty with ingestion
    Feeding disorder
    Psychosocial problems (e.g., apathy, rumination)
    Neurological disorders (e.g., cerebral palsy, hypertonia,
      hypotonia, generalized muscle weakness/pathology)
    Craniofacial anomalies (e.g., choanal atresia, cleft lip and
      palate, micrognathia)
    Dyspnea (e.g., congenital heart disease,
      pulmonary diseases)
    Generalized muscle weakness/pathology
      (e.g., myopathies)
    Tracheoesophageal fistula
    Genetic syndromes
    Congenital syndromes (e.g., fetal alcohol syndrome)
  Unavailability of food
    Inappropriate feeding technique
    Insufficient/inadequate volume of food
    Inappropriate food for age
    Withholding of food (abuse, neglect)

Calorie wasting
  Vomiting
    CNS pathology (increased intracranial pressure)
    Intestinal tract obstruction (e.g., pyloric stenosis,
      malrotation)
    Gastrointestinal reflux
    Metabolic problems
    Drugs/toxins

  Malabsorption
    Primary gastrointestinal diseases: biliary atresia/cirrhosis,
      celiac disease, inflammatory bowel disease,
      enzymatic deficiencies, food (protein) sensitivity/
      intolerance, Hirschsprung disease
    Cystic fibrosis
    Immunologic deficiency
    Infections
    Endocrinopathies
    Drugs/toxins
  Renal losses
    Diabetes
    Renal tubular acidosis

Increased caloric requirements
  Increased metabolism/increased use of calories
    Congenital heart disease/acquired heart disease
    Chronic respiratory disease (e.g., bronchopulmonary
      dysplasia)
    Neoplasms
    Chronic/recurrent infection
    Endocrinopathies (e.g., hyperthyroidism,
      hyperaldosteronism)
    Chronic anemia
    Drugs/toxins (e.g., lead, levothyroxine)
  Defective use of calories
    Metabolic disorders (e.g., aminoacidopathies, inborn
      errors of carbohydrate metabolism)
    Renal tubular acidosis

Altered growth potential/regulation
  Prenatal insult
  Chromosomal abnormality/genetic syndrome
  Endocrinopathies

CNS = central nervous system.
Adapted from Zenel JA: Failure to thrive: a general pediatrician's perspective. *Pediatr Rev* 1997;18:371–378.

from growth failure. A baby's size at birth is significantly influenced by maternal intrauterine conditions, and some downward shifting can occur as the percentile representing the child's true genetic growth potential is achieved. Such shifting generally occurs between 6 and 12 months of age and is associated with a steady, although decreased, rate of weight gain. Downward percentile shifting also can occur due to normal variations in the rate and timing of growth spurts. Because NCHS growth curves were constructed from different samples of children at each age rather than by observing the same cohort over time, they cannot differentiate normal variations in the rate of growth from early pathologic growth. In the normal variant of constitutional growth delay, a child's height and weight are normal at birth, drop off proportionately during the first 2 years of life, eventually parallel the NCHS

growth curves at or just below the 5th percentile for most of middle childhood, and then cross percentiles upward to achieve a final normal adult size that is consistent with genetic potential. Bone age is delayed for the child's chronologic age but consistent with height age (the age at which the child's height is at the 50th percentile). Although delays in early growth spurts can raise concerns regarding growth failure, constitutional growth delay often is recognized first when the shifted adolescent growth spurt results in the delayed appearance of secondary sexual characteristics. Like genetic short stature, constitutional growth delay is familial, and parents frequently report delayed adolescent development themselves ("late bloomer") or similar growth patterns in other offspring. The recent availability of longitudinal growth charts, which provide normative data for early-, average-, and

Table 1–7. Failure to Thrive: Components of Evaluation

Growth data
Current growth parameters
Growth curves over time
Relation of growth parameters to each other

History
  Problem context
  Parents' perception of child's growth and overall health
  When growth problem first became a concern
  Previous interventions attempted
  Medical
  Prenatal care and complications (infection, maternal nutrition, drug exposure)
  Gestational age and growth parameters at birth (SGA, prematurity)
  Perinatal complications (infections, CNS insults, anomalies)
  Previous hospitalizations, illnesses, and surgery
  Current medications
  Review of systems (vomiting, stooling patterns, mechanics of feeding/swallowing, anorexia, distress/tiring with feeds)
  Nutritional
  Caloric intake
    Breast fed: schedule and length of feeds; maternal cues to prefeeding engorgement, milk let-down, and drainage postfeeding; maternal diet, rest, stress, and medications
    Formula fed: type, method of preparation; feeding schedule; amount offered and consumed
    Mixed diet: 3-d diet history (food/beverage type, method of preparation, quantity consumed)
  Schedule and length of feedings
  Cue to infant's/child's hunger and satiety
  Daily feeding/mealtime environment
  Location/positioning during feedings
  Perceptions of suck, swallow, and grasp of nipple
  Caregivers involved with feedings
  Amount and type of mealtime supervision
  Behavior during feeding
  History of progression to solid/table foods
  Favorite/disliked foods
  Parental knowledge/beliefs regarding child/infant feeding
  Family eating practices and beliefs
  Financial constraints affecting food availability
  Psychosocial
  Caregiving environment
  Family support systems
  Family finances

Stability of parents and their relationship
Family/household composition
Parent–child relationship
Attitudes toward parenting
Content/structure of typical day for child
Parents' perceptions of child's needs
  Developmental/behavioral
  Age-related behavior problems (e.g., attachment, autonomy)
  Developmental milestones: gross/fine motor, language, social/emotional, cognition
  Parents' perception of child's temperament/behavior

Physical examination
Physician–child interaction
Skinfold measurements
Complete physical examination

Developmental/behavioral assessment
Neurodevelopmental assessment of gross/fine motor, language, socioemotional, cognitive skills

Observation of a feeding
Feeding environment (home observation)
Type and amount of food offered
Pace and duration of feeding
Child's oromotor and fine motor skills
Child's cues to and parental response regarding readiness to eat and satiation
Parents' use of opportunities for positive reinforcement and social interaction
Parents' awareness and use of child's developmental abilities
Overall parent–child interaction

Laboratory studies
Diagnostic tests directed by positive findings on history, physical, and review of growth date
Consider: complete blood count, serum electrolytes, serum creatinine, urinalysis (±culture), total protein/albumin, bone age (if height growth also poor)

Disposition
Hospitalize if
  Evidence of physical abuse and/or severe neglect
  High risk for abuse and neglect due to very disturbed parent–child interaction, poor parent functioning, and/or an extremely stressful environment
  Severe malnutrition and/or medically unstable
  Outpatient management failure

CNS = central nervous system; SGA = small for gestational age.

Table 1–8. Failure to Thrive: Key Questions

Growth data
Is the child failing to thrive or does growth represent a normal variant?
Do growth parameters and curves suggest a specific etiology?

History (medical, nutritional, psychosocial, developmental/behavioral)
Do caretakers perceive growth to be a problem?
Does the history suggest that growth failure is due to inadequate caloric intake, calorie wasting, increased caloric requirement, or altered growth potential?
Does the history suggest a specific situational, behavioral, interactional, and/or medical problem?

Physical examination
Is there evidence to suggest an underlying organic etiology?
Is there evidence of severe malnutrition and/or nutritional deficiency?
Is there evidence of a disturbed parent–child relationship, including derivational behaviors and/or signs of physical abuse/neglect?

Developmental/behavioral assessment
Is there global or asymmetrical developmental delay?
Are global behavioral problems present?

Observation of a feeding
Is a specific situational, behavioral, interactional, and/or medical problem observed?

Laboratory studies
Are specific diagnostic studies indicated?
Does the extent of malnutrition warrant further laboratory studies?

Disposition
Is inpatient evaluation and management warranted?

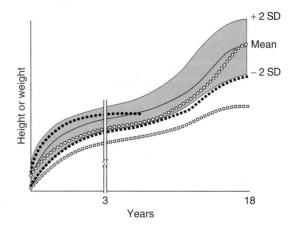

Figure 1–1. Growth curve patterns for children with postnatal onset pathologic growth (solid circles), prenatal onset pathologic growth (open squares), constitutional growth delay (open circles), genetic short stature (solid squares). Shaded area represents mean growth curve ± 2 SD.

late-developing children, allows the physician to identify more readily these constitutional growth variants as normal.

Major discrepancies between growth parameters can indicate a variety of problems. Several characteristic patterns have been described (Figure 1–2). Weight, height, and head circumference that are significantly below those expected for the child's chronologic age suggest an intrauterine insult or genetic abnormality. Relative sparing of the head circumference in relation to weight and height that are significantly below those predicted for chronologic age is more characteristic of the normal variants of constitutional growth delay, genetic short stature, structural dystrophies, and endocrine causes of growth failure. Caloric insufficiency from inadequate intake, increased weight loss, or a hypermetabolic state is suggested when weight is significantly below that expected for chrono-

logic age, with relative sparing of head circumference and height.

When review of growth data shows inadequate growth, the physician must ascertain whether that is due primarily to inadequate caloric intake, calorie wasting, an increased caloric requirement, or alteration in growth potential (Table 1–6). Evidence should support a specific situational, behavioral, interactional, or medical problem. In addition to detailed medical information, a thorough dietary, feeding, social, behavioral, and developmental history is essential. Most cases of failure to thrive result from inadequate consumption of appropriate amounts or kinds of food. Inadequate calorie intake is due most often to psychosocial and/or behavioral problems including parental ignorance and misperceptions regarding appropriate feeding, variations in infant temperament, appetite, and behavioral response (both infant's and caregivers') to progressive stages of infant feeding, a dysfunctional feeling environment or interaction, more global problems with the parent–child relationship, and/or a lack of access to food. However, inadequate intake also can be due to oromotor or other feeding dysfunction or to medical problems that result in secondary anorexia or food refusal. When caloric intake appears to be adequate, evidence should suggest a condition associated with calorie wasting, an increased caloric requirement, or an alteration in growth potential. Excessive caloric losses occur primarily with several gastrointestinal and renal disorders. Children with cardiopulmonary problems, malignant tumors, hyperthyroidism, and chronic or

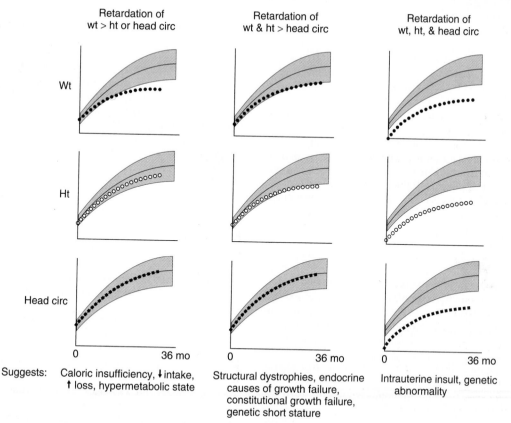

Figure 1–2. Relations between growth parameters (weight, height, and head circumference) and suggested causes.

recurrent infections might have increased caloric needs. A variety of prenatal insults, genetic abnormalities, and endocrinopathies can lead to alterations in the child's growth rate and potential.

Physical examination of a child who is growing poorly should focus on identifying signs of underlying organic disease or syndrome, severity of malnutrition, and important concomitant findings such as evidence of physical abuse or neglect and the presence of deprivational behaviors. Observation of the parent–child interaction should occur throughout the visit. Watching a feeding session is an excellent way to identify specific behavioral and interactional problems occurring during the feeding situation. A psychomotor developmental assessment also should be obtained. Children with severe psychosocial failure to thrive can manifest a variety of gaze disturbances, ranging from hyperalert, wary watchfulness, to total avoidance of eye contact and apathetic withdrawal. Infants might resist cuddling and prefer interactions with inanimate objects, whereas toddlers might demonstrate indiscriminate affection-seeking behaviors. Many of these children also

manifest developmental delays, especially in the areas of language and social adaptive behavior, which depend most on environmental stimulation.

The diagnostic laboratory evaluation should be guided by concerns raised in the history, physical examination, and review of growth data. Organic disease presenting only with growth failure is extremely uncommon. An undirected laboratory evaluation rarely identifies an unsuspected diagnosis and is potentially harmful. Depending on the length and severity of the growth failure, additional laboratory studies might help assess nutrition status and the presence of concomitant problems such as iron deficiency anemia. Most children with failure to thrive should receive a complete blood count, serum electrolytes, serum creatinine, total protein:albumin, urinalysis, urine culture, and determination of bone age (if height growth is also poor) as part of their evaluation.

Most children with growth failure can be evaluated and managed as outpatients, but some will require hospitalization. Among those are children with psychosocial failure to thrive who manifest evidence of, or are at high risk for, physical abuse or severe neglect, who are severely malnourished or medically unstable, or who have failed a trial of outpatient management. The approach to a child with failure to thrive requires time and sensitivity. To facilitate subsequent communication and management, it is important to understand the parents' perspective regarding their child's growth and health and be cognizant of previous efforts to intervene when concerns have been present. Many parents of children who are failing to thrive experience feelings of guilt, inadequacy, and anger when behavioral and/or psychosocial problems are uncovered; subsequent efforts to intercede often are perceived as criticisms of their parental abilities. Focusing concern on the child's health and well-being and the positive goal of enhancing the parent–child relationship might defuse some of those feelings. Ultimately, the success of treatment often depends on establishing a positive and caring long-term alliance with children and their caretakers. Management of the child with psychosocial failure to thrive must be individualized to the specific needs of that child and its family. In addition to nutritional rehabilitation, efforts should focus on correcting any dysfunctional child–parent interactions by addressing areas of parental misinformation, providing and implementing specific feeding guidance, and addressing the larger psychosocial needs of the family. A multidisciplinary team approach involving the primary care provider, nutritionist, social worker, child-behavior specialist, and community-based outreach services is often the most beneficial.

OBESITY

Childhood obesity is one of the most frequent and challenging growth problems faced by the pediatric health care provider. As many as 25% of children in the United States have been estimated to be significantly overweight. Concern for their well-being has focused on several immediate and future issues. Obesity in children and adults has been associated with increased risk of hypertension, diabetes, hyperlipidemia, and cardiovascular disease. The longer children remain obese, the more likely they will continue to be overweight as adults and suffer the long-term cardiovascular consequences. Obesity is most likely to persist when present during middle and late childhood or adolescence and when there is a history of parental obesity. Excessive weight can predispose some children to orthopedic problems, such as Blount's disease and slipped femoral capital epiphyses. Of equal importance to these medical concerns are the psychological consequences of obesity. Despite secular trends in food consumption and physical activity that have encouraged the rising prevalence of childhood obesity, our society puts a high premium on thinness. Children who are overweight frequently are subjected to conscious and unconscious stereotyping and discrimination by adults and other children. They are often less popular with their peers than normal-weight individuals and may find themselves socially ostracized or isolated. Despite the complex causal relationship between biologic, environmental, and psychological factors, many individuals, including parents, simply blame these children for their weight problems by assuming them to be slovenly and lacking in self-control. Several investigators have described a higher incidence of poor self-concept and personality disturbances among obese than among normal-weight children. However, it should be remembered that many overweight children suffer no psychological problems as a result of their obesity.

Childhood obesity is defined in most settings by comparison of indirect measures of body composition and fat distribution with population norms (Table 1–9). Unfortunately, those statistical definitions do not identify the point at which a given child is at risk for present or future morbidity. The simplest way to assess body fatness in children is to compare their weights with those of other children of similar age and sex. However, weight alone is a poor indicator of body fatness because it does not take into account differences in body size and lean body mass. Measurements that incorporate weight and height, such as the body mass index (weight in kilograms divided by height as meters squared), are an improvement in that they allow correction for body size (height) but do not differentiate differences in body composition (adiposity vs. lean body mass). However, due to its ease of calculation, the ready availability of age and sex norms, and its correlation with subsequent complications of obesity, many experts recommend the body mass index as the optimal way to screen for childhood obesity. Skinfold measurements, obtained by gently compressing and measuring with calipers the skin and subcutaneous tissue in the triceps and subscapular areas, are a practical way to assess body adiposity and thereby differentiate the child who is overweight because of excess fat as opposed to lean body mass.

Excess body fat results from energy intake that is in excess of energy expenditure. Although parents frequently are concerned about an underlying organic etiology, this occurs in fewer than 5% of children with excessive weight gain (Table 1–10). Most cases of childhood obesity are caused by a complex interaction between genetic and environmental factors affecting food consumption, activity level, and metabolic rate. The obese child often is the visible result of much broader family patterns of food intake, eating behavior, and physical activity, thereby making intervention extremely challenging. Components of the evaluation of an obese child and its family are presented in Table 1–11. Key questions to be answered by the evaluation and that have relevance to etiology and subsequent management are presented in Table 1–12.

By reviewing past and present growth data and performing skinfold measurements, the physician can assess the extent to which the child's weight exceeds predicted norms based on height and represents an excess of adi-

Table 1–9. Commonly Used Measures and Definitions of Obesity

Measure	Definition of Obesity	Comments/Limitations
Weight[1]	>95th percentile for age/sex norms	Easy to obtain, reliable, does not take into account variations in frame size (height) and body composition (lean vs. fat mass)
% Overweight	≥20% above ideal body weight[2] for age/sex norms	Reliable, easy to obtain. Corrects for variations in frame size (height) but does not take into account variations in body composition (lean body vs. fat mass).
Weight for height[1] Body mass index (weight/height^2)	>95th percentile for age/sex norms >85th percentile for age/sex norms	
Subcutaneous fat thickness (skinfolds)	>85th percentile for age/sex norms	Best office-based, noninvasive method to directly assess degree of adiposity; independent of above anthropometric measures
Densitometry: Air versus hydrostatic (underwater) weighing Radioisotope distribution (K 40 space)		Gold standard for assessing adiposity and body fat; not practical for use in office setting

[1] Using National Center for Health Statistics growth charts.
[2] Ideal body weight = weight at the percentile that corresponds to the patient's height percentile on National Center for Health Statistics growth charts.

Table 1–10. Causes of Secondary Obesity

Central nervous system damage
  Trauma
  Tumor
  Postinfection

Endocrinopathies
  Hypothyroidism
  Insulinoma
  Cushing syndrome
  Exogenous corticosteroids
  Mauriac syndrome (diabetes with excess insulin administration, characterized by short stature and hepatomegaly)

Congenital syndromes
  Prader-Willi
  Laurence-Moon-Biedl (mental retardation, short stature, polydactyly, hypogonadism, retinitis pigmentosa, deafness)
  Alstrom syndrome (deafness, diabetes mellitus, retinitis pigmentosa, short stature, hypogonadism)
  Vasquez syndrome (males with X-linked short stature, mental retardation, hypogonadism, gynecomastia)
  X-Chromosome disorders
  Pseudohypoparathyroidism
  Pseudopseudohypoparathyroidism

From Merritt RJ: Obesity. *Curr Prob Pediatr* 1982;12(11):1–58.

posity as opposed to lean body mass. Knowledge of birth weight and growth curves over time can assist the physician in identifying and exploring events surrounding changes in a previously stable growth pattern. It is also important to assess the adequacy of the child's linear growth. With the exception of hyperinsulinemia, most endocrinopathies and congenital syndromes causing secondary obesity are associated with poor height growth. Children with endogenous obesity are typically average or above average in height.

When the child's weight gain or adiposity is found to be excessive, the physician must seek to understand the child's and parents' perspectives on being overweight, how this problem fits into the larger family dynamic, and previous interventions. In addition to exploring those issues, the history should focus on documenting the amount and type of foods consumed, physical activity, individual and environmental factors influencing food consumption and activity level, the presence of or risk for medical or psychological morbidity, and evidence of an underlying disease process. Blood pressure assessment is an important aspect of the evaluation. Hypertension is a frequent complication of obesity and, when present, underlines the need for intervention. The physical examination might provide important clues to the rare presence of an underlying disease process. Centrifugal fat distribution, abdominal striae, skin and hair changes, dysmorphic features, and advanced or delayed pubertal development should be noted. Because

Table 1–11. The Obese Child: Components of Evaluation

Growth data
Current growth parameters
Growth curves over time
Relation of growth parameters to each other: body mass
   index, pattern of height growth
Skinfold measurements

History
Problem context
   Parents'/child's perceptions of weight/size
   When excess weight first became a concern
   Previous interventions attempted
Medical
   Prenatal care and complications
   Growth parameters at birth
   Perinatal complications: infections, central nervous system
      insults, anomalies
   Previous hospitalizations, illnesses, and surgery
   Current medications
   Review of systems: cold intolerance, constipation, fatigue
      (hypothyroidism); hypoglycemia, hyperphagia
      (primary hyperinsulinemia); pubertal delay
      (hypothalamic problem)
Family history
   Weight problems
   Endocrinopathies
   Cardiovascular risk factors and disease
Nutritional/eating
   3-d diet history: food/beverages consumed, method of
      preparation, quantity consumed
   Feeding/mealtime context
      Schedule and length of feedings/meals
      Cues to infant's/child's hunger and satiety
      Daily feeding/mealtime environment
      Location/positioning during feedings
      Caregivers involved with feedings
      Amount and type of mealtime supervision
      Behavior during feeding/mealtime
   Factors affecting eating behavior
      Availability of foods at home and school and in
         neighborhood
      Parents' knowledge, attitudes, and feelings regarding
         food, eating, and overeating
      Family eating behavior
      Eating environment (e.g., television)
      Non–appetite-driven cues to eat
      Parental reinforcement/mixed messages
Activity level
   Diary of type and amount of daily physical activity
      (especially aerobic)
   Factors affecting exercise behavior and activity level
      Competing daily activities
      Availability of exercise facilities/equipment and
         role models

Family exercise behavior patterns
Peer exercise behavior
Parents'/child's knowledge and attitudes about
   exercise
Environmental cues and reinforcers
Perceived energy level, physical abilities
Perceived reward value of exercise versus sedentary
   activities (e.g., television)
Past experience with exercise
Psychosocial
   Family and household composition
   Parent–child relationship
   Relationships between other family members
   Family stressors
   Role of child's obesity in family dynamics
   Peer relationships
   Child's self-esteem/self-concept
   Content/structure of typical day for child
Developmental/behavioral
   Age-related behavior problems
      (e.g., attachment, autonomy)
   Developmental milestones: gross/fine motor, language,
      social/emotional, cognition
   Parents' perception of the child's temperament/behavior

Physical examination
Observation of parent–child interaction
Assessment of child's interaction with physician
Blood pressure measurements
Skinfold measurements
Complete physical examination with emphasis on fat
   distribution (central may suggest Cushing syndrome),
   presence of dysmorphism (syndromes), neurologic
   examination (primary hypothalamic problems), presence of striae (Cushing syndrome), presence of dry
   coarse skin or hair (hypothyroidism), secondary sexual
   characteristics (delay suggests hypothalamic problem)

Developmental/behavioral assessment
Neurodevelopmental assessment of gross/fine motor,
   language, socioemotional, cognitive skills (delay/
   retardation suggests syndrome)

Assessment of cardiorespiratory fitness
Submaximal step test
Submaximal bicycle ergometer test
12-min run–walk test
Steady-state run test

Laboratory studies
Diagnostic tests directed by concerns raised in history and
   physical examination
Consider thyroid screening (classic physical findings of
   hypothyroidism may be absent)
Depending on severity of obesity and family history:
   cholesterol and lipid screening, glucose tolerance testing

Table 1–12. The Obese Child: Key Questions

Growth data
Is the child's weight growth and adiposity excessive?
Is height growth normal, advanced, or stunted?

History
Do caretakers or child perceive weight to be a problem?
Does the history suggest an underlying disease process or syndrome?
Are there identifiable individual and environmental factors encouraging excessive caloric intake or inadequate physical activity?
Does the history suggest current or future high risk for medical/psychological morbidity?

Physical examination
Is there evidence of an underlying disease process or syndrome?
Is there evidence of current medical/psychological morbidity?

Developmental/behavioral assessment
Is there developmental delay/mental retardation?

Assessment of cardiorespiratory fitness
What is the child's current fitness level?

Laboratory studies
On the basis of history and physical examination, are diagnostic laboratory tests indicated?
Does the severity of obesity and family history warrant screening for additional morbidity and cardiovascular risk factors?

portance of intervention. Treatment efforts that tailor suggestions to individual children and their environments, address controlling factors for food intake and energy expenditure, and focus assessment and management on the family rather than on the individual level have the greatest chance of success (Table 1–13). Older children in particular might benefit from the mutual support and camaraderie provided by group activities with others who are overweight. Because of the potential adverse effects of therapeutic dieting on brain and linear growth in children, caloric restriction is rarely encouraged. Rather than weight loss, the goal is to slow the rate of fat deposition, i.e., allow the child to "grow into" its weight. Emphasis is

Table 1–13. Treating the Child with Endogenous Obesity

Develop an alliance with the child and family regarding the issues involved and the importance of therapy
Focus assessment and management at the family rather than the individual level (e.g., How can the whole family develop healthier eating habits?)
Tailor suggestions to the specific child and its unique family circumstances/environment
Dispel misperceptions and provide accurate factual information regarding the child's nutritional needs
Encourage dietary and activity changes that can be maintained long-term
Address specific controlling factors regarding the type and quantity of food ingested and energy expenditure
  Inappropriate behavioral dynamics such as use of food as a reward
  Vulnerable times such as after school or before bed
  Situational/environmental cues such as watching television or feeling stress, that encourage unhealthy eating habits
Emphasize qualitative changes in diet rather than calorie restriction (dieting), which will slow rate of fat deposition and allow the child to grow into his or her weight
  Decrease fat content
  Remove unhealthy foods from house
  Identify and substitute preferred healthy foods for preferred unhealthy foods
Encourage participation in aerobic activities to increase energy expenditure, increase cardiovascular fitness, and improve self-esteem
Limit television watching
Use specific behavioral techniques
  Self-monitoring
  Contingency training
  Positive reinforcement
Use "groups," if available, especially for older children
Use a team approach (physician, psychologist, nutritionist, case-manager/social worker) for children with significant obesity; may be most beneficial
Provide long-term encouragement and follow-up

of secondary endocrinologic effects, obese children tend to experience the physical changes of adrenarche and pubarche at earlier ages than their lean age-matched peers. Obesity in conjunction with delayed pubertal development suggests a hypothalamic abnormality. Because the obese child's level of physical activity is an important part of the problem and the solution, assessment of the child's overall cardiorespiratory fitness can be helpful. Laboratory evaluation of the obese child should be directed at confirming diagnostic concerns raised by its history and physical examination. Depending on the severity of obesity and family history, screening for concurrent morbidity and cardiovascular risk factors also should be done (e.g., cholesterol and lipid screening). A lower threshold for obtaining thyroid screening tests may be warranted because infants and children with obesity secondary to hypothyroidism might not present with the classic findings.

Once a child's adiposity is identified as a problem, making significant and sustained changes is a difficult but not impossible task. For this to occur, however, it is imperative that the child (if age appropriate) and parents perceive the obesity as a problem and recognize the im-placed on making qualitative changes in diet, such as reductions in fat content, and encouraging participation in aerobic activities, which increase energy use, cardiovascular fitness, and self-esteem. With significantly obese children, a team approach involving a primary care provider, nutritionist, behavior therapist, and family or child counselor might be the most beneficial. Long-term encouragement and follow-up are important because many children and their families return to old behavior patterns once the intense period of treatment is completed. Despite our inability to document long-term success in dealing with many obese children, the potential benefits of establishing more healthful eating and activity patterns warrant our continued efforts to intervene early on and develop more effective therapies.

VARIATIONS IN HEAD GROWTH: SIZE & SHAPE

Head size is obtained by measuring the greatest occipitofrontal circumference and reflects the volume of intracranial contents, including brain, cerebrospinal fluid, and blood, as well as the thickness of the skull and scalp. Macrocephaly and microcephaly are defined statistically as a head circumference greater than 2 SD above and below the mean of those measures for children of near the same age. According to that definition, approximately 5% of the population are considered macrocephalic or microcephalic. As with other growth parameters, the significance of a given measurement is best defined within the context of normal variations, the pattern of past head growth, the relation of head size to other growth parameters, and the presence or absence of associated historical or physical findings.

Although unrelated to intracranial volume, scalp edema or a cephalhematoma might significantly increase the head circumference. The effect of head shape on circumference also should be kept in mind. For the same intracranial volume, a round head has a smaller head circumference than a more oval one. Gestational rather than chronologic age should be used when plotting the head circumference of preterm infants. As a result of catch-up growth, these infants also exhibit accelerated rates of head growth compared with full-term babies, initially exceeding gains in weight and height. The disproportionately enlarging head may raise concerns regarding hydrocephalus. The fact that many premature infants are also at increased risk for this complication emphasizes the need for close observation.

When a child's head size or rate of head growth provokes concern, a thorough history, physical examination, and review of growth curves should be obtained. Knowledge of head size at birth and the pattern of prior head growth is important. A child whose head circumference consistently falls within the same percentile is more likely to be normal than the child whose growth channel is shifting upward or downward across percentiles. Head size

also must be assessed within the context of the child's overall body size. General concordance exists between growth parameters in a given individual, and significant discrepancies between head circumference and body size (height and weight) increase the likelihood of pathology. The influence of benign familial factors as well as specific syndromes and problems often can be identified by evaluating the head circumference of the child's parents and siblings. The history and physical examination should identify signs and symptoms of causal or concomitant problems such as developmental disabilities; mental retardation; neurologic abnormalities such as cerebral palsy, seizures, and focal deficits; dysmorphology; abnormal fontanelles and sutures; and skin findings suggestive of a neurocutaneous disorder. A history of prenatal, perinatal, and postnatal factors with potential import to subsequent central nervous system growth and development should be elicited, including poor prenatal care, maternal drug use or infection during pregnancy, prematurity, perinatal asphyxia, hypoglycemia, hypotension, and central nervous system infection.

Macrocephaly can result from excess cerebral spinal fluid (hydrocephalus), excess brain tissue (megalencephaly), thickening of the skull, or hemorrhage into the subdural or epidural spaces. Each of these problems in turn may be secondary to a variety of inborn and acquired disorders that rarely present exclusively with head growth abnormalities. Hydrocephalus might result from conditions causing increased production, decreased absorption, or obstruction to flow of the cerebral spinal fluid and, among potential causes of macrocephaly at birth, is the only one associated with increased intracranial pressure. *Megalencephaly* refers to the presence of excess brain tissue secondary to an increased size or number of brain cells. This might be a primary anatomic condition with or without concomitant syndromic or neurologic abnormalities or due to a variety of metabolic disorders associated with cerebral edema or brain cell storage of accumulated substances. Infants with anatomic megalocephaly generally are born with large heads, whereas those with metabolic causes of megalocephaly typically have normal head size at birth with subsequent enlargement during the neonatal period. Metabolic megalencephaly frequently is accompanied by developmental regression or delay, signs of increased intracranial pressure, and concomitant neurologic problems, such as seizures.

The widespread availability and use of computed tomography (CT) has resulted in the identification of several benign conditions associated with macrocephaly. Benign enlargement of the subarachnoid space is a relatively common cause of macrocephaly in an otherwise normal infant. These children typically have large but normal-sized heads at birth and provoke concern during infancy when their head circumferences subsequently cross percentiles upward to exceed and then parallel the

98th percentile for children of similar age and sex. A head CT, if obtained, demonstrates an enlarged subarachnoid space, normal to slightly increased ventricular size, and widened sulci and sylvian fissure. A genetic etiology is suspected because of the male predominance of this condition and the frequent concomitant finding of macrocephaly in the identified child's father. Aside from the head growth abnormalities, these children are neurologically and intellectually normal. Genetic megalencephaly (large brain), another common, normal variant causing macrocephaly, might be indistinguishable from the previously described condition unless a head CT is performed. These children may or may not have large heads at birth but subsequently cross percentiles upward to parallel the curve above the 98th percentile. A head CT, if obtained, is normal. The family history is usually positive for megalencephaly and, as with children identified with benign enlargement of the subarachnoid space, neurologic and mental function are normal. A child identified as having one of these two benign conditions does not require further evaluation unless head growth subsequently deviates further from the normal curve or a neurologic abnormality or developmental delay is detected.

Microcephaly is indicative of a small-sized brain and typically the result of a primary or secondary defect in brain development. It is associated frequently with mental retardation, although normal intelligence can occur. *Primary microcephaly* refers to a genetic or chromosomal condition in which bulk or structural brain growth is intrinsically flawed. In *secondary microcephaly,* previously normal brain development is impaired by a variety of prenatal and postnatal infections, toxins, and central nervous system injuries. Because brain expansion dictates skull growth, inadequate brain growth can result in premature fusion of the cranial bones. This cause of premature suture closure usually can be differentiated from primary craniosynostosis by the absence of an abnormally shaped skull and palpably thickened suture lines.

Microcephaly at birth establishes the antenatal timing of impaired brain growth but does not differentiate primary from secondary etiologies. With the exception of some chromosomal disorders, a normal-sized head at birth with subsequent development of growth failure strongly suggests a secondary etiology for the microcephaly. Perinatal insults to the central nervous system rarely result in recognizably impaired head growth before the ages of 3–6 months. When such insults cause microcephaly and mental retardation, they also are associated with motor deficits (cerebral palsy) and frequently with seizures. Cranial CT scans of children with primary microcephaly typically are normal or show dysmorphology characteristic of the specific etiology, whereas CT scans of those with secondary microcephaly usually show abnormalities suggested by a combination of nonspecific findings such as ventricular enlargement and cerebral atrophy.

Plagiocephaly, or asymmetric head growth, is caused by alterations of the normal internal and external forces that influence skull growth and by inherent or acquired abnormalities in bone formation. Most infants born vaginally have some degree of head molding at birth that resolves during the first few weeks of life unless other factors perpetuate it. Deformational flattening due to lack of variation in head positioning pre- and postnatally is the most common cause of asymmetrical head shape and can be exacerbated by factors associated with delayed head control (e.g., prematurity) and conditions that predispose the infant to turning to one side (torticollis, neurologic or ophthalmologic conditions). In recent years, pediatricians have seen a significant increase in the number of infants presenting with posterior plagiocephaly because of to the success of the "Back to Sleep" campaign, which has significantly decreased the incidence of sudden infant death syndrome by promoting the supine sleeping position for young infants. It is most important for clinicians to differentiate this common form of deformational plagiocephaly from asymmetric growth caused by premature closure of one or more of the cranial sutures (synostotic plagiocephaly). Normally most sutures are closed by 12–24 months of age. Most are ossified by age 8 years and fusion is complete by early adulthood. With craniosynostosis, premature closure or absence of one or more cranial sutures results in compensatory growth along the remaining open sutures in a direction parallel to the closed suture. The resultant head shape can be predicted based on the sutures involved (Figure 1–3). Although primarily causing problems with cosmetic appearance, craniosynostosis can be associated with ocular problems, neurologic impairment, and increased intracranial pressure. Craniosynostosis involving only one suture is usually an isolated condition occurring with a prevalence of 1–2 in 1000. Eighty-five percent of cases occur in white children, with a male:female ratio of 3:2. The sagittal suture is involved in almost half the cases, with stenosis of the coronal (1 in 3) and metopic (1 in 10) sutures the next most commonly observed. Most importantly, premature closure of the lambdoidal suture, which causes posterior plagiocephaly, occurs rarely. Craniosynostosis involving more than one suture often is associated with one of several genetic syndromes. Head shape is generally severely distorted and ophthalmologic or neurologic problems and other stigmata of the syndrome are usually present.

The approach to a child with an asymmetric head should include a thorough history, physical examination, and directed laboratory and radiographic evaluations. The physician should ascertain when the asymmetry was first noted and whether it has been progressive. Risk factors for deformational (e.g., favored side or position, torticollis, prematurity, and neuromotor problems) and synostotic (e.g., ventriculoperitoneal shunting of hydrocephalus, microcephaly, and metabolic bone disease) plagiocephalies

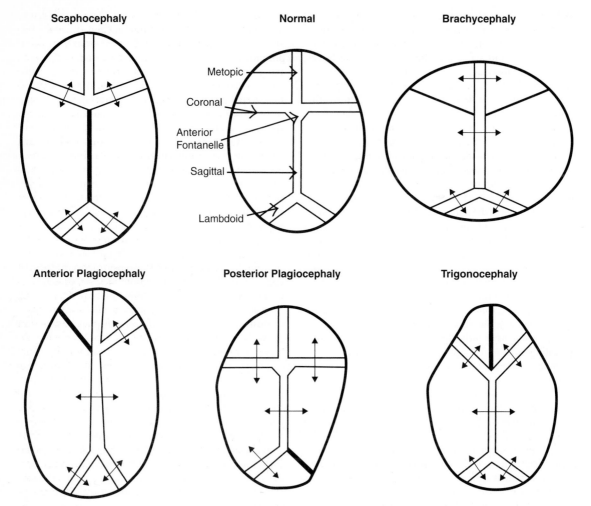

Figure 1–3. Craniosynostosis and corresponding head shapes: Fused or absent sutures are shown as heavy single lines. Arrows indicate compensatory growth along open sutures, resulting in characteristic head shape.

also should be explored. Evaluation of head circumference is important: children with deformational plagiocephaly and single-suture craniosynostosis have normal-sized heads and growth rates. Premature closure of multiple sutures rarely is the cause of restricted brain growth; more often, the absence of the outward pressure of a normally growing brain causes premature closure of multiple cranial sutures. When microcephaly is the primary problem, gross skull malformation and signs of increased intracranial pressure are absent. The physical examination can be very helpful in differentiating deformational posterior plagiocephaly from true craniosynostosis. In synostotic posterior plagiocephaly, occipital flattening might be accompanied by a thick ridge overlying the fused lambdoid suture or the absence of a palpable suture. Compensatory growth causes

frontal and parietal prominence on the side opposite the occipital flattening, resulting in an overall trapezoidal head shape. The ear on the side of the fused suture is displaced downward and backward. In deformational posterior plagiocephaly, the occiput is flattened but the sutures are open and ridging is absent. Occipital flattening results in a prominence of the frontal and temporal areas on the same side, giving the head an overall parallelogram shape and, in contrast to lambdoid synostosis, the ear is pushed forward and down, away from the area of flattening. During the physical examination the provider should focus also on identifying a specific etiology (torticollis, neuromuscular and/or developmental problems, or syndromic stigmata) or complications (increased intracranial pressure or ocular and neurologic problems). If the deformation observed is severe, suggestive of synostosis, progressive after several weeks of conservative treatment, and/or associated with significant parental anxiety, plane skull radiographs are warranted. In most children, skull films interpreted within the context of clinical data will clarify the diagnosis. However, because plain radiographs will not identify all synostotic sutures, when the clinical situation is suggestive and plain films are equivocal, a head CT or three-dimensional CT reconstruction is indicated.

Mild positional posterior plagiocephaly is largely benign and will disappear as the child spends less and less time lying down and in one position. Parents should be counseled to use the supine sleeping position for infants but change the infant's head position when it is asleep. Crib toys can be moved to encourage the infant to turn to a less favored side. Babies also should be given the opportunity to spend time in the prone position when they are awake and can be observed. This "positional therapy" should be combined with physical therapy (stretching exercises to achieve normal neck mobility) in the infant with torticollis. For most children with mild to moderate positional plagiocephaly, implementation of these conservative measures will result in a normal or nearly normal appearance within 2–3 months. For infants with severe positional plagiocephaly and those with a moderate deformity that does not respond to a period of conservative measures, use of helmet molding may be considered. To be effective and avoid potential complications, this therapy requires almost constant use of the helmet (22 hours per day) and involvement of an orthotics expert. Optimal therapeutic results from helmet molding are achieved when treatment is initiated before age 6 months. Treatment for plagiocephaly due to craniosynostosis is surgical. Because the cosmetic outcome of surgery depends on the potential for further skull growth, surgical correction of single-suture synostosis ideally should take place by 6–12 months of age.

■ MOTOR & PSYCHOLOGICAL DEVELOPMENT

To assess their patients' overall developmental progress and functioning and counsel parents regarding a variety of developmentally based issues, physicians must have a firm understanding of the normal patterns and common variations in the developmental process. Knowing the average ages at which children achieve certain neurodevelopmental milestones and encounter specific developmental tasks provides a conceptual framework for normative child development. However, developmental normality cannot be defined in absolute terms. Whereas the sequence of development is similar for all children, the rate of progress differs from child to child, and "dissociation" of performance between developmental fields often can be normal. By

comparing a child's performance with those of others, one can say only that, the further a child is from "average," the less likely he or she will be "normal." It is important to remember that a child's developmental level and progress are the result of different factors, many unrelated to the child's genetic mental endowment, such as acute or chronic illness, physical or sensory handicaps, and the quality of the nurturing environment. Current developmental thinking emphasizes the interactional contributions of "nature" and "nurture" to the child's overall functioning. Developmental assessment should emphasize their equal importance by addressing the child's medical history, physical examination, and psychosocial history, in addition to eliciting specific developmental skills and information. A longitudinal and multidimensional approach to developmental monitoring should be encouraged, and overreliance on isolated developmental scales and tests avoided.

Table 1–14 outlines general areas of developmental observation and the average ages at which common milestones occur. Motor development tends to parallel central nervous system maturation, progressing in a cephalocaudal and proximal-to-distal direction. The disappearance of primitive reflexes must precede the appearance of volitional movements, and generalized mass activity is replaced by specific responses. Controlled use of the upper extremities precedes that of the lower extremities, and truncal coordination occurs before mastery of the extremities. In general, there is greater variation in the timing of gross motor development than in the acquisition of fine motor skills. It must be remembered that some of the most important aspects of developmental assessment, such as alertness, responsiveness, persistence, and concentration, defy objective scoring, whereas some of the most easily scored items, such as gross motor development in infancy, are the least reliable indicators of overall mental ability. Among objective areas of assessment, speech and language development is the best predictor of subsequent cognitive performance. However, problems in this area also might be related to many factors unrelated to mental endowment.

An important aspect of the pediatric health supervision visit is the opportunity for periodic assessment of the child's overall developmental functioning. For this purpose, standardized developmental screening instruments, such as the Denver II, are used frequently. *Developmental screening* implies finding children at high risk for otherwise unsuspected developmental problems. Screening tests by definition are not diagnostic and, when findings are abnormal, must be followed by a thorough diagnostic evaluation. The value of a screening test lies in its ability to decrease morbidity through early detection and treatment (see section on Screening). Definitive diagnostic strategies and effective treatment programs must exist and be supported to achieve this goal. A screening test

Table 1–14. Aspects of Developmental Assessment and Common Developmental Milestones[1]

Perceptions/concerns of others: parents, teachers, and other caregivers	
General responsiveness and alertness	
Symmetry of movement	
Use of eyes and ears	
Follows dangling object from midline through a range of <45 degrees	0–1 mo
Follows dangling object from midline through a range of 90 degrees	1 mo
Follows dangling object from midline through a range of 180 degrees	3 mo
Consistent conjugate gaze (binocular vision)	4 mo
Alerts or quiets to sound	0–2 mo
Lateralizes sound (turns head to sound made on level with ear)	3 mo
Localizes sound well in all directions	7–10 mo
Tone: posture, resistance to passive movement, clonus, deep tendon reflexes, head and truncal control	
Primitive and postural reflexes	

	Present by	Absent by
Moro		3–4 mo
Palmar grasp		2–3 mo
Asymmetrical tonic neck		2–3 mo
Placing/stepping		1.5–2 mo
Landau	3 mo	1 y
Parachute	6–9 mo	

Head control: prone, ventral suspension, pull to sitting	
Prone	
Head rests on table turned to one side	1 mo
Lifts head momentarily	1 mo
Head up 45 degrees	2 mo
Head up 90 degrees	3–4 mo
Weight on forearms	3–5 mo
Weight on hands with arms extended	5–6 mo
Ventral suspension	
Head hangs completely down	newborn
Momentarily holds head in plane of body	6 wk
Head sustained in plane of body	2 mo
Maintains head beyond plane of body	3 mo
Pull to sitting	
Complete head lag, back uniformly rounded	newborn
Slight head lag	3 mo
No head lag, back straightening	5 mo
Lifts head off table when about to be pulled up	6 mo
Raises head spontaneously from supine	7 mo
Rolling	
Rolls front-to-back	4–5 mo
Rolls back-to-front	5–6 mo
Sitting	
Back uniformly rounded, cannot sit unsupported	newborn
Back straightening, sits with propping	5–6 mo
Back straight, sits with arms forward for support	6–7 mo
Sits with no support	7 mo
Fine motor/manipulation	
Hands predominantly closed	1 mo
Hands predominantly open	3 mo
Hand regard	3–5 mo
Hands come together	4 mo
Foot play	5 mo
Voluntary grasp (no release)	5 mo
Transfers objects from hand to hand	6 mo
Ulnar grasp of cube	5–6 mo
Grasps cube against thenar eminence	6–8 mo
Grasps cube against lower thumb	8–10 mo
Mature cube grasp—finger tips and distal thumb	10–12 mo
Index finger approach to small objects and finger-thumb opposition	10 mo
Voluntary release of objects	10 mo
Plays pat-a-cake	9–10 mo
Enjoys putting objects in and out of box	≥11 mo
Casting objects	10–13 mo
Tower of 2 cubes	13–15 mo
Tower of 4 cubes	18 mo
Tower of 6–7 cubes	2 y
Tower of 10 cubes	3 y
Good use of cup and spoon	15–18 mo
Weight bearing and walking	
Some weight bearing	3 mo
Supports most weight	6 mo
Pulls to stand	9 mo
Walks holding onto furniture (cruising)	11 mo
Walks with one hand held	12 mo
Walks without help	13 mo
Walks well	15 mo
Runs well	2 y
Up and down stairs, two feet each step	2 y
Up and down stairs, one foot per step down, two feet per step up	3 y
Up and down stairs, one foot per step	4 y
Jumps off ground with two feet	2.5 y
Hops on one foot	4 y
Skips	5–6 y
Balance on one foot 2–3 s	3 y
Balance on one foot 6–10 s	4 y
Personal/social and cognitive	
Social smile	1–2 mo
Smiles at image in mirror	5 mo
Looks after dropped toy—beginning of object permanence	6 mo
Separation anxiety/stranger awareness	6–12 mo
Interactive games: peek-a-boo and pat-a-cake	9–12 mo

(continued)

Table 1-14. (Continued)

Waves "bye-bye"	10 mo	Imitates sounds made by others	9–12 mo
Rolls ball to examiner	12 mo	First words (~4–6, including *mama, dada*)	9–12 mo
Feeds self with cup and spoon	15–18 mo	Understanding one-step command (without gesture)	15 mo
Dresses self, except for buttons in back	3 y		
Ties shoe laces	5 y	Jargon (i.e., expressive, unintelligible language), recognizable words increase with age	15–24 mo
Autonomy and independence issues often begin	18 mo–2 y		
Parallel play	1–2 y	Vocabulary of 10–50 words	13–18 mo
Cooperative play	3–4 y	Vocabulary of 50–75 words	18–24 mo
Magical thinking and symbolic (pretend) play	18 mo–5 y	Vocabulary of 250 words	3 y
Able to distinguish fantasy from reality	5 y	Two-word sentences	18–24 mo
		Three-word sentences	2–3 y
Speech and language		Four-word sentences	3–4 y
Cooing	2–4 mo	Five-word sentences	4–5 y
Babbles with labial consonants (*ba, ma, ga*)	5–8 mo		

[1] Ages are averages based primarily on the data of Arnold Gesell.

Modified and reproduced, with permission, from Illingworth RS: *The Development of the Infant and Young Child: Normal and Abnormal,* 9th ed. Williams & Wilkins, 1980, 1987.

with sufficient sensitivity, specificity, and predictive value for the population in which it is to be used must be available to minimize the psychological and financial costs of identifying false-positive cases and missing true cases. Each of these areas has provoked considerable controversy with regard to developmental screening. Most moderate to significant disabilities, rather than being identified during routine developmental screening, are suspected and identified because of concerns raised by a parent, teacher, or physician in the context of an ongoing relationship with the child. Information regarding the efficacy of intervention programs for children with a variety of developmental disabilities remains incomplete, and in many communities the availability of subsequent comprehensive diagnostic and treatment programs is limited. Much discussion has focused on the strengths and weaknesses of specific developmental screening tests. Such tests are designed to assess the likelihood of a developmental problem at one point in time. Given the dynamic and multifactorial nature of the developmental process, it is not surprising that developmental screening tests are only weakly predictive of later developmental performance and correlate poorly with subsequent school problems or failure. The sensitivity, specificity, and predictive value of a test changes with the population to which it is applied. Considerable problems in interpretation and validity arise when a test is administered to individuals in populations significantly different from those in which the instrument was standardized. Concern has arisen especially with respect to cross-cultural applications and the screening of developmentally "high-risk" populations, such as premature infants, not originally included in the population used to validate the screening instruments.

Despite the concerns and uncertainties, developmental screening instruments provide a measure of normative development within a given population and a useful framework on which to structure developmental observation and discussion during the health supervision visit. If a screening tool is used, one should be familiar with the specific strengths and weaknesses of the instrument chosen and consider whether its use is appropriate in the intended patient population. When evaluating developmental performance in the office, it is important to allow children to demonstrate their best efforts and abilities. Testing should not occur when the child is sick or frightened. Care must be taken to avoid prognosticating or labeling a child on the basis of a screening test.

The information obtained through screening tests should enhance rather than supplant broader, ongoing developmental monitoring in the context of a primary care relationship with the parents and family. Given the limitations of developmental screening tests, the much broader, time-honored concept of developmental surveillance is receiving renewed attention and growing support. Surveillance, although it requires no less thorough a knowledge of normal and deviant patterns of development, relies less on developmental testing and more on continual monitoring of developmental functioning and well-being by paying attention to parental concerns and making longitudinal observations during all encounters with children and their families.

In the context of such a relationship, pediatric primary care providers frequently face concerns regarding a child's global or selective developmental abilities. The remainder of this section addresses the initial evaluation and management of children with suspected developmental delay and speech or language problems. The approach to the child with school failure and learning disabilities is discussed in Chapter 3.

Common Issues & Concerns

SUSPECTED DEVELOPMENTAL DELAY

Because parents more commonly overestimate than underestimate their child's abilities, developmental concerns, when such concerns are expressed, should be taken seriously. Although parents of children with suspected developmental delays most often worry about the possibility of mental retardation, many factors besides inherent mental ability can affect a child's apparent developmental level. Performance can be artificially lowered if testing occurs when a child is sick, frightened, or uncooperative, or if screening instruments are applied indiscriminately. Otherwise normal premature infants can manifest slight differences in their patterns of development, particularly with respect to gross motor skills, and might be labeled erroneously as abnormal when compared with the performance

of full-term babies. Further, an age correction for the extent of prematurity should be made until the child is 18–24 months old. Developmental disabilities, frequently unrelated to intellectual endowment, can result from cerebral palsy; major sensory deficits such as hearing or vision loss; specific speech or language problems; and emotional or behavioral disturbances such as autism, specific learning disabilities, a neglectful or abusive environment, or chronic illness. Many of these conditions interfere with a child's developmental performance and initially can present as developmental delay. The therapeutic and prognostic implications of differentiating these conditions are great.

When a developmental problem is suspected, a definitive diagnostic evaluation should be undertaken to determine whether a delay is truly present and, if so, whether a specific etiology can be identified with implications for prognosis, therapy, and subsequent offspring (Table 1–15). Key questions to be answered by the evaluation are listed in Table 1–16. A comprehensive developmental assessment, using a standard age-appropriate instrument, should be obtained by trained personnel. If a developmental

Table 1–15. Suspected Developmental Delay: Components of Evaluation

Developmental assessment
  Developmental screening/surveillance
  Definitive developmental test using standardized
    instrument (e.g., Baley's Scales of Infant Development)

History
  Problem context
    Parental concerns/problem perceptions
    Parental expectations
  Developmental history
    Parental recollection of milestones, problem onset
  Family history
    Family history of developmental problems/syndromes
  Medical history
    Prenatal care and complications: infections, toxin/drug
      exposure
    Perinatal complications: problems with delivery, asphyxia,
      infection, central nervous system insults, anomalies,
      postpartum problems
    Gestational age and growth parameters at birth:
      prematurity, small for gestational age, microcephaly
    Previous hospitalizations, illnesses, and surgery
    Current medications
  Review of systems
    Complete review of systems with emphasis on detecting
      symptoms of neurologic disorders (e.g., seizures), and
      chronic illness

Psychosocial/behavioral assessment
  Caregiving environment
  Parent–child relationship

Family stressors
Behavioral problems: "willful" (e.g., tantrums, hitting,
  disobedience), "non-willful" (e.g., hyperactivity,
  impulsivity, distractibility, problems with interpersonal
  interactions)

Physical examination
  Growth parameters (especially head circumference)
  Observations of child's interpersonal interactions, alertness,
    curiosity, persistence
  Complete physical examination, with emphasis on detect-
    ing neurologic abnormalities, dysmorphic features,
    congenital anomalies, skin pigment abnormalities

Sensory evaluation
  Hearing test
  Vision test

Laboratory evaluation
  Diagnostic tests directed by concerns raised in history and
    physical examination
  Newborn/infant: follow-up of state metabolic screen
  Serum lead level
  Idiopathic mental retardation
    Chromosomal testing (cytogenetic)
    Testing for fragile X must be specifically requested
    Based on clinical presentation and philosophy:
      magnetic resonance imaging, metabolic screen

Table 1–16. Suspected Developmental Delay:
Key Questions

Developmental assessment
Is a developmental delay present?
Is the delay global or selective?

History (problem context, developmental, family, medical,
review of systems)
Do caretakers perceive development to be a problem?
Was there a distinct onset to the developmental problem?
Has developmental regression been noted?
Does the history suggest a potential etiology?

Psychosocial/behavioral assessment
What is the nature of the caretaking environment?
Are significant emotional/behavioral problems present?

Physical examination
Is there physical evidence of a potential etiology?
Is growth retardation or microcephaly present?

Sensory evaluation
Is hearing or visual deficit present?

Laboratory evaluation
Are specific diagnostic tests warranted?

problem is confirmed, it is important to ascertain whether the delay is global or selective. For example, a problem primarily with language suggests a hearing problem, inadequate environmental stimulation, or autism. An isolated motor problem can occur with neuromuscular disease, hemiplegia or paraplegia, or cerebral palsy. With confirmation of a delay, a complete history, physical examination, and formal evaluation of hearing and vision are essential. It is important to ascertain from the parents whether their child's developmental problems had a distinct age of onset, suggesting specific causal factors, and whether any developmental regression has been noted. Slow developmental progress might be indicative of a static or progressive process. However, developmental regression, as manifest by loss of previously achieved developmental milestones, always suggests a progressive neurologic disorder. Prenatal, perinatal, and postnatal risk factors for subsequent developmental problems and a positive family history for similar problems should be investigated. A thorough psychosocial and behavioral assessment should be obtained, with an emphasis on exploring the caretaking environment and any concomitant behavioral problems. Nonwillful problems, such as hyperactivity, impulsivity, distractibility, and poor social interactions, should be differentiated from willful behavioral problems, such as tantrums, hitting, and disobedience, which might be indicative of a specific underlying behavioral problem. Overall patterns of growth, with special emphasis on head cir-

cumference, should be noted. A complete physical examination should be performed, with a focus on detecting neurologic problems, dysmorphic features, congenital anomalies, and skin pigment abnormalities suggestive of neurocutaneous disorders. When congenital anomalies or dysmorphic features are identified, evaluation by a dysmorphologist skilled in the identification of specific syndromes is warranted. During the examination, the child's general alertness, curiosity, persistence, and interpersonal interactions can be assessed.

Laboratory evaluation of a child with a confirmed developmental delay in general should be guided by the child's history and physical examination (Tables 1–15 and 1–17). Given our growing awareness of the deleterious effects of relatively low levels of ingested lead and its pervasive presence in our environment, children with unexplained developmental delay should be screened for lead toxicity. A child with significant unexplained mental retardation also should have chromosomal studies performed, including specific cytogenetic testing for fragile X syndrome. The routine use of neuroimaging in the evaluation of idiopathic mental retardation is controversial. The recent availability of high-resolution magnetic resonance imaging has increased our ability to detect different degrees of cerebral dysgenesis and provide parents with at least a partial explanation for their child's disability, although it may not necessarily be the primary etiology. The desire to identify a specific etiology, however, also must be weighed against the cost of the test and the low likelihood of identifying specific findings with relevance to the child's subsequent treatment and prognosis. Routine screening for metabolic disorders in otherwise asymptomatic children with idiopathic mental retardation is usually nonproductive. Most of these conditions present with additional findings such as seizures, failure to thrive, lethargy, hypoglycemia, acidosis, vomiting, and a plateau or progressive loss of developmental skills. When the clinical situation is suggestive, however, appropriate metabolic screening tests should be obtained. In addition, results of state-mandated newborn metabolic screening always should be followed up in the newborn period.

While a developmental evaluation is ongoing, it is important to avoid labeling the child with terms such as *developmentally delayed, disabled,* or *mentally retarded.* If an otherwise unexplained problem is confirmed by definitive testing, it should be pointed out to parents that the delay observed relates to the child's current performance. Although the likelihood of a child's ability being normal decreases the further its performance is from expected norms, present developmental tests are poor predictors of future performance, in particular those used during infancy and toddlerhood.

Perhaps parents' greatest concern during such an evaluation is that their child will be discovered to be mentally retarded. Mental retardation is defined as subnormal

Table 1–17. Suggested Indications for Diagnostic or Screening Tests Recommended in Children with Unexplained Mental Retardation and Specific Findings

Magnetic resonance imaging of the brain	IQ < 50
Cerebral palsy or motor asymmetry	Skin pigmentary anomalies (mosaicism)
Abnormal head size or shape	Suspected contiguous gene syndromes (e.g., Prader-Willi,
Craniofacial malformation	Angelman, Smith-Magenis)
Loss or plateau of developmental skills	
Multiple somatic anomalies	**Metabolic studies**[2]
Neurocutaneous findings	Episodic vomiting or lethargy
Seizures	Poor growth
IQ < 50	Seizures
	Unusual odors
Cytogenetic studies[1]	Somatic evidence of storage
Microcephaly	Loss or plateau of developmental skills
Multiple (even minor) somatic anomalies	Movement disorder (choreoathetosis, dystonia, ataxia)
Family history of mental retardation	Sensory loss (especially retinal abnormality)
Family history of fetal loss	Acquired cutaneous disorders

[1] Because of high prevalence, lack of specific clinical features, and variable developmental manifestations, some experts suggest specific cytogenetic testing for fragile X syndrome in males and females with otherwise unexplained mental retardation.
[2] Basic laboratory screen: fasting plasma amino acids, blood lactate, ammonia, very–long-chain fatty acids, urinary oligosaccharides/mucopolysaccharides. Further metabolic evaluation is usually directed best by a specialist.
From Palmer FB, Capute AJ: Mental retardation. *Pediatr Rev* 1994;15:473–479.

intellectual functioning statistically represented by an IQ less than 2 SD below the population mean on standardized intelligence testing and associated with coexisting delays in adaptive skills such as self-care, home living, communication, and social interactions. This corresponds to an IQ of approximately 70–75 on the Stanford-Binet and Wechsler intelligence tests. Mild mental retardation is generally defined as an IQ of 50–70, and moderate to severe retardation as an IQ less than 50. In more recent definitions, an effort has been made to avoid categorization on the basis of IQ levels and place greater emphasis on descriptions of functional deficits in a variety of adaptive skill areas. Mild mental retardation occurs with an incidence of 20–30 per 1000 individuals, is often familial or polygenic, and is noted more frequently in boys and in groups of lower socioeconomic status. Identifiable chromosomal abnormalities account for only 4–8%. Although the majority of these abnormalities are believed to be idiopathic, a variety of insults and pathogenic processes, such as prenatal substance exposure and postnatal lead toxicity, might be causal. By contrast, severe mental retardation occurs with an incidence of 3–4 per 1000 individuals, is typically sporadic, and, although still more common in boys, shows no socioeconomic predilection. An etiology can be determined in approximately 60–70% of cases. Chromosomal abnormalities are the single largest group of etiologies detected (30%), and among those, Down's syndrome, or trisomy 21, is the most frequent disorder identified. Because of the recent availability of specific molecular and cytogenetic techniques, a syndrome called fragile X has

increasingly been identified as a cause of mental retardation. This X-linked–inherited disorder typically affects males (although approximately one third of female carriers are also affected) and is classically characterized by mental retardation, facial dysmorphism, and macroorchidism. A history of central nervous system injury secondary to teratogens, infection, and prenatal, perinatal, and postnatal insults can be found in 15–20% of cases of severe mental retardation in children. Neuroradiologic imaging studies can identify another 10–15% as having significant cerebral dysgenesis. When found without other anomalies or the stigmata of a specific syndrome, this usually indicates a sporadic and nonprogressive process. Children with multiple congenital anomalies and an identifiable syndrome constitute only 4–5% of cases of severe mental retardation. However, it is important to identify those conditions through a thorough assessment of dysmorphology and family history because many represent single-gene disorders with important implications for parents' subsequent childbearing. Endocrine and metabolic causes of severe mental retardation account for 3–5% of cases.

Many physicians and parents might delay evaluation of a child for whom they have developmental concerns because of the perception that effective interventions are lacking. However, given the many factors that can affect developmental performance, a variety of specific treatable conditions can be detected. The physician also might identify conditions with important implications for parents' future childbearing. Furthermore, although the field of developmental intervention is relatively new and many questions remain, a growing body of data suggests that long-term, comprehensive programs that combine child-focused services with parental education and family support can effectively enhance the developmental abilities of many children with established disabilities and help families to cope better with the many demands of having a child who is developmentally disabled. Helping parents adjust to the realization that their child has a developmental disability can be difficult. Feelings of denial, guilt, anger, and sadness often are exacerbated by the frequent underlying uncertainty regarding cause, subsequent prognosis, and recurrence risk. Pediatric primary care providers can provide the long-term support and coordination of care so important to these families and are also in a unique position to advocate effectively for the needs of these children and their families with schools and other outside agencies.

SUSPECTED SPEECH & LANGUAGE DELAY

Although speech and language problems frequently coexist with more global developmental delays, pediatricians often are faced with specific concerns regarding a child's progress in that area. Approximately 50% of children with delayed language development have delays in other areas. Particularly when more global problems are present, a child's language ability is highly correlated with subsequent cognitive performance. However, problems in that area can be indicative of a variety of primary language disorders and additional factors that are independent of intellectual endowment.

The most frequent causes of inadequate language development are listed in Table 1–18. Sensorineural and recurrent conductive hearing loss can result in abnormal language development. Although deaf infants produce vowel sounds (cooing), progression beyond that point is usually impaired. Formal hearing assessment is essential because parental impressions and crude office testing are notoriously inaccurate. Autism, or autistic spectrum disorder, is an organic brain disorder of unknown and probably multifactorial etiology, characterized by a behavioral symptom complex consisting of abnormalities in socialization and interpersonal interactions (e.g., prefers inanimate objects to people, little affection with caretakers), affect modulation (e.g., mood swings), communication (usually receptive and expressive aspects of language affected), and play (e.g., narrow focus of interest, little interactive or pretend play). It is also frequently associated with cognitive abnormalities, stereotypic motor behaviors (e.g., toe walking, hand flapping, rocking, twirling), sensory abnormalities (e.g., relative pain insensitivity, increased or decreased response to sensory stimuli), and a variety of nonspecific behavioral problems (e.g., attention problems, sleep problems). Developmental language disorders, or dysphasic syndromes, are disorders of higher cerebral functioning resulting in impaired language development. Dysphasia typically is classified into multiple subtypes based on whether primarily expressive, receptive, or a combination of both types of language deficits are present and whether higher-order language processing is impaired (semantics, syntax). Dysarthria (neuromotor abnormalities of the orofacial muscles) and anatomic problems of the oropharynx and larynx also can impair speech. Children who grow up in neglectful or overtly abusive environments frequently manifest language and other developmental delays. *Elective mutism* refers to a child who uses language in some environments but not in others and can be indicative of an underlying language disorder or a significant emotional disturbance.

Early language development can be divided into prespeech, naming, and word-combination stages. During the prespeech period (0–10 months), the infant learns to localize sounds, produce melodious vowel sounds (cooing) first randomly and then in a give-and-take pattern with caregivers, and, beginning at approximately 6 months, add consonants to the vowels to make repetitive syllables (babbling). Although deaf infants will coo, progression to interactional cooing and babbling is impaired. By the end of this period, vocalizations become very interactive, and when random utterances approximate words (*dada, mama*), positive responses from caregivers' begin to reinforce their repeated use. The naming period (10–18 months) is characterized by the rapid acquisition of names and labels for the people and objects around them as children learn the symbolic significance of language. Receptive understanding of words precedes expressive language skills. By 12 months of age, many infants understand 75–100 words, can follow simple commands (with and then without gestures), and can vocalize several "first words." Increasingly complex babbling is interspersed with recognizable words and strung together with an intonation and cadence that resembles mature sentences (jargoning). Pointing also becomes very important during this period as a way to obtain desired objects, gain parental attention, learn the name of specific objects, and communicate a shared experience (e.g., pointing and vocalizing *Airplane!*).

Table 1–18. Causes of Inadequate Language Development

Hearing problem
Mental retardation
Dysphasia (developmental language disorder)
Autistic spectrum disorder
Dysarthria
Structural problems of the oropharynx and upper respiratory tract
Elective mutism
Child abuse and neglect

The word-combination period typically begins near age 18 months. Before then, children might use "giant word" combinations such as "Stop it" and "Let's go" and "holophrases," single words that imply a whole sentence of meaning (e.g., pointing at and saying *book* to mean "this book is mine"). True word combinations generally occur after the child has acquired an adequate expressive vocabulary (at least 50 words). First sentences are telegraphic in nature, with prepositions, pronouns, and articles typically omitted. Vocabulary and syntax and grammar skills progress rapidly after the second year of life.

Because of the influence of individual temperament, social or cultural factors, and the child's verbal and language environments, children manifest greater variability in the acquisition of language than in other developmental areas. This is especially true with respect to expressive verbal skills. Further, the pace of observable development is not constant. Parents frequently become concerned during the beginning of their child's second year of life when the acquisition and use of new words occur rather slowly, only to be amazed by the veritable explosion in vocabulary and comprehension during the second half of the same year. A transient and relative delay in the emergence of expressive language skills might reflect differences in the kinds and extent of opportunities for verbal interaction encountered by children in different families. Children from bilingual families also might manifest transient delays in their expressive language and frequently combine elements of both languages in their early verbalizations. By 2–3 years of age, however, most of those children can separate the languages appropriately and use them in their respective contexts. No long-term language problems have been associated with multilanguage exposure, and there is some evidence suggesting that subsequent language development can actually be facilitated by this experience. As children learn the patterns of their language, rules are often overgeneralized, leading to common developmental "mistakes" (e.g., *sheeps* instead of *sheep, goed* instead of *went*), which must be differentiated from deviant language development. In general, screening instruments rely heavily on the assessment of expressive language abilities. Because of normal variability in this area and the frequently encountered difficulties with obtaining an accurate expressive performance in an office setting, many children may be erroneously labeled as language delayed. A longitudinal perspective regarding the child's language and overall development can put concerns into perspective. Although care must be taken to avoid mislabeling normal children, the availability of effective treatments for a variety of conditions with primary or secondary effects on speech and language development makes prompt evaluation of significant or persistent concerns important.

Initial evaluation of a child with a suspected language delay should include direct assessment of the child's language abilities through the use of informal observation and specific language screening instruments; a thorough developmental history and assessment; formal hearing evaluation; a complete medical, family, psychosocial, and behavioral history; and a thorough physical examination. Table 1–19 lists important expressive and receptive developmental language milestones and specific indications for further evaluation and referral. Key findings that should prompt concern are the absence of apparent response to sound in an infant, the absence of babbling by 9–12 months of age, the absence of any words by 18 months, the absence of meaningful phrases by 24 months, speech that is largely unintelligible to strangers at 3 years, an inability to use language communicatively, and apparent difficulties with language comprehension. To optimize the likelihood of an accurate assessment, attempts to evaluate a child's language ability should take place in a quiet, nonthreatening environment when the child is otherwise well and before other more distressing aspects of the visit are performed. Although observation of children's verbal interaction with their parents and the use of simple toys and picture books to engage them in casual conversation can be very useful, a variety of specific language screening instruments, such as the Early Language Milestone scale and Clinical Linguistic Assessment Measurement, are available for use in the office setting. These scales are designed to differentiate receptive, expressive, and mixed language disorders. It is also important to ascertain, through a thorough developmental assessment, whether the language delay is an isolated problem or part of more global developmental concerns. A formal hearing assessment using behavioral or brainstem-evoked response audiometry always should be performed on a child with suspected speech and language problems. Medical and familial risk factors for hearing or speech and language problems, such as prematurity, perinatal asphyxia, prolonged aminoglycoside use, known central nervous system insults, and a family history of prior syndromes or hearing and language problems, should be elicited. A thorough behavioral assessment is essential, with special emphasis on detecting behaviors suggestive of autism. The nature and quality of the child's psychosocial environment also should be evaluated. Children exposed to neglectful or abusive environments frequently manifest delays in language and personal social skills disproportionate to their motor abilities. The physical examination should focus on identifying abnormal growth patterns (especially microcephaly), congenital anomalies and dysmorphism suggestive of an underlying syndrome or prenatal insult, neurologic abnormalities, ear pathology, and abnormalities of the oropharynx.

Specific therapies are available for a variety of conditions resulting in inadequate speech and language development. Success in treating primary developmental language disorders depends on the type and severity of dysphagia; the age of diagnosis; and the presence of

Table 1–19. Clinical Evaluation of Language Skills

Age	Receptive Skills	Expressive Skills	Specific Indication for Referral
0–1 mo	Recognizes sound with startle; turns to sound and looks for source; quiets motor activity to sound; "prefers" human speech with high inflection	Differentiated crying; body language of positive and negative response	No response to pleasing sound when alert; neonatal sepsis; meningitis; neonatal asphyxia; prematurity; congenital infection; familial deafness; renal abnormalities; aminoglycoside therapy
2–4 mo	Prolonged attention to sounds; responds to familiar voice; watches the speaking mouth; enjoys rattle; attempts to repeat pleasing sounds with objects; shifts gaze back and forth between sounds	*Ed, ih, uh* (hind mouth vowels); cooing, blows bubbles; enjoys using tongue and lips; reciprocal cooing; play dialogues; loudness varies	No response to pleasing sounds; does not attend to voices
5–7 mo	Seeks out speaker; localizes sounds; understands own name, familiar words; associates word with activity (e.g., *bath, car*)	Initiates sounds; pitch varies; babbles with labial consonants (*ba, ma, ga*); uses sounds to get attention, express feeling; sounds directed at object	Decrease or absence of vocalizations
8–12 mo	Begins word comprehension; responds to simple commands—"point to your noise," "say bye-bye"; knows names of family members; responds to a few words, those associated with specific objects	First words, five to six—*mama, dada*; inflected vocal play; repeats sounds and words made by others; *oo, ee* (foremouth vowels); intentional gestures	No babbling with consonant sounds; no response to music
13–20 mo	Single-step element commands; identifies familiar objects	Points to objects with vocalization; vocabulary of 10–50 words; pivot and open class words, rate, and content varies	No comprehension of words; does not understand simple requests
18–24 mo	Recognizes many nouns; understands simple questions	Telegraphic speech; vocabulary of 50–75 words; 20-word sentences, phrases; stuttering common	Vowel sounds, but no consonants; no words
24–36 mo	Understands prepositions; can follow story with pictures	Identifies body parts; vocabulary of 200 words; dependent on phrases, three-word sentences; uses words for expressive needs; pronouns; early grammar	No words; does not follow simple directions; no sentences
30–36 mo	Understands some syntax (difference between *car hit, train* and *train hit car*); understands opposites; understands action in pictures	Sentences of four or five words, three elements; tells stories; uses "what" and "where" questions; uses negation; uses progressive and past tense, all regular form; uses plurals, regular form	Speech largely unintelligible to stranger; dropout of initial consonants; no sentences

(continued)

Table 1-19. (Continued)

Age	Receptive Skills	Expressive Skills	Specific Indication for Referral
3–4 y	Understands three-element commands	Talks about what she is doing; uses *I* with grammar by her own rules; vocabulary of 40–1500 words; speech intelligible to strangers; "why" questions; commands; uses past and present tenses; passive speech in spontaneous speech; nursery rhymes; says colors, numbers 1–4, full name, sex; articulation of *m, n, p, h,* and *w;* four-word sentences	Speech not comprehended by strangers; still dependent on gestures; consistently holds hands over ears; speech without modulation
4–5 y	Understands four-element commands; links past and present events; decreasing ability for second language acquisition	2700-word vocabulary; defines simple words; auxiliary verbs *has* and *had;* conversation mature with "how" and "why" questions in response to others; articulation of *b, k, g,* and *f;* five-word sentences; "normalizes" irregular verbs and nouns; increases in accessibility of forms	Stuttering; consistently avoids loud places
5–6 y	Understands five-element commands; can follow a story without pictures; enjoys jokes and riddles; can comprehend two meanings of a single word	Correct use of all parts of speech; vocabulary 5000 words; articulation of *y, ng,* and *d;* six-word sentences; corrects own errors in speech; can use logic in recounting story plots	Word endings dropped; faulty sentence structure; abnormal rate, rhythm, or inflection
6–7 y	Asks for motivation and explanation of events; understands time intervals (months, seasons); right and left differences	Articulation of *l, r, t, sh, ch, dr, cl, bl, gl,* and *cr;* has formal adult speech patterns	Poor voice quality, articulation
7–8 y	Can use language alone to tell a story sequentially; reasons using language	Articulation of *v, th, j, s, z, tr, st, sl, sw,* and *sp*	
8–9 y		Articulation of *th, sc,* and *sh*	

From Dixon SJ, Stein MT: *Encounters with Children—Pediatric Behavior Development,* 3rd ed. St. Louis: Mosby, 2000, pp. 303–305.

concomitant developmental, behavioral, psychosocial, and other medical disorders.

■ COUNSELING & ANTICIPATORY GUIDANCE

An integral part of child health supervision is the provision of information, support, and anticipatory guidance to parents and children regarding a variety of age-related topics important to the health and well-being of the growing child. Parents increasingly turn to their pediatrician for the advice and support once provided by extended family. The physician, by developing a strong long-term relationship with patients and their families, is in a unique position to respond to specific problems and concerns as they arise and to facilitate health promotion and disease prevention by providing and personalizing information and support.

The pediatric health supervision visit allows for discussion of age-appropriate topics related to nutrition, daily care, behavior and development, injury prevention, family functioning, and the management of minor medical problems. Prevention of specific problems is an important aspect of anticipatory guidance, but an equally important goal is the promotion of health and development by optimizing the parent–child relationship and encouraging positive health behaviors. Helping parents to understand the impact of their child's temperament and environment on growth and development and anticipate abilities, behaviors, and issues that typically emerge at different ages encourages an understanding of how the child is similar to and different from other children.

Despite the potential for benefit, limited and conflicting data exist regarding the optimal content, technique, and overall effectiveness of anticipatory guidance. In this era of cost containment, providers increasingly are being asked to provide tangible cost–benefit data to justify the services they provide. Further research should define the most effective use of the clinician's limited time during the well-child visit and the relative roles of the physician, health educator, and other personnel in the areas of prevention and health counseling. Nonetheless, several general principles should be kept in mind when incorporating anticipatory guidance into child health supervision.

The perceived need to cover a predetermined list of topics at each visit should not overshadow the importance of establishing strong relationships between the doctor, parents, and child. Advice given within the context of such a relationship can have a powerful effect on health behavior choices.

Always address the specific concerns of the parent and child first before covering other topics.

Discussion, using appropriate language and explanations, should be encouraged and advice personalized to the resources and experience of the child and family.

Emphasizing the developmental basis for age-appropriate issues, although enjoyable for some parents, is not essential to providing meaningful information and discussion.

More is not always better. It is important to prioritize the information one wishes to convey and not try to cover too much at each visit.

It is also wise to recognize when scientific evidence regarding a particular approach or issue is unclear and thus avoid being overly dogmatic or judgmental when giving advice. Making an issue over a relatively minor point in the long run might diminish your chances of influencing the parents on matters of importance where data are well established.

Given the time constraints of the health supervision visit, clinicians should make use of "natural" counseling moments as they occur, such as when reviewing the child's growth chart with the parents, when per-

forming the physical examination, or when observing a particular behavior in the office.

Important information should be repeated several times during the visit.

Both children and adults respond best to positive rather than negative reinforcement. It is always important to recognize and acknowledge good parenting and child-parent interactions when observed.

Based primarily on a consensus of expert opinion, the American Academy of Pediatrics (AAP; *Guidelines for Health Supervision III*) and the National Center for Education in Maternal and Child Health (*Bright Futures: Guidelines for Health Supervision of Infants, Children, and Adolescents*) have issued guidelines regarding recommended anticipatory guidance content for child health supervision visits. *Guidelines for Adolescent Preventive Services* is an expansion on issues relevant to the preventive health care needs of adolescents (Table 1–2). These areas are addressed further in Chapter 2. A condensation of suggested topics for discussion at different ages is given in Table 1–20. Selected areas of anticipatory guidance and common age-related issues are expanded in subsequent sections. In-depth discussion on the diagnosis and management of specific behavioral problems occur in Chapter 3.

Common Issues in Nutrition & Feeding

BREAST FEEDING

Infant feeding practices, influenced by a variety of social, cultural, scientific, and commercial factors, have changed widely over the past half century. The availability of nutritionally sound infant formulas has given parents more flexibility and options in the feeding of their infants. However, the nutritional, immunologic, and psychological advantages of breast feeding remain compelling. The decision to breast or bottle feed an infant usually is made before the baby is born and therefore is an important topic for discussion during the prenatal visit. Physicians should promote the benefits of breast feeding by providing information, dispelling misconceptions, and helping parents to clarify their own feelings and attitudes about infant feeding. Once a decision is made, however, it is important to be supportive and nonjudgmental.

Most breast-feeding mothers who wean their infants in the first several weeks postpartum do so because of a lack of information regarding breast-feeding norms and supportive guidance in dealing with a variety of common problems. Postpartum counseling should encourage maternal confidence by providing training in correct nursing technique and anticipatory guidance regarding breast-feeding physiology, norms, and common problems. Because questions commonly arise, it is especially important to offer early follow-up counseling to parents who elect to breast feed their infants.

Table 1–20. Anticipatory Guidance—Suggested Topics at Each Visit

Prenatal			
Injury prevention	Safe baby furniture; car safety restraints; smoke detector; water thermostat set <120°F		rolling; do not leave unattended on bed or table; caution about hot liquids, burns; advise against infant walkers
Feeding/nutrition	Breast vs. bottle	Feeding/nutrition	As above; waiting to introduce solids at 4–6 mo
Medical	Circumcision; what to expect at delivery; schedule of health supervision visits	Daily care/activities	Sleep, crying, and bowel patterns
		Developmental/ behavioral issues	As above
Other	Maternal health issues; social supports; siblings	Medical	Immunizations; URI management: bulb syringe, saline nose drops
Newborn		Other	As above; child care arrangements and support
Injury prevention	Review above. Emphasize: never leave infant unattended, use car restraints	**4 mo**	
		Injury prevention	Review above. Emphasize: keep small objects out of reach
Feeding/nutrition	Issues with breast or bottle feeding: norms, common problems	Feeding/nutrition	Introducing solid foods: iron-fortified cereal, fruits and vegetables
Daily care/activities	Crying, sleeping, sleep position, and SIDS, stooling patterns; bathing and skin care; hiccups, sneezing, "wet burps"	Daily care/activities	Sleep: night awakening; teething/drooling
Developmental/ behavioral issues	Normal reflexes (startle); individuality of infant; importance of close interaction and responding to infant's needs (cannot spoil)	Developmental/ behavioral issues	As above; talk to baby: respond to vocalizations
		Medical	Immunizations; management of mild gastroenteritis
Medical	Care of umbilical cord and circumcision; jaundice; how to take a baby's temperature; when and how to call the doctor: fever, vomiting, diarrhea, decreased feeding; review schedule of health supervision visits	Other	Parent and family functioning; child care arrangements and support
		6 mo	
		Injury prevention	"Child-proofing" house in preparation for mobility; syrup of ipecac/Poison Control Center number; car safety; walkers and stair gates; window guards; bathtub safety; electrical cords and outlets; burn risks
Other	Postpartum adjustment; change in parent and family relationships; sibling reactions		
2–4 wk			
Injury prevention	Review above; bath safety; sun exposure/protection	Feeding/nutrition	Issues with feeding solids; norms regarding caloric needs (volumes); introducing finger foods (7–9 mo); begin practice with cup; discourage milk or juice as pacifier or bottle to bed; discuss when to introduce cow's milk (end of first year, if possible)
Feeding/nutrition	Issues with breast vs. bottle feeding; fluoride supplementation, if indicated		
Daily care/activities	Sleep patterns; crying and "colic"; bladder and bowel habits		
Developmental/ behavioral issues	Emphasize infant's abilities; enjoy holding, cuddling, talking to baby (cannot spoil)	Daily care/activities	Resistance to sleep: suggest favorite toy or possession (transitional objects); teething/dental care; shoes (soft, flexible)
Medical	Reinforce when to call the doctor		
Other	Time to themselves for parents: baby sitters; spending time with siblings; plans for substitute care if mother works outside home	Developmental/ behavioral issues	Separation and stranger anxiety
		Medical	Immunizations
2 mo		Other	As above
Injury prevention	Review above. Emphasize: use car restraints, protect from falls,		

(continued)

Table 1-20. (Continued)

9 mo

Injury prevention	Review above. Emphasize: toddler car restraint when ≥ 20 lb; ingestants (e.g., small objects, peanuts, grapes, hot dogs; burns)
Feeding/nutrition	Finger/table foods; self-feeding: cup and spoon practice; begin to wean from bottle; anticipate decreased food intake; introducing cow's milk
Daily care/activities	Sleep: night awakening, favorite toy or possession; shoes; dental care
Developmental/ behavioral issues	Separation and stranger anxiety; vocalization, communication, imitation; social games; anticipate autonomy issues of toddler period; discipline: setting limits, consistency, distraction
Other	Parent and family functioning; child care arrangements and support

12 mo

Injury prevention	Reinforce: syrup of ipecac/Poison Control Center number; tap water at maximum of 120°F; kitchen, stair, water, and car safety; fences, gates, and latches; burn risks
Feeding/nutrition	Table foods, weaning from bottle; decreased food intake; introducing cow's milk
Daily care/activities	As above
Developmental/ behavioral issues	Speech development; talk to baby; discuss autonomy, limit-setting, discipline; praise desired behavior (positive reinforcement); prohibitions: few but firm
Other	As above

15 mo

Injury prevention	Review above
Feeding/nutrition	Self-feeding, eats meals with family; phase out bottle use, advise against bottle in bed
Daily care/activities	As above
Developmental/ behavioral issues	Review indicators of toilet training readiness; discipline/ temper tantrums: remove from temptation, consistency between parents, time-out, substitution, avoid reinforcing tantrum behavior, praise good behavior; read books together
Medical	Immunizations

Other	Parent and family functioning; child care arrangements and support; sibling rivalry

18 mo

Injury prevention	Review above. Emphasize: supervised play near street, in driveway; yard, pedestrian, and playground safety; dangers of climbing; never leave unattended in car or in house; unsafe toys, plastic bags and balloons
Feeding/nutrition	Wean from bottles; good use of spoon and cup in self-feeding
Daily care/activities	Sleep: short ritual before regular bedtime, night fears, night awakening; self-comforting behaviors: thumb sucking, masturbation, favorite toy or possession
Developmental/ behavioral issues	Discipline; need for autonomy and independence; "rapprochement"— transient return to clinging behavior; may show toilet training readiness at 18–24 mo; play games: praise, show affection; read simple stories to child regularly
Medical	Immunizations
Other	As above

24 mo

Injury prevention	Review above
Feeding/nutrition	Avoid struggles about eating; discourage nonnutritious snacks; encourage social/family aspects of meals
Daily care/activities	Sleep: discuss a move to regular bed; reassure that day napping varies; use of toothbrush
Developmental/ behavioral issues	Autonomy: do not hurry, consistent limits, present choices. Toilet learning: does child show interest and readiness, understand expectations? Curiosity about body parts; provide for play and peer contacts; imaginary friends
Other	Parent and family functioning; child care arrangements and support; sibling rivalry

3 y

(continued)

Table 1-20. (*Continued*)

Injury prevention	Review above. Emphasize: car safety restraints; street and water safety; animals and pets; teach full name, emergency number, and address	Other	Family functioning
		6 and 8 y	
		Injury prevention	Bicycle safety; seat belts; learn to swim; child supervision when away
Feeding/nutrition	Balanced diet, avoidance of junk foods	Feeding/nutrition	Avoid junk food, maintain appropriate weight; encourage social aspects of mealtime
Daily care/activities	First dental appointment; sleep: regular bedtime and routine, napping variability		
		Daily care/activities	Exercise regularly; brush teeth; get adequate sleep; school and academic activities; peer interactions; family interactions
Developmental/ behavioral issues	Discipline; toilet training; nursery school, day care, baby sitters: encourage out-of-home experiences, peer interactions; allow to explore, show initiative, and communicate; talk about activities with child; reserve time alone with child; limit television viewing; watch children's programs with child; masturbation; satisfy curiosity about babies, sex differences	Developmental/ behavioral issues	Establish rules, act as role model; provide allowance; spend time with child; show interest in school; praise, encourage, show affection; limit television viewing
		Other	Library card
		10 y	
Other	Family functioning	Injury prevention	Review above. Emphasize: skateboard and bicycle safety; drugs, alcohol, and tobacco; supervise potentially hazardous activities; sport safety
4 y			
Injury prevention	Review above. Emphasize: bicycle and pedestrian safety; water safety; car seat, booster, or seat belt; refusal of food or rides from strangers; electrical tools, firearms, matches, and poisons; know emergency number and address; home fire safety drills	Feeding/nutrition	As above
		Daily care/activities	As above
		Developmental/ behavioral issues	As above; social interactions: peers, hobbies, social skills; sex education at home, school; discuss pubertal changes; academic activities; family communications: method of resolution, limit setting, sense of responsibility
Feeding/nutrition	Balanced diet, social aspects of meals		
Daily care/activities	Dental care, sleep		
Developmental/ behavioral issues	Toilet training; discipline; provide interactions with other children; assign chores; limit television viewing; sexual curiosity, masturbation; nursery school, day care; issues around school, readiness assessment	**12 y**	
		Injury prevention	Review above
		Feeding/nutrition	Avoid junk food, maintain appropriate weight; encourage social aspects of mealtime
Other	Family functioning		
5 y		Daily care/activities	Exercise regularly, brush teeth, get adequate sleep; school and academic activities; sports, hobbies, and weekend jobs; peer and family interactions
Injury prevention	Review above		
Feeding/nutrition	Balanced diet		
Daily care/activities	Dental care, sleep		
Developmental/ behavioral issues	School readiness; plays well with other children, normal development, endures half-day separation from home; promote interactions with other children; assign chores; discipline; sexual curiosity, masturbation	Developmental/ behavioral issues	Discuss: rapid physical growth and sexual development, body image; sex education; establish rules, communicate with child; respect privacy, allow decision making
Medical	Immunizations		

(*continued*)

Table 1-20. (Continued)

14 y Injury prevention	Review above. Emphasize: risk-taking behaviors; encourage responsibility for health and health behavior choices	Daily care/activities	sports, hobbies, jobs; regular physical exercise; peer and family interactions
Feeding/nutrition	As above	Developmental/ behavioral issues	Goals and values clarification, future plans; fair rules, allow decision making; family and
Feeding/nutrition Daily care/activities Developmental/ behavioral issues	As above Review above. Emphasize: dating, peer pressure; sexuality		peer communication; expect periods of estrangement; respect privacy; encourage independence; serve as role
16–20 y Injury prevention	Review above. Emphasize: responsibility for health; driving safety; substance abuse; CPR training		model; sexuality and activity, contraception and prevention of sexually transmitted diseases
Feeding/nutrition	Healthy diet, maintaining appropriate weight School and academic activities;		

CPR = cardiopulmonary resuscitation; SIDS = sudden infant death syndrome; URI = upper respiratory infection.
Modified, with permission, from American Academy of Pediatrics, Committee on Psychosocial Aspects of Child and Family Health: *Guidelines for Health Supervision III,* 3rd ed. Elk Grove Village, IL: American Academy of Pediatrics, 1997.

The suckling newborn stimulates the mother's pituitary to release prolactin and oxytocin, which in turn stimulate the production and "letdown" of breast milk. During the first several days postpartum, the infant receives antibody-rich colostrum. Suboptimal feeding routines during this time rarely interfere with ultimate breast feeding success. However, once the mother's milk has "come in," usually 2–5 days after delivery, and she begins to produce a significant volume, suboptimal breast emptying or other factors that interfere with the complex hormonal balance may jeopardize the success of continued lactation. Parents who wish to supplement breast feeding with an occasional bottle of pumped breast milk or formula are advised to wait several weeks until the breast-feeding pattern is well established. The mouth and tongue movements used in breast feeding differ from, and generally more effort intensive than, those used with an artificial nipple. Some infants might have difficulty switching back and forth or might prefer the artificial nipple once exposed. Occasionally an older infant who has never used an artificial nipple also might have difficulty transitioning from the breast to the bottle should this becomes necessary or desirable.

Most women find the optimal position for nursing to be one where the infant is cradled at the level of the breast in front of and completely facing the mother. In this position, the mother's free hand can be used to gently squeeze the breast, thereby making the nipple and areola more protractile. Stroking the infant's lips with the nipple will stimulate its mouth to open. When this occurs, the baby should be moved gently but firmly to the breast so that the infant's mouth covers the nipple and as much areola as possible. Once the baby is positioned, symptomatic milk ejection reflex (breast and nipple tingling, milk dripping), slow rhythmic movements of the mandible, and audible swallowing are important indicators that the baby is getting milk. When removing the infant from the breast, the mother should gently insert a finger between the infant's mouth and the breast to break the suction and minimize nipple trauma. Current breast-feeding philosophy discourages rigid schedules for feeding duration and timing. Nipple soreness, once thought to be due to early prolonged suckling, now is believed to be related primarily to poor positioning of the infant and trauma when the infant is removed without breaking suction. Most women work up to feedings of 10–15 minutes or more at each breast with each feeding over the first several days postpartum. In general, the infant will determine when the feeding is over, and parents should be helped to recognize the signs of satiety. To facilitate optimal breast drainage and milk production, it is important that the infant take milk from both breasts at each feeding. Alternating the breast offered first is encouraged for the same reason. Intervals between demand feedings vary, but average every 90 minutes to 3 hours in the first several weeks (8–12 times per day). Newborns should not be allowed to go longer than 4–5 hours between feedings. Most infants omit one of the middle-of-the-night feedings by age 2 months. However, because the protein composition of breast milk results in a more rapid digestion time than occurs with formula, breast-fed infants tend to continue to feed more frequently than bottle-fed infants. Maternal pain, stress, fatigue, and anxiety can have a significant impact on the hormonal milieu necessary for effective lactation. It is important to encourage the lactating mother to get as much rest as possible and to enlist the assistance of the baby's father or other support persons in this regard. Her diet should be nutritious and include plenty of fluids. Suggestions to help facilitate milk let-down during feedings include nursing in a quiet, comfortable place; nursing while lying down; and taking a hot shower or bath just before a feeding.

Sore nipples, engorgement, and maternal fatigue are common problems that can undermine successful breast feeding. Nipple soreness is a frequent and almost always a self-limited condition that diminishes as nipples become conditioned. However, it can be exacerbated by improper nursing technique or factors that interfere with successful milk let-down and flow. Problems with technique most frequently observed include not using the ventral-to-ventral position, so that the infant ineffectively grasps and puts tension on the nipple, not getting enough of the areola in the baby's mouth, and forgetting to break suction before removing the baby from the breast. A warm shower or heating pad might enhance milk let-down and flow. Spreading a thin layer of breast milk on nipples and allowing nipples to air dry with the help of a warm lamp facilitates healing and conditioning. Application and removal of creams and ointments with each feed might increase trauma and abrasion and therefore are generally discouraged. Using different nursing positions to change the pressure points during suckling also might be helpful. Other suggestions to reduce nipple soreness are initiating the feeding and milk let-down on the less sore side and then switching to the sore nipple and manually expressing enough milk to initiate milk let-down so that the most vigorous period of sucking is avoided. However, it is very important that the nursing mother not decrease feeding because of sore nipples because doing so might lead, through inadequate breast drainage, to engorgement.

Engorgement refers to the uncomfortable swelling of the breasts that occurs when regular, effective breast emptying does not take place. Feedings from an engorged breast can be painful and difficult because of decreased nipple protractility. A cycle of decreased feeding leading to increasing engorgement, involution of the milk supply, and possible mastitis can result if adequate drainage does not occur. Engorgement can be avoided with regular, frequent nursing. If it occurs, it is important to counsel mothers that increasing rather than decreasing feedings on the affected side will hasten relief. This can be facilitated initially by manually expressing some milk or using a hand pump until it is easier and less painful for the infant to suckle. Warm compresses to facilitate milk let-down during feedings and cool compresses between feedings also can be helpful.

Breast-feeding mothers frequently worry about whether their milk supplies are adequate and whether their infants are getting enough. Not all women experience fullness or the sensation of milk let-down despite successful breast feeding. Parents should be counseled on ways to assess indirectly whether intake is adequate, such as weight gain, signs of hydration, and satiety behavior (Table 1–21). Breast-fed infants may lose up to 10% of their birth weights before regaining it by 10–14 days of age. Greater or more prolonged weight loss may be a sign of feeding difficulty. During growth spurts (typically at 3, 6, and 12 weeks), the infant might transiently decrease the interval between feedings to stimulate more milk production. It is important to inform parents of this normal phenomenon, so that the change is not perceived as a sign of inadequate milk supply. The use of vitamin and fluoride supplements and the introduction of solid foods in conjunction with breast feeding are discussed below.

The decision about when to begin weaning should take into account the needs and realities of the infant and the mother. Weaning ideally is a gradual process whereby nutritive and psychological needs are increasingly provided by other sources and activities. One can begin by substituting a cup or bottle for the least favorite breast-feeding session at the same time each day. The last feeding to be eliminated should be the one to which the child is most attached. Cuddling and holding without nursing also should be encouraged. In the somewhat older child, periods of separation from the mother and the use of distraction techniques may be helpful. A supportive bra increases the comfort of the mother during the weaning process, and maternal fluid intake should be decreased accordingly.

FORMULA FEEDING

For parents who elect to not breast feed, various manufactured formulas are available. Parents should be informed regarding similarities and differences between formulas, their appropriate preparation and storage, and what to expect in terms of frequency and volume of feedings.

Most of the common commercial formulas designed for healthy, full-term infants are based on cow's milk

Table 1–21. Cues to Assessing Adequacy of Breast Feeding

Nursing frequency no more than 8 feeds/d
Presence of fullness before feeding and relief of fullness after feeding
Presence of symptomatic milk ejection reflex
Audible swallowing by infant
Signs of satiation in infant after feeding
At least 6 wet diapers/d (normally 6–8)
At least 4 stools/d (normally 6–10)
Birth weight loss 10% (birth weight regained by age 2 wk)

and composed of reconstituted skim milk or skim milk with added whey protein. The carbohydrate source is lactose, and the fat content consists of a mixture of vegetable oils that are better digested and absorbed than butter fat. The composition of these formulas is thought to provide an adequate nutritional alternative to breast milk. Differences within this group are relatively small and, in choosing among them, weight should be given to relative cost and the taste preference of the infant. Soy-protein formulas, introduced in the 1920s as hypoallergenic alternatives to preparations based on cow's milk, were initially deficient in several important nutrients. Since then they have undergone a series of refinements and are now considered a nutritionally sound alternative to the milk-based formulas for full-term infants. Soy-based formulas have been found to contain relatively high levels of aluminum. Because of reduced renal function, use in preterm infants has raised concerns about potential aluminum toxicity and reduced skeletal mineralization due to competitive absorption with calcium. Soy-based formulas also have been associated with poorer growth rates in premature infants than have formulas based on cow's milk protein. For those reasons, soy-based formulas are not recommended for preterm infants who weigh less than 1800 g. Despite their origin, formulas based on soy protein are of limited value as hypoallergenic preparations because of the high incidence of cross-reactivity to soy protein among infants with allergy to cow's milk protein and the development of protein hydrolysate formulas for this purpose. The fat composition of soy formulas is similar to that of formulas based on cow's milk. Because the source of carbohydrate is sucrose or corn syrup solids, soy-protein formulas also might be useful as transitional formulas for the infant with transient lactase deficiency that follows significant diarrheal illness. Formula switching for vague constitutional and gastrointestinal symptoms or mild viral gastroenteritis risks inappropriately labeling the child as allergy prone or having gastrointestinal problems should be discouraged. The lack of any evidence linking gastrointestinal symptoms with the concentration of iron in formulas based on cow's milk and soy should be discussed with parents and is addressed further below. Weaning formulas designed for infants older than 6 months have been introduced recently into the market. Although those formulas provide satisfactory nutrient content, they offer no advantage over the currently recommended combinations of breast feeding, infant formula, and iron- and vitamin-containing solids for children of this age.

Most formulas can be purchased in powdered, concentrate, or ready-to-eat forms. Powdered and concentrate preparations are the least expensive but require care in reconstituting to the appropriate concentrations. Unless the family lives in an area where the water supply is potentially unsafe, sterilization of bottle and formula is no longer necessary. Between uses, bottles and nipples should be cleaned with warm, soapy water. Once opened, a can of concentrate or ready-to-eat formula should be refrigerated and used within 48 hours.

As with breast feeding, an on-demand feeding schedule should be encouraged. Most newborns will feed 2–3 oz every 2–3 hours and should not be allowed to go longer than 5 hours between feedings. Formula-fed infants usually lose less than 8% of their birth weight and regain that weight by 7–10 days after birth. After the first week, most infants take 2–4 oz every 2–4 hours, or average approximately 2–3 oz/lb/d. Most bottle-fed infants eliminate the middle-of-the-night feeding by age 2 months. During the second half of the first year, the infant generally should be taking less than 30 oz of formula per day in combination with solids, and calories from formula should not exceed 65% of the total daily intake. Especially with bottle-fed infants, it is important to encourage parents to learn to distinguish crying due to hunger from that due to other causes and to recognize the signs of satiety to avoid the common problem of overfeeding. Putting the older infant to sleep with a bottle should be discouraged because of the risk of nursing-bottle caries and the likely exacerbation of subsequent problems with discontinuing its use. Most parents begin weaning the infant from the bottle at age 9–12 months. Allowing a toddler or preschool child to "roam" with a bottle on demand will make eventual discontinuation much more difficult and can lead to a variety of feeding problems such as inadequate intake and restricted acceptance of solid foods.

Vitamin, Iron, & Fluoride Supplementation

Commercial formulas are fortified with vitamins and minerals. Formula-fed full-term infants require no additional supplementation. Breast milk is naturally rich in vitamins A and C. Although quantitative levels of vitamin D are low in breast milk, clinical rickets is uncommon in full-term breast-fed infants when maternal vitamin D intake during pregnancy and lactation is adequate and when mother and child receive normal amounts of sunlight exposure. Vitamin D supplementation (400 IU/d) is recommended for the nursing infant if the mother's diet is deficient in vitamin D or the infant's sun exposure is limited due to darkly pigmented skin coloration or inadequate sunlight exposure. Vitamin B_{12} deficiency also can occur in breast-fed infants of mothers who are strict vegetarians.

If dietary iron is not provided, full-term infants begin to deplete their iron stores by age 4 months. For all but exclusively breast-fed infants, iron supplementation from one or more sources, such as formula, iron-fortified cereal, or ferrous sulfate drops, should begin at 4–6 months of age in the full-term infant and 2 months of age in the preterm infant. Although the iron content of breast milk is lower than that of formula, exclusively breast-fed infants require no extra source of iron because of its greater bio-availability. However, when solids are started and breast-milk intake is decreased, as with formula-fed children, iron-rich foods are indicated. Early introduction of whole cow's milk can cause iron deficiency anemia because of its low iron content and potential for causing occult gastrointestinal blood loss and should be discouraged before the age of 1 year. Contrary to popular belief, ample evidence now supports the notion that iron-containing formulas do not increase gastrointestinal symptoms such as constipation or gas in most children. It is wise to discuss this with parents and explain the reason iron is important to their child's diet.

The topical and systemic uses of fluoride have dramatically decreased the incidence of dental caries. Excess fluoride, however, can cause fluorosis of the enamel, a cosmetically disfiguring condition. Current recommendations regarding the need for supplementation are based on the concentration of fluoride in the local water supply. The AAP and the American Dental Association Council on Dental Therapeutics recommend beginning fluoride supplementation, if needed, at age 6 months. The dose administered depends on the age of the child and the degree to which the fluoride content of the local water supply is insufficient (Table 1–22). Although levels of fluoride in breast milk are low, the incidence of caries in exclusively breast-fed infants whose mothers drink fluoridated water is similar to that of formula-fed infants living in the same area. Therefore, only breast-fed infants living in areas of inadequate fluoridation need supplementation. It is important to remember to supplement the formula of the rare infant who is ingesting only ready-to-eat formula because these are manufactured with nonfluoridated water. When assisting the toddler in brushing its primary teeth, it is important not to use toothpaste or to use only a very small amount because much of it is swallowed and can lead to excess fluoride intake with subsequent enamel fluorosis.

Table 1–22. Fluoride Supplementation

Age	Water Fluoride Content (ppm)[1]		
	<0.3	0.3–0.6	>0.6
Birth–6 mo	0	0	0
6 mo–3 y	0.25	0	0
3–6 y	0.50	0.25	0
6–16 y	1.00	0.50	0

[1] Fluoride daily doses are given in milligrams.

From Committee on Nutrition, American Association of Pediatrics: Fluoride supplementation for children: interim policy recommendations. *Pediatrics* 1995;95:777.

ADVANCING TO SOLIDS, COW'S MILK, SELF-FEEDING, & A PRUDENT DIET

Current recommendations regarding the introduction of solid foods are based on considerations of developmental readiness, nutrient needs, and the potential for adverse reactions. In the first 4–6 months of life, breast milk or infant formula provides optimal nutrition for the baby, and the use of solid foods should be discouraged. Although they can be force fed, babies younger than 4 months have strong tongue-protrusion reflexes and have not yet developed the mouth and tongue movements necessary for coordinated swallowing of solid foods. By 4–6 months, the infant's head and oromotor control are sufficiently developed to begin to participate actively in exploring the different tastes and textures of solid food and indicate when the baby feels full. Initially, the volume of food consumed is less important than the experience. Parents should be prepared for some fun and mess and allow infants to explore foods with their mouths and fingers. As they get older, infants can be given a second spoon. Many begin by offering solid foods at one or two feedings a day and then advancing to a schedule that gradually approaches the family mealtimes. The order in which foods are introduced is, to a large extent, dictated by tradition. However, because of concerns about the impact of gastrointestinal immaturity on the development of food allergy, it is generally recommended that substances frequently associated with allergic symptomatology, such as egg white, wheat, and fish, be introduced later. Most parents begin with iron-fortified infant cereals and advance to strained or pureed vegetables and fruits, followed by meats and poultry. It is important to remind parents to introduce one new food at a time and wait 3–5 days before adding another to appreciate any adverse effects. With time, a variety of foods should be offered routinely. All infants have food preferences and dislikes, which can and should be respected. However, foods previously refused should be reoffered periodically. It is important to let infants determine when they have had enough and avoid force feeding. When purchasing baby food, one-item foods are preferable to combination dinners. Infant preparations also can be made easily and cheaply at home by cooking foods until tender and then pureeing them with a blender, food mill, or kitchen strainer. Food can be prepared in advance and stored in meal-sized portions by freezing the puree in ice-cube trays. Babies appear to be born with a preference for sweetness. An innate preference for saltiness appears later in the first year of life. However, sweet and salty taste preferences can be exaggerated by dietary exposure. Parents should avoid adding salt or processed sugar to their infant's food.

The early introduction of whole cow's milk, because of its low iron content and potential to cause occult gastrointestinal blood loss, has been associated with iron deficiency in early infancy. Adding cow's milk to an infant's diet should be delayed until after its first birthday. Whole milk rather than skimmed milk is recommended during the first 2 years of life.

By age 6–8 months, most infants can sit, bring objects to their mouths, and begin holding a cup and spoon. With practice, relatively controlled use of the cup and spoon usually occurs between 15 and 18 months of age. Most infants are ready to enjoy finger foods by 7–9 months. Mature chewing skills are usually present by 18 months. In choosing what to offer, it is important to avoid large, hard, spherical, or coin-shaped items that could cause airway obstruction if aspirated. These include foods such as raw carrots, large pieces of raw apple, whole hot dogs or hot dog coins, whole grapes, large cookies, peanuts, and hard candy. Infants and toddlers always should be seated and observed by an adult when eating.

Ample evidence now exists that atherosclerotic disease begins in childhood. Prudent dietary and other life-style practices begun early can prevent or decrease atherosclerotic morbidity in later life. However, excessive dietary fat restriction might lead to impaired growth and nutrition in the developing child. Many expert panels and groups, including the National Cholesterol Education Program (NCEP), the AAP, and the American Heart Association, have issued recommendations regarding a prudent diet for children. These guidelines emphasize the need to eat a varied and nutritionally balanced diet, maintain ideal body weight, decrease total fat intake, increase polyunsaturated fats at the expense of saturated fats and cholesterol, and avoid excessive salt. Children younger than 1–2 years need adequate amounts of dietary fat (30–50% of daily calorie intake) for optimal growth and development. During that time, dietary fat and cholesterol should not be restricted, and whole milk, rather than skim or 2% fat-free milk, should be used. After age 2 years, the child should gradually be transitioned (by age 5 years) to a prudent diet containing (1) no more than 30% and no less than 20% of total calories from fat, (2) less than 10% of total calories from saturated fats, and (3) less than 300 mg/d of dietary cholesterol.

COMMON TODDLER FEEDING ISSUES

Parents of toddlers often become concerned about their children's dietary intake and eating habits. Worry frequently centers around the volume and variety of food consumed. It is important to inform parents that a child's rate of growth slows considerably after its first year of life, and caloric needs per pound decrease even as activity increases. Reviewing the growth chart with parents can be very reassuring. It is also important to point out that otherwise healthy (physically and psychosocially) children will not willfully starve themselves. Parents should be advised to evaluate success at meeting nutritional needs, such as sufficient intake from various food groups, over the course of a week rather than at each meal. Normal

toddler issues of autonomy and self-assertion frequently present themselves around mealtimes. Parental responses to such events often play an important role in exacerbating and/or preventing subsequent feeding problems.

Suggestions to help prevent common toddler feeding and mealtime behavior problems are listed in Table 1–23. Toddlers need consistent mealtime routines and rules. However, mealtimes must not be allowed to become battlegrounds. Parents should strive to create a structured but pleasant and interactive atmosphere in which the social and nutritional aspects of the meal can be emphasized. Families should sit down together and avoid distracting activities such as watching television and reading during the meal. Efforts should be made to include children in table talk and avoid long conversations between adults. The family meal is also an excellent time to find opportunities to praise the child for appropriate mealtime and/or daytime behaviors. With toddlers, it is important to give realistic portions, starting with small, achievable volumes and giving seconds rather than initially overwhelming the child with a seemingly insurmountable mountain of food. It is also helpful to provide the child with opportunities for choice while maintaining control over more

Table 1–23. Preventing Common Toddler Feeding/Mealtime Behavior Problems

Don't make mealtimes a battleground; should be pleasant
Establish mealtime routine and rules
Eat as a family and encourage social aspects
Avoid other concurrent activities (television, reading)
Don't carry on conversations with another adult for longer than a few minutes; include child in table talk
Find opportunities to praise your child for appropriate mealtime/daytime behaviors
Provide opportunities for mealtime choice while regaining control over important issues
Provide variety: praise trying (taste test); offer previously refused types of foods at periodic intervals
Allow and encourage self-feeding (even if messy)
Portion control: give realistic (small) portions, seconds if child finishes
Mealtimes should be of a finite/realistic duration (15–30 min)
When food is refused, avoid routinely preparing a "special" meal for child
Don't make leaving table contingent on cleaning plate
Remove food not finished after the prediscussed time period and, except for routine snacks, avoid additional feedings until next meal
Avoid excessive intake of liquids (juice, milk) and continual "grazing" between meals
Provide nutritious between-meal snacks; avoid excessive snacking
Model good eating behavior as parents

important dietary issues. Self-feeding should be allowed and encouraged, even if messy. Mealtimes should be of a finite duration (20–30 minutes): long, drawn-out battles are rarely productive. Leaving the table should not be contingent on cleaning the plate. Food not finished after the allotted period should be removed, and, except for routine between-meal snacks, parents should avoid additional feedings until the next meal. Excessive intake of liquids such as juice and milk and continual "grazing" between meals should be avoided. All toddlers will have preferred and nonpreferred foods. If a child consumes a reasonable quantity and variety of food, such preferences can be respected. However, a variety of "new" and "old" foods, including those previously rejected, should continue to be offered, and the temptation to prepare routinely a separate meal for the child should be resisted. Children learn by observation: parents should model the same good eating behaviors that they wish their children to exhibit.

Normal Age-related Sleep Patterns & Common Problems

The character and patterns of sleep undergo a normal transition from infancy to adulthood that is influenced by neuromaturational factors and the child's temperament and caretaking environment. Sleep comprises two distinct states: active or rapid eye movement (REM) sleep, characterized by rapid eye movements, motor movements, vocalizations, dreaming, and easy awakening; and the deeper quiet or non-REM sleep. Fifty percent of an infant's sleeptime is spent in the REM state, with non-REM intervals of 50–60 minutes between active phases, whereas only 20% of the adult sleep cycle consists of REM sleep interspersed with 90–100-minute intervals of quiet sleep.

Newborns sleep approximately 18 hours per day, with sleep time distributed evenly over the day and night hours. However, sleep–wake patterns quickly become entrained to a day–night cycle because of inherent circadian rhythms and parental caregiving schedules. Between 6 and 15 months of age, most children sleep approximately 10–12 hours at night and take two daytime naps, each lasting more than an hour, in the midmorning and afternoon. Children usually take only one nap during the day after age 15 months and have discontinued napping altogether by age 4 years. Although individual differences are significant, the 5 year old requires approximately 11 hours and the 10 year old requires 9½ hours of sleep per night. Most adolescents need 8–9 hours of sleep each night.

By inquiring about sleep habits or problems and providing information and anticipatory guidance, pediatric primary care providers are in a unique position to diagnose, manage, and prevent many common age-related sleep problems. Several excellent suggestions to help parents facilitate optimal sleep habits and prevent subsequent

sleep problems in their infants and young toddlers are given in Table 1–24. Parents might inadvertently slow their early infant's adaptation to a day–night sleep schedule by prolonged or frequent periods of nocturnal feeding and attention. Spontaneous awakenings are normal and occur often during periods of REM sleep. The ability of infants to use internal mechanisms to return themselves to sleep usually develops around 3–4 months of age and is referred to as "settling." At this time an infant begins to sleep for 6–8 uninterrupted hours during the night. Although the vast majority of infants "settle" by 6 months of age, some children continue to have frequent and prolonged nighttime awakening. Aside from inherent temperamental differences, several environmental factors might be involved. First, parents can misperceive the movements, vocalizations, and brief awakenings of REM sleep as indicating a need for intervention and, in attending to the infant, inadvertently might cause the child to arouse further. Frequent feedings and prolonged attention at night also can encourage this pattern. Older in-

Table 1–24. Strategies to Encourage Night Settling

Early infancy (birth–4 mo)
During the day, limit the duration of sleep to 3–4 consecutive hours
Place baby to sleep in crib in own room, if feasible
Place baby in crib sleepy but awake
Allow baby to fall asleep alone (e.g., without rocking, feeding, or pacifier)
Allow baby to self-calm (e.g., find his or her own thumb)
Make middle-of-the-night feedings "brief and boring"
Do not respond to normal sounds made during sleep by picking up the baby

Middle infancy (4–6 mo)
Delay response to fussing for several minutes to allow infant opportunity to fall back asleep
Gradually reduce duration and amount of nighttime feeding
Avoid unnecessary stimulation (e.g., picking up) when checking on fussy infant

Later infancy (6–12 mo)
For separation anxiety: provide a transitional object (e.g., blanket, toy) or night light; leave door to bedroom open
Provide extra reassurances and cuddling during day
Make bedtime routine pleasant, predictable, and quiet
Set firm limits after infant is put to bed (e.g., "once in bed, stay in bed")
Further delay response in infant fussing and avoid physical contact and extra stimulation
Promptly respond to nightmares and bedtime fears
Promptly reinstitute strategies after recovery from illness

From Algranati PS, Dworkin PH: Infancy problem behaviors. *Pediatr Rev* 1992;13:16–22.

fants (older than 6–9 months) who are accustomed to receiving several full feedings during the nighttime hours will be hungry and continue to awaken at those times until such feedings are gradually weaned. Infants who always fall asleep while being rocked, fed, or otherwise soothed might be unable to return themselves to sleep when normal nighttime awakening occurs and the same conditions are not present. To avoid this problem, parents should be encouraged to allow infants to fall asleep in their cribs.

Normal separation issues might make going to sleep difficult for the 9- to 18-month-old child. Use of a transitional object, such as a favorite blanket or stuffed animal, that the child can take to bed might make falling and staying asleep easier. The older toddler frequently resists going to bed. A passion for experience and the desire for autonomy and control contribute to this behavior. At this age, it is especially important to have established consistent bedtime routines and rituals that allow the child to "wind down" from more stimulating activities and, at the same time, to take charge of certain aspects of the bedtime process. Transient changes in routine such as travel or a minor illness frequently can unravel a previously stable bedtime pattern. Parents also must be able to assess whether expectations regarding naps, bedtime, and total sleep requirements are age appropriate and whether illness, specific fears, or emotional stress are contributing to bedtime struggles.

During the preschool and school-age years, nighttime fears are frequent and usually transient. Potentially frightening activities such as watching disturbing television programs or reading scary books before bedtime should be avoided. A nightlight or open door can minimize fears. Nightmares are also common during this period. These occur during REM sleep and frequently cause spontaneous wakening with vivid recall. Nightmares are usually easily distinguished from night terrors, which affect approximately 3–5% of young children (peak age: 3–8 years), and occur during deepest non-REM sleep, usually during the first third of the night. During a night terror the child appears extremely frightened and agitated and, although seemingly awake, is actually in deep sleep and difficult to arouse. Upon awakening, the child has no apparent memory of the event. Although frightening to parents, night terrors are believed to be self-limited and benign. A more detailed discussion regarding the diagnosis and management of common sleep problems encountered during infancy and childhood is provided in Chapter 3.

Crying & Fussiness

Crying is a normal physiologic response to distress or discomfort, and it alerts the caretaker to the baby's needs. The quality and duration of an infant's crying might differ with the cause of distress, the temperament of the child, and the caretaking response that it elicits. The results of Brazelton's study of 80 otherwise healthy middle-class infants indicated that a 2-week-old infant cries approximately 2 hours per day. Crying tends to increase to an average of 3 hours per day at 6 weeks and then decrease to 1 hour per day by 3 months of age. Most crying occurs during the evening hours.

Many parents become concerned about what they perceive to be excessive crying. Parents' perceptions of their baby's crying can be affected by prior expectations about what is normal, the duration or character of the crying, the baby's responsiveness to attempts at consolation, and parental functioning in the face of various environmental stresses. Evaluation of such a complaint should involve a thorough history, including a description of the character and pattern of crying, past and current attempts at management, specific parental concerns, environmental stresses, and overall parental coping. A physical examination is important to rule out underlying medical problems and reassure the parents.

Although there is no universally accepted definition, the term *colic* generally refers to excessive, unexplained paroxysms of crying lasting more than 3 hours per day and occurring more than 3 days per week in an otherwise well-nourished, healthy infant. The crying usually occurs at the same time each day, most commonly during the evening hours, and is frequently resistant to simple soothing maneuvers. During these episodes, the infant may have excess flatus and draw the legs up to the chest, leading many parents to believe that the child is having abdominal discomfort. When present, colic typically begins during the first week of life and subsides by 3–4 months of age regardless of the management strategy used.

Approximately 10–30% of infants will be described as having colic. Although many etiologic theories have been proposed, the cause of colic is probably multifactorial. The current interactional model suggests that in most cases excessive crying is the result of a combination of intrinsic and extrinsic factors such as normal neuromaturational events, differences in infantile temperament, and the caretaking environment. Whereas evidence suggests that milk protein allergy or lactose intolerance explains the symptoms in a small subset of infants diagnosed as having colic, the vast majority will not have an identifiable gastrointestinal problem. Formula switching should be discouraged without other evidence of dietary intolerance or before trying a variety of behavioral management techniques.

Just as one etiology cannot be determined, no single intervention will be effective for all infants with colic. It is important to start with a thorough history and physical examination to reassure oneself and the parents that nothing is medically wrong and to individualize management suggestions. Parents should be reassured that infants cannot be spoiled at this age by promptly responding to their crying and that the duration of colic is limited. Caretakers should be encouraged to develop a consistent set of responses to the infant's crying episodes (Table 1–25). A variety of behavioral techniques have been proposed to help soothe the colicky baby; parents should be encouraged to find what works best for them. For some infants, decreasing stimulation by swaddling them or laying them down in a quiet, darkened room is helpful. For others, gentle, rhythmic stimulation is most effective and might include rocking the baby, walking while holding the baby or using a soft front carrier, offering a pacifier, putting the child in a wind-up swing, taking a ride in the car or stroller, and gently rubbing or patting the infant. Soothing sounds like singing or other music might be helpful. Parents should be encouraged to take turns soothing their child during crying episodes and to schedule "quality time" together away from the infant. For those infants with severe colic who appear to be unresponsive to such behavioral interventions, a trial of a formula not based on cow's milk and without lactose (soy or protein hydrolysate formula) or a maternal milk-free diet in breast-fed infants might be warranted. The use of pharmacologic agents, such as dicyclomine hydrochloride, remains controversial and should be avoided except in the most extreme cases, when they may be used as a temporary adjunct to behavioral techniques. Good follow-up is essential in the management of colic to evaluate the success of previous suggestions and provide ongoing support. The time-limited nature of this problem is a relief to parents and physicians. Additional discussion regarding the etiology and treatment of infantile colic is presented in Chapter 3.

Discipline

Parents frequently consult pediatricians for advice regarding discipline. The health supervision visit provides an excellent opportunity to discuss age-appropriate guidelines and help parents understand how normal developmental pressures, parental styles, environmental factors, and individual temperamental differences interact to affect a child's behavior and socialization. Although frequently used to refer to punishment, *discipline* is derived from the word *disciple,* "to teach," and, in its broadest definition, is the structure provided by parents that helps to foster a child's sense of being a lovable and capable human being. Parents who make an effort to listen to and get to know their child and who spend even a short period of uninterrupted "special" time with their child each day are conveying the powerful message that the child is loved and important. By showing interest and caring, complimenting good behavior, providing consistent appropriate limits, and setting a good example, parents can best shape their child's behavior and conscience according to their own values and practices. Punishment, when necessary, should be age appropriate and close in time to the misbehavior and should not be physically or psychologically destructive. Corporal punishment is less effective than positive reinforcement, is potentially harmful, and teaches children that physical aggression is an acceptable means of dealing with anger.

Contrary to common belief, infants younger than 4 months cannot be "spoiled," and parents should be encouraged to respond to their child's needs with unrestricted nurturing and care. By age 4–6 months, infants can begin to use crying in manipulative ways, and behavior modification techniques may be helpful. Care must be taken not to inadvertently reinforce behaviors such as frequent nocturnal awakening or feeding by providing excessive nighttime attention. Setting limits becomes important for the older infant, and the expression of verbal or nonverbal disapproval is an effective form of punishment for individuals in this and older age groups. At all ages, verbal disapproval is most effective when combined with positive instruction regarding appropriate behavioral alternatives and should focus on the misbehavior rather than on personally belittling the child. The older infant and early toddler may respond to constructive distraction or redirecting, techniques that have the added advantage of being useful preventively. As the naturally curious child develops mobility, the parent must take responsibility for structuring an environment that not only is safe but also

Table 1–25. Strategies to Manage Fussy Periods During Early Infancy

To diminish the amount of crying and fussing
Carry and cuddle frequently during both fussy and nonfussy periods
Respond promptly to baby's cry and do not worry about "spoiling" the infant
Help baby to become a self-soother (e.g., help baby to find its own thumb or a comfortable body position)

Develop a routine series of responses to soothe baby
Pick up baby
Change diaper, if soiled
Cuddle
Offer feeding if last feeding was more than 2 h ago
Burp
Offer a pacifier
Check to see that baby is neither too hot nor too cold and that clothing or diaper is not constricting
Place baby in a swing or crib rocker or carry in a front pack
Turn on music or heartbeat simulator
Go for a walk or ride in the car
Put baby in crib and allow to cry and fuss
Repeat routine

From Algranati PS, Dworkin PH: Infancy problem behaviors. *Pediatr Rev* 1992;13:16–22.

minimizes temptations for misadventure. Parents who accommodate their playing toddler's need for frequent, brief, verbal, and nonverbal contact can prevent an escalation of negative attention-seeking behavior, which can occur when a parent is otherwise preoccupied. Toddlers often have difficulty with shifts in their routine and abrupt transitions from one activity to the next and, when possible, should be given advance warning of such changes. Providing toddlers with the opportunity to make choices among acceptable options (e.g., clothing or food) allows them to positively express their growing need for control and independence. Negativism and temper tantrums are common expressions of the toddler's struggle for autonomy and self-control. Harmless behaviors, such as tantrums, sulking, and whining, frequently can be averted by redirecting the child or avoiding excessive fatigue and hunger and are extinguished most effectively by ignoring them. Children engaging in harmful or potentially harmful behavior may need to be manually removed from the situation. The technique of "time-out," described below, is an effective method for dealing with harmful or disruptive behavior. From an early age, it is also important to help children recognize and verbalize their feelings rather than act them out physically. The preschooler and older child often respond to natural and logical consequences whereby, within the bounds of safety, they learn by experiencing the negative natural or social consequences of their actions. For example, the child who is late for dinner is confronted by a plate of cold food, toys that are mishandled are removed, and the child who spills juice helps to clean it up. Family conferences that permit the child to participate in discussion and negotiation are important when establishing rules and responsibilities for older school-aged children. Delaying privileges until other less pleasurable tasks are completed and removing privileges as a consequence of rule infractions are also frequently effective for the older child.

Time-out is an effective method for extinguishing harmful or disruptive behavior and works by temporarily withdrawing social interaction. It can be used as early as 9–12 months of age and should be phased out by 5–6 years. A time-out location, such as a chair in the corner of the room, that is devoid of interesting distractions but not frightening to the child, should be chosen in advance. For young children, this should always be an area in which they can be observed easily by an adult. When a pre-agreed behavior warranting time-out occurs, parents should give one warning and then ask the child to go to the time-out location if the behavior persists. The child who does not go voluntarily may need to be taken there. Parents should maintain calm control and avoid engaging in angry lecturing or negotiations when applying time-out. Behavior that is out of control initially may be exacerbated by attempts to establish control. However, consistency and persistence are essential to the success of

this technique. The length of time-out should be brief, approximately 1 minute for every year of life, up to a maximum of 5 minutes. Use of a kitchen timer might be helpful. Children who leave the time-out location prematurely should be calmly returned, and the clock restarted. It is not important that the child be quiet, only that he or she stay in time-out. Occasionally it may be necessary to gently hold the child in the chair for the prescribed duration while minimizing conversation and interaction. When the period is over, the child should be verbally released from time-out and welcomed back into the social setting, without further mention of the previous infraction. After time-out, it is important to help the child learn socially acceptable alternative behaviors and, as soon as is possible, to recognize and compliment positive behavior.

Safety & Injury Prevention

Injuries, unintentional and intentional, are responsible for more childhood morbidity and mortality than all other diseases and conditions combined. Perhaps not surprisingly, toddlers and adolescents are at highest risk for injury-related morbidity and mortality. Data from the National Center for Health Statistics (1993–1995) show that more than three fourths of all unintentional injury-related deaths among infants younger than 1 year are caused by suffocation (44%), motor vehicle accidents (21%), fires or burns (11%), and drowning (8%). Among preschoolers, motor vehicle accidents (30%), fires (22%), drowning (21%), suffocation (7%), and pedestrian injuries (5%) account for 85% of such deaths. Over half of all unintentional injury-related deaths in the school-age years are due to motor vehicle accidents (53%), with fires or burns and drowning causing 14% and 12%, respectively. Among adolescents 10–14 years, motor vehicle accidents (41%), homicide (16%), and suicide (12%) cause more than three fourths of all injury-related deaths, with motor vehicle accidents alone causing 57% of unintentional deaths. Motor vehicle accidents (39%), homicide (30%), and suicide (18%) are also the leading causes of death due to injury (and death overall) among 15–24 year olds. When looking only at those deaths that were unintentional, motor vehicle accidents were responsible for 75% of injury-related death in this age group. Such mortality statistics underestimate the frequency of injuries that less often result in death. Common nonfatal injuries include falls, cuts, being struck by objects, burns, poisonings, animal bites, solitary (e.g., bicycling or skating) and team sports injuries, and motor vehicle accidents. Many people believe that injuries are random, unavoidable events and that children who incur them are simply "accident prone." However, an growing body of data suggests that, with appropriate personal, community, and legislative actions, many injuries can be prevented or diminished in severity. Further, whereas certain behavioral and environmental characteristics are associated with higher rates of injury, most injuries occur to children without such risk factors.

Recent epidemiologic data suggest that prevention efforts have significantly lowered the incidence of some unintentional injuries in children. However, there has been an alarming increase in intentional injury and violence within the pediatric population. Homicide is currently the second leading cause of death among adolescents and suicide is a close third. Children and teens are increasingly confronted with violence in their homes, schools, communities, and larger society. The causes of these trends are complex and multifactorial. However, disintegration of traditional social networks and institutions, socioeconomic inequities, lack of appropriate adult role models or guidance regarding nonviolent conflict resolution and tolerance of differences, media glorification of violence as entertainment, and the availability of handguns and other weapons contribute to the growing problem with violence.

The pediatrician is in a unique position to become involved in the prevention of injury and violence as an advocate for safety legislation and as a resource and counselor for prevention strategies in which individual families and communities can engage. Getting parents to translate the information provided into actual preventive action and changes in behavior provides a key challenge for the primary care provider. Individuals are much more likely to engage in preventive behaviors if they feel personally susceptible to a given problem and believe that they can favorably alter their risk by modifying their behavior. It is easier to get people to take onetime actions, such as buying a car seat, installing a smoke detector, or turning down the temperature on the hot-water heater, than to engage in behaviors that require regular or frequent action, such as consistent, appropriate use of car restraints. The amount of effort, decrease in comfort, and cost associated with a particular prevention strategy also affect how widely it is adopted. At the health supervision visit, providing an all-inclusive list of potential safety hazards to parents is less important than focusing on the most prevalent problems at each age and facilitating preventive action by personalizing the information provided. An integrated approach to accident prevention involving individual counseling and community-based action has a greater chance of success than either approach alone.

The AAP recommends that all parents be counseled regarding the safety measures outlined in Table 1–26, which focus on the major causes of accidental death and injury in childhood. In addition to these specific topics, the AAP suggests regular discussion during the health supervision visit of age-, season-, and locality-appropriate safety issues and corresponding prevention strategies. Suggested safety topics to cover at each visit are listed in Table 1–20.

A developmental approach to counseling allows the pediatrician to emphasize the normal age-related variations in cognitive, motor, and perceptual skills that significantly affect the frequency and kinds of problems children encounter. Not surprisingly, infants 1–2 years of age have the highest rates of accidental injury. At this age, an insatiable desire for experience and autonomy, coupled with difficult impulse control, outstrip cognitive and motor abilities, leading to unfortunate consequences. Recently acquired mobility, a pincer grasp, and an enjoyment of oral exploration also put children of this age at increased risk. With the achievement of object permanence, the infant and toddler actively search for objects and, as they begin to learn about cause and effect, may engage in dangerous behavior in an attempt to re-create a particularly fascinating event. Children at this age cannot understand or foresee the consequences of their actions and require parents to provide a safe environment, firm limits, and appropriate supervision. This continues to be important for preschoolers who, immersed in magical and egocentric prelogical thinking, have difficulty understanding that cause and effect is not a function of their own desires and intentions. Three-year-olds may believe that, just by not intending or wanting something to happen, an undesirable outcome of their actions can be avoided. At this age, fantasy and reality can be confused. Preschoolers in general cannot empathize with others who might be hurt by their actions. An inability to generalize or learn from past experiences is also common during this period.

To the school-aged child, peer group identification and acceptance become increasingly important. Dangerous or irresponsible behavior can arise out of a desire to be accepted by or not to "lose face" within a peer group. In challenging themselves to do things on their own, children at this age can overestimate their skills and competence. During this period, children develop the capacity for concrete operational thinking. Although they understand the concept of rules, they often challenge them, believing that they know more than their parents. It is important to allow school-aged children to be involved in the rule-making process and, within the constraints of safety, to learn from experience and gradually increasing responsibility. Parents also should be encouraged to help their child develop empathy and problem-solving and conflict-resolution skills by providing opportunities for family discussion and role-modeling tolerance of differences and nonviolent means of resolving disagreements.

After toddlers, adolescents have the highest rate of accidental death during childhood. Motor vehicle accidents are the most common cause of injury and death among teenagers and often involve the concomitant use of alcohol and other mind-altering substances. Homicide, suicide, and violent trauma are the next most common

Table 1–26. Office-based Counseling for Injury Prevention

All children should grow up in a safe environment

Anticipatory guidance for injury prevention should be an integral part of the medical care provided for all infants and children

In addition to below, all physicians caring for children should counsel parents in age-appropriate, season-appropriate, and locality-appropriate prevention strategies that reduce common serious injuries; medical records should reflect this counsel

Infants and preschoolers

Physicians caring for infants and preschool children should advise parents about the following issues

Traffic safety: appropriate use of currently approved child safety restraints (car seats); parental use of their own seat belts

Burn prevention: installation and maintenance of smoke detectors in home; setting of hot-water heater temperature at ≤120–130°F

Fall prevention: use of window and stairway guards/gates in place; use of infant walkers discouraged

Poison prevention: storage of medicines/household products out of sight and reach and in original childproof containers; storage of 1-oz bottle of syrup of ipecac at home for use as advised by pediatrician

Choking prevention: provision of age-appropriate foods; avoidance of running/playing during eating; supervision of mealtime; use of age-appropriate toys

Drowning prevention: supervision of infant/young child in bathtub or wading pool; emptying of all buckets, tubs, wading pools immediately after use; installation of appropriate fencing/safety guards with swimming pools; supervision of preschool-aged child while swimming (irrespective of child's swimming ability)

Cardiopulmonary resuscitation training: training of parents in CPR; knowledge of how to access local emergency care system

School-aged children

Physician advice to parents of elementary school-aged children begins to be more focused on the child's

behavior. The child is included in this process and the parents are reminded of their need to model safe behaviors.

Traffic safety: use of seat belts/booster seats; knowledge of safe pedestrian practices; use of approved bicycle helmets when cycling and protective equipment for inline skating/skate boarding

Water safety: provision of swimming instruction for children older than 5 y; knowledge of appropriate rules for water play; supervision of swimming; use of personal flotation devices with boating activities

Sports safety for adults who supervise children participating in organized sports: importance of appropriate safety equipment and physical conditioning

Firearm safety: removal of any handguns in the home (if parents choose to keep a firearm, gun must be unloaded, and gun and ammunition must be kept in separate locked cabinets)

Adolescents

Injury prevention advice to adolescents should be included in a broader discussion of healthy life-style choices (e.g., alcohol/drug use, sexual activity, diet/physical activity). Specific areas of injury prevention guidance should include the following.

Traffic safety: use of seat belts; role of alcohol in teenage motor vehicle accidents; use of motorcycle/bicycle helmets; use of protective equipment for inline skating and skateboarding

Water safety: alcohol use in water-related activities; use of approved personal flotation devices when boating

Sports safety: importance of proper safety equipment and physical conditioning for adolescents participating in organized sports programs

Firearm safety: knowledge of unique dangers of in-home firearms during adolescence—risk of impulsive, unplanned use resulting in suicide, homicide, or other serious injuries (if parents choose to keep a firearm, unloaded gun and ammunition must be kept in separate locked cabinets)

Modified from the Committee on Injury and Poison Prevention, American Academy of Pediatrics. *Pediatrics* 1994;94:566–567.

causes of death in this age group. Feelings of invulnerability, susceptibility to peer pressure, a need to establish independence, and high rates of substance use and experimentation contribute to these problems. One cannot overemphasize the importance of providing teens with specific situational skills to avoid uncomfortable or potentially dangerous situations with their peer group and to resolve conflicts nonviolently when they arise.

Adolescent risk-taking behavior is discussed in more depth in Chapter 2.

■ SCREENING

Many of the history and physical examination findings at each health supervision visit are directed toward identification of undetected problems and their risk factors. Pediatricians need to be aware of not only current recommendations regarding screening and the specific tests available but also the basic principles and concepts behind screening to evaluate whether a given program does more good than harm for their patients and community. Screening implies the presumptive identification of disease or its precursors in an otherwise asymptomatic individual or population and is, by definition, not diagnostic. It assumes that persons so identified will undergo definitive diagnostic testing and subsequently benefit by the earlier implementation of treatment or prevention programs. The effectiveness of a given screening program can be demonstrated by performing a randomized clinical trial in which all pertinent outcomes are evaluated. Unfortunately, such data are often lacking and difficult to obtain. Without such studies, the value of a given screening program must be defined in relation to certain characteristics of the condition being screened for, the test being used, the population being evaluated, and the larger social context in which decisions regarding the value of detection and the allocation of resources are being made.

When deciding what conditions are worth screening for, one must consider the suffering caused by a particular condition, as defined by its prevalence and severity, and the availability of a specific treatment or prevention strategy that, when implemented early, results in a longer or greater benefit to the individual than would have occurred with diagnosis at the onset of symptoms. The identification of conditions for which no treatment exists, or for which the benefit of existing therapy is unproved, is of questionable value and potentially harmful. Even when effective interventions do exist, one must weigh the potential risks and benefits of the treatment itself with those of the identified condition and consider the impact of public acceptance on compliance with screening and treatment recommendations.

The value of screening also depends on the existence of a good screening test. The accuracy of a test is defined by its sensitivity and specificity when compared with gold-standard measures of the presence or absence of disease and its positive and negative predictive value within a population with a given disease prevalence. It is important to understand how these test characteristics affect the overall value of and implementation strategies for screening programs.

The *sensitivity* of a test refers to the proportion of individuals with a condition who have an abnormal test result. Thus, a highly sensitive test misses few true cases because a large proportion of individuals with the disease have an abnormal test. The *specificity* of a test refers to the proportion of individuals without disease who have a normal test result. A highly specific test identifies few false-positive results because most individuals without the disease have a normal test. The sensitivity and specificity acceptable in a screening test reflect a relative weighing of the risk of missing true cases (sensitivity) compared with the risk of identifying false-positive results (specificity).

The *predictive value* of a test is the probability of the presence or absence of disease given an abnormal or normal test result. *Positive predictive value* refers to the prob-

ability that, given an abnormal result, an individual actually has the condition. *Negative predictive value* indicates the probability of the absence of the condition in an individual whose test result is normal. Predictive value depends on the sensitivity and specificity of the screening test being used and on the prevalence of the disorder in the population being screened. The greater the sensitivity of a test, the greater its negative predictive value, and the greater the specificity of a test, the greater its positive predictive value. Independent of the screening test's sensitivity and specificity, decreasing the population prevalence of the condition being sought diminishes the positive predictive value of the test by changing the proportion of true- to false-positive results. One should be aware of the population on which the test was standardized and whether the group being screened is sufficiently similar so that measures of predictive ability are comparable and application of the instrument is appropriate. For most screening situations, it is important to know the predictive ability of the test in a population with low disease prevalence because this is generally how screening tests are used. In many cases, selective testing of high-risk subgroups may make more sense than mass screening.

The costs associated with a screening program must be broadly defined. These costs include not only the screening itself but also the subsequent diagnostic, therapeutic, and supportive services required. The psychological impact on individuals falsely identified as positive and the costs involved in the definitive evaluation of these individuals can be significant. Early identification through screening does not always imply a better outcome. One must question the ultimate value of the screening program if the health care system or community cannot provide the subsequent, necessary diagnostic and therapeutic services. If persons who are at greatest risk do not avail themselves of the screening program or individuals with abnormal screening tests do not follow through with subsequent diagnostic and therapeutic recommendations, the screening program will not produce the intended benefits.

Current recommendations regarding screening during routine health supervision visits reflect an increasing awareness of the importance of these issues when deciding the value of specific screening programs. They also recognize that different strategies are appropriate for different populations. The following section addresses specific aspects of screening during the health supervision visit. Areas of health screening unique to adolescents are discussed in Chapter 2.

Specific Screening Areas

Newborn Screening for Metabolic Diseases

The number of metabolic diseases that can be diagnosed and treated in the newborn period, before the onset of symptoms or morbidity, is rapidly increasing. Although all states in the United States have initiated neonatal metabolic screening programs, because of the absence of federal guidelines, considerable state-to-state variability exists. Currently, all states screen for congenital hypothyroidism and phenylketonuria. Two thirds also screen for galactosemia. All these disorders are treatable and, if not diagnosed early, lead to irreversible brain damage. A blood sample should be obtained from all full-term neonates just before hospital discharge. In no case should the sample be collected after age 7 days. Special testing arrangements must be made if birth takes place in a nontraditional setting. Identification of some disorders, such as phenylketonuria, requires sufficient build-up of metabolites to be detected. If, because of early discharge, blood was drawn before the infant was 24 hours old, a second sample should be obtained when the child is 1–2 weeks old. Blood transfusions and dialysis, which introduce foreign blood cells and reduce concentrations of circulating metabolites, might produce false-negative and false-positive results when screening newborns for metabolic disorders and hemoglobinopathies. When feasible, samples should be obtained before these procedures are done. However, preterm and sick infants should be screened by 1 week of age regardless of the presence of these or other factors (e.g., parenteral feeding, antibiotic use, or prematurity) that might interfere with specific assays or the interpretation of test results. When such concerns exist, a repeat sample should be obtained at an interval appropriate to resolution of the confounding factors. In addition, due to variability in disease presentation and the technical aspects of screening, some affected infants might test falsely normal on their initial screens. Irrespective of the results of prior screening, specific diagnostic testing should be performed when clinical suspicions warrant. Because the choice of screening test, threshold values, and implementation strategies often differ state to state, providers should be familiar with the methodology, standards, and follow-up procedures for their regional screening programs.

NEWBORN SCREENING FOR HEMOGLOBINOPATHIES

Hemoglobinopathies occur with significant frequency and are a major cause of illness and death in the United States. Sickle cell disease alone (SS, SC, and SB thalassemia) affects approximately 1 of every 400 African-American newborns in the United States, as well as newborns from a variety of other ethnic and racial groups. Although the technology has existed for some time, compelling support for hemoglobinopathy screening in the newborn period was provided when a significant decrease in morbidity and mortality was demonstrated for children with sickle cell disease when diagnosis and initiation of a comprehensive treatment program, including prophylactic penicillin, occurred before symptomatic presentation.

In 1987, a National Institutes of Health Consensus Conference on this subject recommended that universal newborn screening for hemoglobinopathies be provided by each state. Debate continues on the need for universal versus selective screening and the optimal screening procedure. Concern also has been raised over variability in laboratory accuracy and the adequacy of subsequent diagnostic and counseling services for individuals identified as heterozygotes or homozygotes for these conditions. Current screening policies differ widely from state to state. Both heel-stick and cord blood samples may be used. Specimens usually are examined with electrophoresis at an alkaline pH, and abnormal samples are evaluated further with acid electrophoresis.

PHYSICAL EXAMINATION

During routine health supervision visits, a physical examination is performed for diagnostic or case finding (screening) purposes. In addition, it provides a useful framework for parent–child education and reassurance. Although the importance of the latter function should not be overlooked, the case finding value of routine physical examinations, when pathology is otherwise unsuspected, is limited and might not be the most effective use of the limited time available during the well-child visit. Except in the newborn period, among high-risk populations, or without adequate history, the primary aim of the well-visit physical examination should be to rule in or out pathology suspected by history or observation and provide reassurance and guidance to families.

DEVELOPMENTAL SCREENING

See the section on development earlier in this chapter (Motor & Psychological Development).

VISION SCREENING

Routine vision screening is an effective way to identify otherwise unsuspected problems that are amenable to correction. Because normal visual development depends on the brain's receipt of clear binocular visual stimulation and because the plasticity of the developing visual system is time limited (first 6 years of life), early detection and treatment of various problems that impair vision are essential to prevent permanent and irreversible visual deficits. Routine age-appropriate assessments should be incorporated into each health-supervision visit, beginning with the newborn examination. At all ages this should include a review of relevant historical information regarding visual concerns and family history, gross inspection of the eye and surrounding structures, observation of pupillary symmetry and reactivity, assessment of ocular movements, elicitation of the red reflex (to detect opacities and asymmetries in the visual axis), and age-appropriate methods to assess ocular preference, alignment, and visual acuity. A successful ophthalmoscopic examination generally can be accomplished by age 5 years. In the infant, ocular preference, alignment, and visual acuity can be grossly assessed by observing the baby's ability to visually track an object, noting any behavioral cues of an eye preference by alternatively covering each eye while presenting an interesting object, and observing the position and symmetry of the light reflected off the corneas when a light is held several feet in front of the eyes (corneal light reflex). Ocular alignment (conjugate gaze) should be consistently present by 4 months of age. It is especially important to assess the red reflex during infancy. Identification of an absent, defective, or asymmetric red reflex is key to the timely identification and treatment of opacities in the visual axis and many abnormalities at the back of the eye. In the toddler and preschooler, ocular preference and alignment also can be assessed by performing a more sophisticated unilateral cover test. This involves covering and uncovering each eye while the child is looking straight ahead at an object approximately 10 feet away. The observation of any movement of the uncovered eye when the opposite is covered or of the covered eye when the occluder is removed suggests potential ocular misalignment (strabismus) and warrants referral to an ophthalmologist for further evaluation. Regardless of the underlying etiology, strabismus that is left untreated eventually will result in cortical suppression of visual input from the nondominant eye and the absence of depth perception, making early detection and treatment critical. By 3–5 years of age, stereoscopic vision can be assessed using the random-dot–E stereo test or stereoscopic screening machines. Formal visual acuity testing should begin at 3 years of age with age-appropriate methods. Approximately 20% of children will have a refractive error identified, usually myopia (nearsightedness), before adulthood. Use of picture tests, such as the LH test and Allen picture cards, are most effective when screening preschoolers. By 5 years of age, most children can be screened successfully with a standard Snelling alphabet chart, the tumbling E test, or the HOTV test. School-aged children including adolescents should have their visual acuities checked on a yearly basis. Preschoolers should be referred for further testing if the acuity in either eye is $^{20}/_{40}$ or worse. In children 5 or 6 years of age, an inability to read most of the $^{20}/_{30}$ line warrants referral. At all ages, a difference in the acuity measurements between eyes of more than one line necessitates further evaluation.

HEARING SCREENING

Approximately 1–3 of every 1000 infants is born deaf, and in many children sensorineural hearing deficits develop during childhood. Timely detection of these problems allows for earlier initiation of interventions aimed at enhancing the communication, social, and educational skills of these children. Controversy recently has centered around the value of selective versus universal audiologic screening during infancy. Only half the infants with significant hearing impairment are identified with the use of a selective screening strategy based on the presence or absence of risk factors for hearing impairment (family history of childhood hearing abnormalities; history of congenital infection; anatomic malformations of the head, neck, or ears; birth weight less than 1500 g; history of hyperbilirubinemia exceeding exchange levels; severe birth asphyxia; history of bacterial meningitis; significant exposure to ototoxic medications; prolonged mechanical ventilation; and the presence of a syndrome or its stigmata associated with sensorineural hearing loss). Currently the average age at which a child with a significant hearing problem is identified is 14 months. However, the limitations in screening technologies, which lead to inconsistencies in interpretation and high rates of false-positive results, and the logistical problems with availability and implementation have raised concerns about the larger implications of a universal screening policy. In 1995 and 1999, after reviewing those issues, the AAP endorsed a policy of universal hearing screening during infancy with the goal of identifying all infants with significant hearing impairment by 3 months of age so that intervention could be initiated by 6 months of age. Ideally screening would take place before nursery discharge. Infants younger than 6 months traditionally have been screened with the use of brainstem response testing. A newer physiologic measure, otoacoustic emissions testing, holds promise as a simpler screening technique. However, problems with specificity (overreferral) and logistical issues with consistent use and interpretation have raised questions regarding the implementation of this method for universal screening. Some groups have advocated a two-step screening strategy whereby infants failing otoacoustic emissions testing are referred for screening with brainstem response testing. Until a clearly superior screening method emerges, the AAP has not endorsed a specific methodology for newborn hearing screening. Children older than 6 months may be screened by using behavioral, auditory brainstem response, or otoacoustic emissions testing. Regardless of the technique used, screening programs must be able to detect a hearing loss of 30 dB or greater in the 500–4000-Hz region (speech frequencies), the level of deficit at which normal development of speech and language may begin to be impaired. If a hearing deficit is identified, the child should be referred in a timely manner for further evaluation and early intervention services.

In addition to performing a gross hearing assessment and inquiring about hearing concerns at each well visit, the AAP endorses a policy of formal hearing screening for all children at ages 3, 4, and 5 years and every 2–3 years during adolescence. The U.S. Preventive Services Task Force does not recommend routine hearing screening for asymptomatic children older than 3 years. Risk factors warranting formal hearing screening beyond the newborn period are parental concerns regarding hearing and/or language and developmental delay; history of bacterial meningitis; the presence of neonatal risk factors associated with progressive hearing loss; history of significant head trauma, especially involving fractures of the temporal bone; the presence of a syndrome associated with sensorineural hearing loss; significant exposure to ototoxic medications; the presence of a neurodegenerative disorder; and the diagnosis of infectious diseases such as mumps and measles that are associated with hearing loss. Because a variety of transient conditions, such as middle ear effusion, and testing problems, can affect the hearing evaluation of older, otherwise healthy children, the results of audiologic screening must be interpreted within the context of the child's history of ear disease and the results of physical examination.

BLOOD PRESSURE

Routine blood pressure screening during the well-child visit allows identification and potential treatment of children with persistently elevated blood pressure who are at increased risk for hypertension and its subsequent complications as adults. In a minority of patients, an underlying medical etiology may be found. Screening also provides an opportunity to evaluate and potentially modify additional cardiovascular risk factors and provide education regarding prudent dietary and life-style choices.

In 1996, the National High Blood Pressure Education Program issued updated guidelines for pediatric blood pressure norms, screening, evaluation, and treatment. Blood pressure standards change with age, sex, and body size (as reflected by height). Routine blood pressure screening is recommended for all otherwise healthy children aged 3 years and older at least once a year. Blood pressure measurements also should be taken in ill and potentially symptomatic children and children younger than 3 years who are believed to be at increased risk for hypertension due to coexisting medical conditions.

In the child, blood pressure should be measured in the sitting position with the arm held at heart level. The width of the cuff bladder should be approximately 40% of the circumference of the upper arm at its midpoint; when wrapped, the bladder should cover 80–100% of the circumference of the arm to avoid an artificially elevated reading. The cuff is inflated to approximately 20 mm Hg above the point at which the radial pulse disappears and deflated 2–3 mm Hg/s while listening over the brachial artery. The level at which the first tapping sound is heard (Korotkoff sound 1 or K1) is recorded as the systolic blood pressure. The level at which all sounds disappear (K5) represents the diastolic pressure.

Normal blood pressure is defined as systolic and diastolic readings below the 90th percentile for age and sex. High normal and high blood pressure (hypertension) are defined, respectively, as readings between the 90th and 95th percentiles and greater than or equal to the 95th percentile for age and sex, found on at least three separate occasions. Children with persistently elevated blood pressure readings (above the 90th percentile) warrant a thorough history and physical examination to identify underlying causal factors, end-organ damage, and concomitant cardiovascular risk factors, in addition to a long-term surveillance and treatment plan (see Chapter 16: Kidneys & Electrolytes).

CHOLESTEROL & LIPIDS

Epidemiologic data support the hypothesis that atherosclerosis and coronary heart disease have their precursors in childhood and that identifiable risk factors, such as hypertension, obesity, and hypercholesterolemia, are associated with an increased incidence of atherosclerotic disease. Serum cholesterol and other cardiovascular risk factors can be influenced significantly by dietary and life-style choices. Although long-term pediatric data are lacking regarding the risks and benefits of following prudent life-style recommendations during childhood, until more definitive information is available, it seems reasonable that pediatricians should provide preventive counseling to all their patients and families in these areas.

Controversy has centered around the value of selective versus universal cholesterol and lipid screening strategies for children as a part of routine pediatric health supervision. The AAP, the American Heart Association, and the recent NCEP report have endorsed a selective screening strategy for children based on the presence of a high-risk family history and, when this is unknown, the presence of additional risk factors for atherosclerotic disease. Given the current paucity of information regarding the risks and benefits of treatment for hyperlipidemia in childhood, the costs and limitations of available screening tests, and the potential benefit of promoting healthful life-style and dietary choices to all families, these groups do not support universal cholesterol screening for children. On the basis of the recent NCEP report, the AAP recommends that children older than 2 years whose parents or grandparents have histories of early atherosclerotic disease (e.g., a myocardial infarction, angina pectoris, positive coronary arteriogram, or cerebrovascular or peripheral vascular disease before age 55 years) be screened with a fasting (12-hour) serum lipid profile (total cholesterol, high-density lipoprotein cholesterol, triglycerides, and low-density lipoprotein cholesterol). In children whose parents have significantly elevated blood cholesterol levels (above 240), a nonfasting total serum cholesterol level should be obtained followed by the fasting lipid panel, if this is significantly elevated. When family history is unclear or unknown or a child presents with additional cardiovascular risk factors such as obesity, smoking, hypertension, physical inactivity, or diabetes, screening with a nonfasting total serum cholesterol also might be appropriate. The paradigm recommended by the AAP for selective screening and subsequent follow-up of children with elevated cholesterol levels is shown in Figures 1–4 and 1–5.

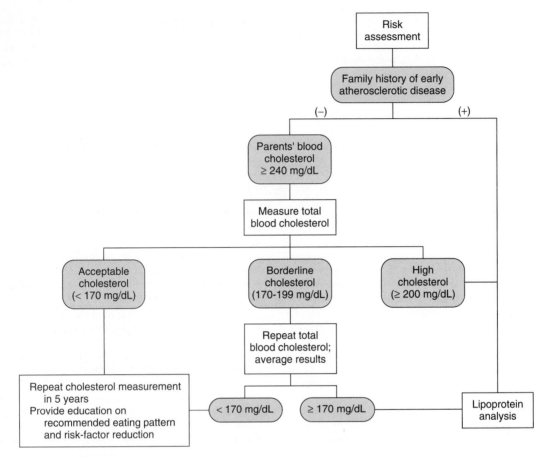

Figure 1–4. Risk assessment for elevated cholesterol and low-density lipoprotein cholesterol. (Reproduced, with permission, from National Cholesterol Education Program. Report of the expert panel on blood cholesterol levels in children and adolescents. *Pediatrics* 1992;89(pt 2, suppl):548.)

IRON DEFICIENCY ANEMIA

The recent decline in the prevalence of iron deficiency anemia in the United States has caused a reevaluation of the standard policy of obtaining screening hematocrits or hemoglobins for all children at ages 9–15 months and 4–6 years and during adolescence. Current thinking favors a selective screening approach including infants (at 9–15 months) and adolescents (at health supervision visits) who belong to groups at increased risk for iron deficiency and any children in whom anemia is suspected by history or examination. Risk factors for iron deficiency during infancy include prematurity, low birth weight, introduction of cow's milk before age 12 months, insufficient dietary iron intake, and low socioeconomic status. At increased risk for iron deficiency are menstruating female adolescents and male and female athletes. Because of the frequent occurrence of mild transient anemia with

acute illness, hemoglobin screening should not be done while a child is ill or within several weeks of a fever or infection. Hemoglobin measurements obtained by venipuncture are more accurate and reproducible than capillary hematocrits obtained by skin puncture. Abnormally low values are defined as being more than 2 SD below the mean for children of similar age and sex.

LEAD SCREENING

The United States has made significant progress toward eliminating ongoing sources of environmental lead contamination. However, lead poisoning remains a significant health problem for children in that country. Although the use of lead-containing paint was effectively banned in the 1970s, ingestion of lead-containing paint chips and dust created by the deterioration or renovation of older homes remains the primary source of lead contamination

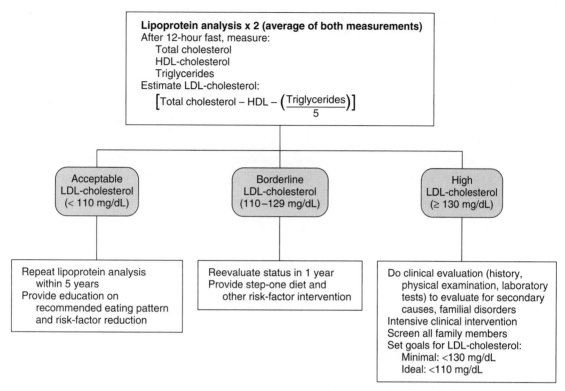

Figure 1–5. Classification, education, and follow-up based on low-density lipoprotein (LDL) cholesterol. HDL = high-density lipoprotein. (Reproduced, with permission, from National Cholesterol Education Program. Report of the expert panel on blood cholesterol levels in children and adolescents. *Pediatrics* 1992;89(pt 2, suppl):549.)

in children. Considerable attention has been focused recently on this issue because of a growing body of evidence that suggests an association between subtle neurobehavioral effects and blood lead levels previously believed to be innocuous. These studies, in combination with national data demonstrating a significant prevalence of low but potentially clinically significant lead levels among children in the United States, prompted the Centers for Disease Control and Prevention (CDC) in 1991 to recommend universal blood lead screening for all children aged 6–72 months and to lower the intervention threshold to levels greater than 10 mg/dL. Since their issue, the CDC recommendations have provoked ongoing debate regarding the risks and benefits of universal versus selective (risk-based) lead screening. Subsequent national prevalence data have suggested that, apart from the presence of known risk factors, the likelihood of lead exposure in a given community can be predicted from local blood lead levels and housing age data. This led the CDC in 1997 to revise their screening recommendations to endorse a regional selective (risk based) or universal screening policy based on local prevalence and

housing data. Specifically, universal screening is still recommended for communities with inadequate prevalence data, those in which at least 12% of 1- and 2-year-old children have blood lead levels of at least 10 μg/dL, and those where at least 27% of the housing was built before 1950. For all other communities, a targeted screening strategy based on the presence or absence of established risk factors is recommended.

Primary care providers should periodically review lead exposure risk for all children, beginning at age 6 months. Risk factors that should be assessed are: (1) whether the child lives in or regularly visits a house that was built before 1950, (2) whether that child lives in or regularly visits a house that was built before 1978 and is being or has recently been remodeled (during last 6 months), and (3) whether that child has a sibling or playmate who has or has had an elevated blood lead level. State and local health departments may add questions to their routine risk assessment based on specific local conditions. Additional risk factors that have been identified are use of lead-containing folk remedies, emigration or adoption from countries with a high prevalence of lead poisoning, known exposure to lead-containing dust or soil, and parental lead exposure secondary to vocation, avocation, or remodeling. Irrespective of age or risk factors, children who exhibit pica or excessive hand-to-mouth activity or have unexplained anemia or iron deficiency, seizures, neurologic symptoms, developmental delay, abdominal pain, or other symptoms consistent with lead poisoning should also have a blood lead level drawn.

In communities where universal screening is recommended, asymptomatic children without identified risk factors should be screened routinely at ages 9–12 and 24 months. Asymptomatic children with one or more identified risk factor should be screened initially at 6 months and then at 12 months. If both levels are normal, the testing frequency is decreased to once a year. Recommended follow-up for children whose levels are elevated are shown in Table 1–27. Due to an increased potential for contamination from environmental sources, venous blood specimens are preferred to capillary (finger-stick) samples. Elevated values obtained from capillary specimens should be confirmed with venous blood testing.

URINALYSES & URINE CULTURES

In the absence of clinical concerns or risk factors, routine surveillance urinalyses and urine cultures are not cost effective. The relatively frequent occurrence of minor abnormalities, such as microscopic proteinuria, is of questionable significance and, in addition to contaminated culture specimens, necessitate costly and inconvenient repeated urine studies. Routine screening rarely leads to the detection of significant asymptomatic renal disease and, when it does, one must ask whether early detection results in benefit to the patient over diagnosis with the onset of symptoms. Urine studies should be obtained

Table 1–27. Recommended Follow-up Services, According to Diagnostic Blood Lead Level

BLL (µg/dL)	Action
<10	No action required

10–14	Obtain a confirmatory venous BLL within 1 mo; if still within this range,
	    Provide education to decrease blood lead exposure and
	    Repeat BLL test within 3 mo

15–19	Obtain a confirmatory venous BLL within 1 mo; if still within this range,
	    Take a careful environmental history
	    Provide education to decrease blood lead exposure and lead absorption
	    Repeat BLL test within 2 mo

20–44	Obtain a confirmatory venous BLL within 1 wk; if still within this range,
	    Conduct a complete medical history (including an environmental evaluation and nutritional assessment) and physical examination
	    Provide education to decrease blood lead exposure and lead absorption
	    Refer the patient to the local health department or provide case management that should include a detailed environmental investigation with lead hazard reduction and appropriate referrals for support services
	    If BLL is >25 µg/dL, consider chelation (not currently recommended for BLLs <45 µg/dL), after consultation with clinicians experienced in lead toxicity treatment

45–69	Obtain a confirmatory venous BLL within 2 d; if still within this range,
	    Conduct a complete medical history (including an environmental evaluation and nutritional assessment) and a physical examination
	    Provide education to decrease blood lead exposure and to decrease lead absorption
	    Refer the patient to the local health department or provide case management that should include a detailed environmental investigation with lead hazard reduction and appropriate referrals for support services
	    Begin chelation therapy in consultation with clinicians experienced in lead toxicity therapy

≥70	Hospitalize the patient and begin medical treatment immediately in consultation with clinicians experienced in lead toxicity therapy
	    Obtain a confirmatory BLL immediately
	    The rest of the management should be as noted for management of children with BLLs of 45–69 µg/dL

From the American Academy of Pediatrics, Committee on Environmental Health: Screening for elevated blood lead levels. *Pediatrics* 1998;101:1075.

when disease is suspected or when the child is at increased risk for specific renal problems.

TUBERCULOSIS

Yearly tuberculin testing is no longer recommended for all children. Although the number of cases of tuberculosis in the United States has increased in recent years, these cases continue to occur primarily within the previously identified high-risk groups. In populations with a low prevalence of tuberculosis, most reactive tests reflect false-positive results, often due to cross-reactivity with nontubercular mycobacterium, leading to unnecessary treatment with isoniazid. The AAP, the American Thoracic Society, and the CDC currently endorse a selective screening strategy based on the presence of risk factors and residence in a community with a high prevalence of tuberculosis (Table 1–28). Routine tuberculin testing is no longer recommended for low-risk, asymptomatic children who live in areas of low disease prevalence. Children with one or more risk factors should be screened on a regular basis, the frequency of which is determined by the degree of risk. Children who do not have risk factors but reside in high-prevalence communities and whose history regarding risk status is unknown or incomplete might be screened on a periodic basis at ages 4–6 and 11–16 years. In all screening situations, intradermal Mantoux testing should replace multipuncture testing, and the results should be read by qualified medical personnel. Prior bacillus Calmette-Guérin vaccination is not a contraindication to placement of a purified protein derivative. Individuals who have received this vaccine can still acquire tuberculosis. Although some previously vaccinated individuals have

Table 1–28. Revised Tuberculin Skin Test Recommendations[1]

Children for whom immediate skin testing is indicated
Contacts of persons with confirmed or suspected infectious tuberculosis (contact investigation); this includes children identified as contacts of family members or associates in jail or prison in the past 5 y
Children with radiographic or clinical findings suggesting tuberculosis
Children immigrating from endemic countries (e.g., Asia, Middle East, Africa, Latin America)
Children with travel histories to endemic countries and/or significant contact with indigenous persons from such countries
Children who should be tested annually for tuberculosis[2]
Children infected with human immunodeficiency virus
Incarcerated adolescents
Children who should be tested every 2–3 y[2]
Children exposed to the following individuals: those with human immunodeficiency virus or homeless individuals, residents of nursing homes, institutionalized adolescents or adults, users of illicit drugs, incarcerated adolescents or adults and migrant farm workers; this would include foster children with exposure to adults in the above high-risk groups
Children who should be considered for tuberculin skin testing at ages 4–6 and 11–16 y
Children whose parents immigrated (with unknown tuberculin skin test status) from regions of the world with high prevalence of tuberculosis; continued potential exposure by travel to the endemic areas and/or household contact with persons from the endemic areas (with unknown tuberculin skin test status) should be an indication for repeat tuberculin skin testing
Children without specific risk factors who reside in high-prevalence areas; in general, a high-risk neighborhood or community does not mean an entire city is at high risk; it is recognized that rates in any area of the city may vary by neighborhood, or even from block to block; physicians should be aware of these patterns in determining the likelihood of exposure; public health officials or local tuberculosis experts should help clinicians identify areas that have appreciable tuberculosis rates
Risk for progression to disease
Children with other medical risk factors, including diabetes mellitus, chronic renal failure, malnutrition, and congenital or acquired immunodeficiencies, deserve special consideration; without recent exposure, these persons are not at increased risk of acquiring tuberculosis infection; underlying immune deficiencies associated with these conditions theoretically would enhance the possibility for progression to severe disease; initial histories of potential exposure to tuberculosis should be included on all of these patients; if these histories or local epidemiologic factors suggest a possibility of exposure, immediate and periodic tuberculin skin testing should be considered in these patients; an initial Mantoux tuberculin skin test should be performed before initiation of immunosuppressive therapy in any child with an underlying condition that necessitates immunosuppressive therapy

[1] Bacillus Calmette-Guérin immunization is not a contraindication to tuberculin skin testing.
[2] Initial tuberculin skin testing initiated at the time of diagnosis or circumstance.
From the Committee on Infectious Diseases, American Academy of Pediatrics: Update on tuberculosis skin testing of children. *Pediatrics* 1996;97:282–284.

positive tuberculin skin test results, there is no reliable way to differentiate this reaction from that resulting from a natural infection with *Mycobacterium tuberculosis;* recommendations regarding screening, test interpretation, and subsequent evaluation and treatment remain the same.

Tuberculin testing relies on skin hypersensitivity to indicate subclinical or clinical infection. Reactivity usually develops within 2–12 weeks of infection. Two forms of tuberculin are currently available: old tuberculin, used in the Tine and Mono-Vacc tests, and the less expensive and more commonly used purified protein derivative. Multiple puncture tests, such as the Tine and Mono-Vacc, have the advantage of easy administration but lack consistency in the amount of tuberculin to be delivered. Reactions cannot be quantified accurately, and the numbers of false-positive and false-negative results are significant. All positive multiple puncture test results must be confirmed by subsequent Mantoux testing. However, some individuals might experience a booster effect when retesting occurs within 10 days to 12 months of the previous tuberculin exposure, thereby falsely enhancing the degree of reactivity. Because of these problems, the intracutaneous test (Mantoux) should be used preferentially in tuberculosis screening, when the disease is clinically suspected, and in the evaluation of persons known to have been exposed to tuberculosis. In the Mantoux test, a standardized dose of tuberculin (5 tuberculin units in 0.1 mL of solution) is delivered intradermally through a 26-gauge needle and has the advantage of allowing quantification of the subsequent response. The Mantoux test should be read at 48–72 hours by tactile measurement of the margins of induration. Erythema alone does not signify a positive reaction. Test interpretation is based on the size of induration, reason for testing, and the presence or absence of other risk factors. Guidelines for interpreting test findings have been defined by the AAP, the American Thoracic Society, and the CDC (Table 1–29). This classification presumes the physician's knowledge of the child's and family's risk factors and the background prevalence of tuberculosis in the community. It should be remembered that skin testing results may be negative early in the course of the disease or in the presence of anergy. A positive Mantoux test result necessitates obtaining posteroanterior and lateral chest radiographs and investigating contacts for disease. Decisions regarding the need for prophylactic or therapeutic treatment are based on the subsequent evaluation.

Table 1–29. Definition of a Positive Mantoux Skin Test Result (Five Tuberculin Units of Purified Protein Derivative) in Children[1]

Reaction ≥5 mm
Children in close contact with known or suspected infectious cases of tuberculosis
  Households with active or previously active cases if treatment cannot be verified as adequate before exposure, treatment was initiated after the child's contact, or reactivation is suspected
Children suspected to have tuberculous disease
  Chest roentgenogram consistent with active or previously active tuberculosis
  Clinical evidence of tuberculosis[2]
Children receiving immunosuppressive therapy[3] or with immunosuppressive conditions, including HIV infection

Reaction ≥10 mm
Children at increased risk of dissemination
  Young age (<4 y)
  Other medical risk factors, including diabetes mellitus, chronic renal failure, or malnutrition

Children with increased environmental exposure
  Born, or whose parents were born, in high-prevalence regions of the world
  Frequently exposed to adults who are HIV infected, homeless, users of illicit drugs, medically indigent city dwellers, residents of nursing homes, incarcerated or institutionalized persons, and migrant farm workers
  Travel and exposure to high-prevalence regions of the world

Reaction ≥15 mm
Children ≥4 y of age without any risk factors

[1] The recommendations should be considered regardless of previous Bacillus Calmette-Guérin administration.
[2] Evidence on physical examination or laboratory assessment that would include tuberculosis in the working diagnosis (i.e., meningitis).
[3] Including immunosuppressive doses of corticosteroids.
HIV = human immunodeficiency virus.

From the Committee on Infectious Diseases, American Academy of Pediatrics: Update on tuberculosis skin testing of children. *Pediatrics* 1996;97:282–284.

■ IMMUNIZATIONS

Routine immunization has dramatically decreased the morbidity and mortality from a variety of infectious diseases and has become an important aspect of pediatric preventive health care. Even though the value of such programs is well established, the field is dynamic and rapidly changing. The number of infectious diseases against which children can be effectively immunized has grown significantly in recent years. Currently, children are routinely immunized against eleven infectious diseases (Table 1–30). All are examples of active immunization, whereby live-attenuated or inactivated organisms, their components, or their products are administered to the recipient to stimulate a protective immunologic response. The Committee on Infectious Diseases of the AAP (*Red Book*) and the Advisory Committee on Immunization Practices (ACIP) of the U.S. Public Health Service (*Morbidity and Mortality Weekly Report*) regularly publish updated recommendations that differ only in minor ways with regard to the administration and schedule of routine immunizations. These guidelines offer a current standard of care that is subject to change as our knowledge continues to evolve (Table 1–31).

To maximize efficacy and minimize toxicity, recommendations regarding schedule, dose, route, and site of administration should be followed for each immunization. Subcutaneous and intramuscular injections usually are given in the anterolateral upper thigh in infants and, when muscle mass is sufficient, the deltoid area in children and adults. The buttock should be avoided as a site of injection because of the potential for sciatic nerve damage and inconsistent intramuscular deposition. For intramuscular injections in infants and children, a 20- or 22-gauge, $\frac{5}{8}$- to $1\frac{1}{4}$-inch needle is used; in adults, the standard needle length is $1\frac{1}{2}$ inches. Subcutaneous injections are administered with a 25-gauge, $\frac{5}{8}$- to $\frac{3}{4}$-inch needle for all ages. To avoid accidental intravascular injection, it is important to pull the syringe plunger back and monitor blood return before injecting any substance.

Table 1–30. Routine Childhood Vaccines: Route and Doses

Vaccine	Type	Route	Dose
DTaP, DTwP, DT, Td 　D = diphtheria 　d = reduced amount toxoid 　T = tetanus 　aP = acellular pertussis 　wP = whole-cell pertussis	Toxoids (D&T) Bacterial components (aP) Inactivated whole bacteria (wP)	Intramuscular	0.5 mL
Hib 　*Haemophilus influenzae* to 　conjugate vaccine	Bacterial polysaccharide conjugated to 　protein	Intramuscular	0.5 mL
Poliovirus vaccines 　IPV = inactivated 　OPV = oral	Inactivated viruses of all three 　serotypes Live viruses of all three serotypes	Oral Subcutaneous	Unit dose 0.5 mL
MMR 　M = measles 　M = mumps 　R = rubella	Live viruses	Subcutaneous	0.5 mL
Hep B 　Hepatitis B vaccine	Plasmid-derived viral antigen	Intramuscular	Varies with preparation 　and recipient's age
Var 　Varicella zoster virus vaccine	Live virus	Subcutaneous	0.5 mL
PCV 　Pneumococcal conjugate vaccine	Bacterial polysaccharides conjugated 　to nontoxic diphtheria toxin	Intramuscular	0.5 cc

Modified from Rudolph AM (editor): *Rudolph's Pediatrics,* 20th ed. Appleton & Lange, 1996, p. 30.

Table 1-31. United States, January–December 2001

Vaccine	Birth	1 mo	2 mo	4 mo	6 mo	12 mo	15 mo	18 mo	24 mo	4–6y	11–12y	14–18y
Hepatitis B[2]	Hep B 1		Hep B 2		Hep B 3						*	
Diphtheria, tetanus, pertussis[3]			DTaP	DTaP	DTaP		DTaP[3]			DTaP		Td
H. influenzae type b[4]			Hib	Hib	Hib	Hib						
Inactivated polio[5]			IPV	IPV	IPV[5]					IPV[5]		
Pneumococcal conjugate[6]			PCV	PCV	PCV	PCV						
Measles, mumps, rubella[7]						MMR				MMR[7]	*	
Varicella[8]						Var					*	
Hepatitis A[9]									Hep A—in selected areas			

Vaccines are listed under routinely recommended ages. ⬜ Bars indicate range of recommended ages.

[1] Vaccines are listed under routinely recommended ages. Bars indicate range of recommended ages for immunization. Any dose not given at the recommended age should be given as a "catch-up" immunization at any subsequent visit when indicated and feasible. Asterisks indicate vaccines to be given if previously recommended doses were missed or given before the recommended minimum age. This schedule indicates the recommended ages for routine administration of currently licensed childhood vaccines, as of November 1, 2000, for children up to age 18. Additional vaccines may be licensed and recommended during the year. Licensed combination vaccines may be used whenever any components of the combination are indicated and its other components are not contraindicated. Providers should consult the manufacturers' package inserts for detailed recommendations. For additional information about these vaccines, please visit the National Immunization Program Home Page at http:/www.cdc.gov/nip/ or call the National Immunization Hotline at 800-232-2522 (English) or 800-232-0233 (Spanish).

2 Infants born to HBsAg-negative mothers should receive the first dose of hepatitis B (Hep B) vaccine by age 2 mo. The second dose should be at least 1 mo after the first dose. The third dose should be administered at least 4 months after the first dose and at least 2 months after the second dose, but not before 6 mo of age for infants. Infants born to HBsAg-positive mothers should receive hepatitis B vaccine and 0.5 mL HBIG within 12 h of birth at separate sites. The second dose is recommended at 1–2 months of age and the third dose at 6 mo of age. Infants born to mothers whose HBsAg status is unknown should receive hepatitis B vaccine within 12 h of birth. Maternal blood should be drawn at the time of delivery to determine the mother's HBsAg status; if the HBsAg test is positive, the infant should receive HBIG as soon as possible (no later than 1 wk of age). All children and adolescents who have not been immunized against hepatitis B should begin the series during any visit. Special efforts should be made to immunize children who were born in or whose parents were born in areas of the world with moderate or high endemicity of hepatitis B virus infection. HBIG = hepatitis B immune globulin; HBsAg = hepatitis B surface antigen.

3 The fourth dose of diphtheria and tetanus toxoids and acellular pertussis vaccine (DTaP) may be administered as early as 12 months of age, provided 6 mo have elapsed since the third dose and the child is unlikely to return at age 15–18 mo. Td (tetanus and diphtheria toxoids) is recommended at 11–12 y of age if at least 5 y have elapsed since the last dose of DTP, DTaP or DT. Subsequent routine Td boosters are recommended every 10 y.

4 Three *Haemophilus influenzae* type b (Hib) conjugate vaccines are licensed for infant use. If polyribosylribotol-phosphate–outer membrane protein (PRP-OMP) (PedvaxHIB or ComVax, Merck) is administered at 2 and 4 mo of age, a dose at 6 mo is not required. Because clinical studies in infants have demonstrated that using some combination products may induce a lower immune response to the Hib vaccine component, DTaP/Hib combination products should not be used for primary immunization in infants at 2, 4 or 6 mo of age, unless approved by the Food and Drug Administration for those ages.

5 An all-inactivated/injected polio vaccine (IPV) schedule is recommended for routine childhood polio vaccination in the United States. All children should receive four doses of IPV at 2 mo, 4 mo, 6–18 mo, and 4–6 y of age. Oral polio vaccine (OPV) should be used only in selected circumstances (see *MMWR* 2000;49(RR-5):1–22).

6 The heptavalent conjugate pneumococcal vaccine (PCV) is recommended for all children 2–23 mo of age. It also is recommended for certain children 24–59 mo of age (see *MMWR* 2000; 49(RR-9):1–35).

7 The second dose of measles, mumps, and rubella (MMR) vaccine is recommended routinely at 4–6 y of age but may be administered during any visit, provided at least 4 wk have elapsed since receipt of the first dose and that both doses are administered beginning at or after 12 mo of age. Those who have not previously received the second dose should complete the schedule by the 11–12 y old visit.

8 Varicella (Var) vaccine is recommended at any visit on or after the first birthday for susceptible children, i.e., those who lack a reliable history of chickenpox (as judged by a health care provider) and who have not been immunized. Susceptible persons 13 y of age or older should receive two doses, given at least 4 wk apart.

9 Hepatitis A (Hep A) is shaded to indicate its recommended use in selected states and/or regions, and for certain high risk groups; consult your local public health authority (see *MMWR* 1999;48(RR-12):1–37).

From the American Academy of Pediatrics, Committee on Infectious Diseases: Recommended childhood immunization schedule—United States, January–December 2001. *Pediatrics* 2001;107:202–203.

The value of and need for a given vaccine depend on the prevalence and severity of the disease targeted, its ability to prevent or ameliorate that disease, and the incidence and severity of vaccine-related morbidity. With the dramatic decrease in disease-related morbidity and mortality brought about by current immunization practices, attention has focused increasingly on the potential adverse effects of the vaccines themselves.

In addition to the active immunizing antigen(s), vaccines contain other materials including suspending fluids such as saline or complex tissue culture, preservatives, stabilizers, antibiotics to prevent bacterial overgrowth, and adjuvants to enhance immunogenicity. These components can contribute to local and systemic side effects attributed to the vaccine. Although rare, anaphylactic allergic reactions are due most frequently to egg antigens in the suspending fluid of vaccines prepared in embryonated egg (influenza and yellow fever), antibiotics used to prevent bacterial overgrowth (streptomycin, neomycin, and polymixin B in oral polio vaccine [OPV] and inactivated/injected polio vaccine [IPV]; neomycin in the measles, mumps, and rubella vaccine [MMR], varicella, and rotavirus; amphotericin B in rotavirus), and gelatin, which is used as a stabilizer (MMR, varicella, and yellow fever). Individuals with histories suggestive of anaphylactic reactions to any of these components should undergo skin testing to determine the safety of subsequent immunization with these vaccines.

Many side effects, such as local tenderness, low-grade fever, and allergic reactions, can be attributed directly to the vaccine because of their temporal relationship, frequency, and unique presentations. These adverse reactions, whether common or rare, are predictable and unavoidable. The relation between vaccination and other uncommon but naturally occurring events, such as seizures, mental retardation, and encephalopathy, is much less well established. Such outcomes, if sometimes vaccine related, occur against a background of indistinguishable idiopathic events, making differentiation between a temporal and a causal relation difficult. Issues pertaining to specific immunizations are addressed below. Current standards regarding valid and nonvalid contraindications to specific vaccines are shown in Table 1–32.

In recognition that some persons are adversely affected by their participation in mass immunization programs and to provide some stability to vaccine supply and cost in the face of escalating liability litigation, the U.S. Congress passed the National Childhood Vaccine Injury Compensation Act in 1986. This act, which was amended in 1987 and became effective in 1988, establishes an optional no-fault system of compensation with a mandatory initial approach for a predefined list of possible vaccine-related reactions. The act also requires that all physicians and health care workers who administer vaccines comply with guidelines regarding record keeping, centralized reporting of potential vaccine reactions, and distribution of standardized pamphlets describing risks and benefits to vaccine recipients and their parents. The *Red Book* should be consulted for more detailed information.

The following section provides specific information about childhood vaccines routinely recommended in the United States. Many other vaccines are available and recommended for use in selected populations based on increased susceptibility or potential for morbidity (e.g., influenza, pneumococcus) and/or the likelihood of exposure (e.g., meningococcus, hepatitis A, yellow fever, typhoid, and rabies for international travelers). The reader is referred to the AAP's *Red Book* and the CDC's *Morbidity and Mortality Weekly Report* for detailed information regarding the use of these vaccines. In addition, the CDC maintains an excellent web site with up-to-date international travel information with regard to regional vaccine recommendations, current infectious disease outbreaks, and other helpful travel tips (http://www.cdc.gov).

Specific Vaccines

DTwP (Diphtheria, Tetanus, Whole-Cell Pertussis) & DTaP (Diphtheria, Tetanus, Acellular Pertussis)

The DTwP vaccine is composed of diphtheria toxoid, tetanus toxoid, and inactivated whole *Bordetella pertussis* cells. Since 1991, several vaccines substituting acellular for whole-cell pertussis (DTaP) became available. These contain one or more pertussis antigens but little or no endotoxin. Because acellular pertussis preparations are associated with fewer side effects than whole-cell vaccine, the DTaP is currently the preferred vaccine for primary and booster doses. Single-antigen products, combinations of diphtheria and tetanus toxoids, and combined DTwP or DTaP/*Haemophilus influenza* type b (Hib) vaccines are also available. Adults and children older than 7 years are not given pertussis vaccine because potential morbidity from wild-type disease is greatly diminished by this age. Because of enhanced local reactivity, these individuals receive a booster vaccine containing one tenth the the concentration of diphtheria toxoid given to younger children. At all ages, a dose of 0.5 mL is delivered intramuscularly with the use of needle sizes and sites as described at the beginning of this section. The recommended DTaP and diphtheria toxoid immunization schedules for children vaccinated at standard ages are given in Table 1–31. The primary series consists of three doses of DTaP separated by 4–8-week intervals beginning at 6 weeks to 2 months of age (usually at 2, 4, and 6 months). A fourth primary dose is given 6–12 months after the third (usually at 15–18 months of age), and a fifth (booster) dose is given at ages 4–6 years. The fifth dose is not necessary if the fourth dose was administered after the child's fourth birthday. Several acellular products are available for use. Until data confirm the interchangeability of these products, the same

Table 1–32. Overview of Valid and Nonvalid Contraindications to Vaccination

True Contraindications and Precautions	Not True (Vaccines May Be Administered)
General for all vaccines (DTwP/DTaP, OPV, IPV, MMR, Hib, HBV, PCV, Var)	
Contraindications	Mild to moderate local reaction (soreness, redness, swelling) after a dose of an injectable antigen
Anaphylactic reaction to a vaccine contraindicates further doses of that vaccine	Mild acute illness with or without low-grade fever
Anaphylactic reaction to a vaccine constituent contraindicates the use of vaccines containing that substance	Current antimicrobial therapy
Moderate or severe illnesses with or without a fever	Convalescent phase of illnesses
	Prematurity (same dosage and indications as for normal, full-term infants)
	Recent exposure to an infectious disease
	History of penicillin or other nonspecific allergies or family history of such
DTwP/DTaP	
Contraindication	Temperature <40.5°C (105°F) after a previous dose of DTwP/DTaP
Encephalopathy within 7 days of administration of previous dose of DTwP/DTaP	Family history of convulsions[2]
Precautions[1]	Family history of sudden infant death syndrome
Temperature ≥ 40.5°C (105°F) within 48 h after vaccination with a prior doses of DTwP/DTaP	Family history of an adverse event after DTwP/DTaP administration
Collapse or shock-like state (hypotonic–hyporesponsive episode) within 48 h of receiving a prior dose of DTwP/DTaP	
Seizures within 3 d of receiving a prior dose of DTwP/DTaP[2]	
Persistent, inconsolable crying lasting ≥ 3 h within 48 h of receiving a prior dose of DTwP/DTaP	
OPV	
Contraindications	Breast feeding
Infection with HIV or a household contact with HIV	Current antimicrobial therapy
Known altered immunodeficiency (hematologic and solid tumors; congenital immunodeficiency; and long-term immunosuppressive therapy)	Diarrhea
Immunodeficient household contact	
Precaution[1]	
Pregnancy	
IPV	
Contraindication	
Anaphylactic reaction to neomycin or streptomycin	
Precaution[1]	
Pregnancy	
MMR	
Contraindications	Tuberculosis or positive skin test
Anaphylactic reactions to gelatin and/or neomycin	Simultaneous tuberculin skin testing[3]
Pregnancy	Breast feeding
Known altered immunodeficiency (hematologic and solid tumors; congenital immunodeficiency; long-term immunosuppressive therapy, severely immunocompromised HIV-infected individuals)	Pregnancy of mother of recipient
	Immunodeficient family member or household contact
	Infection with HIV (except severely immunocompromised HIV-infected individual)
Precaution[1]	Nonanaphylactic reactions to eggs or neomycin
Recent (within 3 mo) immune globulin administration	Anaphylactic and nonanaphylactic reactions to egg
History of thrombocytopenia (see text)	

(*continued*)

Table 1-32. (Continued)

True Contraindications and Precautions	Not True (Vaccines May Be Administered)
Hib	
None identified	
Hep B	
None identified	Pregnancy
Var	
Contraindications	Nonvalid contraindications
History of anaphylactic reaction to neomycin and/or gelatin	Nonanaphylactic reactions to neomycin
Known cellular or combined cellular and humoral immuno-deficiency such as HIV infection with significant immunosuppression; congenital immunodeficiency, long-term immunosuppressive therapy (exception: asymptomatic or mildly symptomatic HIV-infected children meeting criteria of the Centers for Disease Control and Prevention)	Persons with isolated humoral immunodeficiency
Persons with blood dyscrasias, leukemia, lymphomas, and other malignant neoplasms of bone marrow or lymphatic systems (exception: acute lymphocytic leukemia in remission meeting protocol criteria)	Pregnant household member
Children with a family history of congenital or hereditary immunodeficiency in a first-degree relative unless recipient's immune competence has been documented	Immunocompromised household member
Pregnancy	Breast feeding (mother and infant)
	Children receiving inhaled or low-dose oral steroids (see text)
Precautions	
Recent administration of immune globulin or other blood products	
Children requiring long-term salicylate therapy (see text)	
PCV	
None identified	

¹ The events or conditions listed as precautions, although not contraindications, should be reviewed carefully. The benefits and risks of administering a specific vaccine to an individual under the circumstances should be considered. If the risks are believed to outweigh the benefits, the vaccination should be withheld; if the benefits are believed to outweigh the risks (e.g., during an outbreak or foreign travel), the vaccination should be administered. Whether and when to administer DTP to children with proven or suspected underlying neurologic disorders should be decided on an individual basis. It is prudent on theoretical grounds to avoid vaccinating pregnant women. However, if immediate protection against poliomyelitis is needed, OPV, not IPV, is recommended.

² For children with a personal or family (siblings or parents) history of convulsions, acetaminophen should be considered before DTwP/DTaP is administered and thereafter every 4 h for 24 h.

³ Measles vaccination can temporarily suppress tuberculin reactivity. If testing cannot be done the day of MMR vaccination, the test should be postponed for 4–6 wk.

DTwP/DTaP = diphtheria-tetanus toxoid and pertussis vaccine; DTaP = diphtheria and tetanus toxoids and acellular pertussis vaccine; OPV = oral poliovirus vaccine; IPV = inactivated whole-cell poliovirus vaccine; MMR = measles-mumps-rubella vaccine; Hib = *Haemophilus influenzae* type b vaccine; Hep B = hepatitis B vaccine; HIV = human immunodeficiency virus.

Modified and updated from National Vaccine Advisory Committee: Standards for pediatric immunization practices. *MMWR* 42;1993;(RR-5):1. This information is based on the recommendations of the Advisory Committee on Immunization Practices (ACIP) and those of the Committee on Infectious Diseases of the American Academy of Pediatrics (AAP) as of January 2001. These recommendations can differentiate from those contained in the manufacturer's package inserts. For more detailed information, providers should consult the published recommendations of the ACIP, AAP, American Association of Family Practice Physicians, and the manufacturer's package inserts.

vaccine should be used for at least the first three doses. If this information is unknown or the previous product is not available, immunization should continue with any of the licensed acellular vaccines. Additional booster doses with Td (adult-type tetanus and diphtheria) are recommended at 11–12 years of age (not later than 16 years of age) and every 10 years thereafter. If the child is 7 years or older when vaccination is instituted, a primary series is given consisting of two Td separated by 4–8 weeks, followed by a third dose 6–12 months after the second. Booster doses are required every 10 years. The DTaP or DTwP vaccine can be given concurrently (different sites) with all other routine childhood immunizations without diminishing antibody responses. Studies of the immunologic response to DtaP and DTwP vaccinations and side effects in premature infants support the approach of ignoring gestational age and beginning immunization at the usual chronologic age.

Common side effects of the DTwP vaccine, which are attributed primarily to the whole-cell pertussis component, include local redness, swelling, pain at the site of injection, and systemic reactions such as low to moderate fever, fretfulness, drowsiness, vomiting, and anorexia. The incidence of local reactions and fever associated with DTwP administration appear to increase with the number of doses given, whereas the likelihood of other minor systemic reactions decreases. However, for any given child, the risk of a mild systemic reaction is greater with subsequent doses if it occurred with the first dose. More serious but less frequent systemic events have been reported in relation to administration of the whole-cell DTwP vaccine including persistent inconsolable crying for more than 3 hours, temperature above 40.5°C, hypotonic or hyporesponsive episodes, convulsions with or without fever, encephalopathy, and a variety of neurologic defects such as mental retardation and cerebral palsy. Considerable controversy has surrounded the relation between pertussis vaccine and several serious neurologic conditions that, although indistinguishable from otherwise naturally occurring idiopathic events, have at times appeared temporally related to DTwP vaccination. Several recent studies using sophisticated statistical and experimental techniques have found no evidence to support a causal relation between pertussis vaccination and some alleged reactions (e.g., sudden infant death syndrome, infantile spasms, attention-deficit/hyperactivity disorder, learning disorders, and autism) and, with respect to others, have suggested that vaccination accelerates events otherwise destined to occur in a given individual (e.g., seizures). An increased incidence of seizures after DTwP administration has been consistently observed, but most have been associated with fever and have the clinical characteristics of benign febrile seizures. There is no evidence that convulsions after DTwP administration cause neurologic damage or epilepsy. As an outgrowth of the National Childhood Vaccine Injury Act,

the National Academy of Science's Institute of Medicine undertook an extensive analysis of all existing scientific data pertaining to potential adverse effects of the whole-cell pertussis vaccine. It found that evidence was consistent with a causal relation between DTwP vaccination and several rare events including acute encephalopathy, hypotonic or hyporesponsive shock-like episodes, anaphylaxis, and prolonged inconsolable crying. It also found that children experiencing severe, acute neurologic illnesses (e.g., encephalopathy) within 7 days after DTwP vaccination were at increased risk for chronic neurologic dysfunction at levels similar to those seen in children experiencing these same acute neurologic events temporally unrelated to DTwP administration. In these rare children, the committee believed that evidence was consistent with but did not prove a causal relation between DTwP vaccination and some forms of chronic nervous system disorders. Based on their own review of the data, the National Vaccine Advisory Committee concluded that evidence was insufficient to determine whether a history of administration of DTwP before an acute neurologic event independently influenced the potential for subsequent long-term neurologic dysfunction. The ACIP and AAP concurred with that analysis.

Use of acellular vaccine results in significantly lower rates of minor local and systemic reactions, such as tenderness and fever, than does use of the whole-cell product. Prophylactic administration of acetaminophen (15 mg/kg) at the time of injection can further reduce the incidence of those side effects. Decreased frequency of several moderate to severe systemic events (compared with DTwP) also have been documented including hypotonic or hyporesponsive episodes, fever above 40.5°C, and prolonged crying lasting longer than 3 hours. Because of its rarity, the frequency of temporally associated encephalitis after DTaP has yet to be determined.

Current contraindications to vaccination with DTwP and DTaP are listed in Table 1–32.

POLIOVIRUS (ORAL & INACTIVATED/ INJECTED POLIO VACCINES)

Poliovirus vaccines were introduced in the 1950s and 1960s. Their use since that time has dramatically decreased wild-type poliomyelitis worldwide, thus making global eradication of this disease an attainable goal for the near future. Two forms of trivalent poliovirus vaccine are available for use—the enhanced potency, inactivated injectable (introduced at its original potency by Salk in 1954) and Sabin's live attenuated oral vaccine. In addition to the immunizing agents, the IPV and the OPV contain various combinations of neomycin, streptomycin, and polymyxin B to prevent bacterial overgrowth.

In determining the relative advantages and disadvantages of using OPV or IPV, a number of epidemiologic and societal factors need to be considered. For societies with endemic disease or those that receive many immigrants from polio endemic areas where universal immunization cannot be assured, OPV offers several advantages. First, oral vaccination with attenuated live virus is thought to induce lifelong immunity in much the same way as a natural infection, thereby avoiding the need for boosters. Second, because of the induction of mucosal immunity (pharyngeal, intestinal) and systemic immunity, the natural transmission of wild-type virus in the population is interrupted. Third, because of fecal shedding of the vaccine viruses for several weeks after vaccination, indirect immunization or boosting of immunity in contacts also is achieved. The lack of the need for injections, which might prevent some individuals from being vaccinated, and the lower cost of OPV compared with IPV are other advantages. The disadvantage to the use of OPV is its ability, although rare, to cause vaccine-associated paralytic poliomyelitis (VAPP) in the recipient and his or her contacts. Most cases occur in immunocompetent adults. Only 10–15% of afflicted individuals have an underlying immunodeficiency. However, immunodeficient individuals are at increased risk of vaccine-induced disease; therefore, they and their family members should not be immunized with live-virus vaccine. Household contacts are at higher risk for disease than community contacts, and the risk for recipients and contacts is highest after exposure to a first dose.

The inactivated injectable polio vaccine offers the advantage of being unable to cause paralytic poliomyelitis. The current enhanced potency product provides some mucosal immunity, although less than that provided by OPV. At its original potency the IPV required booster doses every 4–5 years. However, the current enhanced potency injected vaccine induces significantly prolonged and possibly lifelong immunity, thereby reducing or potentially eliminating the need for subsequent boosters.

Until recently, the live attenuated oral vaccine was the vaccine of choice for routine childhood vaccination in the United States. Recent changes in the epidemiology of poliomyelitis has caused the ACIP and the AAP to reevaluate the relative advantages and disadvantages of using OPV versus IPV in the United States and led them to revise their recommendations regarding the use of these products in routine childhood immunization. The last case of indigenously acquired wild-type virus poliomyelitis in the United States was reported in 1979. However, between 1980 and 1994, 125 cases of VAPP were reported. Given the fact that the risk of acquiring vaccine-associated polio in the United States, although low, is currently significantly greater than the risk of acquiring the wild-type viral infection, the ACIP and the AAP now recommend an IPV-only regimen for routine vaccination of all children in the United States. A series of four injections are given at ages 2 months, 4 months, 6–18 months, and 4–6 years (Table 1–31). A minimum of 4 weeks should separate the first two doses. If the third dose of

vaccine is given after the child's fourth birthday, the fourth dose is unnecessary. To advance the goal of global eradication, OPV remains the preferred vaccine for use in countries where wild-type poliomyelitis is or has recently been endemic, for controlling outbreaks of wild-type polio virus, and in most developing countries where relative cost issues and inadequate sanitation systems provide compelling reasons for use of OPV rather than IPV.

Other than the risk of VAPP with live virus vaccine, side effects from using OPV and IPV are minimal and consist of rare hypersensitivity and anaphylactic reactions primarily due to trace amounts of neomycin, streptomycin, and polymyxin B. Although concern has been raised about a possible connection between OPV or IPV administration and Guillain-Barre syndrome, recent data do not confirm a causal relation. Valid and nonvalid contraindications to vaccination are listed in Table 1–32.

MEASLES, MUMPS, & RUBELLA

The MMR vaccine combines three attenuated live viruses. Single-agent preparations also are available. Vaccine strains of measles and mumps are grown in chick embryo tissue culture, and rubella is grown in human diploid-cell culture. These vaccines contain minute quantities of neomycin to prevent bacterial overgrowth. A 0.5-mL dose is administered subcutaneously by using needle sizes and sites described previously. The MMR vaccine can be administered concurrently (different sites) with all of the other routinely recommended childhood vaccines without diminishing antibody response. However, it is recommended that injected live-virus vaccines, if not given on the same day, should be spaced 4 or more weeks apart. Measles vaccination might temporarily suppress tuberculin reactivity for 4–6 weeks after immunization but will not interfere with the accuracy of the test placed on the same day. Administration of immunoglobulin interferes with the immune response to MMR vaccination for a dose-dependent period. Ideally, MMR vaccination should be given at least 2 weeks before the administration of immunoglobulin or, if this is not possible, delayed for a period of time appropriate to the dose of immunoglobulin received (see *Red Book*).

Recommendations regarding the optimal timing and frequency of immunization against measles, mumps, and rubella (Table 1–31) reflect a balance between several factors including the duration of maternal antibody protection conferred to the infant, the seroresponse to vaccine at different ages, the rate of primary vaccine failure, the duration of vaccine-induced immunity, and the overall level of vaccination achieved within the population. During the 1980s, when it was recommended that children receive one dose of MMR at age 15 months, several outbreaks of measles were reported. These occurred primarily among three populations: unvaccinated preschool children younger than 15 months, unvaccinated preschool children older than 15 months, and previously vaccinated school-aged children. Cases occurring in children younger than 15 months were believed to be due in part to an earlier decline in levels of protective maternal antibody among infants born to women who themselves had received measles vaccine rather than natural infection. A 2–10% primary vaccine failure rate was believed to be the primary cause of cases occurring in previously vaccinated school-aged children, although waning immunity was a potentially important factor. Outbreaks among unvaccinated children who had not received the MMR at the recommended age represented a failure of the vaccine delivery system to maximize access, catchment, and public acceptance. The AAP and ACIP subsequently changed their policy to recommend a two-dose MMR vaccine schedule and lowered the age for administration of the initial dose from 15 months to 12–15 months for all children. Both groups currently recommend that the second dose be routinely given at school entry, between the ages of 4 and 6 years. This dose, however, can be administered as soon as 1 month after the initial vaccine as long as the first was given at age 12 months or older. To better address problems with vaccine delivery, immunization practice guidelines for health care providers have been issued by the National Vaccine Advisory Committee. Since implementation of these changes, the number of cases of measles reported in the United States has decreased dramatically, with the vast majority occurring in previously unvaccinated children.

A recent increase in the number of mumps cases among adolescents and young adults has been observed and is believed to be caused primarily by the existence of a relatively underimmunized cohort of children born between 1967 and 1977, when mumps vaccine was available but not routinely recommended. Individuals who were not immunized with live mumps virus vaccine on or after their first birthdays or who have not experienced natural infection as diagnosed by a physician or documented by the presence of serum antibody should be vaccinated against mumps. Most people born before 1957 are likely to have been infected naturally and generally can be considered immune even if they do not remember having had a symptomatic case. Unlike the characteristic presentation of mumps, a clinical diagnosis of rubella is notoriously unreliable. Individuals should not be considered immune to rubella unless they have been immunized with live-virus vaccine on or after their first birthdays or have evidence of serum antibody. There is no evidence to suggest that it is harmful to immunize someone against mumps or rubella who has previously received vaccine or had a natural infection.

Contraindications to receiving the MMR vaccine are listed in Table 1–32. Although the MMR is prepared in chick embryo cell culture, it does not contain significant amounts of cross-reacting egg proteins. A history of anaphylactic allergy to chicken eggs is no longer a contraindication to vaccination with MMR. However, a history of anaphylactic allergy to neomycin warrants withholding this vaccine until skin testing can be obtained. Because the incidence of thrombocytopenia with wild-type measles or mumps is much greater and the natural history of vaccine-induced thrombocytopenia is generally benign and self-limited, in most instances the benefits of vaccinating a child with a previous history of thrombocytopenia outweigh the disadvantages. However, if the previous thrombocytopenia occurred after a first dose of MMR, it may be prudent to withhold the second dose. In general, live-virus vaccines should not be given to individuals who are known to be or are suspected of being immunodeficient. An exception to this rule is the recommendation that asymptomatic and symptomatic children positive for human immunodeficiency virus (HIV) who are not severely immune compromised (based on age-specific quantification of CD4 lymphocytes) should receive the MMR vaccine because of their increased risk of morbidity and mortality with the acquisition of wild-type measles infection. Concerns about immunization during pregnancy apply to all live-virus vaccines, although the greatest concern has centered on rubella. The CDC reporting registry shows no evidence of defects consistent with wild-type congenital rubella syndrome among the live-born infants or aborted fetuses of women inadvertently vaccinated against rubella during or just before pregnancy. However, vaccine virus has been isolated from aborted products of conception, proving that the attenuated virus can cross the placenta. Although it is to be avoided, rubella vaccination just before or during pregnancy is not a reason to interrupt pregnancy.

Side effects of measles vaccination include frequent local tenderness and swelling, fever appearing 7–12 days after immunization (5–15%), and a morbilliform rash following the same time course (5%). Recipients of the killed measles vaccine, available between 1963 and 1967, have a higher incidence of local reactions when revaccinated with the live-virus vaccine. However, because of a greater risk of having serious atypical measles if exposed to wild-type virus, these individuals should be revaccinated. Thrombocytopenia presenting in the 2 months after immunization has rarely been reported in association with the MMR. This condition is generally transient and benign and occurs at a rate significantly lower than that associated with wild-type measles or mumps infection.

Encephalitis and encephalopathy occasionally have been reported to follow measles and mumps vaccination, but at an incidence lower than the "background" frequency of encephalitis from unknown etiology, suggesting a temporal relationship only. Although subacute sclerosing panencephalitis, a late complication of wild-type measles infection, has been reported to occur after measles vaccination in the absence of a known natural infection, the incidence of this devastating disease has been reduced dramatically by mass immunization. Side effects of the mumps vaccine include local tenderness, low-grade fever, and, rarely, a mild orchitis or parotitis. In addition to local tenderness and a rubella-like syndrome consisting of rash, fever, and lymphadenopathy, rubella vaccination is associated with transient arthritis and arthralgias occurring 1–3 weeks after vaccination, most commonly among postpubertal women (10–15%). In a recent review of all scientific data pertaining to potential adverse effects of the MMR vaccine, the National Academy of Science's Institute of Medicine found evidence to establish a causal relation between this vaccine and anaphylaxis, thrombocytopenia, febrile seizures, and acute arthritis. Evidence did not support a causal link between this vaccine and other events such as neuropathies, Guillain-Barre syndrome, and thrombocytopenic purpura.

HAEMOPHILUS INFLUENZAE TYPE B CONJUGATE VACCINE

Vaccines against invasive Hib infections have undergone a dramatic evolution since their initial licensure in 1985.

Four conjugate Hib vaccines are currently available for use. Each consists of an Hib capsular polysaccharide linked to a different carrier protein (Table 1–33). Only diphtheria CRM_{197} protein conjugate (HbOC), polyribosylribotol phosphate–outer membrane protein (PRP-OMP), and polyribosylribotol phosphate–tetanus toxoid (PRP-T) are licensed by the Food and Drug Administration for use in infants younger than 1 year. Polyribosylribotol phosphate–diphtheria toxoid (PRP-D) is licensed in children at least 12 months old for booster use and at least 15 months old for primary administration. DTaP–Hib combination vaccines are also available. However, because some of these products can result in suboptimal immune responses when used at 2, 4, and 6 months of age, only those products licensed for this age group should be used in young infants. Conjugate vaccines offer a significant advantage over the original unconjugated polysaccharide vaccine because of their ability to elicit a protective antibody response in young infants when the incidence of invasive *H. influenzae* disease is greatest. As with the original vaccine, the conjugate *H. influenzae* vaccines do not protect against nontypable strains of *H. influenzae*, which are responsible for many recurrent upper respiratory diseases such as otitis media. Conjugate vaccine also should not be considered a protective immunizing agent against their carrier protein (e.g., diphtheria, *Neisseria meningitidis*, or tetanus). For all products, a dose of 0.5 mL is given intramuscularly with the needle sizes and sites described previously. All of the Hib vaccines can be given

Table 1–33. Licensed *Haemophilus influenzae* Type b Conjugate Vaccines Available in the United States[1]

Manufacturer	Abbreviation	Trade Name	Carrier Protein
Lederle Laboratories, Pearl River, NY (distributed by Wyeth-Lederle Vaccines, Wyeth-Ayerst Laboratories, Philadelphia, PA)	HbOC	HibTITER	CRM_{197} (a nontoxic mutant diphtheria toxin)
Merck & Co, Inc. (West Point, PA)[2]	PRP-OMP	PedvaxHIB	OMP (an outer membrane protein of *Neisseria meningitidis*)
Pasteur Mérieux Sérums & Vaccins, SA, Lyon, France (distributed by Connaught Laboratories, Swiftwater, PA, and SmithKline Beecham Pharmaceuticals, Philadelphia, PA)	PRP-T	ActHIB, OmniHIB	Tetanus toxoid
Pasteur Mérieux Connaught (Swiftwater, PA)	PRP-D	ProHIBiT	Diphtheria toxoid

[1] HbOC (diphtheria CRM_{197} protein conjugate), PRP-OMP (polyribosylribotol phosphate–outer membrane protein), and PRP-T are recommended for infants beginning at approximately 2 mo of age. PRP-D is recommended only for children 12 mo of age or older. The U.S. Food and Drug Administration, however, has approved labeling for PRP-D for booster administration beginning at 12 mo of age and for primary administration at 15 mo of age. These vaccines can be given in combination products or as reconstituted products with DTaP (diphtheria and tetanus toxoids and acellular pertussis) or DTP (diphtheria and tetanus toxoids and pertussis), provided the combination or reconstituted vaccine is approved by the FDA for the child's age and administration of the other vaccine component(s) also is justified.

[2] A combination of *Haemophilus influenzae* (PRP-OMP) and hepatitis B (Recombivax, 5 µg) vaccine is licensed for use ages 2, 4, and 12–15 mo (Comvax).

From the American Academy of Pediatrics, Committee on Infectious Diseases: In: *2000 Red Book: Report of the Committee on Infectious Disease*, 25th ed. Pickering L et al (editors). Elk Grove Village, IL: American Academy of Pediatrics, 2000.

simultaneously (at different sites unless a licensed combination vaccine is used) with other routinely recommended childhood without diminishing the immunologic response.

The recommended schedule for administration of *H. influenza* vaccination differs with the preparation used and the age of the child at first immunization (Table 1–31). Recipients of HbOC or PRP-T who are immunized at the recommended times should receive a primary series of three doses at ages 2, 4, and 6 months. Use of PRP-OMP requires only two primary doses, at ages 2 and 4 months. Because seroconversion after a first dose of PRP-OMP is significantly higher than that seen with the other conjugate products (60% vs. 20%), when available, this preparation is preferred for use in populations and regions with an increased frequency of Hib invasive disease (e.g., American Indians and Alaska Natives). When possible, the same preparation should be used to complete the primary series. However, when this is unknown or if this product is unavailable, three doses of any of the conjugate products licensed for use in infants younger than 12 months are considered sufficient to complete the primary series. All children should receive a booster dose at 12–15 months of age with any of the four available preparations. Children not initiating vaccination at the recommended age who are between 2 and 6 months of age should receive a primary series of three HbOC or PRP-T (or two PRP-OMP), each separated by at least 2 months, and a booster dose at 12–15 months of age. Unvaccinated children 7–11 months old require two primary doses with any of the three preparations licensed for this age group separated by at least 2 months and a booster dose (at least 2 months from the last) at 12–18 months of age. Children 12–14 months old should receive two doses of vaccine (given 2 months apart). Individuals 15–60 months old who have not been previously immunized require only one dose with any of the four conjugate vaccines available. Children younger than 24 months who have had invasive *H. influenzae* disease still should be vaccinated because many do not develop adequate immunity after natural infection. Irrespective of age, children who are believed to be at increased risk for invasive *H. influenzae* disease, such as those with functional or anatomic asplenia, also should receive conjugate vaccine.

Side effects attributed to the *H. influenzae* conjugate vaccines are minimal and include primarily local tenderness, swelling, erythema, and low-grade fever in a minority of recipients (25%). There are no specific contraindications to vaccination with Hib vaccines. Premature infants should be vaccinated in accordance with the recommended schedule based on their chronologic, not gestational, age.

HEPATITIS B VACCINE

Acute hepatitis B and its chronic sequelae are the cause of significant morbidity and mortality in the United States.

A plasma-derived hepatitis B vaccine, licensed in 1982, has since been replaced by two recombinant vaccines (Recombivax and Engerix B) that use synthetic hepatitis B surface antigen (HBsAg) produced in yeast by plasmid gene insertion. These vaccines are highly immunogenic, conferring protection against hepatitis B infections in more than 90% of recipients, including infants. Failure of control strategies using selective immunization of high-risk groups and HBsAg screening of pregnant women has led the AAP and ACIP to recommend universal hepatitis B immunization during infancy. Those groups also recommend universal vaccination for older children and adolescents who missed vaccination during infancy and vaccination of adults at high risk for hepatitis B exposure (Table 1–34).

Table 1–34. Persons Who Should Receive Preexposure Hepatitis B Immunization[1]

All infants
Children at high risk for early childhood HBV infection[2]
Adolescents[3]: Hepatitis B vaccination should be given by or before 11–12 y of age; special efforts should be made to vaccinate *all* adolescents, not only those at high risk.
Injection drug users
Sexually active heterosexual persons with more than one sex partner during the previous 6 mo or who have a sexually transmitted disease
Sexually active men who have sex with men
Household contacts and sexual partners of HBsAg-positive persons
Health care personnel and others at occupational risk of exposure to blood or blood-contaminated body fluid
Residents and staff of institutions for developmentally disabled persons
Staff of nonresidential child care and school programs for developmentally disabled persons if the program is attended by a known HBsAg-positive person
Patients undergoing hemodialysis
Patients with bleeding disorders who receive clotting factor concentrates
Members of households with adoptees who are HBsAg-positive
International travelers to areas in which HBV infection is of high or intermediate endemicity
Inmates of juvenile detention and other correctional facilities

[1] HBV = hepatitis B virus; HBsAg = hepatitis B surface antigen.
[2] Alaskan Native and Asian-Pacific Islander children and children born to first-generation immigrants from HBV-endemic areas.
[3] Immunization can be initiated before children reach adolescence.

From the American Academy of Pediatrics, Committee on Infectious Diseases: In: *2000 Red Book: Report of the Committee on Infectious Disease,* 25th ed. Pickering L et al (editors). Elk Grove Village, IL: American Academy of Pediatrics, 2000.

Current recommendations regarding the schedule, dose, and volume of vaccination differ with the preparation used, the age of the child being vaccinated, the mother's HBsAg serologic status, and the presence of relevant underlying disease (Tables 1–35 and 1–36). The vaccine is administered intramuscularly and can be given simultaneously at different sites with all other routinely recommended childhood vaccines. The AAP and ACIP advocate giving healthy infants born to HBsAg-negative mothers their first immunizations before discharge from the nursery, the second when the child is 1–2 months old, and the third at 6–18 months (Table 1–31). Several alternative schedules are acceptable. The minimum intervals between administration of the first and second doses and between the second and third doses are 1 and 2 months, respectively. Not less than 4 months should separate the first and third doses in the series. Infants born to HBsAg-positive mothers should receive hepatitis B immune globulin (HBIG) and their first immunizations at birth. For these infants, the second and third doses are recommended to be given at 1 and 6 months of age, respectively. Although routine testing for postimmunization antibody response is not recommended for all infants, babies born to HBsAg-positive women should be tested for HBsAg and anti-HBs at 9 months of age and revaccinated if measured antibody titers are below 10 mIU/mL. When the HBsAg status of the mother is unknown, the infant should receive the first immunization at birth and HBIG should be given as close as possible to that time (within 1 week) if the mother subsequently is found to be HBsAg positive. Because of concerns regarding diminished antibody responsiveness in small preterm infants immunized at birth, such infants who are born to HBsAg-negative women should not receive their first hepatitis B vaccinations until they are 2 months of age or weigh at least 2000 g. Preterm infants born to HBsAg-positive women should receive HBIG and immunization at birth, as previously described, and an additional three doses (the first dose is not counted) to complete the series (see *Red Book*). The AAP and ACIP also recommend immunization for all older children and adolescents who were not immunized during infancy and for adults at high risk of hepatitis B exposure (Table 1–34). The recommended schedule for administration in these individuals is 0, 1, and 6 months.

Adverse effects associated with hepatitis B vaccination are minimal and limited primarily to local tenderness, although several rare hypersensitivity reactions to yeast and vaccine preservative have been reported. In recent years, several cases of multiple sclerosis and other demyelinating diseases have been reported in adults who had received hepatitis B vaccines within the preceding 2–3 months. In 1998, the Viral Hepatitis Prevention

Table 1–35. Recommended Dosages of Hepatitis B Vaccines[1]

	Vaccine[2]	
	Recombivax HB[3] dose, µg (mL)	*Engerix-B[4] dose, µg (mL)*
Infants of HBsAg-negative mothers, children and adolescents younger than 20 y	5 (0.5)	10 (0.5)
Infants of HBsAg-positive mothers (HBIG, 0.5 mL, also is recommended)	5 (0.5)	10 (0.5)
Adults 20 y or older	10 (1.0)	20 (1.0)
Patients undergoing dialysis and other immunosuppressed adults	40 (1.0)[5]	40 (2.0)[6]

[1] HBsAg = hepatitis B surface antigen; HBIG = hepatitis B immune globulin.
[2] Vaccines should be stored at 2–8°C (36–46°F). Freezing destroys effectiveness. Both vaccines are administered in a three-dose schedule. A two-dose schedule, administered at 0 and 4–6 mo later, is available for adolescents 11–15 y of age using the adult dose of Recombivax HB (10 µg).
[3] Available from Merck and Co, Inc. (West Point, PA). A combination of hepatitis B (Recombivax, 5 µg) and *Haemophilus influenzae* b (PRP-OMP) vaccine is licensed for use at 2, 4, and 12–15 mo of age (Comvax).
[4] Available from SmithKline Beecham Pharmaceuticals (Philadelphia, PA). The U.S. Food and Drug Administration has approved this vaccine for use in an optional four-dose schedule at 0, 1, 2, and 12 mo.
[5] Special formulation for dialysis patients.
[6] Two 1.0-mL doses given in one site in a four-dose schedule at 0, 1, 2, and 6–12 mo.

From the American Academy of Pediatrics, Committee on Infectious Diseases: In: *2000 Red Book: Report of the Committee on Infectious Disease*, 25th ed. Pickering L et al (editors). Elk Grove Village, IL: American Academy of Pediatrics, 2000.

Table 1–36. Recommended Schedule of Hepatitis B Immunoprophylaxis to Prevent Perinatal Transmission[1]

Vaccine Dose[2] and HBIG	Age
Infant born to mother known to be HBsAg positive[3]	
First	Birth (within 12 h)
HBIG[4]	Birth (within 12 h)
Second	1–2 mo
Third	6 mo
Infant born to mother not screened for HBsAg[5]	
First	Birth (within 12 h)
HBIG[4]	If mother is HBsAg positive, give 0.5 mL as soon as possible, not later than 1 wk after birth
Second	1–2 mo
Third	6 mo[5]

[1] HBsAg = hepatitis B surface antigen; HBIG = hepatitis B immune globulin.
[2] See Table 1–35 for appropriate vaccine doses.
[3] See text for recommendations for subsequent serologic testing.
[4] HBIG (0.5 mL) given intramuscularly at a site different from that used for vaccine.
[5] Infants of HBsAg-negative mothers should receive third dose at 6–18 mo of age.

From the American Academy of Pediatrics, Committee on Infectious Diseases: In: *2000 Red Book: Report of the Committee on Infectious Disease*, 25th ed. Pickering L et al (editors). Elk Grove Village, IL: American Academy of Pediatrics, 2000.

Board, a part of the World Health Organization's Center for the Evaluation of Vaccination, undertook a thorough review of existing data to determine whether or not a causal relation exists between those two events. This group found no statistically significant association between hepatitis B vaccination and multiple sclerosis or other central nervous system demyelinating diseases in studies conducted to date. Further, the age and sex distribution of cases of multiple sclerosis has not changed since widespread use of hepatitis B vaccine and does not differ between groups whose diagnosis was and was not temporally related to vaccination. Although additional research is ongoing, this group found no evidence of a causal association between hepatitis B vaccination and central nervous system demyelinating disease and therefore does not warrant changing current recommendations regarding universal childhood vaccination. These findings subsequently were endorsed by other recommending organizations.

VARICELLA VACCINE

Before the availability of a varicella vaccine (licensed in 1995), approximately 4 million cases of chicken pox occurred each year in the United States. Although most of these infections were self-limited, secondary complications, such as bacterial soft tissue infections, pneumonia, and encephalitis, led to more than 10,000 hospitalizations and 100 deaths annually. Although morbidity from varicella is greater in adolescents and adults, 90% of all cases, 60% of hospitalizations, and 40% of deaths occurred in children younger than 10 years. Further, the economic and social costs of this infection, which necessitates prolonged school absence and home care by a parent or other caregiver, are great. After weighing those issues against data regarding vaccine efficacy and safety, the ACIP and the AAP recommended routine varicella vaccination for all children who have not had the clinical disease.

Varicella vaccine is composed of a live attenuated virus and minute quantities of neomycin and gelatin. For individuals no older than 12 years, a single dose of 0.5 mL is delivered subcutaneously with needle sizes and sites as described above. Routine vaccination is recommended at 12–18 months of age (Table 1–31) and can be given concurrently (using separate sites and syringes) with other routine childhood immunizations. If the MMR is not given on the same day, however, these live-virus vaccines should be administered at least 1 month apart. Teenagers and adults with no history of natural infection also should be vaccinated. Ninety-five percent of children 12 years or younger will seroconvert after one dose of vaccine. However, a diminished antibody response is observed in adolescents and adults. Therefore, it is recommended that individuals 13 years or older be given a two-dose (0.5 mL) regimen separated by 4–8 weeks. Because 70–90% of adults who do not recall an episode of varicella will have antibody evidence of prior infection, it may be cost effective to test immune status in adults and older children (if return can be assured) before giving the vaccine. However, there are no problems associated with immunizing an individual who has previously experienced a natural varicella infection. Varicella vaccination is 85% effective in preventing all disease and greater than 95% effective in preventing moderate and severe disease. On the basis of follow-up studies to date (more than 20 years), serologic evidence of immunity appears to be long-lasting and, like many other live-virus vaccines, is likely to be life-long. However the need for subsequent booster doses continues to be assessed.

The varicella vaccine is associated with few side effects. Approximately 20–30% of recipients will experience transient pain and tenderness at the site of injection. Of greater significance, a mild varicelliform skin eruption will develop in approximately 3–5% of children within 1 month of receiving the immunization. Because the vaccine virus has rarely been recovered from these lesions, a very small risk exists for exposing others to the attenuated virus. Relevant precautions are given below. A mild zoster-like disease also has been reported to occur in some vaccine recipients. This is less severe and occurs at a significantly lower rate than that observed with reactivation of the wild-type virus.

Valid and nonvalid contraindications to varicella vaccination are listed in Table 1–32. Based on a review of new risk benefit data, the ACIP recently modified its recommendations regarding the use of this live-virus vaccine in individuals with certain primary or acquired immunodeficiencies. Individuals with selectively impaired humoral immunity, such as hypogammaglobulinemia and dysgammaglobulinemia, can now be vaccinated. Vaccination of individuals with cellular immunodeficiencies and illnesses and therapies (e.g., high-dose steroids) resulting in global immunosuppression is still contraindicated with two exceptions: Although varicella vaccine is not licensed for use in individuals with neoplasms affecting the bone marrow or lymphatic systems, children with acute lymphocytic leukemia who have been in remission for at least a year and who meet strict protocol cell count criteria can be safely and effectively immunized. Vaccine is provided free of charge to this population by the manufacturer as a part of a research protocol. Because of their increased risk for severe wild-type disease, children with HIV who are asymptomatic or mildly symptomatic (see ACIP recommendation) also should be considered candidates for vaccination. For these children and those in the acute lymphocytic leukemia protocol, a two-dose regimen (irrespective of age) is recommended. Otherwise immunecompetent children with asthma or other conditions for which they are receiving inhaled steroids or less than 2 mg/kg of prednisone or its equivalent per day (less than 20 mg/d if body weight is above 10 kg) can be vaccinated. Children living in households with immunodeficient individuals can and should receive the vaccine. If a vaccine-related skin rash develops, contact between the recipient and the immunocompromised individual should be avoided until the rash resolves. Varicella vaccine should not be given to a pregnant woman, and pregnancy should be avoided for at least 1 month after receiving the vaccine because of the potential risk to the fetus. However, a pregnant woman is not a contraindication to vaccinating a child living in the same household. The varicella vaccine also should not be administered to individuals with histories of anaphylactic reactions to neomycin or gelatin. Caution is advised when vaccinating children taking salicylates. Although no cases of Reye's syndrome have been reported in association with the varicella vaccine, the manufacturer recommends that salicylates be avoided for 6 weeks after administration of the vaccine because of the well-established relation between Reye's syndrome and the use of salicylates during wild-type infection.

PNEUMOCOCCAL CONJUGATE VACCINE

Streptococcus pneumoniae currently is the most common cause of invasive bacterial disease, including sepsis, meningitis, and bacteremia, among children in the United States, with a peak incidence of disease occurring between ages 6–23 months. This organism is also the causative agent in many noninvasive respiratory diseases including acute otitis media, sinusitis, and pneumonia. Groups at highest risk for invasive disease are children with sickle hemoglobinopathies, functional or anatomic asplenia, primary and secondary immunodeficiencies (e.g., HIV infection, malignancies), and certain chronic diseases (e.g., cardiac and pulmonary diseases, diabetes, chronic renal failure). Children of Native American (American Indian and Alaska Native) and African American descent have a moderately increased risk for invasive pneumococcal infection when compared with other healthy children. An increased incidence of infection (two- to threefold increase) and nasopharyngeal colonization also have been documented in children attending out-of-home, group childcare compared with their at-home peers. Since the 1980s, a 23-valent pneumococcal polysaccharide (23PS) vaccine has been available for use in adults and children older than 2 years who are at highest risk for invasive pneumococcal infections. However, the vaccine is not effective in children younger than 2 years, and it has not been recommended for universal childhood vaccination.

In February 2000, the Food and Drug Administration licensed a new 7-valent pneumococcal conjugate vaccine (PCV7) that is effective in children younger than 24 months. It is composed of seven serotype capsular polysaccharides coupled to a nontoxic variant diphtheria toxin. (As with other vaccines using diphtheria toxin as their protein conjugate, this vaccine does not protect against diphtheria.) The vaccine also contains a small amount of an aluminum phosphate adjuvant. The serotypes included (of 90 potential ones) are responsible for 80% of the invasive pneumococcal infections seen in children younger than 6 years in the United States and currently encompass the majority of those strains with the highest rates of penicillin resistance. In studies to date, the vaccine has been highly efficacious in preventing invasive pneumococcal disease. Its use also has been associated with a modest decrease in the incidence of acute otitis media, pneumonia, antibiotic usage, and nasopharyngeal carriage of vaccine strains. The duration of protection after primary immunization with PCV7 currently is unknown, although immunologic memory (booster response to subsequent doses) has been documented. Whether or not additional doses will be necessary for high-risk children remains to be determined. In studies to date, adverse effects appear to be minimal and include local erythema, induration, and tenderness at the site of injection, as well as fussiness and low-grade to moderate fever in a minority of recipients. Contraindication to vaccination includes known hypersensitivity to any of the vaccine components. Vaccination also should be deferred in children with moderate or severe illness.

The availability of the new conjugate vaccine has led the ACIP and the Committee on Infectious Diseases of the AAP to recommend that all children younger than 24 months be routinely immunized during infancy. A dose of 0.5 cc is given by intramuscular injection in a four-doses series at ages 2, 4, 6, and 12–15 months. The first dose should not be give before age 6 weeks. The PCV may be administered concurrently with other childhood vaccines using separate syringes and sites. Premature and low-birth-weight infants should receive the vaccine at the chronologic age of 6–8 weeks. Recommendations for "catch-up" dosing in older infants and children are given in Table 1–37. Routine vaccination of children 24–59 months of age at high risk for invasive pneumococcal infection also is recommended. Groups at highest risk and AAP guidelines regarding the use of PCV7 and 23PS vaccine in these populations are shown in Tables 1–38 and 1–39, respectively. Consideration also may be given to vaccinating children 24–59 months of age who are at moderately increased risk for invasive pneumococcal disease (children 24–35 months of age; children of Native Alaskan, American Indian, and African American descent; and children who attend group daycare) using one dose of PCV7. Data are limited regarding the use of PCV7 in adults and children older than

Table 1–37. Recommended Schedule of Doses for PCV7, Including Primary Series and Catch-Up Immunizations, in Previously Unvaccinated Children[1]

Age at First Dose	Primary Series	Booster Dose[2]
2–6 mo	3 doses, 6–8 wk apart	1 dose at age 12–15 mo
7–11 mo	2 doses, 6–8 wk apart	1 dose at age 12–15 mo
12–23 mo	2 doses, 6–8 wk apart	
≥24 mo	1 dose	

[1] Recommendations for high-risk groups are given in Table 1–39.
[2] Booster doses to be given at least 6–8 wk after the final dose of the primary series.
From the American Academy of Pediatrics, Committee on Infectious Diseases: Policy statement: recommendations for the prevention of pneumococcal infections, including the use of pneumococcal conjugate vaccine (Prevnar), pneumococcal polysaccharide vaccine, and antibiotic prophylaxis. *Pediatrics* 2000;106:363.

Table 1–38. Children at High Risk of Invasive Pneumococcal Infection

High risk (attack rate of invasive pneumococcal disease >150/100,000 cases/y)
  Sickle cell disease, congenital or acquired asplenia, or splenic dysfunction
  Infection with human immunodeficiency virus

Presumed high risk (attack rate not calculated)
  Congenital immune deficiency: some B- (humoral) or T-lymphocyte deficiencies, complement deficiencies (particularly C1, C2, C3, and C4 deficiencies), or phagocytic disorders (excluding chronic granulomatous disease)
  Chronic cardiac disease (particular cyanotic congenital heart disease and cardiac failure)
  Chronic pulmonary disease (including asthma treated with high-dose oral corticosteroid therapy)
  Cerebrospinal fluid leaks
  Chronic renal insufficiency, including nephrotic syndrome
  Diseases associated with immunosuppressive therapy or radiation therapy (including malignant neoplasms, leukemias, lymphomas, and Hodgkin's disease) and solid organ transplantation[1]
  Diabetes mellitus

Moderate risk (attack rate of invasive pneumococcal disease >20 cases/100,000/y)
  All children 24–35 mo old
  Children 36–59 mo old attending out-of-home care
  Children 36–59 mo old who are of Native American (American Indian and Alaska Native) or African American descent

[1] Guidelines for the use of pneumococcal vaccines for children who have received bone marrow transplants are currently undergoing revision (Centers for Disease Control and Prevention, personal communication, 2000).
From the American Academy of Pediatrics, Committee on Infectious Diseases: Policy statement: recommendations for the prevention of pneumococcal infections, including the use of pneumococcal conjugate vaccine (Prevnar), pneumococcal polysaccharide vaccine, and antibiotic prophylaxis. *Pediatrics* 2000;106:364.

5 years. Those who are at high risk for pneumococcal disease (e.g., sickle cell disease, HIV infection) may receive 23PS vaccine or PCV7; however, there is some rationale in this age group for using the 23PS vaccine because only 50–60% of invasive pneumococcal infections in older children and adults are covered by PCV7.

ROTAVIRUS VACCINE

In the United States, rotavirus is the most common cause of severe gastroenteritis in children and infants, accounting for 30–50% of all hospitalizations for dehydration due to diarrheal disease in children younger than 5 years. The

Table 1–39. Recommendations for Pneumococcal Immunization With PCV7 or 23PS Vaccine for Children at High Risk of Pneumococcal Disease, as Defined in Table 1–38[1]

Age	Previous Doses	Recommendations
≤23 mo	None	PCV7 as in Table 1–37
24–59 mo	4 doses of PCV7	1 dose of 23PS vaccine at 24 mo, at least 6–8 wk after last dose of PCV7 1 dose of 23PS vaccine, 3–5 y after the first dose of 23PS vaccine
24–59 mo	1–3 doses of PCV7	1 dose of PCV7 1 dose of 23PS vaccine, 6–8 wk after the last dose of PCV7 1 dose of 23PS vaccine, 3–5 y after the first dose of 23PS vaccine
24–59 mo	1 dose of 23PS	2 doses of PCV7, 6–8 wk apart, beginning at least 6–8 wk after last dose of 23PS vaccine 1 dose of 23PS vaccine, 3–5 y after the first dose of 23PS vaccine
24–59 mo	None	2 doses of PCV7 6–8 wk apart 1 dose of 23PS vaccine, 6–8 wk after the last dose of PCV7 1 dose of 23PS vaccine, 3–5 y after the first dose of 23PS vaccine

[1] Children with sickle cell disease, asplenia, human immunodeficiency virus infection, and other high-risk factors. PCV7 = 7-valent pneumococcal conjugate vaccine; 23PS = 23-valent pneumococcal polysaccharide.

From the American Academy of Pediatrics, Committee on Infectious Diseases: Policy statement: recommendations for the prevention of pneumococcal infections, including the use of pneumococcal conjugate vaccine (Prevnar), pneumococcal polysaccharide vaccine, and antibiotic prophylaxis. *Pediatrics* 2000;106:364.

peak age for clinically significant disease is 3–24 months, with virtually all children experiencing at least one rotavirus infection by 3–5 years. Although primary infection provides significant protection, recurrent, usually attenuated, illness is common. In 1998, a live attenuated oral vaccine containing four strains of rotavirus (three human rhesus resortant strains and one rhesus strain) became available for use. Because of the considerable morbidity and social and economic costs associated with this illness, the AAP (December 1998) and the ACIP (March 1999) recommended that all infants be routinely immunized with this vaccine. However, as use became more widespread, an increased number of cases of intussusception were reported in the first few weeks after vaccination. This observation led the AAP and ACIP to recommend suspension of the routine use of this vaccine.

REFERENCES

Physical Growth

Barlow SE, Dietz WH: Obesity evaluation and treatment: expert committee recommendations. Pediatrics 1998;102:E29.

Fenichel GM: Disorders of cranial volume and shape. In: *Clinical Pediatric Neurology: A Signs and Symptoms Approach,* 2nd ed. Philadelphia: WB Saunders, 1993; pp 359–376.

Pollack IF et al: Diagnosis and management of posterior plagiocephaly. Pediatrics 1997;99:180.

Rohan AJ et al: Infants with misshapen skulls: when to worry. Contemp Pediatr 1999;16:47.

Strauss R: Childhood obesity. Curr Probl Pediatr 1999;29:5.

Zenel JA: Failure to thrive: a general pediatrician's perspective. Pediatr Rev 1997;18:371.

Motor & Psychological Development

Blasco PA: Pitfalls in developmental diagnosis. Pediatr Clin North am 1991;38:1425.

Colson ER, Dworkin PH: Toddler development. Pediatr Rev 1997;18:255.

Dixon SD, Stein MT: *Encounters with Children: Pediatric Behavior and Development,* 3rd ed. Chicago: Year Book, 1990.

Illingworth RS: *The Development of the Infant and Young Child: Normal and Abnormal.* New York: Churchill-Livingstone, 1987.

Johnson CP, Blasco PA: Infant growth and development. Pediatr Rev 1997;18:224.

Palmer FB, Capute AJ: Mental retardation. Pediatr Rev 1994;15:473.

Sturner RA, Howard BJ: Preschool development part 1: communicative and motor aspects. Pediatri Rev 1997;18:291.

Sturner RA, Howard BJ: Preschool development part 2: psychosocial/behavioral development. Pediatr Rev 1997;18:327.

Counseling & Anticipatory Guidance

Algranati PS, Dworkin PH: Infancy problem behaviors. Pediatr Rev 1992;13:16.

American Academy of Pediatrics: *Policy Reference Guide, a Comprehensive Guide to AAP Policy Statements Published through January 2000,* 13th ed. Elk Grove Village, IL: American Academy of Pediatrics, 1999.

American Academy of Pediatrics, Committee on Psychosocial Aspects of Child and Family Health: *Guidelines for Health Supervision III.* Elk Grove Village, IL, American Academy of Pediatrics, 1997.

Elster AB, Kuznets NJ: *Guidelines for Adolescent Preventive Services (GAPS).* Baltimore: Williams & Wilkins, 1993.

Green M (ed): *Bright Futures: Guidelines for Health Supervision of Infants, Children, and Adolescents,* rev. ed. Arlington, VA: National Center for Education in Maternal and Child Health, 1998.

Howard BJ: Discipline in early childhood. Pediatr Clin North Am 1991;38:1351.

Report of the U.S. Preventive Services Task Force: Guide to Clinical Preventive Services, 2nd ed. Alexandria, VA: International Medical Publishing, 1996.

Rivara FP: Pediatric injury control in 1999: where do we go from here? Pediatrics 1999;103:883.

Screening

American Academy of Pediatrics: *Policy Reference Guide, a Comprehensive Guide to AAP Policy Statements Published through January 2000,* 13th ed. Elk Grove Village, IL: American Academy of Pediatrics, 1999.

Cadman D et al: Assessing the effectiveness of community screening programs. JAMA 1984;251:1580.

Centers for Disease Control and Prevention: *Screening Young Children for Lead Poisoning. Guidance for State and Local Public Health Officials.* Atlanta, GA: US Department of Health and Human Services, Public Health Service, 1997.

Fletcher RH et al: Clinical Epidemiology—The Essentials. Baltimore: Williams & Wilkins, 1996.

National High Blood Pressure Education Program Working Group on Hypertension Control in Children and Adolescents: update on the 1987 task force report on high blood pressure in children and adolescents. Pediatrics 1996;98:649.

Report of the U.S. Preventive Services Task Force: Guide to Clinical Preventive Services, 2nd ed. Alexandria, VA: International Medical Publishing, 1996.

Sackett DL et al: Clinical Epidemiology: a Basic Science for Clinical Medicine, 2nd ed. Boston: Little Brown, 1991.

Immunizations

Advisory Committee on Immunization Practices: General recommendations on immunization: recommendations of the Advisory Committee on Immunization Practices (ACIP). MMWR 1994;43(RR-1).

Advisory Committee on Immunization Practices, Centers for Disease Control: Update: vaccine side effects, adverse reactions, contraindications, and precautions. MMWR 1996;45(RR-12):1.

American Academy of Pediatrics: Immunization of adolescents: recommendations of the Advisory Committee on Immunization Practices, the American Academy of Pediatrics, the American Academy of Family Physicians, and the American Medical Association. Pediatrics 1997;99:479.

American Academy of Pediatrics, Committee on Infectious Diseases: *2000 Red Book. Report of the Committee on Infectious Diseases,* 25th ed. Elk Grove Village, IL: American Academy of Pediatrics, 2000.

National Vaccine Advisory Committee: standards for pediatric immunization practices. MMWR 1993;42(RR-5):1.

Adolescence

William Adelman, MD, & Jonathan Ellen, MD

HISTORICAL CONTEXT

I would there were no age between ten and three-and-twenty,

or that youth would sleep out the rest;

for there is nothing in the between but getting wenches with child,

wronging the ancientry, stealing, fighting.

William Shakespeare, The Winter's Tale,
Act III, Scene III

Adolescence, from the Latin *adolescere,* "to grow into maturity," is the transition from childhood to adulthood. G. Stanley Hall, in his 1904 treatise, *Adolescence,* introduced the modern concept of adolescence as a time of Sturm und Drang (storm and stress). Hall largely borrowed this concept from the 18th and 19th century German writings of Goethe and Schiller who depicted youth as passionate, idealistic, moody, and full of suffering. This concept was well known in literature and philosophy, but Hall formalized and legitimized it as "scientific." Works published in the 1950s and 1960s by Anna Freud and others on disturbed teens further supported the idea that psychological turmoil is the norm during adolescence. The teenager as an inherently troubled being was the dominant theme in the 20th century until the 1970s, when researchers decided to examine "normal" teenagers and not psychiatric inpatients. Today, the bulk of empirical evidence shows that adolescence is a gradual transition that proceeds without undue upheaval in most teens. Four of five adolescents relate well to their families and peers and are comfortable with their social and cultural values. Conversely, as many as one in five teenagers may have difficulty with this transition and therefore require expert evaluation and treatment.

A thorough understanding of the normal emotional, cognitive, social, and physical development of the adolescent is crucial for implementation of effective health care to this unique segment of our population. Although in no way exhaustive, we hope that this chapter will serve as a guide to the clinical approach to teenagers and so allow delivery of developmentally appropriate health care.

EPIDEMIOLOGY & CURRENT TRENDS

Statistics relating to the epidemiology of adolescence are often confusing because of the different definitions of the ages that comprise this group. Currently, 10–19 year olds comprise 15% of the population in the United States. This percentage has remained stable over the past decade as the absolute number of adolescents continues to rise with that of the general population. Minorities comprise a disproportionate number of adolescents when compared with the general population. One third of adolescents are members of ethnic minority groups. This proportion is expected to continue to rise as the United States sees increases in immigration and birth rates among minorities. In 1993, nearly 17% of adolescents lived below the poverty line. Adolescents living in one-parent households are most likely to live in poverty, and women head 87% of one-parent families with adolescents. Lack of economic resources combined with less support within the family structure reinforces the need for comprehensive health services for adolescents.

Adolescence is a relatively healthy period in the life cycle, with a low incidence of disabling or chronic illnesses compared with other periods of life, fewer short-term hospitalizations, and fewer days in which individuals stay home. Only 1 in 15 teens in the United States is chronically ill, and the illness is usually due to mental, respiratory, or musculoskeletal causes. In the middle of the 20th century, illness and disease accounted for more than twice as many deaths as violence and injury. The reverse is true today, as the rates of death and disability in adolescence have decreased substantially. The "new morbidities" of adolescence are largely preventable entities—homicide, accidents (including motor vehicle accidents), and suicide.

HEALTH CARE DELIVERY SYSTEMS

Adolescents are far less likely than adults to seek and receive medical and dental care. In 1985, U.S. teens 10–18 years old made an average of 1.6 visits to private, office-based physicians compared with the national average of 2.7 for all ages. In 1994, despite comprising 15% of the population, adolescents accounted for only 9% of all office visits. Many barriers to adolescent health care exist. A partial list includes inability to independently navigate through the medical system, lack of transportation, concerns of confidentiality, lack of documented insurance, and lack of funds to pay out of pocket. Child-oriented waiting rooms of pediatricians and unwelcome décor in adult-provider waiting rooms might discourage adolescents. The proliferation of school-based health centers has increased the accessibility to health resources for teenagers. School-based health centers, usually located within or in close proximity to middle and high schools, provide a variety of services such as routine and sports physical examinations, treatment of minor illness or injury, health education, dental care, and counseling with regard to substance abuse, sexuality, and mental health. These centers are increasingly popular because they address the fact that most adolescent health problems are preventable, that health services are underused by teenagers, and that teens want health services to be confidential. Studies show that most visits to these centers are for physical examinations, acute illnesses, and minor illnesses.

■ GROWTH & DEVELOPMENT

SOMATIC GROWTH & DEVELOPMENT

Puberty is the physical hallmark of adolescence and, in its technical sense, refers to the process of becoming capable of sexual reproduction. The sequence of events in puberty is predictable and generally is the same from one female or male to the next. In contrast, the timing and tempo of puberty are not as predictable. All adolescents do not begin puberty at the same time and they do not complete the maturation process in the same period. Compared with their peers, adolescents can be described as maturing early, average, or late. Whereas early maturation may be beneficial to boys, early maturing girls are at greatest risk for adopting health-compromising behaviors.

The physical changes that occur during puberty consist of neuroendocrine changes, rapid skeletal growth, changes in body composition, and sexual maturity. Most aspects of the biology and physiology of adolescents correlate better with pubertal maturation than with chronologic age. For example, boys' hemoglobin levels correlate better with stage of pubertal maturation rather than with chronologic age.

Neuroendocrine Changes

Adrenarche (increase in steroid production by the adrenal glands) occurs approximately 2 years before the onset of the secondary sexual development of puberty. Although not required for puberty to occur, adrenarche is characterized by the development of body odor and, in some individuals, hair formation. A sleep-associated increase in pulsatile gonadotropin-releasing hormone and leutinizing hormone (LH) production is the first step in

puberty. There is a decrease in the sensitivity of the hypothalamus to circulating estradiol and testosterone. This leads to an increased secretion of follicle-stimulating hormone (FSH) and LH. FSH peaks in mid-puberty, whereas LH increases throughout puberty. Among females, ovulation is secondary to a mid-cycle surge of estrogen, with positive feedback to the hypothalamus that results in a burst of gonadotropin-releasing hormone and LH. It is important to recognize that ovulation is not necessary for menstruation because those processes are controlled by two separate mechanisms. The hormonal events of puberty and abnormalities in pubertal development (precocious and delayed puberty) are discussed in greater depth in Chapter 19.

Skeletal Growth

Height growth during puberty accounts for 25% of final adult height (23–28 cm in girls and 26–28 cm in boys). The height spurt lasts 24–30 months and there is seasonal variation, with the greatest height gains in the spring and summer. For girls, peak height velocity averages 9 cm per year and occurs early in puberty. Boys gain 10.3 cm per year at peak height velocity and this occurs later in puberty. Because boys start their growth spurts approximately 2 years after girls do, they start from a taller base. Boys also become taller because of their greater growth during puberty. Weight gain during puberty peaks during the height spurt and accounts for 40–50% of ideal adult body weight.

Body Composition

Significant changes occur during puberty with regard to body composition in the areas of lean body, adipose, muscle, skeletal, internal organ, and erythrocyte mass. In girls, lean body mass decreases from 80–85% of body weight to 75% at maturity as adipose tissue increases. In boys, lean body mass increases from 80% to 90% at maturity as muscle mass increases due to circulating androgens. In girls, adipose tissue increases from 15% of body fat before puberty to 26.7% at maturity. In boys, adipose tissue decreases from approximately 14% to 11% over the course of puberty. Muscle mass peaks 3 months after the height spurt in boys and girls, but the increase in mass is twice as great in boys as in girls. Muscle strength lags behind muscle mass until the final stage of puberty in boys. Skeletal mass and lean body mass undergo parallel alterations. About 40% of adult bone mass accrues during puberty. Epiphyseal maturation of long bones occurs under the influence of estradiol and testosterone. Pelvic remodeling occurs in females with a more rapid widening than in the anterior–posterior dimension. Internal organs also undergo significant growth: heart weight doubles, with a decrease in heart rate and a rapid rise in systolic blood pressure in boys. Blood pressure plateaus in girls. Lung size increases as respiratory rate decreases, and vital capacity increases. Electroencephalography shows an evolution in the brain from low-frequency waves to α waves, although there is no change in mass.

Sexual Maturity

Stages of secondary sexual characteristics (breast, pubic hair, size of male genitalia) are measured by the Sexual Maturity Rating (SMR) scale first described by Marshall and Tanner in 1962 (Figures 2–1 and 2–2). These stages are commonly known as Tanner stages.

The typical timing and sequence of these changes are shown in Figures 2–3 and 2–4. For approximately 85% of girls, the first sign of puberty is breast budding, which generally occurs at age 11 years. However, 10–15% of girls will develop pubic hair before breast buds. Menarche is a late event for girls and usually occurs in SMR stage 4. Most height growth is achieved before the onset of menses, with an average addition of only 7 cm after menarche. Puberty in girls can occur as early as age 8 years, and all girls should have some evidence of secondary sexual characteristics before age 14 years. During puberty, the uterus and ovaries increase in size five- to sevenfold. Uterine length increases from 3.3 to 6.9 cm. Ovarian volume increases from 1.9 to 3.5 cm³. Menarche occurs on average at age 12.6 years (range 9–17 years). It requires about 17% body fat, but regular menses will not occur until the adolescent has about 22% body fat. Menarche generally is achieved about 2 years after the onset of breast buds. At the time of menarche, only 20–30% of cycles are ovulatory. Ovulation with at least 80% of cycles does not occur until 4–5 years after menarche.

On average, males enter puberty approximately 0.5–1.0 years later than girls do. Boys begin puberty at about age 11.6 years, with an increase in testicular volume being the first sign. Boys are considered to be pubertal when the length of their testes is 2.5 cm. They should not begin puberty before age 9 and should have started puberty by age 14. The production of sperm occurs at a median age of 13.4 years, at SMR 2–3, and with little development of pubic hair. Ejaculation occurs at SMR 3 and fertility by SMR 4. The penis does not begin to grow until SMR 3. On average, a boy completes puberty in 3 years (range 2–5 years).

PSYCHOSOCIAL GROWTH & DEVELOPMENT

Adolescence can be divided into three developmental stages: **early, middle, and late.** Specific goals and tasks for normal development characterize each stage. Although the definition and division of such stages are somewhat arbitrary and overlap of stages certainly occurs, the concept of the teenager having different concerns and abilities at each stage is clinically useful as a means to deliver age-appropriate care and advice. Overall, the concerns of adolescence can be simplified as four major areas: independence, body image, peer group, and identity. Each stage of adolescence addresses these areas differently during the normal process of emotional and cognitive development.

The Early Adolescent

Chronologic age: 10–13 or 14 years
Educational age: junior high school
SMR: 2–4

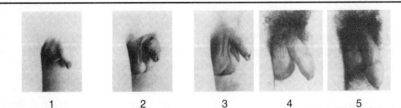

SMR 1 2 3 4 5

Figure 2–1. Male adolescent development. Genital development: SMR 1, prepubertal-sized testes, scrotum, and penis; SMR 2, testes and scrotum begin to enlarge, penile growth is minimal; SMR 3, continued growth of scrotum and testes, penis enlarges especially in length; SMR 4, continued growth of scrotum and testes, continued penile growth especially in width; SMR 5, adult size and shape of genitalia. Pubic hair development: SMR 1, no pubic hair; SMR 2, sparse growth of straighter, lighter, downy hair at the base of the penis; SMR 3, coarse, darker, curly hair, more extensive distribution; SMR 4, continued expansion of adult-type hair but not yet onto thighs; SMR 5, adult consistency, quantity, and distribution of hair (onto thighs and center line of lower abdomen). SMR 1–5 = Sexual Maturity Rating, stages 1–5. (From Wieringen JD et al: *Growth Diagrams 1965.* New York: Walters-Nordhoff, 1971.)

SMR

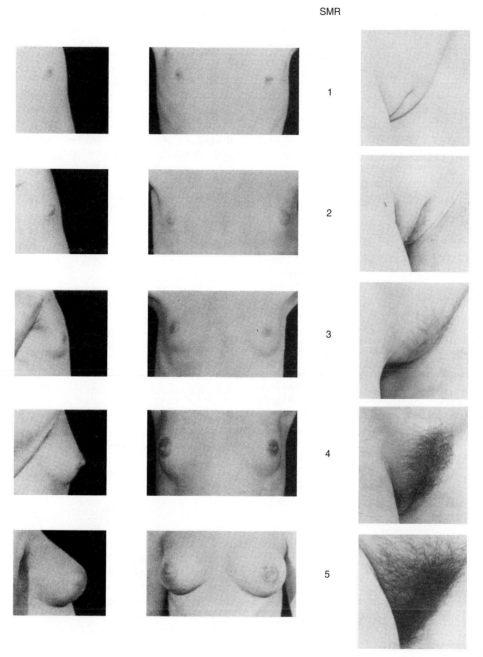

Figure 2–2. Female adolescent development. Breast development: SMR 1, prepubertal breasts; SMR 2, appearance of breast buds; SMR 3, further enlargement of breasts, no break in contour between areola and breast; SMR 4, continued growth of breasts, the areola and papilla form a distinct mound above the remaining breast tissue; SMR 5, adult breast in size and contour, areola is level with the contour of the breast. Pubic hair development: SMR 1, no pubic hair; SMR 2, sparse growth of straighter, lighter, downy hair along the labia; SMR 3, coarse, darker, curly hair, more extensive distribution; SMR 4, continued expansion of adult-type hair but not yet onto thighs; SMR 5, adult consistency, quantity, and distribution of hair (onto thighs). SMR 1–5 = Sexual Maturity Rating, stages 1–5. (From Wieringen JD et al: *Growth Diagrams 1965*. New York: Walters-Nordhoff, 1971.)

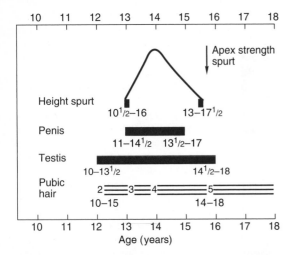

Figure 2–3. Diagram of sequence of events at adolescence in boys. The age range of each event is indicated. (From Tanner JM: *Growth at Adolescence.* New York: Blackwell, 1962.)

GENERAL CONCERNS

Independence. This period is the transition from childhood. It is characterized by a desire for greater privacy and less interest in parental activity. Parents often describe the early adolescent as having more "mood swings" (although studies do not show consistent vacillation in mood unrelated to activity but only an increase in negative moods with age). Although the early adolescent may begin to assert his independence at this age, he is constantly looking for role models. It is a time when parents need to assert more, not less, supervision.

Body image. With the onset of the biologic changes of puberty comes the question, "Am I normal?" Interest in sexual anatomy and physiology comes to the forefront. Dirty jokes are very popular, and issues such as menses and wet dreams hold fascination, excitement, and some anxiety. Early development is advantageous for the self-esteem of boys but detrimental for the self-esteem of girls.

Peer group. At this age, the peer group consists predominantly of intense same-sex friendships, with a strong desire to conform. It is the age of "blood brothers" and "friends 4ever." The opposite sex is usually encountered in groups (consider a junior high school dance where the boys are on one side of the gym floor and the girls—usually a head taller—are on the other).

Identity. As children leave the confines of what Sigmund Freud termed the "latency age," they develop increased self-interest and marked egocentrism. There is an obsession with self, as the teen "feels on stage" and develops the "personal fable" of being the center of the world. This period is marked by the development of fantasy, day-dreaming, and idealism. Most early adolescents have unrealistic expectations for their futures in that they envision becoming professional athletes, singers, or actors. As early teens struggle with these identity issues, they develop an increased need for privacy. Thinking is concrete, described by the Swiss psychologist Jean Piaget as "operational." Usually there is no capability for abstract thought. Early adolescents tend to understand instructions literally.

THE EARLY ADOLESCENT HEALTH CARE VISIT

The interview. The early adolescent health care visit should include private time with the adolescent, as the provider builds a relationship as the patient's advocate. However, discussion with a parent or guardian is mandatory for information about medical history, observations of behavior, and motivating factors for the office visit. The early adolescent characteristically has little insight. Questions must be blunt, without the use of euphemism, and instructions should be concrete to ensure understanding.

The examination. Minor blemishes or changes with puberty are serious threats to the self-identity of the adolescent. The early adolescent perceives these issue as important, so they require careful explanation and handling by the provider. Similarly, many early adolescents are quite modest and easily embarrassed with the physical examination. Therefore, it is important to allow the teen to disrobe in private, describe in simple terms what

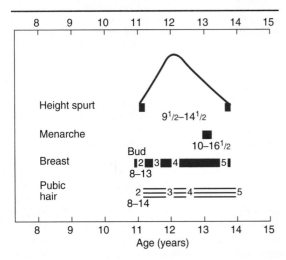

Figure 2–4. Diagram of sequence of events at adolescence in girls. The age range of each event is indicated. (From Tanner JM: *Growth at Adolescence.* New York: Blackwell, 1962.)

will occur during the examination before performing it, make instructions clear as to what clothing is to be removed and what is to be left on, and allow a parent in the room if requested by the child. For example, one might say, "I will step out in a minute and let you get undressed. Please take off all your clothes except for your underpants, then put on this gown opening up in front." It is also important to normalize rather than ignore or belittle the embarrassment: "Teenagers and adults are embarrassed to get undressed for a physical examination, but it is an important part of staying on top of your health."

Anticipatory guidance. A clear delineation of the normality of pubertal changes is required. Relationships and behaviors are "me oriented" to the early teen who usually becomes introduced to opportunities for risk-taking behaviors such as substance use. Upcoming challenges such as peer pressure, experimentation, health risk behaviors, and general safety should be introduced.

Common medical problems
- Eating disorders in girls
- Acne
- Injuries, both overuse and unintentional

The Middle Adolescent

Chronologic age: 15–17 years
Educational age: high school
SMR: 4–5

GENERAL CONCERNS

Independence. Despite the stereotype to the contrary, many teenagers undergo a quiescent period during middle adolescence, as the physical changes of puberty have largely occurred, and increased autonomy with the increased workload of high school offers new challenges. In contrast, the archetypal "rebellious" teen characteristically presents in middle adolescence and usually is one who undergoes major conflicts over control during continued struggle for emancipation. This is the age of "temporary parental disablement." Although the early adolescent recognizes parents as less perfect than previously presumed, she will frequently look to a parent as an important role model and for cues for behavior. In contrast, for the middle adolescent, parents are inherently not cool and the peer group becomes more influential with regard to behavior, dress, personal choice, and activities. Too much distance from the family unit during this period can lead to inappropriate behavior with peers. "Rules apply to everyone else but not me" is how many teens view authority at this age. This period has been described as the period of "experimentation without commitment" and is applicable in the areas of sexuality, life-style, appearance, and morality.

Body image. As puberty progresses, the teen shifts from "Am I normal?" to "Am I attractive?" Concern shifts to general attractiveness and acceptance of physical changes. Middle adolescents may spend hours in front of the mirror, working to appear a certain way, through make-up, piercing, clothes, etc. Similarly, health issues that affect appearance continue to be tantamount. Acne, breast size and development, weight issues, and anything else that may make them different from their peers can cause them distress.

Peer group. Middle adolescence is the peak of peer group influence and conformity. Social behaviors are dictated largely by the behaviors of the peer group, e.g., sexual experimentation and activity, violence, cigarettes, alcohol, and illicit drugs. What the peer group is doing is the best indicator of what the adolescent is doing. Experimentation and taking risks characterize this period. Clubs, religious groups, sports teams, and gangs are manifestations of the desire to bond with a peer group in a meaningful way and help solidify self-identity.

Identity. In most teens, abstract thinking skills and creativity develop. For many, this is the first time they can realistically see themselves in the future. The concept of consequences of actions becomes understandable and thus can alter decisions if thought through. Mental exercises that begin with "What if . . . ?" allows for effective education through role-play. The middle adolescent begins to consider future plans, may have more realistic adult goals, or be faced with indecision. Cognition moves to include abstract reasoning and should include what Piaget termed "formal operational" thinking. However, middle adolescent thinking continues to include a sense of omnipotence and immortality, especially with issues of experimentation. This allows for high risk-taking behavior and high morbidity and mortality from consequences of quick, sometimes inappropriate, decisions.

THE MIDDLE ADOLESCENT HEALTH CARE VISIT

The interview. Most of the visit should be with the patient. All information relayed, education, and anticipatory guidance should be directed to the adolescent with or without the parent or guardian. New patients often require many visits and establishment of personal trust before emotionally charged issues can be uncovered or completely addressed. The provider must be on the lookout for the "hidden agenda"—i.e., presentation with a specific complaint that is not the *real* reason for the visit. This hidden agenda may be revealed after trust has been established during a particular visit or after many visits. The impact of a particular behavior needs to be assessed as to whether an activity is an experiment (normal for developmental age) or has become part of the adolescent's life or identity (abnormal or maladaptive for development), e.g., drug experimentation versus regular use or abuse.

Anticipatory guidance. When risks are identified, in most cases the practitioner can lead the adolescent through a decision-making process to consolidate the teenager's understanding of his control over the outcome of his actions and decisions (e.g., "What happens if you don't take your insulin?" "After you get pregnant, how will your life change?" "If you carry a gun, and we get into an argument, and I make a sudden move . . ."). This is a great advantage over the early adolescent for whom the abstraction of future consequences to present actions is largely unattainable.

Common medical problems
- Sexuality-related problems: pregnancy, sexually transmitted disease
- Drug use: tobacco, alcohol, and other mind-altering substances
- Intentional injury: homicide, suicide
- Unintentional injury: overuse injury, vehicular accidents

The Late Adolescent

Chronologic age: 18–21+ years
Educational age: college, work force
SMR: 5

GENERAL CONCERNS

Independence. This is the final transition to adulthood. During this period, teenagers try to answer the question, "Who am I in relation to society?" The great task is to achieve independence and the ability to operate without parents—financially, socially, and morally. The length of this period is variable. For some, late adolescence may end not long after turning 18 years old if they live independently with paying jobs (e.g., in the military). For others, continued education without meaningful employment (or accruement of debt) arguably extends this period to age 25 or beyond (e.g., medical students?). Return to acceptance of parents occurs during this stage because they no longer threaten independence and are seen in the light of adulthood. The necessary task is to achieve autonomy and adult relations during this stage.

Body image. Most teens move away from concerns of body image to concentrate on a more comprehensive definition of self-image. The pubertal process has ended, and this stage is characterized by acceptance of physical appearance or extreme behaviors to alter appearance (e.g., surgery and eating disorders).

Peer group. Identification with multiple peer groups occurs as the late adolescent recognizes her varied interests. The capacity for intimacy is shown by the adolescent's ability to care enough about another person to alter behavior based on the effect that behavior will have on the sig-

nificant other. More time is devoted to intimate relationships. For some, that relationship might include marriage and beginning a family.

Identity. Formal reasoning with a sense of future and specific vocational goals to achieve financial independence characterize the late adolescent. Refinement of the individual's own moral, religious, and sexual values occurs. There is a shift from decisions based on fear of punishment to decisions that are the "right thing to do." The late adolescent must consolidate identity to avoid "ego diffusion" as described by Erik Erikson. That is, the final shaping of identity dictates adult life, and lack of consolidation of financial, social, and moral identities leads to significant anxiety, stress, and maladaptive behavior.

THE LATE ADOLESCENT HEALTH CARE VISIT

The interview. Virtually all interactions are with the patient. The late adolescent usually has a specific agenda for the visit. The provider's goal is to encourage these patients to take responsibility for their health care decisions and participate fully in their health care plans. Discussion of long-term issues is reasonable.

Anticipatory guidance. Specific, adult-oriented issues should be the routine. Teaching lifelong health care strategies, such as proper diet, yearly Papanicolaou (Pap) smears, breast or testicular self-examination, are important. At this time, depending on age, it is appropriate to consider transferring the patient to a new health care practitioner.

Common medical problems
- Second peak of anorexia nervosa, peak of bulimia nervosa, other eating disorders
- Continued risk of overuse, vehicular, and other unintentional injuries
- Continued risk of intentional injuries through young adulthood
- Stress-induced physical symptoms or illness

■ APPROACH TO THE ADOLESCENT ENCOUNTER

GENERAL ISSUES

The medical interview is the most important clinical tool available to health practitioners. To provide effective care and establish rapport with the adolescent, the health care provider must be comfortable with adolescents. There is no single correct way to interview adolescents or their parents; what works well for some may be inappropriate for others. The adolescent should feel that the provider cares about him or her as a person first, and that the provider is a resource for health issues. Individuals who do not feel comfortable with or who dislike adolescents should not care for them.

When meeting adolescent patients for the first time, providers should introduce themselves, shake hands, and then ask to be introduced to the teens' parents. From the outset, it should be clear that the provider's prime concern is for the teenager and that the interaction will focus on him or her.

Adolescents are concerned about confidentiality and find a lack of assurance of confidentiality a barrier to seeking care. For example, most adolescents claim they would not seek care for problems regarding sexuality if they believed their parents would find out. Unfortunately, most teenagers are not aware that many confidential services may be available. Therefore, assurance of confidentiality is important. However, blanket statements of confidentiality might cause a provider to break a promise, place the patient at risk, or provide less than optimal care. It is most beneficial to approach the issue of confidentiality with the patient and the patient's parents at the initial visit and in a straightforward manner. One can then explain that many teenagers have personal questions that they do not feel comfortable asking their parents or asking the doctor in the presence of a parent or guardian. Similarly, there are questions that providers ask all of their teenage patients that may be personal and more difficult to answer when a parent is in the room. Therefore, time is provided in every visit to see the adolescent alone and this time is increased as the adolescent matures. The provider also should explain that the visit is private and confidential.[1] Providers should state during the initial visit that they will not lie to parents or teenagers and that they will similarly refer the parent to the teenager for questions of a personal nature.

ADOLESCENT HEALTH SUPERVISION

Guidelines for Adolescent Preventive Services

Since the U.S. Preventive Services Task Force (USPSTF) published its seminal report in 1989, many organizations have published guidelines for adolescent health care. Examples are the American Medical Association's (AMA) guidelines for adolescent preventive services, the American Academy of Family Physicians (AAFP) age charts for periodic health examinations, the Maternal and Child Health Bureau of the Health Resources and Services Administration's Bright Futures, and the American Academy of Pediatrics' (AAP) recommendations for pediatric preventive health care. Even though preventive services for infants and children are a mainstay of primary care, a major reason for the development of these guidelines is the fact that physicians provide preventive guidance for adolescents only sporadically and they often avoid emotionally sensitive issues. A summary of recommendations for adolescent preventive services is shown in Table 2–1.

Table 2–1. Adolescent Preventive Health Care[1]: Recommended Components

Health guidance for teenagers
  Normal development
  Injury prevention
  Nutrition
  Physical activity
  Dental health
  Breast or testicular self-examination for middle and
    late adolescents

Health guidance for parents

Screening
  Hearing
  Vision
  Obesity
  Hypertension
  Sexual activity
  Contraception
  Tobacco use
  Alcohol use
  Other substance use
  Abuse (physical, emotional, sexual)
  School problems
  Depression and risk for suicide
  Eating disorders

Tests in populations at risk
  Cholesterol
  Tuberculosis
  Sexually transmitted diseases
  Papanicolaou test
  Human immunodeficiency virus

Tests for all adolescents at least once during adolescence
  Hematocrit
  Urinalysis

Immunizations according to the Advisory Committee on
  Immunization Practices (ACIP) of the U.S. Public
  Health Service.

[1] Yearly preventive visits recommended for ages 11–21 years.

[1] Personal issues will not be disclosed to others without the permission or knowledge of the teenager. However, the patient must be made aware that the responsibility of the provider is the patient's health. Therefore, in extreme circumstances, the provider may need to discuss issues with other medical providers or the patient's parent. In those cases, I guarantee the patient that I will discuss the issue with her first, and together we may proceed as to how best to disclose the information.

The Adolescent Visit

HISTORY

The average practitioner performs 120,000–160,000 interviews in a professional career. The adolescent interview is used to determine problems that need to be addressed, build a strong provider–patient relationship, and act as an effective vehicle for patient education. What sets the adolescent interview apart from other interviews is the need for a complete psychosocial review of systems. Specifically, it allows early identification of problems that might lead to significant morbidity and mortality. One system for organizing the psychosocial history is known by the acronym HEADSS, which stands for home, education/ employment, activities, drugs, sexuality, and suicide/ depression (Table 2–2).

PHYSICAL EXAMINATION

The physical examination is similar in content to that of a child or adult. However, it is common for the teenager not to present with the real reason for visiting the physician ("hidden agenda"). Therefore, it is important to continue probing. Mentioning and explaining findings during the examination that might not be related to the stated reason for the visit should be done. For example, because acne is so prevalent during adolescence, the provider might not even mention it, but the acne might be a significant source of discomfort for the teenager who may

Table 2–2. Sample Questions to Ask During the HEADSS Assessment

Home
- Who lives at home with you?
- Have there been any recent changes at home?
- Who can you talk to at home about personal or private issues?
- What causes stress at home?
- If you could change anything about your home, what would it be?

Education/employment
- What school do you attend?
- What grade are you in?
- Are you in any special classes [e.g., honors or remedial]?
- Has there been any recent change in your grades?
- How are you doing at school this year compared with last year?
- How many days of school have you missed this year?
- Has anyone mentioned to you that they are concerned with your performance at school?
- Have you been suspended?
- Have you gotten in a physical fight at school in the past year?
- Are you involved in any school teams or clubs?
- Do you have a job outside of school?
- What do you do?
- How often do you work?
- How does your work affect your home life? Social life? School?

Activities
- What do you like to do when you are not in school?
- What do you do for entertainment?
- Are you involved in sports? School activities? Religion?
- Do you have hobbies?
- Do you have a best friend?
- Tell me about your friends?
- Do you carry weapons?
- Have you ever been in trouble with the police?

Drugs
- I see you attend _____ high school. You must see students there who smoke cigarettes.
- Do any of your friends smoke cigarettes?
- Tell me what your experience has been with cigarettes?
- Have you ever been concerned with a friend's use of alcohol or other drugs?
- Have any of your friends been concerned with your use of alcohol or drugs?
- Have you ever been concerned about your own use of alcohol or drugs?
- What has your experience been with alcohol? Marijuana? Heroin? Cocaine? LSD? Other drugs?

Sexuality
- Many people become interested in romantic relationships at your age. Is there anyone that you feel that way about? Tell me about that. [This type of neutral questioning allows potential disclosure of both homosexual and heterosexual feelings.]
- Are any of your friends dating?
- What has your experience been?
- What sexual activities have you done with this person?
- How about with previous relationships?
- Have you had sex with men/women/both?
- Have you ever been in a sexual situation that you felt was against your will? That you felt uncomfortable with?
- Have you ever been pregnant? Fathered a child?
- Have you ever had an abortion? Have you ever had a miscarriage?
- Have you ever had a sexually transmitted disease?
- What do you use to protect yourself against sexually transmitted diseases and pregnancy?
- Do you want to become pregnant?

Suicide/mental health
- How do your describe your mood today?
- Do you feel sad?
- Does this get in the way of your usual activities?
- Have you had any sleep disturbances? Changes in appetite, energy, or concentration?
- Have you ever thought of killing yourself?

be too embarrassed to bring it up. Therefore, a casual comment (e.g., "I notice you have some mild acne on your cheeks. Is that something you are interested in talking about?") can be used to start the discussion.

LABORATORY EVALUATION

In general, routine laboratory screening of asymptomatic teenagers is not recommended. Screening studies are indicated for selected adolescents who are at risk for sexually transmitted diseases (STDs), tuberculosis, and elevated cholesterol. The AAP recommends screening for anemia in all adolescents. STD screening in sexually active adolescents is discussed later in this chapter. Recommendations for screening in other areas are discussed in greater depth in Chapter 1.

IMMUNIZATIONS

All adolescents should be immunized according to the recommendations developed by the Advisory Committee on Immunization Practices (ACIP) of the Centers for Disease Control and Prevention. Teenagers who are foreign born and do not attend public school are at increased risk for underimmunization. Indeed, in the absence of a school requirement, population-based data suggest that most adolescents lack documentation of recommended vaccinations. In 1996, the ACIP, AAP, AAFP, and AMA recommended routine health care visits for children aged 11–12 years, with an emphasis on vaccinations with hepatitis B vaccine; measles, mumps, and rubella vaccine if two doses had not been received previously; tetanus and diphtheria toxoids; and varicella vaccine for those without the disease in childhood.

In certain cases, meningococcal, pneumococcal, influenza, and poliomyelitis vaccines may be advisable or indicated. Further information on immunization can be found in Chapter 1.

ANTICIPATORY GUIDANCE

Anticipatory guidance should be performed at the end of every well-child visit. Specific topics to address depend on the age and developmental stage of the patient and the issues identified during the history and physical examination. It is important to point out areas where the teenager has been successful and reinforce healthy choices such as abstinence or refusal to try cigarettes. In addition, providing information on topics discussed in the form of a pamphlet on safe sexual practices and usable resources such as condoms may make behavioral changes easier. Other areas of anticipatory guidance to address are puberty, nutrition, dental care, breast or testicular self-examination, drug-refusal skills, sexuality, coping skills, peer pressure, and safety issues such as personal security and the risks of fighting and carrying weapons. In recognition of the "new morbidities" of adolescence, six priority behaviors have been identified as the most effective and achievable for avoiding the major causes of death: (1) use seat belts, (2) do not drink (or use drugs) and drive; (3) use condoms when having sex, (4) do not smoke, (5) eat a low-fat diet, and (6) engage in regular aerobic exercise.

■ MAJOR ADOLESCENT HEALTH ISSUES

MENTAL HEALTH & COGNITIVE ISSUES

Depression

More than half of teenagers have reported feeling depressed currently or recently, and as many as 17% of all teenagers might meet criteria for a depressive disorder. Epidemiologic data suggest that the prevalence of depression is increasing, and depression and suicide are increasingly recognized as major causes of morbidity among adolescents. Prepubertal children show no gender difference in depression, but rates are twice as high in female teenagers and adults as in male teenagers and adults. Major depression is estimated to have a prevalence of 4–9% among teenagers. It is characterized by depressed mood most of the day nearly every day for at least 2 weeks and is distinguished from the normal vicissitudes in mood of adolescent life by its persistence and inconsistency with life context. For example, it is appropriate for a teenager to report sadness, even for a day or two, after viewing a film in school about the Holocaust. However, if this teenager feels sad at parties, disengages from usual enjoyable activities, and feels guilty or worthless, it is more likely that she is depressed. In teenagers, depression may present as a persistent irritable mood instead of sadness. Adolescents with depression might benefit from antidepressants, individual and family therapy, or psychotherapy. Approximately two-thirds of cases improve with pharmacologic and psychological treatments.

Suicide

Suicide is the third leading cause of death among 15–24 year olds. It claimed at least 4186 lives in this age group in 1997. Of these, 1802 involved individuals between the ages of 15 and 19. The rate of suicide for 15–19 year olds is nearly 11 per 100,000, with boys six times more likely than girls to commit suicide in this age range. Nearly one in four 7th through 12th graders has reported seriously considering suicide, one in five has reported planning for suicide, and one in eleven has made an attempt. However, completed suicide is relatively uncommon among teenagers and is less likely in teens than in adults.

Female adolescents attempt suicide two to nine times more often than their male counterparts, but male adolescents are three to eight times more likely than female adolescents to successfully complete a suicide. For both sexes, firearms, in particular handguns, are the most common method of completed suicide. Firearms are used in 63–67% of all adolescent suicides. Males are next likely to succeed with hanging, whereas females are next successful with jumping from tall heights. Toxic ingestion accounts for most attempts by girls but is rarely successful. Wrist slashing is the second most common means of suicide attempt in the Unites States, characteristically with less than lethal results. Alcohol use has been associated with 50% of suicides.

Native American males have the highest suicide rate. African American females have the lowest suicide rate. Homosexual and bisexual youth have higher rates of suicide than heterosexuals, and 28% of bisexual and homosexual males and 20% of bisexual and homosexual females have reported attempting suicide.

The tragedy of teenage death, with the realization of potential life lost, necessitates the diagnostic imperative for the primary care provider to identify teenagers at risk for suicide. The AAP recommends that pediatricians know the risk factors associated with suicide, routinely ask questions about depression and firearms in the home, and serve as a resource for parents and other community leaders on issues related to suicide.

There is no way to accurately predict a suicide attempt, but many studies have identified factors more prevalent among those who commit suicide than among individuals who died from other means. Risks unique to the act of suicide include a history of suicide attempt, current suicidal ideation especially if accompanied by a plan, impulsive or accident-prone behavior, recent suicide attempt or completion by a friend, and having a handgun in the home. Less specific risk factors include depression, dysfunctional family situation, feelings of hopelessness and worthlessness, social isolation, and substance abuse. Immediately before suicide, the following events and qualities are implicated: suffering a significant or humiliating loss; preoccupation with or excessive talk of death, hopelessness, or suicide; giving away valued possessions; and preoccupation with getting affairs in order. Any of these issues, when identified, should prompt the clinician to completely evaluate suicidal intent. Examples of adolescents at low, moderate, and high risk for suicide are presented in Table 2–3. The simplest way to assess suicidal ideation is to ask. It is important to remember that, even though suicidal youth are unlikely to spontaneously volunteer thoughts of suicide, if asked in an honest and straightforward manner, they are likely to reply similarly. One reasonable approach to this sensitive topic might be to say, "You seem sad (or agitated or confused or upset) to me. Tell me about your feelings. Have you ever thought about hurting yourself or committing suicide? Do you feel like hurting yourself or committing suicide

Table: 2–3. Examples of Adolescents at Low, Moderate, and High Risk for Suicide

Low risk
Took 5 ibuprofen tablets after argument with girlfriend
Impulsive; told mother 15 min after taking pills
No serious problems at home or school
Occasionally feels "down" but has no history of depression or serious emotional problems
Has a number of good friends
Wants help resolving problems and is no longer considering suicide after interview

Moderate risk
Suicidal ideation precipitated by recurrent fighting with parents and failing grades in school
Wants to "get back" at parents
Cut both wrists while home alone; called friend 30 min later
Parents separated, changed school this semester, history of attention deficit/hyperactivity disorder
Symptoms of depression for the last 2 mo, difficulty controlling temper
Binge drinking on weekends
Answers all questions during interview, agrees to see a therapist if parents get counseling, will contact the interviewer if suicidal thoughts return

High risk
Thrown out of house by parents for smoking marijuana at school, girlfriend broke up with him last night, best friend killed in auto accident last month
Wants to be dead; sees no purpose in living
Took father's gun; is going to shoot himself, where "no one can find me"
Gets drunk every weekend and uses marijuana daily
Hates parents and school, has run away from home twice, and has not gone to school for 6 weeks
Hospitalized in the past because he "lost it"
Does not want to answer many of the questions during the interview and hates "shrinks"

Adapted from the American Academy of Pediatrics Committee on Adolescence: Suicide and suicide attempts in adolescents. *Pediatrics* 2000;105:873.

now? What would you do the next time you have these feelings?"

An adolescent who reports suicidal ideation, is depressed, or reveals a history of suicide attempt deserves a prompt and thorough evaluation. If there is any doubt regarding the risk of suicide, a mental health provider should be consulted without delay.

Eating Disorders

Eating disorders are severe disturbances in eating behavior. In anorexia nervosa and bulimia nervosa, eating behavior and perceptions of body weight and shape are disturbed. The significant difference between the two is that those with anorexia nervosa refuse to maintain a normal body weight, whereas those with bulimia nervosa characteristically are of normal weight. Eating disorders may be thought of as addictions to the concept of losing or maintaining weight. Treatment might be frustrating or impossible for those who lack expertise in this area. Referral to an appropriate facility or practitioner is warranted with diagnosis.

ANOREXIA NERVOSA

Anorexia nervosa affects up to 1% of adolescent and young adult females. The prevalence of subthreshold anorexia nervosa, i.e., disordered eating, is higher. Females are 20 times more likely than males to have this condition. The mean age of onset is 17 years, with bimodal peaks at ages 14 and 18 years. Onset of illness often is associated with a stressful life event, such as leaving home for college.

The essential feature of anorexia nervosa is maintenance of a body weight that is below a minimum for age and height. In growing teens, this may present with lack of growth in contrast to marked weight loss. Criteria for the diagnosis of anorexia nervosa are listed in Table 2–4. Suggested parameters include being below 85% of ideal body weight based on height or a body mass index (weight in kilograms/height in meters squared) less than 17.5.

Subtypes of anorexia nervosa are restricting and binge-eating/purging. *Restricting type* refers to those who accomplish weight loss primarily through dieting, fasting, or excessive exercise. The current episode does not include binge eating or purging. *Binge-eating/purging type* refers to those who engage in binge eating, purging, or both, on a regular basis, during the current episode. Effective treatment for eating disorders requires expert supervision. Behavioral, multidisciplinary, and specialized treatment team approaches are more likely to be successful than treatment by the primary care provider alone.

The course and outcome of anorexia nervosa are highly variable. Long-term mortality can be as high as 10%, usually results from starvation, suicide, or electrolyte imbalance, and appears to be highest among those with prior university hospital admissions and recurrent episodes.

BULIMIA NERVOSA

Bulimia nervosa usually begins in late adolescence or early adulthood. Prevalence of bulimia nervosa is 1–3% among adolescent and young adult females and similar in most industrialized countries. This disorder is characterized by binge eating with inappropriate compensatory behaviors to prevent gaining weight. Binge eating commonly begins during periods of dieting, and, like those with anorexia nervosa, bulimia sufferers have an inappropriate focus on body shape and weight. Females are diagnosed with bulimia nervosa 10 times more often

Table 2–4. Diagnostic Criteria for Anorexia Nervosa

Refusal to maintain body weight at or above a minimally normal weight for age and height (e.g., weight loss leading to maintenance of body weight less than 85% of that expected; or failure to make expected weight gain during period of growth, leading to body weight less than 85% of that expected)

Intense fear of gaining weight or becoming fat, even though underweight

Disturbance in the way in which one's body weight or shape is experienced, undue influence of body weight or shape on self-evaluation, or denial of the seriousness of the current low body weight

In postmenarcheal females, amenorrhea, i.e., the absence of at least three consecutive menstrual cycles (a woman is considered to have amenorrhea if her periods occur only after hormone, e.g., estrogen, administration)

Specify types
  Restricting: during the current episode of anorexia nervosa, the person has not regularly engaged in binge-eating or purging behavior (i.e., self-induced vomiting or the misuse of laxatives, diuretics, or enemas)
  Binge-eating/purging: during the current episode of anorexia nervosa, the person has regularly engaged in binge-eating or purging behavior (i.e., self-induced vomiting or the misuse of laxatives, diuretics, or enemas)

Reprinted with permission from the *Diagnostic and Statistical Manual of Mental Disorders,* 4th ed. © 1994 American Psychiatric Association.

than males. Diagnostic criteria for this disorder are presented in Table 2–5.

Subtypes of bulimia nervosa are purging and nonpurging. With purging, there is the regular engagement in self-induced vomiting or misuse of laxatives, diuretics, or enemas during the current episode. With nonpurging, there is use of other inappropriate behaviors, such as fasting or exercise, but no use of vomiting, laxatives, diuretics, or enemas during the current episode.

Most individuals with bulimia nervosa have disturbed eating patterns for many years after diagnosis. Therefore, treatment should be ongoing and supervised by individuals with expertise in bulimia treatment. The course is variable, and the long-term outcome is unknown.

EATING DISORDER NOT OTHERWISE SPECIFIED

This category consists of eating disorders that do not meet the criteria for the other specific disorders. For example, an obese woman who develops anorexia nervosa might not meet the weight criterion. Another example is a woman who meets all criteria for bulimia nervosa except that her binge eating and inappropriate compensatory

Table 2–5. Diagnostic Criteria for Bulimia Nervosa

Recurrent episodes of binge eating; an episode of binge eating is characterized by both of the following:

Eating, in a discrete period of time (e.g., within any 2-h period), an amount of food that is definitely larger than most people would eat during a similar period of time and under similar circumstances

A sense of lack of control over eating during the episode (e.g., a feeling that one cannot stop eating or control what or how much one is eating)

Recurrent inappropriate compensatory behavior to prevent weight gain, such as self-induced vomiting; misuse of laxatives, diuretics, enemas, or other medications; fasting; or excessive exercise

Binge-eating and inappropriate compensatory behaviors both occur, on average, at least twice a week for 3 mo

Self-evaluation is unduly influenced by body shape and weight

The disturbance does not occur exclusively during episodes of anorexia nervosa

Specify types

Purging: during the current episode of bulimia nervosa, the person has regularly engaged in self-induced vomiting or the misuse of laxatives, diuretics, or enemas

Nonpurging: during the current episode of bulimia nervosa, the person has used other inappropriate compensatory behaviors such as fasting or excessive exercise but has not regularly engaged in self-induced vomiting or the misuse of laxatives, diuretics, or enemas

Reprinted with permission from the *Diagnostic and Statistical Manual of Mental Disorders,* 4th ed. © 1994 American Psychiatric Association.

Table 2–6. Criteria for Substance Abuse

A maladaptive pattern of substance use leading to clinically significant impairment or distress, as manifested by one (or more) of the following occurring within a 12-mo period:

Recurrent substance use resulting in a failure to fulfill major role obligations at work, school, or home (e.g., repeated absences or poorwork performance related to substance use; substance-related absences, suspensions, or expulsions from school; neglect of children or household)

Recurrent substance use in situations in which it is physically hazardous (e.g., driving an automobile or operating a machine when impaired by substance use)

Recurrent substance-related legal problems (e.g., arrests for substance-related disorderly conduct)

Continued substance use despite having persistent or recurrent social or interpersonal problems caused or exacerbated by the effects of the substance (e.g., arguments with spouse about consequences of intoxication, physical fights)

The symptoms have never met the criteria for substance dependence for this class of substance

Reprinted with permission from the *Diagnostic and Statistical Manual of Mental Disorders,* 4th ed. © 1994 American Psychiatric Association.

mechanisms occur less frequently than twice a week or for a duration of less than 3 months.

Substance Use & Abuse

Any alcohol or other drug use that leads to clinically significant impairment or distress (i.e., interference with regular activities in life) is problematic and should be of concern to the provider. Terminology related to substance use and differentiation of problem behavior from developmentally anticipated experimentation might be confusing to many practitioners. Criteria for identifying substance abuse and substance dependence are presented in Tables 2–6 and 2–7, respectively.

The pattern of substance abuse among teenagers has increased significantly over the past 30 years. Adults predominantly abused alcohol, tobacco, and other psychoactive drugs in the 1960s. In the late 1960s and 1970s, substance abuse became widespread among adolescents and reached an all-time high. There followed a reduction in use in the 1980s and early 1990s, with an increase since then. Usage is currently alarmingly high among preadolescents. High school students showed a steady increase in the use of alcohol and other drugs during the 1990s.

Most children and adolescents who use alcohol and other drugs will not become problem users of those substances. However, casual use with early onset quickly progresses to problem use for many adolescents. The earlier a young person begins to drink alcohol or use other drugs, the greater the likelihood of future problems in that area.

Genetic influences, household drug use (especially parental use), ongoing disruption of families with persistent chaos, use of drugs within the peer group, antisocial behaviors, and poor parental monitoring and supervision are independent risk factors for adolescent substance abuse. Conversely, protective factors against adolescent substance abuse are a close sense of connection to one's parents or a significant other, consistency of the family structure and family activities, belonging to a non–drug-using peer group, clear parent-defined conduct norms, and siblings intolerant of alcohol or other drug use.

Annual risk behavior screening is recommended by many. In addition to the HEADSS mnemonic previously described, the CAGE mnemonic can be a clinically use-

Table 2–7. Criteria for Substance Dependence

A maladaptive pattern of substance use, leading to clinically significant impairment or distress, as manifested by three (or more) of the following occurring at any time in the same 12-mo period:

Tolerance, as defined by either of the following:
   A need for markedly increased amounts of the substance to achieve intoxication or desired effect
   Markedly diminished effect with continued use of the same amount of the substance

Withdrawal, as manifested by either of the following:
   The characteristic withdrawal syndrome for the substance
   The same (or a closely related) substance is taken to relieve or avoid withdrawal symptoms

The substance is often taken in larger amounts or over a longer period than was intended

There is a persistent desire or unsuccessful efforts to cut down or control substance use

A great deal of time is spent in activities necessary to obtain the substance (e.g., visiting multiple doctors or driving long distances), use the substance (e.g., chain smoking), or recover from its effects

Important social, occupational, or recreational activities are given up or reduced because of substance use

The substance use is continued despite knowledge of having a persistent or recurrent physical or psychological problem that is likely to have been caused or exacerbated by the substance (e.g., current cocaine use despite recognition of cocaine-induced depression, or continued drinking despite recognition that an ulcer was made worse by alcohol consumption)

Specify if
  With physiologic dependence: evidence of tolerance or withdrawal (i.e., either of the first two items above)
  Without physiologic dependence: no evidence of tolerance or withdrawal (i.e., neither of the first two items)

Modified and reprinted with permission from the *Diagnostic and Statistical Manual of Mental Disorders,* 4th ed. © 1994 American Psychiatric Association.

ful tool to screen for substance abuse in teenagers or members of their families: Have you ever . . .

Thought about Cutting down your use?

Felt Annoyed by what others have said about your use?

Felt Guilty about something you said or did during your use?

Used as an Eye opener Early in the morning or to feel normal?

If positive, this initial screen should prompt further investigation with an exhaustive assessment of medical, behavioral, psychological, and social aspects of the patient's environment, with the use of a subspecialty referral if indicated.

Much debate has recently focused on the issue of drug screening to detect, monitor, and deter adolescent substance use. It is important to understand the benefits and limitations of drug testing. Many people misunderstand the information provided by such tests, believing them to be diagnostic of dependency or addiction rather than a spot check for certain drugs or metabolites. Positive drug tests are not mentioned in the definitions of substance abuse or substance dependence in the *Diagnostic and Statistical Manual of Mental Disorders,* 4th edition (DSM-IV). More importantly, drug test results without the appropriate clinical context are useless. For example, false-negative results are common because of technical limitations and many known ways to "beat" the test, and an individual with a negative drug test but a suggestive history may very well have a drug problem. Conversely, a positive urine screening result is not proof of chemical dependency or a maladaptive pattern of use.

TOBACCO

Tobacco is the single most preventable cause of death and disease in the United States; it kills 450,000 Americans and costs the United States more than 100 billion dollars each year. Tobacco use is a pediatric disease. Nine of every 10 adult smokers began smoking as adolescents. Greater than one-third of high school students smokes cigarettes, and half of all teenagers who smoke into adulthood will die of a smoking-related illness. Adolescents comprise the only age group that showed a rise in smoking behavior during the 1990s. Despite this, most teenagers are interested in quitting smoking at some point during adolescence, often after 1–3 years of use. Seventy percent of adolescent smokers regret smoking, and three of four young smokers have tried to quit at least once and failed. Unfortunately, few smoking-cessation options are available to teenagers and most pediatricians are ill equipped to deal with smoking issues among teenage patients.

The AAP's position on drug testing is that it can be used when necessary to determine the cause of a change in mental status, suspicious physical findings, and dysfunctional behavior. However, in adolescents with decisional capacity, involuntary testing is not appropriate and should be performed only if there are strong medical or legal reasons to do so. Drug testing should be seen as a potentially useful laboratory tool; however, the appropriate response to the suspicion of drug abuse in an adolescent is referral to a qualified health care professional for comprehensive evaluation.

The key for the practitioner is identification and persistent follow-up of smoking status. Ask at every visit whether a teen smokes cigarettes. Congratulate every teenager who does not smoke for being smart enough to not pick up the habit. Advise every smoker to quit smoking. Among adults, a simple medical message from the provider that quitting smoking is absolutely recommended leads to a 5% quit rate. Therefore, a statement such as, "As your health provider, I am obligated to tell you that the single best thing you can do for your health is to quit smoking. If you are interested in quitting, let me know so I can help you," is a simple intervention that is worthwhile with every smoker. Keep the message short. Teenagers will disregard lectures and longer explanations, especially if perceived as judgmental or condescending. If the teenager is interested in quitting and requests assistance, the provider should have available a quit-smoking plan to review with the teenager. If the teenager is not interested in quitting, the provider should simply state, "When you are interested in quitting, I am here to help you." It is then crucial that the provider follow up with the teenager at every visit regarding that teen's smoking habits so that the teenager can begin to think about quitting and ask for assistance.

Pharmacologic options for smoking cessation include nicotine replacement in the form of the patch, gum, nasal spray, and inhaler and a non-nicotine option in the drug bupropion, marketed as Zyban and Wellbutrin. To date, the only rigorously evaluated intervention shown to be effective for adolescent smoking cessation is a school-based curriculum that involved group sessions for motivated teenagers.

ALCOHOL

Alcohol is the most common substance of abuse among teenagers. Eighty percent to 90% of high school seniors have used alcohol by that point in their lives. Binge drinking, or consumption of five or more drinks in a row, presumably to achieve intoxication, is reported to have occurred in the past 2 weeks by 16% of 8th graders, 25% of 10th graders, and 30% of seniors. About 10.4 million current alcohol drinkers were 12–20 years old in 1998. Of those, 5.1 million were binge drinkers and 2.3 million were heavy drinkers, meaning they had five or more drinks on the same occasion on at least five different days in the past month. Family history and the CAGE questionnaire can be used to uncover individuals with problems in these areas.

MARIJUANA

Marijuana is the most commonly used illicit drug and accounts for 81% of all illicit drug use in the United States. In 1998 about 8% of 12–17 year olds were current marijuana users. The active ingredient of marijuana is tetrahydrocannibinol, commonly smoked from the leaf or resin of the *Cannabis sativa* plant. Inhalation leads to peak plasma concentration in 10–30 minutes, with 2–3 hours of desired effects such as distortion of time sense, enhancement of special senses, and impairment of learning, judgment, and general cognitive functioning. Toxic and idiosyncratic effects include mood fluctuations, depersonalization, hallucinations, anxiety, panic attacks, paranoia, impaired vigilance, coordination, reaction time, and multiple stimuli attention deficit. Although often termed a "gateway drug" because of its association with the use of other drugs, chronic marijuana use in and of itself can be debilitating.

INHALANTS

One percent to 2% of teenagers are current inhalant users, but inhalants have the second highest lifetime prevalence of use (10–13%) after marijuana. Typically, these are the first consciousness-altering drugs tried. They are popular with early adolescents and discontinued at a young age, after 1–2 years of use.

Volatile solvents such as rubber cement, spray paint, glues, gasoline, lighter fluid, propellants, and refrigerants contain hydrocarbons with different chemical structures. The user's experience is described as one of euphoria and lightheadedness, with various degrees of sedation and derealization, similar to an opiate high. Adverse effects include hallucinations that have led people to jump from high places with tragic consequences, anoxia, and *sudden sniffing death syndrome,* postulated to result from ventricular fibrillation after sensitization of the myocardium by hydrocarbons and elevated catecholamines.

HEROIN

The rate of heroin initiation among 12–17 year olds increased from below 1% during the 1980s to 2.7% in 1996. Newer forms of heroin that allow smoking, sniffing, and snorting have increased its popularity. In 1998, 87% of new heroin users were younger than 26 years and 72% of those had never injected heroin. With the change in means of delivery has come increased use, increased casual use without addiction, and many more deaths. Often the only means of uncovering a heroin addiction is through a careful history in the office setting. Acute symptoms of heroin overdose are depressed mental status, confusion, stupor or coma, bradypnea, decreased response to painful stimuli, miotic pupils, and mottled, cool skin.

COCAINE

The highest rate of cocaine use in 1998 occurred in those 18–25 years old (2.0%). The rate of use for those 12–17 years old is 0.8%. However, the rate of initiation in the 12–17-year-old group has increased from 4.1 per

1000 in 1991 to 10.8 per 1000 in 1997. Rates of cocaine use are twice as high for men as for women. Acute cocaine intoxication presents with hyperalertness, restlessness, and euphoria, often with sweating and elevated temperature. Occasionally, there can be labile affect, anxiety, agitation or paranoia, with delirium and hallucinations. Dilated pupils, hyperreflexia, paresthesias, and tremor are seen on neurologic examination. Hypertension, tachycardia, and arrhythmia are common cardiovascular effects. In overdose, cocaine can cause coma, psychosis, chest pain, myocardial infarction, hyperthermia, rhabdomyolysis, stroke, and seizures.

HALLUCINOGENS

The rate of initiation of hallucinogens among youths 12–17 years old increased from 11.1 to 25.0 per 1000 between 1991 and 1995 and has remained level since then. Intoxication effects include perceptual alterations, loss of time sense, euphoria, depersonalization, and hallucinations. In acute evaluation of an intoxicated individual, characteristic findings include labile affect, anxiety, paranoia, dizziness, ataxia, tremor, anorexia, and nausea. Physical examination might show elevated temperature with flushing and piloerection, elevated blood pressure and tachycardia, dilated pupils with conjunctiva injection and lacrimation, paresthesias, hyperreflexia, and dry mouth.

Attention Deficit/Hyperactivity Disorder in the Adolescent

Attention deficit/hyperactivity disorder (AD/HD) has been reported to be one of the most common disorders of childhood. Most children with AD/HD remain distractible, impulsive, inattentive, and disruptive throughout adolescence. AD/HD is associated with increased risk for many other problems such as major affective disorders, family disturbance and conflict, alcohol and substance abuse, delinquency and criminality, conduct disorders, aggression, job failures, and divorce. What makes AD/HD a challenge during adolescence is that it is more difficult to diagnose. The following section focuses on the presentation of this disorder in adolescence. For a broader discussion of AD/HD, the reader is referred to Chapter 3.

The triad of symptoms in AD/HD comprises inattention, impulsiveness, and hyperactivity. In adolescence, symptoms shift from hyperactivity toward more attentional and impulsivity difficulties and derived or associated problems such as poor motivation, demoralization, and delinquent activities. As a result, the diagnosis commonly is missed. A telling sign of AD/HD in the adolescent is incessant talking and interrupting. Inattention is often the core symptom for adolescent sufferers. Adolescents who are concerned about their grades might bring that issue to the attention of another. If they are smart enough, they might get grades lower than they are capable of (mostly Bs) but, because they are within the acceptable range, their academic performance may not be seen as problematic to others. A prior missed diagnosis of AD/HD by adolescence may have produced a "longstanding underachiever" not particularly interested in school, thus setting the risk for school failure. By high school, concerns and activities are largely social, and impulsiveness often presents a problem. Symptoms like blurting out thoughts or ill-advised actions are very common. Being too impulsive while driving a car, initiating sexual activity, or engaged in a volatile situation with others can have dire consequences. To compound the difficulty in making the diagnosis, other "soft signs" of AD/HD often are attributed to normal adolescence. Those signs are conflict with authority, clumsiness, substance use, and peer relationship difficulty.

Diagnosis can be made with DSM-IV criteria (see Chapter 3) or one of many checklists after ruling out organic problems. Treatment of AD/HD should include pharmacologic therapy and behavior management, school intervention, and social competence training. Some benefit from family therapy has been shown. In summary, AD/HD should not be overlooked in the adolescent because it is an important factor in adolescent scholastic and social failure. If noticed, the adolescent with AD/HD responds well to therapy. Conversely, when missed, the adolescent can develop more injuries, increased substance abuse, more comorbid disorders, and adult failure.

REPRODUCTIVE HEALTH

Issues Related to Sexuality & Sexual Activity

Most of our understanding of sex during adolescence is based on a plethora of research that focuses on the sexual act rather than the feelings, reasons, and ideas behind such actions. In other words, although we understand the prevalence and incidence of sexual intercourse and other behaviors, our understanding of adolescent sexuality remains limited. A sensible approach to adolescent sexuality requires the understanding that development of feelings of sexuality is necessary to achieve adult sexual well-being. The role of the practitioner is to assist the teen in traversing this developmental milestone safely and responsibly.

GAY, LESBIAN, & BISEXUAL YOUTH

An anonymous study of more than 4000 children in grades 9–12 in Massachusetts showed that 2.5% identified themselves as "gay, lesbian, or bisexual" (GLB). Those who self-identify as GLB in high school report disproportionate risk for a variety of health risk and problem behaviors, including suicide, victimization, sexual risk behaviors, and multiple substance use. It is important to phrase questions of sexuality in neutral terms so as not to assume heterosexuality and to ask directly if the teenager has had experience with homosexual feelings or actions. Allowing a safe, nonjudgmental place for teenagers to discuss feelings of sexuality is critical for any practitioner who sees adolescents, so as to identify health issues unique to that population.

PREGNANCY

The rate of teenage pregnancy is decreasing or at least leveling off in every state in the United States. However, the scope of teen pregnancy in the United States remains alarming. The United States has the highest teen pregnancy and birth rates of any industrialized country, and it is nearly double that of the next highest country, Great Britain. Each year, nearly 1 million teenagers become pregnant. Half of those pregnancies result in live births, 30–40% result in abortion, and the remainder result in miscarriage. Teens account for nearly one-fourth of all abortions performed in the United States. Eighty-five percent of teenage pregnancies are unwanted or unplanned, and three-fourths of teenage births are to unmarried teens.

The consequences of teenage pregnancy are well documented. When controlled for socioeconomic status, teenage mothers as compared with those who delay childbearing until age 20 or 21 are less likely to complete high school (33% vs. 50%), more likely to be single parents, and more likely to have multiple births. Children of teen mothers are more likely to be born prematurely and at low birth weight. Despite the inherent morbidity associated with such conditions, they receive less medical care and treatment. They perform worse in school, with a 50% higher chance of repeating a grade, have higher rates of behavior problems and higher rates of not working or attending school, and daughters who are products of teen pregnancy are 22% more likely to become teen mothers themselves.

Prevention of teenage pregnancy should be a primary medical goal. Therefore, frank and open discussion of sexuality should begin with the early adolescent, and resources such as contraception and confidential counseling should be made available to teenagers. Health care providers must have a high index of suspicion regarding the potential for pregnancy and be able to make a prompt diagnosis. Urine pregnancy tests are rapid, cost effective, specific, and almost as sensitive as the serum human chorionic gonadotropin assays. Urine tests will demonstrate a positive pregnancy test within 7–10 days after conception, before the first missed menstrual period, and long before any clinical signs or symptoms. With a diagnosis of pregnancy, the AAP recommends that pediatricians help the adolescent understand her options and act on her decision to continue or terminate the pregnancy. Health care providers who cannot support the adolescent in her decision must refer her care to a physician who can.

CONTRACEPTION

Most teenagers present to the office for contraception after the onset of sexual intercourse. At least half of all teenage pregnancies occur within 6 months of sexual debut, and the mean interval between first intercourse and clinic visit is 9–23 months.

Various methods of contraception and their relative efficacy rates are presented in Table 2–8. The best form of contraception for an adolescent is the method that he or she will use effectively. Optimal use of contraception depends not only on the adolescent but also on the form of contraception and the environment or health system in which it is provided. Important questions to ask the teenager who is interested in contraception are listed in Table 2–9. Several of the most commonly used contraceptive methods are discussed.

Abstinence. Abstinence is an effective form of contraception and prevention of sexually transmitted disease. The abstinent teenager always should be congratulated for making a healthy and positive choice. Few teenagers choose this form of contraception. Because half of all teenage pregnancies occur within 6 months of onset of sexual activity and most of those teens were "practicing abstinence" at the time, this method leaves little recourse after it is discarded. Although promotion of abstinence is a laudable goal and achievable for some teenagers, it is not a realistic choice for many adolescents.

Barrier methods. Barrier methods of contraception include the condom, contraceptive sponge, diaphragm, and cervical cap. Spermicidal agents used as an adjunct increase the effectiveness of the barrier method and independently decrease the rate of pregnancy and STD.

The **condom** is perhaps the best-publicized method of contraception and STD prevention and is given some of the credit for the reduction in unwanted pregnancies throughout the United States.

The male condom, if used perfectly, offers a 3% chance of pregnancy, and the female condom, 5%. Typical use, however, leads to pregnancy rates of 14% with the male condom and 21% with the female condom. A disadvantage of the male condom is that its use may be out of the female's control. The female condom is considered awkward by many teens and has not gained popularity in this age group. Effective condom use also has been shown to protect against acquisition of STDs.

Maximal condom effectiveness is achieved through proper use. Proper use consists of several components: (1) the condom is lubricated with spermicide or a spermicide is added every time; (2) the condom must be placed before any vaginal contact, and, if the male is not

Table 2-8. Methods of Contraception[1]

Method	Mechanism of action	Efficacy: Rate of Pregnancy 1st Year of Use[2]		Coital dependence	Cost	Prescription required	Protection from STD/HIV	Complications	Comments
		Theoretical	Actual						
Abstinence	No intercourse	0%	0%	No	None	No		None	Can encourage See text
Combined OCP	Inhibits ovulation Alters cervical mucus and endometrium	0.1%		No	$15–25/mo	Yes	Some protection against PID	Side effects. SIDs (See text)	
Oral progestin		0.5%	5%		$200–300				
Intrauterine device	Probably prevents implantation	1.2%		No	$100–200	Yes	No	Bleeding, cramping, pain, expulsion, increased risk of PID, ectopic pregnancy	Not recommended for teenagers
Condom (female)	Barrier	5%	21%	Yes	$3 each	No	– +	Slippage	Expensive, difficult
Condom (male)	Barrier	3%	14%	Yes	$6–12/dozen	No	– +	Reaction to latex	Some dislike
Vaginal spermicides (foam, jelly, suppositories)	Spermicidal agent	6%	26%	Yes	$10–12/ container (18 uses)	No		Reaction to spermicide	Some describe as "messy" to use
Condom and foam	Barrier with spermicidal agent	2%	12%	Yes	See above	No	+ –	Reaction to latex or spermicide	Requires using two methods
Diaphragm with spermicide[3]	Barrier with spermicidal agent	3%	18%	Can be inserted up to 6 hours before intercourse	$30–40 + spermicide	Yes	+	Reaction to spermicide, pelvic discomfort, recurrent UTIs ↑ risk of toxic shock syndrome	Requires comfort with body

(continued)

Table 2-8. (Continued)

Method	Mechanism of action	Efficacy: Rate of Pregnancy 1st Year of Use[2]		Coital dependence	Cost	Prescription required	Protection from STD/HIV	Complications	Comments
		Theoretical	Actual						
Coitus interruptus	Withdrawal before ejaculation	4%	18%	Yes	None	No	No	None	Requires self-control Preejaculatory semen contains sperm
Cervical cap with spermicide[4]	Barrier with spermicidal agent	5%	18%	Can remain in place 2–3 days	$35–40 + spermicide	Yes	?	Recurrent UTI. ↑ risk of cervical dysplasia & toxic shock syndrome	Difficult to insert/remove
Periodic abstinence	During peak fertility Abstinence during times of peak fertility	6–10%	20%	No	None	No	No	None	Requires monitoring menstrual cycle
Chance	Chance	89%	89%	Yes	None	No	No	Pregnancy	Can intervene
Depo-medroxy-progesterone	Suppresses ovulation, thickens cervical mucus	<1%	<1%	No	$45/3 mo	Yes	No	(See text)	Requires every 3 month intramuscular injections; must comply with follow-up visits
L-norgestrel implant	Suppresses ovulation, thickens cervical mucus	<1%	<1%	No	$600 with insertion	Yes	No	(See text)	Requires surgical implantation/removal q 5 y
Emergency contraceptive pills	Suppresses ovulation/implantation	N/A	75%	No		Yes	No	Nausea, bleeding	Use within 72 h of intercourse

OCP = oral contraceptive pill; PIC = pelvic inflammatory disease; STD = sexually transmitted disease; UTI = urinary tract infection.

[1] In approximate order of decreasing theoretical efficacy.

[2] Adapted from Hatcher RA, et al, 1992 and Trusser G, et al, 1987; *theoretical efficacy* is defined as the best *estimate* of the accidental pregnancy rate during the first year of use among couples who initiated the use of a method (not necessarily for the first time) and who used it consistently and correctly; *actual efficacy* is defined as a measure of the accidental pregnancy rate during the first year among "typical couples" who initiated the use of a method (not necessarily for the first time) if they did not stop use for any other reason.

[3] Cost exclusive of clinician visit.

[4] Efficacy rates based on use of specific method *without* addition of a spermicide.

Table 2–9. Questions to Ask a Teen Who Wants Contraception

Tell me why you want to start contraception?
What methods have you used previously?
What methods are you using currently?
What methods do your friends use?
What problems have your friends had with those methods?
What have they liked about them?
What methods have you thought about?
What concerns do you have about these methods?
Does your partner know you are here for contraception?
What are your partner's feelings about contraception?
Does your mother know that you are sexually active?
Does she support your choice for contraception?
What questions do you have for me?

circumcised, then the foreskin should be pulled back; (3) condoms should be "burped," i.e., before unrolling the condom, air should be squeezed out of the reservoir tip; (4) after ejaculation, the penis must be withdrawn while still erect; and (5) the base of the condom should be held during withdrawal to prevent spillage or breakage. In the case of leakage, spillage, or breakage, a spermicide should be inserted into the vagina and/or emergency contraception should be employed (see Emergency Contraception, below).

The **diaphragm, contraceptive sponge, and cervical cap** afford independence for decision making by the female because they can be used without male knowledge. However, those methods require planning and forethought for effective use. If a teenager appears capable of using this type of method effectively, it should be encouraged. The diaphragm and cervical cap require fitting by a health professional, and the sponge is relatively expensive. As a result, these forms of contraception are not as popular or realistic for many teenagers.

Hormonal methods. Hormonal contraception can take the form of oral pills, injections, or implants. Currently, the combined oral contraceptive pill and progesterone injections are the most common choices for hormonal contraception among teenagers.

Combined oral contraceptive pills (OCPs) consist of estrogen and progestin components and therefore are referred to as "combined" pills, as distinct from the "minipill," which includes only a progestin component. The combined OCP is safe and effective. It has been extensively studied throughout the world and many countries dispense it over the counter.

Oral contraceptives prevent pregnancy primarily by suppression of ovulation through inhibition of FSH and LH, thereby mimicking pregnancy and preventing pituitary release of ovarian-stimulating hormones. They also alter the structure of the endometrium, thicken cervical mucus, affect sperm abilities, and hamper implantation. In the United States, all pills contain either ethinyl estradiol or mestranol as the estrogen component. Multiple progestins are used, including norethindrone, norethindrone acetate, ethinodiol diacetate, norgestrel, levonorgestrel, norethynodrel, and the "new" or "third-generation" progestins desogestrel, norgestimate, and gestodene.

Perfect use of the pill results in a failure rate of 0.1%. This means that 1 in 1000 women will become pregnant during the first year of use when used perfectly. Typical use results in a 5% failure rate. In other words, 1 in 20 women become pregnant on the pill within the first year of typical use.

Any missed pills or errors that result in an increase in the hormone-free interval decrease the pill's effectiveness. Therefore, missed pills during the first and third weeks of the pill pack are more likely to result in pregnancy than are missed pills in the middle of the active pill regimen.

In addition to the OCP being a safe way to prevent pregnancy, it offers many other benefits to teenagers: (1) menstrual advantages: decreased cramps, elimination of *Mittelschmerz* (midcycle pain due to ovulation), fewer bleeding days, and a 60% decrease in blood loss, so it can be prescribed for dysmennorhea, ovarian cysts, heavy periods, irregular periods, or anemia; (2) improvement in hirsutism due to higher sex hormone binding globulin levels and suppression of ovarian androgens; (3) acne improvement through the above mechanism and lowering of testosterone levels; and (4) once prescribed, it can be used as an emergency contraception after unprotected intercourse (see Emergency Contraception, below). The choice of a specific OCP may be guided by those additional clinical considerations.

Disadvantages for teenagers who use the OCP are: (1) it does not protect against sexually transmitted infections, so barrier protection must still be used; (2) it requires daily dosing that might be difficult for some teenagers; and (3) initial side effects such as nausea from the estrogen might prevent continued use. For most teens, the side effects associated with OCPs use are minimal or nonexistant. The most commonly reported adverse effects are nausea, weight gain (cyclic or persistent), acne, and breakthrough bleeding (Table 2–10). Nausea is infrequent with the use of low-dose estrogen pills. Weight gain, if present, is often cyclical owing to estrogen-induced water retention. However, the progestin component can enhance appetite, leading to a persistent weight gain. Breakthrough bleeding is generally a self-limited problem that resolves after several cycles of OCP use as the hormones exert a suppressive effect on endometrial proliferation. This problem can be minimized by consistent use and taking the pill at the same time each day. Common side effects can often be managed by changing to an OCP

Table 2–10. Hormonal Side Effects

Estrogenic effects
  Nausea
  Increased breast size (ductal and fatty tissue)
  Stimulation of breast neoplasia
  Cyclic weight gain due to fluid retention
  Leukorrhea
  Cervical erosion or ectopia
  Thromboembolic complications (pulmonary emboli,
    cerebrovascular accidents)
  Hepatocellular adenomas and cancer
  Increased cholesterol concentration in gallbladder bile
  Growth of leiomyomata
  Telangiectasia

Progestogenic effects (progestin and/or estrogen related)
  Breast tenderness
  Headaches
  Hypertension
  Myocardial infarction

Androgenic effects (caused by some progestins, minimized
  with new progestins)
  Increased appetite and weight gain
  Depression, fatigue, and tiredness
  Decreased libido and enjoyment of intercourse
  Acne, oily skin
  Increased breast size (alveolar tissue)
  Increased low-density lipoprotein cholesterol levels
  Decreased high-density lipoprotein cholesterol levels
  Diabetogenic effect
  Pruritus
  Decreased carbohydrate tolerance

Adapted with permission from Hatcher RA et al: *Contraceptive Technology*, 1994–1996, 17th ed. Irvington, 1998; p 419.

Table 2–11. Additional Clinical Considerations in Choosing an Oral Contraceptive Pill

To minimize nausea, breast tenderness, vascular headaches
    and estrogen-mediated side effects, prescribe
  Loestrin $1/20$ or a 30-mg pill such as
    Alesse
    Estrostep
    Levlen
    Loestrin, 1.5–30 mg
    Lo-Ovral
    Nordette

To minimize spotting and/or breakthrough bleeding, prescribe
  Lo-Ovral, Nordette, or Levlen
  Estrostep
  Desogen or Ortho-Cept
  Ortho-Cyclen or Ortho Tri-Cyclen

To minimize androgen effects such as acne, hirsutism, oily
  skin, sebaceous cysts, pilonidal cysts, or weight gain,
  prescribe
  Desogen, Ortho-Cept
  Ortho Tri-Cyclen
  Ortho-Cyclen
  Ovcon-35, Brevicon, or Modicon (norethindrone pills)
  Demulen-35 (ethnodiol diacetate pills)

To produce the most favorable lipid profile, prescribe
  Ortho-Cyclen or Ortho Tri-Cyclen
  Desogen or Ortho-Cept
  Ovcon-35, Brevicon, or Modicon (norethindrone pills)

Adapted with permission from Hatcher RA et al: *Contraceptive Technology*, 1994–1996, 16th ed. Irvington, 1994; p. 253.

whose hormonal make-up minimizes the unwanted effect (Table 2–11).

There are few contraindications for OCP use among generally healthy teenagers (Table 2–12). In the United States, pregnancy carries much higher health risks than using the OCP.

Progestin-only contraceptives (Depo-Provera, Norplant, and the minipill) are hormonal alternatives to the combined OCP. *Depo-Provera* is the most commonly used injectable contraceptive. It consists of one 150-mg intramuscular injection of depot medroxyprogesterone acetate (DMPA) given every 12 weeks. It is extremely effective, with a failure rate of only 0.3%, and has been shown to have appeal across ethnic, educational, and age categories.

DMPA has a mechanism of action similar to that of all progestin contraceptives that prevents pregnancy through some or all of the following effects: inhibition of ovulation, thickened and decreased cervical mucus, suppression of midcycle surges of LH and FSH, production of a thinned endometrium, reduction in fallopian tube cilia function, and decreased functioning of the corpus luteum.

Advantages of DMPA for teenagers are that it requires only one dose every 3 months, thereby eliminating daily therapy concerns with the OCP. It also has a long-lasting effect and might eliminate menses altogether after 6 months to 1 year of use. It has the same menstrual advantages as OCPs, with decreased cramping, pain, and bleeding.

A major disadvantage of this method of contraception for teenagers is weight gain. The average user gains 5.4 pounds over the first year of use, 8.1 pounds after 2 years, and 13.8 pounds after 4 years. Weight gain is thought to be secondary to appetite stimulation. Another disadvantage is menstrual irregularity, which is the most common reason for discontinuation among teenagers. Many experience more days of bleeding, with an unpredictable pattern of light bleeding. Amennorhea can be

Table 2–12. Precautions in the Provision of Combined Oral Contraceptives (OCs) to Adolescents and World Health Organization (WHO) Categories

Refrain from providing for women with the following diagnoses
WHO category #4
   Current or history of deep vein thrombosis or pulmonary embolism.
   Current or history of stroke or coronary artery disease.
   Structural heart disease complicated by pulmonary hypertension, atrial fibrillation, or history of subacute bacterial endocarditis.
   Diabetes with nephropathy, retinopathy, neuropathy, other vascular disease.
   Diabetes of more than 20 years duration.
   Breast cancer.
   Pregnancy.
   Lactation (< 6 weeks postpartum).
   Current or history of benign hepatic adenoma or liver cancer.
   Active viral hepatitis.
   Severe liver cirrhosis.
   Headaches, including migraine, with focal neurologic symptoms.
   Major surgery with prolonged immobilization.
   Hypertension of 160+/100+ or with vascular disease.

Exercise caution if OCs are used and monitor for adverse effects
WHO category #3
   Postpartum <21 days.
   Lactation (6 weeks to 6 months).
   Undiagnosed abnormal vaginal/uterine bleeding.
   Use of drugs that affect liver enzymes: rifampicin, rifabutin, griseofulvin; phenytoin, carbamazepine, barbiturates, topiramate and primidone.
   Current biliary tract disease.

Advantages generally outweigh theoretical or proven disadvantages and generally can be used without restriction
WHO category #2
   Severe headaches that start after initiation of OCs.
   Migraine headaches without focal neurological symptoms.

Diabetes mellitus, gestational diabetes or diabetes without vascular disease.
Major surgery without prolonged immobilization.
Sickle cell disease or sickle C disease.
Moderate blood pressure: 140–159/100–109.
Undiagnosed breast mass.
Cervical cancer awaiting treatment and cervical intraepithelial neoplasia.
Family history of hyperlipidemia.
Family history of death of a parent or sibling due to myocardial infarction before age 50.

Do not restrict use
WHO category #1
   Postpartum > 20 days or postabortion.
   Mild headaches.
   Irregular vaginal bleeding patterns and no anemia.
   Current, recent, or past history of pelvic inflammatory disease.
   Current or recent history of sexually transmitted infections.
   Vaginitis.
   HIV positive or AIDS.
   Family history of breast cancer, current benign breast disease.
   Cervical ectropion.
   Endometrial or ovarian cancer.
   Viral hepatitis carrier.
   Uterine fibroids.
   Past ectopic pregnancy.
   Obesity.
   Goiter, hypothyroidism, hyperthyroidism.
   Epilepsy.
   Current use of antibiotics.
   Iron deficiency anemia, severe dysmenorrhea.
   Tuberculosis, malaria, schistosomiasis.

Modified with permission from Hatcher RA, Guillebuud MA: The Pill: Combined Oral Contraceptives. *Contraceptive Technology*, 17th ed. Irvington, 1998; pp. 420–424.

seen as advantageous to some girls and worrisome to others and might be particularly advantageous for girls with developmental delay and hygiene problems.

Norplant is a subdermal implant of levonorgestrel capsules, which is released at a slow, steady rate and offers effective contraception for up to 5 years. The method is reversed by removal of the capsules. Implantable contraception is most popular among teenagers who already have had unplanned pregnancies and is generally not looked on as favorably as DMPA.

The greatest advantage of Norplant is that its typical and perfect user rates are the same, with a remarkably low 0.05% failure rate. Although currently out of favor with many in the United States, the effects on unwanted pregnancy are dramatic. For example, in Colorado, nearly 30% of teens covered by Medicaid in 1992 chose Norplant. The repeat birth rate for Medicaid-covered teens choosing the implant was 2.5% after 24 months, whereas the repeat birth rate for teens not using the implant was nearly 10 times higher at 22.1%.

The *minipill* is a progestin-only pill. It is less effective than combined OCPs. However, it is less confusing because all pills are the same color, and it is a good choice for lactating women and those who cannot tolerate estrogen. Inconsistent use leads to irregular bleeding, so the minipill usually is not a primary choice for the non–breast-feeding teenager.

Emergency contraception, or *postcoital* conception, refers to a method that a woman can use after coitus for prevention of pregnancy. The most commonly used option is use of a combined or progestin-only OCP regimen within 72 hours of unprotected intercourse. This is sometimes referred to as the *morning-after pill.* Several regimens have been shown to work (Table 2–13). Each regimen consists of two doses that are 12 hours apart. The best-tolerated regimen is currently marketed as "Plan B" and consists of two 0.75-mg doses of levonorgestrel. This regimen has no estrogen, so it does not have the associated nausea that interferes with use. It also requires fewer pills.

Emergency contraception reflects the nature of its one-time protection intention. It should be considered with the lapse of any contraceptive method, such as when a condom breaks or a cervical cap or diaphragm dislodges, and in cases of sexual assault. Some providers routinely prescribe emergency contraception for their sexually active patients for immediate availability, if needed. Others prefer to see patients who believe they are candidates for emergency contraception before its provision. It is estimated that in the United States emergency contraception use might prevent 1.7 million pregnancies per year and reduce the abortion rate by 40%.

SEXUALLY TRANSMITTED DISEASES

Adolescents who have had sexual intercourse have the highest STD rates of any age group. When rates are corrected for the percentage in the group who are sexually active, the youngest adolescents have the highest STD rates of any age group. Biologic, behavioral, and developmental factors act together to increase the likelihood of STD acquisition during adolescence.

At puberty, estrogen exposure causes the vaginal and cervical lining to thicken with layers of squamous epithelium. Persistence of cervical columnar epithelium in young women appears to significantly increase their vulnerability to STD. *Chlamydia trachomatis* infects columnar and not squamous epithelium. *Neisseria gonorrhoeae* attaches preferentially to columnar rather than to squamous tissue. Human papillomavirus preferentially attaches to the transition zone between cervical and squamous cell epithelia.

The usual adolescent behavior pattern of "serial monogamy," i.e., many short-term relationships in succession, also increase the risk for STDs. Among high school students in the United States, 16% report having had four or more sexual partners. Simply put, the younger age of sexual debut is associated with more sexual partners, which is an important determinant of STD risk.

Specific organisms. The three most common sexually transmitted diseases in the United States are genital human papillomavirus, herpes simplex, and *Chlamydia trachomatis.* These, in addition to *Neisseria gonorrhoeae,* are discussed in the following section. Specific STDs and their manifestations across the pediatric age spectrum are addressed in Chapter 9.

Genital human papillomavirus. Genital human papillomavirus (HPV) infection is the most common STD in the United States. As many as 20–40% of sexually active adults are infected with HPV, with about 1% of sexually active Americans having genital warts. Of the 100 HPV types identified, approximately 30 cause infection of genital mucosal sites. "High-risk" HPV types (HPV-16, -18, -31, -33, -35, -39, -45, -51, and -52)

Table 2–13. Emergency Contraception—Effective Regimens

Birth Control Pill	Dose[1] (Tablets)	Ethinyl estradiol (μg)	Levonorgestrel (mg)	Comments
Ovral	2	100	0.50	White pills
Lo-Ovral	4	120	0.60	White pills
Nordette	4	120	0.60	Light-orange pills
Levlen	4	120	0.60	Light-orange pills
Triphasil	4	120	0.50	Yellow pills
Trilevlen	4	120	0.50	Yellow pills
Alesse	5	100	0.50	No estradiol,
Levonorgestrel, 0.75-mg pill (Plan B)	1	0	0.75	marketed as Plan B
Ovrette (Levonorgestrel minipill)	10	0	0.75	No estradiol

[1] Two doses are given 12 h apart.

Because of the high prevalence of STDs in the adolescent population and the fact that many of the causative organisms are carried asymptomatically, all sexually active teenagers should be screened for gonorrhea and chlamydia (using culture or rapid molecular detection techniques) during routine, yearly, health examinations. If syphilis exists in the community, screening for this disorder also should be done. Consideration also should be given to testing for human immunodeficiency virus (HIV) based on the teen's risk factors. More frequent STD screening might be indicated if the adolescent is engaging in high-risk behavior, there has been a recent change in sexual partner, or there is a particularly high prevalence of disease in that community.

cause abnormal Pap smears (low- and high-grade squamous intraepithelial lesions) and are etiologically related to cervical, vulvar, anal, and penile cancers. "Low-risk" types of HPV (HPV-6, -11, -42, -43, and -44) cause genital warts, recurrent respiratory papillomatosis, and low-grade Pap-smear abnormalities (low-grade squamous intraepithelial lesions).

The natural history of HPV among women is an area of ongoing study. Prior research demonstrates that approximately 70% of adolescent and young women undergo HPV regression by 24 months after identification, with low-risk HPV significantly more likely than high-risk HPV to regress. Therefore, a more conservative approach to follow-up among teenagers with low-grade Pap-smear abnormalities currently is advocated in place of invasive procedures such as biopsy.

Genital herpes. Genital herpes is caused by the herpes simplex viruses (HSVs) and is one of the three most prevalent STDs in the United States. It is recurrent and incurable. Most cases of genital herpes are caused by HSV-2, although genital infection with HSV-1 is increasingly recognized. The seroprevalence of HSV-2 is rising in the United States and was 21.7% in 1991. Almost all HSV-2 infections are acquired between the ages 15 and 40 years. Among sexually active individuals, no STD, with the possible exception of HIV, causes more concern, as shown by the fact that the Centers for Disease Control and Prevention's National STD Hotline annually receives more calls regarding herpes than any other STD, almost as many as for all other STDs combined.

Many people infected with HSV-2 have asymptomatic or symptomatic but unrecognized disease. Clinical manifestations include the classic vesiculopustular lesions but also can include painless or painful ulcers, dysuria, perianal, scrotal, and vulvar fissures, urethral and vaginal discharge, or nonspecific vulvar irritation. Diagnosis is usually made clinically or by HSV culture or immunoassay.

More than 85% of people with HSV-2 antibodies but no lesions shed virus from the genital tract. Also, many that acquire infection subclinically subsequently develop clinical recurrences. Further, genital ulcer disease is a risk factor for sexual acquisition and transmission of HIV infection, and HSV is by far the most common cause of genital ulcer disease in the United States.

Treatment for genital herpes consists of systemic antiviral medications that help control the symptoms and signs of herpes. Their use, however, will not eradicate latent virus or change the risk, frequency, or severity of recurrences after the drug is discontinued. Acyclovir, valacyclovir, and famciclovir have been shown to provide clinical benefit. Treatment options differ according to medication chosen, goals of management, and whether or not treatment is for a first clinical episode, a recurrent episode, suppressive therapy, or a special situation such as treatment in a pregnant or immunocompromised individual.

Chlamydia trachomatis. *Chlamydia* is the most common bacterial STD. Adolescents are particularly at risk for this disease because age younger than 20 years is the most significant risk factor for contracting *Chlamydia* infection. It is implicated as a major cause of upper genital tract infection, or pelvic inflammatory disease (PID), and causes disease in the newborn (see Chapter 9). Other risk factors for acquisition are history of STDs, multiple sex partners, a new partner within the past 2 months, and use of nonbarrier or no contraception. In the United States, asymptomatic infection is common among men and women, and screening of sexually active adolescents with cultures or rapid molecular detection tests should be routine during annual examinations. When symptomatic, *Chlamydia* may present as mucopurulent cervicitis or superficial mucosal infection. Infections without evidence of upper tract involvement can be treated with a one-time dose of oral azithromycin (1 g) or 100 mg of oral docycycline twice a day for 7 days. Patients do not need to be retested for *Chlamydia* after completing treatment unless reinfection is suspected or symptoms persist. Patients must refer all sex partners in the past 60 days for evaluation, possible testing, and treatment.

Neisseria gonorrhoeae. *Neisseria gonorrhoeae* is a significant cause of STD in adolescents. On Gram stain these organisms appear as gram-negative intracellular diplococci. Sixty percent of cases occur in patients 15–24 years old. Clinical manifestations often are similar to those of *Chlamydia trachomatis* and they frequently occur together in the same individual. Like *Chlamydia,* gonorrhea infections often are asymptomatic and should be screened routinely for using culture or rapid detection techniques.

Symptomatic infections include cervicitis, urethritis, proctitis, pharyngitis, conjunctivitis, and Bartholinitis. Disseminated gonorrhea occurs in up to 1% of those with gonorrhea. Arthritis secondary to infection with gonorrhea is seen in up to 1–3% of infected individuals, usually within 1 month of exposure. These patients generally present with one of two disease patterns: arthritis–dermatitis or monoarticular septic arthritis. Treatment for uncomplicated infection of the cervix, urethra, and rectum include one 400-mg oral dose of cefixime, one 125-mg intramuscular dose of ceftriaxone, or one 500-mg dose of ciprofloxacin or other regimens. In addition, presumptive treatment for chlamydial infection is usually given. Pharyngitis tends to be more difficult to eradicate so ceftriaxone or ciprofloxacin is preferred. Disseminated gonococal infection usually is treated as an inpatient, with 1 g of ceftriaxone, intravenously or intramuscularly, every 24 hours. As with *Chlamydia*, all sex partners must be treated.

Pelvic inflammatory disease. *Pelvic inflammatory disease* refers to upper genital tract inflammation. It is a syndrome with a wide spectrum of presentation and disease and can include any combination of endometritis, salpingitis, tubo-ovarian abscess, and pelvic peritonitis. More than 1 million cases of PID occur in the United States each year; the rate is highest among sexually active teenagers and young adults. Age is an independent risk factor, with estimated rates to be 1 in 8 sexually active 15 year olds versus 1 in 80 sexually active 24 year olds. Amount of sexual activity, a history of prior STDs, not using barrier contraception, use of an intrauterine device, timing of menses and sexual activity, and increased cervical ectopy (as normally is present with adolescents) are risk factors for PID. Gonorrhea and *Chlamydia* are the etiologic agents implicated in most cases, but mixed infections are the rule, with many other organisms associated with PID.

The diagnostic criteria for PID are listed in Table 2–14. A definitive diagnosis can be made on laparoscopy, endometrial biopsy, transvaginal sonography, or other imaging study showing evidence of upper tract disease. These techniques are not readily available, however, so the diagnosis is based largely on clinical grounds, despite its imprecision. Empiric treatment is indicated in every sexually active young woman if all of the minimum criteria are present and no other cause for illness is identified. Additional criteria often are used by clinicians to support a diagnosis and enhance the specificity of the minimum criteria.

Because of the possibly catastrophic results such as ectopic pregnancy or future infertility if PID is missed, treatment regimens must provide empiric, broad-spectrum coverage of likely pathogens such as *N. gonorrhoeae, C. trachomatis,* gram-negative facultative bacteria, and streptococci. Most clinicians favor at least 24 hours of inpatient therapy in patients with tubo-ovarian abscesses, but decisions regarding hospitalization must be made on an indi-

Table 2–14. Criteria for Diagnosis of Pelvic Inflammatory Disease

Definitive criteria (one required for diagnosis)
Histopathologic evidence of endometritis on endometiral biopsy
Transvaginal sonography or other imaging modalities showing thickened fluid-filled tubes with or without pelvic free fluid or tubo-ovarian complex
Laparoscopic abnormalities consistent with pelvic inflammatory disease

Minimum criteria (three required for diagnosis)
Lower abdominal tenderness
Adnexal tenderness
Cervical motion tenderness

Additional criteria (not required but can enhance specificity of diagnosis)
Oral temperature >101°F (>38.3°C)
Abnormal cervical or vaginal discharge
Elevated erythrocyte sedimentation rate
Elevated C-reactive protein
Laboratory documentation of cervical infection with *Neisseria gonorrhoeae* or *Chlamydia trachomatis*

Adapted from Centers for Disease Control and Prevention: 1998 Guidelines for treatment of sexually transmitted diseases. *MMWR* 1998;47(No. RR-1):80.

vidual basis. Hospitalization always should be considered for teenagers because they are more likely to have difficulty following an outpatient regimen. In addition, hospitalization is recommended if a surgical diagnosis cannot be ruled out or the patient does not respond to oral antibiotics, has symptoms of severe illness, nausea and vomiting, and/or high fever, is diagnosed with a tubo-ovarian abscess, or is pregnant or immunodeficient.

Inpatient regimens for treatment may consist of 2 g of cefoxitin (or cefotetan) intravenously every 6 hours plus 100 mg of doxycycline, intravenously or orally, every 12 hours. Outpatient regimens may consist of 400 mg of ofloxacin orally twice a day for 14 days plus 500 mg of metronidazole orally twice a day for 14 days or 250 mg of ceftriaxone intramuscularly plus 100 mg of doxycycline orally twice a day for 14 days.

Some clinical sites use a PID score to monitor the patient's progress. This allows a number to be given to signs and symptoms and, although partly subjectively scored, provides a more objective assessment of improvement. All patients should show improvement within 3 days of starting therapy. If not, the diagnosis and treatment should be reexamined with further testing or surgery, as indicated. Sex partners of patients with PID should be examined and treated if they had sexual contact with the patient during the 60 days before onset of symptoms.

Reproductive Health Issues Unique to Females

BREAST MASSES

Discovery of a breast mass is a concern for a woman of any age. Thankfully, the incidence of breast cancer in the adolescent is very small, with 0–2% of all surgically treated breast masses in adolescents being malignant. Despite the very low risk of cancer, evaluation of a breast mass, found during routine examination or self-examination, should be complete. Most breast "lumps" evaluated in the office setting in adolescents are normal. Among breast masses that are referred and surgically removed, fibroadenoma (a benign neoplasm of mammary gland) accounts for about two-thirds of cases.

The patient's medical history should be investigated for known risk factors for breast disease. Those factors include radiation to the chest, previous breast disease, previous or current malignancy, and family history of breast disease and breast cancer. The current complaint must be investigated fully. The medical history should document size, consistency, mobility, duration, nipple discharge, and constitutional and associated symptoms.

Physical examination should include a complete breast examination, with careful attention to the presence of erythema or warmth (suggestive of mastitis or an abscess), nipple discharge (galactorrhea), size (measure), consistency, and mobility of the lesion. Diffuse thickening and lumps that might become tender and enlarged before menses characterize fibrocystic or proliferative changes. Fibrocystic changes are present clinically in 50% of women and microscopically in 90%. Physical findings tend to change each month, so simply following a mass with repeated examinations may aid in diagnosis and rule out other causes such as cysts or solid tumors.

In most cases, the diagnosis is evident after a history and physical examination. For example, an unremarkable history with cord-like thickening suggests fibrocystic changes, whereas tenderness and erythema are consistent with abscess or infection. If an apparently solid lesion is present, a reasonable approach is to follow the lesion through at least one full menstrual cycle. Seventy-seven percent of fibrocystic changes are expected to change during this time, and cystic lesions may partly or completely resolve. Alternatively, one may wish to perform adjunctive tests such as an ultrasound to help delineate between a solid and cystic mass. Mammography is not a sensitive examination in adolescents and thus not recommended. A persistent solid mass must be evaluated further. Some centers prefer a fine needle aspiration, whereas others prefer an excisional biopsy.

MENSTRUAL ISSUES

Menstrual issues are a major reason for clinical visits by young women. In this section, we discuss normal menses and problems with menstrual cycles from the points of view of too little bleeding (amenorrhea), too much bleeding (dysfunctional uterine bleeding), and too much pain (dysmenorrhea).

Normal menses. Menarche occurs in girls at an average age of 12.6 years, (±2 SD), with an age range of 11–15 years. Most teenagers are at SMR 4 at the time of menarche, about 25% are SMR 3, 10% are SMR 5, and fewer than 5% are SMR 2. Menarche occurs about 3 years after the start of the growth spurt, 2 years after thelarche, and 1 year after peak height velocity. A measurement of 17% body fat is necessary for menses to begin but a measurement of 22% appears necessary to maintain or restore menstruation once periods have started.

A menstrual cycle is the time from the beginning of one menstrual flow to the beginning of the next menstrual flow. Normal cycles usually last 28 ± 4 days (range of 21 to 35–40 days). A typical menstrual period lasts 3–7 days and causes an average blood loss of 35 mL (range = 25–70 mL). Characteristically, menstrual periods are irregular in the first 2 years after menarche, with only 70% of teenagers having ovulatory cycles 3 years after menarche.

The menstrual cycle can be divided into follicular, ovulatory, and luteal phases (Figure 2–5). The follicular phase usually lasts 14 days but is highly variable, with a range of 7–22 days. It ends with ovulation. In this phase, with stimulation from FSH, an ovarian follicle matures. Estradiol levels rise, leading to negative feedback on FSH and, initially, LH secretion from the pituitary. After a dip in LH, a positive feedback mechanism is employed and there is a rise in LH. During that time, the endometrium is regenerating (after having been sloughed off during the menstrual flow), increasing from 0.5 to 5.0 mm in depth with the development of endometrial glands. This phase is sometimes referred to as the *proliferative stage* because of endometrial growth.

Ovulation occurs after a rapid rise in LH secondary to the preovulatory estradiol surge. Final maturation of the follicle occurs with release of an oocyte. *Spinnbarkeit,* or stringiness of the cervical mucus, is seen 24 hours before the LH surge. Ovulation usually occurs 10–16 hours after the LH surge. Once the mature follicle releases an oocyte, it becomes a functioning corpus luteum.

The luteal phase begins with ovulation and ends with the menstrual flow. It is constant at 14 ± 2 days, the life span of the corpus luteum. The corpus luteum produces large amounts of progesterone and higher levels of estrogen. Secondary to progesterone, endometrial glands become coiled and secretory, with increasing vascularity. Thus, this phase sometimes is referred to as the *secretory phase.* If fertilization occurs, human chorionic gonadotropin protects the corpus luteum and keeps steroid hormone levels high to sustain pregnancy. Otherwise, levels of estrogen and progesterone diminish as the corpus luteum

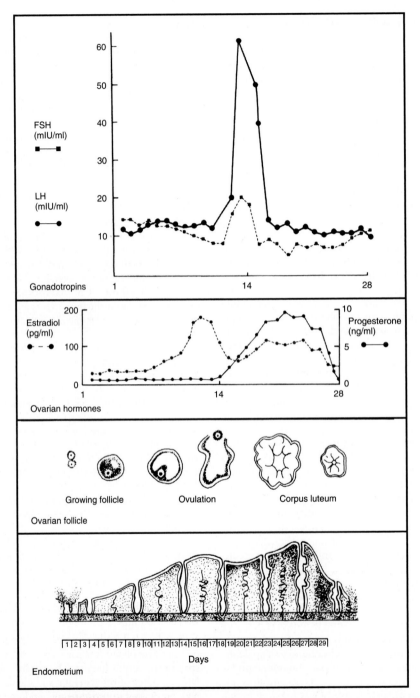

Figure 2–5. Physiology of the normal ovulatory menstrual cycle: gonadotropin secretion, ovarian hormone production, follicular maturation, and endometrial changes during one cycle. FSH = follicle-stimulating hormone; LH = luteinizing hormone. (From Laufer MR: The physiology of puberty. In: Emans SJ, Laufer MR, Goldstein DP [editors]. *Pediatric and Adolescent Gynecology,* 4th ed. Philadelphia: Lippincott Williams & Wilkins, 1998:121.)

involutes at the end of the luteal phase, which leads to endometrial and blood vessel necrosis and bleeding. Local prostaglandins then produce vasoconstriction and uterine contractions. Because of the decreased levels of estrogen and progesterone, LH and FSH are increased, and there is a repetition of the menstrual cycle.

Amenorrhea. Amenorrhea can be primary or secondary. *Primary amenorrhea* refers to never having had a menstrual cycle by the time when one is expected, based on age, sexual maturity, or clinical correlation. The chronologic cutoff is usually 15 or 16 years of age, which is 2 SD past the average age of menarche, or 4 years after the beginning of the development of secondary sex characteristics. Similarly, if no breast budding is present by age 14, it would be anticipated that no menses would occur by age 16, so evaluation for delayed puberty would be indicated. Causes of primary amenorrhea are sensibly thought of as conditions affecting any of the various physiologic sites involved in menstruation: the hypothalamus, pituitary, adrenal cortex, ovary, uterus, or vagina.

Conditions that affect the hypothalamus include stress, anorexia nervosa, obesity, Kallman's syndrome, or physiologic delay. Those who participate in intense athletics also have delayed menses and this is similarly believed to be hypothalamic in origin. Idiopathic hypopituitarism and pituitary tumors also cause primary amenorrhea. Adrenal issues such as congenital adrenal hypoplasia and adrenal tumors can lead to no menses, as can multiple ovarian problems such as Turner's syndrome and mosaic variants, polycystic ovary syndrome, gonadal dysgenesis, gonadal failure, and testicular feminization syndrome. Genital tract anomalies will lead to primary amenorrhea, primarily because of mechanical obstruction and rare entities such as uterine agenesis or Asherman's syndrome (postabortion synechiae) should not be overlooked. Similarly, imperforate hymen, vaginal septa, or Mayer-Rokitansky-Kuster syndrome (congenital absence of the vagina with normal ovaries and rudimentary uterus) can obstruct menstrual outflow and be associated with hematocolpos and cyclic abdominal pain. Any cause of poor nutrition, such as inflammatory bowel disease or malabsorption syndromes, can similarly delay menses.

Secondary amenorrhea is much more common than primary amenorrhea and defined as the absence of menses for at least the length of time of three previous cycles or 4–6 months after at least one prior episode of menstrual bleeding. The most common cause of secondary amenorrhea is pregnancy. Other causes of secondary amenorrhea can be hypothalamic in origin, resulting from a change in diet, weight gain or loss, stress, chronic illness, or increased exercise. Drug effects, including contraception, can change menstrual flow.

The clinical approach to amenorrhea, whether primary or secondary, should begin with a complete history, physical examination, and urine pregnancy test (Figure 2–6). The physical examination must include an evaluation for androgen excess (hirsutism, acne, and clitoromegaly), signs of systemic disease, malnutrition, stigmata of Turner's syndrome, SMR including a breast examination to rule out galactorrhea, and a pelvic examination if the teen is sexually active or her history and physical examination have not uncovered the cause. If specific abnormalities are suggested, such as a Turner's syndrome habitus or genital outflow tract obstruction, then a directed evaluation with specific studies should be performed. If the patient is not pregnant and has normal secondary sexual characteristics without evidence of chromosomal abnormality, then thyroid function tests and a prolactin test should be performed. Hyperprolactinemia requires an evaluation for a prolactinoma. If thyroid disease is found, further specific testing and therapy should follow. If thyroid studies and prolactin are normal, serum LH and FSH levels should be measured. High levels of LH and FSH suggest ovarian failure and should be followed with a karyotype and possibly antiovarian antibodies. An elevated LH:FSH ratio greater than 2.5:1 with androgen excess suggests polycystic ovarian disease. If levels of LH and FSH are normal or low, then a progestational challenge is indicated. Induction of menses should be attempted with the use of Provera, 10 mg by mouth once or twice a day for 5–10 days. If withdrawal bleeding occurs, anovulation with lack of progesterone effect likely was the cause of absent menses and might have been due to anovulatory cycles consistent with hypothalamic immaturity, as commonly occurs in early or middle adolescence, or chronic anovulation secondary to hypothalamic dysfunction, as discussed above. If no withdrawal bleeding occurs after progestational challenge, then an estradiol should be obtained. A normal estradiol suggests an end organ or outflow tract abnormality and specific end organ hormonal studies (free testosterone, androstenedione, Dehydroepiandrosterone (DHEA), Dehydroepiandrosterone Sulfate (DHEAS), 17-OH progesterone) and a pelvic ultrasound would be indicated. If estradiol concentration is low, then an estrogen- and progestin-induced cycle should be attempted. If there is no withdrawal bleeding, then end organ or outflow tract abnormality is most likely. However, if there is withdrawal bleeding, then a head computed tomogram or magnetic resonance imaging should be considered to rule out a central nervous system lesion. If normal, then hypothalamic dysfunction is the likely cause.

Dysfunctional uterine bleeding. Dysfunctional uterine bleeding (DUB), or primarily painless menstrual bleeding that is abnormally heavy or frequent in the absence of an underlying organic lesion, usually results from an anovulatory cycle. Occasionally, DUB can present emergently due to significant blood loss. It is, by definition, a diagnosis of exclusion. In teenagers, 90% of abnormal bleeding is

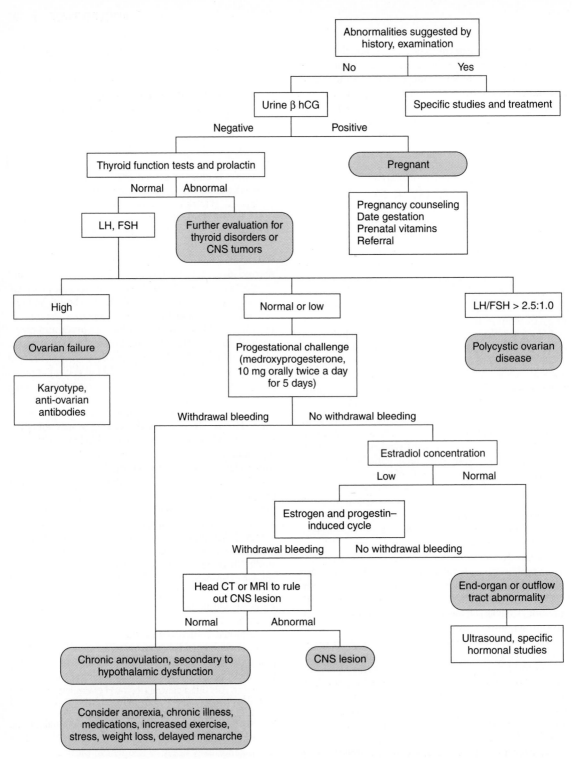

Figure 2–6. Diagnostic approach to amenorrhea. CNS = central nervous system; CT = computed tomography; FSH = follicle-stimulating hormone; hCG = human chorionic gonadotropin; LH = luteinizing hormone; MRI = magnetic resonance imaging; TSH = thyroid-stimulating hormone.

the result of anovulatory menstrual cycles, but in the remainder, an organic problem is present (Table 2–15). Most adolescent cases of anovulatory cycles are due to immaturity of the hypothalamic–pituitary–ovarian axis. As mentioned previously, 30–55% of teenagers may be anovulatory 2–4 years after menarche and as many as 20% may have anovulatory cycles 4–5 years after menarche. In general, the later menarche occurs during adolescence, the longer the time of anovulation.

Organic causes of abnormal vaginal bleeding in adolescence include complications of pregnancy, infection, local trauma or foreign body, systemic illness, or a medication effect. When a teenager presents with vaginal bleeding, pregnancy must be ruled out first. Ectopic pregnancy and threatened, incomplete, complete, or posttherapeutic abortion can present with bleeding. Ectopic pregnancy often will be diagnosed after finding a low level of β-human chorionic gonadotropin (β-hCG) or decreased doubling time (more than 2 days and no intrauterine pregnancy on ultrasound). β-Human chorionic gonadotropin levels of 1500 correspond to the detection of a gestational sac in the uterus by transvaginal ultrasound. If ectopic pregnancy is suspected, then immediate gynecologic consultation is indicated. A threatened abortion will present with bleeding and closed cervical os, without passage of tissue. After a therapeutic abortion, it is normal to have bleeding for 1–2 weeks, with low β-hCG levels.

Bleeding might be a sign of infection due to cervicitis, endometritis, salpingitis, or oophoritis. Pelvic examination showing a friable cervix, uterine, cervical motion, or adnexal tenderness suggests infection. Systemic illnesses leading to bleeding include blood dyscrasias, most commonly von Willebrand's disease; idiopathic thrombocytopenic purpura; platelet disorders; lupus; leukemia; renal or liver disease; and thyroid dysfunction. The chance of a bleeding disorder complicating DUB increases with the severity of the bleeding. Almost one in five patients who require hospitalization, one in four with a hemoglobin level below 10 g/dL on presentation, one of three who require transfusion, and one of two who present with severe abnormal bleeding at menarche have a coagulation disorder. Medications that affect menses include hormonal contraceptives, seizure medications, tranquilizers, anticoagulants, and antineoplastics.

Once pregnancy, infection, systemic disease, and medications have been ruled out, dysfunctional uterine bleeding due to anovulation can be ruled in. Anovulation leads to lack of a corpus luteum and therefore an "overestrogenized" endometrium that sloughs irregularly until the ovarian follicle finally involutes.

An algorithm for the evaluation and treatment of dysfunctional uterine bleeding is shown in Figure 2–7. Evaluation of the adolescent with vaginal bleeding should include a history looking for evidence of an organic etiology and a complete menstrual history. That history should

Table 2–15. Causes of Abnormal Uterine Bleeding in Adolescents

Dysfunctional uterine bleeding (anovulation)

Complications of pregnancy
    Ectopic or molar pregnancy
    Threatened or incomplete abortion
    Spontaneous abortion
    Placental polyp

Bleeding disorders
    von Willebrand disease
    Other hemophilias including factor VIII and IX deficiencies
    Thrombocytopenia—congenital or acquired (including idiopathic thrombocytopenic purpura)
    Platelet dysfunctions—congenital or acquired

Infections
    Endometritis
    Cervicitis
    Pelvic inflammatory disease

Endocrine disorders
    Hypothyroidism or hyperthyroidism
    Adrenal dysfunction (Addison or Cushing disease), congenital adrenal hyperplasia
    Polycystic ovary syndrome
    Hyperprolactinemia
    Premature ovarian failure

Local pathology
    Endometriosis
    Uterine polyp or myoma
    Trauma
    Foreign body
    Tumors—ovarian, uterine, vaginal
    Ovarian cysts

Systemic illnesses
    Systemic lupus erythematosus
    Inflammatory bowel disease
    Chronic renal failure
    Severe liver disease
    Malignancies

Medications
    Oral contraceptives
    Aspirin
    Anabolic steroids
    Others

From Neinstein LS: Menstrual problems in adolescents. Med Clin North Am 1990;74:1190; and Blythe M: Common menstrual problems: part 3: abnormal uterine bleeding. *Adolescent Health Update* 1992;4:2.

include dates of prior cycles, number of pads or tampons usually used and any difference in use with this episode, and where in the cycle the bleeding is occuring. A blood dyscrasia is more likely if bleeding occurs at the expected time of menses but is exceptionally heavy. However, bleeding beyond the normal cycle of 21–35 days is more consistent with anovulatory bleeding. A sexual history including previous STDs and contraception use is needed to assess risk of infection and pregnancy. Also, information about weight changes, exercise, stress, systemic illness, and any history of bleeding problems is helpful to rule out systemic illness. Dysfunctional uterine bleeding is usually painless, so a history of painful bleeding suggests other causes such as infection or complication of pregnancy.

The physical examination should include a breast examination to rule out galactorrhea, a general examination to rule out signs of systemic illness, and a pelvic examination to assess for gynecologic trauma or infection. An early adolescent who is within the first 1–2 years of menarche, is not sexually active by history, is experiencing painless

bleeding, has a negative pregnancy test, and has a nearly normal level of hemoglobin (above 11 g/dL) does not necessarily require a pelvic examination.

The laboratory examination should include a pregnancy test and a complete blood count to assess anemia. Further testing should be guided by the history and physical examination. Additional tests to consider are routine cultures for gonorrhea and chlamydia if a pelvic examination is performed, liver function, renal function, thyroid function, prothrombin time, partial thromboplastin time, von Willebrand factor, and other tests if indicated after the physical exam.

Much of the management and treatment of DUB will be dictated by the blood studies. With mild DUB, if this is a first episode and hemoglobin is normal, reassurance and education are adequate. Consideration of iron supplements is advised because, if the pattern continues, the teenager will be at risk for anemia. Follow-up 2 months after completion of a menstrual calendar is helpful to assess risk for future difficulty. Moderate DUB with

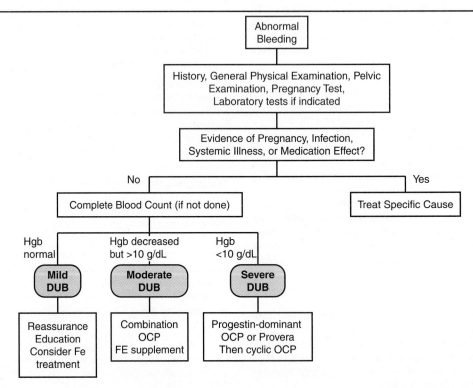

Figure 2–7. Simple algorithm for evaluation and treatment of dysfunctional uterine bleeding. Hospitalization should be considered for any patient with active bleeding, hemoglobin level below 7 mg/dL, or hemodynamic instability. Inpatient treatment might consist of intravenous Premarin with combined oral contraceptive pills and possibly nonsteroidal antiinflammatory drugs. DUB = dysfunctional uterine bleeding; Fe = iron; Hgb = hemoglobin; OCP = oral contraceptive pill.

some anemia but a stable hemoglobin above 10 g/dL can be treated with combined oral contraceptives. In addition, iron supplementation should begin. In severe DUB, the hemoglobin level is below 10 g/dL and there may be active bleeding. In that case, a regimen of progestin-dominant oral contraceptives is given, beginning with one pill four times per day for 4 days, one pill three times per day for 7 days, one pill twice a day for 7 days, and finishing with one pill daily for 7–14 days. After this regimen, cyclic oral contraceptives should be used for 3–6 months, with subsequent reassessment. Alternatively, one can give Provera, 10 mg/day, for 10–14 days.

In DUB requiring hospitalization, there is usually active bleeding, the patient is hemodynamically unstable, or the hemoglobin level is below 7 g/dL. In that case, inpatient therapy with intravenous Premarin and a combined OCP is effective. Nonsteroidal antiinflammatory drugs (NSAIDs) also have been shown to decrease menstrual blood loss in women with DUB and may be beneficial in mild, moderate, and severe cases.

Dysmenorrhea. Dysmenorrhea is the most common of all menstrual complaints, and its prevalence rises with age and sexual maturity (39% of 12 year olds, 72% of 17 year olds, 38% at SMR 3, and 66% at SMR 5). It is the greatest single cause of lost work and school hours in females. *Primary dysmenorrhea* is defined as pain with the menstrual flow without evidence of organic pelvic disease and accounts for 95% of all cases. *Secondary dysmenorrhea* is menstrual pain secondary to organic disease such as endometriosis or ovarian cysts.

Primary dysmenorrhea presents most commonly within 2 years of the onset of menses, between the ages of 14 and 16 years, peaks by age 18 years, and then decreases during the woman's 20s and 30s. The prostaglandin release that occurs after ovulation under the influence of progesterone is believed to be the primary cause for dysmenorrhea. Clinically, pain is described as crampy, spasmodic, and usually most severe in the lower abdomen, with radiation to the back and anterior thighs. About half of females will have associated systemic complaints such as nausea, vomiting, fatigue, diarrhea, headache, or backache.

In contrast to primary dysmenorrhea, secondary dysmenorrhea characteristically presents with onset of pain after age 20 years. It is important to obtain a full sexual history to rule out a sexually transmitted infection and a gastrointestinal and genitourinary history to identify referred pain from those systems. If the patient is sexually active, a pelvic examination is indicated to rule out sexually transmitted infection, pelvic inflammatory disease, endometriosis, cervical, outflow tract, or uterine anomalies, and the rare case of polyps or fibroids in the teenager. If the patient has never been sexually active, then a trial of medical therapy may be prescribed without a prior pelvic examination.

Anti-prostaglandin therapy is the mainstay of treatment for dysmenorrhea. Nonsteroidal antiinflammatory drugs are prostaglandin inhibitors and alleviate menstrual cramps and associated symptoms. Multiple NSAID regimens are effective; 400–600 mg of ibuprofen, three to four times per day, is a good place to start. If the patient requests contraception, cannot take NSAIDs due to allergy or poor response, or is at risk for pregnancy, then OCPs are a good choice. Because combined OCPs inhibit ovulation and therefore prostaglandin release, they are effective in more than 90% of cases.

Reproductive Health Issues Unique to the Male

GYNECOMASTIA

Gynecomastia is glandular enlargement of the male breast. Although usually physiologic, it might be a significant cause for concern and embarrassment to the male teenager. Estrogens strongly stimulate mammary growth and androgens weakly inhibit mammary growth. Gynecomastia signifies a transient or permanent disturbance in steroid hormone physiology that occurs when the male breast is exposed to a decreased androgen:estrogen ratio.

Between the ages 10 and 16 years, about 40% of boys develop transient gynecomastia, with a peak incidence of nearly 65% at age 14 years. It occurs as a result of increased aromatization of plasma androstenedione and testosterone to estrone and estradiol during puberty. Pubic hair development, pigmentation of the scrotum, and testicular enlargement are typically present for at least 6 months before the onset of breast enlargement, making most boys SMR 2 or 3 at diagnosis. Pubertal gynecomastia disappears spontaneously in about 75% of boys within 2 years and in 90% within 3 years.

Pubertal gynecomastia usually has glandular tissue smaller than 4 cm in diameter. The disk of subareolar glandular tissue feels like coiled rope. It is freely movable and nonadherent to underlying tissue. It should not be confused with lipomastia, where the soft subcutaneous fat sometimes makes obese boys look like they have breasts. Asymmetry in development, unilateral development, and tenderness are often seen. Glandular tissue larger than 5 cm in diameter is referred to as *macrogynecomastia*. It can be pubertal or pathologic but is unlikely to regress spontaneously.

Pathologic gynecomastia is breast enlargement that develops as a result of a drug side effect or an underlying disease. A myriad of drugs cause gynecomastia: hormones; psychoactive drugs; cardiovascular drugs; testosterone antagonists such as ketoconazole, spironolactone, and cimetidine; antituberculosis drugs; and nearly all street drugs and alcohol. Diseases that cause gynecomastia include endocrinopathies (e.g., hypogonadism, hyperthyroidism, and adrenal disorders), tumors (e.g., testicular, pituitary, adrenal, liver, or breast), and chronic diseases (e.g., liver disease, malnutrition, renal failure, and nervous system damage). Familial gynecomastia also has been reported.

Most healthy adolescents will require no laboratory work-up for gynecomastia. In those cases, glandular tissue is smaller than 4 cm in diameter and gynecomastia occurs after the onset of pubertal development. There is a negative drug, family, and medical history. Physical examination is normal, with SMR 2 or 3 genitals and an unremarkable testicular examination. Reassurance is all that is required because 90% of cases will resolve within 3 years. Indications for pathologic gynecomastia are onset in SMR 1 or 5, rapid development, or gynecomastia with other symptoms such as testicular enlargement, testicular mass, ascites, dyspnea, or signs of systemic illness. If pathologic gynecomastia is suspected, the underlying cause must be identified and treated. In either case, if the gynecomastia is larger than 4 cm in diameter, treatment should ensue because the condition is unlikely to resolve spontaneously, and boys with gynecomastia of that size have many more problems with regard to anxiety, stress, and other psychological morbidities that might precipitate additional problems. Medical treatments for gynecomastia are tamoxifen, which competes for estrogen binding sites on mammary tissue, testolactone, which inhibits aromatase activity, and surgery. Surgery remains the therapy of choice when breast tissue exceeds 6 cm or has been present for 4 years and has become firm from extensive fibrosis.

Anticipatory guidance regarding gynecomastia is important. Most boys will not complain of gynecomastia because of embarrassment. It is important to reassure the teenager with pubertal gynecomastia that it is not a sign of loss of masculinity (in fact, it is a direct result of increasing male hormones or increasing masculinity), that he is not turning into a girl, and that it is not due to masturbation (a concern of most boys this age).

TESTICULAR PROBLEMS: PAIN, MASSES, & SWELLING

Pain, swelling, and masses are the most common presentations of scrotal or testicular pathology in the adolescent. Teenagers may delay seeking care because of embarrassment, fear, or denial. A logical approach to the adolescent male with genital complaints is to differentiate the painful from painless masses.

Painless testicular masses

Hydrocele. A hydrocele is a scrotal fluid collection between the parietal and visceral layers of the tunica vaginalis. A hydrocele usually presents as a soft, painless, fluctuant, fluid-filled mass that is anterior to the testicle and transilluminates (Figure 2–8). It occurs in about 0.5–1% of males and can appear at any age. Most cases of hydrocele are primary and idiopathic, but the practitioner

must be suspicious of other processes such as orchitis, epididymitis, or testicular tumor. If the hydrocele prevents adequate palpation of the testis, an ultrasound should be performed to define the testicle, differentiate a hydrocele from an inguinal hernia, and rule out a testicular tumor, which appears as a heterogeneous mass sonographically. If a hydrocele is tense, painful, or associated with a hernia (communicating hydrocele), surgical intervention is advised. Otherwise, no treatment is necessary because the hydrocele likely will resolve spontaneously.

Spermatocele. A spermatocele is a retention cyst of the epididymis and has an incidence of much less than 1%. Microscopic examination of aspirated contents shows spermatozoa, usually dead. Grossly, the fluid is thin, white, and cloudy. The etiology of a spermatocele is not known. Usually, a spermatocele is located at the head of the epididymis, posterior and superior to the testis, and presents as a small, freely movable, painless, transilluminating cystic mass (Figure 2–8). Most spermatoceles are smaller than 1 cm in diameter and usually found by the physician during routine examination. However, if the spermatocele is large enough, the patient may present with

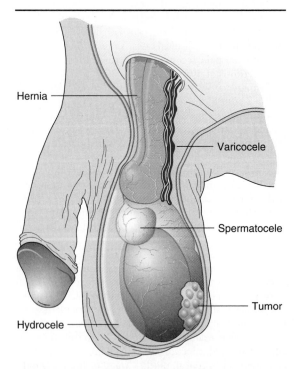

Figure 2–8. Testicular masses. (Reproduced from Adelman WP, Joffe A: adolescent male genital examination: What's normal and What's not. *Contemp Pediatr* 1999; 16(7):76.)

the complaint of a "third testicle." In the case of a large spermatocele, turbidity from increased spermatozoa may prevent transillumination. A spermatocele can be differentiated from a hydrocele in that the hydrocele covers the entire anterior surface of the testicle, whereas the spermatocele is firm and palpable separate from, and superior to, the testicle. On ultrasound examination, a spermatocele appears as an echo-free collection posterior and superior to the epididymis. The spermatocele should be palpable separate from the testis, thereby ruling out testicular tumor. Discovery of a spermatocele requires no therapy unless it is large enough to annoy the patient, in which case referral to an urologist for excision is advised.

Hernia. A hernia is a sac-like protrusion of intestine through the inguinal ring into the scrotum (Figure 2–8). The incidence is 1% or less in teenage boys and can appear at any age. A hernia may resemble a hydrocele but can be distinguished by a number of features. A hernia reduces when the patient is in the supine position, will not descend with traction on the testicle, and may be associated with bowel sounds in the scrotum. The examiner can locate the top of a hydrocele within the scrotum but cannot do so with a hernia. Hernias and hydroceles can coexist. Treatment of a hernia is surgical correction.

Varicocele. Varicoceles are the most common scrotal masses among teenagers, but their treatment remains controversial. Varicoceles are elongated, dilated, tortuous veins of the pampiniform plexus within the spermatic cord (Figure 2–8). Among 10–25 year olds, the incidence varies from 9 to 25.8%. Approximately 15% of adult males have varicoceles. Most cases of varicocele are asymptomatic and therefore discovered on routine physical examination. Occasionally, they might be associated with discomfort such as an ache or a "dragging" sensation. The characteristic physical finding is the palpation of a mass in the spermatic cord, with the sensation of a "bag of worms" that is more prominent in the upright than in the supine position. A varicocele occurs most often on the left side (85–95% of cases), presumably as a consequence of retrograde blood flow from the left renal vein, but it can be bilateral or, less commonly, occur on the right side.

If a varicocele is found, the patient should be examined in the supine position. Doing so can confirm the diagnosis, because varicoceles tend to shrink when the patient is supine. In contrast, a thickened cord due to a lipoma will not change with position. If a varicocele is present, the sizes of both testes should be compared (volume). Current recommendations for varicocele repair are based on abnormalities in testicular volume. Patients with large, symptomatic, or right-sided varicoceles should be referred to a urologist, as should those with testicles not growing as puberty progresses or a difference in testicular volume that is greater than 2 mL.

Testis tumor. Testicular cancer, predominantly of germ cell origin (95%), is the most common cancer in young men between the ages of 15 and 34 years. It accounts for 3% of all cancer deaths in that age group and affects approximately 1 in 10,000 teens. A testicular tumor most commonly presents as a circumscribed, nontender area of induration within the testis itself that does not transilluminate. Bilateral tumors occur in 2–4 % of patients. The patient discovers the tumor in the majority of cases. Patients can present with a sensation of fullness or heaviness of the scrotum. Often there is a history of recent trauma, which draws attention to preexisting pathology in the scrotum. Testicular pain can be a presenting symptom in 18–46% of patients with germ cell tumors. Acute pain might be associated with torsion of the neoplasm, infarction, or bleeding into the tumor. Of particular note in the sexually active adolescent, signs and symptoms indistinguishable from those of acute epididymitis have been observed in up to one-fourth of patients with testicular neoplasms. Less common presentations include gynecomastia secondary to hCG-secreting tumors and back or flank pain from metastatic disease. In most cases of testicular tumor, the epididymis and cord feel normal. When the tumor is more advanced, the testis might be diffusely enlarged and rock hard. Secondary hydroceles can occur. Twenty-five percent of patients with seminoma and 60–70% of those with a nonseminomatous germ cell tumor have metastatic disease at the time of presentation. Because a delay in diagnosis can negatively affect prognosis, the clinician must have a high index of suspicion for this entity. Any of the following symptoms should prompt examination of the testis: back or abdominal pain, unexplained weight loss, dyspnea (pulmonary metastases), gynecomastia, supraclavicular adenopathy, urinary obstruction, or a "heavy" or "dragging" sensation in the groin. Initial evaluation of a testicular mass is ultrasonography, a sensitive and specific test that can discriminate between a testicular neoplasm and nonmalignant processes included in the differential diagnosis. Even if an obvious mass is palpated on physical examination, an ultrasound should be performed on both testicles to rule out bilateral disease. Once a tumor is suspected, further evaluation should be performed in consultation with an oncologist.

Because diagnosis of testicular tumors might be delayed significantly if not noticed by the patient, some researchers advocate testicular self-examination as a simple, potentially life-saving intervention. Prior studies have shown that nearly 90% of young adults are not aware of their risk for testicular cancer and that fewer than 10% of at-risk males have been taught testicular self-examination. However, no data currently exist showing that testicular self-examination reduces morbidity or mortality from testicular cancer, and its universal application remains controversial.

Painful testicular masses & swelling. The painful or acutely swollen scrotum is a potential emergency that requires accurate and timely evaluation.

Testicular torsion. Testicular torsion is a twisting of the testis and spermatic cord that results in venous obstruction, progressive edema, arterial compromise, and, eventually, testicular infarction. It is a surgical emergency. A delay in diagnosis of only 4–6 hours can result in abnormal testicular function and a delay of more than 6 hours often leads to testicular infarction. Testicular torsion is the most common cause of testicular loss in young males. The risk of developing testicular torsion by age 25 years is estimated to be about 1 in 160. It can occur at any age, but two-thirds of cases occur in boys between the ages of 12 and 18 years, with a peak at 15–16 years.

The "bell-clapper" deformity predisposes an individual to testicular torsion and refers to the anatomic appearance of the testis within an abnormally enlarged and engulfing tunica vaginalis, like a clapper in a bell. It generally occurs bilaterally. The bell-clapper deformity often is associated with horizontal orientation ("horizonatal lie" or "transverse lie") of the testicle, causing it to be more mobile and therefore more susceptible to torsion.

The history for testicular torsion consists of the sudden onset of pain and swelling in one testicle, often while the young man is sleeping or otherwise inactive. One-third to one-half of patients might relate previous episodes of such pain, presumably secondary to spontaneous resolution of prior episodes of torsion. Pain may be referred to the abdomen, back, flank, groin, or thigh, so all boys with such complaints deserve careful genital exami-

nations. Nausea and vomiting commonly occur. If testicular torsion is suspected, a urologist should be consulted immediately.

Examination of a standing patient usually shows an elevated, tender testis on the side of the torsion. In some cases, the testis appears to be horizontal. Early in torsion, the epididymis might be felt anteriorly and high in the scrotum. If presentation is delayed, the entire gonad can become so swollen that the epididymis cannot be distinguished from the testis on palpation.

Testicular torsion is often difficult to differentiate from epididymitis (Table 2–16). Alleviation of testicular pain by elevating the testis above the pubic symphysis suggests possible epididymitis (Prehn's sign). Failure to lessen pain with elevation of the testis suggests torsion. An absent cremasteric reflex is the most sensitive physical finding for diagnosing testicular torsion. Contraction of the cremaster muscle can be produced by lightly scratching the skin in the area supplied by the ilioinguinal nerve (the medial aspect of the superior part of the thigh). This results in reflex retraction of the ipsilateral testicle. In the case of intravaginal torsion, the cremaster muscle is prohibited from effectively contracting. Therefore, patients presenting with tender testicles and without cremasteric reflexes are much more likely to have testicular torsion than epididymitis or torsion of the appendix testis. Conversely, the presence of a cremasteric reflex almost always allows the physician to rule out testicular torsion. The presence of urinary symptoms is uncommon in testicular torsion. Signs and symptoms such as low-grade fever, elevated white blood cell count, Prehn's sign, a history of

Table 2–16. Differentiating Features Between Testicular Torsion and Epididymitis

Symptoms and Other Findings	Torsion	Epididymitis
Cremasteric reflex	Usually absent	Usually present
Epididymal abnormality	Obscured or anterior	Palpable and tender
Pain		
Onset	Sudden/abrupt	Hours to days
Prior episodes	50% of cases	Usually not
Position of affected testis	Long axis horizontal Elevated in scrotum	Normal
Prehn sign	Absent: No relief of or increase in pain with elevation of scrotum	Present: Pain relief with elevation of scrotum
Urethral symptoms	Absent	May have dysuria, discharge
Urethral Gram stain	Negative	May be positive for gram-negative intracellular diplococci or white cells
Urinalysis	Usually negative	First-catch urine is positive for white blood cells and/or leukocyte esterase activity

Reproduced from Adelman WP, Joffe A: The adolescent with a painful scrotum. *Contemp Pediatr* 2000;17:115.

pain, elevation of the testicle, and abnormal lie of the testicles may be present in 21–50% of torsion cases. Individually, none of these signs or symptoms is sufficiently sensitive or specific to confirm or exclude the diagnosis of testicular torsion.

If a reasonable suspicion for torsion exists, the primary therapy should be surgical exploration, without delaying to order diagnostic tests. To ensure a timely evaluation, it is imperative that the urologist is involved in the care of the patient from the time of presentation. In consultation with a urologist, diagnostic imaging such as nuclear scintigraphy or color Doppler ultrasonography might be indicated. Surgical exploration remains the best diagnostic tool and is necessary to salvage the testis. If the testis is viable, bilateral orchiopexy is performed to prevent recurrence. Infarcted testes are removed.

Torsion of the appendix testis or appendix epididymis. In contrast to testicular torsion, torsion of the appendix testis or appendix epididymis has a much better prognosis and rarely results in significant sequelae. The incidence of torsion of an appendage peaks between 10 and 14 years of age. The right and left sides are affected equally.

Most commonly, an early adolescent will present with subacute onset of scrotal pain. The pain is usually much less intense than that of a torsed testicle. Early in its natural history, pain is localized to the area of the torsed appendage and a small tender mass can be palpated at its anatomic location. A "blue dot" representing a gangrenous appendix might be seen; it is seen best when the scrotal skin is stretched taught or with transillumination. As the torsion progresses, most patients develop reactive hydroceles and significant edema and erythema, making the examination difficult. White blood cell count and urinalysis are unremarkable. Further studies rarely are required. A torsed appendage often can be left alone to autoamputate. Supportive treatment with analgesics and bed rest is recommended, and pain usually subsides in a few days. Some urologists advocate surgical removal.

Epididymitis. *Epididymitis* refers to inflammation of the epididymis secondary to infection or trauma. It is primarily a problem of sexually active adolescents. Epididymitis is uncommon in prepubertal children and, when present, often is associated with underlying genitourinary anomalies. The urethritis that precedes epididymitis may be asymptomatic. Among males younger than 35, epididymitis is most often caused by *C. trachomatis* or *N. gonorrhoeae*. *Escherichia coli* is a causative agent among men who engage in insertive anal intercourse.

A sexually active middle or late adolescent characteristically presents with the subacute onset of pain in the hemiscrotum, inguinal area, or abdomen (Table 2–16).

Approximately two-thirds of individuals present after 24 hours of pain, which tends to be later than in those who present with testicular torsion. Some will have a history of dysuria or urethral discharge, but these symptoms might be so mild that the patient will not mention them.

Typically, there will be unilateral testicular pain and tenderness on examination. Early on, the affected epididymis alone is tender, swollen, and thickened. Later, swelling of the scrotum, testis, and spermatic cord or a reactive hydrocele might obscure the diagnosis. The scrotal skin becomes erythematous and edematous. Few patients are febrile, but fever is present more often in epididymitis than in torsion. Dysuria and urethral discharge may or may not be present. The affected testis is lower than the contralateral testis and its lie is normal. Elevation of the testicle might relieve pain (Prehn's sign). The cremasteric reflex is usually present. If the swollen epididymis cannot be differentiated clearly from the testicle or if the examination is obscured due to reactive edema and inflammation, immediate urologic consultation and evaluation to rule out testicular torsion is mandated.

Examination of a first void (first 15 mL) of urine for leukocytes and Gram stain and culture of uncentrifuged urine might help identify an infectious etiology. A Gram stain of urethral exudate or an intraurethral swab is recommended for diagnosis of urethritis. A presumptive diagnosis of gonococcal infection can be made if gram-negative intracellular diplococci are found. A culture (urethral exudate or the urethral swab specimen) or nucleic acid amplification test (urethral swab material or urine) should be performed for *C. trachomatis* and *N. gonorrhoeae*. Because epididymitis is an STD, syphilis serology and HIV counseling and testing are also recommended.

Empiric therapy is indicated in all cases of epididymitis. The Centers for Disease Control Sexually Transmitted Disease Treatment Guidelines recommends a single intramuscular injection of 250 mg of ceftriaxone plus 100 mg of doxycycline orally twice a day for 10 days. If suspicion exists for epididymitis caused by enteric organisms or the patient is allergic to cephalosporins or tetracyclines, 300 mg of ofloxacin orally twice a day for 10 days is the recommended regimen. In severe cases or with unreliable follow-up, hospitalization may be required. Supportive care with bed rest, NSAIDs, scrotal support, and ice packs also may be beneficial. Patients should be instructed to refer all sex partners from the prior 60 days for evaluation and treatment. Further sexual intercourse should be avoided until they and their sex partners have completed therapy and no longer have symptoms. Patients should begin to improve within 24–48 hours of starting therapy. Failure to improve within 2 days requires reevaluation of the diagnosis and therapy.

Orchitis. Many viruses and bacteria can cause orchitis (inflammation of the testicle) or epididymo-orchitis (inflammation of the testicle and epididymis). The most common cause of infectious orchitis in the adolescent is mumps: Up to 40% of postpubertal males infected with the mumps virus develop orchitis. Similarly, approximately 40% of all cases of mumps orchitis occur in teenagers. Mumps orchitis remains a problem in the United States among underimmunized adolescents. Therefore, this diagnosis should be considered in any adolescent with testicular pain who has not received two doses of the measles, mumps, and rubella vaccine. Its incidence peaks in mid to late adolescence and early adulthood (15–29 years old).

OTHER ADOLESCENT HEALTH ISSUES

Sports Medicine

PRE-PARTICIPATION SPORTS SCREENING

Sports participation can be valuable to the adolescent as a way to enhance fitness and coordination, self-esteem, and social interaction. The objectives of a preparticipation physical evaluation are primarily to detect conditions that might predispose to injury, be life-threatening or disabling, and meet legal and insurance requirements for sports participation. Secondary objectives include the opportunity to determine the general health of a youngster who might not otherwise present to a physician (78% of athletes have no periodic health examination other than the preparticipation physical), counsel on health related issues, and assess the fitness level of an individual for a specific sport. Optimally, the examination should be performed by qualified health care providers at least 6 weeks before the start of preseason practice to identify, correct, and/or rehabilitate identified problems. The two most common settings for performing the preparticipation sports assessment are in the physician's office and a station-based screening environment. Important questions to ask the teen are listed in Table 2–17. Growth parameters and blood pressure should be measured. A complete physical examination is performed, with an emphasis on the cardiopulmonary and musculoskeletal systems and any relevant issues identified by medical history. The teenager's immunization status also should be documented.

SPORTS INJURIES

Each year in the United States, approximately 3 million injuries (defined as time lost from the sport) occur during sports participation among children and adolescents. The preparticipation physical examination provides an opportunity to review, diagnose, and rehabilitate old musculoskeletal injuries. It is also a time to examine the role that the sport plays in the youngster's life. Psychological injury secondary to sports participation should not be overlooked.

Musculoskeletal sprain and strain are by far the most common sports injuries. Most musculoskeletal injuries seen in the office are nonemergent sprains, strains and contusions. Rarely, these also might be associated with more serious complications such as vascular insufficiency or nerve damage. Indications for immediate consultation with an orthopedic specialist are vascular compromise, nerve compromise, deep laceration over a joint, a dislocation that does not reduce, a complete tear of a muscle–tendon unit, or an angulated, displaced, or open fracture. Few adolescent specialists or pediatricians deal with the acute or emergent phase of injuries. However, most providers need to have a thorough understanding of the four phases of rehabilitation for musculoskeletal injuries: (1) limiting additional injury and controlling pain and swelling, (2) improving strength and flexibility of the injured structures (improving range of motion), (3) progressively improving abilities (strength, flexibility, proprioception, and endurance) until near-normal function is obtained, and (4) returning to exercise and sports without symptoms.

An easy way to remember how to achieve phase 1 rehabilitation is through the mnemonic RICE, which stands for Rest, Ice, Compression, and Elevation. Relative rest, meaning limitation of all painful activity while allowing activity that is pain free, for the first 24 hours after injury is crucial to limit further injury and speed the recovery process. For example, after an ankle sprain, if bearing weight cannot be accomplished without pain, then crutches are indicated until weight bearing is pain free. Ice helps to control pain and decrease swelling after an injury. Ice should be placed in a plastic bag and applied directly to the area of injury for 20 minutes. For the first 48 hours, this can be done three to four times per day and then continued daily as long as pain or swelling persists. Crushed ice allows conformity to joint surfaces. Icing for more than 20 minutes at a time is not recommended because of possible peripheral nerve injury. Compression, usually in the form of an elastic bandage, should be tight enough to promote reabsorption of edema at the injury site yet allow venous return distal to the compression. It also serves as a reminder to the patient against overexertion in this area. Elevation limits swelling. Clear and specific instructions should be given. Elevating the leg as much as possible is recommended during the day and especially at the end of the day, after maximal swelling is likely to occur.

In addition to RICE therapy, analgesia is very important, especially in the short term, to prevent guarding, disuse, and resultant inflexibility, atrophy, and loss of endurance. Nonsteroidal antiinflammatory medications can decrease inflammation and pain. Analgesia should continue for 7–10 days.

Phases 2 and 3 of rehabilitation are best performed under the supervision of a physical therapist or athletic

Table 2–17. Important Health Questions in the Sports Preparticipation Evaluation

1. Have you had a medical illness or injury since your last checkup or sports physical?
   Do you have an ongoing or chronic illness?
2. Have you ever been hospitalized overnight?
   Have you ever had surgery?
3. Are you currently taking any prescription or nonprescription (over-the-counter) medications or pills or using an inhaler?
   Have you ever taken any supplements or vitamins to help you gain or lose weight or improve your performance?
4. Do you have any allergies (e.g., to pollen, medicine, food, or stinging insects)?
   Have you ever had a rash or hives develop during or after exercise?
5. Have you ever passed out during or after exercise?
   Have you ever been dizzy during or after exercise?
   Have you ever had chest pain during or after exercise?
   Do you get tired more quickly than your friends do during exercise?
   Have you ever had racing of your heart or skipped heartbeats?
   Have you had high blood pressure or high cholesterol?
   Have you ever been told you have a heart murmur?
   Has any family member or relative died of heart problems or of sudden death before age 50?
   Have you had a severe viral infection (for example, myocarditis or mononucleosis) within the last month?
   Has a physician ever denied or restricted your participation in sports for any heart problems?
6. Do you have any current skin problems (e.g., itching, rashes, acne, warts, fungus, or blisters)?
7. Have you ever had a head injury or concussion?
   Have you ever been knocked out, become unconscious, or lost your memory?
   Have you ever had a seizure?
   Do you have frequent or severe headaches?
   Have you ever had numbness or tingling in your arms, hands, legs, or feet?
   Have you ever had a stinger, burner, or pinched nerve?
8. Have you ever become ill from exercising in the heat?
9. Do you cough, wheeze, or have trouble breathing during or after activity?
   Do you have asthma?
   Do you have seasonal allergies that require medical treatment?
10. Do you use any special protective or corrective equipment or devices that aren't usually used for your sport or position (e.g., special neck roll, foot orthotics, retainer on your teeth, hearing aid)?
11. Have you had any problems with your eyes or vision?
    Do you wear glasses, contacts, or protective eyewear?
12. Have you ever had a sprain, strain, or swelling after injury?
    Have you broken or fractured any bones or dislocated any joints?
    Have you had any other problems with pain or swelling in muscles, tendons, bones, or joints?
13. Do you want to weigh more or less than you do now?
    Do you lose weight regularly to meet weight requirements for your sport?
14. Do you feel stressed out?
15. Record the dates of your most recent immunizations (shots) for: tetanus, hepatitis B, measles, chickenpox

Females only

16. When was your first menstrual period?
    When was your most recent menstrual period?
    How much time do you usually have from the start of one period to the start of another?
    How many periods have you had in the last year?
    What was the longest time between periods in the last year?

Reproduced from American Academy of Pediatrics, American Academy of Family Physicians, American Medical Society for Sports Medicine, American Orthopaedic Society for Sports Medicine, American Osteopathic Academy of Sports Medicine: *Preparticipation Physical Evaluation*, 2nd ed. 1997.

trainer. Improvement of strength and flexibility often is achieved first with isometric exercises; as pain-free mobility is achieved, improved strength, flexibility, endurance, and stability can be achieved. Once flexibility, strength, and proprioception return, a stepwise return to athletics is indicated. Phase 4 rehabilitation allows for gradual return to full athletic activity. For example, a pitcher with a shoulder injury should return to the team once phase 3 has been completed. However, he should start with lighter pitching at practice, with increased rest, and gradual return to full strength over 7–14 days. In general, ensuring that injuries are properly rehabilitated before return to practice and play will improve overall sports health and prevent reinjury.

Acne

Acne is so prevalent during adolescence that many providers forget to ask the teenager about it, despite the significant emotional discomfort the disease often causes. Studies show that 80–90% of all individuals will develop acne between ages 10 and 20 years. Acne is the most common reason for dermatology visits by adolescents and as many as 75% of acne sufferers are embarrassed by it, with over half feeling socially inhibited.

The lesions of acne develop in the sebaceous follicle, which consists of multilobulated sebaceous glands. Under the influence of androgens during puberty, the sebaceous glands enlarge and discharge oily sebum. Excessive sebum production, bacteria, obstruction of the pilosebaceous canal, androgen effect, and genetic predisposition have been implicated in the pathogenesis of acne. Chocolate, fried foods, nuts, other junk foods, sexual activity, and masturbation have never been shown to influence acne, although acne exacerbation is associated with increased stress.

There are four basic types of acne lesions: open and closed comedones, papules, pustules, and nodulocystic lesions. These lesions can appear alone or in combination. Open comedones, or blackheads, are 2–5-mm papules with dark centers caused by oxidation of lipids and melanin. The orifice is open, so open comedones usually do not progress to inflammatory lesions. Closed comedones, or whiteheads, are 1–3-mm, flesh-colored papules with pinpoint openings. They are precursors to inflammatory acne lesions. The sebaceous follicle is obstructed just beneath the surface of the skin at the follicular opening, resulting in cystic swelling of the follicular duct. On the surface of the skin, a pustule often forms. These pus-filled inflammatory lesions usually will resolve over the course of a few days without scarring. Papules are raised, solid lesions that represent deeper inflammatory reactions. They take longer to heal and can be associated with scarring. The most severe form of this disease is nodulocystic acne. Lesions are tender and firm and represent abscesses within the dermis that may extend to the intradermal fat. They are associated with significant scarring.

The goals of treatment are improvement of appearance and prevention of scarring. Most cases respond to topical treatment, and multiple modes of therapy have been shown to be effective. One classification system and suggested treatment plan is presented in Table 2–18. When using topical agents, the most common side effect and patient complaint is skin erythema with scaling. Therefore, it is beneficial to recommend initial use of topical benzoyl peroxide, retinoic acid, or other topical treatments on an every-other-day basis for the first 2 weeks. It also is suggested that therapy be applied in the evening to prevent unwanted side effects from showing prominently during the school hours.

Systemic antibiotics are effective for acne that is unresponsive to topical therapy and for treatment of significant acne on the chest and back. Tetracycline and erythromycin are inexpensive and inhibit growth of *P. acnes*. Minocycline, a second-generation tetracycline, achieves a high intrafollicular concentration and is effective longer than tetracycline. Its disadvantages are its relatively high cost and rare idiosyncratic reactions. Combined OCPs

Table 2–18. Classification and Treatment of Acne

Grade I (comedones)
  Benzoyl peroxide 2.5–5% gel at bedtime *or*
  Retin-A 0.025–0.05% cream at bedtime

Grade II (comedones and papules)
  Benzoyl peroxide 2.5–5% gel at bedtime *or*
  Retin-A 0.025–0.05% cream at bedtime
  Topical antibiotics once or twice a day if any inflammation
    is present

Grade III (pustules)
  Benzoyl peroxide 2.5–5% gel in the morning *and*
  Retin-A 0.025–0.05% cream or 0.025% gel at bedtime
  Topical antibiotics twice a day
  Systemic antibiotics, 500–750 mg twice a day, if necessary
  Consider trying Azelex 20% cream, twice a day, if pustules
    or scars are hyperpigmented (use instead of Benzoyl
    peroxide and Retin-A)

Grade IV (nodulocystic acne)
  Benzoyl peroxide 2.5–5% gel in the morning *and*
  Retin-A 0.025–0.05% cream or 0.025% gel at bedtime
  Topical antibiotics twice a day
  Systemic antibiotics, 500–1000 mg twice a day
  Referral to a dermatologist—candidate for Accutane

Reproduced from Strasburger V, Brown R: Common medical problems. In: Callaghan P, Strasburger V, Brown R (editors). *Adolescent Medicine. A Practical Guide,* 2nd ed. Philadelphia: Lippincott Williams & Wilkins, 1998:35.

are effective for acne and might be a logical choice for the female who also requests birth control.

In the most severe forms of acne, 13-cis-retinoic acid (Accutane) has revolutionized treatment. It is a sebostatic compound recommended in those with severe cystic acne. Due to its multiple potential adverse effects and well-known teratogenic properties, it should be used only in select cases and under close supervision. Many pediatricians prefer to refer cases requiring Accutane to dermatologists.

REFERENCES

Adelman WP, Duggan Ak et al: Effectiveness of a high-school smoking cessation program. Pediatrics 2001;107(4):50.

Adelman WP, Joffe A: The adolescent male genital examination: what's normal and what's not. Contemp Pediatrics 1999; 16(7):76.

Adelman WP, Joffe A: The adolescent with a painful scrotum. Contemp Pediatrics 2000;17(3):111.

American Academy of Family Physicians, American Academy of Pediatrics, American Medical Society for Sports Medicine, American Orthopaedic Society for Sports Medicine, American Osteopathic Academy of Sports Medicine: *Preparticipation physical evaluation* (monograph). Leawood KS (editor). 1992, 1996.

American Academy of Pediatrics Committee on Adolescence: suicide and suicide attempts in adolescents. Pediatrics 2000;105:871.

American Psychiatric Association: *Diagnostic and Statistical Manual of Mental Disorders,* 4th ed. Washington, DC: American Psychiatric Association, 1994.

Berman SM, Hein K: Adolescents and STDs. In: Holmes KK et al (editors). *Sexually Transmitted Diseases.* New York: McGraw-Hill, 1999.

Centers for Disease Control and Prevention: 1998 Guidelines for treatment of sexually transmitted diseases. MMWR 1998; 47(RR-1):1.

Dahlberg L: Youth violence in the United States. Am J Prev Med 1998;14:259.

Division of STD Prevention: *Prevention of Genital HPV Infection and Sequelae: Report of an External Consultants' Meeting.* Atlanta: Department of Health and Human Services, Centers for Disease Control and Prevention, 1999.

Elster AB: Comparison of recommendations for adolescent clinical preventive services developed by national organizations. Arch Pediatr Adolesc Med 1998;152:193.

Fishman M et al: Substance abuse among children and adolescents. Pediatri Rev 1997;18:394.

Hergenroeder AC: Prevention of sports injuries. Pediatrics 1998; 101:1057.

Neinstein LS: *Adolescent Health Care: A Practical Guide,* 3rd ed. Baltimore: Williams & Wilkins, 1996.

Sobel JD. Vaginitis. N Engl J Med 1997;337(26):1896.

Speroff L et al: *Clinical Gynecologic Endocrinology and Infertility.* Baltimore: Lippincott Williams & Wilkins, 1999.

Strasburger VC, Brown RT: *Adolescent Medicine: A Practical Guide,* 2nd ed. Philadelphia: Lippincott-Raven, 1998.

Whitaker DJ, Miller KS. Parent–adolescent discussions about sex and condoms: impact on peer influences of sexual risk behavior. J Adolesc Res 2000;15:251.

Developmental & Behavioral Pediatrics

3

Daniel L. Coury, MD

The rapid changes in growth and development that occur in the pediatric and adolescent age groups are unrivaled in the rest of medicine. Whereas most other changes in the patient's condition are due to diseases, in pediatrics the major changes are part of the normal developmental process. As a result, the most common subject of parental questions for the physician relate to the child's development and behavior. Many of these concerns focus around normal development and its variations, but at times the child does present with symptoms of a developmental–behavioral disorder. This chapter focuses on understanding those disorders by thoroughly understanding the normal aspects of behavior and their variations.

An important concept is that of *developmental–behavioral* disorders, not simply behavioral disorders. Development and behavior are linked because behavior is so dependent on the child's underlying developmental skills. Some parental concerns regarding the child's behavior are more reflective of a child's delayed development rather than of abnormal behavior. Similarly, some parental concerns about behavior reflect developmental expectations that are inappropriate for a child of that developmental stage and age group. To properly address a parent's concern about a child's behavior or development, the physician must assess the full developmental–behavioral status of the patient.

Children's behavior not only is limited by their developmental abilities but also reflects their environment. The child's behavior provides insights into the family's lifestyle, functioning, and values. Behavior also is likely to show changes when there are changes in this home environment, as can be seen with family illness, divorce, and changes in housing. Although the parents may present with a concern about the child's behavior, the diagnosis may in fact be based more on the family than on the child.

This chapter focuses on childhood development and behavior in a chronologic fashion, beginning with common concerns and problems in infants and toddlers and progressing to adolescence. The concept of developmental–behavioral assessment is emphasized, because a review of normal development was covered in an earlier section of this book. This chapter focuses more on the behavioral aspects of these concerns.

■ INFANTS & TODDLERS

Humans come into this world with limited skills. With minimal mobility and communication skills, principal parental concerns in the first few months of life center around basic body functions—sleeping, eating, and elimination. Communication concerns early in life present to the physician as problems with crying. As motor development progresses during the first year of life and social and language skills appear, other parental concerns arise. These were discussed in their normative states in Chapter 1.

Excessive Crying & Colic

Crying serves several purposes. Although it almost universally indicates distress, in an infant it is used to communicate a variety of needs, ranging from feeding to being held. Infant cries not only communicate distress but also cause distress in others, especially in caregivers. In assessing the significance of an infant's crying, the physician should note the timing in relation to meals and time of day, the lengths of crying episodes, and the response to efforts to console the infant. Most crying problems can be handled through the tactics outlined in Chapter 1.

Although there is no universally accepted definition, excessive crying is defined as crying that persists for more than 3 hours per day and occurs more often than 3 days per week. The term colic generally is used to refer to excessive, unexplained paroxysms of crying in an otherwise well-nourished, healthy infant. The crying usually occurs at the same time each day, most commonly during the evening hours, and is frequently resistant to simple soothing maneuvers. During these episodes, the infant might have excess flatus and draw its legs up to its chest, leading many parents to believe that the child is having abdominal discomfort.

Classically, colic is described as beginning in the first 3 weeks of age and ending by 3–4 months of age, hence the term "3-month colic." It is considered a mysterious ailment, with no apparent cause and no universally effec-

110

tive treatment. As mysteriously as it seems to appear, it disappears regardless of the treatment strategy used; with more than 50% showing improvement by age 3 months and approximately 90% by age 4 months. Colic is a diagnosis that should rarely be made at the first visit for crying. Rather, it often takes many visits over a period of days or weeks to warrant the label.

Approximately 10–30% of infants will be described as having colic. Whereas many etiologic theories have been proposed, the cause of colic is probably multifactorial. The current interactional model suggests that, in most cases, excessive crying is the result of a combination of intrinsic and extrinsic factors such as normal neuromaturational events, differences in infantile temperament, and the caretaking environment.

A common theory is that colic is caused by gas. This theory presumably is related to the fact that after several minutes of crying the infant passes gas and seems to be somewhat relieved, although the infant might continue to cry. Most likely the gas that is passed is a product of swallowed air during the process of crying excessively; it does not appear to be a primary cause of the crying.

The evaluation should involve a thorough history, including a description of the character and pattern of crying, past and current attempts at management, specific parental concerns, environmental stresses, and overall parental coping. If the history has not shed light on a possible cause, a complete and thorough physical examination must be done to rule out underlying medical problems and reassure the parents. Among the identified causes for persistent crying in infants are otitis media, foreign bodies in the eye or oral pharynx, insect bites, oral lesions, medication reactions, and infections such as those in the urinary tract and central nervous system (CNS). The general condition of the infant is also important because it might lead one to consider other possibilities such as child abuse or neglect, inadequate caloric intake, overstimulation, or other parent–child interaction problems.

Parental attitude should be noted during the interview and examination. Are the parents appropriately concerned, frustrated, or angry or resentful toward the child? Who seems most upset by the baby's crying? Are there any incidents or occurrences that seem to coincide with the onset of the crying? A dietary change suggests food intolerance, and association with a change in caregiver might raise concerns of an unreported injury, accidental or otherwise.

After a complete history and thorough physical examination, some additional studies might be recommended. A urinalysis and urine culture should be considered to rule out a urinary tract infection. A chest x-ray might be considered for the infant who is tachypneic, and a skeletal survey is in order if any bruises are noted or abuse is suspected. A careful and complete history and physical examination will find a cause for persistent crying in approximately 30–50% of cases.

For those infants in whom no immediate cause is identified, treatment should be initiated in an empiric fashion. Just as one etiology cannot be determined, no single intervention will be effective for all infants with colic. It is important to start with a thorough history and physical examination to reassure oneself and the parents that nothing is medically wrong and to better individualize management suggestions. Parents also should be reassured that infants cannot be spoiled at this age by promptly responding to their crying and that the duration of colic is limited.

Caretakers should be encouraged to develop a consistent set of responses to the infant's crying episodes. A variety of behavioral techniques have been proposed to help soothe the colicky baby; parents should be encouraged to find what works best for them. For some infants, decreasing stimulation by swaddling them or laying them down in a quiet, darkened room is helpful. For others, gentle, rhythmic stimulation is most effective and might include rocking the baby, walking while holding the baby or using a soft-front carrier, offering a pacifier, putting the child in a wind-up swing, taking a ride in the car or stroller, and gently rubbing or patting the infant. Soothing sounds like singing or other music might be helpful. As with any treatment in medicine, it is best to stick to a single treatment and monitor the infant's response. If there is no improvement in a day or two, switching to another treatment might be indicated. The clinician should avoid embarking on three or more interventions at the same time. Not only is this no more likely to result in helping the child's symptoms, it is perhaps more likely to promote parental breakdown under the strain of the treatment process. Parents should be encouraged to take turns soothing their child during crying episodes and schedule "quality time" together away from the infant.

Adhering to the basics can be very positive because it tends to promote parental involvement despite the difficult situation, and because the recommendations discourage treatment of excessive crying as a behavior problem in need of discipline. Because crying is a universal sign of pain, many parents and physicians assume that the infant is in pain. Remember that crying in infancy is a method of communicating distress or displeasure for a variety of situations but does not necessarily mean that the child is in physical pain. The use of analgesics is not recommended.

For those infants with severe colic that appears to be unresponsive to such behavioral interventions, a trial of a formula that does not contain lactose and is not based on cow's milk (soy or protein hydrolysate formula) or a maternal milk-free diet in breast-fed infants may be warranted. Although evidence suggests that milk protein allergy or lactose intolerance explains the symptoms in a small subset of infants diagnosed as having colic, the vast majority will not have an identifiable gastrointestinal problem. Formula switching should be discouraged without other evidence of dietary intolerance or before trying a variety of behavioral management techniques.

Treatment with medications affecting gastrointestinal motility has been reported to be helpful with some cases. However, there have been reports of respiratory arrests with these agents and for this reason their use is not advised. The use of other pharmacologic agents, such as dicyclomine hydrochloride, remains controversial and should be avoided except in the most extreme cases, when they may be used as a temporary adjunct to behavioral techniques. Good follow-up is essential in the management of colic to evaluate the success of previous suggestions and provide ongoing support. The time-limited nature of this problem is a relief to parents and physicians.

Some have suggested that colic in infancy predicts a difficult temperament later in life. Most studies have not confirmed such a relationship. Regardless, it is generally not helpful to bring up this theory at the time that the colic is being treated. The parents are experiencing enough stress without the belief that their child is going to be difficult to manage for its entire life. It is far preferable to stick with what is well known; colic will pass by 4 months of age. This deadline for improvement offers hope and a clear resolution point for parents. The most useful activities a physician can engage in are to provide this sense of hope and continue to reassure and support the family. Identifying and enlisting the help of others to give the primary caretakers a respite is invaluable.

Toilet Training

Toilet training probably represents a major milestone to parents because it signifies their release from having to deal with a child's soiled diapers. For some parents it also represents another facet of their child's development and a point of pride that their child has achieved a certain skill at an early age. For these and other reasons, perhaps no other developmental milestone is encouraged and promoted as much as toilet training.

An important part of dealing with the issue of toilet training is to educate parents about the signs of readiness for their child to begin. Fewer than 25% of all children achieve toilet training by 24 months, but most will have achieved it by age 48 months. Reassure parents that their child is progressing normally and discourage efforts to hurry the child. Remember that toilet training occurs at the age commonly referred to as the "terrible two's–terrible three's," a time when toddlers are developing autonomy and displaying temper tantrums. The situation is ripe for problems if parents become too intrusive over a matter of no importance to the child.

Signs of readiness include adequate language to describe the need to defecate and for parents to communicate with the child about this need. A child demonstrating an awareness that the diaper needs changing might be ready to learn. The child who likes to please its parents and wants to demonstrate self-care skills might be motivated to use the toilet. The child who is beginning to show some degree of shyness or awareness of its bodily urges by going off to a corner to defecate can be steered into a bathroom to perform this function (Table 3–1).

As with any other skill, repetition is useful and reinforcement for effort is always helpful. Praising the child's efforts is a first step. The behavioral technique of shaping often is useful. Initially, parents can praise the child for going and sitting on the toilet for a few minutes even though there is no bowel movement. Eventually, praise is amplified when there is actual production of stool. At all times it is important for the parents to maintain a positive attitude. Children should never be shamed for failing to use the potty chair or for accidents as they go through the process. The toileting process takes several months, and accidents are frequent. Parents should be prepared for that.

Breath-Holding Spells

Breath-holding spells are one of the more frightening experiences parents encounter with their young children. These episodes involve the sudden cessation of breathing in response to a strong emotional stimulus. A prolonged episode can lead to unconsciousness. However, it is important to reassure the parents that there are no reported adverse outcomes associated with breath holding. This is an important part of the management of the problem.

Children with breath-holding spells fall into two categories. One category consists of cyanotic episodes, which are generally precipitated by a temper tantrum or other instance of frustration or anger. As the child is expressing its displeasure, there is involuntary holding of the breath during expiration. This is initially frightening and will bring a parent rushing to the child's attention. If it persists for several seconds longer, the child may lose consciousness.

Table 3–1. Signs of Readiness for Toilet Training

The child's verbal language, body language, or activity indicates she is about to urinate or defecate
The child's bowel movements are occurring on a predictable schedule
The child's diaper is dry for prolonged periods, indicating some functional bladder capacity
The child can remove his clothes reliably
The child shows an interest in imitating family members
The child shows an interest in pleasing family members
The child can follow instructions

The other category consists of episodes that occur during inspiration in response to a sudden fright or pain experience. The child gasps and turns pale and limp. The mechanism of action in this category appears to be an overresponsive vagal nerve that results in bradycardia. In either type of episode, key points to recall are:

The spells are self-limited and will resolve without any intervention.
The child will spontaneously begin breathing again without intervention.
The child will not die.
The child will not suffer brain damage.

This reassurance is vital. Because these spells can occur as a result of a temper tantrum, some parents will attempt to placate the child to avoid tantrums. This might reduce the breath-holding spells but will encourage more behavior problems because of poor limit setting. On occasion, children having breath-holding spells have an iron deficiency anemia and the spells resolve after treatment of the anemia. The pathophysiology of this association is not well understood.

Temper Tantrums

Virtually every child displays a temper tantrum at some point in its life. Temper tantrums occur when strong feelings of frustration or anger exceed the child's cognitive abilities to manage them. Tantrums generally occur in young toddlers who have limited language for communication and limited behavioral strategies for dealing with these frustrations. The result is a display of crying, jumping up and down, falling on the ground, or other physical display of displeasure. Through maturation and experience, a child develops improved communication and a wider variety of strategies for dealing with these frustrations. As a result, the incidence of temper tantrums decreases as children mature to school age. Studies suggest that up to 80% of toddlers have a tantrum at least once a week. Development of the ability to control one's tantrums does not simply come with age. The parents must teach their child better self control with proper management techniques.

When parents complain of their child's tantrums, a routine history should focus on when the tantrums occur, what appears to be a precipitating event, the behaviors displayed, the parent's response, and the eventual outcome. Tantrums that occur at regular predictable times, such as an hour before meals or at bedtime, can be reduced by parents being more aware of their child's condition. The hungry child may need a snack before dinner; the tired child may need to have an adjustment in the evening schedule so that bedtime is earlier. If the parents interfering with the child's exploration of the home environment frequently set off the tantrum, the home setting might need to be adjusted. Too many items that are off limits to the child suggest a home that is not geared toward children and likely will promote more tantrums than are truly necessary.

A description of the tantrum is helpful because it is important to ensure that the child is not at risk of harming itself during the tantrum. Another aspect of when the tantrum occurs relates to who is present. When tantrums occur more frequently with one parent than the other, examine that relationship more carefully. Is that parent setting more limits and unnecessarily provoking tantrums? Or is this the result of that parent not setting limits, such that tantrums have become a learned mechanism for obtaining what the child wants? Accompanying information to determine is whether the tantrums occur in other settings with other adults. It is important to examine what the tantrum produces for the child. Does the child get its way? If so, caregivers need to learn to set limits more firmly.

Management of temper tantrums begins with setting limits. Parents should not be seen giving in to, and thereby reinforcing, the tantrums. Parental behavior during the tantrum usually consists of some effort at ignoring the child or not speaking to the child. Too many parents attempt to reason with their child; the child has lost control because it does not have the cognitive abilities to control its emotions, much less listen to the parent's reasoning. Some parents who attempt to ignore the child complain that the tantrums become worse. This in fact is true, at least temporarily, as the child might persist with this behavior if it has been effective in the past. The parents should be warned that, when they attempt to ignore any behavior, the first response is for the behavior to increase. However, as the behavior continues to be ignored and is ineffective, the behavior eventually will decrease and disappear. This period generally lasts only a few days, but many parents lack the patience to persist with the strategy for an adequate period.

Indications for referral include those situations where the tantrums are only part of a larger picture of oppositional behavior; tantrums occurring in multiple settings with multiple caregivers, resulting in impairment in functioning in those settings and with peers; and situations of parental mental illness or family dysfunction, where the primary care physician cannot obtain satisfactory cooperation of the adult caregivers.

Fears & Phobias

Fear is the unpleasant feeling that accompanies the anticipation of danger in living organisms. It is a normal response, with cognitive and physiologic changes. In the infant, fear is a part of the Moro, or startle, reflex; the infant's response of rapidly extending the extremities and crying out serves to gain the caregiver's attention, so that the caregiver might attend to and protect the infant. As the infant matures, the startle reflex disappears and cognitive development progresses. By approximately 8 months of age, development has progressed to include visual recognition memory. This is well represented by stranger anxiety, where an infant recognizes regular caregivers but has a wary hesitancy around strangers. Common fears in young children tend to relate to areas they cannot cognitively understand or physically easily master. Examples include fear of the dark, falling, and separation from primary caregivers. As children mature and their cognitive understanding of the world increases, fears change. Fear of the dark is replaced by fear of monsters; fear of separation from a caregiver is refined to fear of loss of a parent by death. To a certain extent, parents can be reassured that their child's fears are appropriate to its development or even a sign of developmental progress. Because fear is a protective mechanism, the goal is not to eliminate all fears. Rather, the goal is to teach the child healthy ways of dealing with common fears. The parents first of all should acknowledge and respect the child's fear. They should not embarrass or humiliate the child through teasing. Initially, it might be necessary to avoid the situation or object provoking the fear, but plans should be made for learning to deal with it. Initially, this often consists of talking about the fear at times when the situation or object is not present. Parents can review methods of dealing with the fear and practice how they will handle it when it arises. Gradual planned exposure to the fear stimulus, with a parent present, can help the child gradually overcome the fear. The child should be praised for progressively mastering the situation.

Parents need to be clearly instructed not to threaten, embarrass, or ignore their child's fears. They also might need education regarding appropriate fears for certain developmental stages in order to dispel any unreasonable expectations of the child's behavior (Table 3–2).

Phobias are fears that are specific and developmentally inappropriate. They clearly impair the person's ability to function. Often the fear has become exaggerated to the point where it lacks credibility, e.g., fear of family members dying in a car accident every time they travel in a car, or fear of entering a dark room because spiders might crawl up the leg. Phobias share much in common with compulsive disorders when the phobia results in the child thinking about all of the awful things that might happen at times when the situation is distant. Phobias require involvement of a mental health professional and may entail the use of behavior modification programs or medications.

Separation is a common time of fearfulness and behavior difficulties with young children. Stranger anxiety and fearfulness are common in children approximately 8–18 months old. When a stranger comes forward, the child will draw closer to the parent and look to the parent for cues regarding the stranger's potential as a threat.

Table 3–2. Common Childhood Fears

Fear	Typical Age of Appearance	Typical Age of Disappearance
Strangers	7–8 mo	18–24 mo
Darkness	12 mo	School age
Severe weather (wind, thunder, lightning)	12–18 mo	School age; may persist to adulthood
Loud objects (vacuum, power tools)	6–12 mo	School age
Separation anxiety	2–3 y	School age; may persist
Nightmares	2–3 y	School age; occur occasionally throughout life
Night terrors	2–3 y	School age
Heights	1–2 y	School age; may persist to adulthood

The parent who smiles, continues speaking in a pleasant voice, and generally shows no fear but a warm attitude toward the stranger will help the child adjust to that person. Similarly, the parent who shows fears and concern of the stranger will quickly impart those apprehensions to the child. Situations where separation is a common problem include leaving the child with baby sitters or at child care centers. Parents can facilitate introducing their child to those other caregivers by staying for a while before leaving. As the new caregivers become known to the child, they enter the circle of known adults and are accepted. The establishment of routines can help facilitate this. For example, the child could hang up the caregiver's coat, put away that person's lunch box, kiss daddy goodbye, and go to the window to wave to daddy outside. All of these actions provide a sameness and reassurance to the child. Parents should be reassured that their upset toddler generally settles down within a few minutes of their leaving. When the child continues to show significant distress for prolonged periods after the parents leave, or if the distress does not decrease or is carried over in the form of negative behaviors at home, the parents should reassess the child care situation. They should think about any other behavioral concerns for their child and consider referral to a mental health professional.

Sleep Problems

Concerns about a child's sleep habits are common, and most of these concerns can be easily handled with guidance, as described in Chapter 1, and many can be prevented by providing this anticipatory guidance through health supervision visits. Those that go beyond normal variation present greater concerns to parents, although even then intervention is not always necessary. Important factors to recall are the normal physiology of sleep and sleep patterns, cultural and socioeconomic factors, and dynamics of the family relationship. The problem of frequent and prolonged nighttime awakening by the infant was discussed in Chapter 1.

SLEEP SCHEDULE PROBLEMS—TOO LATE TO BED, TOO EARLY TO RISE

Problems with delayed onset of sleep or early awakening are disruptive to families. Parents complain that they themselves are not getting enough sleep by being up too late or rising too early with the child. A sleep diary is a very helpful starting point. By reviewing a sleep diary and being aware of normal sleep requirements for the child's developmental stage, one can quickly determine whether the child is getting adequate sleep. The great majority of these children are receiving an adequate amount of sleep in a 24-hour period, but it is not meeting the parent's schedule. It is also important to examine the setting in which the difficulty is occurring. If the problem is one of late onset of sleep, information must be gathered regarding the environment at that time. *Sleep hygiene* refers to the complete milieu surrounding the bedtime process. It consists of an integration of activities intended to prepare one for sleep. These include settling activities such as bathtime, reading from books, lullabies, and tucking into bed and kissing goodnight. Associated environmental changes include an overall quieting of the household and the child's room, low-level lighting such as a nightlight, and providing a favorite item or transitional object such as a stuffed toy.

If appropriate sleep hygiene is in place and the child is receiving an appropriate amount of sleep in a 24-hour period, then adjustments to the sleep schedule can be made. For the child with late onset sleep, reducing the amount of total sleep in the next 24 hours will result in a gradual movement of the bedtime toward an earlier, more appropriate hour. If the child normally takes a nap, avoiding the nap and keeping the child awake will result in an earlier bedtime. In the older child who does not nap, earlier awakening for the next several mornings will gradually move the onset of bedtime to an earlier hour. Similarly, the early riser can be managed by cutting back on a daytime nap or delaying onset of sleep.

Sleep refusal may be part of a generalized problem of oppositional behavior or may be focused on avoiding going to bed. When focused on bedtime, treatment should begin with evaluation of appropriate sleep hygiene. Discussing with the child reasons for not going to bed can be useful in determining the roadblocks to an appropriate bedtime. Additional preparation for sleep, such as guided imagery, may be helpful. The child can be told to close the eyes and think about a pleasant or preferred experience. The parent can guide the child through this exercise for a minute or two, with the instruction for the child to continue to dream about this experience. Favorite trips to vacation spots or other pleasurable activities are common themes. If there are no other sleep difficulties or persistent oppositional behaviors apart from bedtime, a contingency system might be used. This should be initiated with a reward for the next day ("If you go to bed right now, I will fix a special breakfast for you tomorrow morning"). After some initial success, the contingencies can be adjusted ("If you go to bed on time 5 nights in a row, we will rent a video next weekend"). As the preferred behavior of going to bed on time becomes the norm, the contingencies become less frequent and the negative behavior is extinguished.

SLEEP AROUSAL PROBLEMS

Some parents complain that their child awakens regularly at a specified hour in the middle of the night. They often comment that you can set your clock by this, and, indeed, the timing of the awakening coincides with a certain number of complete sleep cycles since falling asleep. These are disorders of sleep arousal and occur when the child is going through a period of light sleep at the end of a sleep cycle. They are easily aroused before entering into the next phase of sleep. At this point, they might sleepily toddle into their parents bedroom seeking comfort, reassurance, or simply parental presence. The child is not frightened and has not had a nightmare. He or she is simply awakening between sleep cycles and is physiologically well prepared to enter into another sleep cycle. For this reason, the best recommendation is to return the child to its own bed without a word and tuck the child back into bed with little more than a verbal good night. Additional talking with the child will only promote further awakening. Other factors to consider focus on the sleep milieu. Is the household noisy? Did the child fall asleep elsewhere and is startled to be in someone else's bed? If these factors are regular occurrences, efforts need to be directed toward changing them and not the child's behavior. Persistent patterns of inappropriate sleep arousal might require additional management (Figure 3–1). Planned night waking consists of awakening the child before the child's awakening anticipated in the middle of the night. The parent is instructed to awaken the child approximately 30 minutes before the child normally arouses. By doing so, it is hypothesized that the normal sleep cycle is disrupted. Because the child is tired and sleepy, the child can go back to sleep and re-initiate the sleep cycles. After the sleep disruption, the child will usually sleep through the rest of the night. Following a planned schedule of night wakening for several nights often will correct this problem.

Algorithm for Sleep Arousal Problems

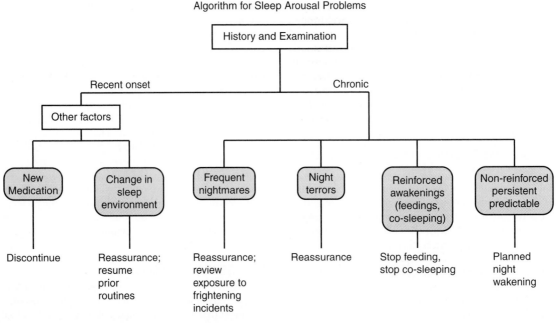

Figure 3–1. Algorithm for sleep arousal problems.

NIGHTMARES, NIGHT TERRORS, SLEEP TALKING, & SLEEP WALKING

Nightmares generally begin around the age of 3 years. Before that, children might awaken frightened but their fear is thought to be related to separation issues rather than to bad dreams. True nightmares involve frightening events, often of people or other events that scare the child. They may be related to an activity that occurred that day, including fictional activities experienced through books or movies. The child is frightened, might cry out or leave the bed and enter the parent's room, and might give a history of the upsetting dream. Treatment consists of reassurance and returning the child to its own bed. Reassuring and calming the child in its own room is an important part of maintaining good sleep hygiene. The child who is reassured and made comfortable in the parent's bedroom is likely to resist returning to its own bed. The child likely will consider the parents' bedroom as the safest place. Reassurance and calming in the child's own room helps confirm that it is a wonderful place to sleep, and that the problem was the nightmare and not the child's bed.

Night terrors are different from simple nightmares. These occur during the deepest, non–rapid eye movement sleep, usually during the first third of the night. These affect approximately 3–5% of young children (peak age 3–8 years). The terror itself presents as crying, perhaps kicking or flailing of arms and legs, all while the child is completely unresponsive to the parents attempting to

help. Although the eyes may be open, there does not seem to be recognition of family members and the child is quite inconsolable. However, upon awakening the child has no apparent memory of the event. Night terrors are far more frightening to parents than nightmares and more likely to result in physician consultation. They generally are benign and will resolve on their own, although they may cause distress to the family for several weeks or months. Medication is rarely recommended in their management.

Somniloquy, or *sleep talking,* is a common occurrence. Sleep talking is most likely a verbal component of normal dreams and varies from mumbling and nonsensible to clearly worded statements. It differs from nightmares in that the child is not in distress. It can persist throughout childhood and into adulthood and requires no treatment. *Somnambulism,* or *sleep walking,* is thought to be the motor equivalent of acting out a dream. It may be accompanied by sleep talking and commonly presents as a child who enters the parents' bedroom, makes a few nonsensical statements, and then returns to its own bed. At other times the episodes might persist for several minutes, with the child wandering throughout the house. The child is not truly awake, does not respond appropriately in conversation, and usually can be led back to bed with no difficulty. In persistent cases there may be a need to ensure the child's safety through changes in the environment. Such changes might include simply shutting the child's bedroom door completely, putting latches on kitchen cupboards to prevent access to sharp objects, and placing gates across stairways.

Evaluation of night terrors and somniloquy also should include investigation into any changes in the household. If onset of these sleep problems has occurred with the beginning of a medication, a change or adjustment in the medication should be considered. In persistent cases, an evaluation in a sleep laboratory might produce useful information. Rarely are these associated with seizures but, if identified, seizure treatment can be useful.

Pervasive Developmental Disorders

Autism is the more commonly known term for the most severe of the spectrum of disorders known as *pervasive developmental disorders* (PDDs). Key features of autism are a clear qualitative impairment in social interaction and skills, impairments in communication, and an overly restricted repertoire of behaviors and activities. In severe cases, the abnormal social interaction might have presented in infancy as a child who seldom smiled or did not want to be cuddled or was difficult to console. Most children with autism are diagnosed based on a presenting complaint of delayed language. As a result, they are most commonly identified late in the second year of life or later. Children identified at age 3–4 years tend to present unusual behaviors, with their delay in language having been considered an isolated problem up to that point. The American Psychiatric Association diagnostic criteria for autistic disorder are reproduced in Table 3–3.

The impairment in social interactions is significant. These children have very poor eye contact and often seem to be in a world of their own. Facial expressions often are inappropriate to the current activity, such as smiling at inappropriate times or during inappropriate activities. Parents may report frustration with a child who does not want to be hugged, or who does not even refer to them as mommy or daddy. The deficit in communication is not restricted to spoken language. Receptive language is also greatly decreased, with children often appearing not to hear or understand statements addressed to them. The communication deficit also extends to nonverbal communication. Autistic children do not adequately use gestures or other signals to communicate their needs. Many behavior problems and temper tantrums are a result of parents' inability to guess what their child is trying to communicate to them.

Many children with autism have repetitive motor movements such as hand flapping that occur during periods of excitement. At other times these repetitive behaviors occur as though the child were bored and might represent a preferred behavior that the child finds stimulating. There is a preoccupation with sameness in their world, and parents report serious behavioral consequences if they change their

Table 3–3. Criteria for Autistic Disorder

A. A total of six or more items from (1), (2), and (3) below, with at least two from (1) and one each from (2) and (3):
  1. Qualitative impairment in social interaction
     a. Marked impairment in nonverbal behaviors, such as eye-to-eye gaze, facial expression, body postures to regulate social interaction
     b. Failure to develop peer relations appropriate to developmental level
     c. Lack of spontaneous seeking to share enjoyment, interests, or achievements with other people
     d. Lack of social or emotional reciprocity
  2. Qualitative impairments in communication
     a. Delay in, or total lack of, development of spoken language
     b. When speech is present, marked impairment in ability to initiate or sustain a conversation with others
     c. Stereotyped and repetitive use of language or idiosyncratic language
     d. Lack of varied, spontaneous make-believe play or social imitative play appropriate to developmental level
  3. Restricted, repetitive, stereotyped patterns of behavior, interest, and activities
     a. Preoccupation with one of more stereotyped and restricted patterns of interest that is abnormal either in intensity or focus
     b. Inflexible adherence to specific, nonfunctional routines or rituals
     c. Stereotyped and repetitive motor mannerisms (e.g., hand flapping)
     d. Persistent preoccupation with parts of objects
B. Delays or abnormal functioning in at least one of the following areas, with onset before age 3 years: (1) social interaction, (2) language as used in social communication, or (3) symbolic or imaginative play
C. Does not meet the criteria for Ret disorder or childhood disintegrative disorder

Adapted from *Diagnostic and Statistical Manual of Mental Disorders*, 4th ed. © 1994 American Psychiatric Association.

routine. Unusual routines regarding diet, clothing, and play activities are common.

Other disorders in the PDD spectrum include Rett's syndrome, which occurs exclusively in girls, and Asperger's disorder. Persons with Asperger's disorder also have been referred to as high functioning autistic persons. Their language is not as impaired as their social skills. These children often do not get along well with others and lack appropriate social skills. When they do interact with others, they are apt to make unusual statements that result in them being teased or shunned.

It is not known what causes autism and the other PDDs. There is clear evidence of familial inheritance, with a variety of genetic causes proposed. Autism is seen more frequently in association with other contributing factors. There is an increased incidence in children with congenital infections such as rubella, and an increased incidence has been reported with fragile X syndrome. Metabolic disorders such as phenylketonuria, genetic disorders such as tuberous sclerosis, and CNS infections also are associated with increased risk for autistic behaviors.

Just as there is no clear etiology for autism, there also is no cure. Multiple treatments have been proposed based on anecdotal reports or proposed theories of etiology, but at this date there is no cure for these disorders. The only proven effective treatment is one of intense behavioral intervention that requires 30–40 hours of involvement weekly with trained professionals. These behavioral intervention programs are most effective when instituted at an early age, so early diagnosis and intervention are vital. Medical involvement is aimed at identifying any possible medical disorders that can otherwise account for the child's features, for purposes of treatment or genetic counseling for the family. Medications sometimes are used to treat problem behaviors. Medications used to treat these behaviors are similar to those used for treating those same behaviors in persons without autism. For example, stimulant medication sometimes is used to treat the symptoms of hyperactivity seen in these children. Anticonvulsants may be needed, as these patients have an increased incidence of associated seizures. The medical evaluation should assess hearing and perform chromosomal studies, a screen for metabolic disorders; and an electroencephalogram if clinical findings suggest it would be helpful.

■ SCHOOL-AGE CHILDREN

Enuresis

The failure to attain adequate bladder control is referred to as *enuresis*. Enuresis is defined according to the child's age to differentiate it from normal variation. A lack of regular daytime bladder control after age 4 years is a widely accepted definition. Nocturnal bladder control often lags behind, so it is considered normal to have nocturnal enuresis through age 6 years. Boys generally obtain bladder control later than girls. The differentiation between diurnal and nocturnal enuresis is also important in terms of prognosis. Nocturnal enuresis is far more common and most often idiopathic, although there are some genetic tendencies. Diurnal enuresis is more likely to have an organic pathology. Enuresis is often classified further as primary or secondary. In primary enuresis, the child has never attained consistent bladder control. In secondary enuresis, the child has a history of at least 3 months of consistent control before the current situation of incontinence. Children with secondary enuresis are more likely to have

an organic problem or psychosocial component. Initial assessment begins with the history (Figure 3–2). Attention should be directed to symptoms suggestive of medical illness. Questions regarding dysuria, polyuria, polydipsia, abnormal urine stream, and constipation are important. Information regarding a family history of enuresis is important for prognostic factors.

The physical examination should focus on the abdomen for any signs of masses, palpation for stool and rectal examination for fecal impaction, assessment of anal sphincter tone and anal wink as markers for neurologic integrity, and deep tendon reflexes in the lower extremities. Examination of the genital region for any urethral malformations is also important.

Laboratory evaluation should include a urinalysis. A urine culture also might be necessary if the urinalysis suggests urinary tract infection. Additional laboratory studies should be done as clinical findings indicate.

Diurnal enuresis is the less common form and occurs in approximately 10% of children. Most fall into one of two categories. The first category consists of children who have repeated accidents but use a toilet regularly and are embarrassed by those accidents. These children tend to have unstable bladders and respond well to bladder control exercises. Also known as stream interruption exercises, the child is instructed to stop urinating at midstream. After a delay of 10–15 seconds, the child is instructed to finish urinating. This exercise is repeated with increasing periods of stream interruption, with an eventual goal of stopping for 2 or 3 minutes. These children are motivated to perform these exercises and have a good prognosis.

The second category of diurnal enuresis consists of children who are voluntary wetters. Many wet themselves for oppositional or defiant reasons, sometimes related to the toileting process and other times simply to struggle with parents. A motivational program focused on acquiring incentives for remaining dry are usually successful with these children; the reason for the child's wetting is ignored and attention is focused on the incentive. Some children have more significant oppositional or emotional problems, and enuresis is a small part of the general behavioral difficulties of the child. These children should be referred to a mental health professional for treatment of their other issues. As those issues resolve, the enuresis often will resolve as well.

Nocturnal enuresis is by far the most common form of incontinence. It accounts for approximately 90% of enuresis, and a family history is found in approximately half. A number of treatments exist for nocturnal enuresis. When one considers that nocturnal enuresis is, in its simplest terms, a failure to awaken and go to the bathroom to void, it seems logical that a technique that would train the child to awaken when the bladder is full would be most effective. Various enuresis alarms serve this purpose. Newer alarms have sensors designed to attach to the child's under-

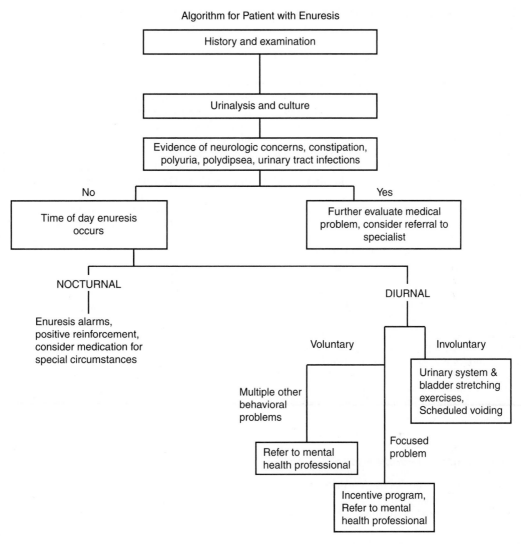

Figure 3–2. Algorithm for the patient with enuresis.

wear that allow only a few drops before setting off the alarm. Initially, the child continues to wet, with the alarm waking the child at some point during urination. Many parents complain that their child sleeps deeply, and that the alarm wakens them but not the child. Parents should be reassured and encouraged to continue with the alarm system. Gradually, through repeated nights of the alarm sounding, a conditioned response develops. Eventually the child's body recognizes that the bladder is full and that the alarm is about to go off, and the child awakens and can go to the bathroom before voiding. Although results may be seen with this method in much less time, it may take as long as 4–6 months to be effective. Parents need to be

informed of this at the beginning because many parents expect this treatment to work within a few days and, as a result, become disenchanted and give up on this system. The enuresis alarm is the only treatment that can truly cure enuresis, whereas medications show significant relapse when discontinued.

Desmopressin acetate has been used to treat nocturnal enuresis. It is highly effective and works by decreasing urine production. Because nocturnal enuresis is not a problem of urine production but rather of not awakening to void, this treatment is not a cure. Discontinuation is accompanied by a very high relapse rate. However, it can be very useful for select social situations when the child needs to spend the night away from home, such as at camp or sleepovers with friends. The cost of this treatment is rather high; a single month's supply costs approximately double the cost of an alarm. Given that the child most likely will require treatment for many months or years, it should be considered primarily for those situations where other treatments have failed or the child is so discouraged that there is some need for immediate success to obtain participation in other ongoing treatments.

Imipramine has been used for many years as a treatment for enuresis. It is fairly effective and works through unknown mechanisms. It is far less expensive than desmopressin acetate but has a greater risk of side effects from overdosage.

Encopresis

Encopresis is the voluntary or involuntary passing of stool in the underwear. Like enuresis, it can be classified as primary or secondary. Primary encopresis is seen more often in persons with developmental disabilities or neurologic compromise. Most cases are secondary. It is also important to rule out organic causes before treatment.

The history should gather information regarding the onset of the problem, its frequency, and when and where it occurs. A child who soils only at school may have a fear of using the school bathrooms. Is there a history of constipation or of enuresis? Nearly all children with encopresis have accompanying constipation. Approximately 25% also have enuresis. At times it is unclear which came first, the child's enuresis or encopresis. A chronically constipated child with large amounts of stool in the colon may have increased pressure on the bladder, thereby reducing capacity and promoting enuresis. Often in these cases treatment of the encopresis also resolves the enuresis. A history of production of large stools, so much so as to clog the toilet, further suggests constipation and an accompanying functional megacolon. A commonly elicited symptom is that the child claims not to feel any urge to use the bathroom and does not know when stool is about to be passed. This concerns parents and physicians alike with the possibility of a neurologic problem. Most commonly, however, this is related to long-standing constipation and overstretching of stretch receptors in the colon.

The physical examination should identify constipation through abdominal palpation or rectal examination. Neurologic examination should focus on identifying any abnormalities in the lower extremities. The child's gait should be evaluated, as should the deep tendon reflexes and motor strength. Sensation, the presence of an anal wink, and sphincter tone should be assessed. Rectal examination is a required part of evaluating the child with encopresis. The rectal vault is generally filled with clay-like stool and distended. Rectal tone may be normal or slightly decreased, in contrast to a child with Hirschprung's disease, who

classically has a history of pencil-thin stools and on rectal examination presents a tight sphincter tone and release of a large amount of stool upon removal of the examining finger.

Treatment of the child with encopresis is similar to reteaching toileting skills (Table 3–4). Initial treatment includes evacuation of the bowel with oral laxatives or, if necessary, enemas. The child is then continued on daily stool softeners for the next 4–6 months. Concurrent with this is the institution of a schedule of toileting. Ideally, the child should be going to the toilet for a 5-minute period approximately 15 minutes after each meal and before bedtime. The timing of this schedule should take advantage of the natural gastrocolic reflex, which helps provide an urge to defecate after meals. Because the colon usually is overdistended from months of impaction, the stretch receptors in the colon do not reliably send the sensation of fullness in the bowel and the need to defecate. The daily stool softener helps facilitate this and the schedule helps the child become attuned to the body's signals. Follow-up should be frequent, approximately every 2 weeks for the first month and then monthly thereafter. Parent and patient alike need to be well informed of the need to continue with the schedule and stool softener for several months. A common mistake is for parents to discontinue treatment after a few weeks, thinking that the problem has resolved. Because the overly distended colon is not yet sending a sensation of fullness, the child quickly falls into old habits of not going to the bathroom regularly and becoming impacted. It is often a good strategy for the physician to take on as much responsibility as possible for the child's treatment. For example, if the child is regularly having additional accidents, one may assume responsibility for not having prescribed adequate amounts of stool softener. With frequent follow-up and a sharing of responsibility, the child's self-esteem can be preserved and

Table 3–4. Management of Encopresis

Initial	Maintenance	Ongoing
Bowel catharsis Hypophosphate enemas twice Biscodyl tablet qhs Repeat daily up to 3 cycles	Mineral oil, 2–4 tablespoons daily for 4–6 mo	In case of relapse, take Biscodyl qhs for 3 days
High-fiber diet	Continue diet	Continue diet
Go to toilet for 10 min after each meal	Continue toilet schedule	Continue toilet schedule

the child better motivated to work harder with the schedule and taking the medications.

School Avoidance

The child who is repeatedly absent from school for vague physical symptoms represents the condition known as *school avoidance.* These children generally miss school due to vague nonspecific symptoms such as abdominal pain or headache or nausea. The symptoms are severe enough so that parents will allow the child to stay home, or school officials will send the child home, but do not seem significant enough to warrant medical attention. As a result, these children often have missed many days of school before being seen by the physician. It is a common problem affecting approximately 5% of school-aged children.

Children with school avoidance tend to fall into two categories. The first category consists of those who demonstrate symptoms of anxiety in addition to repeated absences. They may have a shy personality, show other difficulties with separation such as refusal to attend sleepovers at friends' houses, or be unwilling to attend summer camps. One or both parents are often very protective of the child by insisting that she or he has it difficult and producing many rationalizations for the child's need to stay home.

The second category comprises far few anxiety symptoms. Instead, these children appear to have clear secondary gains for their school absences. Common reasons are a big test for which they have not adequately studied or a desire not to participate in a school activity. School avoidance allows them additional study time or total avoidance of the activity. Family factors in these cases generally include a parent who does not set limits on the child's behavior. Whereas the anxious child presents with common somatic symptoms related to anxiety such as headache or abdominal pain, the school avoider with secondary gains is often more likely to fabricate other symptoms such as leg pains or back aches.

A key point in all cases of school avoidance is the normal physical examination. As with other somatization problems, the child reports clear symptoms but the physical examination and accompanying review of systems do not find anything significant. The history, review of systems, and physical examination are key points in supporting the physician's diagnosis that there is nothing physically wrong with the child.

An excellent question to pose while taking the child's history is "What did you think was causing this problem?" The child usually will have no idea. The worried parent may believe that it is a physical condition affecting another family member or friend. By addressing this concern directly, the physician can initiate management. A common response by frustrated parents is that "it's all in her head." This response is right on target and should

be addressed. A more acceptable way of discussing this is to tell the child and parents that stress can cause many symptoms and that you feel that that is the cause here. Reassure them that this does not mean that the problem is "in your head," as these physical pains are very real. However, it does mean that the treatment for those pains is not with symptomatic medication but rather identification of the cause of the stress.

Treatment consists of sending the child back to school. The family is informed that the child is not to be kept out of school without a visit to the physician's office. If the child has returned to school, the child is not to be sent home without a visit to the school nurse. Physician communication with the school nurse should focus on the school avoidance and discussion of some clear parameters that would warrant the child leaving school. Those parameters include documented, significant fever (above 101°F orally), vomiting, or other documentable sign of illness for the nurse to justify sending the child home. Otherwise, the school nurse can serve as a valuable part of the treatment plan by allowing the child to leave the classroom and come to the nurse's office for a brief period (5–10 minutes) before returning to the classroom. The nurse also can reassure the child that everything is all right and that there is no significant illness occurring. The nurse is also in a position to provide more frequent feedback to the child regarding her progress ("You have been doing so well, I haven't seen you in the office lately").

For those children who have associated anxiety symptoms, consultation with a psychologist or other mental health professional might be useful. Treatment should focus on the child's other anxiety symptoms because school avoidance is only one aspect of a larger problem. Children with school avoidance due to secondary gain usually are identified and managed by their parents. Those who come to medical attention also will quickly respond when their parents are informed of the cause of the children's absences. Should the parents continue to have difficulty setting limits, consultation with a mental health professional might be useful in providing parental training and support. In all cases, insist that the child return to school while being treated.

Attention-Deficit/Hyperactivity Disorder

Attention-deficit/hyperactivity disorder (ADHD) is the most researched and written about of all behavioral disorders, in pediatrics or adult medicine. The complaint of "he's hyper" has become a common one, but the term is used loosely by many parents. It is often misused to describe a child who is disobedient, engages in a lot of fighting, swears, or has other problem behaviors. Even though the child has those behavior problems, the problem is not necessarily ADHD. To appropriately diagnose a child with ADHD, one must refer to the criteria for diagnosis as set forth by the American Psychiatric Association (Table 3–5).

Collecting the information needed to reach a diagnosis is a time-consuming process (Table 3–6). The criteria require information that supports the child having these symptoms in more than one setting, so gathering information from teachers or other care providers is an important part of the process. An efficient use of time is to distribute questionnaires to be completed by the parents and teacher. Such questionnaires are useful because they

Table 3–5. Diagnostic Criteria for Attention-Deficit/Hyperactivity Disorder

A. Either (1) or (2), for at least 6 mo
  1. Six or more of the following symptoms of inattention
     a. Fails to give close attention to work
     b. Difficulty sustaining attention in tasks or play activities
     c. Often does not seem to listen when spoken to directly
     d. Trouble following through on directions or fails to finish schoolwork
     e. Difficulty organizing tasks and activities
     f. Reluctant to engage in tasks that require sustained mental effort
     g. Often loses things necessary for school activities
     h. Easily distracted by extraneous stimuli
     i. Often forgetful in daily activities
  2. Six or more of the following symptoms of hyperactivity or impulsivity
     Hyperactivity
     a. Often fidgets with hands or feet and squirms in seat
     b. Often leaves seat in classroom when remaining seated is expected
     c. Often runs or climbs excessively
     d. Often has difficulty playing or engaging in leisure activities quietly
     e. Often "on the go" or "driven by a motor"
     f. Often talks excessively
     Impulsivity
     g. Often blurts out answers before questions are completed
     h. Often has difficulty awaiting turn
     i. Often interrupts or intrudes on others (in conversation or games)
B. Symptoms present before age 7 years
C. Impairment from symptoms in two or more settings (school and home)
D. Symptoms not accounted for by other diagnoses (e.g., pervasive developmental disorder, schizophrenia, or anxiety disorder)

Modified from *Diagnostic and Statistical Manual of Mental Disorders*, 4th ed. © 1994 American Psychiatric Association.

Table 3–6. Components of an ADHD Assessment

Direct interviews and information gathering
Parent
Child
Other adults who know the child well (e.g., child care provider, teacher)
Standardized questionnaires to assess ADHD and other symptoms
  Parent questionnaires (e.g., Conners, Barkley Home Situations Questionnaire)
  Teacher questionnaires (e.g., Conners, Barkley School Situations Questionnaire)
Evaluation of possible coexisting conditions
  Oppositional-defiant disorder
  Conduct disorder
  Mood disorders
  Learning disabilities
  Other medical conditions (e.g., motor disabilities, vision and hearing problems)
Conformity of symptoms identified with criteria listed for ADHD in the *Diagnostic and Statistical Manual*, 4th ed.

ADHD = attention-deficit/hyperactivity disorder.

require other adults who know the child to answer multiple questions regarding the child's symptoms and behavior. Such questionnaires often uncover problem areas in addition to the ADHD symptoms which are of immediate concern.

The principal features of ADHD are a persistent pattern of hyperactivity and impulsivity and problems of inattention inappropriate for the child's developmental level. Although the criteria are delineated clearly, physicians do not use them consistently. Studies have shown that diagnoses frequently are made with inadequate information. In some cases, a child may have several symptoms but not enough to meet the criteria. In other cases, the physician does not obtain information regarding the child's performance in other settings. There is a great tendency to overdiagnose the problem if physicians do not adhere closely to the criteria.

Medical evaluation includes hearing and cognitive testing in addition to tests focused on any symptoms possibly related to developmental and behavioral problems. Children with fetal alcohol syndrome have an increased incidence of attention and learning problems. Thyroid disorders, especially hyperthyroidism, can present with overactivity. Hypothyroidism may present as a problem of inattention but generally will not have the overactive behavior components. The role of medications in mimicking ADHD is a controversial one. Phenobarbital has been documented to increase activity and problems with attention span. In most other cases, medication such as theophylline and albuterol have an uncertain role in mimicking those symptoms. If the history clearly indicates onset of the symptoms with the initiation of a medication, one should consider discontinuing the medicine.

Although the genetics of ADHD are not clearly understood, a positive family history is seen in about 50% of cases. There is also a close relation with learning disabilities, with some studies suggesting that nearly half of ADHD children also have an accompanying learning disability. A perinatal history suggesting a CNS insult may be found, but most ADHD children have unremarkable medical histories.

There is no single laboratory test or physical finding diagnostic of ADHD. The most important parts of the evaluation are the interview and history.

Psychological testing might be useful because it can identify problems in cognition that are contributing to the child's symptoms or mimicking attentional problems. Psychological or psychiatric consultation also can be helpful as a second opinion in the diagnostic process.

Treatment of ADHD consists of pharmacologic and nonpharmacologic therapies. Behavioral therapy and counseling principally are aimed at refining the parent's skills in behavior management. However, ADHD is not the result of poor parental discipline; the ADHD child is extremely challenging and parents must be as competent as possible in managing their child's behavior.

Medication has been used to treat hyperactivity for more than 60 years (Table 3–7). Medications of choice are in the stimulant class and include methylphenidate, dextroamphetamine, and combinations of dextroamphetamine and levoamphetamine salts. These medications improve attention and concentration and decrease distractibility and impulsivity. As a result, multiple disruptive behaviors and performance problems can be reduced when the child is making efforts to stay on task and follow directions. Adjustments in medication dosage should be made based on the response of core ADHD symptoms. Many parents and teachers might request an increase in medication in an attempt to control symptoms that are not part of the child's core ADHD problem. Studies have shown that the best outcome for these children is seen with a combination of medication and behavioral management. Medication can be most useful with core ADHD symptoms of attention and impulsivity, whereas behavioral management is more useful with secondary symptoms such as oppositionality and poor social skills.

Learning Disabilities

The child who presents with school underachievement is another concern for parents. Initially, the parents might feel that their child is performing adequately or needs to work harder. Persistent underachievement can result in a child developing negative attitudes toward school, school avoidance, or family strife over the child's failures.

The initial evaluation begins with a history of the problem and should include such questions as:

How long has the child been having difficulty in school?

Has this been a concern dating back to preschool years, or has it occurred only this year? If the problem is relatively recent, are there other psychosocial factors such as a recent move, change in family structure, or change in school environment that might be responsible?

Table 3–7. Medications for Attention-Deficit/Hyperactivity Disorder

Medication (brand names)	Format	Half-life	Dosing
Methylphenidate (Ritalin)	5-, 10-, 20-mg tablets	3–4 h	Starting dose of 2.5 mg bid or 0.3 mg/kg; if needed, increase at 2.5-mg intervals to a maximum of 60 mg/day divided bid/tid
	20-mg SR tablets	6–8 h	Same as dose of regular tablets established over 8-h period; *must be swallowed whole*
Dextroamphetamine (Dexedrine)	5-, 10-mg tablets	3–4 h	2.5 mg or 0.15 mg/kg, increase by 2.5 mg weekly, if needed, to a maximum of 30 mg/day divided bid/tid
	5-, 10-, 15-mg spansules (SR)	6–8 h	Once daily
Mixed amphetamine salts (Adderall)	5-, 10-, 20-, 30-mg tablets	4–8 h	2.5 mg–30 mg qd or bid
Pemoline (Cylert)	18.75-mg tablets	5–6 h	>6 y old, 37.5 mg/day-given qam or bid; if needed, increase at 18.75-mg intervals to 112.5 mg/day

Has he missed much school?

Frequent absences can result in a lack of exposure to classroom material and academic difficulty. Absences without medical problems might represent a school avoidance problem that needs to be addressed.

Are there certain subjects that are most difficult?

A child who is having difficulty in all subjects might have cognitive problems such as mild mental retardation or low normal intelligence. A child with problems in specific subject areas is more likely to have a learning disability.

How is everything else at home?

Families undergoing significant change, such as divorce or chronic illness, can have negative effects on the child's school performance.

The differential diagnosis of the child with school failure includes low cognitive abilities, learning disabilities, problems with the home or school environment, and chronic illness. Most often, the physician's role is to screen for medical conditions that might be compromising the child's ability to learn, such as vision and hearing problems or presence of an attention disorder. Accurate diagnosis of a child's learning problems will require psychological testing, which should include general intelligence testing, achievement testing, and projective testing to assess any emotional issues.

For over a quarter of a century, the federal government has identified children with learning disabilities as being entitled to an appropriate education. As a result, psychoeducational evaluations are performed by the public school systems. Such assessments, commonly referred to as *multifactored evaluations,* will assess for learning disabilities, speech and language skills, motor skills, and other areas as suggested by the child's history and presenting symptoms. The treatment of educational problems lies in the educational domain. There are no effective medications for any of the learning disabilities or low intelligence. The pediatrician's role is one of supporting and advising the family and helping to optimize development.

The Gifted Child

In addition to identifying children with learning disabilities, the identification of children with exceptional abilities has begun to make headway in the educational system. The concept of the gifted child encompasses more than exceptional intelligence. The gifted child has a combination of above-average skill, creativity, and ability to stay on task, thereby accomplishing activities well beyond those of other school children. This three-factor model is an important one to remember, as many parents of bright children consider them gifted based on IQ alone. Gifted children generally are not identified until school age, at which time they are achieving beyond their peers and demonstrating additional skills and abilities. In retrospect, many of them achieved higher cognitive skills early, such as early language or reading. However, this is not always the case. More important than past milestones is the status of current achievement.

As with the child with learning disabilities, the physician's role in managing the gifted child is to support and advocate for services that will promote optimal development. Parents should be advised not to push their child because these children generally have enough intrinsic motivation. Instead, the parents should be supportive and minimize roadblocks to the child's activities. They do not need to provide additional stimulation so much as they need to provide a fertile environment in which the child can grow and develop.

Sibling rivalries can pose problems in families with gifted children. Parents should be advised to emphasize that each family member has unique strengths and qualities, and that all are loved and appreciated in the family.

REFERENCES

American Psychiatric Association: *Diagnostic and Statistical Manual of Mental Disorders,* 4th ed. Washington, DC: American Psychiatric Association, 1994.

Elia J et al: Treatment of attention-deficit hyperactivity disorder. N Engl J Med 1999;340:780–788.

Levine MD et al: *Developmental-Behavioral Pediatrics,* 3rd ed. Philadelphia: WB Saunders, 1999.

Loening-Baucke V. Encopresis and soiling. Pediatr Clin North Am 1996;43:279–298.

Schmitt BD: Nocturnal enuresis. Pediatr Rev 1997;18:183–190.

Wolraich ML et al (editors): *The Classification of Child and Adolescent Diagnoses in Primary Care: Diagnostic and Statistical Manual for Primary Care (DSM-PC) Child and Adolescent Version.* Elk Grove Village: American Academy of Pediatrics, 1996.

Zametkin AJ, Ernst M: Problems in the management of attention-deficit hyperactivity disorder. N Engl J Med 1999;340:40–46.

The Perinatal Period

4

Augusto Sola, MD, Marta R. Rogido, MD, & John Colin Partridge, MD, MPH

■ PERINATAL HISTORY

The care of the newborn, in particular the sick newborn, has evolved significantly over the past 20 years. Eighty percent to 90% of infants admitted to hospitals in the United States are healthy. Nonetheless, the neonatal period is important because many conditions that originate during this period can have a major impact, not only on infant mortality but also on future development of the infant.

Infant mortality, the death of infants from birth to 12 months of age, is now fewer than 7 per 1000 live births in the United States. More than 60% of these deaths occur during the neonatal period; the more frequent causes of neonatal death are perinatal asphyxia, prematurity, respiratory distress syndrome (RDS), congenital malformations, and infections. Infant mortality is inversely proportionate to birth weight. Even though the specific rate of infant mortality for any birth weight category under 2500 g is lower for blacks than for whites, the overall mortality among black infants is twice that among white infants because of the higher percentage of black low-birth-weight (LBW) infants. The interplay between multiple factors—environmental, behavioral, psychosocial, biologic, and clinical—affects birth weight and prematurity.

Morbidity is also higher in the neonatal period than during the first 12 months of life. Many neurologic abnormalities that manifest themselves during infancy or childhood, such as hearing deficits, vision deficits, cerebral palsy, and mental retardation, are secondary to injuries to the nervous system that occurred during labor and delivery or during the neonatal period.

At the time of birth, many physiologic changes must occur for the fetus to adapt from intrauterine to extrauterine life. Among these changes, the most immediate is the transfer of the function of gas exchange (oxygen uptake and carbon dioxide removal) from the placenta to the lungs. This requires that rhythmic ventilation of the lungs and an adequate pulmonary blood flow be established.

To evaluate the newborn completely, a detailed prenatal history should be elicited (Table 4–1); this includes paternal and maternal histories and a history of the neonate during intrauterine life. Risks to a neonate often can be identified during pregnancy or labor. About 20% of all pregnancies are considered to be "high risk," and they account for approximately 55% of fetal and neonatal (perinatal) morbidity and mortality. An additional 10% of high-risk infants can be identified during labor and represent 20–25% of perinatal morbidity and mortality. Thus, 75–80% of perinatal morbidity and mortality could be identified before birth; the remainder occurs with apparently normal pregnancy and labor.

■ ADAPTATION TO BIRTH

EFFECTS OF LABOR

During labor, repetitive stresses are placed on the fetus because uterine contraction temporarily reduces uterine blood flow, thus interfering with oxygen supply to the fetus. The more severe and prolonged the contraction, the greater is the effect on oxygen delivery. Although the normal fetus can tolerate considerable reductions in oxygen delivery for fairly prolonged periods, labor may have a deleterious effect on the fetus that is already compromised because the placenta is abnormal or because the mother has a condition further influencing uterine blood flow. Fetal hypoxemia and acidemia develop, resulting in changes in fetal heart rate, blood pressure, and distribution of blood flow to the fetal body and organs. Uterine contraction during labor also can produce adverse effects on the fetus by causing head compression in the pelvis and, possibly, by compressing the umbilical cord if it is in the pelvis.

Fetal bradycardia occurs during uterine contraction, probably because of chemoreceptor stimulation by the hypoxemia or because of head compression if the fetal head is in the pelvis. Although deaths before labor outnumber those occurring during labor by approximately 3 : 1, no other comparable period contributes as heavily to fetal mortality and morbidity. The occurrence of intrapartum fetal deaths is usually stated as 1.5–4 per 1000 fetuses, but a specific cause can be identified in only about 50% of cases. Fetal scalp blood sampling to measure acid–base status and continuous monitoring of fetal heart rate and uterine contractions have been useful in assessing fetal well-being during labor. Recently, Doppler ultrasound studies of umbilical blood flow velocity and cerebral arterial blood flow, percutaneous blood sampling from the umbilical cord, and fetal electrocardiographic (ECG) changes have contributed significantly to fetal assessment.

125

Table 4–1. Neonatal Risks Associated With Various Prenatal and Perinatal Factors

Family history
  Genetic abnormalities, congenital malformations, multiple pregnancies
 	
History before this pregnancy
  Lower socioeconomic class: Prematurity, fetal growth retardation, infection
  Maternal history: Diabetes; infections; hypertension; renal, cardiovascular, or pulmonary disease; smoking; alcohol intake; medications; street drugs; Rh disease
  Maternal age: Adolescent, fetal growth retardation; older age (>36 y), chromosomal anomalies
  Previous pregnancies: Abortions, prematurity, neonatal deaths, malformations
 	
History of labor and delivery
  Medications during labor: Prolonged anesthesia or analgesia may cause hypotension, hypothermia, CNS or respiratory depression
  Prolonged labor: Fetal distress, trauma, or death
  Rapid labor and delivery: Hemorrhage, trauma
  Cord prolapse, tight nuchal cord, real knot of the cord: Fetal distress, anemia, death
  Uterine tetany: Fetal distress, death
  Abnormal signs of fetal well-being (ultrasound, fetal monitoring, scalp pH): Fetal distress, death
  Meconium-stained amniotic fluid: Fetal distress, intrapartum death, meconium aspiration syndrome, persistent pulmonary hypertension syndrome
  Premature birth: All problems associated with prematurity
  Post-term birth: Fetal distress, meconium, hypoglycemia, polycythernia, hyperthermia, prenatal or postnatal death
	History of this pregnancy
	  Prenatal visits: Optimum is 8–10
	  Urinary tract infection: Prematurity, neonatal sepsis
	  Hemorrhage: Prematurity, fetal distress, fetal death, neonatal anemia
	  Isoimmunization (Rh and others): Fetal death, fetal hydrops, neonatal anemia, hyperbilirubinemia
	  Prolonged rupture of membranes: Chorioamnionitis, prematurity, neonatal sepsis, oligohydramnios, pulmonary hypoplasia
	  Multiple pregnancy: Prematurity, fetal growth retardation, fetal distress, anemia, hypovolemia, obstetric trauma
	  Medications during pregnancy: Many congenital anomalies can be ascribed to various drugs (see Chapter 5)
	  Polyhydramnios: Anencephaly, gastrointestinal obstruction, omphalocele, gastroschisis, renal tumors, fetal hydrops, chromosomal abnormalities, diaphragmatic hernia, fetal anemia
	  Oligohydramnios: Placental insufficiency, renal malformations, fetal growth retardation, pulmonary hypoplasia
	  Abnormal fetal position: Cord prolapse, placenta previa, obstetric trauma, congenital malformations
	  Decreased fetal growth: Small-for-gestational-age infants, congenital malformations
	  Increased fetal growth: Obstetric trauma, neonatal hypoglycemia, polycythernia, infant of diabetic mother, congenital malformations
	  Decreased fetal movements: Death before or during labor, CNS and neuromuscular diseases

CNS = central nervous system.

Drugs administered to the mother during labor can have significant effects on both the fetus and on the newborn infant. Ritodrine, a β_2-receptor antagonist, can decrease uterine blood flow and cause fetal tachycardia. Magnesium sulfate tocolysis, used to inhibit uterine contractions during premature labor, can induce vasodilatation, hypotonia, hyporeflexia, and apnea in the neonate. However, it also can provide some protection for serious, long-term neurologic abnormalities.

Indomethacin therapy for premature labor has been shown to cause constriction of the ductus arteriosus in approximately 50% of fetuses. Local anesthetics used for epidural analgesia are rapidly transferred across the maternal circulation to the fetus and may cause fetal or neonatal seizures. In addition, most analgesic or hypnotic drugs administered to the mother cross the placenta and may result in central nervous system (CNS) depression in the newborn, with respiratory compromise.

TRANSITION TO NEONATAL LIFE

In most cases, the fetus changes from the intrauterine environment to the extrauterine one and becomes a normal neonate without any difficulty. However, this transition is a fairly complex physiologic process involving many changes in organ and system function. The most significant of these changes are summarized in Table 4–2. The most important fetal physiologic functions necessary for normal growth and development are to pump blood to the placenta and to collaborate in some endocrine functions. Most of the organic functions, such as respiration, nutrition, metabolism, excretion, and even defense against infection, are performed by the placenta and the mother. To survive after birth it is mandatory that the neonate, regardless of degree of maturity, adapts satisfactorily to the new demands that are imposed by the extrauterine environment.

Table 4–2. Changes During
Fetal–Neonatal Transition

Cord clamping
  Placental circulation disappears
  Hormonal concentrations increase
  Peripheral vascular resistance increases

Breathing
  Increased alveolar P_{O_2}
  Release of vasoactive substances
  Decrease of pulmonary vascular resistance
  Increase of pulmonary blood flow

Decrease of pulmonary fluid
  During labor and after birth; mostly through capillary
    circulation

Circulatory changes
  Closure of ductus arteriosus: Bidirectional shunt initially
    followed by functional closure and complete closure
    (term neonate, 10–12 d for anatomic closure)
  Closure of foramen ovale: Immediate closure due to
    changes in right and left atrial pressures
  Closure of ductus venosus: Closes within 2–7 d after birth

Endocrine changes
  Increase in catecholamine concentration
  Increase in vasopressin and renin–angiotensin
    concentrations
  Decrease in prostaglandin concentration

INTRAUTERINE STATUS

Early in pregnancy, the lungs start to produce a fluid similar to plasma but with significantly less protein. Toward the end of gestation, the volume of this lung fluid is approximately the same as the functional residual capacity found soon after extrauterine spontaneous respirations (30–35 mL/kg). The secretion of pulmonary fluid decreases during the hours that precede birth. During labor, a significant portion of this fluid is resorbed into the circulation in preparation for birth; this resorption of fluid continues after birth. The lymphatic drainage of this fluid is minimal, as is the quantity of fetal pulmonary fluid that is eliminated through the compression of the thorax during the fetal passage across the birth canal. In birth by cesarean section without preceding labor, plasma colloid oncotic pressure is low. Infants born by cesarean section without labor do not reabsorb pulmonary fluid as rapidly as those born by vaginal delivery or those born by cesarean section after preceding labor. In some infants, this slow resorption of fetal lung fluid causes transient respiratory distress.

The fetus exhibits rapid, oscillatory thoracic respiratory movements in utero. These movements are impor-
tant for adequate lung growth and development. Fetal breathing movements are a useful clinical tool to assess fetal well-being (respiratory activity increases after meals or administration of glucose to the mother): Smoking and alcohol intake decrease fetal breathing movements.

The fetal circulation and its changes after birth are discussed in Chapter 17.

PULMONARY ADAPTATION AFTER BIRTH

Respiratory movements after birth appear in response to multiple stimuli. During normal labor, partial pressure of arterial carbon dioxide ($PaCO_2$) increases modestly, and partial pressure of arterial oxygen (PaO_2) and serum pH decrease. Through the peripheral and central chemoreceptors, there is stimulation of the respiratory center. Further, there are sensory stimuli from light and noise, pressure at various sites of the body, and a rapid decrease in body temperature. The first inspiration originated by a rapid descent of the diaphragm generates a negative intrapleural pressure of approximately 35–40 cm of water. These initial high transpulmonary pressures are needed to overcome the resistance generated by the elevated surface tension at the air–fluid interface and the high viscosity of the fluid that fills the airways. In addition, those negative pressures cause alveolar fluid to move into the interstitial space. For air to be distributed appropriately in the lung and for a normal functional residual capacity to develop, surface tension in the alveoli needs to be low, and the pulmonary fluid has to be eliminated. Pulmonary surfactant decreases surface tension during expiration, thereby maintaining alveolar stability and avoiding collapse; subsequent inspirations therefore require significantly less transpulmonary pressures. The lack of surfactant causes RDS or hyaline membrane disease (HMD), in which alveolar stability is decreased and interstitial fluid passes into the alveoli.

Expansion of the lungs and removal of alveolar fluid significantly decrease pulmonary vascular resistance. Mechanical expansion of the lung causes a decrease of pulmonary vascular resistance by release of prostaglandin I_2 (PGI_2; prostacyclin). Oxygen or air causes pulmonary vasodilation through release of endothelial-relaxing factor (EDRF), or nitric oxide (NO). This release induces a massive increase in pulmonary blood flow. Simultaneously, systemic pressure increases as a result of umbilical cord clamping, release of hormones, and possibly other mechanisms. During fetal life, pulmonary blood flow is low (approximately 20 mL/[kg/min]) and increases 5–10 times with adequate alveolar ventilation after birth. When pulmonary vascular resistance does not decrease and the normal increase in pulmonary blood flow does not occur after birth, the infant is said to have the syndrome of persistent pulmonary hypertension of the neonate (PPHN), or **persistent fetal circulation.**

PERINATAL ENDOCRINE RESPONSES

Concentrations of several hormones increase during the transition from the intrauterine to extrauterine environment. This increase might be due to physiologic stress secondary to the mild to moderate fetal hypoxia, uterine contractions, and compression of the fetal head in the birth canal. These hormonal responses may help the fetus to tolerate the stress of labor and promote neonatal adaptation to the extrauterine environment.

Corticotrophic hormone and glucocorticoid concentrations increase 2–3 days before birth in some species, and this increase probably is responsible for maturation of many enzyme systems. During labor, antidiuretic hormone (vasopressin) and renin and angiotensin concentrations increase; these hormones assist in achieving the increase in vascular resistance that occurs after birth.

Catecholamine concentrations increase after birth. The fetus responds to stress with an increase in norepinephrine concentrations, with a minor increase in epinephrine concentrations. Catecholamines are important in increasing the energy supply for maintenance of body temperature after birth by stimulating release of fatty acids into the circulation from brown fat. Furthermore catecholamines stimulate the conversion of T_4 to T_3. Thyroid stimulating hormone (TSH) increases in concentration at the time of birth because of an increase in thyrotrophin releasing hormone (TRH). The increase in TRH is mediated through α-adrenergic stimulation. TSH concentrations return to low basal levels within 2–3 days after birth. In congenital hypothyroidism, when concentrations of thyroid hormones are low, TSH levels remain elevated. Growing preterm infants, with low metabolic rates, have lower than normal serum concentrations of T_4 and T_3 but their TSH concentrations are not elevated. This is usually a transient, self-resolving condition; in some instances, however, treatment with thyroid hormones is indicated to avoid poor long-term outcome.

TEMPERATURE REGULATION

In the intrauterine environment, the fetus does not need to produce heat to maintain body temperature. The fetus is surrounded by amniotic fluid with a temperature only 0.2°C less than fetal body temperature. Thus, there are no losses by radiation or evaporation, and losses of heat by conduction and convection from the fetal skin are minimal. Fetal temperature does not increase because heat produced is lost by convection through blood flow in the placenta. A decrease of placental blood flow can produce an increase in fetal temperature. This may occur in small-for-gestational-age (SGA) infants who have low placental blood flows and, as a result, are often born with rectal temperatures of 38.0–38.5°C. Fetal temperature may also increase with maternal fever because heat loss to the mother is reduced. The fetus does not possess defense mechanisms against temperature increases, and severe prolonged maternal hyperthermia could be dangerous for fetal survival and development.

Thermal instability of newborn & premature infants. Environments with temperatures that are comfortable for adults may be inappropriate for newborn infants. At 22°C (72°F) there is a significant and rapid decrease in the neonate's body temperature because neonates lose heat easily and have limited ability to increase heat production in cold environments. Part of the rapid heat loss is associated with their large body surface to body volume ratio. A term infant with a birth weight of 3 kg has a body surface to body volume ratio three times greater than that of an adult, and a premature infant with birth weight of 1500 g has a ratio four times greater. The neonate also has thinner skin and subcutaneous fat layer; this is even more marked in premature infants. The skin of the newborn and premature infant has greater thermal conductance than that of the adult; they consequently lose more heat per unit of surface area than does the adult.

In addition to producing heat by movement, as in the adult, the neonate has a well-developed mechanism to increase the production of heat in cool environments through energy metabolism in brown fat. Nevertheless, the thermal-regulating ability of the neonate is less efficient than in the adult and can be impaired further by hypoxia, sedatives, and anesthetic drugs. In suboptimal environments, newborn body temperature can decrease rapidly (up to 0.3°C/min), reaching 33–35°C. Therefore, newborn infants should be kept in a **neutral thermal environment,** which is defined as that environment in which heat losses are equivalent to the minimum metabolic needs of the infant. In this environment, oxygen consumption is minimal, as is the thermal regulatory water loss. This environment usually is achieved with a relative humidity of 50% and an environmental temperature of 31–34°C when the infant is naked. When the infant is dressed, the necessary environmental temperature is about 25°C in term infants. The level of neutral thermal environmental temperature decreases with postnatal age and is always higher in infants of lower gestational age.

Infants exposed to temperatures below the neutral thermal environment might have cold stress, which induces increased oxygen consumption and elevated circulating catecholamine concentrations. Cold stress may cause a rapid decline in a neonate's health status (Table 4–3). To prevent cold stress, infants should be dried immediately after birth, with particular attention to the head and face, which represent a large proportion of total body surface area. Body temperature should be checked soon after birth, at least twice in the first hour and then every 1–2 hours in the first 8 hours. During physical examination, the neonate should not be placed on a cold surface or exposed to air conditioning or air currents. A radiant source of heat should be used if the environment is not warm enough. Normal neonatal body temperature should be 36–37.5°C.

Table 4–3. Effects of Cold Stress

Increased O$_2$ consumption	Increased circulating
Increased fat metabolism	catecholamines
Increased surfactant	Increased fatty acids
consumption	Metabolic acidosis
Hypoxia	Hypoglycemia
Pulmonary vasoconstriction	Peripheral vasoconstriction
Persistent pulmonary	Apnea
hypertension	Cyanosis
Respiratory distress	

The neonate also should not be exposed to environments in which the temperature is much higher than neutral thermal environment. Newborn infants cannot lose heat efficiently; premature neonates cannot sweat, and full-term neonates have limited capacities to perspire. Therefore, with temperatures above the neutral thermal environment, skin temperature increases. Environmental hyperthermia is a common cause of hyperthermia in the neonate; usually rectal temperature does not increase significantly. Thus, rectal temperature is a useful parameter in excluding nonenvironmental causes of hyperthermia. Neonates lose large amounts of water through their thin skin by evaporation and, if exposed to heat, can become dehydrated.

■ ASSESSMENT OF NEWBORNS

Apgar Scores

In 1953, Virginia Apgar introduced a simple, systematic assessment of intrapartum stress and neurologic depression at birth. Five variables—heart rate, respiratory effort, muscle tone, reflex irritability, and color—are evaluated at 1 and 5 minutes after birth, and each one is scored from 0 to 2, as described in Table 4–4A. The final score is the sum of the five individual scores, with 10 representing the optimal score. Although the Apgar score is useful in evaluating the acute status of the infant at birth, it has limitations because several factors other than asphyxia can affect the score; these are summarized in Table 4–4B. Regardless of the cause, a persistent, very low score indicates the need for resuscitation. Scoring should continue every 5 minutes until a final score of 7 or more is reached.

The Apgar score should not be used to establish long-term prognosis. Only the clinical neurologic status at the time of hospital discharge has been clearly associated with poor prognosis related to asphyxial encephalopathy.

Maturity Gestational Age

Several clinical methods have been used to assess gestational age in the neonate on the basis of external physical

Table 4–4A. Apgar Scoring System

	Score		
Variable	**0**	**1**	**2**
Heart rate	Absent	<100 beats/min	>100 beats/min
Respiratory effort	Absent	Slow, irregular	Good, crying
Muscle tone	Limp	Some flexion of extremities	Active motion
Reflex irritability (in response to catheter in nose)	Absent	Grimace	Grimace and cough or sneeze
Color	Blue, pale	Body pink, extremities blue (acrocyanosis)	Completely pink

From Apgar A: A proposal for a new method of evaluation of the newborn infant. *Curr Res Anesthesiol* 1953;32:260.

characteristics and neuromuscular evaluation. Although there may be an error of 1–2 weeks, trained and experienced physicians can closely estimate gestational age. External characteristics include the plantar creases, skin texture, skin opacity, lanugo, nipple formation and breast size, and evaluation of the ears and genitalia. Neurologic status is not always easy to evaluate and can change in relation to the state of the infant (quiet sleep, crying, etc), if there is CNS depression due to drugs or asphyxia or the infant is critically ill. Ballard devised a simplified method that includes six parameters of neuromuscular maturation and six physical characteristics (Figure 4–1). Each

Table 4–4B. Causes of Low Apgar Scores

Asphyxia
Maternal drugs: Anesthetics, sedatives, opiates, drugs of abuse
Central nervous system disease
Congenital muscular disease
Prematurity
Fetal sepsis

Neuromuscular maturity

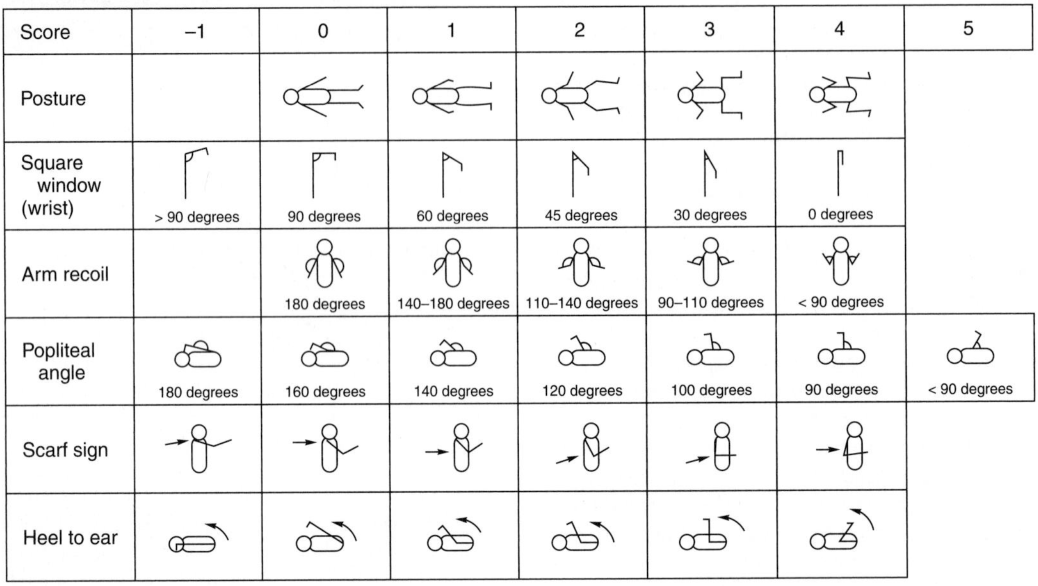

Score	−1	0	1	2	3	4	5
Posture							
Square window (wrist)	> 90 degrees	90 degrees	60 degrees	45 degrees	30 degrees	0 degrees	
Arm recoil		180 degrees	140–180 degrees	110–140 degrees	90–110 degrees	< 90 degrees	
Popliteal angle	180 degrees	160 degrees	140 degrees	120 degrees	100 degrees	90 degrees	< 90 degrees
Scarf sign							
Heel to ear							

Physical maturity

Score	−1	0	1	2	3	4	5
Skin	Sticky, friable, transparent	Gelatinous, red, translucent	Smooth pink, visible veins	Superficial peeling or rash, few veins	Cracking, pale areas, rare veins	Parchment, deep cracking, no vessels	Leathery, cracked, wrinkled
Lanugo	None	Sparse	Abundant	Thinning	Bald areas	Mostly bald	
Plantar surface	Heel–toe 40–50 mm: −1 < 40 mm: −2	> 50 mm no crease	Faint red marks	Anterior transverse crease only	Creases anterior two thirds	Creases over entire sole	
Breast	Imperceptible	Barely perceptible	Flat areola, no bud	Stippled areola, 1–2 mm bud	Raised areola, 3–4 mm bud	Full areola, 5–10 mm bud	
Eye/ear	Lids fused Loosely: −1 Tightly: −2	Lids open, pinna flat, stays folded	Slightly curved pinna; soft; slow recoil	Well-curved pinna; soft but ready recoil	Formed and firm; instant recoil	Thick cartilage, ear stiff	
Genitals (male)	Scrotum flat, smooth	Scrotum empty, faint rugae	Testes in upper canal, rare rugae	Testes descending, few rugae	Testes down, good rugae	Testes pendulous, deep rugae	
Genitals (female)	Clitoris prominent, labia flat	Clitoris prominent, small labia minora	Clitoris prominent, enlarging minora	Majora and minora equally prominent	Majora large, minora small	Majora covers clitoris and minora	

Maturity rating

Score	−10	−5	0	5	10	15	20	25	30	35	40	45	50
Weeks	20	22	24	26	28	30	32	34	36	38	40	42	44

Figure 4–1. Newborn maturity rating and classification. (Adapted from Ballard JL, et al: New Ballard Score, expanded to include extremely premature infants. *Pediatr* 1991;119:417.)

receives an individual score; gestational age is determined from the sum of these scores. When the gestational age—determined from the first day of the last menstrual period—is 37–42 weeks (259–294 days), the newborn infant is considered to be at term. **Preterm** infants are those with less than 37 completed weeks (<258 days), and **postterm** infants those with gestational age greater than 42 weeks (>294 days).

Normal weight, length, and skull circumference at different gestational ages are shown in Figure 4–2. When fetuses grow normally, birth weight for a particular gestational age lies within 2 SD of the mean, and the infant is considered **appropriate for gestational age (AGA).** Infants can be born preterm, at term, or postterm and be AGA. **Small for gestational age (SGA)** is defined as birth weight less than 2 SD below the mean, and it suggests intrauterine growth retardation. **Large for gestational age (LGA)** is defined as birth weight greater than 2 SD above the mean. Infants born at term with appropriate weight for gestational age have the lowest neonatal risk. Morbidity and mortality rates are higher with LGA and SGA infants (see section entitled 'Abnormalities of growth' in this chapter).

Regardless of gestational age, an infant with a birth weight less than 2500 g is considered an LBW infant. An LBW infant (e.g., 2000 g) can be AGA, SGA, or LGA, according to the gestational age at birth. Infants born at less than 1500 g are considered **very-low-birth-weight (VLBW),** and infants born at less than 1000 g are considered **extremely low-birth-weight (ELBW).** By definition, regardless of gestational age, an infant with a birth weight greater than 4000 g is considered a high-birth-weight infant. As discussed later, infants with abnormalities of **maturity** (premature or postmature infants) are clinically very different from infants who have abnormalities of **growth** (SGA and LGA infants).

Physical Examination of the Newborn Infant

INITIAL EVALUATION

The changes in practice that have led to early hospital discharge of mothers and newborn infants after birth pose a new challenge to pediatricians, namely how to make sure that the newborn is healthy. When the newborn's health cannot be ensured by observation and detailed physical examination at different postnatal ages in the hospital, arrangements must be made for providing the same outside the hospital setting. The transitional period from fetal to neonatal life is one of many changes. Some abnormal conditions can and must be recognized during this period to improve outcome, but others will not become apparent until later. For these reasons, there is a need to observe and examine newborn infants, as summarized in Table 4–5 and described in the subsequent section. The

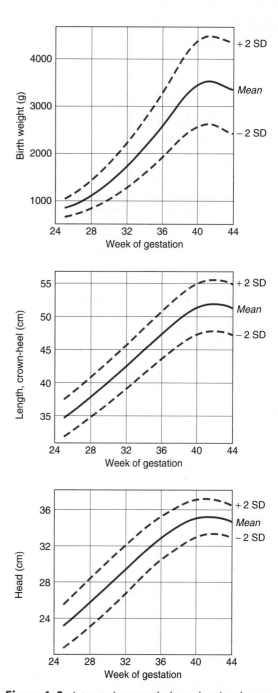

Figure 4–2. Intrauterine growth charts showing the normal values of body weight, length, and head circumference for infants born at different gestational ages at sea level (Montreal). (Data from Usher R, McLean F: Intrauterine growth of live-born Caucasian infants at sea level: Standards obtained from measurements in 7 dimensions of infants born between 25 and 44 weeks of gestation. *J Pediatr* 1969;74:901).

Table 4–5. Observation and Examination of
Newborns During the First Postnatal Week

Initial examination at birth
Apgar scores
Rule out major anomalies that are detectable at birth, e.g.,
choanal atresia, major limb defects, omphalocele, congenital diaphragmatic hernia, meningomyelocele, anal
atresia, ambiguous genitalia, hypospadias
Detailed observation: skin, craniofacial, neck, chest, back,
extremities; rule out cyanosis and respiratory distress
Vital signs: length, weight, head circumference

Detailed examination: first 6–12 h after birth
Include all details of neonatal examination, from craniofacial
to extremities; establish successful early transition; rule
out early jaundice, gastrointestinal obstructions, abdominal masses, hip abnormalities, some cardiac diseases;
verify pulses in lower extremities

Another detailed examination: 36–48 h
Same as before; rule out exaggerated jaundice and weight
loss; complete neurologic examination if not done before

Observation at 72–96 h
Appropriate weight loss and intake; rule out exaggerated
jaundice; check pulses in lower extremities, vital signs

Another detailed examination: 6–10 d
Include neurologic examination

---

neurologic examination completes the evaluation of the
infant.

In the first few minutes after birth, a partial physical
examination is performed when Apgar scores are assigned.
Subsequently, within 24 hours after birth, a detailed
physical examination must be performed to confirm the
presence or absence of congenital malformations, traumatic injuries, or any other manifestation of neonatal disease. Before the first physical examination at birth, one
should be familiar with the prenatal and perinatal histories. The examination should be performed after the
infant has been dried and stabilized; heat loss should be
minimized during this examination.

SPECIFIC FINDINGS

General appearance. The general appearance of the
neonate is observed to assess spontaneous activity, passive
muscle tone, respirations, and abnormal signs such as cyanosis, retractions, or meconium staining. Vital signs should
be included in the examination, and accurate measurements of weight, length, and head circumference are plotted according to gestational age to determine whether the
infant is appropriately grown (Table 4–5).

Skin. Skin texture differs with gestational age, being
softer and thinner in premature infants. Postterm infants

can have dry, scaly skin. The skin is covered with lanugo
hair in preterm infants; this is minimally present in term
babies. The skin may be covered in some areas by **vernix
caseosa,** a thick, white, creamy material in term babies.
In preterm infants, vernix caseosa covers large areas of the
skin; it is absent in postterm infants. The normal color of
the skin a few hours after birth is pink, but **acrocyanosis**
(cyanosis of the hands and feet) is frequent during the
first 48 hours and can last in some babies throughout the
first month of life, particularly when the infant is cold.
Acrocyanosis and **cutis marmorata** (mottling of the skin
with venous prominence) are frequent intermittent signs
of the vasomotor instability characteristic of some infants. However, mottling could be a serious sign in some
instances, such as with infection. Pallor can be a sign of
neonatal asphyxia, shock, or chronic anemia. Jaundice is
always abnormal if detected within the first 24 hours after
birth. Subsequently, it is frequently seen during the first
few days after birth but usually is not associated with serious disease.

Mongolian spots, dark blue areas over the lumbosacral area and buttocks, are transient, hyperpigmented
macules that have no pathologic significance and occur
predominantly in Asians, blacks, and Latinos. **Erythema
toxicum,** a rash resembling flea bites, is noted in up to
50% of full-term infants but is found much less frequently in preterm infants. It can be found on the trunk,
on the arms and legs, but not on soles and palms. It occurs
more frequently in the first 72 hours after birth but can
last up to 10–15 days. No treatment is required. **Milia,**
tiny, whitish papules that are seen over the nose, cheeks,
forehead, and chin, are very small cysts formed around
the pilosebaceous follicles or sudoriparous glands. The
condition is frequent and usually disappears in a few weeks
without treatment.

"Birth marks," or **nevus simplex,** are pink macular
hemangiomas on the neck, upper lip, and eyelids and
above the nose. They are usually transient. Capillary
hemangiomas of more significance are the so-called port-
wine stains, or **nevus flammeus.** These are usually located over the face and trunk, become darker with advancing postnatal age, and may be associated with intracranial
or spinal vascular malformations, seizures, and intracranial calcifications. **Cavernous hemangiomas** occur in
approximately 10% of infants and are often first noticed
a few days after birth. They increase in size after birth and
usually resolve within 18–24 months (see Chapter 12).
Pustular melanosis consists of small, dry vesicles over a
dark macular base. These are also benign lesions, which
occur more frequently in black infants, but must be differentiated from viral infections, such as herpes simplex,
or bacterial infections, such as impetigo.

Craniofacial. The skull may show molding; this is seen
particularly after prolonged labor with vertex presentation,
in which the vertical diameter of the head becomes elon-

gated and the parietooccipital area becomes prominent. **Caput succedaneum** is diffuse edema or the swelling of the soft tissue of the scalp that crosses the cranial sutures and usually the midline. With bruising, the area of caput will have a bluish discoloration. Caput succedaneum usually disappears in 2–3 days, and molding in 5–6 days. In general, head circumference immediately after birth is 1–2 cm different than it is 3–4 days later. **Cephalhematomas** are subperiosteal hemorrhages, usually involving the parietal or occipital bones. The head is typically elongated in its anterior posterior diameter in breech presentation and fairly round in those infants born by cesarean section without labor. The posterior portion of the skull often is depressed in infants born by persistent occipitoposterior delivery.

The **anterior fontanelle** is situated between the coronal and sagittal sutures, has a diamond shape, and measures approximately 1.5–2 × 1.5–2 cm. At birth, the anterior fontanelle might not be evident because of overriding of skull sutures or, less often, an abnormality such as premature fusion of the sutures or cranial synostosis. Causes of large fontanelles are listed in Table 4–6. Infants with intrauterine growth retardation (IUGR), in whom the skull grows more slowly than the brain tissue, may show widely split sutures and large fontanelles. These findings may become more noticeable a few days or weeks after birth. This does not represent an abnormality and does not indicate hydrocephalus. The posterior fontanelle, located between the sagittal and lambdoid sutures, is usually barely palpable at birth. In some infants, the metopic suture can be felt over the frontal bone as an extension of the sagittal suture.

A head circumference below the 10th percentile can be due to a familial trait but can represent fetal–neonatal pathology (Table 4–7). **Craniotabes,** soft areas with a ping-pong ball feel, may occur in the parietal bones parasagittally; they are not related to rickets and disappear in weeks or months. In infants in whom a scalp electrode was applied for intrauterine monitoring during labor, this area should be inspected carefully and cleaned appropriately. Other signs of trauma or lacerations should be detected at the time of birth.

The face should be examined in detail. The infant delivered by a face presentation might have edema of the eyelids and face, and, if bruising is severe, an ecchymotic mask may be present. This feature also might be present

Table 4–6. Causes of Large Fontanelle

Hydrocephalus	Osteogenesis imperfecta
Rickets	Cleidocranial dysplasia
Hypothyroidism	Hypophosphatasia
Achondroplasia	Intrauterine growth retardation

Table 4–7. Causes of Neonatal Microcephaly

Familial: Autosomal dominant trait (normal intelligence); autosomal recessive; X-linked (e.g., Paine syndrome)
Structural brain malformations (i.e., lissencephaly)
Chromosomal and malformation syndrome (e.g., trisomy 13, deLange syndrome)
Maternal: Radiation exposure, alcoholism, phenylketonuria, infections (toxoplasmosis, cytomegalovirus)
Posthypoxic encephalopathy

in infants who have had the umbilical cord wrapped tightly around the neck. The presence of dysmorphic features allows for diagnosis of genetic anomalies or classic chromosomal syndromes (see Chapter 5). An asymmetric facies may be due to seventh cranial nerve palsy or, if the asymmetry occurs only with crying, to congenital absence or hypotonia of the depressor muscle at the angle of the mouth.

Ears. The ears should be examined to assess maturity. By term, the ears are firm and have assumed their characteristic shape. Low-set ears can be normal but frequently are a feature of genetic syndromes. Normal infants hear at birth and may startle or have a complete Moro reflex with a sudden noise. The ears should also be inspected for preauricular tags or sinuses.

Eyes. The eyes open spontaneously soon after birth, particularly when the infant is awake and in the upright position. After several hours, the eyelids might develop edema, which can make spontaneous opening difficult. Subconjunctival hemorrhage due to rupture of scleral capillaries is common and results from compression of the head during labor and delivery; the lesion disappears in a few weeks. Epicanthal folds, slanted palpebral fissures, and hypertelorism may be normal variations; however, they should alert the examiner to the possibility of other anomalies. Nystagmus or fixed strabismus should be excluded; the pupils should be symmetric and respond to light.

The iris, in general, is hypopigmented at birth, often presenting a grayish or bluish color. By 6 months of age, the eyes of most infants have a more definite color. The iris should be examined to rule out coloboma, which may be associated with intrauterine infections or malformations.

Aniridia is rare but may be associated with Wilms' tumor. Nonfixed strabismus that persists more than 30–45 days requires careful ophthalmologic evaluation. Microphthalmia suggests other malformations or intrauterine infections such as rubella or toxoplasmosis.

A mucous ocular drainage is common in the first 2 days after birth; it should not be confused with conjunctivitis. However, if the eyelids are swollen and red, ocular infection is likely. Constant tearing a few days after birth usually represents a blockage of the nasolacrimal duct. In general, this resolves spontaneously; however, sometimes recurrent conjunctival infections develop, and probing of the duct is necessary.

The red reflex of the retina is easily observed when examining with the ophthalmoscope 10–20 cm from the infant's eye. If there is obstruction to the passage of light, the red reflex will not be seen, and a white reflex will be present. This is abnormal and may be due to corneal opacification, crystalline opacification (cataracts), retinoblastoma, or severe chorioretinitis; if it appears a few weeks after birth, it might be due to retinopathy of prematurity.

Cataracts, in which the iris is seen clearly and the pupil appears whitish, are frequent in congenital rubella and other intrauterine infections. When there is corneal opacity, the iris is partly occluded; this may occur in glaucoma of any etiology. Corneal diameter larger than 11–12 mm suggests congenital glaucoma.

Nose. The nose should be examined immediately to rule out unilateral or bilateral choanal atresia. If this is suspected, it can be excluded by passing a nasogastric tube through each nostril. The tube also should be advanced to the stomach to exclude the presence of esophageal atresia. In the neonate, nasal obstruction of any origin can result in serious respiratory distress, not only because the diameter of the upper airway is normally small, but also because neonates have difficulty breathing through the mouth. The nose may be compressed or deformed by pressure before birth. Rarely, the nasal septum is dislocated. Correction should be performed to prevent permanent deformities. A flat and broad nasal bridge, a beaked nose, or anteversion of the nostrils and a long philtrum may be normal but could be part of a congenital syndrome.

Mouth. The mouth should be examined with the infant at rest and while crying. The newborn infant may open the mouth when gentle digital pressure is applied on the lower lip or chin. Micrognathia should be noted. If there is cleft lip, a dimple in the lower lip indicates an autosomal-dominant condition. This increases the risk of cleft palate in future offspring from 4% to 50%. Clefts of the soft and hard palates are easily noted by inspection, but submucous clefts in the soft portion of the palate should be ruled out by digital palpation. These clefts may be isolated or associated with other dysmorphic features. A high-arched palate is, in general, an isolated finding. Retrognathia and/or micrognathia, together with cleft palate, glossoptosis, and obstruction of the upper airway, can be found in Pierre–Robin anomaly or sequence. Macroglossia is characteristic of the Beckwith–Wiedemann syndrome, which presents with omphalocele, macrosomia, and hypoglycemia. Although not as significant, macroglossia can be present in Down syndrome, hypothyroidism, and gangliosidosis G_{M1}.

Rarely, neonatal teeth may be seen, usually in the area of the medial lower incisors. Sometimes they are not white but covered with pink, membranous tissue. Such teeth should be removed because of the risk of aspiration when they fall out spontaneously. White, small epidermoid–mucoid cysts on both sides of the hard palate (Epstein pearls) are found normally; they also may be present in the gum or the floor of the oral cavity and disappear in a few weeks. Salivary secretion is scant in the neonate; therefore, saliva should not accumulate in the oral cavity unless there is an abnormality in swallowing or esophageal atresia. Some infants have a short lingual frenulum; this does not usually interfere with feedings or speech, and treatment usually is not necessary. A strong cry is a sign of well-being in neonates. A high-pitched cry can be present in CNS conditions and some congenital syndromes; a cat-like cry is seen in cri du chat syndrome; and a dysphonic cry with inspiratory stridor suggests upper airway problems.

Neck & clavicles. The neck in an infant at term is short and symmetric. To examine the neck, the head should be extended and rotated to observe the lateral border of the sternocleidomastoid muscle. Cysts or sinuses may be due to branchial clefts. The sternocleidomastoid muscle may be shortened due to a fixed position in utero or a postnatal hematoma resulting from birth injury. This produces neonatal torticollis. Clefts or masses in the midline may be due to cysts of the thyroglossal duct, goiter secondary to maternal antithyroid medication, or transplacental passage of long-acting thyroid stimulating antibodies. Edema and webbing of the neck suggest Turner syndrome, but other syndromes, such as Noonan, Klipper–Feil, and pterygium-multiplex, are associated with a short neck. Both clavicles should be examined routinely to rule out fractures. Cystic hygromas occur in the supraclavicular area.

Cardiothoracic. During examination of the chest, inspection of the breast tissue aids in determining gestational age. Accessory nipples, which might be present along the anterior axillary or midclavicular lines, should be noted because they may later grow due to the presence of glandular tissue. In some term infants, breast engorgement develops, unilaterally or bilaterally, at 3–5 days after birth as a result of stimulation by maternal estrogen. Sometimes there is milk secretion. Male and female infants can be affected; no treatment is necessary. Milk expression should not be attempted because it enhances the risk of infection.

Congenital deformities of the thorax, such as pectus-carinatus and pectus-excavatus, and asymmetry due to absence of the formation of ribs or to the agenesis of the pectoralis muscle (Poland syndrome), should be ruled out. The thorax may be small in some skeletal dysplasias and thus cause respiratory distress.

Evaluation of the lung and upper airway requires detailed inspection of respiratory mechanics. Tachypnea, deep respirations, cyanosis, expiratory grunting, and intercostal or sternal retractions are signs of respiratory distress.

The respiratory rate is normally 40–60 breaths/minute, but most neonates, particularly preterm infants, breathe irregularly with short, apneic bursts that last less than 5–10 seconds and have no clinical significance. Breath sounds should be equal in both sides of the chest, and, after the first 2–4 hours, rales should not be present. A scaphoid abdomen and decreased breath sounds on one side suggest the diagnosis of congenital diaphragmatic hernia. Soon after birth, bowel sounds may be heard over the involved side of the chest. Other causes of diminished or absent breath sounds on one side are pneumothorax, pleural effusion, or agenesis of the lung. In all these conditions, the chest may appear asymmetric on inspection.

The cardiac impulse is usually maximal at the fourth intercostal space between the sternum and the midclavicular line, but it shifts in cases of pneumothorax, pneumomediastinum, diaphragmatic hernia, and dextrocardia. The normal heart rate varies between 95 and 180 beats/minute and changes when the infant is feeding, sleeping, or crying. If the heart rate exceeds 200 beats/minute at rest, an ECG should be performed to exclude arrhythmias (see Chapter 16). If the heart rate is less than 70–80 beats/minute, an ECG is useful to differentiate between pathologic sinus bradycardia (as seen in CNS lesions, severe perinatal hypoxia, etc.) and specific bradycardias, such as atrioventricular block.

The second heart sound is normally loud and not split in the first 3 hours after birth because pulmonary arterial pressure is still high; it becomes split in 75% of neonates by 48 hours. A single second sound persists in PPHN, pulmonary atresia, and transposition of the great vessels. Frequently, systolic heart murmurs are heard immediately after birth and during the first 2 days, but they disappear within a few days. Many infants with severe congenital heart disease do not have heart murmurs soon after birth. Peripheral pulses should be palpated in all four extremities. In the neonate in whom symptoms develop, symptoms that could be associated with congenital heart disease or cardiac failure, and in the neonate with a persistent heart murmur, blood pressures should be measured in all four extremities. The infant with coarctation of the aorta or arch interruption may have consistently high upper extremity blood pressure.

Abdomen. The abdomen in the neonate is prominent because of poor development of the abdominal wall muscles, the relatively larger liver, and diaphragmatic movements during respiration. The lack of this normal abdominal prominence is seen in diaphragmatic hernia or esophageal atresia without tracheoesophageal fistula. Lack of abdominal prominence also is noted in SGA and postterm infants. The liver edge is usually felt about 2 cm below the right costal margin, and the kidneys may be palpable. Normally, peristaltic movements are observed on the abdominal wall. If the liver is felt in the midline or to the left, situs inversus, asplenia, or polysplenia syndrome is suggested. Abdominal masses may represent hydronephrosis, multicystic kidneys, ovarian cysts, or other lesions (see this chapter, Approach to Abdominal Masses, for a detailed discussion). Midline abdominal defects, such as diastasis-recti or an umbilical hernia, usually require no therapy. More significant lesions such as **omphalocele** (a herniation of the abdominal contents through the umbilicus) or **gastroschisis** (herniation of the bowel through the abdominal wall 2–4 cm lateral to the umbilicus) are readily apparent. A flaccid abdominal wall, associated with complete or almost complete absence of abdominal muscle, is part of the prune-belly syndrome. These infants also have bladder dilation, hydroureter, hydronephrosis, and cryptorchidism.

The **umbilical cord** should be inspected to confirm the presence of two arteries and one vein and the absence of a urachus. The presence of only one umbilical artery can indicate other, particularly renal, congenital malformations. Infants of diabetic mothers tend to have a thick umbilical cord with increased Wharton jelly; a thin cord is frequently noted in infants with IUGR. Postmature infants and those that have had fetal distress may have a meconium-stained cord. Bleeding from the cord suggests a coagulation disorder. The umbilical cord usually dries and falls off about 7–14 days after birth. When this is delayed or if there is erythema around the umbilicus, omphalitis can develop. Sometimes when the cord falls off, granulation tissue may be noted in the umbilical base, with minimal amounts of secretion. Usually no treatment is required. A chronic discharge suggests a granuloma of the umbilical stump or, on rare occasions, a draining omphalomesenteric cyst. A persistent omphalomesenteric duct usually drains a pink, mucoid, or fecoid secretion over a shiny red polyp. In cutaneous umbilicus the skin of the abdominal wall extends 2–3 cm or more around the cord; when the cord falls off, a prominent cutaneous area is left, but this tends to disappear slowly. With persistent urachus, urine may drain from the umbilicus, particularly when pressure is applied over the bladder.

The **anus** should be examined for patency; on rare occasions, an imperforate anus may not be visible. Anal patency can be confirmed with careful introduction of a soft rubber catheter into the anus or by using a rectal thermometer to determine the initial temperature. Intestinal obstruction should be suspected if there is a history of polyhydramnios; if, soon after birth, gastric content exceeds 15 mL or is bilious stained; or if there is abdominal distention associated with vomiting or decreased number of meconium stools. A nasogastric tube should be passed immediately, and further studies performed. Meconium peritonitis is the result of prenatal intestinal perforation due to intrinsic or extrinsic congenital mechanical obstructions. Calcification in the abdomen is a characteristic finding on the abdominal radiograph. Pneumoperitoneum can occur in infants with necrotizing enterocolitis (NEC) or in-fants with pulmonary air leaks in which the air dissects into the abdomen.

Hirschsprung disease does not usually present im-mediately after birth but can cause abdominal disten-tion in the neonate. Meconium plug and meconium ileus, which can be the first manifestations of cystic fibrosis, delay the elimination of meconium, resulting in abdomi-nal distention. Normally, meconium stool is passed within 24 hours after birth in 90% of term infants and within 48 hours in 99%.

Genitalia. The genitalia should be examined to assess gestational age and exclude anomalies. At term, the labia majora covers the labia minora and the clitoris, but in preterm infants the labia minora and the clitoris are evi-dent. A hymenal appendix may protrude externally from the vaginal floor. This and mucoid cysts, which may be present around the vaginal orifice, disappear within a few weeks after birth. Associated with maternal hormone with-drawal is the presence of a milky-white vaginal discharge, sometimes stained with blood, during the first week after birth; it usually disappears in 1–2 weeks. A hypertrophied clitoris can result from virilization due to androgen excess associated with virilizing adrenal hyperplasia; ambiguous genitalia is a real medical and social emergency. Hydro-metrocolpos is due to an imperforate hymen with reten-tion of vaginal secretions; it presents as a lower midline abdominal mass or as a small cyst between the labia.

In male infants at term, the testes should be descended into a well-formed and pigmented scrotum. In preterm infants, the testes may be in the abdomen or the inguinal canal, and the scrotum will be small with less rugae and pigmentation. In most cases of undescended testes, the testes descend spontaneously before 12 months of age. Undescended testes or cryptorchidism must be differenti-ated from retractile testes, which are intermittently absent from the scrotum but always distal to the inguinal ring. Cryptorchidism may be associated with inguinal hernia, genitourinary malformations, hypospadias, and other syn-dromes. The prepuce in normal newborns is tight and should not be retracted. The penis may be small or, more frequently, appears small because of pubic fat. Micropenis is frequently associated with chloacal extrophy or may be due to primary or secondary hypogonadism; it is also asso-ciated with Prader–Willi syndrome. The urethral meatus should be at the end of the penis. In epispadias, the mea-tus is in the dorsal area of the penis and usually associated with bladder extrophy. In hypospadias, the meatus is on the ventral part of the penis in different locations along the shaft; it is not associated with increased incidence of urinary malformations. Perineal hypospadias presents as ambiguous genitalia; if both testes are within the scrotum, there is no doubt about the genetic sex (see Chapter 20). Scrotal swelling may be present in hydrocele or cases of testicular torsion. Hydroceles can be unilateral or bilateral and are more frequent in term infants. They are caused by persistence of the processus vaginalis; they also may be associated with inguinal hernia. The hydrocele may com-municate with the abdominal cavity, and its size may change. Isolated hydroceles usually cause no clinical prob-lems and often disappear spontaneously in a few weeks. Inguinal hernias are usually easily reducible, but, because the internal inguinal ring is narrow, the risk of strangula-tion is high and surgery should be performed early.

Extremities & back. The extremities should be exam-ined to detect anatomic and functional abnormalities. The lack of spontaneous movements in the upper extrem-ities suggests fractures, infection, or brachial plexus injury. When the upper extremity is moved by the examiner, the infant will show signs of pain in cases of fracture or con-genital syphilis. Partial or complete absence of the clavi-cles, as in cleidocranial dysostosis, allows the shoulders to be flexed forward without limitation. Congenital abnor-malities of the elbow, radioulnar synostosis, and absence or hypoplasia of the radius are usually unilateral and limit pronation and supination movements. Absence or hypo-plasia of the radius may be associated with syndromes such as thrombocytopenia, Fanconi anemia, and Holt–Oram syndrome. The hands and fingers should be inspected carefully for indications of chromosomal malformations. Polydactyly can occur as an isolated anomaly or as part of a syndrome. Rudimentary fingers are often adjacent to the fifth finger. Syndactyly is frequently an isolated find-ing of the second or third fingers and may be inherited as an autosomal dominant trait. Normally, the tibias are curved laterally and internally rotated, and the toes may overlap, which does not require treatment. Edema of the feet with hypoplastic nails is characteristic of Turner and Noonan syndromes. Rocker-bottom feet are frequently seen in trisomy 18.

The hips should be examined for congenital dyspla-sia. In about 1–1.5% of infants, there will be an unstable hip (much more frequent) or a completely dislocated hip (see Chapter 22).

The spine should be examined for hair tufts, nevus, or even lipomas in the lumbar–sacral area, which suggests spina bifida. If there is a sacrococcygeal pilonidal dimple, a careful attempt to identify the base should be made to rule out a neurocutaneous sinus tract. Myelomeningo-celes are usually obvious at the time of birth.

Neurologic & Behavioral Examinations

Newborn infants demonstrate considerable cortical con-trol. They show directed responses in social interaction with a nurturing adult or in response to an attractive audi-tory or visual stimulus. When positive rather than intru-sive stimuli are used, neonates have amazing capacities for alertness and attention. They can respond and interact with the environment from birth with very predictable behavior and can suppress interfering reflex responses to attend to more "interesting stimuli," such as a human face or voice, a soft rattle, or a light caress. This complex interaction of visual, auditory, and motor behaviors to respond to a human stimulus is managed by normal neonates despite the enormous physiologic demands of labor and transition to neonatal life.

BEHAVIORAL STATES

Observation of the spontaneous state of consciousness or "state" of the infant is an important part of the neurologic and behavioral examination. Sleep is categorized as quiet or active sleep or a drowsy state. Wakefulness is classified as quiet alert, active alert, fussing, and crying. Full-term infants spend about 80% of the time in a sleep state and rise to light sleep in a cyclic fashion every 3–4 hours. Active, or rapid eye movement (REM), sleep is predominant in the healthy term newborn. Preterm infants spend more time sleeping, and a higher percentage of this is REM sleep. State also depends on physiologic variables such as hunger, nutrition, degree of hydration, and illnesses, but it is also clearly related to the time within the wake–sleep cycle of the neonate.

Optimal sensory responses are best exhibited during the state of quiet alertness. Neonates respond to a bright light not only with a pupillary response but also with withdrawal. Repeated stimulation is likely to result in neurologic habituation; this explains the lack of response of infants housed in noisy, brightly lit nurseries to sound or light stimuli. Sharply contrasting colors, large squares, and bright objects appeal to neonates and keep them in a prolonged alert state of fixation.

The neonate's auditory responses are specific and well organized. The infant may respond to auditory stimuli with changes in respirations and eye blinks and with more obvious behavioral startles. In addition, alerting and head turning are likely to occur in response to the source of sound. Habituation to repeated auditory stimuli also occurs normally and can be a good test of CNS function because behavioral inhibition is not likely to occur when the cortex is damaged.

Newborn infants can differentiate taste and smell; they respond differently to acetic acid or alcohol than to sweet odors such as milk and sugary solutions. By 5 days, they can reliably distinguish their own mother's breasts from those of other lactating mothers.

Infants are very sensitive to touch. A quiet baby becomes alert with a rapid, intrusive tactile stimulus. When the infant is upset, a slow, modulated tactile stimulus can reduce activity. A lack of response to soothing tactile stimuli in the neonate should raise suspicion of irritability due to CNS disturbance.

Important information about the neonate's status can be gleaned from simple observation of how the infant

Table 4–8. Movement Patterns Suggestive of Central Nervous System Disturbance in the Neonate

Constant lateralized asymmetry of reflex motor responses
Athetoid movements
Obligatory tonic neck responses
Constant strabismus of eyes
Hypertonic/hypotonic muscular responses
Obligatory thumb in fist
Persistent abnormal reflexes (e.g., sucking, Moro)

moves the extremities, the kind of movements made, and, in particular, whether the movements are random startles or seem to be purposeful. Careful assessment of resting muscle tone and responsive motor activity may be the best evidence of CNS disorder. Table 4–8 summarizes movement patterns that are significant in predicting risk in CNS development. They can all be assessed by careful observation.

Assessment of the neonate's behavioral responses should be part of every pediatric examination because it reflects the capacity for integration of the CNS and, therefore, is an accurate way of assessing the well-being of the newborn. The Brazelton Neonatal Behavioral Assessment Examination is a detailed behavioral examination that includes 26 behavioral items that are assessed during specific states of sleep or wakefulness.

NEUROLOGIC EXAMINATION

Neurologic function changes considerably during the last 3 months of gestation. Increase in flexor tone begins in the lower extremities and progresses cephalad between 28 and 40 weeks of gestation. This progression correlates with increasing myelination of subcortical pathways originating in the brainstem. For example, the infant at 28 weeks lies with upper and lower extremities fully extended, and there is little or no resistance to passive movement of the extremities. By 34 weeks the lower extremities are flexed at the knees and the hips. By 36 weeks, there is flexion of the upper extremities. After 40 weeks, a gradual loss of the resting flexion posture begins in the upper extremities. Deep tendon reflexes, such as the biceps and the patellar, can be elicited in normal term infants. Ankle clonus is normally present but not sustained in the neonate.

The neurologic examination should be performed in detail with newborn infants. A screening test designed by Prechtl (Table 4–9) is useful to identify obvious disturbances.

The baby should be examined in a warm environment, preferably 2–3 hours after feeding. The state of sleep or wakefulness and the resting posture should be observed. In the supine position, the posture is normally

Table 4–9. Minimal Neurologic Examination of the Newborn

State at beginning of examination
Posture: Limbs, trunk, head
Overall assessment of tone
Eyes: Centered, constant deviation, constant strabismus
Spontaneous motor activity: Symmetry, intensity, speed, tremors, overshooting, jerks, convulsions
Resistance to passive movements: Neck, trunk, arms, legs
Flexion tests: Resistance in arms and legs; head control
Suck reflex
Moro response: Complete, symmetric, without tremors
A careful assessment of resting muscle tone and responsive motor activity may be the best way to detect evidence of central nervous system disorder

symmetric, with the limbs semiflexed and the lower limbs in slight abduction at the hips. Abnormal signs include opisthotonos, constant turning of the head toward one side with asymmetric body posture. Spontaneous motor activity, athetoid postures and movements, jitteriness, rhythmic twitching of the face or tongue, or frank convulsions should be noted. Skull examination should include head circumference and inspection of the fontanelles and sutures.

Reflexes. Reflex responses should be tested. The **lip reflex,** protrusion of the lips with tapping of the upper or lower lip, is elicited readily in normal sleepy babies. The **glabella reflex,** brisk closure of the eyes of short duration, is elicited by tapping sharply on the glabella. In facial paresis, an asymmetric response is noted. A strong response occurs in hyperexcitable infants, and the reflex is absent or barely discernible in babies with CNS injury. Constant strabismus is abnormal, as is sustained nystagmus after slight movement of the head. Pupils should be of equal shape and size and reactive to light. Asymmetry of the pupils or poor response to light suggests neurologic dysfunction. The **optical blink reflex,** quick closure of the eyelids, is elicited by suddenly shining a bright light into the eyes. An absent response suggests impaired light perception or CNS dysfunction. The **acoustic blink reflex,** elicited by clapping the hands about 30 cm away from the infant's head, may be absent with impaired auditory system. The **corneal reflex,** closure of the eyes on touching the cornea, is absent in lesions of the fifth cranial nerve. The **dolls' eyes test** is performed by turning the head slowly to the right and left; normally, the eyes do not move with the head but lag behind. With CNS anomalies the eyes will move with the head, and in abducens nerve paresis there is asymmetry in the response. This reflex disappears as fixation develops.

Tonic neck reflex is best examined in the supine position by turning the face slowly to the right side and holding it in the extreme position with the jaw over the right shoulder. The arms and leg of the face side will extend, and the "occipital" arm will flex at the elbow. The reflex is then performed toward the left. The response may or may not be present in the newborn, but a constantly present, well-marked tonic neck reflex, even at rest, may be a sign of neurologic dysfunction. The resistance against passive movements, power of active movements, and range of movement should be examined in the supine position, with the head in the midline to avoid the tonic neck reflex. This can be evaluated by moving the upper and lower limbs rhythmically and simultaneously through their full range of movement. During this examination, no undue force should be used.

The palmar grasp is elicited by placing the index fingers into the infant's hands and pressing the palmar surface; the dorsal side of the hands should not be touched. The normal response is flexion of all fingers around the examiner's finger. Difference of intensity of grasp between the two sides suggests an anomaly. If the grasping reflex is absent or weak, sucking should be stimulated because this facilitates grasping. If sucking has no effect, the cause of the absent palmar grasp is probably peripheral and not central. In Erb's palsy or clavicular fracture, for example, asymmetry is present; in infants with CNS depression, the response is weak or absent bilaterally.

The rooting response is produced by stroking one corner of the mouth while the head is kept midline to avoid the asymmetric tonic neck reflex. The normal response is a directed head turn toward the stimulated side. With stimulation of the upper lip at the corner of the mouth there is opening of the mouth and retroflexion of the head. After stimulation of the lower lip, the mouth opens and the jaw drops. In all instances, the infant tries to suck the finger applying the stimulation. This reflex is absent with generalized CNS depression. The sucking reflex is elicited by introducing the index finger 2–3 cm into the infant's mouth; the normal response is a rhythmic sucking movement. All phases of sucking should be evaluated, including the stripping action of the tongue, forcing upward and back, the rate of suctioning, the negative pressure developed, and the grouping of the sucks. Premature infants and those with CNS depression, which may be induced by drugs such as barbiturates, will have poor or absent sucking.

The Moro response should be obtained with the infant in a symmetric position and the head in the midline. The back is supported by one of the examiner's hands, and the head is held by the other. The head is then lowered a few centimeters when the neck muscles are relaxed. A complete Moro response consists of abduction of the upper limbs at the shoulder, extension of the forearms at the elbow, and extension of the fingers followed by adduction of the arms at the shoulder. The threshold for the Moro response should be noted because the reflex may be elicited very easily but may have a medium or high threshold. An absent or constantly weak Moro response indicates serious CNS disturbances; asymmetries occur with Erb's palsy and clavicular fractures.

The infant should also be turned onto the stomach to be examined in the prone position. The vertebral column should be palpated with the first and second fingers, and the skin should be inspected. Normally, the head may be lifted off the table for a few seconds and turned from side to side. Lifting of the head several centimeters for 10 seconds or longer suggests hypertonia or opisthotonos. Crawling can be observed spontaneously or with reinforcement by pressing the hands gently on the soles of the feet (Bauer response). If a stimulus is applied along the paravertebral line, about 3 cm from the midline from the shoulder down to the buttocks, the trunk normally curves with the concavity on the stimulated side; this is the normal incurvation of the trunk response. This response is absent below the level of a lesion of the spinal cord.

One should note whether the thumb is held in an adducted position, buried in the hand, in the so-called thumb-in-fist position. If this is persistent, it represents an unfavorable CNS sign. Babies with different types of neurologic abnormality cry differently than do normal infants. High-pitched or weak cries are almost certainly abnormal, as are whining and a catlike cry.

The infant should be examined upright to test the placing response, which is elicited by holding the baby with both hands under the arms and around the chest and stimulating the dorsal part of the foot by making it touch a protruding edge such as a table top. The feet will be lifted by simultaneous flexion of the knees and hips. This response is absent in paresis of the lower limbs. Subsequently, by allowing the soles of the feet to touch the surface of the table, the infant will show alternating stepping movements. This response is also absent with paresis of the lower limbs, in infants born by breech presentation, and in infants with CNS depression.

The cremasteric reflex is absent in spinal cord lesions. The anal reflex, elicited by scratching the perianal skin with a pin, is characterized by a contraction of the external anal sphincter. An absent reflex may be associated with damage to the sacral cord.

A normal neurologic assessment within the first week of life of the term newborn is a strong predictor of later normalcy. Similarly, for the premature newborn who has reached 40 weeks' postconceptual age, a normal neurologic assessment is a better guarantee for a normal outcome than the absence of visible damage on brain imaging. Further details of neurologic disturbances in the neonate are presented in Chapter 21. Some of the reflexes present in the neonate and their changes during maturation are shown in Table 4–10.

Prechtl proposed clustering abnormal neurologic signs into diagnostic syndromes. **Hyperexcitable** infants are characterized by tremor of low frequency and high amplitude, very active tendon reflexes, and low threshold to the Moro reflex. The **apathy syndrome** is characterized by reduced responsiveness, decreased resistance to passive movements, and long periods of quiet wakefulness. Hyperexcitability is associated with mild sequelae in a small percentage of infants who have had perinatal asphyxia, but apathy is followed by moderate sequelae in a larger percentage of infants. The **hemisyndrome** is characterized by at least three findings of asymmetry in motility, posturing, or response to stimulation; this correlates with unilateral neurologic findings in childhood. The syndrome of severe CNS **depression or coma** is associated with slow or abnormal respiration and depressed response to stimuli; seizures are frequently present. More than 50% of survivors with this syndrome have severe sequelae.

■ ABNORMALITIES OF GROWTH

Adequate fetal growth depends on provision of substrates for fetal consumption, but tissue growth also depends on an appropriate fetal endocrine milieu. Insulin has been implicated as the growth hormone of the fetus; because it does not cross the placenta, it must be secreted by the fetus. In the absence of fetal insulin production, as in transient neonatal diabetes mellitus, congenital absence of the islets of Langerhans, or pancreatic aplasia, fetal growth is impaired. Hyperinsulinism in utero, as occurs in infants of mothers with diabetes, is associated with increased adipose and muscle tissue mass and excessive birth weight. C peptide, a cleavage protein of proinsulin, is also reduced with IUGR and increased with fetal macrosomia. Growth hormone and thyroid hormones do not affect fetal growth. Other hormones, such as insulinlike growth regulatory factor 2, have anabolic and growth functions.

Small-for-Gestational-Age Infants

Infants that are born with a weight below the 5th percentile for corresponding gestational age are considered SGA. This is a sign that intrauterine growth has stopped or slowed significantly some time during pregnancy. Growth failure can be symmetric; that is, the weight, length, and head circumference are approximately in the same percentile. IUGR can also be asymmetric; the head circumference can be normal or less affected than length or weight. The length, in turn, may be affected similarly or less than the weight. Causes and types of SGA infants are shown in Table 4–11. When growth is affected early in gestation, type I SGA, the growth retardation will be symmetric. In many of these infants,

Table 4–10. Strength of Eight Reflexes in Infants Between 28 and 40 Weeks' Gestation

	Weeks						
	28	30	32	34	36	38	40
Sucking	Weak, not really synchronized with swallowing		Stronger and better synchronized with swallowing		Perfect		
Palmar grasp	Present but weak			Stronger		Excellent	
Response to traction	Absent		Begins to appear	Strong enough to lift part of body weight		Strong enough to lift all of body weight	
Moro reflex	Weak, obtained just once, incomplete		Complete reflex				
Crossed extension	Flexion and extension in random pattern, purposeless reaction		Good extension but no tendency to adduction		Tendency to adduction, but imperfect	Complete response with extension, adduction, fanning of toes	
Automatic walking	—		Begins tiptoeing with good support on sole and righting reaction of legs			An infant born prematurely who reaches 40 wk walks in toe–heel progression on tiptoes	
				Quite good; very fast tiptoeing		A full-term newborn of 40 wk walks in heel–toe progression on whole sole of foot	
Root	Good with reinforcement		Good (no reinforcement)		Good	Good	Good
Pupillary response			Present	Present		Present	Present

cell number is decreased in most organs. Head circumference is smaller than in other types of IUGR, and these infants typically have poor long-term outcomes. Infants that are SGA because they were subjected to chronic intrauterine hypoxia associated with uterine placental insufficiency (type II) have a normal number of cells that are reduced in size; they are at increased risk for perinatal problems (Table 4–12). Type III SGA (late intrauterine malnutrition) infants usually do well in long-term follow-up. In addition, if an infant is small because family members are small, outcome is good.

The ponderal index measures the relationship between weight (kg) and length (cm): (weight/length) × 100. In normal infants, it is approximately 5.5–6.5. In type I SGA infants, this index is normal; however, in type III, it is less than 5.5. The lower the index, the more significant the asymmetry in intrauterine growth.

Large-for-Gestational-Age Infants

Infants may be large for gestational age but not show high birth weight (>4000 g). LGA infants, with or without high birth weight, frequently demonstrate hypoglycemia and polycythemia. Infants of diabetic mothers (IDMs) also have a higher incidence of RDS and sudden intrauterine death. Inappropriately increased weight for gestational age often is associated with congenital malformations. The more common causes of increased weight and LGA infants are listed in Table 4–13.

INFANTS OF DIABETIC MOTHERS

Infants of diabetic mothers are large because of increased body fat and visceromegaly, primarily of the liver, adrenals, and heart. The skeletal length is increased in proportion to weight, but the head and face appear disproportionately small. The umbilical cord and placenta are also enlarged. Maternal hyperglycemia causes fetal hyperglycemia and fetal hyperinsulinemia. This causes increased hepatic glucose uptake and glycogen synthesis, accelerated lipogenesis, augmented protein synthesis, and macrosomia. In women with severe vascular complications, however, infants may be SGA secondary to placental insufficiency. Infants of diabetic mothers appear plethoric with round facies. They are at considerable risk for the

Table 4–11. Etiology of Intrauterine Growth Retardation

Type I: Early interference with fetal growth (from conception to 24 wk gestation)
Chromosomal anomalies (trisomies 21, 13–15, 18, etc.)
Fetal infections (cytomegalovirus, toxoplasmosis, rubella, herpes)
Maternal drugs (chronic alcoholism, heroin)
Maternal chronic hypertension; severe diabetes

Type II: Chronic intrauterine malnutrition (24–32 wk gestation)
Inadequate intrauterine space (multiple pregnancies, uterine tumors, uterine anomalies)
Placental insufficiency: Maternal vascular disease (renal, chronic essential hypertension, collagen diseases, pregnancy-induced hypertension)
Small placenta with abnormal cellularity

Type III: Late intrauterine malnutrition (after 32 wk gestation)
Placental infarct or fibrosis
Pregnancy-induced hypertension
Maternal hypoxemia (lung disease, smoking)
Postmaturity
Maternal small stature or malnutrition

Table 4–13. Causes of Large-for-Gestational-Age Infants

Genetic/racial	Functional β-cell hyperplasia
Infants of diabetic mothers	Maternal drugs,
Beckwith–Wiedemann	such as tocolytic
syndrome	sympathomimetics
β-Cell nesidioblastosis	Rh immunization
spectrum	Prader–Willi syndrome

perinatal difficulties summarized in Table 4–14. Hypoglycemia occurs frequently after birth in these infants, and prompt recognition and treatment is important (see Chapter 19).

Evaluation of fetal lung maturity is very important in mothers with diabetes because RDS develops in many with a normal lecithin: sphingomyelin (LS) ratio; evaluation of amniotic fluid phosphatidylglycerol concentration is a more reliable predictor of lung maturity (see later in this chapter, Respiratory Distress Syndrome). High fetal insulin concentrations delay the appearance of lamellar bodies in type 2 cells and increase glycogen content of the alveolar lining cells. If they do not lack pulmonary surfactant, many of these infants have respiratory distress because of transient tachypnea or PPHN. In some infants, hypertrophic cardiomyopathy develops; this is often manifested on ECG by asymmetric septal hypertrophy and thickening of the ventricular wall. This condition is usually benign and resolves spontaneously, but the findings could be interpreted as idiopathic hypertrophic subaortic stenosis.

A condition occurring exclusively in IDMs is the neonatal small left colon syndrome. This presents with failure to pass meconium, abdominal distention, and, in some infants, bile-stained vomitus. Barium enema shows a decreased caliber of the left colon. The syndrome is transient, but some infants improve slowly and require a transient colostomy. Congenital anomalies are two to four times more frequent in IDMs than in normal infants (Table 4–14). Maternal glycohemoglobin concentration (HbA_{1C}) has been correlated with poor diabetic control and an increased incidence of congenital malformations. When maternal HbA_{1C} concentration is less than 8.5% in the first trimester of pregnancy, there is a low incidence of congenital malformations. Many of the problems in IDMs are related to less than adequate diabetic control during the preconceptual period and throughout pregnancy.

Treatment of IDMs includes careful monitoring of blood glucose concentrations, early feeding, and treatment of respiratory or cardiac insufficiency. Many infants require intravenous fluids with glucose for several hours after birth to prevent hypoglycemia. In infants of well-controlled diabetic mothers, not only is the neonatal morbidity rate significantly decreased, but also physical

Table 4–12. Perinatal Problems in Small-for-Gestational-Age Infants

Perinatal asphyxia	Hypocalcemia
Hypothermia	Meconium aspiration syndrome
Hypoglycernia	Intrauterine fetal death
Polycythemia	Hypermagnesemia (maternal MgSO₄
Thrombocytopenia	therapy)

Table 4–14. Problems in Infants of Diabetic Mothers

Sudden intrauterine death	Hypocalcemia
Large for gestational age	Hypertrophic cardiomyopathy
Birth trauma	Persistent pulmonary hyper-
Increased rate of cesarean	tension of the newborn
section	Respiratory distress syndrome
Asphyxia	Congenital malformations:
Hypoglycernia	Cardiac, central nervous
Polycythernia	system, musculoskeletal

and mental development is essentially normal in long-term follow-up. The incidence of subsequent overt diabetes in women who have diabetes during pregnancy is 0.5–1% in most studies, but rates as high as 10% have been reported.

ABNORMALITIES OF MATURITY

Prematurity

A **preterm** delivery is defined as one occurring before 37 completed weeks of gestation from the first day of the last menstrual period. Approximately two thirds of neonates with birth weights less than 2500 g are preterm; few premature infants weigh more than 2500 g. The incidence of preterm delivery is higher in lower socioeconomic populations and in women who do not receive prenatal care. Approximately 7% of births are preterm, but this figure varies widely across the country and across the world. Very-low-birth-weight infants (those weighing less than 1500 g) constitute approximately 1.2% of all births in the United States but account for more than 40% of neonatal deaths. Perinatal care and improved survival rates of these VLBW infants have had a major impact on total neonatal and infant deaths. Further, the decreasing mortality rate has not been associated with a significantly increased morbidity rate. The problems that the premature infant may face from the time of birth to the first several weeks of life are listed in Table 4–15.

Respiratory insufficiency is very common in preterm infants because they have less pulmonary compliance, qualitative and quantitative surfactant deficiency, increased compliance of the airway and rib cage, incomplete development of respiratory muscles, and immaturity of mechanisms involved in respiratory control. Many of these infants require intubation and ventilation immediately after birth. The issues of temperature regulation and many other difficulties faced by preterm infants are discussed elsewhere in this chapter.

Table 4–15. Frequent Problems in Preterm Infants

Increased incidence of neonatal death	Patent ductus arteriosus
Perinatal asphyxia	Intracranial hemorrhage
Hypothermia	Necrotizing enterocolitis
Hypoglycernia	Infection
Hypocalcernia	Retinopathy of prematurity
Respiratory distress syndrome	Bronchopulmonary dysplasia
Fluid and electrolyte abnormalities	Disrupted mother–father–infant interaction
Indirect hyperbilirubinemia	

Postmaturity

The other extreme of maturation is the **postterm** pregnancy, lasting more than 42 weeks beyond the onset of the last menstrual period. The fetus of the postterm pregnancy may continue to grow in utero and therefore may become unusually large. If the uterine environment is unfavorable for fetal growth, the infant at birth may have significant loss of subcutaneous fat and muscle mass. In severe cases, meconium staining of the skin, nails, and umbilical cord; loss of vernix caseosa; and patchy or scaly skin are evident. The term **postmature** has been applied to these infants. **Dysmaturity** refers to infants who are born after sustaining placental insufficiency. The smaller, postmature infants are at great risk for fetal death and distress in labor; by 43 weeks' gestation, perinatal mortality rate doubles, and by 44 weeks it triples, compared with full-term infants at 39–41 weeks' gestation. Neonatal morbidity is also high because of fetal asphyxia, meconium aspiration syndrome (MAS), polycythemia, and hypoglycemia. Prolonged gestation may be secondary to anencephaly or to placental sulfatase deficiency. Because of the high perinatal morbidity of postmaturity, induction of labor is suggested after 42 weeks and definitely recommended after 43 weeks.

APPROACHES TO COMMON NEONATAL CLINICAL PROBLEMS

Cyanosis

Cyanosis is a bluish discoloration of the skin and mucous membranes. Some ancient cultures considered it a sign of divinity. In the neonate, it always constitutes an emergency, requiring immediate diagnosis and treatment. Clinical detection of cyanosis depends on the experience and ability of the observer and on the environmental lighting. Cyanosis does not always indicate hypoxemia (low PaO_2). More important, infants may be severely hypoxic (low oxygen delivery to the tissues) without showing clinical cyanosis.

The interactions between hemoglobin (Hb) and oxygen are well described in physiology texts. Hemoglobin combines rapidly and reversibly with oxygen as long as its iron is in the ferrous state. Cyanosis is directly related to an absolute concentration of unoxygenated or reduced Hb. It is evident when more than 3 g/dL of Hb in arterial blood or more than 5 g/dL in capillary blood is reduced. Fetal and adult Hb differ in their binding capacities for oxygen. The P_{50}, or PaO_2 at which Hb is 50% saturated with oxygen, in adult human blood is about 27 mm Hg. The P_{50} for fetal Hb is about 20 mm Hg.

The Hb oxygen dissociation curve for HbF is thus shifted to the left, so that at the same PO_2 oxygen saturation is higher in fetal than in adult blood. In venous blood, in which PO_2 is about 30–35 mm Hg, Hb oxygen saturation in the neonate is about 80%; however, in the adult it is 70% or less. The PaO_2 necessary to produce oxygen desaturation of a degree to show cyanosis in the neonate is approximately 38–39 mm Hg, but in the adult it is 52–54 mm Hg.

Thus, cyanosis will develop in neonates at a lower PaO_2 than that necessary to produce cyanosis in older children or adults. The Hb dissociation curve can shift to the left or right for reasons other than Hb type (Table 4–16).

With low total Hb concentration, as in anemia, a higher percentage of desaturation is needed to cause cyanosis. In the normal neonate, the usual Hb concentration is 17 g/dL. When oxygen saturation is approximately 82%, more than 3 g/dL of Hb is reduced (18% of 17 g/dL), and cyanosis is evident. (The PaO_2 necessary to produce cyanosis in this case is approximately 38–39 mm Hg.) Many infants, particularly those who are premature, have Hb concentrations of 12 g/dL or less. In such cases, the desaturation needs to be 25% (saturation as low as 75%, PaO_2 30 mm Hg) to produce a reduced Hb concentration greater than 3 g/dL and, therefore, cyanosis.

When the total concentration of Hb is increased, as in polycythemia, the amount of reduced Hb in arterial blood will be higher even with only small reductions of oxygen saturation; cyanosis may be evident at saturations of 85–92%. In polycythemia, hyperviscosity may decrease the velocity of capillary blood, which may increase reduced Hb to more than 5 g/dL in the capillary bed even with normal arterial oxygen saturation, and cause peripheral cyanosis.

The major pathophysiologic mechanisms for cyanosis are shown in Table 4–17. In some conditions, several pathophysiologic mechanisms may be responsible for cyanosis. Oxygen saturation, PaO_2, and $PaCO_2$ differ according to the cause of cyanosis. For example, if an infant's blood is dark with a very low saturation but with a normal PaO_2, the diagnosis is a decreased affinity of Hb

Table 4–16. Causes of Shift in Hemoglobin Dissociation Curve

To the Left (lower P_{50}, more O_2 affinity)	To the Right (higher P_{50}, less O_2 affinity)
HbF	HbA
Alkalosis	Acidosis
Hypocarbia	Hypercarbia
Decreased 2,3-DPG concentration	Increased 2,3-DPG concentration
Hypothermia	Hyperthermia
Carbon monoxide	Anemia
Hexokinase deficiency	Hypoxia
	Increased catecholamine concentration
	Pyruvate kinase deficiency

DPG = diphosphoglycerate; Hb = hemoglobin.

Table 4–17. Pathophysiologic Mechanisms of Cyanosis and Corresponding Clinical Entities

Alveolar hypoventilation
  Lung parenchyma: RDS, pulmonary edema, pulmonary hypoplasia, MAS
  Space-occupying lesions of the chest: Pneumothorax, interstitial emphysema, congenital lobar emphysema, congenital diaphragmatic hernia, pleural effusion, abdominal distention
  Obstructive lesions: Choanal atresia, vocal cord paralysis, vascular rings, stenotic lesions, membranes, and cysts, Pierre Robin syndrome
  Central nervous system: Infection, hemorrhage, asphyxia, seizures, apnea, malformations, tumors
  Neuromuscular: Phrenic nerve palsy, thoracic dystrophies
  Metabolic: Hypoglycemia, hypocalcemia
  Cardiovascular: Heart failure (PDA, supraventricular tachycardia, congenital AV block)

Right-to-left shunt
  Intrapulmonary: MAS, respiratory distress syndrome; also may have alveolar hypoventilation
  Persistent pulmonary hypertension of the newborn: May have alveolar hypoventilation
  Cardiac: Decreased pulmonary blood flow (tetralogy of Fallot, tricuspid atresia, pulmonary atresia), normal or increased pulmonary blood flow (transposition of the great vessels, truncus arteriosus, anomalous pulmonary venous return)

Abnormal ventilation-perfusion ratios
  Lung parenchyma: Atelectasis, MAS, infections, pulmonary hemorrhage

Abnormal diffusion
  PIE, aspirations, pulmonary hemorrhage

Decreased hemoglobin O_2 affinity
  Methemoglobinemia (nitrites, sulfonamides, other drugs, congenital)

Decreased peripheral circulation (peripheral cyanosis)
  Low cardiac output (hypocalcemia, pneumopericardium, cardiomyopathies, etc), shock of any etiology, polycythemia, hypothermia, hypoglycemia

AV = atrioventricular; MAS = meconium aspiration syndrome; PDA = patent ductus arteriosus; PIE = pulmonary interstitial emphysema; RDS = respiratory distress syndrome.

for oxygen (e.g., methemoglobinemia). When an infant is cyanotic and the $PaCO_2$ is increased, cyanosis is likely to be respiratory in origin.

Immediate treatment of cyanosis may be necessary; this includes administration of oxygen and rapid correction of abnormalities of temperature, hematocrit, and glucose and calcium concentrations. In severely cyanotic infants, intubation and mechanical ventilation may be necessary.

Although the cause of cyanosis is usually apparent, it may be difficult to differentiate between a pulmonary and a cardiac condition. A low PaO_2 with a low or normal $PaCO_2$ suggests a right-to-left shunt that can be associated with congenital heart disease, pulmonary disease, or PPHN. In most infants with pulmonary disease, the $PaCO_2$ will be elevated. An **oxygen** test may be useful in differentiation.

In infants who have cyanotic congenital heart disease with reduced pulmonary blood flow, administering 100% oxygen will increase the PaO_2 only slightly, usually less than 10–15 mm Hg. With lung disease, the PaO_2 usually increases considerably, often reaching levels greater than 150 mm Hg. In infants with cyanotic congenital heart lesions associated with normal or increased pulmonary blood flow, PaO_2 usually increases more than 15–20 mm Hg with 100% oxygen, but levels above 150 mm Hg are unusual. Some infants with severe lung disease or PPHN may have large right-to-left shunts through the foramen ovale or ductus arteriosus, and PaO_2 therefore may not increase by more than 10–15 mm Hg with 100% oxygen.

Simultaneous measurement of oxygen saturation in the right arm and the leg may be useful. This can be done with skin surface oxygen saturation measurement or by direct sampling from a right radial artery and an umbilical arterial catheter in the descending aorta to measure PaO_2. Right-to-left shunting through the ductus arteriosus results in a lower oxygen saturation in the lower body. This can occur in congenital cardiac lesions such as interrupted aortic arch, in pulmonary diseases, and commonly in PPHN. In PPHN, the difference in PaO_2 may increase dramatically with 100% oxygen administration, reaching levels considerably higher than 100–150 mm Hg in the right radial artery, whereas descending aortic PaO_2 increases only slightly.

Respiratory Distress

Respiratory problems are among the most significant causes of morbidity and mortality during the neonatal period. Meconium aspiration syndrome and PPHN in the full-term infant and RDS or HMD in the preterm infant are the more common pulmonary causes of respiratory distress. In general, infants with respiratory distress have tachypnea, decreased air entry or gas exchange, retractions (which may be intercostal, subcostal, or suprasternal), grunting, stridor, flaring of the alae nasae, and cyanosis.

Many of these signs are nonspecific responses of the newborn to serious illnesses, and any of the conditions listed in Table 4–18 can cause respiratory distress. Thus, many conditions that produce neonatal respiratory distress are not primary diseases of the lungs. The differential diagnosis involves multiple organ systems.

The prenatal and perinatal histories must be reviewed in detail, particularly in relation to diabetes, the presence of oligohydramnios or polyhydramnios, Rh or blood group incompatibility, maternal hemorrhage, premature rupture of the membranes (PROM), perinatal asphyxia or acidosis, and the need for resuscitation. Oligohydramnios secondary to renal disorders or amniotic leakage could lead to pulmonary hypoplasia, Potter's facies, malposition of the extremities, and growth retardation. Esophageal atresia or atresia of the upper gastrointestinal tract should be suspected with polyhydramnios. However, congenital diaphragmatic hernia, Rh incompatibility, mesoblastic nephroma, and nonimmune hydrops are also associated with polyhydramnios. The possibility of infection or pneumonia should be considered with prolonged rupture of membranes. Respiratory distress is more likely to occur in infants born by cesarean section. The risk of respiratory distress is 11 times greater in infants born by cesarean section than in those delivered vaginally. When a cesarean section is performed without preceding labor, more fluid remains in the lungs after birth; its absorption results in lower plasma colloid oncotic pressures compared with those of infants born by cesarean with previous labor. Further, pulmonary vascular resistance is increased in these infants. Thoracic gas volume is diminished during the first 6 hours after birth, and less pulmonary surfactant is secreted.

The time of onset of respiratory distress is important. Absence of respiratory distress during the first few hours excludes RDS, MAS, transient tachypnea, severe diaphragmatic hernia, choanal atresia and other congenital anomalies, and most cases of PPHN. Table 4–19 classifies respiratory distress according to the time of onset of symptoms and clinical course.

In the infant with respiratory distress, an attempt should be made to differentiate between intrathoracic and extrathoracic causes. Intrathoracic causes include abnormalities of lungs, heart, diaphragm, rib cage, or airways. Extrathoracic causes include neurologic, abdominal, hematologic, and metabolic abnormalities; shock; infection; drugs; and those related to the upper airway obstruction. Extrathoracic causes usually can be excluded readily from the history, physical examination, hematocrit, and blood pressure values. Abdominal causes usually can be diagnosed by inspection and palpation of the abdomen. Neurologic causes can be detected by history, examination, and imaging procedures. Extrathoracic obstruction of the airway usually causes inspiratory difficulty and stridor because the normal reduction in extrathoracic

Table 4–18. Differential Diagnosis of Respiratory Distress in Neonates

Respiratory

Lung	Respiratory distress syndrome, meconium aspiration syndrome, persistent pulmonary hypertension of the newborn, pneumonia, transient tachypnea, pulmonary air leaks, pleural effusions, chylothorax, tumors, pulmonary hypoplasia, congenital lobar emphysema, congenital cystic adenomatoid malformation of the lung, lymphangiectasia, bronchopulmonary dysplasia
Airway	Nasal or choanal atresia, Pierre Robin syndrome, laryngotracheomalacia, membranes or stenosis of larynx or trachea; vocal cord paralysis, hemangiomas, lymphangiomas, massive aspirations, bronchopulmonary dysplasia

Cardiovascular

Heart failure (congenital heart disease, cardiomyopathy)
Myocarditis
Tachyarrhythmias or bradyarrhythmias
Patent ductus arteriosus
Peripheral: Shock

Nervous system

Central	Meningoencephalitis, intracranial hemorrhage, congenital lesions, tumors
Peripheral	Phrenic nerve paralysis, vocal cord paralysis

Muscular–skeletal

Malformations	Thoracic dystrophies (dysplasias, osteogenesis, hypophosphatasia, Jeune syndrome, trisomies D and E)
Diaphragm	Eventration, hernia, paralysis

Hematologic

Anemia
Polycythemia

Metabolic

Hypoglycemia (infants of diabetic mothers)
Hypocalcemia
Hypothermia
Inborn errors of metabolism
Acidosis (organic, lactic, glycogenesis)

Infections

Sepsis, bacteremia
Pneumonia
Meningitis

Drugs

Any that depress central nervous system or induce acidemia or tissue hypoxia

Abdominal

Omphalocele
Gastroschisis
Ascites
Significant distention
Tumors
Congenital anomalies

Other

Erythroblastosis fetalis
Nonimmune hydrops

Table 4–19. Causes of Respiratory Distress According to Time of Onset and Clinical Course

Onset of Symptoms	Acute Course	Progressive Course
At birth	Pneumothorax, apnea, asphyxia, maternal drugs, choanal atresia and other congenital anomalies, diaphragmatic hernia, pulmonary hypoplasia	Respiratory distress syndrome, transient tachypnea, persistent pulmonary hypertension of the newborn, pneumonias, meconium aspiration; aspiration of clear or bloody amniotic fluid; rarely, CHD
0–7 d	Pulmonary air leaks (pneumothorax, pneumomediastinum, pneumopericardium) apnea, sepsis, hypoglycemia, intracranial hemorrhage, pulmonary hemorrhage, aspiration	PIE, pneumonias, congenital intrathoracic lesions; some CHD; abdominal distention, omphalocele, gastroschisis, neuromuscular disease, metabolic acidosis, PDA
After 7 d	Same as above	PIE, pneumonias, PDA, bronchopulmonary dysplasia, diaphragmatic eventration, phrenic palsy, congenital lobar emphysema, congenital cystic adenomatoid malformation of the lung, other intrathoracic abnormalities, some CHD

CHD = congenital heart disease; PDA = patent ductus arteriosus; PIE = pulmonary interstitial emphysema.

airway diameter during inspiration is exaggerated. Suprasternal retraction also may be noted. Obstruction of the intrathoracic airways is unusual in the immediate neonatal period and is related to anatomic or spasmodic narrowing of the small airways during expiration; therefore, it is associated with a prolonged expiratory phase and wheezing. This usually occurs with bronchopulmonary dysplasia (BPD), bronchiolitis, and, occasionally, massive aspiration of meconium. If the obstruction is located in the intermediate segment of the airway, inspiratory and expiratory stridor can occur.

Although a chest radiograph may not be diagnostic soon after birth, it might document such conditions as pneumothorax, pulmonary agenesis or hypoplasia, diaphragmatic hernia, and thoracic cysts. It is useful to classify intrathoracic causes of respiratory distress in the newborn by chest radiograph according to the intrathoracic volume (Table 4–20).

Table 4–20. Chest Radiograph Classification According to Intrathoracic Volume

Increased intrathoracic volume
  Transient tachypnea of the newborn
  Aspiration
  Pneumothorax and other pulmonary air leaks
  Cystic malformations
  Congenital lobar emphysema
  Diaphragmatic hernia
  Some congenital heart diseases
  Some cases of PPHN
  Bronchopulmonary dysplasia

Decreased intrathoracic volume
  Respiratory distress syndrome
  Atelectasis
  Other: Pulmonary edema, hemorrhage, hypoplasia

Normal intrathoracic volume
  Pneumonias
  Some congenital heart diseases
  Asymmetric intrathoracic volume
  Pleural effusions
  Chylothorax
  Diaphragmatic eventration and paralysis
  Congenital lobar emphysema
  Pulmonary cysts
  Diaphragmatic hernia
  Pneumothorax

Variable intrathoracic volume
  Pulmonary edema
  Congenital heart disease
  PPHN
  Mediastinum tumors

PPHN = persistent pulmonary hypertension of the newborn.

EVALUATION

Assessment of the infant with respiratory distress includes a detailed history and examination; a chest radiograph; and measurement of arterial blood gases, Hb, hematocrit, and glucose and calcium concentrations. Depending on the clinical features, blood cultures and leukocyte and platelet counts should be included. An ECG, echocardiogram, and neurologic imaging procedures also may be indicated.

MANAGEMENT

As with all sick newborns, infants with respiratory distress should be placed in a neutral thermal environment with humidification; intravenous fluids and glucose should be administered. Oxygen should be given for hypoxemia. Heart rate and respirations, as well as oxygen maturation or PaO_2, should be monitored continuously by noninvasive methods. Serial blood gas determinations may be indicated; if repeated measurements are necessary, an indwelling radial arterial or umbilical arterial catheter should be placed. Infants whose condition continues to deteriorate, with increasing respiratory acidosis or significant hypoventilation or apnea, require endotracheal intubation and mechanical ventilation. Respiratory acidosis (decreased pH with elevated $PaCO_2$ and no reduction in the bicarbonate concentration) is frequently noted in infants with pulmonary insufficiency associated with lung disease, upper airway abnormalities, malformations of the thoracic rib cage or diaphragm, neurologic abnormalities, and phrenic nerve palsy. Treatment requires assisted ventilation and *not* intravenous alkali such as sodium bicarbonate. Some infants with pulmonary insufficiency have increased $PaCO_2$ and decreased pH but also have reduced bicarbonate concentration (mixed metabolic and respiratory acidosis). In addition to mechanical ventilation, tris (hydroxymethyl) aminomethane (THAM) may be used to correct the metabolic component in these infants. Hypoventilation due to central depression from transplacental passage of narcotics used during labor should be treated by assisted ventilation and narcotic antagonists, such as naloxone.

In the immediate neonatal period, the normal blood pH is greater than 7.30 and the normal base excess is about −4. Metabolic acidosis is considered to be present when pH is less than 7.30 and base excess is −5 or greater. The $PaCO_2$ will decrease if the lungs and CNS are functioning appropriately to compensate for the decrease in pH. In general, bicarbonate should not be given intravenously unless the infant is critically ill, the pH is less than 7.25, and the base deficit is greater than 10.

Continuing management of acidosis should be determined on the basis of the pathophysiologic mechanisms involved. If the infant has respiratory distress with a low PaO_2 and low $PaCO_2$, the problem is likely to be cardiac. If the PaO_2 is normal and the infant is hypotonic or hyporeflexic, the cause may be infectious or, less commonly, an inborn error of metabolism. There are also nutritional, renal, hematologic, or iatrogenic causes of metabolic acidosis during the neonatal period.

Additional therapeutic procedures may be necessary. Blood volume expansion should be instituted for hypovolemic shock, and packed red blood cells should be provided for anemia. Inotropic cardiac support also might be indicated. If metabolic acidosis persists and the pH is less than 7.25, sodium bicarbonate in a solution that contains 0.5 meq/mL may be given by slow intravenous infusion. The dose of bicarbonate in milliequivalents in neonates is derived from the following formula:

$$0.7 \times \text{body weight (grams)} \times \text{base excess}$$

where 0.7 is an estimated constant for the distribution space of bicarbonate. Only half the calculated dose should be given initially; the acid–base status is then reviewed, and additional amounts of sodium bicarbonate may be given. Sodium bicarbonate may cause complications, particularly hypervolemia and hypernatremia. When sodium bicarbonate is used, the serum calcium and particularly ionized calcium concentrations should be monitored carefully, and calcium administered as needed.

Neonatal Anemia

HEMATOPOIESIS

Hematopoiesis begins in the embryo by approximately the 20th day of gestation in blood islands in the yolk sac. The site of erythropoiesis changes during gestation; in the second trimester it occurs primarily in the liver and spleen, and toward the end of the last trimester the bone marrow becomes the predominant site of erythropoiesis. The Hb concentration is usually 8–10 g/dL by 12 weeks' gestation and continues to increase until approximately 33 weeks in male fetuses and 38–39 weeks in female fetuses. Newborn girls normally have lower values of Hb than do boys between 30 and 38 weeks. A full-term male infant with an Hb of 13 g/dL or less at birth should be considered to have anemia, but this is within normal limits for a female infant born at 30 weeks' gestation. The following formula is useful for estimating Hb concentration in relation to gestational age in female infants at birth: Hb concentration = lunar months of gestation + 7. For example, if the duration of gestation was 32 weeks (8 lunar months), the approximate value for a normal Hb concentration would be 15 g/dL. By this time, male fetuses have almost achieved values that are normally accepted for term infants (at 33 weeks the normal value for male infants is already 16.5–17.5 g/dL).

After birth, Hb levels increase transiently by 6–12 hours because of loss of water from the intravascular space. Sub-sequently, Hb concentration decreases, achieving a nadir by 3–6 months in full-term infants and 6–10 weeks in preterm infants. Fetal and neonatal red blood cells are larger than adult cells, with a mean corpuscular volume of 110–120 fL, and they have a shorter half life of 70–90 days versus 120 days for adult cells. By 2 months after birth, normal full-term infants maintain a hematocrit of about 35%, with a red blood cell mass of only 80% of that at birth. However, a premature infant born at 1500 g would require a red blood cell mass of 130% of that at birth to achieve a hematocrit of 35% by 2 months. Premature infants cannot increase the red blood cell mass so that their hematocrits are much lower at 2 months of postnatal age. Clinical signs of anemia are evident only when it is severe enough to affect oxygen delivery to the tissues. Hematocrit and Hb values differ with the site from which they are obtained. In general, values are higher in central venous than in arterial samples, and during the first few days after birth, capillary samples obtained by heel stick have higher values than central venous samples. In edematous infants, values are lower in the capillary samples.

Fetal Hb represents 65–90% of total Hb concentration at birth but normally decreases to less than 5% by 4 months of age. Fetal Hb values decline rapidly in infants that receive multiple transfusions or exchange transfusions. Hemoglobin F is composed of two α chains and two γ chains; adult HbA is composed of two α-globin and two β-globin chains. Hemoglobin F has a lower P_{50} than HbA. The release of oxygen to the tissues is less with HbF than with HbA. For this reason, at the same total Hb concentration and oxygen content of arterial blood, tissue oxygen uptake will be more impaired with higher concentrations of HbF.

The blood volume of the term infant is approximately 85 mL/kg, and it is greater than 90 mL/kg in the preterm infant. The total fetal–placental blood volume is 25–35 mL/kg greater. At the time of birth, the relative blood volumes in the placenta and the infant can change with position and time of cord clamping. Thus, if the baby is above the level of the placenta and the umbilical cord is clamped early, neonatal blood volume will be relatively lower. It is recommended that the infant be kept at the level of the placenta and the cord clamped about 30 seconds after delivery to avoid hypovolemia with subsequent anemia.

ETIOLOGY

Anemia is suspected by pallor, a heart murmur, poor peripheral perfusion, and tissue hypoxia with metabolic acidosis or, more frequently, is detected by a low hematocrit value or a low Hb concentration. The diagnosis of anemia from Hb and hematocrit values must take into account gestational age, sex, and postnatal age.

The common causes of neonatal anemia are blood loss and isoimmune hemolytic conditions. Table 4–21 lists the

Table 4–21. Causes of Neonatal Anemia

	Blood Loss	Hemolysis	Decreased Production	Other
Common	Fetal–maternal transfusion Placenta previa Abruption of placenta Twin–twin transfusion Organ hemorrhage (cranial, hepatic, adrenal) Blood withdrawal	ABO incompatibility Minor group incompatibility	Intrauterine congenital infection	Anemia of prematurity (multifactorial)
Uncommon	Vasa previa Cord accidents (knots, nuchal rupture) Placental severage during cesarean section	Rh incompatibility Enzyme deficiency Abnormal hemoglobin Membrane abnormalities Lupus and other maternal autoimmune conditions Disseminated intravascular coagulation	Congenital aplasia Congenital leukemia Neuroblastoma Osteopetrosis	

causes of neonatal anemia. Severe minor group incompatibilities, severe Rh disease, α-thalassemia, and congenital perinatal infections present soon after birth. ABO hemolytic disease (when the mother's blood type is O, and she carries high IgG titers of either anti-A or anti-B) usually presents more than 48–72 hours after birth with hyperbilirubinemia and decreasing Hb and hematocrit. β-Thalassemia major and sickle cell disease do not commonly manifest anemia during the neonatal period. The cause of blood loss differs in term and preterm infants, as does the time of manifestation of anemia. Early anemia in the term infant due to blood loss usually is related to obstetric conditions (e.g., fetal–maternal bleeding, placenta previa, and cord conditions), whereas in the preterm infant the anemia is usually due to blood withdrawal for laboratory studies or organ bleeding (e.g., intracranial hemorrhage). The most common cause of anemia in a full-term 2–6-month-old infant is an undetected obstetric blood loss.

Early anemia of premature infants usually is associated with repeated blood sampling for laboratory tests; it usually presents with respiratory distress. Because the blood volume of a 1000-g infant is about 85–90 mL, the infant often loses almost half the blood volume in the first 3–7 days of hospitalization. Loss of 1 mL of blood in a 1000-g infant is equivalent to a loss of 55–70 mL in an adult. Other forms of blood loss, such as intracranial or gastrointestinal hemorrhage or disseminated intravascular coagulation, can cause anemia during the first month in premature infants. In preterm infants 2–4 months after birth, the most common cause of late anemia is the so-called anemia of prematurity.

CLINICAL FEATURES

The signs of anemia differ with the cause and the rapidity with which it occurs. Acute blood loss due to a fetal–maternal hemorrhage, rupture of the umbilical cord, or any other obstetric accident presents immediately after birth with pallor and signs of shock (e.g., decreased peripheral pulses, poor peripheral perfusion, and metabolic acidosis). In addition, red cell size, Hb concentration, and hematocrit may be normal. Chronic blood loss is not associated with shock, but Hb and hematocrit values are reduced, and red cell morphology may be abnormal. Hepatic and splenic enlargement are also common, as is presence of a cardiac systolic murmur. Fetal–maternal hemorrhage occurs in more than 50% of pregnancies, but the fetal blood loss varies widely, from 1 to 100 mL. Diagnosis of fetal–maternal bleeding is confirmed by an acid elution test on the mother's blood. Because HbF is resistant to acid elution but HbA is not, the maternal cells are discolored and the fetal blood cells remain pink in the maternal peripheral blood smear. This test (Kleihaur-Betke) is currently available as a kit (Fetal Dex).

Reticulocyte counts are normally 4–12% during the first few days after birth, representing the active erythropoiesis present in utero. After birth, with the increase in arterial blood oxygen, erythropoietin concentrations decrease, as do erythropoiesis and reticulocyte counts. Hemolytic anemias are classically recognized by reticulocytosis and high bilirubin concentration. In all patients with hemolysis or anemia of indefinite cause, a complete blood count, peripheral blood smear, reticulocyte count, red blood cell indices, blood type, direct Coombs test, and bilirubin concentration should be performed in the initial evaluation. Reticulocytosis and anisocytosis are found with isoimmune Rh incompatibility in which hyperbilirubinemia and anemia develop within the first 24 hours after birth. Spherocytes are commonly observed with ABO incompatibility. Determination of the blood type and Coombs test and, in some cases, indirect Coombs or circulating antibody titer determination will help to establish an accurate diagnosis by identifying the antigen and antibody responsible for the hemolysis in isoimmune conditions. If the antibodies are not readily identified, rare cases of nonisoimmune hemolysis must be explored. This necessitates a more extensive workup, including red cell enzyme assays, Hb electrophoresis, red cell membrane tests, and autoimmune testing in mother and infant. Blood loss also may be associated with reticulocytosis, and, in cases of internal hemorrhage, jaundice may be present as the hemorrhage is reabsorbed. An algorithm for a diagnostic approach to neonatal anemia is shown in Chapter 13.

MANAGEMENT

Transfusion with cross-matched red blood cells is the treatment for severe acute blood loss. If isoimmune hemolysis is present and the infant needs a transfusion or an exchange transfusion, the cells must be cross-matched against maternal and neonatal plasmas. All blood used for transfusions should be screened for human immunodeficiency virus (HIV), hepatitis B, and syphilis; for small neonates, cytomegalovirus (CMV)-negative blood is used. In infants with severe hydrops with hemolysis and anemia, it is advisable, as a first step, to do an exchange transfusion with packed red blood cells to increase the Hb concentration without increasing blood volume. Later, exchange transfusions may be necessary if severe hyperbilirubinemia develops. With ABO incompatibility, the blood for exchange should consist of type O red cells suspended in type AB plasma. Blood is irradiated to prevent graft-versus-host disease.

Premature infants who are very ill in the early neonatal period may be anemic and hypovolemic. In addition, the lower the birth weight, the lower the Hb concentration. It is common practice to provide transfusions with 10 mL/kg of packed red cells to maintain the hematocrit at about 45%. An accurate record should be kept of all blood extracted from the infant to replace the blood volume. As the infant improves and can tolerate feeding, rapid growth occurs and iron stores may be inadequate. It is important to provide all elements needed for erythropoiesis, such as folic acid, vitamin E, and iron. These should be provided no later than 30–45 days after birth. By 3–6 weeks after birth, hematocrit and Hb concentrations decrease in growing infants. Normally, this stimulates endogenous erythropoietin production; however, if transfusions are provided (with adult Hb), this will be suppressed, and reticulocytosis will not occur. The greater the number of transfusions, the more the Hb concentration will decrease, because with a higher percentage of HbA there is more oxygen available to the tissues, and symptoms of anemia are therefore less likely to occur. In preterm infants in the first few postnatal weeks, symptoms of anemia include apnea and bradycardic episodes, abnormal weight gain, poor feedings, and tachycardia. The appearance of a heart murmur also can be associated with early signs of anemia. A blood transfusion with packed red blood cells should be provided only when these signs are present in association with a low Hb concentration. Trials with human recombinant erythropoietin (500 mg/[kg/wk]) have been conducted in premature infants, with the aim of decreasing the number of blood transfusions and preventing severe intermediate and late anemia of prematurity.

All premature infants should receive at least 50 mg of folic acid and 5 IU of vitamin E per day. Iron needs for full-term infants are 1 mg/(kg/day) continuing throughout the first year. Premature infants should receive at least 2 mg/(kg/day), and premature infants with ELBW (<30 weeks' gestation) should receive at least 4 mg/(kg/day) of iron. In the trials with erythropoietin, it has been shown that for erythropoiesis to be maintained adequately, 6 mg/(kg/day) of iron is needed in VLBW infants.

Bacterial Infections

Compared with the adult, neonatal immune function is deficient in several aspects: types of specific antibodies, phagocytic and bactericidal function, opsonization, circulating complement, and ability to increase neutrophil production in response to infection. Therefore, the neonate should be considered a "compromised host." The incidence of infections during the newborn period is 1–2 per 1000 live births. Neonatal infections have three temporal patterns of presentation: early, intermediate, or late onset. The causative organisms and the primary site of involvement vary somewhat in relation to the time of onset and whether the infant acquires the infection at home or in hospital (Table 4–22). **Early-onset** infections most frequently involve bacteremia with or without pneumonia and are caused by group B hemolytic streptococci (GBS) and *Escherichia coli.* Urinary tract infections and meningitis are unlikely in these early-onset infections. Infections that appear after 2 weeks in the hospital often are caused by *Staphylococcus epidermidis,* fungi, or some gram-negative organisms. In the infant at home, **late-onset**

Table 4–22. Organisms, Risk Factors, and Choice of Initial Antibiotics in Relation to Time of Onset and Place of Occurrence of Neonatal Sepsis

Onset	Early 0–3 d	Intermediate 4–14 d	Late 14–28 (or more) d	
Place of occurrence	Hospital (home unusual)	Hospital or home	Home	Hospital
Type	Early-onset syndrome	Systemic Urinary tract Skin/joints	Of late onset; 85% will have meningitis	Systemic Pneumonia
Organisms involved	GBS, *Escherichia coli* Other gram-negative organisms *Listeria monocytogenes*	Gram-negative *Staphylococcus* *aureus/epidermidis*	GBS *L. monocytogenes* (Other)	*Staphylococcus* *epidermidis* Fungus (Gram-negative)
Risk factors	Perinatal	Unusual perinatal Other: GU anomaly Surgical procedures Very low birth weight	Unusual	Prolonged central IV access Repeated courses of antibiotics Very low birth weight
Initial treatment	Ampicillin and gentamicin	Ampicillin and gentamicin	Ampicillin and gentamicin	Ampicillin and gentamicin
Possible alternatives (positive blood culture, sensitivities, no response to treatment)	Individualized	First to third generation cephalosporins Vancomycin		Vancomycin Amphotericin B Second to third generation cephalosporins

GBS = group B streptococcus; GU = genitourinary; IV = intravenous.

syndrome is usually caused by GBS or *Listeria monocytogenes;* 85% of these infants have meningitis. Most neonatal infections occur early or in hospitalized infants, particularly in LBW infants. Fatality rates are 15–40%, and there is substantial morbidity in surviving infants. Prompt diagnosis and appropriate medical management are essential.

Several perinatal conditions are associated with increased risk of early-onset sepsis (Table 4–23). These factors are used to select infants to be evaluated and treated until infection is ruled out. Maternal risk factors include vaginal streptococcal colonization, intrapartum fever, prolonged rupture of the membranes (>18–24 hours), prolonged second stage of labor, and chorioamnionitis or a history of urinary tract infection. Early-onset sepsis is also more frequent with prematurity, twin gestation, congenital anomalies, perinatal asphyxia, and male sex. Perinatal risk factors are unusual in late-onset infections, but other factors, such as prolonged intravascular access and prolonged or repeated courses of antibiotics, are frequently noted in nosocomial infections.

SIGNS OF NEONATAL SEPSIS

Early diagnosis is usually made when there is a high index of suspicion. The early signs of neonatal sepsis are subtle and nonspecific; a common early presentation is that the infant "does not look well" and has poor feeding or intolerance to feedings, irritability or lethargy, and temperature instability. By the time the infant manifests multiple and overt signs of sepsis, the morbidity and mortality have increased significantly. Various signs are listed in Table 4–24. Meningitis occurs in 10–30% of early-onset infection. In late-onset sepsis, particularly with GBS or *L monocytogenes,* the incidence of meningitis is about 85%, in contrast with the low rate in early-onset infections. Newborn infants do not usually manifest the classic signs of meningitis described in older children and adults (see Chapter 9).

Many neonatal conditions can mimic the clinical presentation of neonatal sepsis. These include viral infections, congestive heart failure, congenital heart disease, NEC, and metabolic, endocrine, or chromosomal disorders.

Table 4–23. Risk Assessment in Neonatal Sepsis

Clinical Risk Factor	Incidence of Proven Sepsis (%)	Incidence of Proven and Suspected Sepsis (%)
Early-onset		
PROM >18–24 h	1	1–2
Maternal GBS colonization	0.5–1	1–2
PROM + maternal GBS	4–6	7–11
Maternal GBS + fever	3–5	6–10
PROM and chorioamnionitis	3–8	6–10
PROM or GBS in preterm infant	4–6	7–11
PROM and Apgar <6 at 5 min	3–4	6–10
Male sex	4-fold ↑	4-fold ↑
Nosocomial		
Low birth weight, intravascular access, multiple courses of antibiotics, etc	10–15	25

GBS = group B streptococcus; PROM = prolonged rupture of membranes.

WHEN TO EVALUATE FOR SEPSIS?

Because the initial clinical manifestations often are non-specific, the early clinical diagnosis of neonatal sepsis is difficult. The decision to perform a partial or extended evaluation and to institute antimicrobial therapy remains a matter of clinical judgment. The presence of risk factors, inadequate treatment of maternal infection, and whether the infant is preterm should be noted when considering the diagnosis of early-onset sepsis. As shown in Figures 4–3 and 4–4, some infants may require careful observation with or without a sepsis screen, whereas others require an immediate, complete sepsis workup, and still others are given antibiotics pending results of studies. Indications for performing a sepsis workup and for instituting empiric therapy depend on the relative risk. Most clinicians recommend starting antibiotic treatment in infants with neonatal respiratory distress requiring oxygen or ventilatory support, particularly in infants older than 34 weeks' gestation, in whom RDS is unlikely. Symptomatic infants with signs consistent with sepsis, regardless of risk factors and gestational age, should be promptly evaluated and started on antibiotic therapy (see Figures 4–3 and 4–4).

THE SEPSIS WORKUP

The perinatal history, physical examination, and course should be evaluated carefully. Complete blood and differentials counts are often useful; although not specific for sepsis, the association of leukopenia (<6000 µL), neutropenia (<1700/µL, according to postnatal age), and left shifts defined by an immature:total neutrophil ratio of greater than 0.2, have a very good negative predictive value. If none of these is present, the likelihood of sepsis is small. Predictive accuracy is significantly improved by repeat analysis in 8–24 hours. Thrombocytopenia, toxic granulation, vacuolization, and Döhle bodies are other nonspecific alterations that help to exclude sepsis if they are absent. Leukocytosis and neutrophilia are *not* good indicators of neonatal sepsis.

Latex agglutination testing for the presence of GBS antigens usually is done on urine. However, false-positive results can occur in more than 10% of cases. Micro-sedimentation rate, C-reactive protein, fibronectin, and haptoglobin measurements have low positive predictive accuracy and specificity.

A more complete sepsis workup includes chest radiograph and blood culture. When an infant is at risk for infection, younger than 72 hours, and **asymptomatic,** a urine culture and a spinal tap need *not* be performed. An infant in these circumstances is unlikely to have meningitis without having positive blood cultures. However, if the blood culture is positive, cerebrospinal fluid (CSF) should be analyzed. If CSF culture is positive or if there are clear signs of meningitis even with negative cultures, the antibiotic therapy must be prolonged. After the first 72 hours after birth or when there is a strong suspicion of sepsis, a suprapubic bladder tap and a spinal tap must be performed. Some critically ill infants, particularly those with LBW, may be given antibiotics before a spinal tap is performed. If antibiotics are started, the cultures should be incubated for 72 hours to provide

Table 4–24. Clinical Signs in Neonatal Sepsis and Meningitis

Early Onset	Later Onset
"Infant does not look well"	
Grunting	Temperature instability
Tachypnea	Poor feeding
Cyanosis	Weak suck
Poor perfusion	Vomiting or gastric residual
Hypotonia	Abdominal distention
Lethargy/apnea	Lethargy/apnea
Jaundice (<24 h)	Tense fontanelle/convulsions
Shock	Shock

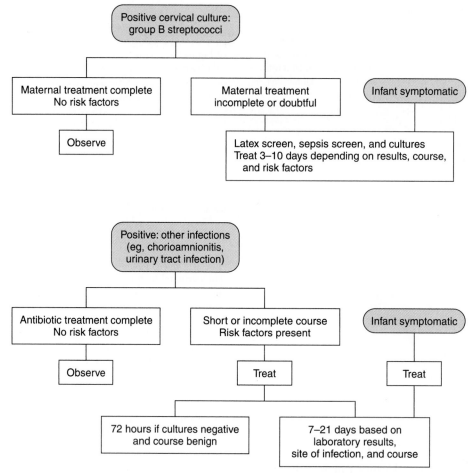

Figure 4–3. Approach to evaluation of neonate when mother has been infected and treated for sepsis.

enough time for the organism to grow before the culture is considered negative and the intravenous antibiotic therapy discontinued. Blood cultures are only 82–90% sensitive in neonates. Therefore, with strong clinical suspicion of sepsis and an abnormal white cell count, the infant may need to be fully treated with antibiotics even with negative blood cultures (see Figures 4–3 and 4–4).

Cerebrospinal fluid examination often is difficult to interpret in the newborn. A normal CSF may have up to 32 white cells per microliter, with up to 60% polymorphonuclear cells. The CSF glucose concentration is variable in neonates but, in general, is greater than 40% of serum glucose concentrations. Protein content may be as high as 180 mg/dL normally or even higher in preterm infants. Organisms should be looked for on Gram stain.

MANAGEMENT

When sepsis is strongly suspected, some tests should be performed promptly and intravenous antibiotic therapy started immediately. Antibiotics are continued until the results of cultures are available and the clinical response to intervention is evaluated. Initially, the infection is treated empirically with a penicillin and an aminoglycoside to provide broad-spectrum coverage against both gram-positive and gram-negative organisms (see Table 4–22). When an organism is identified, antibiotic coverage may need to be changed. The duration of therapy differs with the focus and etiologic agent, the infant's clinical status, and the response to therapy. Sepsis and bacteremia without a focus are usually treated for 7–10 days; pneumonia, 10 days; and meningitis, 14–21 days. Cultures should be repeated to document adequate response; persistent positive cultures

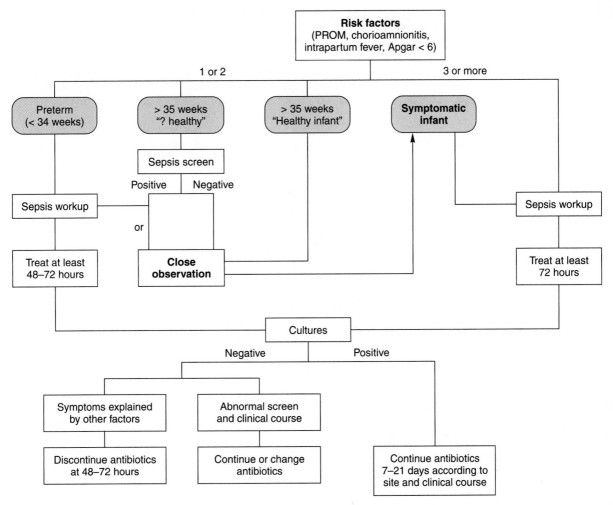

Figure 4–4. Steps in the evaluation of suspected early neonatal infections. PROM = premature rupture of membranes.

warrant an investigation for occult foci, such as abscesses, ventriculitis, or a recurrent portal of entry such as a pilonidal sinus.

Because of the difficulty in diagnosis and the high risk of neonatal sepsis, many infants are overevaluated and empirically overtreated on the basis of "possible infection." Although approximately 10% of all newborns receive some antibiotics, only 1 in 11–25 treated infants eventually has infection documented by a positive culture. Therefore, if cultures prove to be negative at 48–72 hours and the clinical assessment (examination, blood count, and risk factors) suggests low risk for infection, antibiotics may be discontinued (see Figures 4–3 and 4–4). Infants with high risk factors, abnormal sepsis screen, and a strong clinical

suspicion of sepsis may be treated for 7–10 days even if cultures are negative (see Figures 4–3 and 4–4).

All infants with suspected sepsis should be hospitalized and monitored continuously. Some therapies have been proposed as adjuncts to antibiotic therapy; these include administration of blood products, such as fresh frozen plasma, white cell transfusions, whole blood transfusions, exchange transfusions, and, recently, intravenous γ-globulin. These therapies are controversial and have not been proven effective in controlled studies.

Prolonged or repetitive antimicrobial administration increases the risk of altering normal flora and the development of superinfection with resistant bacterial organisms or with fungi, especially in LBW infants.

In infants receiving aminoglycosides or vancomycin, serum concentrations should be monitored and maintained in the safe and therapeutic ranges by modifying the dose and dosage interval as needed. All infants with prolonged aminoglycoside therapy or meningitis should undergo hearing assessment.

Abdominal Mass

Palpation of the abdomen during physical examination of the newborn is not difficult. Allowing the infant to suck or flexing the infant's hips decreases abdominal tone. If the abdomen is distended, nasogastric suction may be indicated to relieve possible functional or anatomic obstruction of the gastrointestinal tract. In the normal newborn, the liver may be palpated 1–3 cm below the right costal margin. The spleen tip is felt less frequently; it is enlarged if it extends 1 cm or more below the left costal margin. The lower poles of both kidneys are usually palpable; the right kidney is typically lower than the left. Uncommon renal anomalies that may be diagnosed by palpation are horseshoe kidney, pelvic kidney, and unilateral agenesis. Other structures that normally may be palpable in the newborn are the aorta, feces in the colon, and a full bladder.

Etiology

Abdominal enlargement may be due to abdominal distention from obstruction to the gastrointestinal tract. Associated signs are vomiting, distention, and absence of stool. Possible causes of intestinal obstruction include atresia (duodenal, jejunal, ileal, or colonic), meconium ileus, malrotation with midgut volvulus, Hirschsprung disease or imperforate anus, annular pancreas, and, at a later age, pyloric stenosis and intussusception. Compressive external abdominal masses or functional obstructions also may lead to abdominal distention.

Clinical Features

Evaluation of an abdominal mass not associated with obstruction includes definition of its mobility, location, characteristics, and associated symptoms. Mobility of the mass distinguishes intraperitoneal from retroperitoneal lesions. Masses in the flank tend to arise from the urinary tract, although adrenal hemorrhage or, rarely, neuroblastoma may displace the kidney. One half of all abdominal masses discovered in the newborn are of renal origin; hydronephrosis and multicystic kidney are the most frequent abdominal masses in the newborn. Obstruction early in renal development results in multicystic kidney, whereas obstruction, unilaterally or bilaterally, after nephron development results in hydronephrosis. The hydronephrotic kidney is smooth and firm, whereas the multicystic kidney, which is usually nonfunctional, is irregular and cystic. Review of the prenatal history may help determine the cause of an abdominal mass, e.g., when there is a history of in-

herited kidney disease (infantile polycystic disease). Renal vein thrombosis, rarely bilateral, usually occurs in the IDM or after polycythemia and severe dehydration; it is often associated with hematuria. Mesoblastic nephroma, a renal hamartoma, is the most common solid tumor in the infant kidney and may be associated with polyhydramnios. It must be distinguished from Wilms' tumor, which is rare in the newborn.

Masses in the right upper quadrant must be distinguished from liver enlargement. Masses involving the liver may be associated with a history of jaundice (choledochal cyst) or birth trauma (subcapsular hematoma). A smooth lower midline abdominal mass may be due to hydrometrocolpos in a female infant (from an intact hymen or lower vaginal atresia) or bladder distention. A distended bladder in a male infant most commonly is due to posterior urethral valves. Neuroblastoma, the most common congenital malignant tumor, arises from the adrenal cortex or along the sympathetic chain. The mass is stony hard and frequently crosses the midline.

Mobile midline cysts may be due to gastrointestinal duplication or lymphatic abnormalities in the mesentery. In the female infant, stimulation by circulating hormones from the mother or chorion may result in ovarian, follicular, or theca lutein cysts. All these mobile cysts are smooth. Ovarian tumors are rare and usually solid and fixed.

The investigation of choice after clinical evaluation is ultrasonography. Plain radiographs of the abdomen may be performed if there is concern for intestinal obstruction. In the past, because of the high incidence of renal lesions, the study of choice for an abdominal mass was intravenous pyelography. Today, such studies with contrast materials can be avoided or delayed when ultrasound is used to identify a mass that arises outside the urinary tract. Nuclear scanning of kidney function, computed tomography (CT), or magnetic resonance imaging (MRI) may be indicated. Laboratory evaluation depends on the nature of the mass (e.g., cystic vs. solid). Many of the abdominal masses reviewed above require surgical intervention.

Seizures

The identification and classification of seizures is a difficult but important clinical problem in the newborn period. The typical unambiguous tonic–clonic seizure pattern seen in older children and adults is not evident, perhaps because of the immaturity of the newborn nervous system. Neonatal seizures frequently are subtle and difficult to distinguish from common, benign newborn activities, such as jitteriness or clonus. It is important to identify seizures correctly because they are frequently associated with underlying disorders requiring specific, prompt treatment. Recent evidence suggests that seizure activity that is allowed to persist without treatment can result in brain injury.

In the newborn, jitteriness may be confused with seizures. Many of the metabolic problems that underlie neonatal seizures, such as hypoglycemia, hypocalcemia, asphyxia, and drug withdrawal, also are associated with jitteriness. Premature infants and IDMs, even those without any of the previously mentioned metabolic problems, frequently have jitteriness. Several characteristics that can help distinguish jitteriness from seizures are presented in Table 4–25.

The prenatal, perinatal, and postnatal histories and a detailed physical examination often provide the necessary information for establishing the etiology of neonatal seizures. Emphasis should be placed identifying any family history of "unexplained" infant death, such as inherited metabolic disorders, in utero exposure to drugs of abuse (methadone, heroin, barbiturates, cocaine, and ethanol), inadvertent injection of local anesthetic agents into the fetus after paracervical or pudendal blocks for maternal analgesia, hypoxic events and perinatal asphyxia, maternal or perinatal infection, neonatal medications such as high doses of aminophylline, or rapid withdrawal after administering narcotics liberally. It is important to note the type and age of onset of the seizure (see below). Clinically, there are four major seizure types in the newborn period: subtle, tonic, clonic, and myoclonic. The additional adjectives focal, multifocal, and generalized describe the site(s) involved in the seizure activity. When several sites are involved, the activity can be synchronous (generalized) or asynchronous (multifocal). Examination revealing a tense or bulging anterior fontanelle suggests intracranial hemorrhage or meningitis, and pupils may be fixed or asymmetric as a result of significant intracranial pathology. Posture, muscle tone, and reflexes should be evaluated carefully and frequently. A significant decrease in hematocrit may result from intracranial hemorrhage, and a high hematocrit (>70%) may be associated with cerebral infarction. Hypoglycemia and hypocalcemia are the most frequent metabolic disorders that cause neonatal seizures. Extreme sodium imbalance also can cause seizures. Significant hypernatremia increases CNS irritability and thus may induce seizures. Hyponatremia decreases CNS excitability, but if sodium concentration decreases rapidly, cerebral edema and seizures may result. Hypernatremia therefore must be corrected slowly to avoid a rapid decrease in serum sodium concentration. A lumbar puncture is necessary to obtain CSF to diagnose meningitis usually caused by group B streptococcus or *E. coli*. Examination of the CSF also may help to diagnose encephalitis resulting from viruses such as herpes simplex, enterovirus, or rubella or parasites such as toxoplasmosis. Evaluation of serum pH and base deficit may lead to the diagnosis of amino or organic acidopathies; in addition to seizures, these present with recurrent or persistent metabolic acidosis and signs of neurologic dysfunction. When early neonatal seizures are resistant to all usual therapeutic medications, pyridoxine dependency should be ruled out by a therapeutic trial with intravenous injection of 50–100 µg of pyridoxine while an electroencephalogram (EEG) is being performed. Normalization of the EEG immediately after the injection confirms the diagnosis. If it is apparent that seizures are not readily attributable to asphyxia, a metabolic problem, drugs, or infection, it is then necessary to perform imaging procedures. Head ultrasound examination can be used to diagnose intraventricular hemorrhages, but CT or MRI scans are usually necessary for diagnosing other lesions and cerebral cortical malformations, such as disorders of neuronal migration. In some infants with neonatal seizures an EEG can be very useful; it may determine the diagnosis in paralyzed or "jittery" newborns and provide information regarding the prognosis. (When the interictal EEG is abnormal, the risk of poor neurologic outcome is high with most seizure types.) The EEG findings differ in relation to the different convulsive clinical types (Table 4–26), and several of the clinical phenomena classified as seizures in the newborn are not associated with synchronous EEG seizure activity. This may occur with many subtle seizures, particularly in the full-term infant, and with focal clonic and generalized tonic seizures when the electrical discharges do not accompany the clinical seizures (Table 4–26). Whether some of these seizures are associated with neural electrical discharges that are not recorded by the surface electrodes of current EEG equipment is unclear.

The clinical seizure type and the postnatal age at which the seizures are first detected bear a strong association with the possible etiology. The most important etiologies with the associated common seizure types and usual age of onset are shown in Table 4–27. Hypoxic-ischemic encephalopathy, usually after perinatal asphyxia, is a very common cause of early neonatal seizures. These seizures can be very difficult to control and often evolve into status

Table 4–25. Comparisons of Jitteriness and Seizure

Characteristic	Jitteriness	Seizure
Abnormal eye movements	No	Yes
Elicited with stimulation or passive stretch	Yes	No
Ceases with passive flexion	Yes	No
Dominant movement	Very rapid, rhythmic	Fast and slow components
Electroencephalogram	Normal	May be abnormal

Table 4–26. Classification of Neonatal Seizures

Type	Manifestation	Common EEG Findings
Subtle	Paroxysms of ocular, oral, buccal, or lingual movements; apnea	Frequently abnormal
Focal clonic	Rhythmic twitching of one extremity	Focal sharp activity
Multifocal clonic	Sequential twitching of several limbs	Multiple foci of sharp activity
Focal tonic	Sustained asymmetric extensor posturing	Typically abnormal
Generalized tonic	Mimics decerebrate or decorticate posture	Discharges do not accompany clinical seizures
Focal myoclonic	Rapid, rhythmic jerks of flexion	Discharges do not accompany clinical seizures
Generalized myoclonic	Asynchronous jerking of several limbs	Burst suppression pattern

EEG = electroencephalogram.

epilepticus despite adequate doses of anticonvulsant medication.

TREATMENT

Urgent treatment of metabolic disorders such as hypoglycemia or hypocalcemia is crucial to prevent complications and sequelae. Hypoglycemia is treated with intravenous glucose solution, 10%, in a dose of 200 mg/kg followed by continuous glucose infusion. Hypocalcemia is treated with 200 mg/kg of calcium gluconate in a 10% solution intravenously. If the diagnosis of pyridoxine deficiency is established (see above), treatment requires sufficiently high doses of vitamin B_6.

Inadvertent injection of local anesthetic agent into the fetus with resultant early seizures, usually at less than 6 hours after birth, has been described most commonly after paracervical or pudendal blocks for maternal analgesia. These seizures require vigorous treatment with anticonvulsants, and the infants usually recover completely and have a perfectly normal long-term follow-up.

For intracranial hemorrhage, meningitis, and any case in which the cause of the seizure is not both readily apparent and amenable to specific treatment, anticonvulsant medication should be initiated promptly. Phenobarbital is the most common first-line therapy, given intravenously

as a loading dose of 20 mg/kg. When seizures are difficult to control, as is often the case in hypoxic-ischemic seizures, repeated doses up to 40–50 mg/kg of the total dose may be necessary in the first 4–24 hours of therapy. Maintenance doses are usually 3–4 mg/(kg/day). When this single therapy is inadequate, phenytoin is usually considered next, with a loading dose of 20 mg/kg and a maintenance dose of 3–4 mg/(kg/day) intravenously. Diazepam and lorazepam, two benzodiazepines, are not used for maintenance therapy and are of limited usefulness in the management of neonatal seizures. For seizures that are refractory and difficult to manage, there has been some success with short-term use of intravenous lorazepam, 0.05 mg/kg.

■ DISORDERS OF THE NEWBORN

RESPIRATORY DISORDERS

Apnea in the Premature Infant

Apnea is defined as a respiratory pause without airflow lasting more than 20 seconds or as a pause of any duration accompanied by bradycardia and cyanosis or oxy-

Table 4–27. Relation of Etiology to Seizure Type and Age of Onset

Etiology	Seizure Type	Age of Onset
Hypoxic-ischemic	Subtle, tonic (premature), or clonic (full-term)	First 24 h
Intracranial hemorrhage	Subtle or focal clonic	First 3 d
Metabolic	Clonic or generalized tonic	First 3 d or >5 d (late hypocalcemia or acidopathy)
Infection	Focal tonic or clonic	>3 d
Cerebral malformation	Focal clonic or myoclonic	Any time from birth on
Drug withdrawal	Clonic or generalized tonic	>2 d but depends on drug(s) of abuse
Systemic injection of local anesthetic agents	Generalized tonic	First 6 h

gen desaturation, as shown by pulse oximetry monitoring. Apnea in neonates can be **central,** with a complete cessation of chest wall movements and no airflow. Apnea also may be due to **airway obstruction;** in this circumstance, chest wall movements of respiratory efforts continue, but there is no airflow. The commonly available monitors do not record obstructive apnea because they continue to detect chest wall movements. A combination of central and obstructive apnea constitutes **mixed apnea,** the most frequent type encountered in premature infants.

When apnea is diagnosed, an immediate evaluation must be made to determine the etiology. Possible causes of apnea in preterm infants are listed in Table 4–28. The incidence of apnea increases with decreasing gestational age. **Idiopathic apnea of prematurity** occurs without any identifiable cause. It usually appears after 24 hours' postnatal age and during the first week after birth; it usually resolves by 38–44 weeks of postconceptual age (gestational age at birth plus weeks of postnatal age).

MANAGEMENT

An approach to the management of apnea is shown in Table 4–29. Recurrent apnea can be treated with continuous positive airway pressure (CPAP) of 3–6 cm of water. Methylxanthines stimulate central inspiratory drive and increase sensitivity of the respiratory center to carbon dioxide. Caffeine is the drug of choice because there is a wide separation between therapeutic (4–18 μg/mL) and toxic (≥50 μg/mL) serum concentrations. The usual oral dose is as follows: loading, 10 mg/kg of caffeine base; maintenance, 2.5 mg/(kg/day). The caffeine citrate loading dose is 20 mg/kg, and maintenance is 5 mg/(kg/day), given once daily. Theophylline can be used, but the toxic and therapeutic concentrations are much closer. Toxic manifestations include tachycardia, irritability, tremors, seizures, and fever. Gastric residual may increase with vomiting; in addition, hyperglycemia and polyuria may occur. If apnea is associated with seizures, methylxanthines are contraindicated because they can increase the risk of seizures.

Table 4–28. Causes of Apnea in Preterm Infants

Infection	Hypoglycemia
Lung disease	Airway obstruction
Hypothermia/hyperthermia	Feedings
Patent ductus arteriosus	Bowel movement
Seizures	Intraventricular hemorrhage
Maternal drugs	Drug withdrawal
Gastroesophageal reflux	Anemia
Idiopathic apnea of prematurity	

Table 4–29. Management of Apnea in Premature Infants

Search for specific etiology

Temperature	Avoid low temperature and rapid warming Maintain neutral thermal environment (lowest normal)
Oxygen	Do not use routinely Treat hypoxia (but avoid hyperoxia)
Airway	Put infant in prone position Place head and neck in neutral position Suction secretions as needed Remove orogastric or nasogastric tubes
Stimulation	Proprioceptive (e.g., rocking or waterbeds) Cutaneous
Medications	Caffeine Theophylline Phenytoin Doxapram
Ventilation	Bag-mask (for a severe apneic episode) Continuous positive airway pressure Intermittent mechanical ventilation

Respiratory Distress Syndrome

LUNG DEVELOPMENT DURING FETAL LIFE

Knowledge of lung development allows an understanding of the preterm infant's ability to maintain adequate respiratory function at different gestational ages. At 3–4 weeks of gestation, the trachea develops from the esophagus, and pulmonary arteries originate from the sixth aortic arch. By 14 weeks, the lung develops as an outpouching of the embryonic gut. By 16 weeks, bronchial segmentation is complete, and the canalicular stage begins with acinar formation and cuboidal cells in the epithelium. A vascular network develops in the mesoderm and proliferates around the potential airspaces. By 20–22 weeks, osmophilic lamellar inclusion bodies appear in the epithelial cells. The development of terminal air sacs begins at 24 weeks, and there is a closer approximation between the respiratory epithelium and the capillaries. The epithelial type II cells have an active endoplasmic reticulum in which phospholipids are synthesized, mainly dipalmitoylphosphatidylcholine (DPPC). Also by this time, the type II cells begin to differentiate into thinner type I epithelial cells. During this stage of lung development, gas exchange is possible, but the distance between the capillaries and the airspaces is still three times greater than in adults. By 26 weeks' gestation, there are larger airspaces in close contact with capillaries but still no true alveoli; gas exchange, however, may be adequate during air breathing.

By 28 weeks, alveolar ducts and respiratory bronchioles are easily distinguishable, with an increase in the area for diffusion. By 30 weeks, the subdivision of terminal bronchioles into respiratory bronchioles has almost ended, and alveoli are actively formed; this stage is completed by 34 weeks. Pulmonary surfactant, the surface-active material that decreases surface tension and prevents atelectasis, is first noted at approximately 23–24 weeks' gestation, with the appearance of the osmophilic inclusion bodies in the type II alveolar cells. However, a sufficient quantity of surfactant is produced only after 30–32 weeks' gestation; beyond this period, the incidence of RDS decreases significantly. Pulmonary surfactant is composed of phospholipids, mainly DPPC, and surfactant proteins A (SPA), B (SPB), and C (SPC). It is secreted into the alveolar lumen and the tracheal fluid, which flows out of the nose and mouth into the amniotic cavity. Pulmonary maturity can be assessed before birth by determining the presence of surfactant in amniotic fluid obtained by amniocentesis. In the "shake" test described by Clements, diluted amniotic fluid is shaken in a test tube; the stability of the bubbles is directly related to the presence of surface-active material. A ratio of lecithin (DPPC) to sphingomyelin (L:S ratio) greater than 2:1 or the presence of phosphatidylglycerol (a minor phospholipid in surfactant) is another indicator of fetal lung maturity.

CLINICAL MANIFESTATIONS

Respiratory distress syndrome occurs in approximately 0.5% of neonates and is the most frequent cause of respiratory distress and insufficiency in preterm infants. The incidence is as much as 50% before 30 weeks' gestation but less than 10% at 35–36 weeks. The risk factors for RDS are summarized in Table 4–30. The syndrome results from deficiency of pulmonary surfactant, resulting in atelectasis with decreased functional residual capacity, lung compliance, and lung volume. The alveolar collapse causes abnormalities in ventilation–perfusion relationships with intrapulmonary right-to-left shunt with hypoxemia. In severe cases, alveolar ventilation is greatly decreased with resultant hypercarbia and respiratory acidosis.

Clinical signs of RDS may develop at birth or a few hours after birth. The infants usually show increasing distress during the first 24–48 hours, with tachypnea, retraction of the chest wall, expiratory grunting, and cyanosis. The chest radiograph may show diffuse atelectasis with an increased density in both lungs and a fine, granular, "ground-glass" appearance of the lungs. The small airways are filled with air and are clearly surrounded by the increased density of the pulmonary field, the so-called air bronchograms. Lung volume usually is decreased, and the diaphragms are somewhat elevated. These radiographic findings may be more noticeable by 24 hours after birth. Arterial blood gases show decreased PaO_2, with elevated $PaCO_2$ in more severe cases.

The clinical features are more severe and prolonged in preterm infants before 31 weeks' gestation. Hyperkalemia and metabolic acidosis develop in many of these infants. Peripheral edema commonly develops. Hypoxia, hypercapnia, and acidosis combine to act on the function of the type II cells, further decreasing surfactant production. Respiratory insufficiency develops in infants with severe RDS, and mechanical ventilation becomes necessary. Pulmonary arterial hypertension may result from hypoxic and acidemic pulmonary vasoconstriction.

With active and adequate treatment in an intensive care nursery, most infants with RDS survive. Clinical improvement may be evident by 48–72 hours after birth, when oxygen and respirator requirements stabilize, diuresis occurs, and edema diminishes. The clinical course of RDS has changed dramatically since the advent of exogenous surfactant. Clinical features and physiologic disturbances in RDS are summarized in Table 4–31.

Several complications may occur during the course of RDS (Table 4–32). Infants with RDS frequently have a left-to-right-shunt across a patent ductus arteriosus (PDA), usually when the lung disease begins to improve. Some infants are very ill for 2–3 weeks, and chronic complications, such as BPD, may develop.

Table 4–30. Risk Factors for Respiratory Distress Syndrome

Asphyxia	Prematurity
Cesarean section without labor	Previous preterm infant
Hypothermia	with RDS
Immature L:S ratio	Second of twins
Infants of diabetic mothers	White race
Male sex	

L:S = lecithin:sphingomyelin; RDS = respiratory distress syndrome.

Table 4–31. Clinical Features and Physiologic Disturbances in Respiratory Distress Syndrome

Tachypnea	Atelectasis
Nasal flaring	Ground-glass appearance in chest
Retractions	radiographs
Expiratory grunting	Decreased compliance
Cyanosis	Increased physiologic dead-space
Hypotonia	Decreased lung volume
Decreased urine output	Hypoxemia/hypercarbia
Edema	Acidemia
Hyperkalemia	Hypotension

Table 4–32. Complications in Respiratory Distress Syndrome

Pneumothorax	Endotracheal tube related
Pulmonary interstitial emphysema	Extubation: misplacement
	Mucous plugs
Intraventricular hemorrhage	Vocal cord damage
Sepsis	Subglottic stenosis
Patent ductus arteriosus	Bronchopulmonary dysplasia
	Retinopathy of prematurity

MANAGEMENT

Since 1991, two products to replace deficient surfactant have been approved for use in the United States. One is synthetic (Exosurf); the other is a natural product obtained from bovine lungs (Survanta). Other natural products have been approved more recently (Curosurf, Infasurf), and newer synthetic ones are being researched. The use of these products has significantly decreased mortality associated with RDS and long-term morbidity such as BPD and intraventricular hemorrhage. These exogenous surfactants are administered into the trachea; even in the smallest infants, they can be administered prophylactically immediately after birth, before respirations are established. Currently, however, surfactant is used more frequently very soon after RDS has become established. The dose is approximately 3–5 mL/kg/dose given at 12-hour intervals; at least two doses must be administered. Even though this replacement therapy has greatly improved survival and morbidity, infants with RDS continue to require intensive care with general supportive measures and skillful ventilatory management.

Larger premature infants with mild to moderate disease can be stabilized by providing an increased concentration of oxygen, administered by hood using warm, humidified gas. Skin surface oxygen saturation or PaO_2 should be monitored continuously, and arterial blood gases measured intermittently. In larger infants, the PaO_2 should be maintained at 50–70 mm Hg, but in smaller infants a PaO_2 of 45–60 mm Hg is acceptable. The pH should be maintained above 7.25 and the $PaCO_2$ between 45 and 55 mm Hg. In some infants, metabolic acidosis with a base excess of −5 to −8 develops; this does not require treatment with alkaline solutions such as sodium bicarbonate or THAM. If hypercarbia with respiratory acidosis develops, mechanical ventilation should be instituted promptly. If the $PaCO_2$ and pH are normal but the infant has hypoxemia with a fraction of inspired oxygen (FiO_2) greater than 0.7, CPAP should be added by nasal prongs, nasopharyngeal tubes, or endotracheal intubation using end-expiratory distending pressures of 6–10 cm

of water. If mechanical ventilation is needed, it is usual to start with an FiO_2 of 0.5–1, peak inspiratory pressures of 20–28 cm of water, a positive end-expiratory pressure (PEEP) of 4–6 cm of water, and a respiratory rate of 30–60 breaths/minute. The inspiratory time should be about 0.25–0.35 seconds. Even though there has been extensive debate in the literature, it seems more prudent to use faster respiratory rates with smaller tidal volumes. Newer techniques of mechanical ventilation, include high-frequency ventilation, which provides 150–600 breaths/minute, and oscillator ventilation, which provides up to 3000 breaths/minute. Even though these techniques may be useful for infants with severe hypercarbia resistant to conventional ventilation and for infants with pulmonary interstitial emphysema, they have not proved to be better than conventional ventilation for most infants.

Mechanical ventilation for long periods can cause lung damage. Furthermore, high concentrations of oxygen in inspired air can result in severe lung damage when used over prolonged periods. For this reason, it may be advisable to accept blood gas values that are considered borderline, rather than increasing ventilation or FiO_2, with risk of lung injury. PaO_2 and $PaCO_2$ can be manipulated by altering ventilator settings to satisfy the needs of each infant. Thus, PEEP, respiratory rate, tidal volume, inspiratory duration, and FiO_2 can be altered for optimal effect.

In infants with RDS, lung compliance changes with the clinical course, postnatal age, and the use of exogenous surfactant. The ventilator settings—and particularly the mean airway pressure and respiratory rate—should be adjusted promptly to adjust for these changes. Failure to do so could result in pneumothorax, decreased venous return, hypoxemia, and hypercarbia.

Most clinicians obtain cultures and administer antibiotics in infants with RDS (usually ampicillin and gentamicin) because some pneumonias, particularly group B streptococcus infection, are difficult to differentiate from RDS. In general, antibiotics are administered for 3 days until the culture results are negative.

Meconium Aspiration Syndrome

Meconium staining of amniotic fluid is noted at delivery in about 15% of pregnancies. The amniotic fluid may remain watery and be stained slightly green, or it may become thick and dark green. Meconium often is passed during intrauterine stress but not before 34–35 weeks' gestation because meconium does not reach the rectal ampulla until that time. If the fetus becomes hypoxic and deep respiratory movements or gasps develop, meconium can reach the distal airway and alveoli in utero. However, most infants with MAS aspirate meconium at the time of birth when taking their first inspirations. The usual clinical symptoms are those of mild to moderate respiratory distress, but some infants have severe symptoms, requiring

Table 4–33. Clinical Signs and Physiologic Changes in Meconium Aspiration Syndrome

Clinical	Lungs	Blood Gases	Other
Term/postterm	Mechanical obstruction	Hypoxemia	Extrapulmonary shunt
Pallor/cyanosis	Chemical inflammation	Hypocarbia/hypercarbia	Myocardial dysfunction
Barrel chest	Air trapping	Acidemia	Renal failure
Tachypnea/retractions	Atelectasis		Coagulopathy
Diffuse rales/ronchi	Uneven ventilation		Seizures
Air leaks	Intrapulmonary shunting		
Persistent pulmonary	↑ Expiratory resistance		
hypertension of the newborn	↓ Surfactant function		
	Mismatched V̇/Q̇		

V̇/Q̇ = ventilation/perfusion.

vigorous respiratory support or extracorporeal membrane oxygenation (ECMO). The clinical signs and physiologic changes in MAS are summarized in Table 4–33.

During birth, suctioning the upper airway before the shoulders are delivered and performing endotracheal suctioning immediately after birth decrease the incidence of MAS in infants born with meconium-stained amniotic fluid. This approach is recommended for all infants with thick, particulate, or "pea-soup" meconium, regardless of the Apgar score or need for resuscitation at birth. When the infants have a 1-minute Apgar greater than 8, with thin, watery meconium, endotracheal suctioning usually is not recommended. The overall reported incidence of MAS in infants born with meconium-stained amniotic fluid is 2–10%; however, the incidence is 2–4% in infants in whom endotracheal suctioning is performed immediately. The reported mortality for MAS varies from 0% to 30%. The wide variability is related to delivery room care. In our center, every infant with moderate or thick meconium-stained amniotic fluid is intubated and suctioned immediately. In the past 11 years (1989–1999), with more than 20,000 deliveries, no infant died or required ECMO for treatment of MAS.

Infants with severe MAS often have PPHN, which usually presents with cyanosis and tachypnea. Pulmonary vascular resistance is increased, and pulmonary blood flow is decreased. Untreated hypoxemia or acidosis accentuates these problems (see below).

Persistent Pulmonary Hypertension of the Newborn

Several structural anomalies of the heart cause pulmonary hypertension. Total anomalous pulmonary venous return sometimes poses a difficult differential diagnosis with PPHN; in certain cases, color flow Doppler studies, cardiac catheterization, or angiography are needed to localize the pulmonary veins. Perinatal asphyxia and meco-

nium aspiration are common causes of PPHN, but there are many other causes (Table 4–34). There is often a large right-to-left shunt through the ductus arteriosus in these infants; therefore, there is a large difference in the PaO2 between blood obtained from preductal aortic branches, such as the temporal or radial arteries, and postductal (descending aortic) blood as obtained from the umbilical arterial catheter or femoral artery. Right-to-left shunting through the foramen ovale is also common. The clinical and laboratory signs of PPHN are summarized in Table 4–35. Characteristic of these infants is respiratory lability, with large shifts in PaO2. This is related to acute changes in pulmonary blood flow with changes in the degree of pulmonary vasoconstriction. This lability may persist even after the condition of these patients begins to improve, requiring prompt increase in respiratory settings and FiO2. The chest radiograph is variable because of the many causes of this syndrome. Usually, pulmonary vasculature markings are decreased initially in infants with idiopathic PPHN without MAS or perinatal asphyxia.

Treatment is summarized in Table 4–36. The cornerstone of therapy is to prevent hypoxemia, maintain a high-normal PaO2 and a normal or above-normal pH, while avoiding extreme hypocarbia. Pulmonary vasodilator drugs (e.g., tolazoline and prostaglandin E1) have been tried, but no drug has been effective. Recently, promising results have been achieved with inhalation of NO in some infants with PPHN. Nitric oxide is released from endothelial cells and has a vasodilator action on pulmonary vessels. Several controlled multicenter trials have shown that inhaled NO (iNO) is useful to decrease the need for ECMO but not to decrease mortality. The dose of iNO varies between 5 and 20 ppm. Long-term follow-up studies have not shown a deleterious effect of this treatment, which has been approved recently for clinical use in refractory hypoxemic respiratory failure of term or near-term infants. In those infants who do not respond to these approaches, ECMO has been instituted. Criteria for starting

Table 4–34. Causes of Persistent Pulmonary Hypertension Syndrome in the Newborn

Increased development in smooth muscle of pulmonary vessels	**Decreased pulmonary blood flow with normal pulmonary vascular bed (with or without vasoconstriction)**
Chronic fetal hypoxia	Perinatal and postnatal asphyxia
Fetal systemic hypertension with associated pulmonary hypertension	Meconium aspiration syndrome
Intrauterine constriction of the ductus arteriosus	Upper airway obstruction
Decreased cross-sectional area of pulmonary vascular bed	Lung disease
Pulmonary hypoplasia	Pneumonia (group B streptococcus)
Diaphragmatic hernia	Central nervous system depression (hypoventilation)
Pulmonary cysts	Polycythemia
Drugs and congenital infections	Hypothermia
Abnormal levels of vasoactive agents	Infant of diabetic mother
Increased availability of pulmonary vasoconstrictors before or after birth	Postmature infants
Decreased availability of vasodilators before or after birth	Cardiomyopathies (ischemic, viral)
	Shock
	Pulmonary microthromboembolism
	Hypovolemia-anemia

ECMO are still not definitive and differ in different institutions. Extracorporeal membrane oxygenation requires insertion of large catheters into a carotid artery and jugular vein; the frequency of complications attributable to this procedure differs from one institution to another. The procedure has proved effective in managing selected patients.

Perinatal Asphyxia

Asphyxia (lack or absence of pulse) is defined as hypoxemia with subsequent metabolic acidosis. However, the consequences of perinatal asphyxia are secondary to the decrease in blood flow and oxygen delivery to different organ systems and not to a particular low level of PaO_2 or a high level of $PaCO_2$. The risk factors for asphyxia are summarized in Table 4–1. Neonates may have difficul-

ties in the delivery room because of problems that occurred in utero or during the transition period from intra- to extrauterine life. Antepartum and intrapartum asphyxias are much more frequent than postpartum asphyxia. During labor, placental gas exchange may be disturbed by reduction of uterine or umbilical blood flow and cause fetal asphyxia. Hypercarbia may occur in the fetus when the placental blood flow is affected. The healthy fetus uses several mechanisms to respond to hypoxia and asphyxia. However, when maternal, placental, or fetal problems compromise those responses, the fetus cannot respond

Table 4–36. Treatment of Persistent Pulmonary Hypertension

General Measures	**Specific Measures**
Avoid hypothermia	Maintain oxygenation
Correct promptly any abnormalities in glucose, calcium, potassium, hematocrit	Avoid hypoxia
	Maintain preductal PaO_2 100–150 mm Hg
Correct acidosis (sodium bicarbonate or THAM)	Initiate mechanical ventilation early
Maintain systemic arterial blood pressure (volume or vasoactive drugs)	Sedation—muscle paralysis
	Maintain normal or alkalotic pH
	Administer pulmonary vasodilators (inhaled nitric oxide)
Avoid unnecessary stimulation, agitation, or crying	Trial of HFV
	Begin ECMO

ECMO = extracorporeal membrane oxygenation; HFV = high frequency ventilation; THAM = tris(hydroxymethyl) aminomethane.

Table 4–35. Features of Persistent Pulmonary Hypertension of the Newborn

Perinatal history of fetal distress	S_2 loud and not split
Term or postterm pregnancy	Preductal and postductal difference in PaO_2
Cyanosis	Chest radiograph: variable lung parenchyma; ± cardiomegaly
Tachypnea (±tachycardia)	
Spontaneous swings in PaO_2	ECG: RV overload
Significant decreases in PaO_2 in response to FiO_2 changes or stimulation	Echocardiography: shunting, RV dilation, tricuspid and pulmonic valve regurgitation
Systolic murmur (50%)	

ECG = electrocardiogram; RV = right ventricle.

adequately and needs immediate treatment before and/or after birth. When asphyxia occurs after birth, it is usually secondary to inadequate pulmonary gas exchange, which leads to hypercarbia and hypoxemia.

During the initial stage of asphyxia, the cardiac output remains stable but is redistributed. Vasoconstriction of the skin and the renal and mesenteric vascular beds results in a marked decrease in blood flow to these organs. In contrast, blood flow to the myocardium, brain, and adrenal glands is increased. This redistribution of blood flow and the increase in systemic arterial pressure and bradycardia result from chemoreflex response, adrenal catecholamine release, and angiotensin and vasopressin response.

Redistribution of cardiac output is an attempt to maintain oxygen supply to vital organs. As oxygen delivery decreases to below critical levels, metabolism becomes increasingly anaerobic; anaerobic glycolysis results in increased lactic acid production with development of metabolic acidemia. Hypoxemia also results in marked pulmonary vasoconstriction. Metabolic acidemia greatly exaggerates the increase in pulmonary vascular resistance associated with hypoxemia.

The redistribution of cardiac output and the increase in systemic vascular resistance are responsible for many of the clinical signs observed in asphyxiated patients (pallor, decreased urine production, or intestinal necrosis). With severe asphyxia, myocardial function may be depressed; this can compromise umbilical–placental flow and thus further interfere with gas exchange. The decreased myocardial performance may persist into the newborn period.

Asphyxial events are better tolerated during the fetal and neonatal periods than during any other period of life. A possible explanation for this increased tolerance is that a large proportion of fetal and neonatal oxygen demand is facultative or nonessential for survival functions such as growth and thermoregulation. In organs with high metabolic activity, such as the heart and brain, the amount of oxygen expended for growth is a very small percentage of the total oxygen requirement. Because the heart has little reserve in terms of increasing oxygen extraction, it depends on increased blood supply during asphyxia to sustain normal function. Table 4–37 summarizes the effects of asphyxia on various organ systems. The CNS effect of asphyxia or ischemia can be of varying degrees and usually begins during the final stages of a severe episode or after repetitive episodes.

During the early stages of asphyxia, the fetus and newborn may make vigorous breathing efforts; however, if hypoxia continues, the ventilatory center becomes depressed. During terminal stages of asphyxia, gasping efforts can be seen, but they are not useful to establish adequate inflation of the lungs. Absence of breathing (apnea) is a frequent finding in asphyxiated newborns.

Cardiopulmonary Resuscitation of the Newborn

Whether the process that causes asphyxia is initiated during intrauterine or extrauterine life, the objective of resuscitation is to reverse ongoing events and ensure respira-

Table 4–37. Effects of Asphyxia on Organ Systems

Cardiovascular
  Regional blood flow redistribution (selective ischemia)
  Hypertension (by increased peripheral vascular resistance)
  Diminished glycogen reserves in myocardium
  Myocardial ischemia—cardiogenic shock (hypotension)
  Myocardial necrosis (subendocardial, papillary muscle)
  Massive tricuspid valve regurgitation
  Conduction abnormalities (bradycardia, first- and second-degree heart block)
  Persistent pulmonary hypertension
  Hypervolemia (less frequently hypovolemia)

Gastrointestinal system
  Necrotizing enterocolitis
  Perforation—mucosal ulceration

Kidney
  Medullar and tubular necrosis
  Stimulation of renin–angiotensin system
  Oliguria
    Renal failure
    Bladder paralysis

Central nervous system
  Loss of autoregulation of blood flow
  Cytotoxic and vasogenic edema
  Ischemia—necrosis
  Hypoxic—ischemia encephalopathy (irritability, hypotonia, seizures, coma)
  Intracranial hemorrhage

Respiratory system
  Increased pulmonary vascular resistance
  Decreased pulmonary surfactant
  Edema (alveolar edema, interstitial/perivascular)
  Hypoventilation (secondary to central nervous system depression)
  Apnea
  Meconium aspiration (prenatal or postnatal)
  Persistent pulmonary hypertension

tory and circulatory sufficiency so that death or survival with permanent CNS damage can be prevented.

The goal of cardiopulmonary resuscitation (CPR) is therefore to protect the CNS during asphyxia. This is possible by reversing the pathophysiologic events that occurred during asphyxia. The first step in CPR is anticipation: This includes knowledge of the maternal personal and obstetric histories; history of the pregnancy, including labor; preparation of the delivery room (e.g., materials, equipment, and, drugs); and, most important, a trained team in the delivery room at the moment it is needed.

Immediately after birth, the infant's skin should be dried vigorously with prewarmed towels, and the baby placed in a radiant warmer to avoid loss of body temperature. This also provides external tactile and sensorial stimulation that can help to initiate ventilation after birth. The immediate use of suction catheters to clear the airways is not recommended unless there is obstruction by meconium, blood, or amniotic fluid. Evaluation of the baby should begin immediately after birth rather than waiting for the 1-minute Apgar score. Figure 4–5 summarizes the steps of evaluation-action-reevaluation recommended by the American Heart Association (AHA) and the American Academy of Pediatrics (AAP).

Most infants are blue at birth and become pink after effective ventilation is established. If central cyanosis persists when the baby is breathing adequately and the heart rate is normal, 100% free-flowing oxygen over the nose and mouth should be administered. If the newborn is apneic or fails to sustain effective ventilation (heart rate <100 even when ventilatory movements are present), intiating artificial ventilation with mask-and-bag at 40–60 breaths/minute is mandatory. Special attention should be paid to the position of the head and neck to ensure adequate lung expansion. An increase in heart rate and reperfusion of the skin signal the adequacy of ventilation, unless severe metabolic acidosis and myocardial failure are present. An orogastric tube must be inserted after 2 minutes of mask-and-bag ventilation to eliminate accumulated gastric air. Mask-and-bag ventilation is contraindicated when congenital diaphragmatic hernia (CDH) is suspected. Endotracheal intubation should be performed in the presence of CDH and in all infants in whom

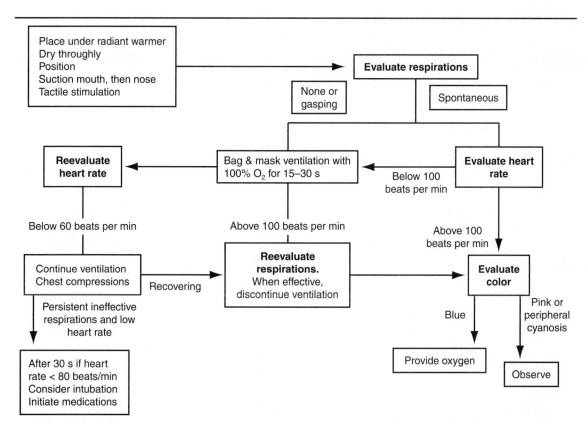

Figure 4–5. Steps of evaluation, action, and reevaluation in perinatal asphyxia.

mask-and-bag ventilation is not effective, or when it is required for more than 2–3 minutes.

If the heart rate remains low after 30–60 seconds of effective ventilation, the infant requires external cardiac massage at a rate of 90 times per minute. According to recent recommendations of the AAP and AHA: "Provide 90 compressions per minute with a pause after every third compression for a ventilation." This represents 30 ventilations per minute and a total of 120 "events" per minute. However, several animal and clinical studies have not shown any detrimental effect of performing cardiac massage and ventilation simultaneously. In addition, hypocarbia during resuscitation should be avoided because it can injure the brain and lungs of newborn infants. The effectiveness of cardiac massage must be evaluated by palpation of femoral or carotid pulses or by measuring arterial blood pressure. If the cardiac massage and ventilation are effective, the pupils will be in the midposition or constricted. If the pupils are dilated and no atropine has been given, cerebral blood flow and oxygenation are inadequate. In the unusual case that bradycardia persists after all these resuscitation efforts, further measures are instituted. Ventilation, cardiac massage, and drugs should be initiated at once when the newborn has asystole. Table 4–38 summarizes the drugs most frequently used during CPR. It has recently been suggested that resuscitation with 100% oxygen is detrimental to the newborn and that the outcome of infants resuscitated with 100% oxygen is no better than with lower concentrations of oxygen or even room air. As the levels of oxygen in the blood increase, oxygen radicals are produced by the hypoxanthine–xanthine system, which increases lipid peroxidation of membranes and causes neuronal damage. Therefore, perfusion–reperfusion of the CNS with blood that has a high oxygen concentration may exacerbate tissue damage and lead to neuronal dysfunction. This is best prevented by rapidly reducing the FiO_2 and maintaining the PaO_2 at 45–75 mm Hg and the SaO_2 at 90–95%. These oxygen levels are sufficient in most cases to meet tissue oxygen demands if the cardiac output, tissue perfusion, and hemoglobin concentrations are adequate. Recent evidence also suggests that, in selected cases, selective cooling of the head can prevent brain injury after hypoxia-ischemia, prevent secondary cell membrane dysfunction, and reduce cytotoxic and oxygen-free radical-induced cell injury. Deep hypothermia also may prolong the time in which measures can be instituted to treat or prevent hypoxic-ischemic encephalopathy. However, although promising, the use of hypothermia is experimental and should not be used routinely.

OTHER DISORDERS

Polycythemia

Polycythemia, defined as a central venous hematocrit greater than 65%, is present in 2–4% of infants born at sea level. It may result from increased placental transfusion (delayed cord clamping) or increased red blood cell production by the fetus in response to hypoxemia and increased erythropoietin secretion caused by placental insufficiency. Polycythemia is associated with several complications of pregnancy (Table 4–39) and with SGA and LGA infants.

Table 4–38. Medications Used During Neonatal Resuscitation

Drug	Indications	Dosage	Route	Effect
Epinephrine	Asystole	0.01 mg/kg (0.1 mL/kg) 1 : 10,000 dilution	ET, IV	↑ Heart rate ↑ Myocardial contractility ↑ Arterial pressure
Sodium bicarbonate	Metabolic acidosis (documented)	1–2 meq/kg diluted 1 : 2 (very slowly)	IV	Corrects metabolic acidosis Improves cardiac output and peripheral perfusion
Naloxone	Maternal administration of opiates + apneic infant	0.1 mg/kg	ET, IV, SC, IM	↑ Ventilatory rate
Fluids (packed red cells, albumin 5%, normal saline)	Hypovolemia	10–20 mL/kg	IV slowly	↑ Blood pressure Improves tissue perfusion

ET = endotracheal; IM = intramuscular; IV = intravenous; SC = subcutaneous.

Table 4–39. Infants at Risk for Neonatal Polycythemia

Small-for-gestational-age infants
Large-for-gestational-age infants
Infants with birth weight >4000 g
Infants of diabetic mothers
Infants born at high altitude
Infants born to hypertensive mothers (even if average for gestational age)
Infants with Down syndrome
Rarely, infants with congenital heart disease; adrenogenital syndrome

Table 4–40. Signs and Symptoms of Polycythemia

Skin	**Renal**
Plethora	Hematuria
Cyanosis	**Hematologic**
Gastrointestinal	Thrombocytopenia
Poor feeding	**Cardiovascular**
Feeding intolerance	Poor perfusion
Respiratory	Ventricular failure
Tachypnea	Acidosis
Respiratory distress	
Persistent pulmonary hypertension	
Central nervous system	
Lethargy	
Hypotonia	
Jitteriness	

The pathophysiologic effects of polycythemia are related to blood hyperviscosity or hypervolemia. Blood viscosity depends on hematocrit values, blood flow velocity, and protein content of plasma (especially fibrinogen). The relation of viscosity to hematocrit is exponential. Below a venous hematocrit of 65%, viscosity changes only modestly with red blood cell mass. Above 65%, increases of hematocrit result in dramatic increases in viscosity. This increased viscosity leads to a slower blood flow in tissues. At any given hematocrit, viscosity is higher with lower flow rates or higher protein content of plasma. Premature infants who have lower concentrations of plasma proteins have higher flow rates than do term infants, even at the same hematocrit values. After birth, fluid is redistributed between plasma and tissues, so that plasma water content decreases. Hematocrit values are highest at 2–6 hours after birth and decrease thereafter.

DIAGNOSIS

Clinical features of hyperviscosity are shown in Table 4–40. Capillary hematocrits should be obtained routinely approximately 4 hours after birth for screening purposes, but infants with known perinatal risk factors for neonatal polycythemia (see Table 4–39) should be screened within 2 hours. If hematocrits exceed 65%, a venous blood sample should be obtained with minimal or no tourniquet or compression and free-flowing blood. If the values are borderline, measurement should be repeated after 2–4 hours. Coulter counter hematocrits are usually lower (5–6 points) than spun values. Infants with hematocrits of 60–65% and symptoms attributable to polycythemia should be considered polycythemia and managed accordingly.

TREATMENT

Standard accepted treatment for neonatal polycythemia is partial exchange transfusion. Blood is removed and replaced by the same volume of plasma or plasma substitutes in a stepwise manner. Hematocrit is thus reduced without further compromising blood flow. Simple phlebotomy or volume infusions alone are not recommended for polycythemic infants, because they will decrease or increase total blood volume.

To establish the volume of blood to exchange, the following formula is used:

$$\text{volume (mL)} = \left(\frac{\text{initial Hct} - \text{desired Hct}}{\text{initial Hct}} \right)$$
$$\times \text{ wt (kg)} \times 90 \text{ (mL/kg)}$$

(Hct = hematocrit; wt = body weight)

Desired hematocrits are 50–55%, and 90 represents the average blood volume (in mL/kg) for most newborn infants. Partial exchange transfusion can be performed safely with crystalloid solutions (e.g., normal saline).

Infants with polycythemia should be observed carefully for 24–48 hours after partial exchange transfusion. Repeat hematocrits should be obtained 2–4 and 12 hours after the partial exchange transfusion. In infants with perinatal risk factors and with Down syndrome, hematocrits should also be obtained 24 and 48 hours after treatment because they may continue to have increased red blood cell production. Occasionally, more than one partial exchange transfusion may be required to maintain appropriate hematocrits.

Hypoglycemia, hypocalcemia, and hyperbilirubinemia may be associated with polycythemia and require management (Table 4–41).

Table 4–41. Potential Complications of Polycythemia

Hyperbilirubinemia	Transient feeding intolerance
Hypocalcemia	Necrotizing enterocolitis
Hypoglycemia	Irritability
Thrombocytopenia	Intracranial hemorrhage/infarct
Transient hematuria	Abnormal development
Renal failure (thrombosis)	

OUTCOME

Short-term outcome of polycythemic infants is usually good; the most troubling complication is NEC, although its exact relationship to polycythemia is not known.

Long-term outcome is still controversial. In reported studies, no attempt has been made to separate "normal" infants from those with IUGR, or to separate infants who receive treatment from those who do not. In some recent studies, no difference in long-term outcome has been found between treated and untreated polycythemia, suggesting that there is no advantage to treating this condition. However, until more reliable studies are conducted, exchange transfusion remains the standard treatment.

Congenital Infections

Perinatal viral, bacterial, or protozoal infections of the mother can be transmitted to the fetus or the newborn infant. The acronym TORCH was coined in 1974 to cover toxoplasmosis, rubella, CMV, herpes simplex virus (HSV), and other agents. However, more maternal pathogens have been found that can infect the fetus and newborn infant transplacentally, hematogenously, or via contact with the colonized birth canal (Table 4–42). Transmissibility and the severity of the disease in infected infants differ according to the pathogen and the timing of the maternal infection during gestation. Many of the pathologic agents cause abortion or stillbirth; some lead to congenital anomalies (see Chapter 5).

CLINICAL FEATURES

Maternal infections with TORCH agents often are asymptomatic, despite the frequency with which these organisms attack pregnant women. Similarly, most congenital infections are asymptomatic in the newborn infant. The clinical manifestations that suggest congenital infection are similar for many infecting agents. Some congenital infections may have recognizable patterns in the neonate (Table 4–43).

Clinical suspicion should be based on specific data from the maternal history and a combination of physical signs in the mother and the infant. Laboratory studies, including specific cultures and serologic testing, are re-

Table 4–42. Organisms Causing Congenital Infections

Transplacental fetal infections	**Ascending infections**
Cytomegalovirus	Bacteroides
Enteroviruses	β-Hemolytic streptococci
Herpes simplex virus, types 1 and 2	Candida
	Enterobacteriaceae
HIV	Escherichia coli
Listeria monocytogenes	**Natal acquisition from maternal birth canal**
Measles	
Mumps	Candida
Plasmodium	Chlamydia trachomatis
Rubella	Cytomegalovirus
Staphylococcus aureus	Hepatitis B virus
Toxoplasma gondii	Herpes simplex virus
Treponema pallidum	L. monocytogenes
Varicella zoster	Neisseria gonorrhoea

HIV = human immunodeficiency virus.

quired to confirm the diagnosis and identify a specific pathogen.

DIAGNOSTIC EVALUATION

Diagnostic workup (Table 4–44) includes viral culture (oropharynx, urine, and rectum), serologic testing for antigens or antibodies to specific congenital pathogens, and microscopic examinations for herpes or syphilis (dark field, fluorescent antibody stain, or Tzanck preparation) from skin lesions. Cytomegalovirus and HSV infections are diagnosed predominantly by culture; syphilis, toxoplasmosis, and hepatitis B virus (HBV) predominantly by serologic tests; and rubella by serologic and culture techniques. The presence of thrombocytopenia or hemolytic anemia suggests the diagnosis of a congenital infection. Radiographic indications of congenital infections include cerebral calcifications and abnormal ossification of long bones (celery-stalking, periostitis, and metaphyseal lucencies). Cerebral CT or MRI also may demonstrate white matter alterations, hydrocephalus, cortical atrophy, and cystic lesions of the cortex. Ophthalmologic evaluation is important in detecting chorioretinitis, as are cataracts and glaucoma caused by congenital infections. Brainstem auditory-evoked responses may detect early hearing deficits that progress after congenital infection by rubella or CMV. Lumbar puncture should be performed on all infants being evaluated for congenital infection. Elevated protein concentration and pleocytosis in the spinal fluid are important confirmatory findings of meningoencephalitis in congenital syphilis and rubella or in natally acquired herpes simplex encephalitis.

Table 4–43. Patterns of Fetal and Infant Morbidity in Some Congenital Infections

Pathogen	Fetus	Congenital Defects	Neonatal Disease	Late Sequelae
Treponema pallidum	Stillbirth, hydrops fetalis	—	Skin lesions, rhinitis, hepatosplenomegaly, jaundice, hemolytic anemia, bone lesions	Interstitial keratitis, frontal bossing, saber shins, tooth changes
Toxoplasma gondii	Abortion	Hydrocephalus, microcephaly	Low birth weight, hepatosplenomegaly, jaundice, anemia, intracranial calcifications	Chorioretinitis, mental retardation
Rubella	Abortion	Heart defects, microcephaly, cataracts, microphthalmia	Low birth weight, hepatosplenomegaly, petechiae, osteitis	Deafness, mental retardation, diabetes, degenerative brain lesions
Cytomegalovirus	—	Microcephaly, microphthalmia, retinopathy	Anemia, thrombocytopenia, hepatosplenomegaly, jaundice, encephalitis, cerebral calcification	Deafness, psychomotor retardation
Varicella zoster virus	—	Limb hypoplasia, cortical atrophy, cicatricial skin lesions	Low birth weight, chorioretinitis, congenital chickenpox or disseminated neonatal varicella	Potential for fatal outcome due to secondary infection
Herpes simplex virus	Abortion	Possible microcephaly, retinopathy, intracranial calcifications	Disseminated disease, multiple organ involvement (lung, liver, CNS), vesicular skin lesions, retinopathy	Neurologic deficits
Hepatitis B virus	—	—	Asymptomatic HBsAg-positive infection, low birth weight, rarely acute hepatitis	Chronic hepatitis, persistent positive HBsAg, cirrhosis, hepatocellular carcinoma
HIV	—	—	Pediatric AIDS	Pediatric AIDS
Enteroviruses	Abortion	Myocarditis, possible congenital heart disease	Mild febrile disease, exanthems, aseptic meningitis, gastroenteritis or multiple organ involvement (CNS, liver, heart)	Neurologic deficits

AIDS = acquired immunodeficiency syndrome; CNS = central nervous system; HBsAg = hepatitis B surface antigen; HIV = human immunodeficiency virus.

Antibody titer determination in perinatal infections is complicated by transplacental passage of maternal IgG and the technical difficulties of specific IgM tests. Total serum IgM concentration has been used as a screening test for congenital infection but is neither sensitive nor specific. Specific IgM titers for toxoplasmosis, rubella, syphilis, and CMV exhibit excellent specificity but are not highly sensitive.

General Management

Universal body substance precautions obviate isolation or separation of the neonate from the mother in most cases. However, untreated tuberculosis, infectious syphilis, and intrapartum varicella may be indications for temporary separation from the mother. Neonates with congenital rubella and possibly HSV should be admitted to isolation rooms to prevent nosocomial spread; other infections are not likely to be spread if universal body substance precautions are followed. In all cases, special care must be taken by pregnant health care providers when handling infants with congenital infections.

Breast feeding is not recommended in HIV-infected mothers or untreated mothers with tuberculosis. Also, CMV and HBV can be transmitted by breast feeding

Table 4–44. Diagnostic Tests in Congenital Infection

Nonspecific Tests	Specific Tests
Complete blood count and platelets	Viral culture
	Oropharynx, urine, rectum
Lumbar puncture	Blood for HIV
Large bone radiographs	Cerebrospinal fluid or
Cerebral imaging	conjunctiva are optional
Computed tomography	Smears of skin lesions (herpes,
Magnetic resonance	syphilis)
imaging	Fluorescent antibody stain
Ultrasound	Darkfield examination
Ophthalmologic evaluation	Tzanck smear
Audiologic evaluation	Serologic tests for
	Rubella
	Toxoplasma
	Syphilis
	Hepatitis B and HIV

HIV = human immunodeficiency virus.

during the acute infection. No consensus exists regarding the risks of chronic HBV carriers. Otherwise, maternal infection does not preclude breast feeding.

Recognition of congenital infections, such as varicella, HIV, syphilis, gonorrhea, tuberculosis, and HBV, should initiate the investigation of other family members at risk.

TREATMENT

Perinatal bacterial infection may be treated with appropriate antibiotics (see Chapter 9). Congenital syphilis or neurosyphilis is treated with penicillin for a 10-day course. Toxoplasmosis can be treated with pyrimethamine and sulfadiazine. Herpes simplex virus infection should be treated promptly with acyclovir. Ganciclovir treatment for CMV infections is still under investigation. The infant born to an HIV-infected mother should receive specific diagnostic testing and, once proved infected, be treated with zidovudine, immunoglobulin, and prophylactic trimethoprimsulfamethoxazole.

PREVENTION

Cesarean delivery is indicated for women experiencing primary herpetic infection at the time of delivery, except when the fetus has been exposed to the birth canal after rupture of membranes for more than 4–6 hours. Recurrent herpes is not an absolute contraindication to vaginal delivery and carries a low risk of HSV infection in the neonate. Maternal chickenpox infection in the last 5 days of pregnancy or the first 2 days after delivery is an indication for treatment with varicella zoster immunoglobulin. Neonatal chlamydia exposure after vaginal delivery

may be an indication for prophylaxis with erythromycin. Natal acquisition of hepatitis B can be prevented to a significant degree by passive immunization with hepatitis B immunoglobulin and active vaccination with recombinant hepatitis vaccine. Neonatal acquisition of tuberculosis can be prevented by isoniazid or by passive immunization with bacillus Calmette–Guérin (BCG) vaccine.

Other methods to prevent congenital infections include maternal education about infectious exposures during pregnancy, rubella vaccination of all nonimmune women in their childbearing years, screening of blood products (for CMV, HIV, HBV, and syphilis), and universal neonatal eye prophylaxis (with silver nitrate or erythromycin ointment).

Birth Trauma

Mechanical forces applied to the fetus during labor and delivery can produce traumatic lesions, such as hemorrhage, edema, tissue laceration, fractures, or organ damage, at different sites. Risk for obstetric trauma is increased in primigravidas, abnormal presentations, fetal–maternal disproportion, multiple pregnancies, forceps and vacuum extraction, oligohydramnios, and internal version maneuvers. Very-low-birth-weight infants (<1500 g) with breech presentation are subject to high risk because the cranium is easily deformable and is large in proportion to the body.

SUBDURAL HEMORRHAGE

Subdural hemorrhage should not occur with obstetric improvements of the past decade: subarachnoid hemorrhage is much less severe and more frequent in preterm infants. Spinal cord lesions may occur in frontal and face presentation or when shoulder dystocia is present with cephalic presentation. The incidence of spinal cord damage is very high in cases of breech presentation with neck hyperextension. High spinal cord or brainstem lesions may be associated with severe respiratory depression and shock from the time of birth. The lesion may be epidural or intraspinal edema or hemorrhage, or even complete cord transection. Usually the cervical vertebrae are normal on routine radiographs; the brachial plexus is affected in about 20% of cases. The differential diagnoses include intraspinal or extraspinal tumors, such as neuroblastoma, spina bifida with tethering cord, and severe hypoxic-ischemic encephalopathy.

FACIAL PALSY

Facial palsy usually is due to excessive pressure over the nerve, which can be induced by the maternal sacrum, a forceps blade, or the fetal shoulder. In complete peripheral palsy, the affected side shows no movement, the palpebral fissure remains open, and the facial folds are less noticeable. With crying, there is muscular contraction only on the healthy side, and the angle of the mouth deviates toward that side. Rarely, facial palsy may be of central origin. In these cases, frontal and ocular muscles are not affected, and there are usually other associated manifestations of intracranial lesions. Peripheral lesions recover partially or completely within weeks. To protect the eye from damage, artificial tears should be used.

BRACHIAL PLEXUS PALSY

Brachial plexus palsy is secondary to difficult delivery in cephalic or breech presentations of mature infants. Clinical presentations are related to sites of injury. **Superior brachial palsy** (C5 and C6: Duchenne-Erb syndrome) is the most frequent and affects the shoulder and arm muscles. The affected upper extremity remains in abduction, extension, and internal rotation; the forearm is in pronation, and the wrist flexed, with very few spontaneous movements. The fingers move normally, and the palmar grasp reflex is normal. Moro reflex is abnormal, and movements of the shoulder are absent or diminished; phrenic nerve palsy can be associated with this lesion. **Inferior brachial palsy** (C8, T1: Klumpke syndrome) is rare. In this condition, wrist drop is present, and the fingers are separated. Frequently, Horner's syndrome occurs on the same side (myosis, ptosis, and enophthalmos) because of lesions of the cervical sympathetic fibers of the first thoracic root. A **complete brachial palsy** is usually serious. The extremity is flaccid with no movement, all reflexes are absent, and there is also a sensory deficit. Superior brachial palsy shows good recovery in approximately 80% of cases, and inferior palsy shows recovery in around 40% of cases; however, in complete palsy, total recovery is rare. Other lesions, such as cerebral lesions, cervical column lesions, clavicle fracture or dislocation, and fracture of the head of the humerus, need to be excluded. Treatment for brachial plexus palsy is symptomatic, keeping the extremity in physiologic position over the chest during the first 2–3 weeks. Subsequently, physical therapy to maintain mobility of joint and avoid contractures and deformities is instituted.

Phrenic nerve palsy is associated with lesions of the nerve roots of C3, C4, and C5 usually after lateral hyperextension of the neck in complicated labors (usually breech presentation). The lesion is unilateral, is associated with superior brachial palsy, and presents with apnea, cyanosis, chest retractions, and asymmetric respiration. Atelectasis is common, and pneumonia may develop. Chest radiograph shows a raised hemidiaphragm, with deviation of the mediastinum and heart. Ultrasound or fluoroscopy shows paradoxical movement of the paralyzed diaphragm, which ascends in inspiration and descends in expiration. Treatment includes oxygen if necessary, and some infants require CPAP; in severe cases, mechanical ventilation may be indicated. A surgical procedure to stabilize the diaphragm is required in some infants.

TRAUMA TO OTHER SITES

Intraabdominal structures, particularly the liver or spleen, may rupture during traumatic deliveries, particularly in infants with breech presentation, in large fetuses, or in those with enlarged viscera due to hydrops fetalis or congenital infections. The clinical features are abdominal distention with progressive hypovolemic shock.

Lesions in the skull include caput succedaneum, which is of no clinical consequence and disappears in the first few days after birth, and **cephalhematoma** which is a hemorrhagic collection caused by subperiosteal vascular rupture. This lesion appears after 24–48 hours, is unilateral, and is found over the parietal area. Cephalhematomas are limited to the area of the affected bone, do not cross the cranial sutures, and, in 15% of cases, are associated with an underlying skull fracture. Complications such as anemia and hypovolemic shock are rare, but large cephalhematomas can induce disseminated intravascular coagulation, hyperbilirubinemia, infection with osteomyelitis, sepsis, or meningitis. Most cases of cephalhematoma resolve spontaneously over the first few months of life, some with some degree of calcification. If there are signs of local infection or abscess formation, the cephalhematoma should be drained for appropriate treatment and to obtain cultures.

Trauma to the sternocleidomastoid muscle may cause an intramuscular hematoma, which subsequently leads to fibrosis and muscle contractures. Necrosis and edema can also develop in this muscle because of venous obstruction during labor. Clinically, the infants have torticollis with a small mass felt medial to the border of the muscle, becoming evident by 10–20 days after birth. Neck movement becomes increasingly limited. The typical position for these infants is with the chin rotated toward the contralateral shoulder and the head tilted over the contractured muscle. If physical therapy is not provided, the face may become asymmetric because of flattening on the facial side of the lesion.

Fractures are infrequent except for clavicular fracture. This type of fracture occurs in vertex or breech presentation but is more common in large fetuses. In general, the movement of the shoulder and arm are not affected, and the Moro reflex could be entirely normal. Often it is noted in a chest radiograph obtained for other reasons. Treatment consists of decreasing pain by immobilizing the arm in a physiologic position. The prognosis is good.

Intracranial Hemorrhage

Intracranial hemorrhage, a significant cause of neurologic morbidity in the newborn, can be classified according to the anatomic space involved (Table 4–45). Subdural, subarachnoid, and intracerebellar hemorrhages are rare in full-term infants and result from birth trauma.

Table 4–45. Classification of Neonatal Intracranial Hemorrhage

Type of Hemorrhage	Clinical Setting	Clinical Presentation	Complications
Subarachnoid	Asphyxia, coagulopathy	Asymptomatic with bloody CSF, seizures	Rarely problems but possible hydrocephalus
Subdural	Birth trauma, difficult delivery	Early—shock, stupor Late—macrocephaly	Subdural effusion requiring surgical evacuation
Intracerebellar	Breech delivery, forceps extraction, asphyxia, prematurity	Blood loss, apnea, or incidental finding on ultrasound or CT scan	Motor deficits, possible hydrocephalus
Periventricular–intraventricular	Trauma, asphyxia, prematurity	Neurologic dysfunction	Posthemorrhagic hydrocephalus

CSF = cerebrospinal fluid; CT = computed tomography.

PERIVENTRICULAR–INTRAVENTRICULAR HEMORRHAGE

Periventricular–intraventricular hemorrhage (PV-IVH) is a frequent cause of neonatal morbidity and mortality in preterm infants. It occurs in approximately 40% of infants with birth weights less than 1500 g but is uncommon in infants born after 34 weeks' gestation. Its incidence appears to have declined over the past decade. The risk of PV-IVH is highest in the most immature infants.

The typical site of bleeding in PV-IVH is the subependymal germinal matrix, a highly cellular region immediately ventrolateral to the lateral ventricle in the developing brain. This tissue is gelatinous with an elaborate, but immature, capillary bed. From 10 to 20 weeks' gestation, the germinal matrix is the source of neuroblasts that migrate to the cerebral cortex. After 20 weeks, this tissue begins to involute over the next 12–15 weeks but remains a source of cerebral glial precursors until near term. During this involution, the capillary bed of the germinal matrix apparently is prone to disruption and hemorrhage, which frequently extends locally from the matrix through the ependyma into the lateral ventricles. The quantity of blood determines whether there is acute ventricular dilation. Blood can spread throughout the ventricular system and potentially obstruct ventricular CSF outflow or impair its absorption by arachnoid villi. Hydrocephalus, acute or chronic, may then result. In approximately 15% of cases of PV-IVH, blood is found in the parenchyma of the cerebral cortex. Experimental and clinical evidence suggests that intraparenchymal hemorrhage is not merely an extension from the initial germinal matrix bleeding but results from a venous infarction believed to follow the same event causing PV-IVH.

PATHOGENESIS

The pathogenesis of PV-IVH is related to sudden disturbances in cerebral blood flow and increases in central venous pressure. The premature infant with less than 34 weeks' gestation appears to be particularly vulnerable to alterations in systemic blood pressure, which may be associated with a number of conditions, including breech delivery and prolonged labor. Mechanical ventilation, asphyxia, RDS, pneumothorax, overzealous volume expansion, PDA, and agitation are considered to be risk factors.

CLINICAL FEATURES

The initial bleeding of PV-IVH usually occurs 12–72 hours after birth. The clinical manifestations are related to blood loss and neurologic dysfunction. These include hypotension, bradycardia, apnea, lethargy, fixed pupils, seizures, and coma. In addition, coagulopathy, thrombocytopenia, and hyperbilirubinemia can occur. Many infants with small hemorrhages are totally asymptomatic, whereas others show intermittent hypotonia, apnea, or changes in heart rate and blood pressure; this has been called the "saltatory" presentation.

DIAGNOSIS

Real-time cranial ultrasound scanning through the anterior fontanelle is the diagnostic tool of choice for evaluation of LBW infants and others at risk for PV-IVH. Several different schemes to grade the severity of PV-IVH have been proposed, but a **severe hemorrhage** is one with intraventricular hemorrhage, ventricular dilation, or intraparenchymal hemorrhage. Because 90% of cases of PV-IVH are evident within the first 4 days, one or two ultrasound scans typically are performed in the first week. Repeat ultrasound scans are used to follow progress and assess subsequent neuropathology. This is important in prognosis and further management. For example, if posthemorrhagic hydrocephalus is progressive, agents to decrease CSF production, such as furosemide and acetazolamide, or serial lumbar punctures, may be indicated.

OUTCOME

The outcome associated with PV-IVH is not universally poor. The incidence for major neurodevelopmental handicaps at 2 years of age for premature infants with grade 1 or grade 2 hemorrhage is about 10%, which is similar to that for comparable infants with no hemorrhage. With increasing severity of hemorrhage, the risk of poor neurologic outcome increases; this appears to depend largely on the extent of associated parenchymal lesions. Posthemorrhagic hydrocephalus, however, does not appear to increase the risk of poor outcome independent of the severity of hemorrhage.

PREVENTION

Recently, major efforts have been directed toward preventing PV-IVH. Several approaches have been evaluated: Fresh frozen plasma to correct coagulopathy; muscle relaxants or phenobarbital to reduce fluctuation in cerebral blood flow and blood pressure; vitamin E for potential antioxidant properties; and ethamsylate to stabilize capillaries in the immature vascular bed. None has been found truly effective. The most promising approach has been the use of prophylactic indomethacin, which induces cerebral vasoconstriction and decreases severe IVH. The potential decrease in cerebral blood flow does not cause long-term adverse effects.

Infants of Drug-Abusing Mothers

Drug exposure of a developing fetus is thought to occur in approximately 15% of pregnancies in the United States, but the true number of pregnancies with substance abuse is perhaps higher. Although cocaine use by women has decreased in the past 7 years since the introduction of crack cocaine, opiate use by women appears to have increased. Most women who use illicit drugs use multiple drugs; thus, a causal relationship between a specific drug exposure and outcome is difficult to establish.

Drugs (particularly illicit drugs) can have serious consequences for the pregnant woman and her fetus. Risks include maternal drug and obstetric complications, impaired fetal somatic and brain growth, congenital malformations, clinical intoxication, and withdrawal symptoms. Use of alcohol, cocaine, amphetamines, phencyclidine (PCP), and narcotics can compound the fetal risk of tobacco, caffeine, and other illicit or prescribed drugs. Perinatal morbidity and mortality rates are higher for drug-exposed infants, as are long-term neurodevelopmental sequelae, later growth abnormalities, and increased risk for sudden infant death. Clinical manifestations in the neonate include irritability, tremulousness, feeding intolerance, and wakefulness. Because they are difficult to take care of, infants of drug-abusing mothers are at risk for child neglect or abuse when discharged home. Because of these increased risks for perinatal complications, pregnancies in which drugs are used should be identified prenatally and attempts made to control the exposure of the fetus. Infants born to women using drugs should be identified early in the neonatal period and observed for complications and withdrawal effects. A summary of the com-

Table 4–46. Perinatal Complications Associated with Substance Abuse

Neonatal Effects	Pregnancy/Mother
Intrauterine growth retardation	Inadequate prenatal care
	Anemia
Prematurity	Endocarditis/hepatitis
Birth defects	Urinary tract infection/
Microcephaly	pneumonia
Antenatal cerebral infarctions	Tuberculosis/HIV
Small central nervous system bleeds	Venereal diseases
	Low self-esteem/depression
Respiratory depression at birth	Low maternal weight gain
	Abruptio placentae
Infections/necrotizing enterocolitis	Possible precipitous delivery
	Preterm labor and delivery
Poor feeding	
Abstinence/withdrawal syndrome	
Neurobehavioral abnormalities	

HIV = human immunodeficiency virus.

plications associated with substance abuse in both mother and infant is presented in Table 4–46.

NEONATAL IDENTIFICATION OF DRUG EXPOSURE

Because mothers frequently deny their drug use and the onset of effects in the neonate can be delayed (depending on the specific drug, time of exposure, and half-life of the drug), identification of the exposed infant can be difficult. All women should be assessed for substance use during pregnancy by standardized interview techniques; the yield in identification improves with the depth of the risk assessment of a drug history. The substance-using woman and her exposed infant also can be identified from physical signs and reported symptoms in the mother.

Screening for drugs may identify drug exposure in the neonate and mother. This is usually performed on urine; the method provides quantitative information about recent substance use but has high rates of false-negative results and misses cases in women who abstain in the days before delivery. Use of newly devised techniques to test for drugs in meconium or in neonatal or maternal hair may improve the likelihood for an accurate diagnosis because those techniques can detect earlier exposure during gestation. Thus, negative toxic screening results and denial of substance abuse during pregnancy do not exclude exposure of the infant. Screening is recommended in conditions in which there is suspicion of toxic abuse in the mother and the neonate. Mothers should be informed whether screening is to be done on their urine because they have the right of refusal. Because many mothers deny substance abuse, we do not advocate obtaining consent for testing the

Table 4–47. Representative Criteria for Considering Toxic Screening

Maternal and family history	
Abruptio placentae	History of incarceration
Limited or no prenatal care	Maternal history of sexually
Intrauterine growth retardation	transmitted disease
History of substance use or alcohol use	Maternal history of prostitution
Maternal psychiatric history	
Neonatal history—three or more of the following:	
Tremulousness/jitteriness	Sneezing, sweating, yawning
Hypertonia, hyperreflexia	
Irritability, incessant crying	Temperature instability
Unexplained depression, lethargy	Apnea
Increased sucking	Seizures or other neurologic signs
Vomiting, diarrhea	Fetal alcohol syndrome

infant, although informing the mother is necessary. Testing is best performed on the mother's and the infant's urine to obtain as many positive results as possible. A summary of the factors that should alert the clinician to perform toxic screening is presented in Table 4–47.

NEONATAL SIGNS

The signs of drug effects differ with the specific drug, some of which cause intoxication and a withdrawal syndrome. The most common signs are jitteriness and hyperreflexia; their presence in neonates should alert the clinician to the possibility of drug exposure.

Mortality rates range from 3% to 10%, and fetal demise can occur in utero from withdrawal. Causes of morbidity include perinatal asphyxia and congenital anomalies. Neurodevelopmental delay, specific neurologic deficits, and sudden infant death syndrome (SIDS) occur with increased frequency in opiate-exposed infants.

Cocaine is currently the illicit drug most commonly used during pregnancy. Symptoms usually are less severe than those with opiate exposure. Infants may be SGA with CNS, skull, eye, gastrointestinal, and genitourinary abnormalities; they may also be at increased risk for SIDS.

Fetal alcohol syndrome is characterized by IUGR, microcephaly, and dysmorphic features, including short palpebral fissures, microphthalmia, and flat nasal bridge. Congenital heart disease occurs in up to 40% of these infants. Chronic alcohol exposure causes neonatal depression and hypoglycemia in addition to a mild withdrawal syndrome in chronically exposed infants. Neurodevelopmental delay and growth failure usually are also noted.

Phencyclidine is associated with abnormal limb and eye movements and disordered regulation of sleep–wake states.

Recently, fine motor control and subsequent behavioral disturbances have been reported in PCP-exposed infants. Microcephaly also has been noted.

PERINATAL MANAGEMENT

Attempts should not be made to detoxify women who use opiates during pregnancy because of the risk of fetal withdrawal syndrome. These women should be maintained on methadone at the lowest dose tolerated. Neonatal care should be provided for the potential intrapartum complications, such as meconium aspiration, perinatal asphyxia, prematurity, IUGR, neonatal depression from maternal opiate use, or shock or asphyxia associated with abruptio placentae. Naloxone is not recommended because it may abruptly induce acute withdrawal in opiate-habituated infants, thereby producing seizures. When neonatal respiratory depression is associated with unknown substance exposure or known opiate exposure, ventilation should be supported to allow for gradual withdrawal from drug after birth.

NEONATAL MANAGEMENT

Supportive care of the drug-exposed infant includes swaddling, limited sensory stimulation, and other comforting measures such as rocking, cuddling, pacifiers, warm baths, and gentle massage. The increased metabolic demands and oxygen consumption of the infant during withdrawal may require a caloric intake greater than 120 cal/(kg/day) to establish appropriate weight gain. Careful evaluation of symptoms (every 2–4 hours) is necessary to make decisions about pharmacologic therapy. The drugs most frequently used to treat withdrawal symptoms are listed in Table 4–48.

Several other issues need to be considered in caring for infants of drug-abusing mothers. Because breast milk contains drug, breast feeding may prolong the withdrawal phase. In addition, there is an increased risk for HIV or hepatitis B infection in these infants because drug-abusing mothers also may have these infections. It is often necessary to provide careful home follow-up because of the adverse social circumstances associated with drug abuse.

Necrotizing Enterocolitis

Necrotizing enterocolitis is the most common acquired gastrointestinal disorder encountered in the neonatal intensive care unit. It predominantly affects premature infants and usually occurs as a complication of conditions such as RDS and PDA, but it occasionally occurs in full-term infants stressed by cyanotic congenital cardiac defect, asphyxia, anemia, or polycythemia.

EPIDEMIOLOGY

The incidence of NEC varies widely. In a collaborative study including several neonatal centers, the prevalence of

Table 4–48. Pharmacologic Treatment of Drug Withdrawal Symptoms

	Phenobarbital	Diluted Tincture of Opium[1]	Diazepam
Comments	Useful but does not control diarrhea. Predictable decrease in serum levels when discontinued (10–20%/d)	Pharmacologic "replacement"; controls diarrhea; requires very slow tapering	Works poorly alone; does not control diarrhea
Dosage	Loading: 10–20 mg/kg Maintenance: 4–12 mg/kg/day orally ($\div$ q 8 h)	0.8–2.0 mL/kg/day orally ($\div$ q 4–6 h)	1.5–3.0 mg/kg/day orally or intramuscularly ($\div$ q 6 h)

[1] Tincture of opium diluted in a concentration of 1 : 25 with H_2O.

proven NEC was 10.1%, and an additional 17.2% of infants had suspected NEC. The risk was greater in black boys and in infants with birth weights less than 1500 g. Significantly increased risk was associated with prolonged rupture of membranes, birth weight less than 1000 g, asphyxia, and maternal hemorrhage, whereas good prenatal care was associated with reduced risk. Ninety percent of cases occur in infants born at less than 36 weeks' gestation. The disease usually develops during the first 2 weeks after birth; it is uncommon before 5 days or after 1 month. The more immature the infant, the later is the onset of NEC.

PATHOGENESIS

The cause of NEC is not known. The most likely factors contributing to NEC are bowel/blood flow, feeding disturbances, and infection.

Hypoxic-ischemic injury. Interference with gastrointestinal blood flow has been considered an important potential initiating factor in NEC. This may result from vasoconstriction caused by severe fetal or neonatal hypoxemia or from hypotension, shock, sepsis, PDA, congestive heart failure, and congenital heart disease with aortic arch obstruction. Vasospasm or thrombosis of the mesenteric circulation also can occur with umbilical arterial catheterization. Mucosal injury with necrosis and ulceration may ensue. Recently, it has been suggested that tissue damage is aggravated by free oxygen radicals released during reperfusion after ischemia.

Bacterial colonization. The gastrointestinal tract is usually sterile at birth. Within the first postnatal week, the gut normally becomes colonized with aerobic and anaerobic bacteria. However, colonization may be delayed by early antibiotic therapy, cesarean birth, or delayed enteric feeding; alternatively, the gut may become colonized with pathogenic bacteria in these conditions.

The role of bacterial infection in NEC is not resolved. Damaged bowel may be secondarily infected. However, epidemic occurrences of NEC have suggested that infection may be the primary etiology. Epidemics have been associated with *E. coli, Klebsiella pneumoniae, Staphylococcus epidermidis, Clostridium butyricum,* and some viruses (e.g., enterovirus, coronavirus, and rotavirus).

Luminal substrate. More than 90% of infants in whom NEC develops had received enteral feedings. Excessive and rapid increases of volume have been suggested as risk factors for NEC but might merely contribute to an already damaged bowel.

Inflammatory mediators. The physiologic events of NEC can be explained by the effects of inflammatory mediators such as tumor necrosis factor produced by endotoxin-stimulated macrophages, platelet-activating factor, and leukotrienes. The role of these mediators in endotoxin-induced ischemic bowel necrosis has been confirmed in an animal model.

CLINICAL MANIFESTATIONS

The earliest clinical manifestation of NEC is evidence of increased gastric residual volume during gavage feeding. Necrotizing enterocolitis also should be suspected if an infant has abdominal distention or tenderness, bilious vomiting, and occult or frank blood in the stool. Other signs are nonspecific: apnea, bradycardia, cyanosis, lethargy, thermal instability, poor peripheral perfusion, hypoglycemia, jaundice, and shock.

The most common laboratory findings are metabolic acidosis, leukopenia, thrombocytopenia, anemia, electrolyte disturbances, reducing substances in stool, and, in severe cases, evidence of disseminated intravascular coagulation. The diagnosis of NEC is confirmed by evaluation of erect and recumbent abdominal radiographs. Bowel distention may be the earliest radiologic sign of NEC; other nonspecific findings are air–fluid levels within the intestine, thickening of the bowel wall, and a fixed dilated loop of intestine that persists in the same location in serial radiographs. **Pneumatosis intestinalis,** bubbles of subserosal air in the bowel wall that result from bacterial gas production, is considered pathognomonic of NEC. Pneumoperitoneum is a sign of intestinal perforation and indicates the need for immediate surgical intervention. The clinical staging criteria for NEC developed by Bell

Table 4–49. Modified Bell Staging Criteria for Necrotizing Enterocolitis

Stage	Classification	Systemic Signs	Intestinal Signs	Radiologic Signs
I	Suspected NEC	Temperature instability, apnea, bradycardia, lethargy	Increased gastric residuals, mild abdominal distention, emesis, guaiac-positive stool	Normal; dilation; mild ileus
IIA	Proven NEC—mild	Same as above	Same as above, plus absent bowel sounds, with or without abdominal tenderness	Pneumatosis intestinalis, intestinal dilation, ileus, edema of bowel wall
IIB	Proven NEC—moderate	Same as above, plus mild metabolic acidosis and mild thrombocytopenia	Same as above, abdominal tenderness, with or without abdominal cellulitis or right lower quadrant mass	Same as above with or without portal venous gas and ascites
IIIA	Advanced NEC—severe; bowel intact	Same as above, plus hypotension, bradycardia, apnea, metabolic acidosis, thrombocytopenia, neutropenia, with or without DIC	Same as above; generalized peritonitis with marked distention of abdomen	Same plus ascites
IIIB	Advanced NEC—severe; bowel perforation or gangrene	Same plus DIC	Same as above	Same plus pneumoperitoneum or fixed bowel loop

DIC = disseminated intravascular coagulation; NEC = necrotizing enterocolitis.

and coworkers are a useful guide to establish severity, treatment, and prognosis (Table 4–49).

TREATMENT

The goals of medical treatment are to stabilize the infant and prevent progression of the disease. When NEC is suspected, enteral feedings should be discontinued immediately and the intestinal tract decompressed by nasogastric or orogastric suction. Fluid and electrolytes should be administered to maintain urine output, blood pressure, and tissue perfusion. In addition, intravenous broad-spectrum antibiotics should be provided promptly. Frequent clinical and radiographic assessments are needed to recognize clinical deterioration early. Serial abdominal radiographs, including left lateral decubitus films to detect free air from intestinal perforation, should be repeated every 4–8 hours until the infant is stable. Parenteral nutrition should be initiated because oral intake usually is withheld for at least 10–14 days.

The timing and extent of surgical intervention in NEC are controversial. Definite indications are pneumoperitoneum, fixed loop on serial radiographs, or brown discoloration or presence of bacteria in peritoneal fluid withdrawn by paracentesis. Less definitive indications include abdominal erythema, abdominal mass, severe gastrointestinal bleeding, marked abdominal tenderness, thrombocytopenia, and clinical deterioration.

The most common late complication of NEC is colonic stricture, which occurs in 15–35% of recovered patients. Adhesions, abscesses, or fistulas may occur. Malabsorption or cholestasis also may occur. Short gut syndrome is a serious problem if a long segment of small bowel had to be removed surgically. It may require long-term parenteral nutrition. Mortality in NEC is high, approximating 10% in stages I and II and 55% in stage III.

Thoracic & Gastrointestinal Neonatal Surgical Conditions

Approximately 1 of every 200 newborns requires a surgical procedure because of anomalies in the thorax, gastrointestinal tract, genitourinary system, or nervous system. Immediate neonatal care has been improved considerably by prenatal diagnosis of many of these anomalies. The more common thoracic and gastrointestinal conditions that require surgical repair during the neonatal period are reviewed.

ESOPHAGEAL ATRESIA & TRACHEOESOPHAGEAL FISTULA

Esophageal atresia and tracheoesophageal fistula are characterized by a separation between the proximal and distal ends of the esophagus. The anomaly presents as five different types (Figure 4–6). The most common (type III) is associated with a tracheal fistula of the distal esophagus;

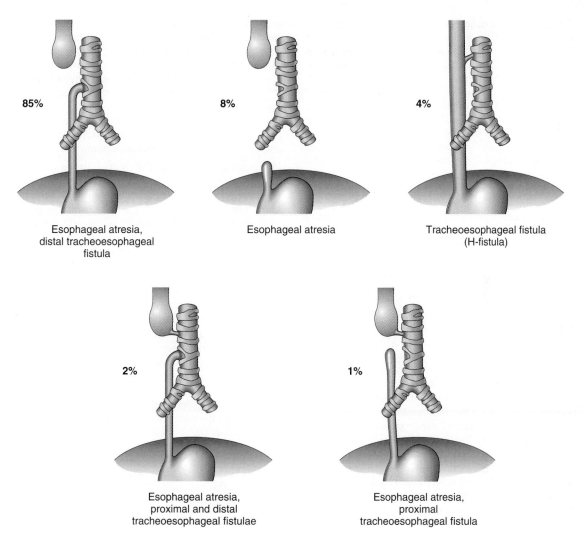

85%

Esophageal atresia,
distal tracheoesophageal
fistula

8%

Esophageal atresia

4%

Tracheoesophageal fistula
(H-fistula)

2%

Esophageal atresia,
proximal and distal
tracheoesophageal fistulae

1%

Esophageal atresia,
proximal
tracheoesophageal fistula

Figure 4–6. The major types and approximate incidence of tracheoesophageal malformations in newborn infants. (Reproduced from Rudolph AM [editor]: *Rudolph's Pediatrics*, 19th ed. Appleton & Lange, 1991:996.)

it occurs in 1 of 3000 infants and often is associated with polyhydramnios. Due to the esophageal obstruction, oropharyngeal secretions are copious because saliva cannot be swallowed. Choking and aspiration pneumonia may occur, particularly if feeding is attempted. In addition, air from the lungs crosses through the fistula to the distal esophageal segment, thereby inducing gastric distention, which in turn can stimulate regurgitation of gastric contents through the fistula into the lungs. Aspiration from the upper airway or gastric contents entering the lungs through the fistula will cause respiratory distress.

To establish the radiographic diagnosis with certainty, no radiopaque substances are needed. An oral gastric tube is inserted until a stop is felt. A chest and abdominal radiograph will show the tube in the upper part of the thorax; air is seen in the stomach crossing through the distal fistula to the trachea.

Approximately 50% of infants with esophageal atresia have associated malformations, including congenital heart disease, anorectal, skeletal, and renal malformations, and the VACTERL association; the latter, present in 5–10% of infants, includes vertebral, anorectal, cardiac, tracheoesophageal, renal, and limb malformations.

General management. Before surgery, the infant should be placed in an infant seat or the head and trunk elevated to avoid gastric reflux into the airway. Attempts to feed the infant should be stopped immediately, and continuous, gentle suction of the proximal esophageal pouch instituted. If the infant has respiratory distress due to aspiration, antibiotics should be started promptly. Cardiac and abdominal ultrasound studies should be performed to rule out associated anomalies. Surgical repair consists of closure of the fistula and anastomosis of the two esophageal segments. In the immediate postoperative period, infants are kept on mechanical ventilation for at least 24–48 hours, and parenteral nutrition is provided until appropriate calories can be administered enterally.

Complications include stenosis at the anastomotic site and prolonged difficulty in instituting oral feeding because of disturbed esophageal motility. Many of these infants also have respiratory distress and stridor because of associated tracheomalacia. The prognosis is most favorable in mature infants who have no associated congenital anomalies, who do not have respiratory distress, and who have no other severe congenital anomalies.

CONGENITAL DIAPHRAGMATIC HERNIA

The diaphragm develops between the fourth and eighth weeks of gestation. Abnormalities in its development may allow herniation of the abdominal contents into the thorax, which in turn impairs appropriate growth and maturation of the lungs. Most cases are in the left diaphragm in the posterior and lateral areas. This condition occurs in 1 per 4000–5000 live births. The diagnosis can now be made in utero by ultrasound; if the lesion is found before 25 weeks' gestation, the prognosis is poor. Fetal surgery may become a solution for these cases.

The newborn with abdominal contents in the thorax and pulmonary hypoplasia has severe respiratory insufficiency from birth, with severe hypoxemia and acidosis. The diagnosis can be made clinically by the presence of a scaphoid abdomen because of abdominal organ displacement into the chest. Chest radiograph shows little or no gas in the abdomen, absence of the diaphragmatic dome, significant mediastinal shift to the contralateral side (usually to the right), and bowel loops in the thorax, usually on the left side. In addition, PPHN occurs frequently.

Management. If the diagnosis has been made before birth, the infant should be intubated immediately, preferably before spontaneous respiratory efforts or crying occur, to avoid gastrointestinal distention. A nasogastric tube should be inserted for continuous suction. *Bag-and-mask ventilation should not be used* because this may distend the bowel and increase compression of the lung. Some infants do not improve with aggressive ventilatory treatment but may be helped by high-frequency or oscillatory ventilation; some require ECMO before surgery. If lung immaturity has been documented, artificial surfactant may be useful. Because the lung is hypoplastic, ventilatory pressures should be as low as possible to achieve adequate blood gases. Slow lung reexpansion is important to

avoid sudden mediastinal shifts and pneumothorax. Once the infant is stabilized, the condition is managed surgically by reduction of the hernia and closure of the diaphragmatic defect. This is usually performed by an abdominal or combined thoracoabdominal approach. When the defect is large, it may be necessary to place a plastic membrane over the abdomen to contain the reduced abdominal organs temporarily. The most serious complications, before or after surgery, are PPHN, pneumothorax, and gastrointestinal or hematologic complications.

Differential diagnosis. Differential diagnoses of diaphragmatic hernia include congenital lobar emphysema and congenital cystic adenomatoid malformation of the lungs. The prognosis of infants with congenital diaphragmatic hernia is related to the size of the defect, the volume of the hernia inside the thorax, and the duration of the hernia in utero; these factors are associated with the degree of pulmonary hypoplasia. Clinical signs that have been associated with poor prognosis include early fetal diagnosis at less than 25 weeks' gestation, presence of liver and stomach in the thoracic cavity, significant polyhydramnios, early and severe neonatal symptoms, severe hypoxemia and acidosis, development of pneumothorax, and lack of improvement after surgery. With appropriate and aggressive neonatal and surgical care, survival has improved and is now greater than 80%. However, fetal and neonatal mortality is much higher for infants in whom the condition is diagnosed before 25 weeks' gestation, and many infants born with severe diaphragmatic hernias die before they are transported to a tertiary care facility.

ABDOMINAL WALL DEFECTS

By the 10th week of gestation, the midgut enters the abdomen. If this process is disturbed, an abdominal wall defect associated with a decrease in intraabdominal volume results. The more common defects are **omphalocele, umbilical cord hernia, and gastroschisis.**

Omphalocele occurs in approximately 1 per 6000–8000 live births. The defect is localized centrally in the abdomen, the umbilical ring is missing, and the umbilical cord is inserted at the vertex of the sac. Abdominal organs other than bowel, such as liver, spleen, and pancreas, can be found in the hernia. It is frequently associated with other anomalies. Umbilical cord hernia has a diameter of less than 4 cm, and the sac contains only bowel.

Gastroschisis is a congenital fissure of the anterior abdominal wall; the umbilical cord is to the left of the defect and separated from the defect by a bridge of skin. In gastroschisis there is no true hernia sac; the small bowel herniates and becomes thickened with adhesions because of contact with the amniotic fluid. In some cases, the intestine is infarcted and may be atretic. The abdominal cavity often is developed better than with large omphaloceles. Table 4–50 lists the principal differences between omphalocele and gastroschisis. Extraintestinal

Table 4–50. Differences Between Omphalocele and Gastroschisis

	Omphalocele	Gastroschisis
Position	Central abdominal	Right paraumbilical
Hernia sac	Present	Absent
Umbilical ring	Absent	Present
Umbilical cord insertion	At the vertex of the sac	Normal
Herniation of other viscera	Common	Rare
Extraintestinal anomalies	Frequent	Rare
Intestinal infarction, atresia	Less frequent	More frequent

Table 4–51. Intestinal Obstruction in Neonates

Mechanical
  Congenital
    Intestinal atresia or stenosis
    Meconium ileus
    Meconium plug
    Malrotation (with or without volvulus)
    Duplication
    Incarcerated hernia
    Annular pancreas
    Preduodenal portal vein
    Intestinal cysts
  Acquired
    Intussusception
    Adhesions
    Stenosis from necrotizing enterocolitis
    Lactobezoar

Functional
  Hirschsprung disease
  Hypoplastic left colon
  Other neuronal dysplasias or muscular diseases

anomalies associated with omphalocele include imperforate anus with colon agenesis; pentalogy of Cantrell with sternal, pericardial, and cardiac defects; and Beckwith–Wiedemann syndrome. Congenital heart anomalies can occur in association with omphalocele; tetralogy of Fallot and atrial septal defects are the most common defects. Some cases are associated with trisomy 13 or, less frequently, trisomy 18.

Treatment is surgical. Sometimes primary closure is not possible because forcing abdominal contents into the small cavity displaces the diaphragm, causing respiratory distress. In addition, bowel ischemia may occur when introducing the bowels under tension into a small abdominal cavity, sometimes resulting in compromised venous return and bowel ischemia. In such cases, a Silastic pouch is sutured to the skin around the defect. The size of this sac is decreased progressively every 1–3 days to introduce the bowel slowly into the abdominal cavity; this may take 10–15 days. Infection is a frequent complication.

Intestinal Obstruction

Intestinal obstruction may be acquired or congenital, and mechanical or functional (Table 4–51). The prenatal history may reveal polyhydramnios. In the immediate neonatal period, there may be abdominal distention, bilious vomiting, and lack of meconium passage. However, passage of meconium does not rule out the presence of obstruction. In more proximal obstructions, vomiting is the earliest sign; in distal obstruction, abdominal distention is marked.

Diagnosis. When intestinal obstruction is suspected, a gastric tube should be placed for immediate decompression, and abdominal radiographs obtained. Anteroposterior views should be taken with the infant supine and in

right or left lateral decubitus; a cross-table lateral view is also useful. Intestinal distention with air–fluid levels and, sometimes, the level of the obstruction may be seen. Air reaches the rectum by 12 hours in term neonates and before 48 hours in preterm infants. Therefore, lack of distal air suggests intestinal obstruction. A barium enema is sometimes indicated; this will define the position of the cecum and thus detect malrotation. It also can be useful in cases of Hirschsprung disease or in congenital left microcolon syndrome.

Causes. Intestinal atresia is the most common cause of obstruction in the neonatal period. It can occur in the small or large bowel. Duodenal atresia may be intrinsic or extrinsic and is caused by malrotation, annular pancreas, or abnormal preduodenal portal vein. More than 50% of infants with duodenal atresia are SGA and have an increased incidence of cardiac, renal, and anal–rectal anomalies. Down syndrome is associated in 30–40% of cases. The diagnosis can be made prenatally by ultrasound or abdominal radiograph, on which the typical "double-bubble" sign is noted. Treatment consists of resection of the area with duodenal–duodenal or duodenal–jejunal anastomosis.

Infants with jejunum–ileal atresias usually have no associated malformations. The cause is probably linked to a mesenteric vascular ischemic accident in utero. Bilious vomiting and abdominal distention differ with the level of obstruction. The abdominal radiograph shows multiple fluid–air levels without distal air. A barium enema may show a very small colon. There are four different anatomic types of atresia. Type 1 is a simple atresia of the mucosa. In type 2, the most frequent, there is interruption of the mesentery and the bowel wall, but the intestinal length is usually normal. Type 3 refers to multiple intestinal atresias. In type 4, the so-called apple peel form, there is significant shortening of the bowel, with a large mesenteric defect and ischemia of the small bowel.

Management. Treatment of jejunum–ileal atresias is surgical. The prognosis is related to the remaining length of intestine and the presence or absence of the ileocecal valve after surgery. Morbidity and mortality are greatest in types 3 and 4 because short bowel syndrome and malabsorption are likely to develop in these infants. Parenteral nutrition has been a great aid in the management of these infants.

Meconium ileus. Meconium ileus is a manifestation of cystic fibrosis during the neonatal period. Abnormal accumulation of intestinal secretions and deficiency of pancreatic enzymes presumably cause increased viscosity of meconium, which leads to occlusion of the distal ileum. Clinical features include abdominal distention, lack of meconium passage, and vomiting. Abdominal radiograph shows distention with minimal or narrow air–fluid levels. Air remains trapped in the meconium; thus, there is no definite air–fluid interface. Fine gas bubbles may be seen mixed with meconium, producing a characteristic "soap-bubble" appearance. A barium enema may show a small colon secondary to the ileal obstruction. Early diagnosis and treatment are important to avoid perforation, meconium peritonitis, and volvulus. In some cases, however, these complications are present at the time of birth. Many newborns may respond to hyperosmolar enemas with iodine radiopaque substances, which are used in diagnosis and treatment. These substances introduce water into the gastrointestinal tract, soften the meconium, and facilitate its elimination. If this procedure is performed, intravenous fluids should be provided appropriately to avoid dehydration and serum hyperosmolarity. If this approach is not successful, surgery is indicated to perform an ileostomy and, sometimes, ileal resection. N-acetylcysteine irrigations into the ileum may be useful for meconium dilution and bowel cleansing.

Intestinal malrotation. Intestinal malrotation causes symptoms because of volvulus or intestinal obstruction secondary to bands. Circulation to the rotated segment is restricted, leading to intestinal gangrene. Volvulus presents with sudden onset of bilious vomiting with abdominal distention, profuse rectal hemorrhage, peritonitis, and shock. The cecum is displaced from its normal location in the right lower quadrant. When a diagnosis of intestinal volvulus is suspected, immediate surgical treatment is required: the volvulus is reduced by rotating the bowel loops counterclockwise, and the gangrenous bowel is resected. Anastomosis may be performed and the intestine fixed in position surgically.

Anorectal malformations. Anorectal malformations occur in approximately 1 per 5000 live births; the incidence is higher in male infants. Half these infants have associated anomalies, esophageal atresia, and genitourinary, skeletal, or cardiovascular malformations. If the defect is **low** it can produce anal stenosis, anal cutaneous fistula, anterior perineal anus, and, in girls, a vulvar anus. When the lesion is **intermediate,** the intestine ends above the elevator of the anus. These lesions include anal agenesis with or without rectal vaginal fistula and anal–rectal stenosis. When the defect is **high,** it produces anal–rectal agenesis and rectal atresia. Fistulas may be rectourethral, rectovaginal, or rectocloacal. The best diagnostic study is perineal examination; x-ray studies are useful to determine the level of the lesion. When there are fistulas, a fistulogram is useful before surgery. The initial treatment in the high and intermediate types is colostomy. By 1–2 years of age a final repair is performed to preserve the function of the sphincter. In the low lesion, perineal anoplasty is performed.

Hirschsprung disease. Hirschsprung disease, or congenital aganglionic bowel disease, is rare, occurring in approximately 1 per 5000 live births. It is five times more frequent in male infants, and in 80% of cases there is a family history. The condition is due to lack of caudal migration of the ganglion cells from the neural crest; this produces contraction of a segment, causing obstruction with proximal dilatation. Vomiting, abdominal distention, and constipation are the classic clinical signs.

Frequent Electrolyte & Metabolic Abnormalities

HYPOGLYCEMIA

Hypoglycemia is common in newborn infants. The actual serum glucose concentration defining hypoglycemia is debatable but is generally agreed to be below 40 mg/dL. It is common practice to measure whole blood glucose concentration with test strips using a glucose oxidase method. Plasma glucose levels are approximately 14% higher than those of whole blood; therefore, a low glucose concentration by test strip should be confirmed by measuring the serum concentration. Hypoglycemia is suggested by an abnormal cry, diaphoresis, jitteriness, and seizures; other features are tachypnea, tachycardia, hypothermia, feeding problems, and, rarely, myocardial failure.

Hypoglycemia may be caused by conditions resulting in insulin excess, defective mechanisms of glucose homeostasis, defective carbohydrate or amino acid metabolism, or diminished substrate for gluconeogenesis (see Chapter 19).

INSULIN EXCESS

Insulin excess occurs most commonly as a transient finding in the IDM. Maternal hyperglycemia results in fetal hyperglycemia and β-cell hyperplasia, with elevated fetal insulin concentration. When the maternal–placental source of glucose is removed at the time of birth, hypoglycemia occurs in about 50% of IDMs in the first 24 hours after birth. β-Cell hyperplasia is also implicated in the hypoglycemia observed with erythroblastosis fetalis and Beckwith–Wiedemann syndrome. β-Sympathomimetic drugs used for tocolysis cross the placenta and stimulate insulin release, causing transient hypoglycemia. Persistent hypoglycemia may result from insulin-producing tumors and usually requires subtotal or total pancreatectomy.

DIMINISHED GLUCOSE PRODUCTION OR SUBSTRATE SUPPLY

Growth-retarded and preterm infants frequently have hypoglycemia because hepatic glycogen stores are limited and gluconeogenesis is poorly developed. Hypoglycemia also can occur after stress of asphyxia, polycythemia (hyperviscosity), congestive heart failure, infection, and cold. Inborn errors of metabolism causing hypoglycemia include galactosemia, hereditary fructose intolerance, glycogen storage disease type I (von Gierke disease), and aminoacidopathies. Endocrine causes of hypoglycemia include growth hormone deficiency, panhypopituitarism, adrenal insufficiency, hypothyroidism, and glucagon deficiency.

The most important aspect of the medical management of neonatal hypoglycemia is appropriate anticipation and prevention in the infant at risk. Treatment is directed at increasing oral feeding, if possible. In the acute situation, glucose should be administered intravenously as a bolus (200 mg/kg as 2 mL/kg of 10% dextrose) followed by 5–8 mg/(kg/min) as a continuous infusion. If hypoglycemia persists, an endocrine evaluation should be instituted (see Chapter 19).

HYPERGLYCEMIA

Hyperglycemia, defined as a blood glucose concentration greater than 150 mg/dL, often results from excessive parenteral glucose administration but may occur with infection, during acute asphyxia or cold stress, and after surgery. Some drugs, such as theophylline and corticosteroids, can cause hyperglycemia. Transient diabetes mellitus occurs during the first 2 postnatal weeks in some SGA babies. Insulin therapy is usually required, although recovery in the first year is expected.

The major problems associated with hyperglycemia are hyperosmolarity and osmotic diuresis. Increased risk of PV-IVH and dehydration may result. If plasma glucose concentration is greater than 300 mg/dL or there is glycosuria, parenteral glucose infusion should be decreased 10–20% every 4–6 hours while plasma glucose concentration and urine are checked frequently. Insulin therapy is rarely required except in diabetic states. Insulin infusion, in very low doses (0.04–0.07 U/[kg/h]), has been used with reported success to increase early caloric intake without resulting hyperglycemia in VLBW infants.

HYPOCALCEMIA

Hypocalcemia in the newborn is defined as a total calcium serum concentration less than 7.0 mg/dL (1.75 mmol/L) or an ionized calcium concentration less than 4.4 mg/dL (1.1 mmol/L). The clinical features of hypocalcemia are nonspecific and include irritability, jitteriness, tetany, and seizures. Infants may have a high-pitched cry, and apnea may occur. The ECG characteristically shows a prolonged QT interval and flat T waves. Neonatal hypocalcemia is usually evident in the first few postnatal days. It is common in preterm infants, in IDMs, and after asphyxia. It also can result from infection or maternal hyperparathyroidism. Later onset may be related to use of furosemide for diuresis.

Treatment of hypocalcemia depends on the clinical setting. Calcium gluconate, 10%, can be added to the intravenous solution. Each milliliter of 10% calcium gluconate (100 mg) provides 9 mg of elemental calcium. The dose ranges from 3 mL/(kg/24 h) to 12–15 mL/(kg/24 h). With severe symptoms such as seizures, 10% calcium chloride is given by slow intravenous infusion in a dose of 25 mg/kg, or 10% calcium gluconate in a dose of 200 mg/kg, while the ECG and heart rate are monitored closely. Bradycardia or other cardiac arrhythmias can occur with rapid calcium infusion. A potentially serious complication of parenteral calcium chloride administration is extravasation into subcutaneous tissue, with skin sloughing. For chronic conditions, once the infant is feeding, oral calcium gluconate can be used.

ABNORMALITIES IN SERUM SODIUM CONCENTRATION

In full-term infants, hypernatremia occurs occasionally in breast-fed infants who have had very little intake over 5–7 days. However, hypernatremia and hyponatremia are more common in sick premature infants. In these infants, serum sodium concentration is the best indicator of water balance during the first 7–14 days. It increases with water deficit and decreases with water excess; for this reason, serum sodium concentration may not accurately reflect total body sodium. **Hyponatremia** by definition is a serum sodium level below 130 meq/L. If hyponatremia develops acutely, cerebral edema and seizures may result. However, hyponatremia usually develops progressively, with clinical manifestations of hypotonia, hyporeflexia, and apneic episodes. The mechanisms responsible for hyponatremia and an approach to diagnosis are outlined in Figure 4–7. The treatment of hyponatremia is outlined in Table 4–52.

Hypernatremia, by definition, is a serum sodium concentration above 150 meq/L associated with excessive sodium intake or negative water balance. Usually in the neonate, excessive sodium intake is associated with an excess in total body water; thus, serum sodium concentration is normal. When hypernatremia is due to excessive sodium intake, sodium intake should be restricted and diuretics administered. When it is due to water deficit, it is associated with weight loss and negative water balance. The clinical manifestations of hypernatremia include hyperexcitability and hyperreflexia. One of the most serious risks in hypernatremia is the rapid correction of the serum sodium concentration. The brain cells contain osmols that prevent intracellular dehydration. If the serum sodium is decreased rapidly, these intracellular osmols draw water into the cells and generate edema, resulting in seizures. This complication is avoided if the serum sodium concentration does not decrease more than 10 meq/L in 6–8 hours. When there is water deficit, the treatment consists of adequate administration of free water to correct the negative water balance slowly (see Table 4–52).

ABNORMALITIES IN SERUM POTASSIUM CONCENTRATION

Hypokalemia may be due to excessive loss, as occurs with diuretics, or with inadequate K^+ intake or metabolic alkalosis. Treatment consists of increasing K^+ in the intravenous fluids and correcting alkalosis.

Hyperkalemia can occur in full-term infants with adrenogenital syndrome. It is very common in ELBW infants; as many as 50% of neonates less than 28 weeks' gestation show serum potassium concentrations greater than 6.5 meq/L. The cause has not been defined but might be due to low urinary output in the first 24–48 hours after birth, tissue damage at birth, acidosis, intracranial hemorrhage, and hemolysis. Neonates are more resistant to cardiac arrhythmias associated with hyperkalemia than are older children. Treatment is indicated when the serum potassium concentrations exceed 7 meq/L. Acidemia, if present, should be corrected, because this increases transfer of potassium from the extracellular to the intracellular compartment. In addition, the serum calcium concentration should be maintained at normal levels to reduce the risk of arrhythmia. Potassium exchange resins, given by enema, may be indicated. Diuretics and dopamine infusion increase urinary output, and thus augment potassium excretion. Glucose and insulin are useful in decreasing serum potassium concentration, but can cause serious problems in VLBW infants. Peritoneal dialysis or continuous arterial venous hemofiltration are rarely required in neonates.

Electrolyte abnormalities usually can be prevented in VLBW infants by careful administration of fluids without sodium and potassium during the first 48–96 hours after birth, with frequent assessments of the glucose and fluid balance.

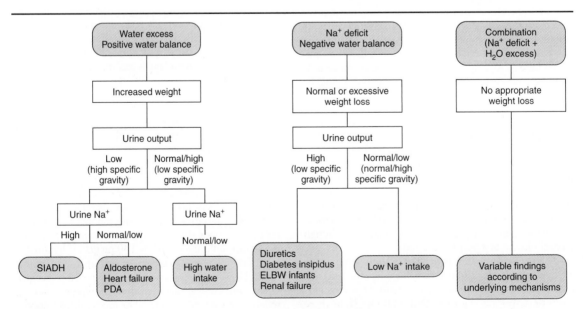

Figure 4–7. Mechanisms and diagnostic steps in hyponatremia. ELBW = extremely low birth weight; PDA = patent ductus arteriosus; SIADH = syndrome of inappropriate antidiuretic hormone secretion.

Table 4–52. Treatment of Sodium Imbalance[1]

Symptomatic hyponatremia
  Fast correction (when serum [Na$^+$] below 120 meq/L)
    (125 − serum [Na$^+$]) × 0.8 × weight (kg) = total Na$^+$ (meq)
      to be given over 2–3 h

Asymptomatic hyponatremia
  Na$^+$ deficit
    (140 − serum sodium) × 0.8 × weight (kg) = total meqs
      of Na$^+$ to be given over 12–36 h (added to
      Na$^+$ maintenance)
  Water excess
    Calculate by weight curve or: 0.8 × weight (kg)
      × (1 − serum [Na$^+$]/140) = H$_2$O liters in excess
    Provide negative water balance, with sodium
      maintenance

Hypernatremia
  Calculate water deficit by weight curve or 0.8 × weight (kg)
    × [(serum Na$^+$/140) − 1] = H$_2$O deficit (liters)
  Provide free water plus maintenance fluids to decrease
    serum sodium not faster than 10 meq/(L/6 h)

[1] The constant 0.8 in the formulas estimates the space of distribution of sodium.

REFERENCES

Perinatal History

Phibbs RH: The newborn infant. Neonatal mortality and morbidity. In: Rudolph AM et al (editors): *Rudolph's Pediatrics,* 20th ed. Appleton & Lange, 1996:197.

Effects of Labor

Marsal K, Lindblad A: Fetal and placental circulation during labor. In: Polin R, Fox WW (editors): *Neonatal and Fetal Physiology.* Saunders, 1998.

Transition to Neonatal Life

Bland R: Formation of fetal lung liquid and its removal near birth. In: Polin RA, Fox WW (editors): *Neonatal and Fetal Medicine, Physiology and Pathophysiology.* Saunders, 1998.

Rudolph AM: Circulation in the fetal-placental unit. In: Cowett RM (editor): *Principles of Perinatal–Neonatal Metabolism.* Springer-Verlag, 1998.

Temperature Regulation

Bruck K: Neonatal thermal regulation. In: Polin RA, Fox WW (editors): *Neonatal and Fetal Medicine: Physiology and Pathophysiology.* Saunders, 1998.

Saver PJJ: Neonatal thermoregulation. In: Cowett RM: (editor): *Principles of Perinatal–Neonatal Metabolism.* Springer-Verlag, 1998.

Assessment of Newborns

Apgar Scores

Apgar V: A proposal for a new method of evaluation of the newborn infant. Curr Res Anesthesiol 1953;32:260.

Nelson KB, Leviton A: How much of neonatal encephalopathy is due to birth asphyxia? Am J Dis Child 1991;145:1325.

Goodwin TM: Clinical implications of perinatal depression. Obstet Gynecol Clin North Am 1999;26:711.

Maturity & Gestational Age

Ballard JL et al: A simplified score for assessment of fetal maturation of newborn infants. J Pediatr 1978;95:769.

Dubowitz LMS et al: Clinical assessment of gestational age in the newborn. J Pediatr 1970;77:1.

Physical Examination of the Newborn Infant

Charlton VE, Phibbs RH: Examination of the newborn. In: Rudolph AM et al (editors): *Rudolph's Pediatrics,* 20th ed. Appleton & Lange, 1996:208.

Neurologic Examination of the Newborn

Amiel-Tison C: Newborn neurologic examination. In: Rudolph AM et al (editors): *Rudolph's Pediatrics,* 20th ed. Appleton & Lange, 1996:218.

Brann AW, Schwartz JF: Assessment of neonatal neurology function. In: Fanaroff AA, Martin RJ (editors): *Neonatal–Perinatal Medicine.* Mosby-Year Book, 1997.

Abnormalities of Growth

Cowett RM: Hypo and hyperglycemia in the newborn. In: Polin RA, Fox WW (editors): *Neonatal and Fetal Medicine: Physiology and Pathophysiology.* Saunders, 1998.

Kliegman R: Intrauterine growth retardation: Determinants of apparent fetal growth. In: Fanaroff AA, Martin RJ (editors): *Neonatal Perinatal Medicine.* Mosby-Year Book, 1997.

Abnormalities of Maturity

Clifford SH: Post-maturity with placental dysfunction. J Pediatr 1954;44:1.

Stubblefield G, Berek JS: Perinatal mortality in term and post-term births. Obstet Gynecol 1980;56:676.

Westgren M et al: Intrauterine asphyxia and long-term outcome in preterm infants. Obstet Gynecol 1986;67:512.

Approaches to Common Neonatal Clinical Problems

Cyanosis

Hoffman JIE: Right-to-left shunts. In: Rudolph AM et al (editors): *Rudolph's Pediatrics,* 20th ed. Appleton & Lange, 1996:1493.

Kitterman JA: Cyanosis in the newborn infant. Pediatr Rev 1982; 4:13.

Tooley W, Stanger P: The blue baby. Circulation or ventilation or both. N Engl J Med 1972;2878:983.

Respiratory Distress

Hazinski TA: The respiratory system. In: Rudolph AM et al (editors): *Rudolph's Pediatrics,* 20th ed. Appleton & Lange, 1996:1569.

Swischuk L: Radiology of pulmonary insufficiency. In: Thibeault DW, Gregory GA (editors): *Neonatal Pulmonary Care,* 2nd ed. Appleton & Lange, 1986.

Neonatal Anemia

Shannon KM et al: Enhancement of erythropoiesis by recombinant human erythropoietin in low birth weight infants: a pilot study. J Pediatr 1992;120:586.

Brown MS, Keith JF III: Comparison between two and five doses a week of recombinant human erythropoietin for anemia of prematurity: a randomized trial. Pediatrics 1999;104(2, pt 1):210.

Doyle JJ: The role of erythropoietin in the anemia of prematurity (review). Semin Perinatol 1997;21:20.

Bacterial Infections

Gerdes JS: Clinicopathologic approach to the diagnosis of neonatal sepsis. Clin Perinatol 1991;18:361.

Klein JO: Current antibacterial therapy for neonatal sepsis and meningitis. Pediatr Infect Dis 1990;9:783.

McCracken GH Jr, Frei BJ: Perinatal bacterial diseases. In: Feigin RD, Cherry JD (editors): *Textbook of Pediatric Infectious Diseases.* Saunders, 1987.

Abdominal Mass

Hartman GE, Shochat SJ: Abdominal mass lesions in the newborn: diagnosis and treatment. Clin Perinatol 1989;16:123.

Koop CE: Abdominal mass in the newborn infant. N Engl J Med 1973;289:569.

Wilson DA: Ultrasound screening for abdominal masses in the neonatal period. Am J Dis Child 1982;136:147.

Seizures

Maytal J et al: Lorazepam in the treatment of refractory neonatal seizures. J Child Neurol 1991;6:319.

Painter MJ, Gaus LM: Neonatal seizures: diagnosis and treatment. J Child Neurol 1991;6:101.

Volpe JJ: Neonatal seizures: Current concepts and revised classification. Pediatrics 1989;84:422.

Disorders of the Newborn

Apnea

Gerhardt T et al: Effects of aminophylline on respiratory center and reflex activity in premature infants with apnea. Pediatr Res 1983;17:188.

Miller MJ, Martin RJ: Pathophysiology of apnea of prematurity. In: RA Polin, WW Fox (editors): *Neonatal and Fetal Physiology.* Saunders, 1998.

Respiratory Distress Syndrome

Avery ME, Merritt TA: Surfactant replacement therapy. N Engl J Med 1991;324:910.

Hazinski TA: Acute respiratory distress syndromes in the newborn. In: Rudolph AM et al (editors): *Rudolph's Pediatrics,* 20th ed. Appleton & Lange, 1996:1597.

Phibbs RH et al: Initial clinical trial of EXOSURF, a protein-free synthetic surfactant, for the prophylaxis and early treatment of hyaline membrane disease. Pediatrics 1991;88:1.

Meconium Aspiration Syndrome & Persistent Pulmonary Hypertension of the Newborn

Bartlett RH et al: Extracorporeal circulation in neonatal respiratory failure: a prospective randomized study. Pediatrics 1985;76:479.

Fox WW, Duara S: Persistent pulmonary hypertension in the neonate: diagnosis and management. J Pediatr 1983;103:505.

Gregory GA et al: Meconium aspiration in neonates: a prospective study. J Pediatr 1974;85:848.

Wiswell TE, Henley MA: Intratracheal suctioning, systemic infection, and the meconium aspiration syndrome. Pediatrics 1992; 89:203.

Wiswell TE, Fuloria M: Management of meconium-stained amniotic fluid (review). Clin Perinatol 1999;26:659.

Perinatal Asphyxia & Resuscitation

Gregory GA: Resuscitation of the newborn. In: Rudolph AM et al (editors): *Rudolph's Pediatrics,* 20th ed. Appleton & Lange, 1996:237.

Gunn AJ et al: Dramatic neuronal rescue with prolonged selective head cooling after ischemia in fetal lambs. J Clin Invest 1997; 99:248.

Jacobs MM, Phibbs RH: Prevention, recognition and treatment of perinatal asphyxia in critical issues in intrapartum and delivery room management. Clin Perinatol 1989;16:785.

Saugstad OD: Resuscitation with room-air or oxygen supplementation (review). Clin Perinatol 1998;25:741.

Neonatal Cardiopulmonary Resuscitation Manual. American Heart Association, American Academy of Pediatrics, 1997.

Polycythemia

Black V et al: Developmental and neurologic sequelae of neonatal hyperviscosity syndrome. Pediatrics 1982;69:426.

Hathaway WE: Neonatal hyperviscosity. Pediatrics 1983;72:567.

Kurlat I, Sola A: Risk of neonatal polycythemia in infants of hypertensive mothers. Acta Paediatr 1992;81:662.

Wiswell TE et al: Neonatal polycythemia: frequency of clinical manifestations and other associated findings. Pediatrics 1986;78:26.

Congenital Infections

Alford CA et al: Congenital and perinatal cytomegalovirus infections. Rev Infect Dis 1990;12:S745.

Alpert G, Plotkin SA: A practical guide to the diagnosis of congenital infections in the newborn infant. Pediatr Clin N Am 1986; 33:465.

Freij BJ et al: Maternal rubella and the congenital rubella syndrome. Clin Perinatol 1988;15:247.

Perlman JM, Argyle C: Lethal cytomegalovirus infection in preterm infants: clinical, radiological, and neuropathological findings. Ann Neurol 1992;31:64.

Sever JL et al: Toxoplasmosis: maternal and pediatric findings in 23,000 pregnancies. Pediatrics 1988;82:181.

Toltzis P: Current issues in neonatal herpes simplex virus infection. Clin Perinatol 1991;18:193.

Birth Trauma

Boome RS, Kaye JC: Obstetric traction injuries of the bracheal plexus. Natural history, indications for surgical repair and results. J Bone Joint Surg Br 1988;70:571.

Mangurten HH: Birth injuries. In: Fanaroff AA, Martin RJ (editors): *Neonatal Perinatal Medicine: Diseases of the Fetus and Infant,* 5th ed. Mosby-Year Book, 1997.

Intracranial Hemorrhage

Allan WC et al: Antecedents of cerebral palsy in a multicenter trial of indomethacin for intraventricular hemorrhage. Arch Pediatr Adolesc Med 1997;151:580.

Ment LR et al: Outcome of children in the indomethacin intraventricular hemorrhage prevention trial. Pediatrics 2000; 105(3, pt 1):485.

Papile L et al: Relationship of cerebral intraventricular hemorrhage and early childhood neurologic handicaps. J Pediatr 1983;103:273.

Volpe JJ: Intraventricular hemorrhage in the premature infant—current concepts. Part I. Ann Neurol 1989;25:3.

Volpe JJ: Intraventricular hemorrhage in the premature infant—current concepts. Part II. Ann Neurol 1989;25:109.

Infants of Drug-Abusing Mothers

Lester B (editor): Prenatal drug exposure and child outcome. Clin Perinatol 1999;26:1.

Hoegerman G et al: Drug-exposed neonates. Addiction Medicine (special issue). West J Med 1990;152:559.

Khalsa JH, Gfroerer J: Epidemiology and health care consequences of drug abuse among pregnant women. Semin Perinatol 1991; 15:265.

Ostrea EM Jr, Welch RA: Detection of prenatal drug exposure in the pregnant woman and her newborn infant. Clin Perinatol 1991; 18:629.

Necrotizing Enterocolitis

Bell MJ et al: Neonatal necrotizing enterocolitis. Therapeutic decisions based upon clinical staging. Ann Surg 1978;187:10.

Kleinhaus S et al: Necrotizing enterocolitis in infancy. Surg Clin North Am 1991;72:261.

Uauy RD et al: Necrotizing enterocolitis in very low birth weight infants: biodemographic and clinical correlates. National Institute of Child Health and Human Development Neonatal Research Network. J Pediatr 1991;119:630.

Thoracic & Gastrointestinal Neonatal Surgical Conditions

Hazebroek F et al: Congenital diaphragmatic hernia, impact of preoperative stabilization. J Pediatr Surg 1988;12:1138.

Meller JL et al: Gastroschisis and omphalocele. Clin Perinatol 1989; 16:113.

Reyes H et al: Management of esophageal atresia and tracheoesophageal fistula. Clin Perinatol 1989;16:79.

Frequent Electrolyte & Metabolic Abnormalities

Costarino A, Baumgart S: Modern fluid and electrolyte management of the critically ill premature infant. Pediatr Clin North Am 1986;33:153.

Loughead J et al: Serum ionized calcium concentrations in normal neonates. Am J Dis Child 1988;142:516.

Ogata ES: Carbohydrate metabolism in the fetus and neonate and altered neonatal glucoregulation. Pediatr Clin North Am 1986; 33:25.

Schaffer SG, Weismann DN: Fluid requirements in the preterm infant. Clin Perinatol 1992;19:233.

An Approach to Clinical Genetics

5

Cynthia R. Curry, MD

Clinical genetics is a rapidly expanding field that is broad in its scope and diversity and has wide applicability to health and disease in pediatrics. From the principles of human heredity set forth by Gregor Mendel in 1865, which went unrecognized for several decades, and intense scientific efforts that soon will have mapped the entire human genome, we have witnessed the growing impact of genetics on all fields of medicine. Nowhere is this more important than in pediatrics, as fully one third of hospitalized children are admitted as the consequence of genetic disease. With attention focused on the prenatal status of the fetus and causes of its death before birth, the fetus also has become a patient. As our technologic capabilities increase, we are aware of the many ethical and practical issues surrounding screening for prenatal, newborn, and childhood inherited disorders. We recognize the importance of accurate determination of risks and recurrence risks for children and their parents. In the following section, a categoric approach to genetic disease is presented, with an emphasis on disorders likely to be encountered in pediatrics.

■ ELEMENTS OF THE GENETIC EVALUATION

A genetic evaluation consists of three principal elements:

1. Determination of the correct diagnosis
2. Estimation of risk
3. Supportive counseling that allows the family to use the information provided

The Pedigree

The first step in the collection of appropriate information is the construction of a family tree, or pedigree. Underused by most medical personnel, the pedigree is a valuable record of genetic and medical information, which is much more useful in visual form than in list form. The use of uniform symbols is helpful, and common ones are denoted in Figure 5–1. An example of a family pedigree is shown in Figure 5–2.

Tips for pedigree preparation include the following:

- Start in the middle of the page to allow enough room for expansion. Start with a proband—his or her siblings

and parents. The proband is the individual through which the family genetic history was ascertained and should always be indicated by an arrow. Concentrate on one side of the family at a time to avoid confusing yourself and the person providing the history.

- Inquire about miscarriages, stillbirths, and neonatal deaths. This information is frequently overlooked and may provide crucial information.

- Always ask about consanguinity. Sometimes the question "Are you (the parents) related by blood?" will result in laughter but produces often potentially useful clues suggesting autosomal-recessive inheritance. Families with multiple marriages or consanguinity can complicate pedigree preparation, but understanding these pedigrees is still simpler and visually clearer than trying to explain the situation in words.

- Even if the disease in question appears to be coming from one side of the family, always get the basic facts about the other side of the family. Sometimes unrelated data may be very important in interpreting the family's overall situation. In addition, obtaining data from both sides can avoid an inference of blame being placed on one family member.

- Obtain the maiden names of women in the family, particularly when investigating an X-linked pedigree.

- Ascertain the ages of living persons and dates of death for deceased family members.

- Place the name of the person obtaining the pedigree and the date recorded at the bottom of the sheet.

The Diagnostic Process

The diagnostic process may be complex and is somewhat different from that used with general pediatric problems. When an infant or child is the proband, obtaining complete prenatal and perinatal history and information regarding developmental milestones is an important part of the medical history. Special attention should be placed on elements of the prenatal history such as maternal illnesses, onset and quality of fetal movements, presence of oligohydramnios or polyhydramnios, fetal presentation (vertex versus breech), and ultrasound abnormalities in the pregnancy. Licit or illicit drug use and alcohol and tobacco use should be queried. In dealing with the family with a

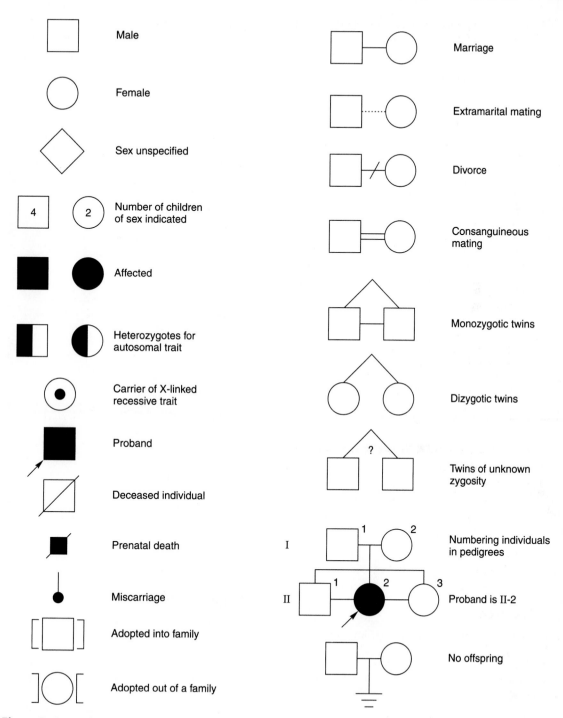

Figure 5–1. Symbols commonly used in the preparation of pedigrees.

Name _____

Date _____

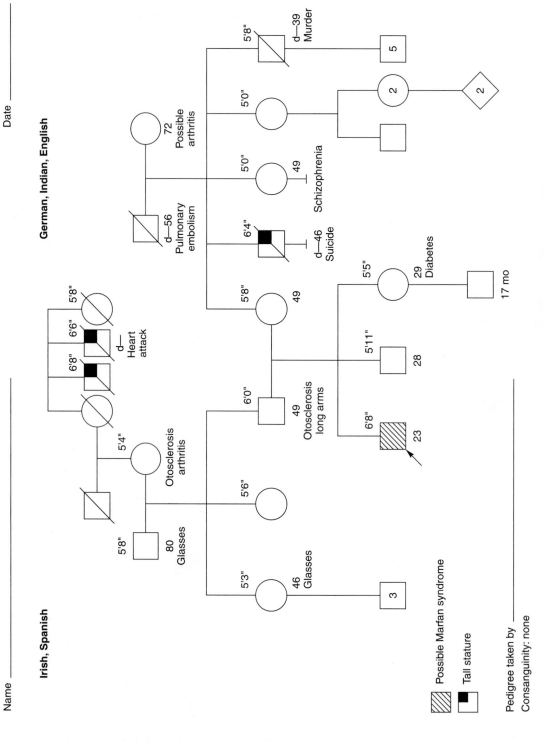

Figure 5–2. Pedigree chart of a family in which the proband (**arrow**) is being evaluated for possible Marfan's syndrome. d = deceased.

disorder such as Duchenne muscular dystrophy or adult-type polycystic kidney disease, it may be difficult to verify the exact diagnosis. The individuals of interest may be long since deceased or may have died without appropriate investigation. In that case, medical records should be requested whenever possible. Even in living affected individuals, a diagnosis can be difficult. For biochemical and DNA studies, samples of urine and blood including newborn screening blood spots sometimes can be obtained and shipped for analysis to appropriate reference laboratories even when relevant family members live far from the evaluation site or are deceased.

A complete genetic evaluation emphasizes components beyond the routine pediatric physical examination. Key elements include the following:

1. Growth parameters (height, weight, and head circumference) need to be plotted on the appropriate growth curves and, if possible, compared with earlier parameters.

2. Features that can be measured should be measured! There are established standards for inner canthal distance, interpupillary distance, ear length, hand length, middle finger length, foot length, penis length, etc.

3. The child's features should be compared with those of parents and siblings (use photographs, if available).

4. The child's features can be meaningfully analyzed over time by examining earlier chronologic photographs.

5. Clues should be sought that help date the onset of the problem, e.g., altered palmar and phalangeal creases (see below).

Approach to the Child with Structural Defects

When confronted by a child with single or multiple birth defects, the physician may be perplexed and unsure how to proceed. The diagnostic process, however, is not mysterious, and a correct diagnosis usually can be made by observing the patient's findings carefully and knowing where to look for additional information.

The first step in the diagnostic process is to determine the type of problem in morphogenesis. Is it an error in embryogenesis (i.e., a **malformation**)? Is it a **deformation,** in which extrinsic forces have altered previously normally formed body parts? Is it a **disruption,** in which a normal fetus has been altered by a destructive process that may be mechanical, infectious, or vascular in etiology? Is the problem prenatal or postnatal in origin? Is there a single localized defect in morphogenesis or are there secondary anomalies? When a single error causes a cascade of subsequent defects, the pattern is known as a **sequence** (Figure 5–3). Patients with multiple structural defects that cannot be explained on the basis of a cascade of events (sequence) are said to have a **malformation syndrome.** Usually such patterns are secondary to single causes, such as chromosomal abnormalities, single congenital defects, or teratogens. Many syndromes, however, have no known cause. Examples of malformations, deformations, disruptions, and syndromes are given in Table 5–1. By using these descriptors, pediatricians can categorize most structural defects.

Minor malformations are found in fewer than 4% of the normal population and usually of no cosmetic or functional importance to the individual. Examples of minor

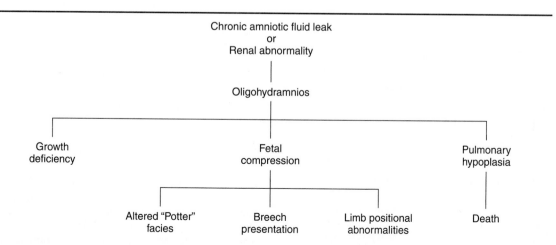

Figure 5–3. A sequence is a cascade of events with a single initiating problem, as exemplified by the condition of oligohydramnios.

Table 5–1. Examples of Structural Defects Caused by Different Mechanisms

Malformations	Deformations	Disruptions	Syndromes
Cleft lip and cleft palate	Plagiocephaly	Amniotic bands	Down
Transposition of great vessels	Torticollis	Jejunal atresia	Cornelia de Lange
Polydactyly	Limb bowing	Congenital rubella	Williams
Anencephaly	Prune belly	Unilateral limb reduction defects (some)	Noonan
Omphalocele	Scoliosis (some)	Gastroschisis	Fetal alcohol
Renal agenesis			

congenital anomalies are presented in Table 5–2. Despite their lack of significance by themselves, the pattern of such abnormalities may be crucial in the recognition of specific syndromes. Many important syndromes with major functional significance for the individual involved are recognized primarily by their distinctive pattern of minor anomalies. For example, most of the features seen on physical examination in Down syndrome, Williams syndrome, and Smith–Lemli–Opitz syndrome are minor anomalies. In general, minor anomalies in an otherwise normal child probably are not significant and do not warrant further investigations, but when the anomaly is one of several or when there are growth or developmental problems, further studies usually are indicated.

It is important to be familiar with several principles and concepts that are useful in evaluating the child with birth defects. A discussion of these follows.

CONCEPT OF VARIABILITY

Structural defects and their associated patterns are highly variable among individuals who have the same condition. Within a given syndrome, it is rare to find a specific feature in 100% of affected patients. In Down syndrome, for example, mental retardation is seen in all patients, and hypotonia is very frequent; however, other specific features, such as Brushfield spots and redundant neck skin, are seen in fewer than 80% of these patients. The diagnosis is based on the overall pattern of abnormality. In addition, some patients with the same condition are severely affected, whereas others are very mildly affected, and the condition is therefore sometimes difficult to recognize. This is particularly true with teratogenically induced

Table 5–2. Minor Malformations

Darwinian tubercle	Preauricular pits
Double occipital hair whorls	Single umbilical artery
Flat nasal bridge	Supernumerary nipples
Micrognathia	Syndactyly: two to three toes
Nevus flammeus	Transverse palmar crease

syndromes, such as fetal alcohol syndrome, in which the effects may range from neonatal death to mild neurologic dysfunction without physical stigmata.

CONCEPT OF CHANGING PHENOTYPE

The presentation of specific conditions and syndromes can change with time, and the diagnosis may be relatively easy or more difficult to determine as the child ages. For example, in mucopolysaccharidosis, facial coarsening and organomegaly are progressive with time. In Noonan syndrome, the face changes rather dramatically in infancy through middle childhood and into adulthood. In Beckwith–Wiedemann syndrome, the appearance of a child who has been severely affected in infancy may appear normal by the time he or she reaches middle childhood.

CONCEPT OF HETEROGENEITY

Similar clinical phenotypes may result from different etiologies. This is obviously very important in terms of diagnosis, prognosis, and recurrence risk counseling. For example, the phenotype of Noonan syndrome can be caused by an autosomal-dominant gene or exposure to alcohol or phenytoin. A Marfan-like phenotype can be seen not only with true Marfan syndrome, which is autosomal dominant, but also with homocystinuria, which is autosomal recessive. A similar Marfanoid phenotype also can be seen in some X-linked syndromes. The history and overall pattern of abnormalities need to be considered carefully before rendering a specific diagnosis.

CONCEPT OF MOST OBVIOUS VERSUS THE MOST FREQUENT ABNORMALITIES

Certain syndromes are distinguishable by their striking features, but if one relies only on these features, most patients with the syndrome will be missed. For example, the white forelock and heterochromia of Waardenburg syndrome are distinctive but not nearly as common as lateral displacement of the inner canthi and hypoplastic alae nasi. Similarly, although cleft lip and palate and scalp defects are easily recognizable features of trisomy 13, they are much less common than the characteristic nose that is nearly always present.

CONCEPT OF DATING THE ONSET

Frequently, a specific diagnosis may not be possible. It is not rare for the child's problems to be ascribed to some perinatal event. Attempts should be made to date the onset as prenatal, perinatal, or postnatal. For example, abnormalities in hair patterning date from approximately the 10th to 15th week of fetal life. Similarly, palmar crease and dermal ridges date from the 13th to the 19th fetal week. If significantly altered and not present in other family members, these minor malformations offer valuable clues to the timing of the insult affecting the child. Problems occurring after 20 weeks' gestation, no matter how severe, will not affect the dermal crease patterns because they are already formed. The presence of a thumb held in the palm (i.e., "cortical thumb") may be seen in cases of birth asphyxia, but when thumb positioning is prenatal in origin, a web of skin will have formed and the thumb may be hypoplastic. This type of observation may be particularly important in the current legal climate, in which families may seek compensation for their damaged child by blaming events around the time of the delivery. Metabolic errors occasionally can present with structural defects, but children with inborn errors usually appear normal at birth, with only gradual development of a specific phenotype. Examination of serial photographs may be particularly useful in documenting that facial changes are postnatal.

CONCEPT OF USING RAREST FEATURE FOR QUICK IDENTIFICATION

Common functional abnormalities, such as short stature and mental retardation, are seen in a vast array of conditions and syndromes and thus are almost diagnostically useless. Features that are uncommon or rare are much more likely to lead to the correct diagnosis. The appendices in *Smith's Recognizable Patterns of Human Malformation* (1998) are useful. The rarer the finding, the more likely this resource is to be helpful. For example, the findings of scalp defects, lens dislocation, or choanal atresia yield relatively short lists of possible diagnoses. The same principle holds true when using any of the diagnostic computer programs in common use today. Research on computer-aided diagnoses in the field of malformation syndromes began in the 1980s and at first was restricted to relatively few users. More recent versions have brought these facilities to a broad audience. The programs most widely in use include OMIM (McKusick's Catalogue of Mendelian Inheritance in Man, http://www3.ncbi.nlm.nih.gov/omim/), the London Dysmorphology Database (LDDB), which soon may be available on line, and pictures of standard syndromes and undiagnosed malformations (POSSUM). In patients in which a diagnosis is suspected, the availability of specific testing can be accessed through the on-line service GENE TESTS (genetests.org). Detailed information on relatively common conditions for which there is DNA-based testing is available through GENE CLINICS (geneclinics@geneclinics.org). Because of the proliferation of syndromes, computer-assisted diagnosis has been welcomed by clinical geneticists as an extremely valuable diagnostic tool. The concept that the rarer the abnormality the more likely one is to make a diagnosis is equally valid with computer-assisted diagnosis. Unfortunately, for the patient with mental retardation, short stature, and a flat nasal bridge as the only identifiable features, this means that a specific diagnosis may be unlikely unless laboratory testing provides additional clues.

The Counseling Process

After the initial pedigree preparation and review of the history and physical examination, it is often necessary to obtain additional records or order specific tests. Indicated testing frequently can include cytogenetic studies (i.e., chromosomes), skeletal radiographs, and urine or serum biochemical studies (i.e., organic acids, lysosomal enzymes, etc.). During the initial visit, it is important to indicate to the family how long it may take to obtain a diagnosis, how many visits may be needed, and how likely it is that a diagnosis actually will be established. It is also important to relieve guilt at this initial meeting, even though no diagnosis may yet be apparent. Parental anxiety is usually great, and almost all parents fear that something they have done, real or imagined, has caused the child's problems. Only rarely is this true.

In clear-cut situations, counseling and recurrence risk information can be given at the initial visit; even in those situations, however, parents may be overwhelmed and require a second visit. Usually during a second visit, issues of recurrence risk need to be dealt with as objectively as possible. In addition, information on modalities that may be available to help them monitor for, or modify, those risks should be discussed. In the initial and subsequent visits, it is important to determine how the family perceives the child (i.e., do they love and accept him or her, or is the child an intolerable burden?). It is important to understand how the family will view the concept of risk. For some families, risks are best presented as high or low. For others, detailed explanations, including derivation of empiric risks, is appropriate. Usually, risks are given as odds or percentages. Some counselors quote odds, such as 1 in 10, 1 in 50, or 1 in 100, whereas others use figures such as 10%, 2%, or 1%. These methods sometimes are used interchangeably and adapted to the requirements of the individual family.

In conveying the risk information, certain points need to be kept in mind:

- It is important to emphasize that "chance has no memory." Odds refer to future occurrence, not to past occurrence. For example, when there is a 1 in 4 chance of recurrence, the fact that the first child was normal does not guarantee that the next three will be normal, nor does the fact that one family has had two affected children in a row make it more or less likely that the next will be affected.

- Parents may reverse the risks in their head when told that they have a 2% chance of recurrence risk and may interpret this as a 2% chance of having a normal child.

- Each family has its own idea of what constitutes a high or low risk, and the interpretation of risk often has more to do with the disease in question than the actual risk. For example, parents may readily accept a 3% chance for recurrence for cleft lip and cleft palate, whereas the same risk for having a child with mental handicap and some associated physical abnormalities may be viewed as intolerable.

- The baseline risk for congenital anomalies facing any couple needs to be stressed and spelled out for the parents.

- It is important that genetic counseling information be given in a nondirective manner.

Although physicians may think that they know what is best for the patient, this usually is not the case. The physician's role is to ensure that families have the facts that will permit them to make their own decisions. Such facts include a knowledge of the disorder, the genetic risks involved, and the possible steps that can be taken to ameliorate the condition or detect it in utero. Although some patients may beg for advice, and in these instances it may often be tempting to comply, it is almost always inadvisable. Certainly, there are genetic counselors whose orientation toward genetic risks is more positive or more negative. For example, some may tend to stress the 25% chance of recurrence, whereas others may stress the 75% chance that the child will be normal. Usually, the approach is tempered by the counselor's knowledge of the disease in question. In the end, however, it is important that parents and individuals make their own decisions and understand that there is no right or wrong answer. Moreover, support should continue to be offered to families regardless of their decisions regarding future childbearing.

LONGITUDINAL FOLLOW-UP

Part of the process of a genetic evaluation involves referral of the child and family to appropriate subspecialists and agencies for follow-up treatment or support. Consequently, geneticists often find themselves in the role of care coordinators. Follow-up contact with families is almost always necessary because the stress of receiving prognostic and genetic information often renders recall difficult or impossible.

Once a diagnosis is established, it is important to give the family available resource information and referrals to local and national support groups. Often these groups have rapid access to new developments in the disorder. An important goal is to have parents or the affected individual become "experts" on their disorder because their care providers often will have only minimal experience with rare disorders. Being given the diagnosis of a rare syndrome is often a great motivator. Pediatricians and consultants can encourage this attitude because it empowers parents and affected individuals and usually improves the physician–patient relationship. Empowering our patients is ever more important, given the complexity of modern medical practice. We should welcome the ready access of many families to the internet and encourage them to contact the specialist with questions, e.g., the availability of specific molecular diagnostic testing.

In those patients with unknown diagnoses and those with disorders requiring regular surveillance routine, reevaluation is important. Families, however, also have the responsibility to contact the consultant or pediatrician with changes in their family situation such as a new or planned pregnancy, new knowledge of similarly affected relatives, or new symptoms that may require further evaluation.

Families in which the diagnosis is "unknown" often are desperate for a diagnosis and will go to almost any length to achieve one. Medical professionals are often equally determined to achieve a diagnosis. It is important to recognize that in about one half of all cases a diagnosis will not be made despite extensive testing. Anxiety usually can be relieved by reassuring parents that the individual's care will not by compromised by lack of a diagnosis and stressing the importance of not making an incorrect diagnosis. "Pounding a round peg into a square hole" just to achieve a "name" for the condition often has unintended negative consequences for the family including an end to diagnostic pursuit and giving possibly incorrect recurrence risk information. Reevaluation in "unknowns" has been shown to result in about a 5% rate of new diagnoses. Often these are based on repetition of testing such as chromosomal analyses done years earlier, the emergence of a more specific clinical or behavioral phenotype, or the development of specific molecular diagnostic testing.

Options such as adoption, sterilization, and artificial insemination by a donor need to be discussed when appropriate. Families should be asked to contact the genetic counselor should they again become pregnant because new information may drastically alter pregnancy monitoring.

■ MENDELIAN INHERITANCE PATTERNS & COMMON PEDIATRIC DISORDERS

As of January 2000, Victor McKusick's catalog, *Mendelian Inheritance in Man,* listed more than 6500 entries in which the mode of inheritance was presumed to be autosomal dominant, autosomal recessive, X-linked dominant, or

X-linked recessive. These disorders are caused by single genes, determined by a single allele at a single locus on one chromosome or a pair of chromosomes. When both alleles in a pair are identical, the individual is **homozygous.** When the alleles differ at the same locus, the individual is **heterozygous.** The inheritance pattern usually is diagnosed by (1) recognition of the condition and knowledge of its mode of inheritance and (2) analysis of the pedigree and the pattern of transmission in the family. When the case is "isolated" and no diagnosis is apparent, several possibilities need to be considered (Figure 5–4). When more than one family member is affected, the pedigree can be analyzed and decisions made regarding the likely mode of inheritance. This process is outlined in Figure 5–5.

Autosomal-Dominant Inheritance

Disorders showing autosomal-dominant inheritance generally are expressed when only one gene in the pair is altered (i.e., the individual is heterozygous). Homozygous states of autosomal-dominant disorders are rare and usually severe or lethal (i.e., homozygous achondroplasia). Rarely, homozygosity may be indistinguishable from heterozygosity (e.g., Huntington disease). In typical autosomal-dominant disorders, counseling is straightforward (Figure 5–6). The risk for the affected individuals' offspring is one half or 50/50, regardless of sex. However, risks alone do not tell the whole story in autosomal-dominant disorders. Several factors can modify the clinical presentation, and descriptions follow.

Age of onset. Certain important genetic diseases, such as adult-type polycystic kidney disease, hemochromatosis, inherited forms of breast and ovarian cancers, and Huntington disease, do not usually manifest until later in life. Thus, individuals have often passed their reproductive years before they become aware that they have the disease. Molecular diagnostic methods might provide information early in life, or even prenatally, but the ethical issues raised by presymptomatic testing are serious and must be approached with caution.

Lack of penetrance. Some dominantly inherited disorders may show absolutely no evidence of the disorder by conventional clinical tools, but clearly the patient must have the gene if he or she has an affected parent and has transmitted the disorder to an offspring. Occasionally, a disorder can be found to be penetrant if one looks carefully with biochemical or radiologic studies. For example, adult-type polycystic kidney disease may appear to be nonpenetrant on the basis of clinical examination, but a renal ultrasound study may show renal cysts indicating the presence of the gene. In some situations such as hemochromatosis or inherited breast cancer, specific molecular testing may allow determination of the presence or absence of the gene, thus defining penetrance at a different level.

Variability. Dominant disorders are characterized by marked variability, and this factor has to be taken into account when the physician assesses an individual for the presence or absence of the condition and in the provision of accurate genetic counseling. For example, the individual with tuberous sclerosis who has seizures, ash leaf spots, and mental retardation is unlikely to be missed. An intellectually normal parent may be erroneously assumed to be unaffected, yet careful ophthalmologic, dermatologic, and radiologic studies may show subtle evidence of the gene's presence (e.g., renal hematomas or subtle skin changes such as ash leaf spots, adenoma sebaceum, or a shagreen patch). Individuals who are mildly affected are much more likely to reproduce. Their chances of having a moderately or severely affected child need to be explored in the counseling setting, and the entire spectrum of the disorder explained. Because more than half the listings in McKusick's catalog are autosomal dominant in etiology, it is not possible to discuss these disorders in detail. Table 5–3 presents information on some of the more common autosomal-dominant disorders. Table 5–4 lists some malformation syndromes displaying autosomal-dominant inheritance.

Autosomal-Recessive Inheritance

Autosomal-recessive phenotypes account for about one third of mendelian disorders. They occur when both parents are heterozygous carriers. Each parent passes a normal or an altered gene to the child who will be affected in 25% of conceptions. Consanguinity increases the risk for autosomal-recessive disorders, as does reproduction among genetically isolated populations, particularly for rare recessive disorders such as Tay–Sachs disease. In an individual family, it may be difficult to determine whether a condition is autosomal recessive because often the affected child is the only one in its family with the disorder. When the diagnosis is definite, counseling is relatively clear-cut (Figure 5–7). The recurrence risk for each sibling of the proband is 25%, or one in four. Male and female siblings are equally affected. Recurrence risks for other relatives are very low. When one's sibling is affected with an autosomal-recessive disorder, one's risk of being a carrier is two thirds. In contrast to autosomal-dominant disorders, many recessive disorders involve aberrant enzyme activities that block pathways crucial to normal metabolic function. Important autosomal-recessive disorders in pediatrics are listed in Table 5–5. Syndromes that are inherited in an autosomal-recessive fashion are probably also caused by alterations in basic regulatory or metabolic pathways, even though the exact cause in many of these syndromes is not known (Table 5–6). Autosomal-recessive metabolic disorders with known abnormalities in mucopolysaccharide, amino acid, or organic acid metabolism are discussed in Chapter 6.

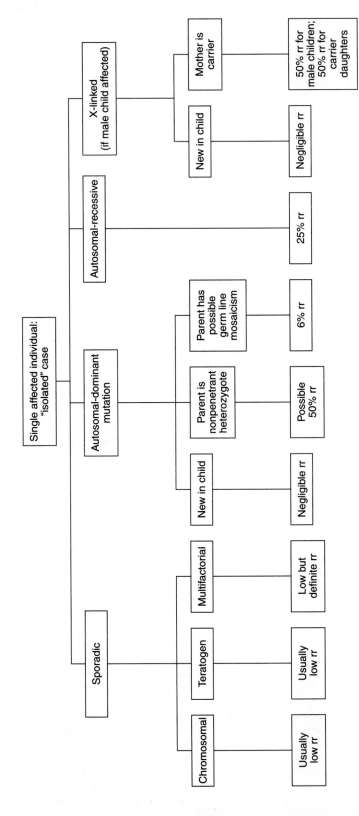

Figure 5–4. Recurrence risks (**rr**) for parents of a child who is the only affected family member.

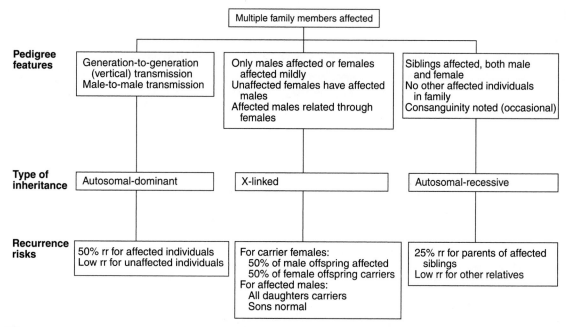

Figure 5–5. Possible modes of inheritance and recurrence risks (**rr**) when multiple family members are affected.

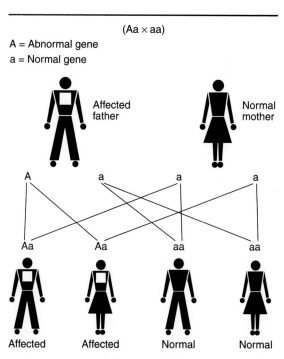

Figure 5–6. Counseling in autosomal-dominant disorders.

X-Linked Inheritance

More than 300 genes have been mapped to the X chromosome. X-linked mutations are fully expressed in male carriers. Female carriers are functionally mosaic, with two cell populations—one carrying the normal X chromosome and the other carrying the altered X chromosome. This characteristic is due to X inactivation that occurs randomly early in embryonic development. As a result of X inactivation, male and female carriers have only one X chromosome active in each cell. X inactivation is random and, therefore, by chance female carriers may have more of their normal X chromosomes inactivated and display some symptoms of an X-linked disorder, clinically or biochemically.

In general, X-linked–recessive disorders affect boys much more frequently than girls. An affected man will transmit the gene to all of his daughters and none of his sons. Affected men or boys in a family are related through women in the family. Male-to-male transmission never occurs. Female carriers usually are asymptomatic, but, as discussed, some may have mild symptoms of the disorder. The approach to counseling is diagrammed in Figure 5–8.

X-linked–dominant disorders are regularly expressed in females, although the distinction between X-linked–dominant and X-linked–recessive disorders blurs as our

Table 5–3. Clinical Features in Several Common Diseases With Autosomal-Dominant Inheritance

Disease	Gene Localization	Disease Incidence	Clinical Features	Prenatal Diagnosis
Neurofibromatosis type I	17q11.2	1:3000–5000 (many cases are new mutations)	Café-au-lait spots, neuro-fibromas; malignancy (5%); mental retardation (5%); learning disabilities (15%)	Possible in some families using DNA
Myotonic dystrophy	19q13	New mutations rare	Muscular weakness: myotonia onset childhood → adult Endocrine abnormalities; cardiac conduction defects; cataracts Congenital presentation: hypotonia, clubfeet, respiratory problems	DNA
Familial hypercholesterolemia	19q13	Heterozygotes 1:500 Homozygotes 1:1,000,000	Elevated LDL, xanthomas, early coronary artery disease, homozygotes; death due to coronary disease in childhood	? DNA techniques
Tuberous sclerosis	9q 16p	High mutation rate	Hypopigmented skin macules; seizures; mental retardation; renal, cardiac, and CNS hamartomas	DNA techniques in appropriate families
Huntington disease	4p16	4–8:100,000 (new mutations rare)	Dementia; chorea; usually onset in 5th decade	DNA
Marfan syndrome	15q	1–2:100,000 (new mutations 15–30%)	Tall stature, arachnodactyly; lens dislocation; aortic root dilatation, mitral valve prolapse	Possible in future using DNA

CNS = central nervous system; LDL = low-density lipoprotein.

Table 5–4. Clinical Features in Several Common Malformation Syndromes With Autosomal-Dominant Inheritance

Syndrome	Primary Features	Gene	Location
Stickler	Marfanoid habitus, myopia, cleft palate arthritis	COL2A1, COL11A1	12q14
Noonan (some cases)	Short stature, ptosis, pulmonary valve stenosis, learning disabilities	N/A	12q24
Nail-patella	Absent patellas, nail dysplasia, renal disease	Lmxib	9q34.1
Treacher Collins	Downstarting palpebral fissures, ear malformations, malar hypoplasia, lid colobomas	TCOFI	5q32
Holt–Oram	Cardiac defects, radial defects	TBX5	12q24
Waardenburg I	Increased inner canthal distance, heterochromia, white forelock, congenital hearing loss	PAX3	2q25
Van der Woude	Cleft lip ± cleft palate; lip pits	N/A	1q32

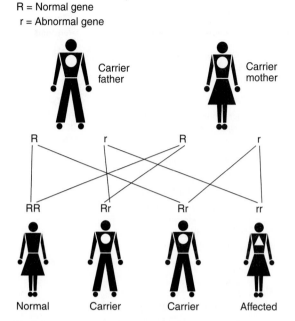

(Rr × Rr)

R = Normal gene
r = Abnormal gene

Carrier father

Carrier mother

R   r   R   r

RR   Rr   Rr   rr

Normal   Carrier   Carrier   Affected

Figure 5–7. Counseling in autosomal-recessive diseases.

ability to detect manifestations in female carriers improves. Pedigrees of X-linked–dominant disorders demonstrate that affected men have daughters who are affected and sons who are never affected. This feature distinguishes X-linked–dominant inheritance from autosomal-dominant inheritance. Women with X-linked–dominant disorders will transmit the trait to half their offspring regardless of sex. X-linked–dominant disorders are rare. One example is X-linked hypophosphatemic rickets. Although classified as a dominant disorder, the rickets is much less severe in female than in male offspring. There are several examples of probable X-linked–dominants that are lethal in male offspring. A classic example is ornithine transcarbamylase deficiency, which leads to lethal hyperammonemia in affected male offspring. Female carriers may show protein intolerance and episodes of lethargy and occasionally present with symptoms resembling those of Reye syndrome. Rett syndrome, characterized by severe mental retardation and seizures, is seen only in female children and is thought usually to be the result of a new mutation occurring only in the affected child. Another syndrome affecting only female children is Aicardi syndrome, in which there are no corpus callosum, severe seizures, hemivertebrae, and unusual lacunarlike defects in the retina. Several important X-linked disorders are presented in Table 5–7.

■ CHROMOSOMAL ABNORMALITIES

Chromosomal disorders form a very important category of genetic disease and are responsible for a high percentage of pregnancy loss, congenital malformations, and mental retardation in surviving children. Whereas approximately 60% of first-trimester pregnancy losses are secondary to chromosomal imbalance, only about 0.6% of liveborn children have chromosomal abnormalities.

Advances in cytogenetic technology and molecular cytogenetics have blurred to some extent the distinctions between mendelian and chromosomal disorders, and this trend is likely to continue. Several malformation syndromes previously thought to be due to inherited single genes have now been found to be secondary to loss of genetic material not usually detectible with routine cytogenetic techniques.

Chromosomal abnormalities may be numeric or structural and involve autosomes, sex chromosomes, or both. When there are too many or too few chromosomes, an individual is said to have **aneuploidy.** The most common form of aneuploidy is trisomy, in which there are three rather than the normal two of any one particular chromosome. Monosomy for specific chromosomes is rare, except monosomy X (i.e., Turner's syndrome). Structural rearrangements account for about 40% of all chromosomal abnormalities, and most of these are balanced (i.e., there is no detectable loss or gain of chromosomal material). These rearrangements, however, when transmitted at conception in an unbalanced form, may cause miscarriage, stillbirth, or offspring with abnormal phenotypes and mental retardation. The nomenclature used to describe various chromosomal abnormalities can be confusing.

In general, the following rules are applied when describing a karyotype:

- The total chromosome number is given first, e.g., 46.
- The sex chromosome constitution is written next (usually either XX, female, or XY, male).
- The arms of the chromosomes are indicated by the letters *p* (petite) for short arm and *q* for long arm.
- Missing chromosomal material is designated *del* (deletion), followed by the chromosome and the breakpoint(s) of the missing segment, e.g., del(11)(p13p14). Additional material of unknown origin attached to a chromosome is designated *add* (addition), followed by the known chromosome with the extra material and the breakpoint(s).
- A translocation is indicated by the letter *t*, with a description of the involved chromosomes in parentheses (e.g., t[13;14]). A derivative chromosome is used to indicate an unbalanced translocation, e.g., der(10)t(10;13)(q21;q32).

Table 5–5. Clinical Features in Several Diseases With Autosomal-Recessive Inheritance

Disease	Gene Localization	Incidence	Clinical Features	Prenatal Diagnosis
Cystic fibrosis	7q31; single mutation in 70% (Δ F508)	1:2000 in whites	Pulmonary disease; pancreatic insufficiency	Yes: DNA
Tay–Sachs disease	15q23–q24	1:3600 in Ashkenazi Jewish populations; rare in other populations	Severe mental retardation and CNS deterioration; death by age 2–3 y	Yes: enzyme analysis (hexosamini-dase A) or DNA
Sickle cell anemia	11p	1:400–600 African-Americans	Severe hemolytic anemia; splenomegaly; infections	Yes: DNA
α-Thalassemia	16p13.3	1:1600 Southeast Asians; frequent in descendents of Mediterranean countries, the Philippines	Deletion of all four alpha chains; hydrops fetalis (death) Three gene deletions: hemoglobin H disease Two gene deletions: silent carrier	Yes: DNA
Werdnig-Hoffmann disease	5q12–q13	1:10,000	Severe hypotonia; anterior horn cell disease; death by age 1–2 y Some forms have later onset and slower progression	Yes: DNA

CNS = central nervous system.

Table 5–6. Clinical Features in Selected Malformation Syndromes With Autosomal-Recessive Inheritance

Syndrome	Clinical Findings	Clinical Outcome	Prenatal Diagnosis
Zellweger	Deficiency of peroxisomes, hypotonia, hepatomegaly, stippled epiphyses, hydrocephalus	Lethal by 1–4 mo	Yes: analysis of amniotic fluid; very long chain fatty acids in amniotic fluid; ultrasound
Meckel–Gruber	Encephalocele, polydactyly, polycystic kidneys, congenital heart disease	Lethal soon after birth	Yes: ultrasound and α-fetoprotein in amniotic fluid
Ellis–van Creveld	Short limbs, natal teeth, congenital heart disease, polydactyly	About 50% die in infancy	Yes: ultrasound second trimester
Smith–Lemli–Opitz	Mental retardation, two- to three-toe syndactyly, genital abnormalities, polydactyly, cleft palate	Some neonatal deaths; some long-term survivors	Yes: 7-dehydrocholesterol levels in amniotic fluid
Seckel	"Bird-headed" dwarfism; primordial short stature, severe microcephaly	Survival	Yes: no good data; ultrasound third trimester
Ataxia-Telangiectasia	Ataxia, immune deficiency, elevated risk for lymphoreticular malignancy, chromosome breakage	Death in 20s–30s, usually secondary to malignancy	Yes: DNA

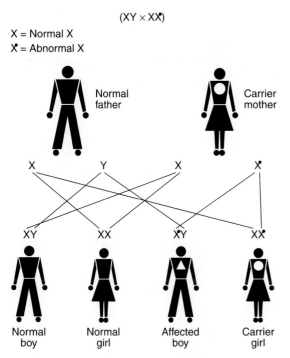

$(XY \times X\cancel{X})$

X = Normal X
$\cancel{X}$ = Abnormal X

Normal father

Carrier mother

X   Y   X $\cancel{X}$

XY   XX   X̄Y   XX̄

Normal boy

Normal girl

Affected boy

Carrier girl

Figure 5–8. Counseling in X-linked recessive disorders.

Autosomal Trisomies

The autosomal chromosome abnormalities of trisomies 21, 18, and 13 are described below, and details are presented in Table 5–8 and depicted in Figure 5–9.

DOWN SYNDROME

As the most common of the autosomal trisomies, this disorder should be familiar to the clinician. This syndrome usually is recognized at birth, although, rarely, diagnosis can be delayed. Hypotonia is universally present, and there are characteristic craniofacial features, including brachycephaly, small ears, upslanting palpebral fissures, Brushfield spots in light-eyed children, flat nasal bridge, underdeveloped midface, and protruding tongue. The hands and feet usually are distinctively broad, with transverse palmar creases, fifth finger clinodactyly, and an increased space between the first and second toes. Despite significant intellectual limitations, individuals with Down syndrome are usually happy and productive and, occasionally, can live semi-independently. In addition, antibiotics and cardiac surgery have increased the life spans of these individuals. Findings of senility characteristic of Alzheimer disease affect individuals with Down syndrome much earlier than the usual age of onset of Alzheimer disease in the general population.

Molecular studies of Down syndrome have localized a Down syndrome "critical region" to 21q22.2 to q22.3. Most of the characteristic phenotypic findings are produced by an extra dose of chromosomal material in that region, as exemplified in some patients with partial trisomy 21.

Prenatal diagnostic efforts (chiefly amniocentesis) have been targeted at women older than 35 years who are at an increased risk to have a fetus with Down syndrome. Currently, more accurate identification of fetuses at risk through serum marker studies, including α-fetoprotein (AFP), human chorionic gonadotropin (hCG), and unconjugated estriol ("triple screen"), should help identify women of all ages who may be at increased risk to have a child with Down syndrome. First-trimester screening using a combination of the ultrasound finding of increased nuchal translucency with serum markers such as placenta associated protein A (PAPP-A) are currently under evaluation as a means to provide even earlier prenatal diagnosis.

TRISOMY 18

Trisomy 18 is much rarer than trisomy 21. It is more frequently identified prenatally on the basis of abnormal ultrasound findings including intrauterine growth retardation, choroid plexus cysts, and congenital anomalies, such as omphalocele and congenital heart disease. In the newborn, the characteristic triangular face, small mouth, short sternum, abnormal hand positioning, absent distal phalangeal flexion creases, and nail hypoplasia aid in the diagnosis of this disorder. Infants with this problem are almost always transferred to tertiary care centers because of problems in neonatal adaptation or congenital abnormalities. The mortality rate in the first 48 hours is more than 50%. A specific pattern of abnormal serum triple screen results detects many fetuses at increased risk for trisomy 18 in the second trimester. Genetic counseling, ultrasound, and amniocentesis are used to give families accurate information after abnormal serum screening results.

TRISOMY 13

Infants with trisomy 13 almost always die in the early neonatal period, and the phenotype of such infants tends to be dominated by severe congenital anomalies, including bilateral cleft lip and cleft palate, congenital heart disease, microphthalmia, and central nervous system defects, especially holoprosencephaly. The face of an infant with trisomy 13 is notably different from that of an infant with trisomy 18. The bulbous nasal tip is particularly distinctive. Other helpful diagnostic findings, when present, can include polydactyly and punched-out scalp defects at the vertex.

Autosomal Deletions

Most autosomal deletions are quite rare or their phenotypes are poorly delineated. An exception is **5p- (cri du chat**

Table 5–7. Clinical Features in Several Important X-Linked Disorders

Disease	Gene Localization	Incidence	Clinical Findings	Prenatal Diagnosis
Hemophilia A	Xq28 (large gene; many mutations)	1:10,000 male carriers (rare in female carriers)	Prolonged bleeding; bruising; joint and muscle hemorrhages; deficiency of factor VIII	Yes: DNA in most cases
Duchenne muscular dystrophy	Xp21 (large gene; many mutations)	1:3000–3500 (one third are new mutations; two thirds have carrier mothers)	Progressive muscle weakness; calf pseudohypertrophy; elevated CPK; death in teens to 20s; absent protein, dystrophin in muscle	Yes: DNA or linkage
Becker muscular dystrophy	Xp21 (gene allelic to Duchenne dystrophy)	Rare	Milder course, but similar to Duchenne dystrophy; survival to middle age; elevated CPK	Yes: DNA or linkage
Ocular albinism	Xp21	Rare	Decreased visual acuity, nystagmus, strabismus, iris transillumination defects; female carriers show tigroid mosaic pattern in retina	Yes: DNA, but most families would not use
Lesch–Nyhan syndrome	Xq26–27	Rare	Mental retardation; choreoathetosis; self-destructive biting of fingers and lips; uric acid stones	Yes: enzyme (HPRT) in chorionic villus biopsy, amniocentesis, or preimplantation diagnosis

CPK = creatine phosphokinase; HPRT = hypoxanthine phosphoribosyl transferase.

syndrome). This condition was given its name because affected infants have a peculiar high-pitched cry similar to that of a mewing cat. The craniofacies is characterized by microcephaly and hypertelorism. Most infants are small at birth, and all exhibit slow postnatal growth and mental deficiency. The distinctive cry becomes less pronounced with age; thus, this diagnosis is less likely to be made in the older child. The critical deleted region missing in all patients with cri du chat syndrome includes the chromosome band 5p1.5.

Sex Chromosome Abnormalities

Sex chromosomal aneuploidy is relatively common, with an overall frequency of about 1 in 500 births. These disorders are, in general, less severe than autosomal aneuploidy. The reasons are probably related to X chromosome inactivation and the relatively low number of genes thought to be carried on the Y chromosome. Only XO Turner syndrome is associated with an increased frequency of spontaneous abortion. More than 99% of all XO conceptions end in pregnancy loss related to severe fetal hydrops. This is of great interest because the clinical phenotype in surviving XO female infants is relatively mild (Figure 5–10). Nearly all sex chromosome abnormalities tend to occur as isolated events without predisposing factors, although some are related to maternal age and errors in maternal meiosis I.

TURNER SYNDROME (45,X & OTHERS)

About 50% of girls with Turner syndrome have a 45,X karyotype. The rest have other karyotypes or mosaicism. Approximately 10% of these girls have 46,X,iso(Xq). Mosaic Turner syndrome may have a somewhat milder phenotype, whereas ring X patients have a higher incidence of mental retardation. The characteristic pheno-

Table 5–8. Clinical Features in Trisomies 21, 18, and 13

	Incidence (in live births)	Mean Birth Weight (g)	Prenatal Survival	Life Expectancy	Clinical Features	Chromosome Findings	Recurrence Risk
Trisomy 21	1:800	2900	Spontaneous abortion in 75%	25% with congenital heart disease die before age 1 y (without surgery); 50% live to >50 y	Hypotonia, typical face, congenital heart disease (40%, AV canal, VSD), IQ 25–50; Alzheimer disease in older patients	Trisomy 21 (95%) Translocation (4%) Mosaicism (1%)	Trisomy: ~1% overall Age-specific risk: >35 y Translocation: (4;21): maternal 5%, paternal 2%
Trisomy 18	1:8000	2240	Spontaneous abortion in 95%	90% die first month	Hypertonia, typical face, clenched hands with second and fifth overlapping third and fourth fingers, short sternum, nail hypoplasia	Trisomy 18 (>90%) Translocation (<5%) Rarely mosaicism	<1%
Trisomy 13	1:25,000	2600	Spontaneous abortion in most	>95% lethal by 6 mo	Severe CNS abnormality; microphthalmia, cleft lip and palate, polydactyly	Trisomy (75%) Unbalanced translocation (20%) Mosaicism (5%)	<1%

AV = atrioventricular; CNS = central nervous system; VSD = ventricular septal defect.

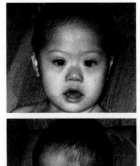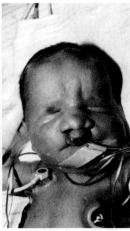

Figure 5–9. Facial appearance in Down syndrome in a Southeast Asian boy, age 19 months (**upper and lower left**), and trisomy 13 (**right**) in newborns.

type of Turner syndrome includes short stature, infertility with gonadal dysgenesis or streak gonads, and an increased frequency of renal and cardiac anomalies, especially coarctation of the aorta (20%). There are mildly unusual facial features, with laterally protruding ears, uplifted lobules, and lower canthal folds; neck webbing; and a low posterior hairline. Edema of the hands and feet is often present at birth and may persist into early childhood. Approximately 18% of all chromosomally abnormal spontaneous abortions are found to have a 45, X karyotype.

Short stature and infertility are the constant sequelae of an XO karyotype. Hormonal treatment at puberty will produce adequate feminization and menstruation. However, stature remains a difficult clinical problem, as does infertility. Multiple studies of growth in patients with Turner syndrome have used growth hormone injections and androgens singly and in combination. Results have been inconclusive, although all methods seem to have short-term positive effects on growth velocity. Intellectual function is nearly always normal in Turner syndrome, although spatial relations and perceptual motor organization skills are frequently impaired, thereby lowering nonverbal IQ.

KLINEFELTER SYNDROME (47,XXY)

Usually this disorder is not diagnosed until puberty, when hypogonadism becomes apparent. Long legs, a thin habitus, and small testes may raise suspicion for this diagnosis in the prepubertal male. The IQ in Klinefelter syndrome is consistently reduced only mildly, with about two thirds of patients exhibiting learning problems such

as dyslexia. Psychosocial adjustment problems are frequent, and infertility is to be expected. New reproductive techniques may make it possible for some men with Klinefelter syndrome to father children.

47,XYY

Accurate assessment of the phenotype of XYY has been complicated by the early observation of an increased frequency of XYY individuals in maximum security prisons. Analysis of prospective data suggests that XYY boys are tall and have an increased risk of psychosocial adjustment problems despite intelligence in the low normal range (usually about 15 points below that of normal siblings). Although aggressive behavior and temper tantrums are definitely increased in XYY boys, the exact risk of deviant behavior in the individual identified with XYY prenatally or postnatally is difficult to predict.

XXX (47,XXX)

The phenotype of XXX remains incompletely understood, although there seems to be a significant risk of developmental and learning problems in these individuals. The exact prevalence of mental retardation is not precisely known, but prospective studies have shown that the mean IQ of XXX girls is 10–25 points below that of their normal siblings. Both receptive and expressive language development are delayed. The phenotype of the triple X female is usually normal, although stature is increased as compared with that of normal siblings. In some instances, the head circumference is reduced. Most XXX women are probably fertile, but menstrual abnormalities, sterility, and early-onset menopause have been commonly reported.

Microdeletion Syndromes

High-resolution chromosome banding techniques and the technique of fluorescence in situ hybridization (FISH) have greatly increased the ability to find abnormalities too small to be seen in ordinary chromosome preparations. These improved techniques have led to delineation of several clinical dysmorphic syndromes. Evolving molecular information has brought closer to reality correlations between genotype and phenotype. Several examples of microdeletion syndromes are shown in Table 5–9.

PRADER–WILLI & ANGELMAN SYNDROMES

These two prototype microdeletion syndromes involve chromosomal deletions of bands 15q11 through 15q13. These deletions appear indistinguishable in cytogenetic and FISH studies. At the molecular level, it is likely that Prader–Willi and Angelman syndromes are caused by two closely linked, but distinct, genes or gene clusters. These very different clinical syndromes were the first two human diseases demonstrating the principle of genomic imprinting. *Genomic imprinting* refers to the process whereby specific genes are differentially marked during parental game-

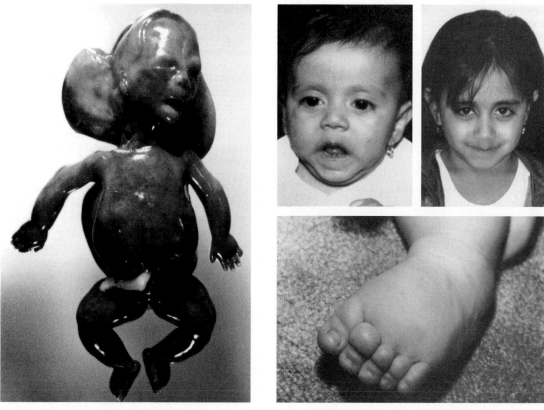

Figure 5–10. XO Turner syndrome. **Left:** Fetus that spontaneously aborted at 16 weeks and had a large cystic hygroma. **Upper right:** Child with XO Turner syndrome as an infant and at age 6 years. She has a relatively mild phenotype but has had coarctation of the aorta and a horseshoe kidney. Note very mild ptosis and laterally protruding ears. Lower right: Note the edema of the toes and nail hypoplasia.

togenesis, resulting in the differential expression of these genes in the embryo and adult. This concept is difficult because we are accustomed to the rules of mendelian inheritance. Imprinting implies that there is differential modification of genetic material depending on whether the genetic material is passed from the mother or the father. This concept is exemplified in Prader–Willi and Angelman syndromes.

Prader–Willi syndrome, first described clinically more than 30 years ago, is characterized by significant hypotonia in infancy followed by an evolving pattern of overeating and obesity that appears between ages 6 months and 2 years, variable mental retardation, characteristic facies, small hands and feet, and hypogonadism. Twenty-eight years ago, Angelman described children with severe mental retardation, seizures, ataxia, and a "puppet-like" gait who had happy dispositions and were prone to episodes of unprovoked laughter. Recently, the P gene, which is involved in the biosynthesis of melanin, has been found to

be responsible for the hypopigmentation that is seen in some patients with Prader–Willi and Angelman syndromes and for oculocutaneous (tyrosinase-positive) albinism. This gene is not imprinted, probably explaining its presence in these syndromes. Mutations or disruption of Ubeza, a gene in which imprinting is restricted to the human brain, are likely responsible for Angelman syndrome.

Both syndromes are associated with abnormalities in the inheritance of chromosomes 15q11 through 15q13. In Prader–Willi syndrome, a cytogenetically or molecularly demonstrable paternal deletion is responsible for 75% of cases. Twenty-five percent of patients with this syndrome have two normal copies of chromosome 15, but there is no paternal chromosome 15 because of nondysjunction or an error in early embryonic development. This is termed *maternal uniparental disomy.* In Angelman syndrome, a deletion accounts for 75% of cases, and paternal uniparental disomy accounts for only 2%. The end result is the loss of a functional paternal

Table 5–9. Well-Recognized Chromosomal Microdeletion Syndromes

Deletion	Chromosomal Segment Deleted	Clinical Features
Prader–Willi syndrome	15q11–q13	Hypotonia, obesity, hypogonadism, developmental retardation
Angelman syndrome	15q11–q13	Seizures, ataxia, inappropriate laughter, developmental retardation
Smith–Magenis syndrome	17p11.2	Abnormal behaviors, developmental retardation
Miller–Dieker syndrome	17p13.3	Lissencephaly, seizures, dysmorphic, developmental retardation
Chondrodysplasia punctata (XL)	Xp21	Bone dysplasia, short stature, cataracts, ichthyosis, developmental retardation
Retinoblastoma	13q14	Retinoblastoma, thumb hypoplasia, developmental retardation
DiGeorge, velocardiofacial syndromes	22q11	Congenital heart disease, immune deficiency, hypocalcemia, developmental retardation

gene(s) for Prader–Willi syndrome or a functional maternal gene(s) for Angelman syndrome. In Angelman syndrome, a mutation of the maternally active gene can cause this syndrome to occur sporadically. This group of patients includes a significant number of familial cases. Rarely, such mutations also can occur in Prader–Willi syndrome.

The concept of genomic imprinting may help explain unusual pedigrees in which parents with apparently balanced chromosome rearrangements have abnormal children with the same rearrangements. In addition, genomic imprinting eventually might explain some family histories in which a disease skips generations or is assumed to be multifactorial. Preliminary work indicates an important role of imprinting in tumorigenesis, particularly of childhood tumors, such as Wilms' tumor and retinoblastoma. The concept of imprinting challenges our understanding of traditional mendelian inheritance and suggests the need to ask how many other diseases or syndromes also might be caused by this mechanism.

22q11 DELETION SYNDROMES (VELOCARDIOFACIAL, DiGEORGE, & CONOTRUNCAL FACE SYNDROMES)

The velocardiofacial syndrome (VCFS) was first described in 1978 by Robert Shprintzen. This is the most common syndrome associated with cleft palate and is estimated to have an incidence of 1 in 5000. Patients with VCFS exhibit a wide spectrum of anomalies, the most frequent of which are cleft palate and velopharyngeal insufficiency, seen in about 90% of patients. Conotruncal heart defects (truncus arteriosus, interrupted aortic arch, tetralogy of Fallot, and ventricular septal defect) are seen in about 30% of these patients. A characteristic facial appearance (Figure 5–11), learning disabilities, and mild retardation are common. Some patients have more complex phenotypes, with delayed growth, immunologic deficiencies, hypocalcemia, microcephaly, and psychiatric disorders. Newly recognized features of VCFS occurring in greater than expected frequencies include growth hormone deficiency and juvenile rheumatoid arthritis.

Several years ago, the spectrum of abnormalities in VCFS, particularly the conotruncal heart defects, suggested to investigators a possible link between the DiGeorge sequence, in which this type of heart defect predominates, and VCFS. Indeed, there are several instances of VCFS and DiGeorge sequence occurring in the same family in an autosomal-dominant pattern of transmission. It is now established that VCFS and DiGeorge sequence are associated with submicroscopic deletions of 22q11, diagnosed with the use of a specific FISH probe. Patients with VCFS likely represent the mild end of the phenotypic spectrum, and those with DiGeorge sequence the more severe end, with more serious heart defects and a higher incidence of thymic and parathyroid hypoplasia. To date, there is no clear molecular distinction between the various clinical phenotypes described in 22q11 deletions. The clinical spectrum of 22q11 deletions and their molecular correlates will continue to demand much attention from clinical and molecular geneticists for some time into the future. Pediatricians should be aware of the wide clinical variability in patients with 22q11 deletions. In patients with conotrun-

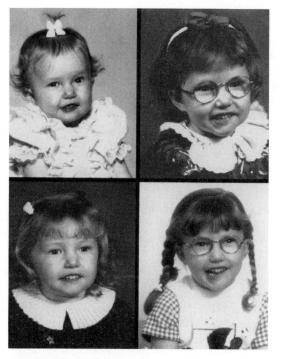

Figure 5–11. Characteristic facial appearance in velo-cardiofacial syndrome.

cal heart lesions or cleft palate, a high degree of suspicion is warranted to rule out this important microdeletion syndrome.

Fragile X Syndrome

For years, investigators have noted an excess of male children among the mentally retarded population. This finding is due primarily to an excess of X-linked genes causing mental retardation. Overall, about 25% of mental retardation is thought to be X linked. Fragile X syndrome, the most common of the X-linked disorders, was so named because of the appearance of a specific cytogenetically detectable heritable fragile site at the end of the long arm of chromosome Xq27.3 in affected individuals. A fragile site is a specific region on a chromosome that does not condense normally during mitosis and is characterized by a nonstaining gap or constriction. Fragile X is the most common cause of mental retardation and the second most common chromosomal cause of mental retardation after Down syndrome. Its incidence is slightly greater than 1 in 2500, with a frequency of 1 in 1500 in female carriers.

The fragile X phenotype is subtle and usually unremarkable to those who are not familiar with the syndrome. Lack of phenotypic clarity has contributed to the failure to appreciate this syndrome fully as a major cause of inherited mental retardation. The features are difficult to recognize in infancy and usually evolve with time. Most male children are bigger than their normal siblings and have prominent foreheads and mandibles and large ears. Macroorchidism is detected usually only after puberty. Hyperextensibility, high-arched palate, flat feet, and mitral valve prolapse are relatively common features, suggesting that this syndrome has components of a connective tissue dysplasia. IQ is usually reduced to the 30–65 range, and behavior may be dominated by hyperactivity, attention deficit disorder, or, occasionally, autism. Approximately 20% of fragile X male carriers are clinically and intellectually normal and have no obvious cytogenetic abnormality but can transmit the disorder to their daughters.

Female carriers may be normal (one third), learning impaired (one third), or mildly retarded (one third). Approximately 30% of female carriers also show some features similar to those in male carriers, such as a long narrow face and large ears.

Before 1991, the usual diagnostic test for fragile X was a cytogenetic study using specific cell culture conditions to enhance identification of the fragile site. Almost all affected fragile X males exhibit the fragile site, as do affected females and a small proportion of female carriers. In the past, unfortunately, accurate genetic counseling of families with this disorder frequently was complicated by inconclusive cytogenetic results.

In 1991, the mutation response for the fragile X syndrome was identified as an expansion of the trinucleotide sequence CGG within a gene designated as fragile X mental retardation 1 (FMR1). This CGG repeat in normal human beings ranges in size from 6 to 52 repeats. In affected patients with fragile X, this repeat has expanded to hundreds and sometimes thousands of CGG repeats. If the trinucleotide repeat of the FMR1 gene exceeds approximately 230 repeats, the DNA of the entire coding region of the gene becomes abnormally methylated, resulting in lack of transcription of FMR1 messenger RNA and the absence of its encoded protein. The length of the amplified CGG segment predicts relatively accurately the severity of the clinical phenotype (e.g., affected male, affected female, female carrier, male carrier). Understanding the molecular basis of fragile X has allowed us to understand the unusual patterns of inheritance seen in this condition. When a mother carries a premutation (a CGG repeat length of 50–230 repeats), this expansion can change in meiosis to a different and usually larger expansion, expanding to the full mutation and causing the full expression of the syndrome in an affected male child. In contrast, a male who carries the premutation (50–230 repeats) will transmit a repeat size only in the premutation range, which will not expand to cause the disorder in offspring. This explains why the condition may appear to skip generations. Knowledge of the size of the mutation in the individual at risk can allow for more accurate predictive counseling. The larger the mutation, the more likely it is to expand in the mother's children. Prenatal diagnosis is available for the fragile X syndrome; many laboratories now perform appropriate DNA testing (Southern blot and polymerase chain reaction) and can determine an individual's status with regard to fragile X with great accuracy. Cytogenetic testing for fragile X may still be appropriate in X-linked pedigrees when molecular studies for FMR1 are normal. At least two other recently identified fragile sites on the X chromosome near the site associated with fragile X are associated with syndromes that are phenotypically similar to those in classic fragile X.

The fragile X syndrome should be considered in any child with developmental delay or mental retardation in which the diagnosis is unknown. The clinician evaluating such a child should order "DNA for Fragile X" but should also order routine chromosomal analysis because the phenotype of several other chromosomal disorders such as XXY can be somewhat similar. The clinical phenotype may be so mild that exclusion of fragile X on clinical grounds alone is not warranted. Once an individual is identified with fragile X, relevant family members should be evaluated with the use of molecular studies. An approach to a child with possible fragile X or another X-linked cause of mental retardation is presented in Figure 5–12.

■ MULTIFACTORIAL INHERITANCE

Although advances in the molecular genetics of single-gene disorders have been "headline grabbers" and progress has been dramatic in understanding cytogenetic disorders, most birth defects and common diseases that run in families are not caused by single-gene errors or chromosome imbalance and are poorly understood genetically. These are termed **multifactorial disorders,** indicating that they are caused by multiple factors, genetic and environmental. These disorders recur in families but do not show particular patterns in the pedigree. Because they are common, epidemiologic studies have allowed estimation of empiric recurrence risks for individual defects. Some multifactorial traits, such as tall and short statures, are merely extreme variations of normal, and others, such as neural tube defects and congenital heart disease, are not thought to manifest until a certain threshold is exceeded. This threshold can differ by the sex of the affected individual, the severity of the defect, the number of family members affected, and several other factors. Another group of multifactorial disorders includes those diseases common to adult life, such as diabetes mellitus, hypertension, common psychiatric disorders, and many forms of cancer and coronary artery disease. Major genetic factors are undeniable in several of these diseases. The contributions of major genes to these disorders are being indentified through the Human Genome Project, but environmental risk factors are also important.

Common multifactorial birth defects are listed in Table 5–10 along with the approximate recurrence risks for first-degree relatives (siblings, sons, or daughters). Many of these traits have a strong predilection for one sex, i.e., fewer genetic factors are needed to cause the defect in the sex that is affected more often. Therefore, when a child with a particular disorder is of the sex that is affected usually less often, more genetic factors are presumed to be present. Recurrence risks for first-degree relatives of this child are higher. For example, boys are five times as likely as girls to have pyloric stenosis. When a girl is affected, her parents' risk of having another affected child is much higher than if a boy had been affected. The severity of the defect also affects recurrence risks. For example, the recurrence risk is less when a child has unilateral rather than bilateral cleft lip. Pertinent information on important multifactorial defects is discussed below.

NEURAL TUBE DEFECTS

Neural tube defects, e.g., anencephaly and spina bifida, are considered to have a common pathogenesis—failure of neural tube closure between 23 and 28 days' gestation. Failure of the neural tube to close in the cranial region results in anencephaly with absence of the forebrain, meninges, and vault of the skull and skin. Spina bifida results from failure of the fusion of the arches of the vertebrae, typically in the lumbar region. The severity depends on whether the defect is open or closed, the involvement of neural elements, and the location of the defect. Spina bifida is a major cause of developmental retardation and motor handicap in surviving infants. The incidence differs significantly between populations, occurring in nearly 1% of live births in Ireland and fewer than 0.2% in the United States. Certain ethnic populations, such as the Sikhs in British Columbia and Hispanics in rural counties in the United States, have an increased risk.

Several studies have suggested the important role of nutritional factors, and much attention has focused on the possible preventative action of folate. Folate supplementation (4 mg/d) has been recommended beginning before conception and continuing for the first 3 months of pregnancy in women who have already had a child with a neural tube defect. The Centers for Disease Control and Prevention recommend that all

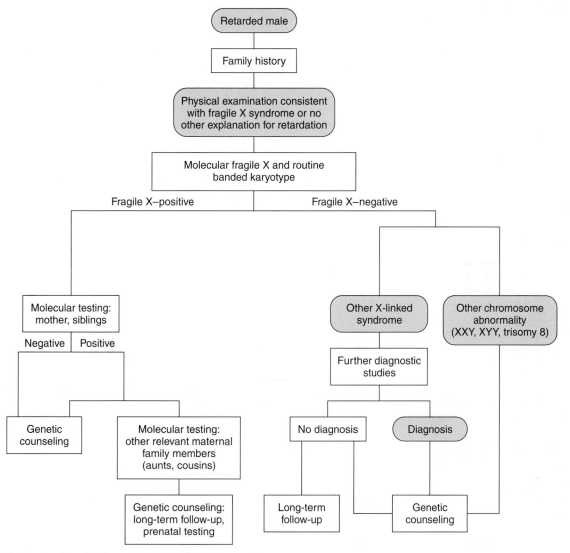

Figure 5–12. An approach to the evaluation of the male child with possible fragile X syndrome.

women of reproductive age take supplemental vitamins containing small amounts of folate (0.4 mg) on a daily basis. As a public health measure, this seems to be a much more reasonable approach to the prevention of neural tube defects because most children with neural tube defects are born into families with an entirely negative history. It is extremely difficult to achieve adequate folate intake from food alone and current supplementation of most cereals and grains provides only about one fourth of the recommended 0.4 mg/d of folic acid. The likely importance of folic acid in the prevention of other common birth defects, including oral clefts and some forms of congenital heart disease, is being studied.

Neural tube defects occasionally are associated with chromosome disorders and, when a neural tube defect is detected prenatally, especially when other defects are present, amniocentesis may be appropriate. Women receiving the anticonvulsants valproic acid (Depakene), Lamotrigene (Lamictol), and carbamazepine (Tegretol) have an increased risk for having children with a neural tube defect as do women with diabetes mellitus. In general, however, neural tube defects are isolated, with presumed multifactorial inheritance.

Table 5–10. Recurrence Risks in First-Degree Relatives in Common Multifactorial Birth Defects

Defect	Sex Ratio (M : F)	Recurrence Risks (%)
Pyloric stenosis	5 : 1	Male affected: 2–5 Female affected: 7–20
Cleft lip ± cleft palate	1.6 : 1	Unilateral: 4 Unilateral + P: 4.9 Bilateral: 6.7 Bilateral + P: 8
Cleft palate	1 : 1.14	3.5
Anencephaly/spina bifida	1 : 1.5	2–3
Congenital heart disease	1 : 1	
Ventricular septal defect		3
Patent ductus arteriosus		3
Hypoplastic left heart syndrome		6

Neural tube defects are detectable prenatally in several ways: by detection of an elevated maternal serum AFP on serum screening, ultrasound, and finding an elevated AFP in the amniotic fluid.

CLEFT LIP & CLEFT PALATE

Cleft lip, with or without cleft palate, is genetically distinct from cleft palate alone. In families in which a child has been born with cleft lip and cleft palate, there is a recurrence risk for cleft lip, alone or with cleft palate, but not for cleft palate alone. Parents of children with isolated cleft palate have a recurrence risk for cleft palate but not for cleft lip. Cleft lip with or without cleft palate is a heterogeneous defect. Numerous single-gene syndromes and chromosome disorders are associated with oral clefting. Teratogens, such as phenylhydantoin, can cause this defect. In contrast to the multifactorial model, several researchers have proposed that there are major genes for these defects. Most data, however, fit best within the multifactorial threshold trait model, and empiric recurrence risks are appropriately used when more complex patterns of malformation have been ruled out.

Cleft palate also occurs frequently as a component of syndromes. The Pierre Robin sequence is not a specific syndrome but a feature of more than 90 conditions. The Pierre Robin sequence consists of a small mandible, which is thought to the primary defect, and a U-shaped cleft palate, which is caused by the tongue falling back and preventing palatal closure. The Pierre Robin sequence is a frequent feature of the autosomal-dominant Stickler syndrome. Because Stickler syndrome is common, many geneticists recommend that all infants with isolated cleft palate be screened ophthalmologically for the severe myopia that is often characteristic of this syndrome. Cleft palate is also a common feature of the velocardiofacial syndrome (see Microdeletion Syndromes).

CONGENITAL HEART DEFECTS

Congenital heart abnormalities are very common and are seen in 4–8 per 1000 livebirths. Heart defects are also common components of multiple syndromes and are increased in frequency in nearly all chromosome disorders. It is therefore important to determine whether the child has an isolated heart defect before using empiric recurrence risks. Certain heart defects, such as patent ductus arteriosus and patent foramen ovale, are essentially normal in premature infants and do not represent real birth defects. Congenital infections, such as rubella, maternal diabetes, and anticonvulsant drugs, also significantly increase the risk for congenital heart disease. Most defects, however, are isolated. Recurrence risks have been subdivided by type of defect and are generally low. Hypoplastic left heart syndrome, coarctation of the aorta, atrial septal defect, and pulmonary valve stenosis may have a stronger predisposition to family recurrence. Mothers who have had a previous child with congenital heart disease, who have a positive family history of congenital heart defects, or who are in a high-risk group (e.g., those with insulin-dependent diabetes and those who are receiving anticonvulsant drugs) should be offered fetal echocardiography during the second trimester of pregnancy to monitor for occurrence or recurrence. Major structural defects of the heart can be detected on fetal echocardiography, although subtle lesions may be missed.

■ APPROACH TO DISPROPORTIONATE SHORT STATURE

Pediatricians are usually rightfully confused when confronted with the differential diagnosis of the disproportionately short infant or child. This confusion stems from the nomenclature, which is a mixture of eponyms, Greek terminology, and a classification based on the part of the skeleton that is affected radiographically. There are also clinical classifications based on the location of shortening (i.e., limb or spine), the age of onset, the presence of associated anomalies, and the mode of inheritance. The confusion has been compounded by the growing recognition of the genetic, molecular, and clinical heterogeneities of many bone dysplasias. There are more than 100 distinct bone dysplasias recognized today. Obviously no pediatrician can be an expert on all these! The purpose of this section is to introduce the classification and suggest an approach to these children.

Most experts rely on radiographic abnormalities as the basis of classification. This method notes which parts of the long bones are abnormal and whether the spine is involved. Thus a disorder may be classified as primarily involving the epiphyses, the metaphyses, the diaphyses, or the spine (**spondylo-**). Various combinations are possible, such as spondyloepiphyseal and spondylometaphyseal. Clinically, there are discrepancies between the lengths of the limbs and trunk in disproportionate short stature. Limb shortening can be defined further by noting which segment of the limb is primarily involved. If the shortening is chiefly proximal (i.e., humerus and femur), it is termed **rhizomelic;** if it involves the middle segment (i.e., radius, ulna, tibia, and fibula), it is termed **mesomelic;** and if the distal segments (i.e., hands and feet) are involved, it is termed **acromelic.** Some bone dysplasias combine elements of altered bone growth with true malformation syndromes. For example, in Campomelic dysplasia, there are abnormalities of the brain and heart in association with sex reversal in genetically male infants. An International Nomenclature of Constitutional Diseases of Bone was proposed in 1970 and most recently updated in 1992. On the basis of this system, skeletal disorders have been divided into five major groups.

1. **Osteochondrodysplasias,** in which there is abnormal growth and development of cartilage and/or bone. The osteochondrodysplasias include disorders evident at birth, such as achondroplasia; those that may manifest before birth or be delayed in onset, such as osteogenesis imperfecta; and those that appear in early childhood such as hypochondroplasia.
2. **Dysostoses,** in which there are malformations of individual bones, alone or in combination.
3. **Osteolytic disorders,** in which there is multiple or focal resorption of bone.
4. **Skeletal abnormalities,** which are associated with chromosome disorders.
5. **Primary metabolic disorders,** such as the Morquio and type I Gaucher syndromes.

With the increased routine use of ultrasonography, evaluation of the patient with disproportionate short stature often begins before birth with the recognition of short limbs in utero. The diagnostic process in the fetus and newborn are similar and complex. Molecular testing plays an increasingly important diagnostic role in these conditions.

To determine an accurate diagnosis, clinicians will require the assistance of a radiologist and a geneticist, who, because of the individual rarity of these conditions, often will need to consult with experts in the skeletal dysplasias. Gathering appropriate data so that the diagnosis can be made is crucial. Appropriate radiographs must be obtained (e.g., long bones, the spine, the skull, and the hands and feet). As in other genetic evaluations, the family history, developmental history, and age when the problem of short stature was first noticed are important. This physical examination should include measurements of arm span and upper:lower segment ratio (measured from the level of the symphysis pubis). Short-limbed dwarfs will have increased upper:lower segment ratios (normal is approximately 1.7 at birth and decreases to 1.0 by age 8 years), and their arm spans will be less than their heights. Short-trunk dwarfs will have decreased upper:lower segment ratios and increased arm spans. Assessment of the primary location of shortening (i.e., rhizomelic, mesomelic, acromelic) can be important. Nonskeletal clinical abnormalities may also be helpful to note, such as cleft palate and myopia in Kniest dysplasia, natal teeth and preaxial polydactyly in Ellis–van Creveld syndrome, and "hitchhiker's" thumbs and swollen ear pinnae in diastrophic dysplasia.

Several dwarfing conditions are fatal before or shortly after birth. Additional diagnostic studies can be of crucial assistance in making an appropriate diagnosis and providing for family counseling when an infant with dwarfism has died. These studies require obtaining bone specimens for biochemical and ultrastructural analysis. Usually a piece of costochondral junction should be flash frozen, a piece fixed for electron microscopy, and sections prepared for routine histologic studies. Bone or skin should be grown in tissue culture for molecular analysis. In prenatal life, testing for the specific genetic mutations associated with achondroplasia, thanatophoric dysplasia, and campomelic dysplasia may influence clinical management.

A virtual explosion of knowledge in the general field of the chondrodysplasias has been based in large part on advances related to the human genome project. Although a full discussion of the molecular basis of these defects is beyond the purview of this chapter, pediatricians should be aware of the rapid advances in this field, which allow children and adults with disproportionate short stature to be classified much more precisely and their specific molecular error identified. Eventually, knowledge of the specific gene defect in each individual should allow for more precise counseling regarding etiology and natural history. The original classifications of bone dysplasia based on such factors as radiologic features and time of onset have been redefined substantially on the basis of our current knowledge of the mutated genes involved.

The first of these disorders delineated on a molecular basis was osteogenesis imperfecta (OI). Previously, OI had been divided clinically into four types, all characterized by increased fracturability. In type I there was normal stature with little deformity, blue sclera, and a high frequency of hearing loss. Type II, lethal in the perinatal period, presented thickened bones, beaded ribs, and marked long-bone deformity. Type III was characterized by progressively deforming long bones, variably blue sclera, dentinogenesis imperfecta, and extreme short stature. Type IV was characterized by normal sclera, mild to moderate bone deformity, and variable short stature. Work in many different laboratories has identified more than 150 specific gene mutations that cause OI. All the mutations are in the gene for the pro-a-1(I) chain of type I procollagen or the pro-a-2(I) chain for the same protein. Ninety percent of patients with OI have mutations in one of these two genes. In more than one third of the mutations that cause the mildest form of OI (type I), there is decreased expression of the gene for the pro-a-1(I) chains. Most mutations in the more severe forms of the disease cause synthesis of structurally abnormal but partly functional pro-a-chains. In general, these abnormal chains exert their effects by changing the configuration of procollagen or by forming abnormally thin and irregular fibers. Any mutation that drastically reduces the amount of collagen or distorts the normal geometry of collagen fibers weakens the entire collagen structure, which is responsible for the structural strength of bone. For all four clinical forms of OI, the most likely inheritance is autosomal dominant. Rarely, types II and III may be caused by autosomal-recessive genes. In counseling families, therefore, it is extremely important to obtain a complete family history and examine relatives. Molecular analysis can clarify this process and allow for refinement of recurrence risks. For parents who are clinically normal but have an affected child, the recurrence risk for OI in a subsequent pregnancy is approximately 6% based on the possibility that one of the parents is carrying a germ-line mutation for the defect.

It has recently been recognized that three quite dissimilar disorders—thanatophoric dysplasia, achondroplasia, and hypochondroplasia—are caused by defects in fibroblast growth factor receptor 3 (FGFR3). It is of great interest that more than 98% of cases of achondroplasia analyzed to date show the same amino acid substitution. This situation is remarkably different from the molecular heterogeneity seen in other disorders. Several different mutations in FGFR 3 have been described in thanatophoric dysplasia and hypochondroplasia.

Several years ago, it was predicted that defects in type II collagen would be found primarily in disorders affecting cartilage, the nucleus pulposus, and the vitreous humor of the eye. Indeed, these molecular defects of type II collagen, termed the *type II collagenopathies,* have been found in a large group of patients with phenotypes ranging from severe achondrogenesis type II to hypochondrogenesis, to the spondyloepiphyseal dysplasias and the spondylometa-

physeal dysplasias through Kniest dysplasia, and Stickler syndrome. Other identified gene defects in the bone dysplasias are abnormalities in the sulfate transporter gene on the long arm of chromosome 5, causing diastrophic dysplasia, atelosteogenesis II, and achondrogenesis IB. The X-linked form of chondrodysplasia punctata, which is mapped to the short arm of the X chromosome (Xp22.3), has been found to contain mutations in previously unrecognized enzymes of sulfate metabolism termed aryl sulfatases E (ARSE), D, and F. Several patients with X-linked recessive chondrodysplasia punctata have been found to have mutations in aryl sulfatase E. Campomelic dysplasia, a disorder associated with sex reversal, was localized to an area on chromosome 17q24.1-225.1 in 1993. In 1995, the gene SOX 9 was characterized and mutations identified in a number of patients with classic campomelic dysplasia who were chromosomally normal. These patients were therefore found to be heterozygous for their mutations, invalidating the previously proposed autosomal-recessive inheritance pattern for this disorder. This, therefore, appears to be a dominant disorder with a very low recurrence for normal parents with an affected child. The pathogenetic mechanism of the SOX 9 mutation in campomelic dysplasia is still unknown.

We can expect that rapid progress in identifying the genes responsible for many other skeletal dysplasias will continue. It will be increasingly important for pediatricians caring for children with disproportionate short stature to be in close communication with a tertiary-level genetic center to provide families with the most current information regarding their child's defect and its likely recurrence risk.

In the surviving child with a bone dysplasia, all efforts usually are warranted to allow the child to lead as normal a life as possible. This requires considerable knowledge of the natural history of the disorder so that appropriate anticipatory guidance can be provided. For example, avoidance of early sitting and weight bearing in children with achondroplasia can reduce the chance of significant gibbus formation and spinal cord compression later in life. Vision and hearing screening are extremely important in children with the spondyloepiphyseal dysplasias because severe myopia and hearing loss are frequent. Surgical bone-lengthening procedures, although associated with very significant morbidity, may greatly increase the self-esteem, employability, and even general health of individuals with bone dysplasias. To date, these procedures have been used mostly in achondroplasia but are likely to be extended to other bone dysplasias. Referral of individuals with bone dysplasias to support groups is of inestimable help. The largest of these, Little People of America, provides an educational, social, and employment network for parents and affected individuals. Provision of accurate genetic counseling is a crucial element to the complete evaluation of a dwarfed individual and is sometimes overlooked because of the complexities of daily management.

Clinical details on several important lethal and nonlethal skeletal dysplasias are presented in Tables 5–11 and 5–12.

■ APPROACH TO THE STILLBORN INFANT

The birth of a stillborn infant is often an unexpected event for the pediatrician who may be unprepared with strategies to help the family cope and may be unsure of the appropriate diagnostic approach. Pregnancy loss is no longer an easily accepted consequence of childbearing. Families now expect answers to such questions as "Will it happen again?" and "Did I do something to cause this to happen?" Too often the answers to these questions are not available, and families then make reproductive decisions with little knowledge of real recurrence risks or understanding of possible prenatal monitoring in subsequent pregnancies. Given a uniform rational approach to the stillborn infant, a diagnosis can be anticipated in a high percentage of cases. The diagnostic and counseling process requires advanced planning and should involve the obstetrician, pathologist, nurses, geneticist, radiologist, and laboratory personnel.

Ideally, complete studies should be performed on all stillborn infants; however, practical issues, such as the

Table 5–11. Clinical and Radiographic Features in Selected Lethal Skeletal Dysplasias

Diagnosis	Mode of Inheritance	Clinical Features	Radiographic Features	Gene	Location
Achondrogenesis IA	AR ?	Extremely short limbs, frequent hydrops	Incomplete spine ossification		
Achondrogenesis IB	AD			DTDST	5q32
Achondrogenesis II (hypochondrogenesis)	AD	Short limbs, fetal hydrops	Poor spine ossification, metaphyseal abnormalities	COL2AI	12q14
Thanatophoric dysplasia	AD	Relatively large cranium, short limbs, spatulate fingers	"Telephone-receiver" femurs	FGFR3	4p16.3
Campomelic dysplasia	AD	Bowing of tibias with skin dimples, sex reversal in XY males, cleft palate, CNS and cardiac malformations	Bowing of the long bones	SOX9	17q24.3
Rhizomelic chondrodysplasia punctata	AR	Cleft palate, cataracts, occasional ichthyosis, short limbs	Punctate epiphyseal calcifications; vertebral, coronal clefts	PEX7	6q22–24
Atelosteogenesis syndromes	?	Very short proximal limbs, depressed nasal bridge, cleft palate, deviation of fingers	Short ribs, flat vertebrae, coronal clefts	N/A	
Short-limb polydactyly syndromes	AR	Short limbs, polydactyly, heart and renal defects	Short horizontal ribs; wide, flat vertebral bodies	N/A	
Jarcho–Levin syndrome	AR	Very short trunk, camptodactyly	Multiple vertebral segmentation defects, "crab-like" appearance of ribs	DLL3	19q13
Osteogenesis imperfecta congenita	AD (usual)	Very short bowed limbs, blue sclera, flat facies, hydrops	Multiple fractures, thick bones, beading of ribs	COL1A1; COL1A2	17q21–22; 7q22.1

AD = autosomal dominant; AR = autosomal recessive; CNS = central nervous system.

Table 5–12. Clinical and Radiographic Features in Selected Nonlethal Bone Dysplasias

Bone Dysplasia	Mode of Inheritance	Age at Recognition	Clinical Features	Radiographic Features
Achondroplasia	AD	Birth	Relatively large head, characteristic face, rhizomelic shortenings of limbs, spinal stenosis, trident hand	Small sacrosciatic notches, decreased interpedicular distance, short pedicles, short, broad long bones
Asphyxiating thoracic dystrophy (Jeune syndrome)	AR	Birth	Narrow chest, occasional polydactyly, variable limb shortening, respiratory insufficiency, renal disease	Short ribs, square, short ilia, acetabular spurs, broad proximal femurs
Spondyloepiphyseal dysplasia congenita	AD	Birth	Short barrel chest, normal hands, slightly short limbs, myopia, retinal detachment, hearing loss, subluxation C1–2	Odontoid hypoplasia; flat, pear-shaped vertebrae; delayed ossification of epiphyses, hips, and knees
Hypochondroplasia	AD	About 2 y	Normal face; rhizomelic shortening of limbs; short, broad hands; mild short stature	Short, wide long bones; lumbosacral interpedicular narrowing; short pedicles
Pseudoachondroplasia	AD	About 2 y	Normal face; long trunk; very short limbs; severe joint problems; small, broad hands	Platyspondyly, epiphyseal, and metaphyseal dysplasia; marked hand involvement

AD = autosomal dominant; AR = autosomal recessive.

yield of the test, the cost, and the impact on the family, need to be considered when choosing diagnostic studies. Sometimes the cause of fetal death is apparent (e.g., cord accident, placental abruption, or acute infection). Even in these obvious cases, however, an autopsy and other studies can be reassuring to families regarding the absence of other anomalies and the anticipated pathologic findings. Such studies are increasingly important in medicolegal defense. Often the cause of fetal death is not clear. In these cases, appropriate focused studies should be routine.

Fetuses that appear to have died soon before delivery are much more likely to have died acutely from a nonrecurring event, such as an ascending infection, cord accident, or placental abruption. These fetuses should be examined carefully, and, if no external malformations are apparent and there is no history of recurrent loss, appropriate studies may consist of an autopsy, an examination of the placenta and cord, and photographs.

Macerated fetuses, which are precisely those least likely to be studied, are more likely to have such findings as malformations, syndromes, and chromosome abnormalities. A complete evaluation should always be performed on these infants. Complete studies also should be performed on infants with an external or suspected internal structural malformation (e.g., cleft lip, with or without cleft palate, ear anomalies, extra or missing digits, or imperforate anus) or those with abnormal prenatal ultrasound examinations. Other infants who warrant complete investigation are those with intrauterine growth retardation because these infants are significantly more likely to have chromosomal errors or severe placental abnormalities. When no cause of death is apparent or with a history of previously unexplained fetal or neonatal loss, a full investigation should be conducted.

The Stillborn Protocol

An algorithm for the evaluation of a stillbirth or neonatal death is shown in Figure 5–13. A complete protocol for the investigation of a stillborn infant includes the following:

1. History of the unsuccessful pregnancy
2. Family history
3. External clinical examination of the infant
4. Photographs
5. Chromosome cultures (via cord or cardiac blood, skin biopsy, or placenta and fetal membranes)
6. Skeletal radiographs (mandatory when short limbs or a dwarfing condition is suspected)
7. Fetal autopsy
8. Examination of the placenta and cord

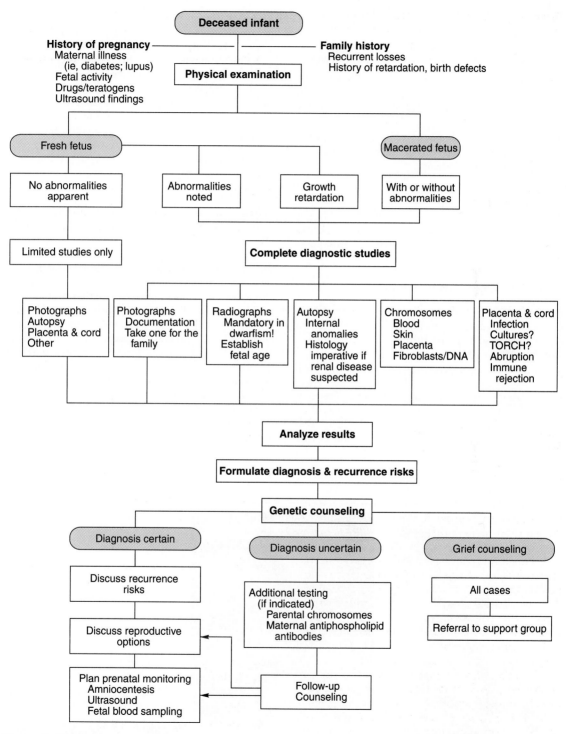

Figure 5–13. Evaluation of stillbirth/neonatal death.

9. Special studies such as cord blood TORCH (Toxoplasmosis, Rubella, Cytomegalovirus and Herpes) titers and cord immunoglobulin M (IgM) levels in suspected in utero infections, hemoglobin electrophoresis in cases of suspected hemoglobinopathy or thalassemia, and skin biopsy for enzymatic and DNA studies in suspected storage or metabolic disorders

10. Counseling, which may be provided by the pediatrician in straightforward situations or by a geneticist or genetic counselor

All the data should be reviewed with the family and appropriate options for prenatal monitoring in subsequent pregnancies discussed. The family should have a clear idea of the recurrence risks involved. Supportive grief counseling and referral to pregnancy loss support groups are appropriate in all cases.

Common Diagnoses in Stillborns

Although it is beyond the scope of this chapter to discuss the myriad conditions presenting as stillbirth, certain conditions are so common to the pediatric experience that they deserve additional discussion.

Chromosome disorders frequently result in stillbirth and neonatal death. About 6% of stillborns and 5.5% of neonatal deaths are chromosomally abnormal. Presentation of the fetus with a chromosome disorder may differ greatly from that seen in newborns or older infants. Relatively small fetal size may make appreciation of dysmorphic features difficult. This is particularly true for Down syndrome. The overturned ear helices, upslanted palpebral fissures, and midface hypoplasia are often not obvious. Fetal maceration also can obscure subtle dysmorphic features as can fetal hydrops or swelling, which is relatively common in Down syndrome and trisomy 18. Fetal swelling is the hallmark of XO Turner syndrome, in which it is associated with nuchal cystic hygroma. Chromosomally abnormal stillborns tend to have more severe and obvious malformations than those seen in liveborn infants. For example, neural tube defects are rather common in stillborn fetuses with trisomy 18 but rare in liveborn infants with trisomy 18.

AMNIOTIC BANDS

Amniotic bands in the liveborn child usually consist of characteristic asymmetric involvement of limbs and digits with occasional facial clefting. Frequently, vestigial fibrous bands remain on the digits at the time of birth and are helpful diagnostically. These children usually are entirely normal apart from their disruptive and deformational defects. This is in marked contrast to the phenotypic picture in the stillborn, which tends to be much more severe and in which body wall defects (the so-called limb–body wall complex), exencephaly, acrania, scoliosis, short cord, and internal malformations may occur (Figure 5–14). Often in these situations, there is no direct evidence of amniotic bands, but examination of the placenta can help establish the diagnosis because the chorial plate is mostly devoid of amnion. These bizarre body wall defects are frequently diagnosed prenatally and probably result from very early disruption of the amnion, although the exact pathogenesis remains somewhat obscure.

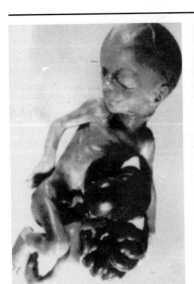
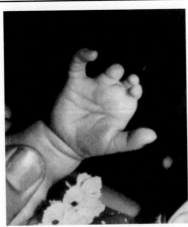

Figure 5–14. Early amnion rupture sequence may result in severe limb and wall defects (**left**) or be limited to distal limb amputations (**right**).

POTTER PHENOTYPE

Severe oligohydramnios, from whatever cause, produces Potter phenotype, which is characterized by an aged facial appearance, lower canthal folds, depressed nasal tip, micrognathia, loose skin, and limb abnormalities secondary to chronic in utero constraint. Death occurs postnatally because of pulmonary hypoplasia. Infants are severely depressed at birth and cannot be ventilated successfully. The overall pattern of the anomalies may not become evident for several hours, when the lack of response to mechanical ventilation becomes progressively apparent. Although Potter phenotype can occur secondary to a chronic amniotic fluid leak or severe intrauterine growth retardation, renal causes are frequent and mandate evaluation of renal histology. Possible renal findings include bilateral renal agenesis or cystic dysplastic kidneys, obstructive uropathy, and type 2 autosomal-recessive infantile polycystic kidney disease. Rarely, type 1 autosomal-dominant adult-type polycystic kidney disease may present with Potter phenotype. These disorders carry different genetic recurrence risks, which may vary from 3.5% for bilateral renal agenesis in parents with normal renal ultrasounds to 25% for type 2 infantile polycystic kidney disease.

After complete evaluation, an accurate diagnosis can be anticipated in most stillborn infants and children dying neonatally. Advances in prenatal diagnosis, especially use of DNA techniques, make accurate investigation of fetal or neonatal death increasingly relevant.

■ IMPORTANT TERATOGENS IN PEDIATRICS

A **teratogen** is an agent that can cause abnormalities in form and function (i.e., birth defects) in an exposed fetus. Teratogens act in a relatively limited number of ways by producing cell death, altering tissue growth, or interfering with differentiation. Because these are basic functions of growing cells and developing organisms, there is commonly more than one effect observed in the developing fetus. Certain characteristics are common to teratogenic agents: infertility or fetal wastage, prenatal onset growth deficiency, alterations in morphogenesis, and alterations of organ system function, including central nervous system performance.

There is a wide variability in the effect of the teratogenic agent on the fetus; this undoubtedly has delayed recognition of many human teratogens. Factors accounting for variability include the dose of the agent, the timing of the exposure, the host's susceptibility (i.e., maternal and fetal genetic factors), and interactions with other environmental agents.

Teratogens include infectious agents; drugs and chemicals; physical agents, such as radiation; and maternal metabolic disorders, such as insulin-dependent diabetes mellitus and phenylketonuria. Major teratogens and their effects are presented in Table 5–13.

Infectious Agents

Recognized effects of viruses, bacteria, and parasites include fetal death, growth retardation, birth defects, and mental retardation. In most instances, the fetus is directly invaded with secondary inflammation of fetal tissues and cell death. Symptoms characterizing prenatal infections include microcephaly, mental retardation, cerebral palsy, seizures, and visual and hearing defects (see Chapter 4). In general, structural defects such as polydactyly are not seen.

RUBELLA VIRUS

Rubella virus is the best studied infectious agent. The severity of fetal effects differs significantly according to the month of gestation at the time of infection. Of infants infected during the first trimester, 15–25% are found to have symptoms of congenital rubella syndrome. After the first trimester, the incidence of severely affected children decreases; however, hearing loss and mental retardation can occur in children exposed in the fourth and fifth months of pregnancy. Congenital rubella syndrome is characterized by growth retardation; failure to thrive; congenital anomalies, including cataracts, pigmentary retinopathy, microphthalmia, and glaucoma; cardiovascular malformations, especially patent ductus arteriosus, pulmonary valvar and arterial stenoses, atrial septal defect, and ventricular septal defect; neonatal myocarditis; and central nervous system abnormalities. Sensorineural hearing loss is frequent. Hepatosplenomegaly, thrombocytopenia, chronic rash, chronic diarrhea, and immune defects are also seen. Prevention of congenital rubella is possible through the routine use of effective rubella vaccines. Attenuated live rubella vaccines are known to cross the placenta, and the virus has been recovered from abortus material. However, inadvertent vaccination of a pregnant woman appears to pose a very low risk to the fetus.

CYTOMEGALOVIRUS

Possibly 5–6% of all pregnant women become infected with cytomegalovirus. Risks to the fetus appears to be confined mainly to those women with primary infection. The overall risk for a woman with primary infection to have an infected fetus is approximately 30–40%. Approximately 10–15% of these infants show some symptoms, although most infants are clinically asymptomatic. Severe congenital cytomegalovirus infection causes diffuse central nervous system damage, including microcephaly, associated with paraventricular calcifications; rarely hydrocephalus; hearing loss; mental retardation; and seizures.

Table 5–13. Important Human Teratogens and Their Major Clinical Effects

Teratogen	Susceptible Period (trimester)	Fetal Effects
Infections		
Rubella	First	Cararacts, congenital heart disease, hearing loss, mental retardation
Cytomegalovirus	First and second	Microcephaly, mental retardation, chorioretinitis, seizures, hearing loss
Toxoplasmosis	First to third	Hydrocephalus, mental retardation, microcephaly, chorioretinitis
Drugs		
Warfarin	First	CNS defects, nasal hypoplasia
Isotretinoin	First	Cardiac, ear, and CNS
Lithium	First	Cardiac (Ebstein anomaly), overgrowth
Anticonvulsant drugs		
Diphenylhydantoin	First to third	Characteristic face, nail hypoplasia, ↑ risk cleft lip ± palate, developmental problems
Valproic acid	First to third	Neural tube defects, characteristic face, learning problems
Carbamazepine	First to third	Neural tube defects, learning problems
Chemical/physical agents		
Hyperthermia	First	Neural tube defects, microcephaly
Radiation	First month	Therapeutic radiation only; microcephaly Diagnostic: low risk
Alcohol	First to third	Wide spectrum of effects; CNS functional impairment most important

CNS = central nervous system.

Ocular involvement with chorioretinitis, optic atrophy, and microphthalmia can produce severe visual impairment. Infants may present with the so-called blueberry muffin syndrome, with hepatosplenomegaly, jaundice, thrombocytopenia, petechiae, or hemolytic anemia.

HERPES SIMPLEX VIRUS

Most of the risk associated with the herpes simplex virus has been attributable to infants acquiring infection at or around the time of birth. Nevertheless, herpes simplex infection in early pregnancy may result in fetal loss and, rarely, microcephaly and microphthalmia. Intracranial calcifications, retinal dysplasia, patent ductus arteriosus, vesicular cutaneous lesions, and hypoplastic distal phalanges also have been reported. Perinatal transmission can often be avoided by appropriate obstetric precautions.

CONGENITAL VARICELLA

Congenital varicella (chickenpox) syndrome resulting from infection of the pregnant mother appears to occur infrequently (±2%). The crucial period for fetal infection appears to be the third and fourth month. Affected children may show growth deficiency, microcephaly, peripheral nerve palsy, ocular involvement, and limb anomalies, including distal phalangeal hypoplasia or hypoplasia of an entire limb. Cutaneous abnormalities include scars, vesicles, and underdevelopment of the skin, possibly secondary to in utero ulceration.

HUMAN IMMUNODEFICIENCY VIRUS

Human immunodeficiency virus has been suggested as a cause of altered growth and development and as a cause of dysmorphic facial features. The bulk of evidence suggests, however, that the virus is not teratogenic, although it may be transmitted transplacentally, causing acquired immunodeficiency syndrome in fetuses and infants.

PARVOVIRUS B19

Since its discovery in 1975, human parvovirus (B19) has been shown to cause a diverse spectrum of clinical manifestations, including the childhood illness fifth disease (erythema infectiosum), aplastic crises in patients with chronic hemolytic anemia, chronic anemia in immunodeficient patients, and arthritis. In 1984, reports appeared of intrauterine death associated with B19 infections. Approximately 50% of adult women are immune to parvovirus. The transplacental infection rate has been estimated to be about 33%, although precise information on fetal risk has been difficult to obtain because B19 infection rarely persists throughout the pregnancy. Therefore, measuring B19 IgM in cord blood of surviving infants is not a reliable method for detecting intrauterine infections. Maternal B19 infection, usually asymptomatic, most often is followed by the delivery of a normal infant. However, fetal loss can occur at all stages of pregnancy; the highest risk occurs during the first 20 weeks, especially between weeks 10 and 20, with hydrops and ascites developing rapidly. Various studies have reported overall fetal risk to be approximately 4–16%.

In the fetus, B19 infection causes a maturational arrest in the development of red blood cells. Because the fetus is rapidly expanding its red blood cell volume and has a short red blood cell life span, it is particularly vulnerable to this type of insult. Anemia results, which is thought to cause cardiac failure, ascites, pleural effusions, and edema of the skin. Myocarditis and liver disease also have been reported, as have meconium peritonitis and, rarely, congenital malformations, although this association has not been proved.

When a mother is known or thought to have been exposed to parvovirus, the first step is to determine her immune status. If her parvovirus IgG findings are positive and her IgM negative, she can be assumed to be immune. If her IgG and IgM findings are negative, testing should be repeated serially to rule out newly occurring infection. In a woman whose IgG and IgM results are positive, the mother should be assumed to be infected and the fetus monitored appropriately. Serum AFP has been suggested as a means of detecting early fetal involvement. However, weekly ultrasound examinations are currently recommended between 6 and 14 weeks' gestation, which represents the maximum interval between maternal illness and fetal death. Early detection of fetal ascites should lead to prompt referral to a center specializing in intrauterine blood transfusions, which have been a life-saving approach in this form of anemia. In some situations, the ascites and hydrops caused by B19-induced anemia resolve spontaneously. Many issues have not been defined, including the role of intrauterine transfusion and the best method for monitoring women at risk.

BACTERIAL AGENTS

Among bacterial agents, only syphilis and possibly mycoplasmas are thought to have significant teratogenicity. Syphilis is the oldest of the known prenatal infectious teratogens, and, although rare, its frequency may be increasing. It is generally thought that infection of the fetus with syphilis does not occur until about the fourth month of pregnancy. If untreated, about 50% of infants will be affected with congenital syphilis, and the remainder will be stillborn or die in the perinatal period. Late infection with syphilis results in only about a 10% risk of fetal infection. Infants with early congenital syphilis may present with fetal hydrops and evidence of generalized infection, as well as with hepatosplenomegaly, lymphadenitis, anemia, thrombocytopenia, rhinitis, and rashes. Inflammation of bone may be manifested by Parrot pseudoparalysis, which may mimic an Erb palsy or present as an irritable infant. Meningitis, nerve palsies, and progressive hydrocephalus may occur. Eye problems are frequent with chorioretinitis, uveitis, optic atrophy, glaucoma, and occasional chancres

of the eyelid. Late manifestations of congenital syphilis, which occur after age 2 years, include Hutchinson teeth, interstitial keratitis, deafness, mulberry molars, and Clutton joints. Saddle nose deformity and linear facial scars around body orifices (rhagades) are late manifestations.

TOXOPLASMOSIS

Toxoplasmosis is the major parasitic teratogen of concern to pediatricians. The major risk to the fetus occurs from acute toxoplasmosis infection during pregnancy. First-trimester infection is associated with a 15–20% risk of fetal transmission, whereas second- or third-trimester infections are associated with a 75% risk. Later infections most often result in clinically asymptomatic disease. Manifestations in the infant include microcephaly or hydrocephalus and a range of systemic symptoms associated with generalized sepsis. Long-term follow-up of involved children shows a high percentage of mental retardation, cerebral palsy, and visual and hearing deficits.

Physical Teratogens

The nuclear disaster in Chernobyl and episodes such as the Three Mile Island accident have raised concern regarding the role of radiation in human malformations. Experimental animal and epidemiologic studies suggest that high doses of radiation (>200 rad) can produce prenatal onset growth deficiency, central nervous system damage, microcephaly, and ocular defects. The sensitive period for such abnormalities appears to be about 2–5 fetal weeks. Therapeutic doses of radiation carry a significant risk of anomalies for the fetus only when delivered to the region of the developing embryo during the first month of pregnancy. Lower doses of radiation appear to have a low risk for malformations or functional abnormalities in humans at any time in pregnancy. There is also the theoretic risk of mutagenesis and carcinogenesis, but the magnitude of risk is quite low. Exposures to radiation should be avoided, but women undergoing diagnostic x-ray studies generally can be given significant reassurance regarding the risks to their fetuses.

HYPERTHERMIA

There appear to be real risks to the fetus from sustained increases in body temperature from whatever cause. The most obvious cause of hyperthermia is maternal fever, but other sources are saunas, hot tubs, bathing, and prolonged exertion. Human data are limited, although laboratory animal data strongly support the role of heat as a teratogenic agent at critical stages in neural tube development. There are several anecdotal reports regarding the association of anencephaly and spina bifida with hyperthermia. In addition, microcephaly, mental retardation, and cerebral palsy have been reported in women who have had sustained, uncontrolled febrile episodes.

Drugs & Chemical Agents

Much attention was focused on drugs as a cause of malformations after the thalidomide disaster in the early 1960s. Good data on most drugs to which pregnant women may be exposed are not available. Unfortunately, because exposures may be rare and outcomes not reported, recognition of potential human teratogens may take years. Only a few of those drugs recognized as teratogens are discussed here.

The recognition of the adverse affects of **alcohol** on fetal growth and development was delayed for many years, in part because the effects on the fetus are diverse and the major effects are functional (i.e., on the central nervous system). Infants with full-blown fetal alcohol syndrome are typically born to chronically alcoholic women who have a 40–50% risk of having infants with severe problems in growth and development. The full-blown syndrome is characterized by a distinctive facial appearance, with short palpebral fissures and long philtrum; prenatal onset growth deficiency; and an increased frequency of congenital abnormalities of the heart, skeleton, joints, and palate. The face, which may be characteristic in the young child, tends to normalize with time, making recognition in the adult difficult. Mental deficiency and learning disabilities, however, do not disappear with time. Consumption of alcohol by pregnant women is a significant public health concern and has led to warning labels on alcoholic beverages and in restaurants and bars. These warnings are perhaps effective for some portions of society, but for those women in which a pattern of heavy drinking has long been established, such measures may have little effect.

Pregnant women usually receive **anticoagulants** because of the presence of prosthetic heart valves or thrombophlebitis. Coumadin derivatives, in particular warfarin, are associated with an approximately 33% risk of death or malformations in infants exposed in the first trimester. The crucial period appears to be 6–9 weeks after conception. The facial and skeletal features resemble those seen in chondrodysplasia punctata, with stippling (like paint spatters) seen radiographically. Children may have severe nasal hypoplasia, occasional choanal atresia, microcephaly, no corpus callosum, and ocular defects. Some survivors with major craniofacial involvement are mentally normal. The use of heparin is not thought to be teratogenic, but there is an increased risk of fetal loss, with an approximate 15% rate of stillbirth and a 20% rate of prematurity. Overall, carefully monitored heparin administration is probably safer for the woman who must have continuous anticoagulation.

Women treated with **anticonvulsants** during pregnancy are clearly at increased risk for serious adverse fetal effects. How much of this risk is attributable directly to anticonvulsants is not clear because the underlying seizure disorder or the mother's reason for seizures may contribute to the risk. Nonetheless, the pattern of anomalies associated with individual anticonvulsants supports the concept that these drugs are directly related to the adverse outcome. All of the anticonvulsant drugs, with the possible exceptions of phenobarbital and Mysoline, have been associated with significant teratogenic risks. The best studied of these, diphenylhydantoin (Dilantin), produces a recognizable pattern of defects in approximately 10% of exposed infants. Findings include underdevelopment of the midface, flat nasal bridge, occasional growth deficiency, increased risk of cleft lip or cleft palate, and hypoplasia of the distal phalanges with notably small nails. Overt mental deficiency is rare, but learning disabilities are frequent.

Valproic acid (Depakene) and carbamazepine (Tegretol) are associated with an approximately 1% risk of neural tube defects. A specific pattern of minor facial anomalies, genital abnormalities, cardiac defects, and learning problems also has been recognized. Trimethadione (Zarontin) and related anticonvulsant drugs are significantly teratogenic. Exposed children have characteristic faces with V-shaped eyebrows, overturned ear helices, and a short upturned nose. Although no anticonvulsant drugs are "safe," this particular class of drug should be rigorously avoided during pregnancy.

Excessive doses of **vitamin A** and other **retinoids** have long been known to cause birth defects, but the recently released drug isotretinoin (Accutane) has been clearly established as a new human teratogen. Isotretinoin is used for cystic acne. The group most likely to use this drug consist of teenagers who are also at an increased risk for unplanned pregnancy. The highest fetal risk is associated with exposure at 2–5 fetal weeks. Miscarriage rates are significantly increased. About 25% of surviving infants show a pattern of characteristic anomalies, including microcephaly with serious central nervous system abnormalities, conotruncal cardiac abnormalities, and malformations of the ear. Death in infancy is common, and survivors have a high incidence of mental retardation. Isotretinoin has a relatively short half-life, but another related drug, etretinate, has a half-life of weeks to months. Children born long after this drug has been discontinued show characteristic birth defects. Use of reliable contraceptive is imperative in women being treated with these agents, and etretinate should be avoided entirely in women of reproductive age.

Cocaine is the most widely used illicit drug in the reproductive age group. Numerous adverse effects have been demonstrated in human pregnancy, including increased rates of spontaneous abortion, abruptio placenta, and premature delivery. The effects on the newborn include an increased incidence of intraventricular hemorrhage, gastrointestinal and genitourinary abnormalities, and limb reduction defects. Long-term neurologic and behavioral sequelae of maternal cocaine abuse have been reported. There may be a fetal cocaine dysmorphic phenotype consisting of periorbital and eyelid edema, flat nasal bridge with transverse crease, short nose, and large fontanelles. It is thought that most prenatal problems associated with cocaine relate to vasospasm from the sympathomimetic effects of cocaine and subsequent vascular disruption.

Maternal Conditions

MATERNAL DIABETES

Maternal diabetes is a known human teratogen. It has been assumed that only women with insulin-dependent diabetes have an increased risk for fetal anomalies, but recent evidence suggests that women with gestational diabetes also may have some increased risk. When women have diabetes at the time of their first prenatal visit, it is difficult to know the status of their glucose control during the critical first few weeks of embryonic development. The specific defects of caudal regression and sirenomelia are definitely increased in infants of mothers with diabetes. The risk of neural tube defects, holoprosencephaly, congenital heart disease, and cleft lip and cleft palate is also significantly increased in these infants. Although available data are inconclusive, careful glucose control during the early weeks of pregnancy is thought to lower the risk of fetal malformations.

MATERNAL PHENYLKETONURIA

Maternal phenylketonuria poses a definite risk to the fetus. Women who were treated for phenylketonuria with diet restriction as children are now of reproductive age, and, in many, dietary restriction was discontinued after age 10 years. Thus, in the pregnant mother with phenylketonuria, the fetus is exposed to very high serum levels of phenylalanine, phenylpyruvic acid, and other metabolites. Twenty-five percent of exposed fetuses have congenital abnormalities, and 90% are mentally retarded and microcephalic. Women with phenylketonuria should be treated with dietary restriction before and throughout pregnancy. Early follow-up studies have suggested greatly improved pregnancy outcomes with appropriate dietary management.

■ PRENATAL DIAGNOSIS

Prenatal diagnosis offers parents and physicians an assessment of the status and well-being of the fetus before birth. Advances in cytogenetic and DNA technology, the development of high-resolution ultrasonography, and new obstetric technologies are allowing parents an ever increasing range of informed choices regarding the unborn child. In the past, families could accept the risk of a handicapped child or avoid childbearing altogether. Prenatal diagnosis offers reassurance to parents in high-risk groups and provides couples who might otherwise not attempt a pregnancy with information about the presence or absence of the genetic disorder in question. When the fetus is found to have a serious defect, the parents may elect to terminate or continue the pregnancy. Even when termination is not an option, parents may use the information to be fully prepared for their child's birth and postnatal care. They may wish to meet with other families who have similarly affected children and are often referred to surgeons or other neonatal specialists who will be involved in their newborn's care. In more than 98% of cases, however, prenatal diagnostic studies provide reassuring information that the baby is not affected by the condition under study.

INDICATIONS

The prenatal diagnosis of many disorders, including cystic fibrosis, the hemoglobinopathies, and inborn errors of metabolism, is now possible with the use of molecular techniques. However, the primary reason for a woman to seek prenatal diagnosis remains the detection of Down syndrome. With advancing maternal age, the risk of a chromosomally abnormal fetus increases. For example, the chance for a 35-year-old woman to have a child with Down syndrome is about 1 in 250 at the time of amniocentesis. At age 40, this risk increases to 1 in 75. Because chromosomally abnormal fetuses have an increased risk of loss during pregnancy, the birth incidence of Down syndrome is somewhat less than the risk cited above.

Other indications for prenatal diagnosis include the following.

A previous child with a chromosome abnormality. When a mother has had a child with Down syndrome and is younger than 35 years, her recurrence risk may be very slightly increased as compared with other women her age. A general recurrence risk of 1% is usually quoted. Parents who have had children with other chromosome abnormalities, such as trisomy 18, trisomy 13, and deletions, also might seek the reassurance that prenatal testing can provide, even though recurrence risks are usually low.

One parent carries a structural chromosomal abnormality. In these situations, the risk of having a child with birth defects and mental retardation significantly increases. For example, if a mother carries a 14/21 translocation, her chance of having a child with Down syndrome is about 5%. The risk is less (about 2%) when the father carries this translocation. Many other translocations carried in balanced form pose a risk to produce children with phenotypic abnormalities and retardation. The exact risk for each specific translocation is different, but in all cases, parents carrying these rearrangements are at a significantly increased risk and eligible for prenatal testing.

Family at risk for a genetic disorder that can be diagnosed by biochemical or DNA testing. This category includes multiple disorders, many of which are inborn errors of metabolism. Most are single gene defects, with risks of 25–50%. The list of defects for which enzymatic or DNA testing is possible is presented in Table 5–14.

Family history of an X-linked disorder for which there is no precise prenatal testing. Fetal sex determination

Table 5–14. Examples of Prenatal Diagnosis of Metabolic Disorders With Enzyme and DNA Analysis

Diagnosis by Enzyme Analysis	Diagnosis by DNA Analysis
Galactosemia	Cystic fibrosis
Glycogen storage disease (II, III, and IV)	Duchenne muscular dystrophy
Citrullinemia	Hemophilia A & B
Maple-syrup urine disease	Sickle cell disease
Methylmalonic aciduria	Ornithine transcarbamy-lase deficiency
Propionic aciduria	
Tay–Sachs disease	α_1-Antitrypsin deficiency
Hurler syndrome	Lesch–Nyhan syndrome
Hunter syndrome	Charcot–Marie–Tooth disease
Adenine deaminase deficiency	
Hypophosphatasia	Huntington disease
	Myotonic dystrophy

may help families make decisions or plan delivery strategies. Fortunately, the list of X-linked disorders for which DNA diagnosis is now possible is increasing so that families do not need to make decisions solely on the basis of knowledge of the fetal sex. However, it may save time and expense if fetal sex is determined before proceeding with DNA diagnostic studies in disorders such as Duchenne muscular dystrophy and hemophilia A and B. Fluorescence in situ hybridization can expedite determination of sex after amniocentesis or chorionic villus biopsy and decrease the overall turn-around time for results.

Family has a risk for a neural tube defect. In general, only first- and second-degree relatives of infants with spina bifida or anencephaly are considered candidates for amniocentesis and determination of amniotic fluid AFP. Most infants with neural tube defects are born to parents with no positive family history. Testing modalities for neural tube defects are discussed below.

TECHNIQUES

Chorionic villus sampling (CVS). In CVS, fetal trophoblastic tissue is aspirated from the villus area of the chorion transcervically or transabdominally. It is usually performed at 10–12 weeks' gestation. This earlier test offers a family more time to make decisions regarding possible abnormal results. Concerns regarding limb reduction defects as a complication of CVS have been raised in several centers. This risk, although very low, may be related to operator inexperience and hemorrhagic lesions in the developing fetus. Most of these complications have occurred in procedures done before 9 fetal weeks. A disadvantage of CVS is that the amniotic fluid AFP value

cannot be provided and mothers will need to undergo later maternal serum AFP screening.

Fetal blood sampling (periumbilical fetal blood sampling or cordocentesis). This procedure is used to obtain samples of fetal blood directly from the umbilical cord. Indications for fetal blood sampling include rapid karyotyping in late gestational age fetuses with abnormalities, obtaining a fetal hematocrit or white count in selected disorders, and obtaining antibody titers in suspected fetal infection. This procedure usually is not done until after 18 weeks' gestation and carries an increased risk of miscarriage (approximately 4%).

Ultrasonography. This procedure has become increasingly important in prenatal diagnosis for assessment of morphologic abnormalities that cannot be detected by amniocentesis, CVS, or AFP testing. Fetal age, multiple pregnancy, fetal viability, and fetal sex can be identified with a high degree of accuracy. It is the procedure of choice for the diagnosis of most skeletal dysplasias, several renal diseases, congenital heart defects, and cleft lip and cleft palate. Ultrasound screening is often a part of routine prenatal care and in experienced hands this may detect unsuspected abnormalities. It is especially useful in the presence of a specific increased risk for a structural birth defect or when abnormalities of fetal growth, amniotic fluid volume, or abnormal serum screening are noted in the pregnancy. A list of selected defects detectable by ultrasound is provided in Table 5–15.

SERUM SCREENING FOR NEURAL TUBE DEFECTS & CHROMOSOME ABNORMALITIES

Maternal serum screening is a noninvasive method of obtaining information about the fetus. As in all medical

Table 5–15. Indications for Ultrasound Prenatal Diagnosis

Previous child with abnormality
  Skeletal dysplasia
  Congenital heart disease
  Renal disease (absence/polycystic)
  Central nervous system abnormalities
  Neural tube defects
  Cleft lip ± palate
  Syndromes without chromosomal or biochemical marker

Abnormal pregnancy
  Polyhydramnios
  Oligohydramnios
  Twins
  Decreased fetal activity
  Abnormal fetal growth
  Maternal illness (e.g., diabetes)

screening, the object is to identify in a healthy population those who are at a sufficiently increased risk of having a particular disorder to be offered specific diagnostic testing. In prenatal screening, the biochemical screening markers are used to select women who may be offered ultrasound examinations, amniocentesis, and other studies to clarify their positive screen test results. Prenatal screening was initially confined to detect neural tube defects on the basis of elevated levels of AFP. α-Fetoprotein is produced in the fetal liver and found in small amounts in the maternal serum and amniotic fluid. With the use of additional analytes, maternal serum screening has been expanded to include risk screening for fetal chromosome abnormalities and third-trimester obstetric complications. The combinations of three different markers are currently measured in maternal serum: AFP, hCG, and unconjugated estriol.

Maternal serum AFP has been used to screen for fetal abnormalities since 1972 or so. The basis for this screening test is that the level of AFP, which is strictly a fetal protein, is elevated when there is an open or non–skin-covered defect, such as meningomyelocele, omphalocele, or gastroschisis. In these situations fetal AFP leaks across the exposed capillaries into the amniotic fluid and across the placenta into the maternal circulation. Normal ranges for AFP have been well established for the gestational ages between 15 and 22 weeks, the time during which most women undergo prenatal testing. Considerable efforts have been undertaken to define cutoff points at which a relatively low number of open neural tube defects or abdominal wall defects are missed so that large numbers of women do not undergo unnecessary testing for false-positive results. In general, a woman who has a high AFP level is referred for high-resolution ultrasonography, which can determine the presence or absence of a neural tube defect with great reliability, as well as detect other defects, such as omphalocele and gastroschisis. When a high maternal serum AFP level is unexplained, there remains an increased risk for prematurity and late fetal death. Maternal serum AFP screening detects about 85% of cases of open fetal neural tube defects, including about 80% of fetuses with open spina bifida and 90% of those with anencephaly. A combination of AFP screening and ultrasound will detect more than 99% of anencephaly.

Some years after the association between neural tube defects and elevated AFP was reported, investigators noted the association between low maternal serum AFP and fetal chromosome abnormalities. Using the maternal serum AFP alone, about 20% of all fetuses with Down syndrome could be detected prenatally. During the past several years, other serum analytes have been reported to improve detection of chromosome abnormalities, in particular Down syndrome. The most useful is hCG, which is elevated in pregnancies of fetuses with Down syndrome. The addition of the serum analyte unconjugated estriol has helped reduce the false-positive rate and detect trisomy 18. With the use of all three markers, the overall detection rate for Down syndrome is 60%; this rate increases with advancing maternal age to approximately 75–90%. This screening method, if applied on a population basis, could reduce the incidence of amniocentesis in women older than 35 years; at present, however, serum screening misses a number of affected pregnancies. Amniocentesis therefore remains the "gold standard" for women of advanced maternal age.

The use of additional serum markers in the first trimester is being explored as a means of providing even earlier identification of mothers who have an increased risk for Down syndrome. These markers combined with first-trimester ultrasound may offer additional options for anxious families.

Much effort has been devoted to the isolation of fetal cells in the maternal circulation. In pregnancy, small numbers of nucleated fetal red blood cells enter the maternal circulation and can be separated by sorting techniques. Once perfected, this procedure would allow determination of fetal chromosome abnormalities and some DNA diagnostic testing in the very early stages of pregnancy without the use of invasive testing.

In Utero Fetal Treatment

Technologies for detection of fetal abnormalities have greatly exceeded our abilities to treat the fetus successfully. However, there have been numerous successful attempts at treating various conditions, and these are likely to increase in the coming years. Most of the conditions for which treatment can be considered are rare and, if untreated, the usual outcome is fetal or neonatal death. Fetal treatment modalities are of several types, and the availability of these treatments underscores the need for early and accurate prenatal diagnosis.

Drugs. Occasionally, medications given to the mother can effectively treat a fetal condition. For example, in the fetus with supraventricular tachycardia, digitalization of the mother may convert the arrhythmia. Other antiarrhythmic agents have been tried with some success. Treatment of the mother with massive doses of vitamin B_{12} has been effective in prenatally detectable vitamin B_{12}–responsive methylmalonic aciduria. There are several other rare examples of treatment of this general type.

Transfusion. Fetal anemia is a common cause of hydrops fetalis and fetal death. Fetal anemia can result from several causes, the most common of which is fetal–maternal hemorrhage. Another relatively recently identified cause is hemolytic anemia secondary to maternal infection with human parvovirus B19. These fetuses are usually identified by ultrasound as having fetal ascites or hydrops. Direct transfusion of packed maternal cells via fetal vessels may be lifesaving. Such techniques are used only in settings with specialists highly experienced in reproductive genetics and fetal–maternal medicine.

Removal of amniotic fluid. Severe polyhydramnios may occur in a variety of clinical settings, and usually removal of fluid is indicated only for reasons of maternal comfort. Polyhydramnios is frequent in monozygotic twin pregnancies affected with twin-to-twin transfusion syndrome. When severe, this condition is lethal for both twins. Several centers have reported improved survival rates with repeated removals of amniotic fluid from around the polyhydramniotic twin. Reasons for the success of this treatment are not entirely clear.

In utero transplantation. Bone marrow transplantation has been tried in the treatment of several genetic disorders in children. Unfortunately, transplantation after birth is often unsuccessful because of rejection phenomena. In addition, the transplantation may not have the desired effect because damage, especially to the central nervous system, may be irreversible. Before 22 weeks' gestation, the fetus lacks immunocompetence and therefore might be considered an ideal target for selected efforts in transplantation. In theory, intraperitoneal transfusion of stem cells could genetically reconstitute fetuses affected with α-thalassemia, various mucopolysaccharidoses, and several other rare genetic disorders. To date, international attempts at in utero stem cell transplantation have been infrequent and successes rare.

Fetal surgery. During the past several years, several centers have attempted direct surgical intervention for selected conditions—specifically, hydrocephalus, obstructive uropathy, diaphragmatic hernia, and, most recently, meningomyelocele. Treatment for fetal hydrocephalus has been abandoned with the recognition that many infants with prenatally detected hydrocephalus have severe abnormalities in general brain development. Thus, even when their hydrocephalus is treated, mental deficiency remains. Surgical approaches for fetuses with urinary tract obstruction have included the placement of catheters into the fetal bladder to relieve distal obstruction and open surgery with the direct placement of small catheters into the ureters. Although these techniques are associated with significant morbidity and fetal mortality, there are several long-term survivors with good renal function. Carefully controlled and long-term studies are required to assess the efficacy of these heroic interventions, which may be appropriate in selected circumstances.

REFERENCES

Cassidy SB, Allanson J (editors): *Management of Genetic Syndrome.* John Wiley & Sons, 2001.

Curry CJR: Pregnancy loss, stillbirth, and neonatal death. A guide for the pediatrician. Pediatr Clin North Am 1992;39:157.

De Grouchy J, Turleau C: *Clinical Atlas of Human Chromosomes,* 2nd ed. John Wiley & Sons, 1984.

Dieck D et al: Prenatal diagnosis of congenital parvovirus B19 infection: value of serological and PCR techniques in maternal and fetal serum. Prenat Diagn 1999;19:1119.

Ferencz C, Boughman JA: Congenital heart disease in adolescents and adults. Teratology, genetics, and recurrence risks. Cardiol Clin 1993;11:557.

Gorlin RJ et al: *Syndromes of the Head and Neck,* 3rd ed. Oxford University Press, 1990.

Graham JM Jr (editor): *Smith's Recognizable Patterns of Human Deformation,* 2nd ed. Saunders, 1988.

Hall JG et al: *Handbook of Normal Physical Measurements.* Oxford University Press, 1989.

Hanson JW: Teratogenic agents. In: Emery AE, Rimion DL (editors): *Principles and Practices of Medical Genetics,* 3rd ed. Churchill Livingstone, 1996.

Harper PS: *Practical Genetic Counselling.* Butterworth, Heinmann, 1998.

Harrison MR, Golbus MS, Filly RA: *The Unborn Patient: Prenatal Diagnosis and Treatment,* 2nd ed. Saunders, 1990.

Jones KL: *Smith's Recognizable Patterns of Human Malformations,* 5th ed. Saunders, 1997.

McDonald-McGinn DM et al: The 22q11.2 deletion: screening, diagnostic workup, and outcome of results; report on 181 patients. Genet Test 1997;1:99.

McKusick VA: *Mendelian Inheritance in Man: A Catalog of Human Genes and Genetic Disorders,* 12th ed. Johns Hopkins University Press, 1998.

Nigro G et al: Prenatal diagnosis of fetal cytomegalovirus infection after primary or recurrent maternal infection. Obstet Gynecol 1999;94;909.

Nora JJ, Nora AH: Update on counseling the family with a first degree relative with a congenital heart defect. Am J Med Genet 1988;29:137.

Pelz J, Arendt V, Kunze J: Computer assisted diagnosis of malformation syndromes: an evaluation of three databases (LDDB, POSSUM, and SYNDROC). Am J Med Genet 1996;63:257.

Rimoin DL: Molecular defects in the chondrodysplasias. Am J Med Genet 1996;63:106.

Seaver LH, Hoyme HE: Teratology in pediatric practice. Pediatr Clin North Am 1992;39:111.

Shepard TH: *Catalog of Teratogenic Agents,* 9th ed. Johns Hopkins University Press, 1998.

Sherer DM, Manning FA: First-trimester nuchal translucency screening for fetal aneuploidy. Am J Perinatol 1999;16:103.

Spencer K: Second trimester prenatal screening for Down's syndrome using alpha-fetoprotein and free beta hCG; a seven year review. Br J Obstet Gynaecol 1999;106:1287.

Spranger J: International classification of osteochondrodysplasias. The International Working Group on Constitutional Diseases of Bone. Eur J Pediatr 1992;15:407.

Stevenson RE et al: *X-Linked Mental Retardation.* Oxford University Press, 2000.

Thompson MW et al: *Thompson & Thompson Genetics in Medicine,* 5th ed. Saunders, 1991.

Warren FT, Nelson DL: Advances in molecular analysis of Fragile X syndrome. JAMA 1994;271:536.

Wigglesworth JS: *Perinatal Pathology.* Saunders, 1984.

Winter RM et al: *The Malformed Fetus and Stillbirth: A Diagnostic Approach.* John Wiley & Sons, 1988.

A Clinical Approach to Inborn Errors of Metabolism

John Christodoulou, MB, BS, PhD, FRACP, CGHGSA

Inborn errors of metabolism are genetic diseases that disrupt normal metabolic function. Although the primary biochemical defect might not be known, there must be some knowledge of the metabolic abnormalities associated with a disease for it to have been included in this group of conditions. This chapter describes the common clinical situations in which inborn errors should be considered and shows that the clinical recognition of these conditions does not depend on sophisticated biochemical analysis. Once laboratory corroboration of a suspected inborn error is obtained, optimal treatment often requires an uncommon degree of diagnostic precision, usually at the biochemical level.

More than 450 biochemically diverse inborn errors have been identified, but despite their diversity, these diseases share a number of features. First, most patients with inborn errors present clinically with one of five general phenotypes (Table 6–1). Although the five major phenotypes are a useful clinical guide, there are other clinical presentations, and some are virtually specific to a single disease or group of disorders; a few of the most important of these distinctive phenotypes are listed at the end of Table 6–1. Second, almost all inborn errors are recessive in inheritance, and most of these conditions map to one of the 22 autosomes; unless otherwise stated, the diseases reviewed in this chapter are assumed to be autosomal recessive. Third, specific and effective treatment of inborn errors often is made possible by our understanding of their biochemical basis. Because inborn errors are genetic diseases, families with affected children can be made aware of the risk of recurrence through genetic counseling. In many instances, presymptomatic treatment of affected relatives, carrier testing, and prenatal diagnosis can be offered.

Which Patients Might Have an Inborn Error?

The critical step in diagnosing any disease is considering the possibility that the patient has the disorder. For the inborn errors of metabolism, this step is particularly difficult for most physicians because few will have encountered a patient with one of these uncommon conditions. Nevertheless, the patient or parents of a patient with an uncommon disease do not care about the rarity of the condition; they are interested only in correct diagnosis and treatment. These two difficulties can be largely reconciled if the physician recognizes that there may be a genetic basis to the patient's illness and that the clinical presentation is one commonly associated with an inherited metabolic disease (Table 6–1).

Genetic Evidence Suggesting an Inborn Error

There are two genetic clues that should make one aware of the need to exclude a genetic disorder. First, a history of a similarly affected sibling or other affected relative strongly suggests a genetic disease. However, because the great majority of genetic metabolic diseases are autosomal recessive in their inheritance, there usually will not be any history of other affected members, apart from siblings. Second, if the parents are consanguineous (or if they come from the same small town or village or have the same surname), an autosomal recessive disease must be carefully excluded. Although some cultures attach a stigma to consanguineous relationships, marriages between cousins are commonplace in many ethnic groups. Marriages between first cousins almost doubles the risk of having a child affected with a genetic disease, from approximately 2% to approximately 4%, an increase due entirely to autosomal recessive diseases.

Less often, metabolic genetic diseases are inherited in an X-linked or autosomal dominant manner or manifest maternal inheritance. Disorders of the latter type are due to a mutation in the mitochondrial genome because only the mitochondria from the ovum—not the sperm—contribute to the mitochondrial DNA of the zygote, and mutations in the mitochondrial DNA are thus passed from one generation to the next strictly through the maternal line.

■ THE FIVE COMMON PRESENTATIONS OF INBORN ERRORS

There are five common clinical presentations (Table 6–1) that always should suggest an inborn error of metabolism. An important sixth category consists of disorders

Table 6–1. Common Clinical Presentations of Inborn Errors of Metabolism[1]

Encephalopathy
  Acute encephalopathy
    Diseases of small diffusible molecules
      Amino acid disorders (maple syrup urine disease)
      Organic acid disorders (methylmalonic aciduria)
      Fatty acid oxidation defects (medium-chain acyl-CoA dehydrogenase deficiency)
      Hyperammonemias (ornithine transcarbamylase deficiency)
      Lactate and mitochondrial disorders (cytochrome oxidase deficiency)
      Encephalopathy with seizures (nonketotic hyperglycinemia)
  Chronic encephalopathy
    Diseases of small diffusible molecules
    Diseases of organelles
      Mitochondrial disorders: defects in pyruvate and electron transport bioenergetics
        Electron transport chain defects (cytochrome c oxidase deficiency)
        Defects of pyruvate metabolism (pyruvate dehydrogenase deficiency)
      Lysosomal storage disorders
        Mucopolysaccharidoses (Hurler disease)
        Glycoproteinoses (α-mannosidosis)
        Gangliosidoses (G$_{M2}$ gangliosidosis)
        Other sphingolipidoses (Gaucher disease)
        Leukodystrophies (metachromatic leukodystrophy)
      Peroxisomal disorders
        Defects of peroxisomal biogenesis & β-oxidation (Zellweger syndrome)
        Rhizomelic chondrodysplasia punctata
        X-linked adrenoleukodystrophy
        Other defects of single peroxisomal enzymes (oxalosis)
    Disorders of protein glycosylation—includes enzyme defects localized to
      Cytosol: carbohydrate-deficient glycoprotein syndrome types Ia and Ib
      Golgi body disorders: carbohydrate-deficient glycoprotein syndrome type II
      Endoplasmic reticulum: carbohydrate-deficient glycoprotein syndrome types Ic and V

Diffuse hepatocellular disease
  Acute or chronic liver disease
    Defects of carbohydrate metabolism (galactosemia)
    Defects of amino acid metabolism (tyrosinemia)
    Defects of metal transport (Wilson disease)
    Defects of protease inhibitors (α1-antitrypsin deficiency)

Myopathy
  Skeletal myopathy
    Acute rhabdomyolysis (muscle phosphorylase deficiency)
    Chronic myopathy (mitochondrial electron transport chain defects; fatty acid metabolism defects)
  Cardiomyopathy
    Lysosomal storage disorders (Pompe disease: α-glucosidase deficiency)
    Disorders of fatty acid metabolism (long-chain 3-hydroxyacyl-CoA dehydrogenase deficiency)

Renal tubular disease
  Glomerular tubular disease
    Lysosomal storage disorder (cystinosis)
    Enzyme defect (oxalosis)
  Transport defects
    Defective transport of individual or groups of similar molecules (cystinuria)

Disorders with distinctive phenotypes
  Hepatomegaly without dementia
    Defects of gluconeogenesis (glucose-6-phosphatase deficiency)
    Lysosomal storage disorders (Gaucher disease non-neuronopathic variant)
  "Cerebral palsy" without a history of perinatal distress
    Five different enzymopathies (Lesch–Nyhan syndrome [HPRT] deficiency)
  Stroke or thrombosis
    Increased risk of thrombosis (homocystinuria)
    Other diverse conditions (MELAS syndrome)
  Disorders causing facial dysmorphism or congenital malformations
    Due to teratogenic metabolites (maternal phenyl-ketonuria)
    Impairment of cellular bioenergetics (pyruvate dehydrogenase deficiency)
  Premature atherosclerosis
    Defects of lipoprotein metabolism (familial hyper-cholesterolemia)
  Menkes' disease
    A disorder of copper metabolism with a unique phenotype

[1] Examples are shown in parentheses. CoA = coenzyme A; HPRT = hypoxanthine phosphoribosyltransferase deficiency; MELAS = mitochondrial myopathy, encephalopathy, lactic acidosis, and stroke-like episodes.

with distinctive phenotypes that ought invariably to suggest an inborn error (Table 6–1).

ACUTE ENCEPHALOPATHY: DISEASES OF SMALL MOLECULES

Encephalopathy is by far the most common clinical manifestation of inborn errors of metabolism. The encephalopathy can be acute, intermittent, chronic, or even nonprogressive, but only the inborn errors of small (i.e., diffusible) molecules cause acute encephalopathy (Figure 6–1). Patients with an acute encephalopathy most often are newborns or infants who have a *severe* enzyme defect that results in the accumulation of toxic metabolites early in life, although the small molecule diseases can cause acute encephalopathy at any age (Figure 6–1). Consequently, the small molecule defects must be excluded in any patient, even adults, with unexplained acute encephalopathy.

The Classic Clinical Presentation of Acute Encephalopathy in the Newborn & Infant

Acute encephalopathy due to genetic metabolic disease usually results from the accumulation in the brain, to a critical level, of a small diffusible metabolite or substrate, or from the deficiency of an essential product or transport process. Sometimes, the substrate accumulation can inhibit other metabolic pathways to produce unexpected pathophysiologic and clinical effects. Typically, the affected neonate will be well for several days to a week after birth because the offending metabolite takes this time, or longer, to accumulate to toxic levels. Such infants are frequently discharged from the newborn nursery, apparently healthy, only to return, sometimes within 24 hours, with poor feeding, vomiting, lethargy, irritability, seizures, and, if metabolic acidosis is also present, tachypnea and hyperpnea. Cerebral edema is a frequent consequence of these conditions. Not surprisingly, given the disruption of metabolism, failure to thrive is invariably present in newborns and infants with "small" molecule metabolic diseases that are severe enough to cause encephalopathy early in life. Hepatomegaly often is also present. The most common alternative diagnoses are infection, perinatal hypoxia, trauma, intoxications, malformations, and malignancies. Failure to diagnose and treat the small molecule inborn errors and reverse the acute encephalopathy will result in a child with severe neurologic damage or death.

PATHOGENESIS

Accumulation of toxic metabolites. The intoxicating molecules that accumulate in inborn errors include amino acids, organic acids, fatty acids, and ammonium (Figure 6–1). Most small molecule diseases affect "housekeeping"

enzymes in catabolic pathways. Consequently, catabolic events, such as infections, will increase the amount of substrate delivered to the mutant enzyme. Other small molecule diseases are due to defects in the transport of small molecules across cell membranes. Although the enzymes implicated in these diseases usually are found in most or all tissues, they are generally most active in the liver, and hepatomegaly and signs of generalized hepatic dysfunction, in particular increased serum glutamic-oxaloacetic transaminase, or aspartate aminotransferase, and abnormalities of clotting function, are often seen. The involvement of the brain in the disease process reflects its vulnerability to metabolic disturbance and not necessarily the fact that the enzymatic activity is greater in the brain.

Product deficiency. The most significant group of disorders that result from product deficiency are those that impair energy production, i.e., the diseases due to defects in pyruvate metabolism or the function of the mitochondrial electron transport system. In contrast to most inborn errors that lead to acute encephalopathy, these conditions probably produce most of their pathophysiologies, not from metabolite accumulation, but from intracellular depletion of the product of energy pathways, adenosine triphosphate (ATP).

CATABOLIC STRESS INITIATES SMALL MOLECULE METABOLIC CRISES

Inborn errors frequently present in the newborn period because this is a time of substantial catabolism; the normal newborn generally loses weight for several days before anabolism dominates. The catabolic breakdown of protein and fat results in increased delivery of the metabolite to the pathway blocked by the mutation and consequent elevations of the metabolite levels. Infants who escape a newborn presentation (often because they have slightly more residual enzyme activity, with a less severe metabolic block) may present after the postnatal period, when they are exposed to increased protein intake (e.g., by a switch from breast milk to formula) or to catabolic stress leading to breakdown of body protein due to infection, starvation, or trauma (including surgery). Moreover, most of the encephalopathic metabolic crises that periodically affect even well-treated patients with inborn errors are precipitated by catabolic stress. The parents of older patients often recognize subtle signs (such as changes in behavior) of impending metabolic decompensation early enough to prevent progression of the episode to acute encephalopathy.

Acute Encephalopathy in Children or Adults Due to Small Molecule Inborn Errors

A child or adult with a small molecule disease may have good health for years or decades and then unexpectedly

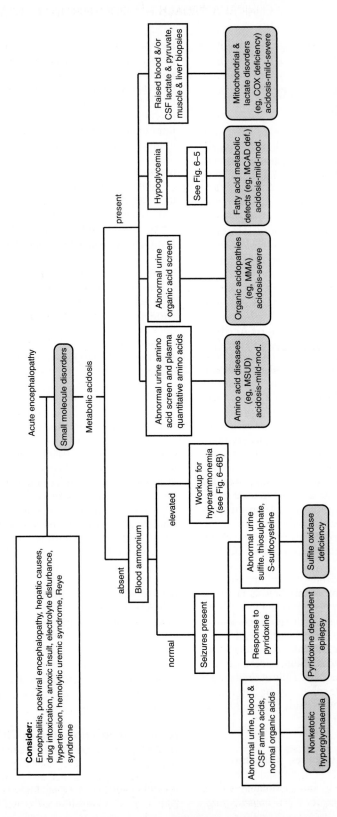

Figure 6–1. Biochemical evaluation of inborn errors causing acute encephalopathy. The five types of small molecules associated with metabolic defects that cause inborn errors are shown, with the laboratory studies required to identify each disease type. Because the clinical presentation of these disorders is often similar, a series of screening investigations (highlighted in the boxes) should be performed in all such children. CSF = cerebral spinal fluid; mod. = moderate; COX = cytochrome c oxidase; MCAD = medium chain acyl-CoA dehydrogenase; MMA = methylmalonic acidemia; MSUD = maple syrup urine disease.

manifest the metabolic defect, presenting with an acute encephalopathy. These patients have sufficient residual enzyme activity to catabolize the substrate when they are in good health, but in the face of a catabolic stress, the residual enzyme activity is insufficient to prevent substrate accumulation. How these patients escape the metabolic crisis in the catabolic newborn period or on other occasions in childhood is unknown, particularly because the later episodes are invariably precipitated by catabolic events, such as viral infections, that the patient tolerated previously without developing a metabolic crisis. One example is the **intermittent variant of maple syrup urine disease (MSUD),** in which the child is biochemically normal except when challenged by the catabolism of intercurrent illness, at which time ataxia and decreased consciousness, due to accumulation of the branch-chain α-ketoacids, develop.

Occasionally a patient with a disease of this type will not present until adult life. For example, the initial presentation of the X-linked urea cycle disorder **ornithine transcarbamylase deficiency** in female carriers of the disease may be after they have given birth, a time of great catabolism. Older patients with small molecule diseases may present with ataxia, disorientation or frank psychosis, and loss of consciousness.

The intermittent or late-onset forms of the small molecule inborn errors are commonly misdiagnosed as **Reye syndrome** because of encephalopathy, cerebral edema, and mild liver dysfunction (increases in aspartate aminotransferase with fatty degeneration of the liver, hypoglycemia, and hyperammonemia). Thus, the diagnosis of Reye syndrome should be made only after the exclusion of small molecule inborn errors.

Inborn errors can affect adults in other ways:

- Disorders resulting in reduced fertility in the affected individual, e.g., galactosemia (direct effect on the ovary) and homocystinuria (possible increased early fetal loss)
- Disorders exacerbated by pregnancy, e.g., glycogen storage disease type I (deterioration in renal function) or type III (worsening cardiomyopathy), cystinosis, and homocystinuria (increased risk of thrombosis)
- Disorders in the fetus that can compromise the health of its carrier mother, e.g., a fetus with long-chain 3-hydroxyacyl-coA dehydrogenase deficiency (see section "Fatty Acid Oxidation Defects" can cause the acute fatty liver of pregnancy or hemolysis, elevated liver enzymes, low platelets (HELLP) syndrome in the carrier mother

Laboratory Studies to Exclude Small Molecule Diseases

Any newborn or infant with acute encephalopathy must quickly undergo investigations to exclude genetic metabolic conditions because aggressive treatment is required to minimize permanent brain damage. The difficulty in remembering to consider genetic metabolic diseases is well illustrated here: unresponsive and seizing newborns are common, and in most such neonates, the cause is not a genetic metabolic defect. Nevertheless, inborn errors must be excluded quickly by initiating the investigations outlined in Figure 6–1. Despite the variety of metabolic defects that can produce acute encephalopathy in the newborn and infant, the clinical presentations often are so similar that it is not possible to make a specific diagnosis without the aid of laboratory studies (Figure 6–1).

The Small Molecule Inborn Errors that Cause Acute Encephalopathy

AMINO ACIDOPATHIES

One group of inborn errors results from abnormalities in the metabolism or transport of amino acids. Amino acids are essential for protein synthesis, but once anabolic needs are met, the surplus is degraded and used for energy. Intake of the amino acid in excess of anabolic needs and at a rate that exceeds the capacity of the pathway affected by the mutation will lead to accumulation of the toxic metabolite. A classic disease of amino acid catabolism that causes acute encephalopathy is MSUD, the unusual urinary odor deriving from the accumulation of urinary α-ketoacids due to the deficiency of the α-ketoacid dehydrogenase (Figure 6–2). The increased levels of the α-ketoacids rather than of the amino acids are the cause of the encephalopathy; for this reason, this disease can be regarded as an amino acidopathy or an organic acidopathy. Patients present with the classic acute encephalopathy phenotype described above. Ketoacidosis (the three accumulating branch-chain ketoacids are shown in Figure 6–2) is the predominant biochemical abnormality, and occasionally patients are hypoglycemic. A widely used but nonspecific test that detects the presence of ketoacids, including those accumulating in MSUD (Figure 6–2) is the 2,4-dinitrophenylhydrazine test, which also can detect ketonuria of any cause. Although screening tests of this type are of historical significance, the diagnosis of inborn errors causing encephalopathy requires the specific tests indicated in Figure 6–1.

ORGANIC ACIDOSES

A defect in an enzyme that degrades an organic acid will result in accumulation of the acid, often producing acidosis. The major clinical difference between amino and organic acidopathies is the metabolic acidosis that often results from the accumulation of organic acids in organic acidopathies. An organic acidopathy should be considered in any patient with a metabolic acidosis. The acidosis causes hyperpnea, a compensatory physiological response. Most organic acidopathies are caused by enzyme defects

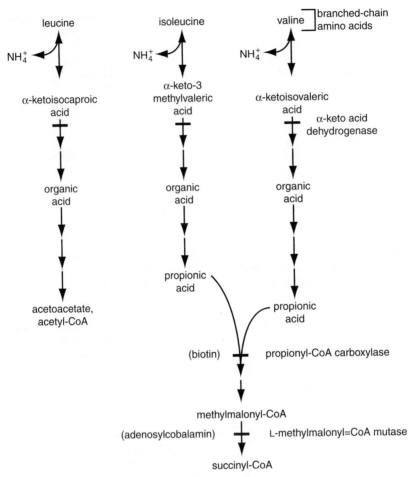

Figure 6–2. The enzyme defects in maple syrup urine disease and the organic acidopathies propionic acidemia and methylmalonic aciduria. Defects of many of the enzymes in these pathways cause organic acidopathies, all of which are autosomal recessive in their inheritance. The branch-chain amino acids are leucine, isoleucine, and valine. The relevant α-keto acids in this context are simply the amino acids from which the amino group has been removed. Biotin is a cofactor of propionyl-CoA carboxylase, and adenosylcobalamin, a vitamin B$_{12}$ derivative, is a cofactor of methylmalonyl-CoA mutase.

in the catabolic pathways of amino acids, as shown in the later steps of the breakdown of the carbon chain of the branched-chain amino acids (Figure 6–2). The different catabolic pathways of the various amino acids result in the formation of many different organic acid intermediates. Two classic inborn errors of organic acid metabolism are due to defects in enzymes active in the metabolism of propionic acid (Figure 6–2), namely propionyl-CoA carboxylase (a defect of that causes **propionic acidemia**), and L-methylmalonyl-CoA mutase (whose deficiency leads to **methylmalonic acidemia**). Propionic acid is a catabolic product of the amino acids isoleucine, valine, threonine,

and methionine; odd-chain fatty acids; and cholesterol. In addition to having the classic encephalopathic phenotype described above and a metabolic acidosis, patients with either of these enzymopathies often have moderate to severe hyperammonemia, the result of a secondary inhibition of the urea cycle by the accumulating organic acids. Less commonly seen are hypoglycemia, leukopenia, and thrombocytopenia.

The anion gap. A clue to the presence of organic acid accumulation is an increase in the anion gap (Figure 6–3). A modest increase in the anion gap (up to 20 mEq/L)

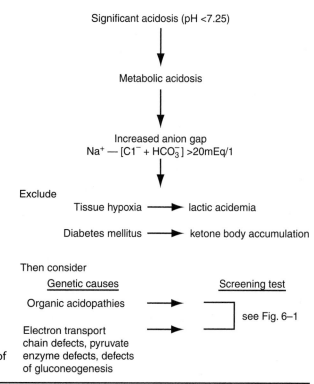

Figure 6–3. Identification and investigation of an increased anion gap in metabolic acidosis.

usually is not significant in a patient who is seriously ill from any cause, but an increase greater than 20 mEq/L requires that organic acid defects be excluded. Of course, most patients with an increased anion gap do not have an inborn error of metabolism but rather an acquired acidosis from lactic acid accumulation secondary to hypoxia or ketone body accumulation (ketoacidosis), as occurs in diabetes mellitus. However, a normal anion gap does not exclude significant lactic acidemia because it can remain normal until blood lactate exceeds approximately 6 mmol/L.

FATTY ACID OXIDATION DEFECTS

A genetic defect of fatty acid β-oxidation (Figure 6–4) should be suspected in any child with fasting coma or lethargy and vomiting associated with fasting hypoglycemia; acute hepatomegaly is often noted. Alternatively, skeletal or cardiomyopathy may be the predominant clinical feature (see the following section on myopathy). A small but important proportion (in the order of 1–2%) of **sudden infant death syndrome (SIDS)** also can result from defects in fatty acid oxidation, and this group of metabolic disorders must be excluded in families with a history of SIDS or in patients in which near-SIDS has occurred. As a consequence of prolonged fasting, hepatic

glycogen stores become depleted, resulting in a shift by brain and muscle to increased use of the fatty acids liberated by lipolysis. Ketone bodies, which can be used directly by brain and muscle, are the product of fatty acid β-oxidation (Figure 6–4), but the decrease in their production in this group of diseases leads to hypoketotic hypoglycemia. Therefore, defects of fatty acid oxidation usually are exposed by fasting, a time when brain and muscle normally rely on ketone bodies as an alternative energy substrates. Because there are a number of other metabolic causes of hypoglycemia, a diagnostic algorithm (Figure 6–5) can be helpful in arriving at a diagnosis. It cannot be stressed how important it is to collect all the appropriate samples during the hypoglycemic episode to maxamize the chance making the diagnosis rapidly and efficiently.

Impaired fatty acid oxidation may result from a deficiency of the very-long-chain, long-chain, medium-chain, or short-chain acyl-CoA dehydrogenases or in any one of several other mitochondrial enzymes or transport functions essential for the transport of carnitine or long-chain fatty acid across the plasma membrane or one of the mitochondrial membranes (Figure 6–4). The most common defect in fatty acid oxidation, with an incidence (*text continues on page 230*)

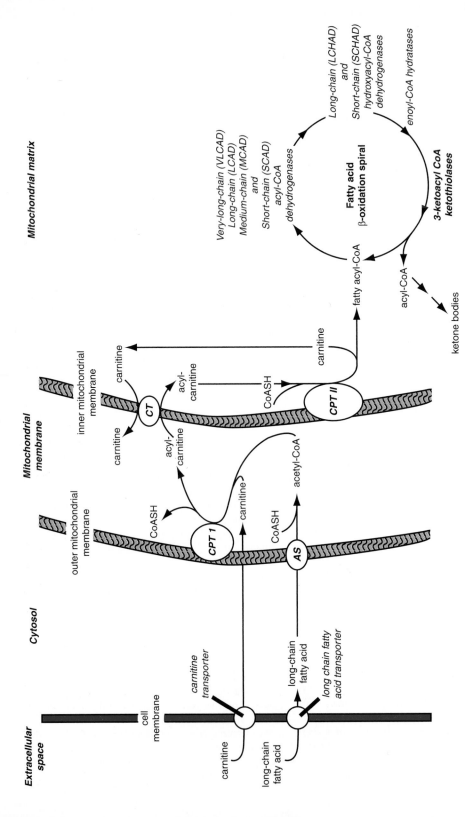

Figure 6–4. Transport and metabolism of fatty acids. To cross the mitochondrial membrane, long-chain fatty acids must be ligated to carnitine by carnitine palmitoyltransferase I (CPT I) and transferred by a translocase. Carnitine palmitoyltransferase II (CPT II) releases the acyl group from carnitine into the mitochondrial matrix. Medium- and short-chain fatty acids can freely enter the mitochondria and do not require the carnitine system. Fatty acids are oxidized in a cycle that removes one acetyl-CoA moiety per turn. Dehydrogenases specific to very-long-, long-, medium-, and short-chain fatty acids catalyze the first reaction. Defects have been found in many of the transporters and enzymes shown. Ketone bodies are formed in the liver from acetyl-CoA moieties. All defects of fatty acid oxidation are inherited as autosomal recessive diseases. AS = acyl-CoA synthetase; CT = carnitine-acylcarnitine translocase.

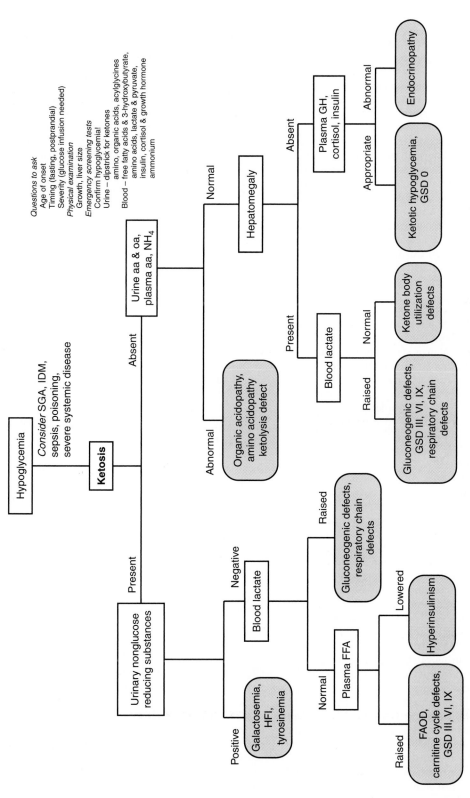

Figure 6–5. Diagnostic algorithm for patients presenting with hypoglycemia. In determining the etiology, it is important to consider a number of questions, shown in the boxed panel. In addition, it is essential that a number of biochemical investigations are undertaken at the time of the hypoglycemic episode. It is sometimes necessary to subsequently perform other investigations to confirm the diagnosis, e.g., controlled fasting study, fasting, and/or postprandial glucagon stimulation test. aa = amino acids; FAOD = fatty acid β-oxidation defect; FFA = free fatty acids; GH = growth hormone; GSD = glycogen storage disease; HFI = hereditary fructose intolerance; IDM = infant of a diabetic mother; NH$_4^+$ = ammonium; oa = organic acids; SGA = small for gestational age.

of approximately 1 per 10,000–20,000 births, is **medium-chain acyl-CoA dehydrogenase (MCAD) deficiency.** The key diagnostic features of this disease, in addition to recurrent episodes of fasting hypoglycemia that usually first occur before age 2 years, are inadequate ketosis relative to the level of total serum free fatty acid levels (although some patients may produce moderate amounts of ketones in the fasting state), reduced levels of carnitine in body fluids, and abnormal fatty acid metabolites (organic acids, acylcarnitines, and acylglycines) in urine, detected by organic acid screening, acylglycine analysis, and plasma acylcarnitine analysis (Figure 6–1). Treatment consists of the avoidance of prolonged starvation. The value of a low-fat diet is uncertain. Carnitine administration may be beneficial because the increased formation of acylcarnitines (Figure 6–4), an enhancement of a normal reaction, may augment the urinary excretion of toxic fatty acyl-CoA intermediates.

HYPERAMMONEMIA

An elevated blood ammonium level mandates that an inborn error of metabolism be excluded as a matter of urgency because ammonium is a potent neurotoxin. Moderate to severe hyperammonemia often is seen in the organic acidoses and fatty acid oxidation defects, reflecting a secondary inhibition of the urea cycle by the accumulating metabolites of those disorders. Genetic defects of ureagenesis (Figure 6–6A) most often present in the first week of life. The most common such defect is **ornithine transcarbamylase (OTC) deficiency,** an X-linked disorder that often manifests in carrier females and is generally very severe in affected males. Affected infants are well for the first day of life but then develop acute encephalopathy, often within 24–48 hours, but sometimes not for as long as a week. Figure 6–6B provides an algorithm to aid in the rapid diagnosis of specific metabolic disorders causing hyperammonemia.

Two clinical clues of hyperammonemia in neonates are **respiratory alkalosis,** due to stimulation of the respiratory center by ammonium, and **pulmonary hemorrhage,** of unknown mechanism but possibly related to an abnormality in nitric oxide homeostasis. Late-diagnosed survivors are invariably neurologically impaired and are at risk of further encephalopathic episodes after excessive protein intake or during catabolic periods. Long-term treatment is directed to reducing protein intake, giving urea cycle intermediates to replenish the cycle (e.g., arginine administration in patients with argininosuccinate synthase and lyase deficiencies; Fig. 6–6A), and providing alternative pathways of ammonium excretion. Sodium benzoate and sodium phenylbutyrate are two such compounds, which are conjugated to glycine and glutamine, respectively, the latter of which must be synthesised de novo to maintain normal body levels, thereby consuming ammonium.

An acquired form of newborn hyperammonemia of unknown cause, **transient hyperammonemia of the newborn,** is observed in premature or low-birth-weight newborns, often in the presence of pulmonary disease. The other major clue to the diagnosis is the early postnatal onset of the hyperammonemia and encephalopathy, usually within 24 hours of birth, in contrast to the urea cycle defects. The elevation of ammonium can be as high as that seen in the most severe urea cycle defects (up to 2500 μM). There are no specific biochemical markers. The condition must be treated in the short term like a urea cycle defect (see below).

LACTIC ACIDOSIS: DEFECTS IN THREE CLASSES OF ENZYMES

Inherited defects of pyruvate metabolism or of the mitochondrial electron transport chain should be suspected in any infant with the combination of acute encephalopathy and lactic acidosis, if poor tissue perfusion due to cardiac or pulmonary disease or some other cause of shock can be excluded as the acquired cause of increased lactate (Figure 6–7). Three classes of inherited diseases may be associated with encephalopathy (acute or chronic) and elevated levels of lactate. Any metabolic defect severe enough to cause acute encephalopathy also usually will be severe enough to elevate the lactate to levels that will cause metabolic acidosis and an increased anion gap, although occasionally the acidosis may be mild and the anion gap normal.

Class I: Disorders of pyruvate & citric acid cycle enzymes. Defects in enzymes that link glycolysis with the citric acid cycle, such as pyruvate dehydrogenase (PDH in Figure 6–7) or pyruvate carboxylase (PC), or enzymopathies of the citric acid cycle itself usually are associated with severe impairment of neurological function. Pyruvate dehydrogenase or PC deficiency must always be considered in the presence of elevated blood (or cerebrospinal fluid [CSF]) lactate. A clue to these may be a normal lactate:pyruvate ratio and in some cases of PC deficiency an elevated plasma citrulline level. Defects in the enzymes of the citric acid cycle are suggested by metabolic acidosis, and urine organic acid screen will reveal the identity of the accumulating organic acid (e.g., fumarate in fumarase deficiency; Figure 6–7). Enzymatic assay is required to confirm the specific diagnosis.

Class II: Defects of gluconeogenesis. The second group is comprised of abnormalities in the enzymes of gluconeogenesis (Figure 6–7). Many of the reactions of glycolysis can be reversed for gluconeogenesis, but five enzymes are unique to gluconeogenesis: PC, phosphenolpyruvate carboxykinase, fructose 1,6 diphosphatase glycogen synthase, and glucose-6-phosphatase (Figure 6–7). Because gluconeogenesis (the formation of glucose from noncarbohydrate sources) is particularly important during fasting, the hypoglycemia that occurs

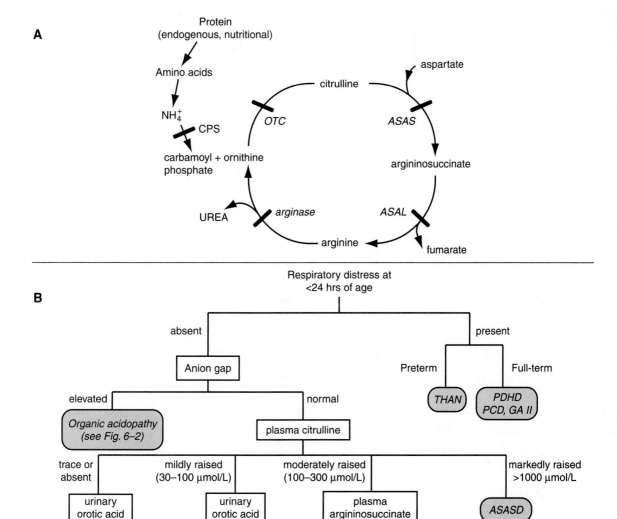

Figure 6–6. **A:** The urea cycle. The urea cycle converts ammonium, which is neurotoxic, to urea, which is nontoxic and excretable. In carbamoyl phosphate synthase (CPS) deficiency and ornithine transcarbamylase (OTC) deficiency, none of the amino acid intermediates of the cycle are increased. Citrullinemia is characteristic of argininosuccinate synthase (ASAS) deficiency, argininosuccinic aciduria of argininosuccinate lyase (ASAL) deficiency, and hyperargininemia of arginase deficiency. All defects of the urea cycle are autosomal recessive, except for OTC deficiency, which is X-linked recessive. OTC carrier females may be affected. *N*-acetylglutamate synthase (NAGS) generates *N*-acetylglutamate, which is a cofactor for CPS (not shown). **B:** Diagnostic algorithm for the hyperammonemic disorders. The hyperammonemic disorders can be biochemically distinguished by measuring the anion gap, plasma amino acids (including citrulline and argininosuccinate), and urinary orotic acid. ASALD = argininosuccinic acid lyase deficiency (argininosuccinic aciduria); ASASD = argininosuccinic acid synthase deficiency (citrullinemia); CPSD = carbamylphosphate synthase deficiency; GA II = glutaric aciduria type II; LPI = lysinuric protein intolerance; NAGSD = *N*-acetylglutamate synthase deficiency; OTCD = ornithine transcarbamoylase deficiency; PCD = pyruvate carboxylase deficiency; PDHD = pyruvate dehydrogenase deficiency; THAN = transient hyperammonemia of the newborn.

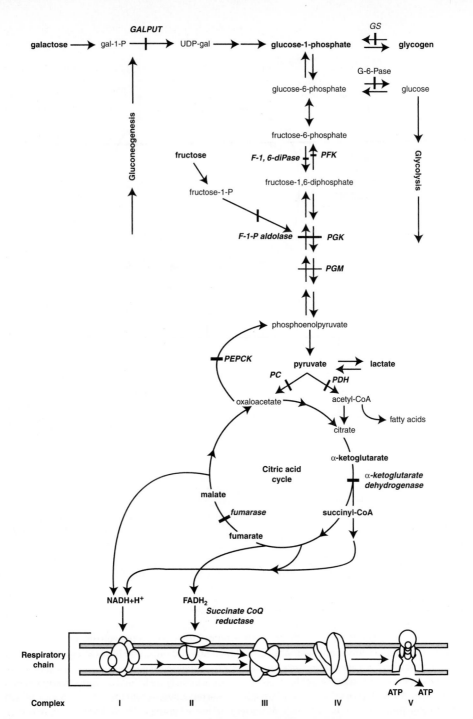

Figure 6–7. Inborn errors of energy metabolism. All of the defects shown are autosomal recessively inherited, except for deficiency of the E subunit of pyruvate dehydrogenase deficiency and phosphoglycerate kinase, which are X-linked, and defects in the mitochondrial DNA, which are maternally inherited. Pyruvate carboxylase (PC), phosphoenolpyruvate carboxykinase (PEPCK), fructose-1,6 diphosphatase (F-1,6-diPase), and glucose-6-phosphatase (G-6-Pase) are enzymes unique to gluconeogenesis. F-1-P = fructose-1-phosphate; FADH = flavin adenine dinucleotide reduced; GAH-3-P = glyceraldehyde-3-phosphate; Gal-1-P = galactose-1-phosphate; GALPUT = galactose-1-P uridyl transferase; GS = glycogen synthase; NADH = nicotinamide adenine dinucleotide reduced; PDH = pyruvate dehydrogenase; PFK = phosphofructokinase; PGK = phosphoglycerate kinase; PGM = phosphoglyceromutase; PK = pyruvate kinase; UDP-gal = uridine diphosphate-galactose.

with the defects of gluconeogenesis occurs after a relatively short period (6–12 hours) of fasting (although hypoglycemia is rare in PC deficiency). Impaired gluconeogenesis leads to the accumulation of pyruvate (the initial compound in the gluconeogenic pathway) and therefore of lactate (Figure 6–7). Acute hepatomegaly is present (not in glycogen synthase deficiency, however), partly due to lipid accumulation from the increased fatty acid synthesis that is secondary to increased formation of acetyl-CoA from pyruvate (Figure 6–7). Ketoacidosis is often present, perhaps reflecting increased formation of acetyl-CoA and ketone body synthesis.

The most common of these disorders is **glucose-6-phosphatase deficiency (von Gierke disease or type 1 glycogen storage disease).** These patients may present in the neonatal period with symptomatic hypoglycemia and pronounced hepatomegaly but only mild ketosis (a newborn with significant ketosis invariably has another serious genetic metabolic disease, such as an organic acid defect). Some patients present later in the first year with enlarged livers, failure to thrive, and doll-like facies. Despite the presence of hypoglycemia, these patients may be asymptomatic because their brains have adapted to the use of ketone bodies rather than of glucose as the primary source of energy. The diagnosis should be suspected on the basis of the hepatomegaly, increased fasting lactate (usually with acidosis), hyperlipidemia, hypercholesterolemia, and hyperuricemia and can be confirmed directly by enzyme assay of liver tissue. Indirect confirmation can be obtained by a glucose load test (resulting in a fall in the plasma lactate level) or the parenteral administration of glucagon; as shown in Figure 6–7, glycogen breakdown will increase the formation of glucose-6-phosphate and ultimately of lactate, but free glucose cannot be released in the face of this enzyme defect. Thus, the designation of von Gierke disease as a glycogen storage defect is actually misleading because it is really the prototypic gluconeogenic defect. Deficiencies of the other gluconeogenic enzymes share many of the features of glucose-6-phosphatase deficiency, although they may not be as dramatic in their presentation. Their diagnosis rests ultimately on specific enzyme assays.

Treatment of the gluconeogenic disorders during acute episodes centers on correction of hypoglycemia and acidosis. Long-term management aims to prevent hypoglycemia (and its attendant metabolic abnormalities) by frequent feeding, particularly of a slow release glucose preparation such as uncooked cornstarch. With good metabolic control, the biochemical abnormalities return toward normal, and growth is improved. The long-term prognosis is reasonably good, but hepatomas and glomerular insufficiency may develop in von Gierke disease.

Class III: Disorders of mitochondrial respiratory chain proteins. The proteins of the respiratory chain (Figure 6–7) mediate energy production by mitochon-

dria. Genetic abnormalities of these polypeptides may be associated with severe lactic acidosis and encephalopathy early in life, whereas less severe defects in electron transport can lead to chronic encephalopathy and other neurologic disturbances. This entire group of diseases is described below (see the section on encephalopathy due to organelle diseases).

ENCEPHALOPATHY WITH PREDOMINATING SEIZURES

Four disorders, nonketotic hyperglycinemia, pyridoxine-dependent epilepsy, sulfite oxidase deficiency, and the molybdenum cofactor deficiency, are characterized by early seizures as the predominant feature and can be reminiscent of perinatal asphyxia, but without a supportive history. These disorders differ from the preceding ones in which seizures often occur as a later and less predominant part of an acute encephalopathy. The screening tests for the other encephalopathic metabolic disorders are normal (Figure 6–1).

Nonketotic hyperglycinemia typically presents in the newborn period as a rapidly progressive disorder with profound hypotonia, progressive obtundation, seizures, and apnea, which is fatal without resuscitative treatment. Hiccups are a clue to the diagnosis. Survivors usually have profound intellectual handicap and poorly controlled seizures. This autosomal recessive disorder results from defects in one of the four proteins of the glycine cleavage system. Variant forms of the disease have been recognized, including a rapidly progressive disorder that first presents after the newborn period, and an early-onset but slowly progressive disorder with moderate to severe intellectual handicap, with or without seizures, and a spinocerebellar degeneration phenotype with onset in the second or third decade. The diagnosis is strongly suggested by an elevated urinary glycine in the absence of organic aciduria, and an elevation in the CSF:plasma glycine ratio. The diagnosis can be confirmed by measuring the activity of the glycine cleavage system in liver or transformed lymphoblasts. Plasma glycine may be normal. There is no effective treatment, although the *N*-methyl-D-aspartate receptor channel antagonist, dextromethorphan, may improve seizure control.

The classic form of pyridoxine (vitamin B_6)–dependent epilepsy is a relentless seizure disorder that begins in the first week of life (or even in utero). The seizures are poorly or not controlled by traditional anticonvulsants. Vitamin B_6–dependent epilepsy should be excluded in any infant or child with an unexplained seizure disorder. The diagnosis is based on the clinical and electroencephalographic (EEG) responses to pyridoxine, which may be rapid (within minutes). Even if there is no immediate improvement clinically or in the EEG, however, the patient should be maintained on vitamin B_6 (75 mg twice a day bid for newborns) for a trial of at least 3 weeks. The site of the primary biochemical defect(s) is unknown.

A second group of children with vitamin B_6–dependent epilepsy have other phenotypes. They may have a later onset, as late as 18 months of age; they may be initially or partially responsive to other anticonvulsants; or they may have seizure-free periods on no medications.

The outcome is variable. Some patients have had good seizure control and normal development, but many others have been intellectually impaired, although this may reflect late diagnosis.

A defect in an enzyme of cysteine catabolism, sulfite oxidase, or in the biosynthesis of its molybdenum cofactor, produce a remarkably similar phenotype, which most often has its onset in the neonatal period. Typical clinical features in the first week or two of life include refractory tonic–clonic seizures, axial hypotonia with peripheral hypertonia, and feeding difficulties. Infants who survive beyond the neonatal period develop progressive destructive brain changes including marked intracerebral calcification, choreoathetoid movements, and dislocation of the lens. Milder variants have been described, with later onset of symptoms and less severe neurologic and somatic abnormalities.

Routine biochemical screening may miss these disorders, but dipstick screening of fresh urine for sulfite is highly suggestive. Specific testing of urine for raised *S*-sulfocysteine and thiosulfite levels are virtually diagnostic. In addition, patients with the molybdenum cofactor defect also have low urinary and blood levels of uric acid because the functional abnormality of another molybdenum cofactor-requiring enzyme, xanthine oxidase. The diagnosis of these autosomal recessive disorders can be confirmed by enzyme assay in liver samples or cultured cells. There is no effective treatment for these disorders.

Treatment of Acute Encephalopathies Due to Inborn Errors of Small Molecules

ACUTE RESUSCITATIVE THERAPY

The initial resuscitative phase of management must be initiated immediately, while the diagnostic workup is in progress. Initial treatment should include:

1. Good hydration and provision of fluid, electrolytes, and glucose (administration of glucose will help reduce catabolism). A useful initial fluid protocol is 10% dextrose in 0.2% saline, run at 150% of maintenance, supplemented with the daily requirement of potassium. This regimen generally supplies approximately 9–10 mg/kg/min of glucose in neonates and infants. Fluid restriction may be necessary if cerebral edema is present.

2. Correction of the metabolic acidosis by sodium bicarbonate administration, if the serum bicarbonate is less than 15 mEq/L. Beware of overcorrection: stop once the bicarbonate level has reached 15 mEq/L. Also beware of producing hypernatremia, although this may be unavoidable and require dialysis.

3. Once these measures have been instituted and even before a precise biochemical diagnosis has been made, hemodialysis or hemofiltration should be begun if the patient is semicomatose or comatose to remove the offending small molecule as quickly as possible.

4. Therapy specific to the disease. For example:
    a. *Nutritional modification,* such as appropriate caloric supplements (e.g., intralipid), and intravenous amino acid supplements free of the offending precursor amino acids (e.g., leucine, isoleucine, and valine in MSUD; Figure 6–2)
    b. *Cofactor administration,* which sometimes will improve the function of a genetically defective enzyme (e.g., vitamin B_{12} in some cases of methylmalonic aciduria, because adenosylcobalamin is a cofactor for methylmalonyl-CoA mutase; Figure 6–2)
    c. *Metabolic manipulation,* such as the administration of sodium benzoate in hyperammonemias, to divert a toxic substrate to a benign excretable form

DIETARY THERAPY FOR SMALL MOLECULE DISEASES

Once the acutely elevated levels of the toxic small molecule have been lowered, dietary modification is instituted to maintain low levels of the toxic metabolite(s). For example, for MSUD patients, leucine, isoleucine, and valine (all essential amino acids) are provided in amounts sufficient to allow normal growth. Levels in excess of those amounts will be catabolized to form the toxic ketoacids. The objective of therapy therefore is to balance anabolic needs and catabolic capacity. Such diets are composed of an artificial formula of the other essential amino acids mixed together with other critical nutrients (vitamins, minerals). The required amounts of leucine, isoleucine, and valine are provided by giving very small amounts of normal protein-containing foods such as milk. Blood must be taken regularly to monitor the levels of the relevant amino acids. For many well-managed and compliant patients, the neurologic outcome may be normal or near normal, depending on the degree and duration of the perinatal encephalopathy, the severity of subsequent encephalopathic episodes, and the quality of the chronic metabolic control.

CHRONIC ENCEPHALOPATHY: SMALL MOLECULE DISEASES & DISEASES OF ORGANELLES

The dramatic clinical presentation of the acute encephalopathies makes it relatively easy to keep genetic metabolic diseases in mind when confronted with such patients. More common and difficult is the problem of the diagnosis of a child with slowly progressive or nonprogressive developmental delay, mental retardation, or another chronic neurologic disorder. Although the etiology often is not determined in such patients, genetic causes must be excluded.

The inborn errors that can produce chronic encephalopathy can be assigned to two broad groups, small molecule diseases and diseases of organelles. The small molecule diseases that cause chronic encephalopathy are of two types: the less severe variants of enzymopathies that also are associated with acute encephalopathy (discussed above) and a quite distinct group of conditions, exemplified by phenylketonuria (PKU), that lead to chronic encephalopathy. The organelle diseases include the lysosomal storage diseases, diseases of mitochondrial energy metabolism, and peroxisomal disorders (Figure 6–8).

Chronic Encephalopathy Due to Small Molecule Diseases

SMALL MOLECULE DISEASES THAT CAN CAUSE ACUTE OR CHRONIC ENCEPHALOPATHY

Patients with mild forms of many small molecule diseases may present with static or relatively nonprogressive devel-opmental delay or mental retardation. Such patients have managed to escape the extreme accumulations of metabolites that are found in the more severely affected cases, generally because they tend to have more residual enzyme activity than more severely affected subjects. The investigations outlined in Figure 6–1 for disorders of amino acid, organic acid, and ammonium metabolism should be completed on such patients. For example, with the intermediate variant of MSUD, the amino and keto acids are chronically increased to a level that damages the brain but does not alter consciousness (except with a catabolic stress). Patients with less severe forms of organic acidopathies may never accumulate enough of the abnormal organic acid to become overtly acidotic, and in those with mild urea cycle defects (e.g., some carrier females with OTC deficiency), blood ammonia may be increased only postprandially (2–3 hours after finishing a protein-containing meal). Exclusion of a mitochondrial defect and disorders of pyruvate metabolism also must be made, particularly if there is any evidence of muscle weakness, by measuring serum pyruvate and lactate. This latter group of conditions is discussed further below. Depending on the disease, patients with this group of chronic encephalopathies may have intellectual handicap, dementia, or motor deficits.

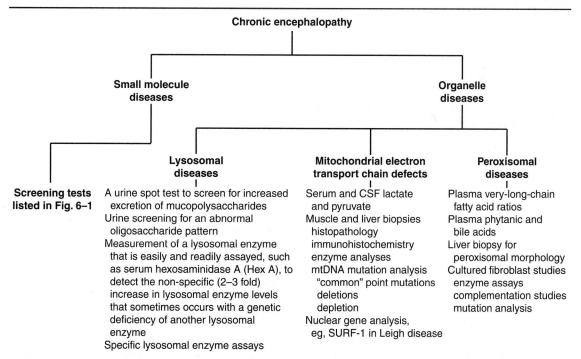

Figure 6–8. Biochemical evaluation of inborn errors of metabolism causing chronic progressive encephalopathy. Hex A = hexosaminidase A.

Phenylketonuria. Some small molecule inborn errors never cause acute encephalopathy but produce developmental delay and mental retardation. The classic example is PKU, due to mutations in the gene encoding phenylalanine hydroxylase. Affected infants are normal at birth, but within the first 48 hours of life the plasma concentration of phenylalanine rises to high levels. This increase has no clinical effects in the short term, but the persistent elevation of phenylalanine or its metabolites is neurotoxic, and the result is profound intellectual handicap, often with seizures and aggressive behavior. There are no other serious clinical manifestations. A diet restricting phenylalanine intake to the minimum necessary for normal growth prevents the intellectual handicap, provided treatment is instituted within the first weeks of life.

Newborn screening programs are used widely to detect PKU within the first weeks of life, with a dramatic reduction in the incidence of severe intellectual handicap. (Newborn screening has been initiated for other metabolic disorders, in particular congenital hypothyroidism, which is genetic in origin in 10–15% of cases). Not all infants with increased postnatal phenylalanine will have classic PKU. About half have less severe disruption of phenylalanine hydroxylase function, and, provided that the blood phenylalanine does not exceed a critical threshold (approximately 400 μmol/L; normal <200), intellectual development will be normal. Such patients are said to have **benign hyperphenylalaninemia.**

About 2% of hyperphenylalaninemics have defects in the synthesis of the cofactor tetrahydrobiopterin or its resynthesis from the oxidized form quinonoid dihydrobiopterin by 4α-carbinolamine dehydratase and dihydropteridine reductase. Patients with hyperphenylalaninemia are routinely screened to identify this group of tetrahydrobiopter in deficient subjects because the treatment is very different from that for classic PKU.

Homocystinuria. Another important small molecule disease that causes nonprogressive encephalopathy is the amino acidopathy homocystinuria, due to a defect in the enzyme cystathionine β-synthase. The clinical features of this disorder include eye abnormalities (high myopia, lens dislocation), skeletal anomalies (osteoporosis, Marfan syndrome–like habitus), and intellectual handicap; in addition, homocystinuric patients are at increased risk of spontaneous venous or arterial thrombosis. In half of the cases, the blood level of homocystine can be normalized or greatly reduced by giving pharmacologic doses (up to 1 g/d in adults) of oral pyridoxine. Because the diagnosis (unlike PKU) usually is not made until the second year of life or later, attempts at dietary restriction of methionine usually are met with poor compliance because the older child finds the diet unpalatable. Supplementation with betaine, a methyl group donor that participates in the normal recycling of homocysteine to methionine, reduces the homocystine level. Treatment should include folic acid because of the risk of folate deficiency.

Chronic Encephalopathy Due to Organelle Diseases

The diseases of organelles that must be considered in patients with slowly deteriorating or static neurologic dysfunction are those that impair the ability of mitochondria to produce energy, lysosomal storage diseases, and peroxisomal disorders (Table 6–1 and Figure 6–8). As indicated in preceding sections, diseases of mitochondrial energy metabolism often present as acute encephalopathy, in addition to being responsible for much chronic neurologic disease. The lysosomal and peroxisomal diseases and Golgi disorders (most notably the carbohydrate-deficient glycoprotein syndrome), in contrast, usually are associated only with chronic neurologic abnormalities.

The major function of mitochondria is to produce energy in the form of ATP. Consequently, patients with defects in the respiratory chain and other key proteins of energy metabolism, in particular PDH and PC (Figure 6–7), often have abnormalities in organs that are heavily energy dependent, particularly brain and skeletal muscle; heart, kidney, retina, and other organs are affected less commonly. The mitochondrial respiratory chain consists of five major protein complexes (Figure 6–7) that together include about 70 different polypeptides. Abnormalities in the function of each of these complexes of the chain (Figure 6–7) have been demonstrated. Most respiratory chain proteins are encoded by the nuclear genome, and defects in these genes are therefore autosomal recessive or X linked in inheritance. Defects in mitochondrial DNA, in contrast, are maternally inherited or sporadic.

A wide range of clinical phenotypes has been observed in patients with diseases that impair bioenergetics (Table 6–2), but encephalopathy is by far the most common and obvious feature. **Leigh disease (subacute necrotizing encephalomyopathy)** is the most frequent of the severe bioenergetic disorders affecting the brain in infancy or later in childhood. A progressive dementia begins within the first year of life in association with pyramidal signs, ataxia, movement disorders (dystonia, tremor), eye abnormalities (optic neuropathy, ophthalmoplegia, nystagmus, ptosis), and respiratory dysfunction (episodes of hypo- or hyperventilation). In addition, some affected individuals have a later age of onset and a more slowly progressive course. The neuropathology is characteristic, with symmetric regions of necrosis involving basal ganglia, pons, midbrain, thalamus, and optic nerves.

Table 6–2. Clinical Findings in Patients with Defects of Mitochondrial Bioenergetics

General
  Small stature
  Anorexia

Central nervous system
  Neonatal acute encephalomyopathy, with severe lactic acidosis
  Leigh disease (subacute necrotizing encephalo-myelopathy)
  Developmental delay
  Dementia
  Myoclonic seizures
  Ataxia
  Stroke-like episodes (often reversible)
  Dysphagia
  Progressive external ophthalmoplegia
  Sensorineural hearing loss
  Retinal degeneration
  Optic atrophy
  Peripheral neuropathy

Skeletal & muscle
  Hypotonia
  Weakness
  Exercise intolerance
  Rhabdomyolysis

Cardiac muscle
  Cardiomyopathy
  Cardiac conduction defects

Kidney
  Renal Fanconi syndrome

Liver
  Progressive hepatic failure

Endocrine
  Diabetes mellitus
  Diabetes insipidus

Hematologic
  Sideroblastic anemia
  Neutropenia

Gastrointestinal
  Malabsorption
  Diarrhea

Many different biochemical defects of energy metabolism have been found to produce the Leigh syndrome phenotype, including abnormalities of the respiratory chain (e.g., cytochrome c oxidase [COX] deficiency), mitochondrial (mt) DNA-encoded ATPase subunit 6, and PDH (Figure 6–7). It was recently discovered that most cases of COX-deficient Leigh's syndrome are not due to a defect of one of the 13 COX subunits but rather to mutations in a nuclear encoded gene, SURF-1, which is thought to be involved in assembly of the COX complex.

Mitochondrial DNA mutations. Several more specific and memorable phenotypes have been found to result from mutations in mtDNA. The mitochondrial genome encodes 13 of the subunits found in four of the electron transport chain complexes, a complete complement of mitochondrial-specific tRNAs, and two mitochondrial-specific RNAs. Generally speaking, defects in the mitochondrial genome should be suspected in any infant or child with unexplained multisystem disease. The most notable phenotypes include myoclonic epilepsy and ragged-red fiber disease, a syndrome with mitochondrial myopathy, encephalopathy, lactic acidosis, and stroke-like episodes (MELAS), Leber hereditary optic neuropathy (late-onset optic nerve death, cardiac dysrhythmias), Pearson syndrome (sideroblastic or aplastic anemia, pancreatic exocrine insufficiency, and progressive liver failure), Alper disease (progressive infantile poliodystrophy: seizures in association with progressive brain and liver failure), and Kearns–Sayre syndrome (KSS; encephalopathy, ophthalmoplegia, ataxia, pigmentary retinopathy, and heart block). Some patients may have only progressive external ophthalmoplegia (CEO), but in others one phenotype can evolve into another (e.g., from CEO to KKS and from Pearson syndrome to KSS). Single nucleotide substitutions of genes encoding respiratory chain subunits have been described in Leber hereditary optic neuropathy and Leigh disease, as have point mutations of one of the tRNAs in the myoclonic epilepsy and ragged-red fiber disease and MELAS syndrome. Large deletions (>1 kb) of the mtDNA are the cause of Pearson syndrome, KSS, and CEO. Small deletions (usually fewer than 25 base pairs) and point mutations of the 16S rRNA also have been described. Diseases due to substitutions of mtDNA are inherited maternally, whereas almost all cases of single deletions in the mtDNA are sporadic.

Blood & CSF lactate. Many neonates with defects in the electron transport chain present with overwhelming lactic acidosis, whereas in others, particularly those presenting later with chronic disease, the increase in blood lactate often is too low to produce acidosis or a noticeably increased anion gap. Thus, any persistent increase in blood lactate (normal <2.2 mM/L) may be significant, and an increase in CSF lactate virtually always signifies a metabolic defect (except with meningitis); in some cases, only the CSF lactate may be increased. Thus, normal blood and CSF lactate effectively exclude almost all bioenergetic defects.

Detection of an increased blood or CSF lactate requires that attempts be made to identify the precise biochemical and genetic defects. This information may allow treatment, and it offers the possibility of precise genetic counseling and prenatal diagnosis. Muscle (usually of skeletal muscle, but of the myocardium if only cardiac involvement is suspected) or liver biopsies provide tissue for biochemical and ultrastructural analysis. Structural abnormalities of the mitochondria are commonly found in these conditions including, in the skeletal muscle of some patients, "ragged-red fibers," which contain peripherally situated clumps of mitochondria that stain red with the modified Gomori trichrome stain used for light microscopy. Tissue-specific defects have been described, sometimes necessitating biopsies of liver and skeletal muscle before the diagnosis can be established.

LYSOSOMAL STORAGE DISEASES

The lysosomal storage diseases are caused by enzyme defects that impair the degradation of macromolecules in lysosomes or disruptions in the efflux of molecules from the lysosome to the cytoplasm. Cell death results from the consequent intralysosomal "storage" of the undigested macromolecule or the accumulation of a nontransportable substrate. Macromolecules are integral structural components of cells. The major function of the lysosome is to degrade such molecules, including glycosaminoglycans, glycoproteins, gangliosides, and glycolipids (the latter two are known collectively as sphingolipids), into their small molecule components, which can then be recycled in metabolism and biosynthesis. In contrast to diseases that disturb the metabolism of small diffusible molecules, the pathology of the lysosomal diseases is restricted to tissues in which the macromolecule is normally degraded. Examples of lysosomal storage diseases are the mucopolysaccharidoses, the oligosaccharidoses, and the gangliosidoses (Figure 6–9). These conditions are recessive and autosomal or X linked in their inheritance.

Clinical features. Most of these diseases are associated with clinically detectable "storage" in many organs and tissues. Clinical features often found (Figure 6–9) include neurologic deterioration culminating in dementia, coarse facial features, hepatosplenomegaly, retina and peripheral nerve degeneration, and bony abnormalities collectively termed **dysostosis multiplex.** The nervous system is affected in most of these conditions, and in many of them it is the only affected system. Virtually any neurologic activity can be disrupted, and the presentations

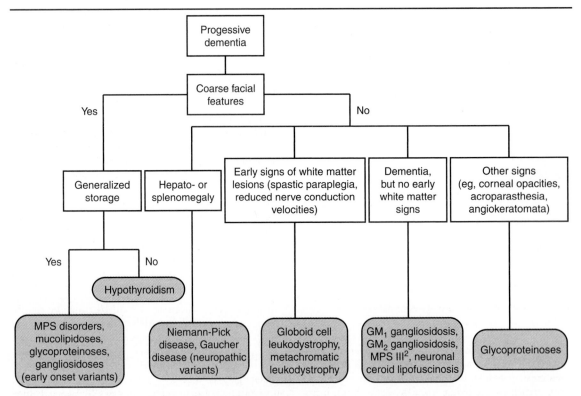

Figure 6–9. Biochemical evaluation of inborn errors causing progressive dementia. All these defects are autosomal recessive in their inheritance except Hunter syndrome, which is X linked. Patients with Sanfilippo syndrome have coarsening of facial features later in the course of their disease.

commonly include seizures, dementia, blindness, deafness, ataxia, and hypotonia. Macrocephaly occurs in some of the conditions that affect the brain, but it is not a predominant or early feature in most of them.

The single invariant characteristic of the lysosomal storage diseases is their progressive nature. In many of these diseases, the deterioration is obvious from early on in the course of the disease. In other instances, the deterioration may be much less evident, progressing with almost imperceptible slowness over years, but eventually being undeniable. In taking the history, it is important to document the loss of developmental milestones or of intellectual or other neurologic functions, to be sure that the condition is not static. A common diagnosis that can masquerade as progressive neurologic deterioration is uncontrolled seizures (pseudodementia). A complicating factor in considering this possibility is that many of the storage diseases are themselves associated with seizures.

Abnormalities diagnostic of storage diseases are often seen in the retina, and because it is the only clinically visible part of the central nervous system, it should always be carefully examined, generally by an experienced ophthalmologist. Typical retinal abnormalities include the "cherry-red spot" (seen in Tay–Sachs disease and a few others), optic nerve atrophy, and macular degeneration.

White matter degeneration is suggested by loss of peripheral nerve function (e.g., hyporeflexia or areflexia), delayed nerve conduction velocity, abnormal auditory brainstem responses, visual evoked potentials (VEPs), and elevated CSF protein. Gray matter degeneration is associated more often with seizures and earlier loss of intellectual function, but white and grey matter diseases eventually lead to intellectual deterioration. The EEG does not show a specific abnormality in these diseases.

Radiographs of the bones show changes of "dysostosis multiplex" in some conditions, most commonly in the mucopolysaccharidoses, such as Hurler syndrome. Features include thickened bones with coarse trabeculations and characteristic bone dysplasia, including the "beaked" vertebra, which results from hypoplasia of the anterior part of the vertebra.

If the clinical presentation and any of the screening tests (Table 6–3) suggest a storage disease, then specific enzymatic assays are performed, guided by the specific clinical findings.

Specific lysosomal storage diseases

Mucopolysaccharidoses. The mucopolysaccharidoses (MPS disorders) should be considered in a child with coarse facies, mental retardation, or dysostosis multiplex (Figure 6–9 and Table 6–4). Other common features are hepatosplenomegaly, thickening of skin and subcutaneous tissues, and reduced joint mobility. The six disorders are due to abnormalities in enzymes that degrade glycosaminoglycans, macromolecular components of connective tissue. Phenotypic heterogeneity in the MPS dis-

Table 6–3. Screening Tests for Lysosomal Storage Diseases

Radiologic examination of skull, hands, vertebral column, and long bones
Careful inspection of the retina and cornea, preferably by slit-lamp examination
Nerve conduction velocity, ABRs, and CT or MRI scan for white matter diseases
Biochemical screening tests (see Figure 6–1)

ABRs = auditory brainstem responses; CT = computed tomography; MRI = magnetic resonance imaging.

eases is broad (Table 6–4), ranging from a severe relentless neurodegenerative and physically debilitating disease with progressive coarsening of facial features, as seen in Hurler's syndrome; to disorders where intellectual deterioration predominates, with initially little in the way of overt physical signs, as in Sanfilippo disease, to disorders where intellectual function is unaffected but lead to severe physical effects, as in Maroteaux–Lamy disease and Morquio disease. Analysis of the urinary MPS pattern, followed by specific enzyme assay of leukocytes or fibroblasts, will establish the diagnosis. No effective therapy is currently available, although bone marrow transplantation has met with limited success in Hurler, Hunter, and Maroteaux–Lamy diseases. All these disorders are autosomal recessive in inheritance, except for Hunter's disease, which is X-linked recessive.

Glycoproteinoses. In general, the glycoproteinoses resemble MPS disorders, with coarsening of facial features, dysostosis multiplex, mental retardation of variable severity, and hepatosplenomegaly (Figure 6–9). In addition, some of these conditions have characteristic clinical features, e.g., cherry-red spot and myoclonic seizures in **sialidosis** (sialidase deficiency), deafness in **α-mannosidosis** (α-mannosidase deficiency), and a telangiectatic skin rash, angiokeratoma corporis, in fucosidosis (α-fucosidase deficiency). Glycoproteins, which are distributed widely throughout the body, have a protein backbone, with oligosaccharide side chains covalently attached; a series of enzymes systematically removes the oligosaccharides one by one. The urine of a patient with suspected glycoproteinosis should be screened for an abnormal oligosaccharide pattern, followed by specific enzyme assay in leukocytes or cultured fibroblasts. No specific treatment is available.

Gangliosidoses. The gangliosidoses highlight the important clinical principle that defects in a single biochemical function can be associated with extremely variable clinical phenotypes, although their common feature is progressive neurodegeneration (Figure 6–9). Neonates

Table 6–4. Clinical and Biochemical Features of the Mucopolysaccharidoses

Syndrome	Clinical Features	Accumulated Substances	Enzyme Defect
Hurler	Coarse facies, corneas cloudy, dysostosis, dementia, hepatosplenomegaly	Dermatan sulfate Heparan sulfate	α-L-iduronidase
Scheie	As above but no dementia, normal intelligence	As above	As above
Hunter	Coarse facies, corneas clear, dysostosis, dementia (mild form has no dementia), hepatosplenomegaly, sensorineural deafness	Dermatan sulfate Heparan sulfate	Iduronate sulfatase
Sanfilippo (4 types)	Signs of "storage" only mild, difficult behavior (hyperactivity), dementia	Heparan sulfate	A heparan-*N*-sulfatase B α-*N*-acetylglucosaminidase C acetyl-CoA:α-glucosaminide acetyltransferase D *N*-acetylglucosamine 6-sulfatase
Morquio (2 types)	Skeletal dysplasia (including odontoid hypoplasia), normal intellect	Keratan sulfate Chondroitin 6-sulfate	A galactose 6-sulfatase B β-galactosidase
Maroteaux–Lamy	Skeletal dysplasia, normal intellect, corneal clouding	Dermatan sulfate	*N*-acetylgalactosamine 4-sulfatase
Sly	Coarse facies, corneas cloudy, dysostosis, mental retardation, hepatosplenomegaly Rarely, presents as neonatal hydrops; milder form has normal intellect	Dermatan sulfate Heparan sulfate Chondroitin 4-sulfate Chondroitin 6-sulfate	β-Glucuronidase

with G_{M1} gangliosidosis (β-galactosidase deficiency) have coarse facies, hepatosplenomegaly, dysostosis, cherry-red spot, and dementia, with death by the age of 2 years. Patients presenting in later infancy or adolescence do not have facial coarseness or hepatosplenomegaly (Figure 6–9) and have only mild dysostosis; the neurodegenerative component remains prominent. Similarly, in G_{M2} gangliosidosis, the clinical phenotype is broad, ranging from infantile forms (Tay–Sachs disease [hexosaminidase A deficiency] and Sandhoff disease [hexosaminidase A and B deficiencies]) to adult onset variants. Specific clues suggesting infantile Tay–Sachs disease are an exaggerated response to sudden sounds (hyperacusis) and a cherry-red spot in the retina. In contrast to the other storage diseases discussed to this point, coarse facies and hepatosplenomegaly are not usual features of the G_{M2} gangliosidoses (Figure 6–9). In the later presenting forms, the course is milder, and the cherry-red spot is an inconsistent finding. The adult-onset form may have a psychiatric presentation or clinical features of a spinocerebellar disorder. Urinary oligosaccharides are not consistently

abnormal, so that the diagnosis must be excluded by specific enzyme assays of serum, leukocytes, or cultured fibroblasts.

Other classic sphingolipidoses: Gaucher disease & Niemann–Pick disease. Two diseases that are biochemically related to gangliosidoses (they are all sphingolipidoses) and have variants that can also cause progressive dementia are Gaucher disease and Niemann–Pick disease. However, unlike many of the other spinoglipidoses, these conditions are not associated with coarse facial features (Figure 6–9). **Gaucher disease** (glucocerebrosidase deficiency), the most common of the lysosomal storage disorders, has non-neuronopathic (most patients) and neuronopathic forms. The clinical features of the non-neuronopathic form result from accumulation of glucocerebrosides in the reticuloendothelial system. Consequently, the clinical signs, which can be extremely variable, include hepatosplenomegaly (massive splenomegaly may occur), pancytopenia, and degenerative bony changes. More severely affected patients have life-threatening anemia, thrombocytopenia, or liver disease and bony "crises" similar to those seen in sickle cell anemia. In infants, the neuronopathic form of Gaucher disease is suggested by the triad of strabismus, trismus, and opisthotonus that occurs in association with a progressive spastic and seizure disorder. In both forms of Gaucher disease, the lipid-laden cells of the reticuloendothelial system have a characteristic "wrinkled tissue" appearance. The diagnosis can be confirmed by enzyme assay of leukocytes or cultured fibroblasts.

Bone marrow transplantation has been used to treat the non-neuronopathic and the subacute neuronopathic forms of Gaucher disease, and trials are underway in the infantile neuronopathic form. An alternative treatment involves regular infusions of a chemically modified form of glucocerebrosidase purified from human placenta. More recently, a genetically engineered form has become available, although both forms are very costly. This therapy has ameliorated the abnormalities in many patients, but further study is needed to determine whether this form of treatment will be of prophylactic value. In addition, gene therapy trials for Gaucher disease have recently commenced.

Niemann–Pick disease is a second sphingolipidosis that has neuronopathic and non-neuronopathic forms, but hepatosplenomegaly and lipid-containing "foam" cells in bone marrow are characteristic of both types. In the neuronopathic form, the neurologic deterioration is progressive but of variable severity and age of onset (Figure 6–9). Affected infants often have a neonatal "hepatitis" that is sometimes fatal. One group of patients have a defect in the enzyme sphingomyelinase, which can be assayed in leukocytes or cultured fibroblasts, whereas the defect in other patients is due to mutations in a gene critical for intracellular cholesterol trafficking. There is no specific treatment for either form.

Leukodystrophies. The white matter degeneration of the leukodystrophies is reflected initially by upper motor neuron signs and peripheral neuropathy (first evident from reduced deep tendon reflexes; Figure 6–9). In the most common form of **metachromatic leukodystrophy** (arylsulfatase A deficiency), which has a late infantile onset between 1 and 2 years, early features include gait abnormalities, ataxia, clumsiness, weakness, behavioral changes, and developmental delay. Within a few years of onset, patients subsequently develop spastic quadriplegia, optic atrophy and blindness, and dementia with seizures. Later-onset forms of the disease have a similar constellation of features, but the rate of progression varies. A second leukodystrophy, **globoid cell leukodystrophy or Krabbe disease** (galactosylceramidase deficiency), has a similar array of clinical features, but the onset of symptoms is usually within the first 6 months of life, with rapidly progressive mental and motor dete-

rioration, severe spasticity culminating in a severe vegetative state with seizures, optic atrophy and blindness, and microcephaly in later stages. An unforgettable sign is that these infants are inconsolably irritable or "crabby."

In both leukodystrophies, nerve conduction velocity is delayed, and CSF protein is elevated, although it may be normal in the early stages of the disease or in later-onset patients. Computed tomography and magnetic resonance imaging show atrophy of white matter. There are no screening tests, and confirmation of the diagnosis rests with enzyme assay of leukocytes or cultured fibroblasts. Treatment is largely symptomatic. Bone marrow transplantation may ameliorate the natural course of the disease, if performed early, but it is not curative. The γ-aminobutyric acid transaminase inhibitor vigabatrin has been found to be effective in reducing the severe spasticity experienced in the terminal stages.

PEROXISOMAL DISEASES

Peroxisomes participate in a number of unique anabolic processes, including bile acid and plasmalogen (ether phospholipids found in almost all membranes, most notably myelin) biosynthesis, and catabolic processes including the oxidation of very-long-chain fatty acids (VLCFA) and pipecolic acid. Over a dozen peroxisomal disorders have been identified, and on biochemical grounds they can be assigned to three groups, genetically to two, and clinically to four (Figure 6–10). Unfortunately, these diseases are almost uniformly untreatable. They are all autosomal recessive in their inheritance, except for X-linked adrenoleukodystrophy.

Clinical presentation. The cardinal feature of most peroxisomal diseases is severe, progressive central nervous system dysfunction, usually evident in infancy. Other features that should raise suspicion of these diseases in early life are facial dysmorphism, hepatomegaly and liver dysfunction, hypotonia, renal cysts, and various ocular abnormalities. In older patients, the phenotype is more variable and can include, in addition to the above findings, diverse manifestations of neurodegeneration including ataxia and other signs of white matter disease. The classification outlined below is based on the current clinical groupings.

Group 1: Defects of peroxisomal biogenesis & β-oxidation. These disorders are associated with more severe, early-onset clinical phenotypes. The defects of peroxisome biogenesis largely or completely impair the synthesis of structurally normal peroxisomes. As a consequence, the activities of multiple peroxisomal enzymes are severely reduced. The classic member of this group is the **cerebrohepatorenal (Zellweger) syndrome.** Affected newborns have profound neurologic impairment, severe hypotonia and weakness, seizures, a typical facial appearance (including dolicocephaly, high narrow forehead, large fontanelle, epicanthic folds, external ear deformities),

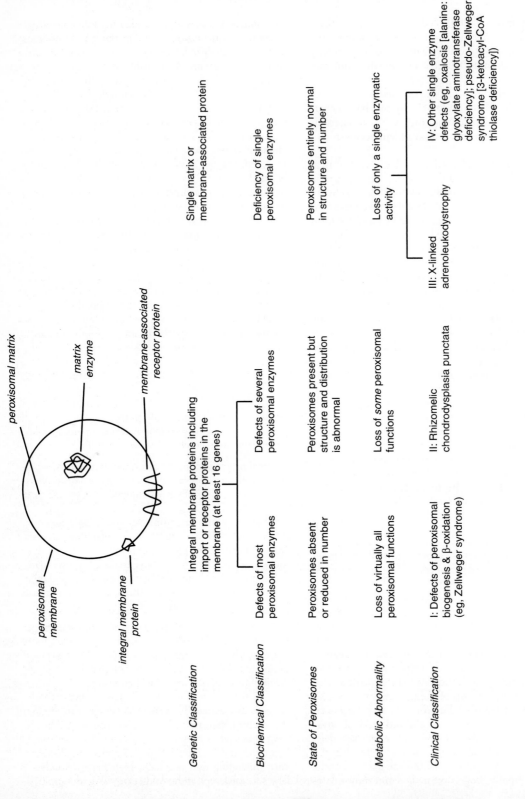

Figure 6–10. Pathogenesis of peroxisomal disorders. All defects are autosomal recessive in their inheritance, except for adrenoleukodystrophy, which is X linked. VLCFAs = very-long-chain fatty acid ratios.

eye abnormalities (including cataracts and corneal opacities), hepatic dysfunction (in particular cholestatic jaundice), and renal cysts. More than half of the affected infants have stippled calcification of the patella. Most die within the first 6 months. Other defects of peroxisomal biogenesis may have little in the way of facial dysmorphism or congenital malformations but nonetheless have a severe neurologic outcome as in neonatal adrenoleukodystrophy. Mutations in at least 14 genes interfere with peroxisomal biogenesis, and 10 have been identified.

Some of these so-called PEX genes (the name is derived from genes of identical function isolated from a yeast model system) encode proteins responsible for cytosolic transportation of newly synthesized proteins, docking or translocation proteins, or release/recycling proteins. More than 20 PEX genes have been identified in the yeast system, so it is likely that at least that many genes will be identified in humans.

Some infants are clinically very similar to those with Zellweger syndrome, yet have a defect involving only one of the peroxisomal β-oxidation enzymes. One example is an abnormality of peroxisomal VLCFA oxidation, 3-ketoacyl-CoA thiolase deficiency, or pseudo–Zellweger syndrome. Figure 6–11 shows a diagnostic algorithm for

group I disorders. In addition, electrophysiologic studies (electroretinography, visual evoked potentials, and brainstem auditory voked potentials (BAEP) are almost always abnormal in this group of patients.

Group II: Rhizomelic chondrodysplasia punctata. In some cases peroxisomes are present, but their distribution and structure are abnormal, and many, though not all, peroxisomal enzymes are deficient. This group is characterized by **rhizomelic chondrodysplasia punctata (RCP)** and its variants. Classical RCP presents in neonates with proximal limb shortening, cataracts, and severe dysplastic changes of endochondral cartilage; ichthyosis may also appear. Seizures may be prominent, and the condition is often fatal in early infancy. This disorder is caused by mutations in the PEX7 gene, which encodes the PTS2 receptor. The enzymes defective in RCP (alkyl-dihydroxyacetone phosphate [DHAP] synthase, DHAP acyltransferase, 3-keto-acyl-CoA thiolase, and phytanoyl-CoA hydroxylase) have peroxisomal targeting sequences that recognize the PTS2 receptor. Hence, the biochemical defect in classic RCP is in the correct targeting of these otherwise normal enzymes to the peroxisome. Unlike most peroxisomal diseases, VLCFA oxidation is normal; hence, plasma VLCFAs are normal. Biochemical screening for this disorder is

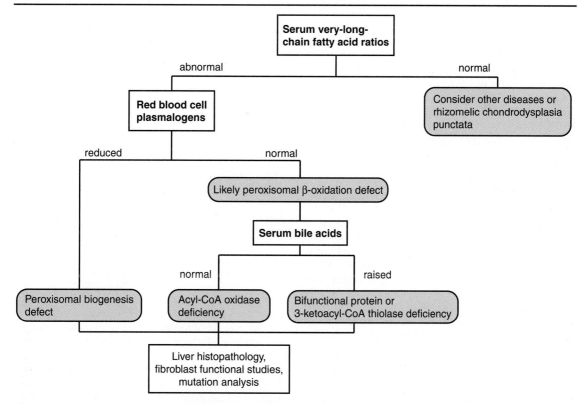

Figure 6–11. Diagnostic approach for patients suspected of having a defect of peroxisome biogenesis.

performed by measuring plasma levels of phytanic acid and red blood cell plasmalogens, both of which are abnormal. Therefore, the incomplete pattern of enzymatic abnormalities differentiates this condition biochemically from the comprehensive defects of peroxisome biogenesis.

Group III: X-linked adrenoleukodystrophy.

This disorder, the most common of the peroxisomal disorders, is in a category of its own because clinically it is quite different from the other disorders in this section. There are at least six clinically distinct phenotypes. The most common type is the childhood cerebral ALD, with its onset between ages 2 and 10 years, and it is characterized by adrenal insufficiency (sometimes the first presenting feature) and rapidly progressive neurologic dysfunction similar to that seen in metachromatic leukodystrophy. Other forms are the adolescent cerebral form (onset between 11 and 20 years), the adult cerebral form (onset after 20 years), adrenomyeloneuropathy (mainly involves the spinal cord initially, with adrenal and cerebral function affected later in the course), and an Addison disease only form (10–20% of ALD patients). More than half of women who are ALD heterozygotes have clinical symptoms similar to those of adrenomyeloneuropathy, with an onset of symptoms in the fourth decade.

All patients can be screened for this disorder by measuring VLCFA ratios. Most perplexing is the fact that some males with the genetic defect of ALD remain free of any clinical problems, despite having raised plasma VLCFA. The primary genetic defect is in an ATP-binding cassette transporter protein that is probably involved in the transport of very-long-chain fatty acyl-CoAs across the peroxisomal membrane. There do not appear to be any definite genotype–phenotype correlations in ALD. Further, the various clinical presentations can be found within the same pedigree, suggesting that epigenetic factors (environmental factors and/or modifying genes) are involved in the pathogenesis.

Diagnostic assessment also should include testing of the adrenal axis and magnetic resonance imaging of the brain (with contrast). Treatment of affected individuals must include adrenal replacement therapy. With regard to specific treatment of the neurologic disease, it is now clear that a diet high in glyceryl trioleate and glyceryl trierucate (Lorenzo's oil) is of only limited value. Bone marrow transplantation is of value in the childhood cerebral form, if it is implemented at the first signs of progression neurologically or on magnetic resonance imaging. In addition, trials currently are underway to determine the efficacy of lovostatin and 4-phenylbutyrate, which lower plasma VLCFA by different mechanisms.

Group IV: Defects of a single peroxisomal enzyme.

Some patients have a deficiency of only a single peroxisomal enzyme, with peroxisome number and structure being normal. Other single-enzyme defects have different clinical phenotypes. For example, Refsum disease (phytanoyl-CoA hydroxylase deficiency) is characterized by childhood or adolescent onset ichthyosis, progressive ataxia, sensorineural deafness, retinitis pigmentosa, and peripheral neuropathy. The only biochemical abnormality is an elevation of phytanic acid, and treatment centers on a diet restricting phytanates.

Other examples of single-enzyme defects are hyperoxaluria type I (alanine:glyoxylate aminotransferase), glutaric aciduria type III (glutaryl-CoA oxidase), mevalonic aciduria (mevalonate kinase), and acatalasemia. These disorders have very characteristic clinical and biochemical features, which should allow specific diagnosis. Some cases of RCP may have *isolated* defects of alkyl-DHAP synthase or DHAP acyltransferase.

Chronic Encephalopathy Due to Abnormalities of Protein Gycosylation

THE CARBOHYDRATE-DEFICIENT GLYCOPROTEIN (CDG) SYNDROMES

This is a relatively newly recognized group of multisystem disorders caused by defects in the synthesis of *N*-linked oligosaccharides. These critical biological compounds are integral components of the posttranslational modification processes of key secretory or membrane-bound glycoproteins, which take place in the cytosol, Golgi apparatus on endoplasmic reticulum. *N*-linked oligosaccharides are essential for the function of cell surface receptors, as protein targeting signals, and for cell-to-cell interactions.

Biochemical or functional defects that are seen as a consequence of this synthesis include low serum haptoglobin and apolioprotein B, decreased levels of a number of coagulation factors, such as hypoalbuminemia, hypocholesterolemia, low thyroxine-binding globulin, and increased liver transaminases, although in many patients only some of these are abnormal.

Given the range of biochemical abnormalities that can be encountered, it is not surprising that clinical presentations include multisystem disorders, with a dynamic clinical course. The most common variant, type Ia, due to a defect of the enzyme phosphomannomutase, is characterized in infancy by failure to thrive, hypotonia, congenital abnormalities (including long fingers and toes, esotropia, inverted nipples, and buttock and pubic area fat pads), and psychomotor retardation. Imaging of the brain may show cerebellar hypoplasia and brainstem atrophy. Some infants may also develop stroke-like episodes or pericardial effusions. With age, moderate to profound intellectual disability becomes apparent, as does progressive retinitis pigmentosa, and the unusual fat pads disappear. Adults have been noted to have ataxia, seizures, or peripheral neuropathy. Other clinical phenotypes have been described and there is a biochemical classification based on the isoelectric focusing pattern of transferrin isoforms in plasma, in addition to the enzyme defect.

The N-glycosylation pathways normally result in the oligosaccharide side chains of transferrin having four, five, or six sialic acid residues. Reproducible deviations from the normal pattern arise as a consequence of specific defects in this process.

The type I profile (reduced tetrasialotransferrin and increases in the disialo and asialo forms) is the most common, with 80% of these patients having a defect of the enzyme phosphomannomutase (CDG type Ia).

Because the 35 enzymes are known to be essential for the synthesis of N-linked oligosaccharide chains, it is likely that genetic defects will be identified in many of these in due course.

Treatment is supportive for all types of the CDG syndrome, although recent studies have suggested that mannose therapy may be of benefit with type Ib, due to phospomannose isomerase deficiency.

DIFFUSE HEPATOCELLULAR DISEASE

Diffuse Liver Disease in the Newborn

A small group of inborn errors present with diffuse hepatocellular disease (Table 6–5). Three of these diseases, galactosemia, hereditary fructose intolerance, and tyrosinemia type I, generally manifest in the newborn period or infancy, but their presentation can appear later. Patients have hepatomegaly, jaundice (direct and indirect hyperbilirubinemia), a marked reduction of clotting factors (reflecting severe impairment of hepatic synthetic functions), increased liver enzymes (reflecting hepatocellular damage), and, often, hypoglycemia. Renal Fanconi syndrome is a feature of these three enzymopathies, as is Wilson disease (see below). This syndrome is characterized by the impaired proximal renal tubular transport of glucose, phosphate, amino acids, protein, bicarbonate, electrolytes, and other solutes and can be detected by their increased urinary concentration, often simply by using a urine "dipstick" test. It is especially important not to miss the diagnosis of these four diseases because they are genetic and treatable. In addition, defects of the mitochondrial respiratory chain, fatty acid β-oxidation, and Niemann–Pick disease may have neonatal hepatic dysfunction as a presenting feature.

Galactosemia. A large proportion of galactosemic neonates present with gram-negative sepsis well before the metabolic diagnosis is suspected; consequently, all septic newborns should have biochemical screening for this disease (Table 6–5). Delayed treatment will result in mental retardation. The absence of galactose in urine (as a reducing substance) does not exclude the diagnosis, which can only be done by the red cell metabolic or enzymatic assays. Galactosemia is managed effectively by dietary restriction of galactose-and lactose-containing products, but, despite early diagnosis and good dietary compliance, subtle defects in intellectual function frequently are present, and ovarian failure occurs in more than 80% of affected females.

Fructose intolerance. Vomiting is the common presenting sign of fructose intolerance, and in the infant or small child it is associated with hypoglycemia, gastrointestinal discomfort, failure to thrive, and rickets. The diagnosis is easily missed if a careful dietary history is not taken to establish that the symptoms began with the ingestion of fructose or sucrose (the most common sources being fruit, some proprietary formulas, and honey or sugar added to food). Older children with fructose intolerance invariably develop an aversion to sweet foods. Fructose loading tests to demonstrate typical biochemical effects such as hypoglycemia are potentially dangerous and may not be diagnostic; assay of the liver enzyme or mutation analysis of the fructose 1-phosphate aldolase gene (Figure 6–9) is required because more than 95% of affected individuals have one of four mutations in the gene (Table 6–5).

Tyrosinemia. Patients with tyrosinemia type I who do not have acute liver disease in the first month present later, even after 1 year, with chronic liver disease or rickets due to the renal phosphate loss. The deficient enzyme (Table 6–5) is in the tyrosine catabolic pathway. Dietary phenylalanine-tyrosine restriction improves the hepatic dysfunction in the short term but liver transplantation offers the only cure at present. The drug 2-(2-nitro-4-trifluoromethylbenzoyl)-1,3-cyclohexanedione, which inhibits the enzyme three steps proximal to fumarylacetoacetate hydrolase, namely 4-hydroxyphenylpyruvate dioxygenase, has been very effective in improving renal tubular and hepatic function. This drug should be used until liver transplantation is possible.

α1-Antitrypsin deficiency. In contrast to the three conditions described above, α1-antitrypsin deficiency usually is associated with cholestatic jaundice, and the liver disease improves without treatment in most patients, although about 5% progress to cirrhosis (Table 6–5). α1-Antitrypsin is a major protease inhibitor, and the most common disease-causing genetic variant, or protease inhibitor type, is the ZZ allele, a mutant polypeptide whose aggregation in the hepatocyte appears to cause the liver disease. The reduced secretion of the ZZ protein into plasma permits the unimpeded activity of neutrophil elastase into the lung. This process slowly destroys the alveoli, causing the most common presentation of α1-antitrypsin deficiency, premature emphysema in adults. Apart from hepatic transplantation, there is no treatment for the liver disease. Evaluation of the effect of regular injections of α1-antitrypsin on the progression of the pulmonary disease is underway.

Table 6–5. Important Inborn Errors Presenting With Diffuse Hepatocellular Disease[1]

Disease	Primary Biochemical Defect	Hepatocellular Disease	Renal Fanconi's Syndrome	Other	Laboratory Diagnosis
Galactosemia	Galactose-1-P uridyl transferase deficiency (see Fig. 6–9)	Invariable	Frequent	Retardation, cataracts,[2] hemolysis, *Escherichia coli* sepsis in neonates; hypoglycemia	RBC screening test & enzyme assay; urine reducing substances often negative[3]
Fructose intolerance	Fructose 1,6-diP aldolase deficiency (see Fig. 6–9)	Invariable after fructose ingestion	Frequent	Vomiting; hypoglycemia; diagnosis often missed because history of fructose intake unrecognized	Enzyme assay of liver biopsy; loading tests are dangerous mutation analysis
Tyrosinemia type I	Fumaryl acetoacetate hydrolase deficiency	May or may not manifest in neonates; inevitable	Inevitable; may be presenting feature in later-onset form	Occasionally no symptoms until teens; rickets	Detection of succinylacetone in urine; often extreme elevation of serum α-fetoprotein mutation analysis
α1-antitrypsin (α1AT) deficiency	Mutations in the α1AT gene impair its hepatic synthesis or secretion	Cholestasis in some affected newborns; no liver disease in many patients	None	Adult-onset emphysema	PI typing of serum α1AT
Wilson disease	Liver-specific copper transporter protein	Presents after ~6 y, not necessarily with liver disease	Variable occurrence & severity	Kayser–Fleisher corneal ring,[2] hemolytic anemia; basal ganglia disease in teens & later	Low plasma ceruloplasmin; elevated urine and liver copper mutation analysis

[1] These diseases are all autosomal recessive in their inheritance.
[2] Detectable only by slit-lamp examination in the early stages.
[3] These tests must be done before blood transfusion or at least 3 mo after any previous transfusion. Urine screening for reducing substances is an unreliable method for excluding the diagnosis of galactosemia.
PI = protease inhibitor; RBC = red blood cell.

Acid lipase deficiency (Wolman's disease). This disorder of lipid metabolism also presents with severe progressive liver failure within the first few weeks of life in association with progressive neurological deterioration and, almost pathognomonically, with adrenal gland calcification, detectable on radiography. It is usually fatal by 6 months of age. The enzyme defect leaves patients unable to hydrolyse cholesterol esters to free cholesterol:

glucose-1, 6-glucosidic linkages

Diagnosis of this disorder hinges on having a high index of suspicion because routine screening tests are not helpful. Liver histopathology shows characteristic abnormalities and the diagnosis can be confirmed by specific enzyme assay in liver or cultured skin fibroblasts. Liver transplantation is effective in tyrosinemia, but has been of no benefit in Wolman's disease.

Diffuse Liver Disease Beyond the Newborn Period

Conditions associated with acute or chronic hepatocellular disease. The five disorders discussed in the previous section (galactosemia, fructose intolerance, tyrosinemia, α1-antitrypsin deficiency, and Wolman disease) can present as acute or chronic hepatopathy. Wilson disease, a defect in copper metabolism, also may present with acute or chronic liver disease, but unlike the other four conditions, the hepatic abnormalities in Wilson disease are rarely evident clinically before age 6 years (see Table 6–5). The primary defect is now known to be in a liver-specific protein required for the biliary excretion of copper. The result is a damaging accumulation of copper in the liver and a secondary copper "spillover" to other tissues. Patients may present acutely in childhood with fulminant liver failure and hemolytic anemia or, more insidiously, in the second or later decades with cirrhosis. After the age of 12 years the presentation may be neurologic, with extrapyramidal or neuropsychiatric signs. The Kayser–Fleischer ring, a dull copper-colored granular deposit at the limbus of the cornea, often is seen. The diagnosis is made by finding low serum ceruloplasmin, high urinary copper excretion, and increased hepatic copper levels and can be confirmed by mutation analysis of the Wilson disease gene.

Conditions associated only with chronic hepatocellular disease. Several inborn errors of glycogen and lipid metabolism are not associated with acute liver disease but cause a chronic process that ultimately produces cirrhosis. The classic example is **brancher enzyme deficiency** (glycogen storage disease type IV)

glucose-1, 4-glucosidic linkages

which presents in infancy with progressive liver failure and portal hypertension, failure to thrive, severe hypotonia, and absent deep tendon reflexes, with most patients dying before the age of 3 years. Cardiomyopathy occasionally may be a prominent feature. The brancher enzyme is responsible for the transfer of glucosyl units from an α-1,4 to a 1,6 position in the glycogen molecule. Liver transplantation has been helpful in some cases.

MYOPATHY

Acute rhabdomyolysis, muscle cramps, muscle weakness and wasting, or cardiomyopathy and the common presenting features of inherited metabolic diseases of muscle. Skeletal muscle relies on glucose as the major fuel for short-lived bursts of intense exercise, whereas resting muscle or muscle during sustained exercise use free fatty acids as the main energy source. Consequently, defects preventing the normal production or transport of these fuels (Figures 6–4 and 6–7) impair the function of skeletal muscle, the myocardium, or both. Myoglobinuria and elevated serum creatine kinase are the biochemical hallmarks of these events. Skeletal myopathy may be prominent in mitochondrial electron transport chain defects and, infrequently, might be the only clinical problem.

Acute Skeletal Myopathy (Rhabdomyolysis)

McArdle disease & defects of muscle glycolysis. Recurrent rhabdomyolysis with myoglobinuria occurs with enzymopathies that reduce energy production from carbohydrate fuels. Major examples include the glycogen storage disorder, muscle phosphorylase deficiency (McArdle disease)

glycogen glucose-1-phosphate,

and defects of glycolysis including phosphofructokinase, phosphoglycerate mutase, and phosphoglycerate kinase deficiencies (Figure 6–7). The initial symptoms usually develop in childhood, with pain, cramps, weakness, and myoglobinuria developing early in the course of intense exercise. Patients often learn to pace themselves until their "second wind" develops. The precise basis for the "second wind" phenomenon is not known but may be due to the use of free fatty acids as fuel when exercise is sustained. Oliguric renal failure secondary to severe myoglobinuria must be prevented by good hydration and alkalinization of urine. Mitochondrial respiratory chain defects occasionally may present with rhabdomyolysis.

Carnitine palmitoyltransferase II deficiency. In contrast to defects of muscle carbohydrate metabolism, the initial symptoms of patients with CPT II deficiency (see Figure 6–4) generally occur later in the course of exercise (when fat becomes the preferred fuel) and later in life. Patients with the milder form of CPT II deficiency (severe CPT II deficiency is discussed later in this chapter) usually present after adolescence, when weakness and myoglobinuria occur after prolonged exercise, particularly if there has been an inadequate caloric intake; other precipitating factors are cold exposure, infection, and emotional stress. Muscle cramps are unusual, and the "second wind" phenomenon does not occur. In most patients, for both groups of disorders, physical examination between episodes is entirely normal, although some patients with CPT II deficiency have muscle weakness. Other disorders of fatty acid β-oxidation, such as deficiencies of long- and short-chain 3-hydroxyacyl-CoA dehydrogenase or very-long-chain acyl-CoA dehydrogenase (Figure 6–4), also may cause intermittent rhabdomyolysis, but these conditions (see below) usually have persistent muscle symptoms.

Diagnosis of glycolytic defects (see Figure 6–7) and McArdle disease can be made by demonstrating that the serum lactate fails to rise normally during exercise, e.g.,

during forearm exercise when the arterial blood supply is blocked by a blood pressure cuff (the ischemic forearm test). CPT II deficiency has no effect on lactate, but about half of patients have a delay or reduction in ketone body formation during a prolonged fast. The diagnosis of these disorders is confirmed by specific assays in muscle or other cells (cultured skin fibroblasts in the case of fatty acid oxidation defects). Avoidance of extreme exercise is advocated for all of these myopathic defects. Treatment of CPT II deficiency includes avoidance of ketosis and other precipitating factors, and some patients benefit from supplements with MCT oil.

Isolated Skeletal Muscle Weakness

Patients who present with muscle weakness alone or with a static or chronic progressive myopathy without myoglobinuria may have one of the glycolytic defects, CPT II deficiency, a defect of one of the mitochondrial respiratory chain components, childhood or adult Pompe disease (see below), or one of a group of disorders that impair fatty acid oxidation and often also cause cardiomyopathy (Table 6–6).

Table 6–6. Defects of Fatty Acid Oxidation that Cause Cardiomyopathy

Defect impairing fatty acid oxidation[1]	Presenting Abnormality						Biochemical Abnormalities	
	Cardiac myopathy		Skeletal myopathy		Fasting coma		Abnormal urine organic acids, acylglycines, or acylcarnitines	Plasma carnitine
Carnitine cycle								
Plasma membrane carnitine transporter defect	+	&/or	+	&/or	+		No	↓↓↓
Carnitine-acylcarnitine translocase deficiency	+	&/or	+	&/or	+		No	↓↓
Carnitine palmitoyl-transferase II deficiency (severe form)	+	&/or	+	&/or	−[2]		No	↓
β-Oxidation cycle								
Very long-chain acyl-CoA dehydrogenase (VLCAD) deficiency	+	&/or	+	&/or	Yes		Yes	N or ↓
Long-chain 3-hydroxyacyl-CoA dehydrogenase (LCHAD) deficiency	+	&/or	+	&/or	+		Yes	↓

[1] Each of these biochemical functions is depicted in Figure 6–4.
[2] Fasting coma has been reported only in severe deficiency.
N = normal.

Cardiomyopathy

Heart muscle is the principal tissue affected in Pompe disease, a classic disorder of glycogen metabolism. Dilated cardiomyopathy also may be a predominant feature of several inborn errors of fatty acid metabolism, although in these conditions other features also may be seen initially, as described above. The numerous diseases that may be associated with cardiomyopathy include glycogen storage disease types III (debrancher deficiency) and IV (brancher deficiency), defects of the mitochondrial respiratory chain, organic acidopathies (including propionic and methylmalonic acidemia), certain mucopolysaccharidoses, and the carbohydrate-deficient glycoprotein deficiency syndrome (discussed earlier in the chapter).

Pompe disease (glycogen storage disease type II). This glycogen storage disease is associated with the accumulation of glycogen within the lysosomes of many organs, particularly the myocardium, skeletal muscle, and brain, due to lysosomal α-glucosidase deficiency. Glucose homeostasis is normal. The classic infantile form of this disease is characterized by the development of congestive heart failure and extreme cardiomegaly, muscle hypotonia, weakness, and an enlarged tongue; the muscles are often hypertrophic and "rubbery" in consistency. The electrocardiogram is characteristic, showing a short PR interval, very large amplitude QRS complexes, and inverted T waves. Death usually occurs in the first year of life. Trials of recombinant human α-glucosidase are currently under way. In contrast to the infantile form, the childhood and adult variants of α-glucosidase deficiency are slowly progressive disorders in which skeletal myopathy is the predominant feature.

Fatty acid oxidation defects. Cardiomyopathy also may be a presenting feature of disorders (Table 6–6) that interfere with the cycling of carnitine back and forth across the inner mitochondrial membrane (Figure 6–4) or impair long-chain fatty acid oxidation. The existence of these disorders reflects the heavy dependence of the heart on fatty acids as a fuel. Affected infants generally are noticed before the age of 5 years, and the cardiomyopathy can be fatal. All these conditions may also present with skeletal myopathy, fasting coma, or the metabolic abnormalities characteristic of fatty acid oxidation defects in general, such as MCAD deficiency: hypoketotic hypoglycemia, hyperammonemia, and metabolic acidosis (Table 6–6). Why MCAD deficiency does not generally affect heart muscle is unclear. Unlike MCAD deficiency, however, the urine organic acid profile of defects of carnitine cycling (Figure 6–4) is normal; for long-chain β-oxidation defects, the urinary profile is almost invariably abnormal. The enzymes or transport proteins involved in these diseases are required for the delivery of carnitine or long-chain fatty acyl-CoA into the mitochondrial matrix or for fatty acid oxidation (Figure 6–4). Treatment of these conditions has had limited success, apart from the reversal of the cardiomyopathy obtained with carnitine supplementation in the carnitine transporter defect. For the other diseases, the benefits of strategies such as the prevention of fasting or dietary supplementation with medium-chain fatty acids have been of variable effectiveness.

RENAL TUBULAR DISEASE

Loss of renal glomerular and tubular function can occur in many inborn errors in which other systems are the primary focus of clinically evident disease, including mitochondrial respiratory chain defects and peroxisomal diseases. Several inborn errors, however, are associated with more specific defects in renal function. For example, a decrease in most of the reabsorptive functions of the proximal tubule, i.e., a renal Fanconi syndrome, occurs commonly in four of the disorders associated with diffuse liver disease (galactosemia, tyrosinemia, fructose intolerance, and Wilson's disease). In other diseases, represented by cystinosis, the renal Fanconi's syndrome is the major initial clinical problem. A final group of renal tubular disorders result from the defective transport of an individual solute, such as phosphate (in X-linked hypophosphatemic rickets) or bicarbonate (in one form of renal tubular acidosis), or a group of chemically similar solutes, such as cystine and the basic amino acids in cystinuria.

Cystinosis. This lysosomal storage disease is caused by an abnormality in the transport protein that mediates cystine efflux from the lysosome. Lysosomal cystine accumulation occurs in virtually all tissues but damages the renal tubule the most quickly, thus producing the renal Fanconi's syndrome. Renal parenchymal destruction gradually leads to renal failure by as early as age 6 years. Most patients present in the first year of life with failure to thrive, dehydration, weakness due to electrolyte losses, acidosis, and rickets. Cystine crystal deposition in the cornea results in photophobia and in the retina to a pigmentary retinopathy. The diagnosis can be established in the appropriate clinical setting by the demonstration of cystine crystals in the cornea or bone marrow, or in rectal biopsies, or direct measurement of leukocyte cystine content with the identification of the gene responsible; definitive prenatal diagnosis is now possible. Symptomatic treatment includes the management of the electrolyte imbalances that occur. Renal transplantation corrects the renal defect, but the later development of hypothyroidism, diabetes mellitus, central nervous system and liver diseases is not prevented. Specific therapy to reduce the intracellular accumulation of cystine using cysteamine improves growth and delays the onset of renal failure if started early in the course of the disease; cysteamine eyedrops can lead to total clearance of cystine crystals from the cornea. Inside the lysosome, cysteamine and cysteine form a mixed disulfide that uses an efflux carrier distinct from that used by cystine.

Cystinuria. This relatively common disease, with a prevalence of approximately 1 per 7000, is due to impaired renal transport of the structurally similar amino acids cystine, ornithine, arginine, and lysine, which share a common carrier (a protein encoded by the *rBAT* gene) in the proximal renal tubule and gastrointestinal epithelium. The only clinical consequence of this defect results from the low solubility of cystine, which causes renal stones. The stones may be multiple and can lead to infection and progressive renal damage, late complications being hypertension and renal failure. The diagnosis must be excluded in any patient with nephrolithiasis, by quantification of urinary cystine (stone analysis is inadequate because some stones in cystinurics contain only trace amounts of cystine). Treatment is aimed at increasing the solubility of cystine and includes increased fluid intake and alkalinization of urine with regular doses of bicarbonate or citrate to keep the urine pH above 7.5. In those patients in whom stones have already formed or where there is already significant renal damage, penicillamine or captopril are advocated. These drugs form soluble mixed disulfides with cysteine, and their use may lead to the dissolution of preexisting stones.

DISORDERS WITH DISTINCTIVE PHENOTYPES

A number of important inherited metabolic disorders have distinctive phenotypes that should immediately suggest the possible diagnosis (Table 6–1). The diagnosis may be missed, however, because many of the clinical features associated with these diseases are found in other diseases. Examples are the apparent "cerebral palsy" that results from a number of enzymopathies and the dysmorphism and malformations that occur with a small number of inborn errors. One classic disease, Menkes disease, a defect of copper metabolism, requires astute clinical observation to be recognized.

Hepatomegaly without Dementia

As seen in many lysosomal storage diseases, metabolic disorders causing hepatomegaly often are associated with a neurodegenerative course. Two notable exceptions are the non-neuronopathic forms of Niemann–Pick disease and Gaucher disease, the neuronopathic variants of which were reviewed above; in Gaucher disease, splenomegaly is predominant. Hepatomegaly is also a prominent feature of defects of gluconeogenesis and in particular of glucose-6-phosphatase deficiency (glycogen storage disease type I or von Gierke's disease; Figure 6–7) and debrancher deficiency (glycogen storage disease type III), as discussed earlier.

"Cerebral Palsy" without a History of Perinatal Distress or Other Neurologic Insult

Cerebral palsy is the term used to describe a variety of nonprogressive neurologic syndromes with disordered movement or posture; mental retardation and seizures also may be present. The condition results from damage to the developing brain from causes such as hypoxia or infection, but in many cases no definitive cause can be ascertained. The four enzymopathies reviewed below should be considered in patients with this clinical presentation, if no other clear cause has been established. In addition, infants with nonketotic hyperglycinemia who survive infancy have spastic cerebral palsy, and this disease also must always be excluded. Although the neurologic disability of these inborn errors often cannot be improved, recognition of the correct diagnosis will allow appropriate genetic counseling.

The Lesch–Nyhan syndrome is a rare X-linked disorder due to a deficiency of hypoxanthine phosphoribosyltransferase, an enzyme of purine metabolism. Affected boys have delayed motor development apparent in the first 6 months of life and develop a movement disorder characterized by athetoid and choreiform movements, poor head control, and hypotonia within the first year. The degree of intellectual handicap, which may seem worse because of dysarthria, probably has been overestimated. Although some patients are definitely cognitively impaired, others are apparently normal. An unforgettable behavior, self-mutilation (e.g., severe biting of lips, ear banging) develops in most, but not all, affected patients. Hyperuricemia is not consistently present in all patients, but a normal urine uric acid:creatinine ratio will exclude the disease. The diagnosis can be confirmed by enzyme assay of erythrocytes or cultured skin fibroblasts. Gout and uric acid renal stones can be prevented by the administration of allopurinol, a drug that reduces the synthesis of urate. There is no therapy for this neurologic disorder.

Deficiency of the urea cycle enzyme arginase (Figure 6–6A), usually causes progressive spastic diplegia, intellectual handicap, and seizures. Acute hyperammonemic encephalopathy is a less common feature. The diagnosis is made by quantification of plasma arginine, and the management is similar to that of the other urea cycle defects.

Fumarase deficiency is a rare defect of the citric acid cycle (Figure 6–7) that may present in early infancy as a severe progressive encephalopathic disorder, with acidosis, leading to death in the first year of life, or as a static disorder with intellectual handicap and dysarthria that mimics cerebral palsy. A urine organic acid screen will detect increased fumarate levels. There is no specific treatment.

Glutaric aciduria type I is an organic acidopathy due to a deficiency of glutaryl-CoA dehydrogenase, an enzyme of the lysine catabolic pathway. The main clinical features are dysarthria, dystonic "cerebral palsy," choreoathetosis, macrocephaly, and mental retardation. Episodes of keto-acidosis and vomiting may be seen (particularly during periods of catabolic stress). Urinary organic acid analysis will usually, although not always, show an elevation of glutaric acid and related compounds. A diet restricting lysine intake appears to be of limited value, but it is generally agreed that aggressive treatment of acute catabolic episodes may ameliorate the often progressive neurodegenerative course.

Stroke or Thrombosis

Cerebrovascular accidents are sometimes seen as a complicating feature of homocystinuria due to cystathionine β-synthase deficiency, organic acidopathies (e.g., methylmalonic acidemia, propionic acidemia, isovaleric acidemia, and glutaric aciduria type I): defects of the mitochondrial electron transport chain (MELAS syndrome), the urea cycle disorders (particularly OTC deficiency), the carbohydrate-deficient glycoprotein deficiency syndrome, sphingolipidosis, Fabry disease (α-galactosidase deficiency), and inherited disorders of coagulation such as antithrombin III deficiency, protein C or protein S deficiency. It should not be forgotten, however, that about 50% of strokes (particularly ischemic strokes) in children and young adults are due to congenital or acquired heart disease; in certain ethnic groups, hemoglobinopathies (particularly haemoglobin SS [HBSS] and haemoglobin SC [HbSC]) need to be considered.

Premature Atherosclerosis

The mendelian disorders of lipid metabolism are important and potentially treatable causes of premature atherosclerosis and myocardial infarction. They are characterized by elevations in cholesterol, triglyceride, or certain plasma lipoproteins. Familial hypercholesterolemia is a particularly important example of this group because it was the first genetic disorder shown to predispose to myocardial infarction and it is the prototypic genetic defect of receptor molecules. It is characterized biochemically by elevated total plasma cholesterol and low density lipoprotein (LDL) cholesterol (giving a type 2 lipoprotein pattern with electrophoretic studies). Familial hypercholesterolemia is inherited in an autosomal dominant fashion and has a heterozygote frequency of 1 per 500, making it one of the most common mendelian defects. It is caused by mutations in the LDL receptor, which takes up LDL cholesterol from the extracellular fluid.

In the second decade heterozygotes often develop xanthomata due to cholesterol deposition, particularly on the extensor tendons of the hands, the Achilles tendon, and the extensor surfaces of the elbows and knees. Cholesterol accumulation around the peripheral margins of the cornea (arcus corneae) and the eyelids (xanthelasma) is seen later. Premature coronary artery disease and myocardial infarction may first become evident in the 30s and 40s. Homozygotes (prevalence, approximately one per million) have a much more severe form of the disease, with cutaneous xanthomas often being present at birth and in all patients by 4 years. The earliest recorded myocardial infarction in a homozygote is at 18 months, and few homozygotes survive beyond the age of 30 years.

The clinical diagnosis in homozygotes is confirmed by finding a plasma cholesterol level above 17 mmol/L in a nonjaundiced child. Both parents will, of course, be heterozygotes. The diagnosis in heterozygotes is more difficult because only 5% of patients with an elevated plasma cholesterol and a type 2 lipoprotein pattern have familial hypercholesterolemia. The diagnosis should be strongly suspected in any individual with a type 2 lipoprotein pattern who also has tendon xanthomata. The diagnosis can be confirmed by assaying LDL receptor function in cultured skin fibroblasts or by mutation analysis of the LDL receptor gene.

Heterozygotes are treated with a combination of dietary cholesterol restriction, enhancement of intestinal bile acid excretion using resins such as cholestyramine, and inhibition of the rate-limiting step in cholesterol biosynthesis (3-hydroxy-3-methylglutaryl-CoA reductase) with inhibitors such as lovostatin. These maneuvers are much less effective in homozygotes, who may respond partially to portocaval shunting (for reasons that are unclear) and regular plasma exchange. Liver transplantation has cured at least one child. Trials to assess the efficacy of LDL-receptor gene transfer into the liver are underway.

Disorders with Facial Dysmorphism or Congenital Malformations

Inborn errors of lysosomes, peroxisomes, and the carbohydrate-deficient glycoprotein syndromes are well-recognized causes of facial and other physical abnormalities in the newborn. In addition, defects in the metabolism of small molecules also may lead to facial dysmorphism and congenital malformations, familiar examples being the disorders of hormone biosynthesis, congenital hypothyroidism, and congenital adrenal hyperplasia. More recently, it has been recognized that small molecule diseases may cause facial dysmorphism or other malformations. These conditions impair fetal development because they lead to the accumulation of teratogens or impair cellular bioenergetics.

One such situation is illustrated by women with untreated phenyketonuria. When such women become pregnant (maternal PKU), the high maternal level of phenylalanine acts as a teratogen on the fetus, causing mental retardation, microcephaly, poor growth, and congenital heart defects, particularly ventricular septal defect (VSD). Most such children are heterozygotes for phenylalanine hydroxylase deficiency. Compliance with a low-phenylalanine diet by PKU women before conception prevents the fetal abnormalities. Examples of inborn errors that probably lead to malformations because they impair fetal energy production include PDH deficiency (see Figure 6–7; facies like that in fetal alcohol syndrome, brain malformations) and severe CPT II (see Figure 6–4; brain malformations, renal cysts).

More recently, another dysmorphic/malformation syndrome has been identified for which the pathogenesis remains uncertain. Smith–Lemli–Opitz syndrome, with an estimated incidence of 1 in 20,000 births, is an autosomal recessive disorder notable for microcephaly, a dysmorphic facies, ptosis, cleft palate, polydactyly, two to three toe syndactyly, hypospadias, renal, brain, lung, gastrointestinal, and heart malformations, cataracts, and intellectual disability. It is now known to be due a defect in the last step of cholesterol biosynthesis, at the level of 3β-hydroxysteriod-Δ⁷-reductase (7-dehydrocholesterol reductase). The pathogenesis is uncertain, but the recent recognition that cholesterol plays an essential role in embryonic development through the sonic hedgehog proteins is being investigated further in Smith–Lemli–Opitz syndrome. With regard to treatment, a cholesterol-rich diet improves growth, development, and behavior and certainly is worth trying.

Small molecule disorders therefore should be considered in infants with dysmorphism or malformations. These and other conditions can be excluded in the infant by examining blood amino acids, lactate, glucose, ammonium, CSF lactate, urine organic acids, and if indicated, plasma phenylalanine in the mother. Screening for Smith–Lemli–Opitz syndrome should include measurement of plasma cholesterol (although this is often "normal" depending on the assay system used) and 7-dehydrocholesterol (using gas chromatography mass spectrometry).

Menkes Disease

The hallmarks of this X-linked defect of copper metabolism in infants are seizures, facial dysmorphism (abnormal eyebrows, pudgy cheeks, sagging jowls), hair fragility, connective tissue abnormalities (including ligamentous laxity, hernias, bladder diverticuli, and arterial rupture), osteoporosis and fractures, a progressive neurodegenerative course, episodic hypothermia, and skin depigmentation. The basic defect is in a membrane copper-transporting ATPase present in most tissues except liver, which is similar in structure to the copper-transporting protein that is defective in Wilson disease. In Menkes disease, copper uptake into the cell is normal, but it cannot be transported to sites of synthesis of copper-dependent proteins such as lysyl oxidase (giving rise to the connective tissue abnormalities), dopamine β-hydroxylase (contributing to the autonomic dysfunction), and cytochrome c oxidase (possibly contributing to the neurologic disturbance). Copper accumulates in the gastrointestina mucosa and kidney, but, paradoxically, copper levels are low in most other tissues, including liver. The diagnosis is established by demonstrating very low levels of serum copper and ceruloplasmin. Treatment with parenteral copper-histidinate makes little difference to the clinical course if brain damage has occurred but may be of benefit if given to affected brothers in whom the disorder is diagnosed early, before the onset of symptoms.

REFERENCES

Fernandes J et al (editors): *Inborn Metabolic Disorders: Diagnosis and Management,* 2nd ed. Springer-Verlag, 1995.

Nussbaum RL, McInnes RR, Willard HF (editors): *Thompson and Thompson Genetics in Medicine,* 6th ed. WB Saunders, 2001.

Scriver CR et al (editors): *The Metabolic Basis of Inherited Disease,* 7th ed. McGraw-Hill, 1995.

Immunologic Disorders

Anna Huttenlocher, MD, & Diane Wara, MD

Infections are commonly seen in children. These infections usually are self-limited and respond promptly to appropriate treatment. Some children present with recurrent infections that are difficult to treat and immediately recur when antibiotics are discontinued, suggesting immunodeficiency. It may be difficult for the primary care physician to determine which of these children require evaluation for immunodeficiency and the extent of this evaluation. The primary immunodeficiencies are relatively rare disorders and occur in the population with a frequency of approximately 1 in 10,000; however, immunoglobulin (Ig) A deficiency can occur as frequently as 1 in 500. More than 50 disorders of the immune system have been described. These disorders reflect the heterogeneity of primary immunodeficiency disorders (Table 7–1). In recent years, the most common form of immunodeficiency in children has been an acquired infection with human immunodeficiency virus (HIV) type I. Pediatric HIV is discussed later in this chapter.

Early detection of immunodeficiency, whether primary or secondary, is increasingly important. Therapy is available for many primary immunodeficiencies and usually is most effective when initiated before the onset of severe clinical disease. In the past few years, remarkable progress has been made in our understanding of the molecular mechanisms underlying primary immunodeficiencies. This progress has implications for new approaches to diagnosis and genetic counseling and the potential development of new therapeutic interventions such as gene therapy.

■ APPROACH TO THE PRIMARY IMMUNODEFICIENCY DISORDERS

The immune system has four main components: the B lymphocytes, or humoral immunity; the T lymphocytes, or cellular immunity; the phagocytic system; and the complement system. These components work together to produce an effective immune response (Figure 7–1). Dysfunction of the immune system may manifest itself as susceptibility to infections or, in the other extreme, autoimmune disease. Although immunodeficiencies are best categorized according to the primary component of the immune system that is abnormal, dysfunction of one component of the immune system can disrupt normal functioning of other components, eg, normal B-cell function requires the participation of T cells.

Clinical Features

The clinical manifestations of primary immunodeficiency are variable in terms of the nature of the symptoms and the age of onset (Table 7–2). Patients with serious immunodeficiency usually present at an early age with recurrent infections. When to suspect an immunodeficiency in a child with frequent infections often is difficult to determine. Normal children can have one or more episodes of upper respiratory tract infection or otitis media per month, particularly during the winter months. Concerning features might include difficulty clearing infections with prescribed treatment or immediate recurrence of symptoms when antibiotic treatment is discontinued. In this era of aggressive antibiotic treatment, patients with immunodeficiency often present at older ages with different symptoms such as arthritis, chronic diarrhea, or failure to thrive. In fact, immunodeficiency should be a diagnostic consideration in the child presenting with failure to thrive or chronic diarrhea. Particular immunodeficiencies might have unique symptoms suggestive of their diagnosis, including thrombocytopenia and eczema in Wiskott–Aldrich syndrome and ataxia and telangiectasia in ataxia–telangiectasia (Table 7–3).

The infections seen in patients with underlying immunodeficiency usually are common, eg, otitis media, sinusitis, and pneumonia. Organisms also are typically the commonly occurring encapsulated organisms such as *Streptococcus pneumoniae* and *Haemophilus influenzae*. More severe infections, such as mastoiditis, bacteremia, osteomyelitis, and meningitis, also can occur. With major primary immunodeficiency, one of the infections usually is quite severe, involving unusual organisms or resulting in unexpected complications. The presence of opportunistic infections, such as *Pneumocystis carinii* pneumonia (PCP) or *Candida* esophagitis, is suggestive of a child with T-cell abnormality. Another consideration is the onset of complications from immunization with live-virus vaccines, including paralytic polio after immunization with oral poliovirus vaccine (OPV), in patients with B- and T-cell defects. In contrast, patients

Table 7-1. Primary Immunodeficiency Disorders

B-Lymphocyte Abnormalities
Selective IgA deficiency
X-linked agammaglobulinemia
Common variable immunodeficiency

T-Lymphocyte Abnormalities
DiGeorge syndrome
Chronic mucocutaneous candidiasis
Purine nucleoside phosphorylase deficiency

Combined T- and B-Lymphocyte Abnormalities
Severe combined immunodeficiency
Ataxia–telangiectasia
Wiskott–Aldrich syndrome

Phagocytic Cell Abnormalities
Chronic granulomatous disease
Neutropenia
Leukocyte adhesion defect
Chédiak-Higashi syndrome

Complement Deficiencies
C1 deficiency
C4 deficiency
C2 deficiency

with phagocytic disorders typically present with recurrent abscesses and distinctive organisms such as *Staphylococcus aureus* and gram-negative organisms such as *Serratia*. Patients with complement deficiencies present with recurrent infections involving encapsulated organisms such as pneumococcus and meningococcus. Several distinguishing features on history and physical examination should be emphasized when differentiating primary immunodeficiency from pediatric HIV (summarized in Table 7–4). Features on physical examination include the presence of lymphadenopathy and splenomegaly in HIV and their absence commonly in deficiencies of antibody or cell-mediated immunity.

Laboratory Evaluation

The complete evaluation of a patient with suspected immunodeficiency may be difficult to determine, but the initial screening tests are straightforward (Table 7–5). Substantial information can be obtained from a complete blood count (CBC) and erythrocyte sedimentation rate (ESR). For instance, an elevated ESR may be consistent with chronic infection. In the immunodeficient child, the CBC may show anemia of chronic disease, thrombocytopenia suggestive of Wiskott–Aldrich syndrome, or a low absolute lymphocyte count (ALC) indicative of a possible T-cell–mediated defect. Normal values for ALC differ

with age; an ALC below 3000 is abnormal in infancy, whereas an ALC below 1200 is abnormal in older children. Neutropenia or neutrophilia might suggest specific immunodeficiencies such as cyclic neutropenia or leukocyte adhesion deficiency, respectively. Additional laboratory tests to include in a screening evaluation are HIV antibody, CH50, delayed hypersensitivity skin tests, and isohemagglutinin and quantitative immunoglobulin levels. Low immunoglobulin levels suggest a specific immunodeficiency, whereas high levels suggest HIV or chronic granulomatous disease. Determination of isohemagglutinin levels, which are IgM antibodies to A and B polysaccharide antigens, also is a useful screening test in children older than 2 years; this information assesses the ability to make specific IgM antibodies. Skin testing for specific antigens (mumps, *Candida,* and tetanus), which is useful only in children older than 2 years, is performed by intradermal injection and interpreted by determining the extent of induration. Induration greater than 10 mm at 48 hours makes a primary T-cell defect very unlikely. More extensive evaluation of immune function might be indicated when the screening tests yield abnormal results or if the clinical index of suspicion for immunodeficiency is high (Table 7–6).

The clinical and laboratory features of the disorders of immunity are summarized in Table 7–7.

■ DISORDERS OF ANTIBODY-MEDIATED IMMUNITY

Development of Antibody-Mediated Immunity

B-cell–mediated immunity develops in two stages. The first stage is antigen independent and involves rearrangement of activated immunoglobulin genes. This stage occurs in the fetus by 8 weeks of gestation. By 13 weeks, the fetus has B cells capable of undergoing the second stage of differentiation, which is antigen dependent and requires the binding of a specific antigen to a surface immunoglobulin. The second stage usually occurs after birth and requires multiple signals, including T-cell participation (Figure 7–1). Ultimately, B cells differentiate into plasma cells that can secrete specific antibodies that act with activated complements to coat or opsonize foreign antigens. Activated phagocytes engulf this complex through immunoglobulin and complement receptors on their surfaces, thereby eliminating the foreign antigens.

Distinct classes of antibody play unique roles in the immune response and appear at different stages of development (Table 7–8). Immunoglobulin G, the only immunoglobulin class capable of transplacental passage, plays an important role in protecting the full-term new-

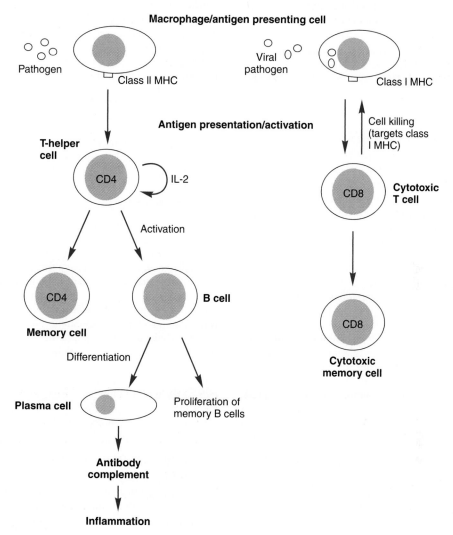

Figure 7–1. Schematic representation of a normal immune response. IL-2 = interleukin-2; MHC = major histocompatibility complex.

born from infection during the first few months. This protective feature delays the onset of clinical symptoms in patients with hypogammaglobulinemia until after they lose maternal immunoglobulin at 4 to 6 months after birth. Transplacental passage of IgG occurs at 30 to 32 weeks of gestation; therefore, premature infants might be deprived of the protective advantage of maternally acquired IgG. Because the half-life of IgG is approximately 25 days, normal infants might have significant decreases in IgG concentrations (as low as 200 mg/dL) at approximately 3 to 4 months of age before they synthesize their own IgG. Premature infants who lack maternally acquired IgG may have significant decreases to concentrations as low as 60 mg/dL at age 4 months. Transient hypogammaglobulinemia of infancy (THI) must be considered in the differential diagnosis of a patient presenting with low immunoglobulin levels in infancy. Unlike infants with hypogammaglobulinemia, those with THI can make specific antibodies to diphtheria and tetanus toxoids by age 6 to 10 months. There are four IgG subclasses, which may be selectively deficient and result in disordered immunity. Immunoglobulin G_1 and G_3 subclasses follow the pattern of total IgG in the infant, with a decrease during the first 3 to 6 months and a subsequent

Table 7–2. Clinical Features Consistent with Primary Immunodeficiency

Chronic or recurrent infection (more than expected for age)
Incomplete response to treatment
Unusual infections (opportunistic: e.g., *Pneumocystis carinii*)
Chronic thrush
Chronic diarrhea
Failure to thrive
Recurrent abscesses

Table 7–3. Features of Specific Primary Immunodeficiencies

Ataxis or telangiectasia (ataxia–telangiectasia)
Eczema or thrombocytopenia (Wiskott–Aldrich syndrome)
Tetany (DiGeorge syndrome)
Endocrinopathy (chronic mucocutaneous candidiasis)

gradual increase to adult concentrations. Immunoglobulin G_2 and G_4 subclasses increase more slowly and do not reach physiologic concentrations until 2 to 3 years of age. Immunoglobulin G_1 antibodies are produced in response to protein antigens, whereas IgG_2 antibodies are produced in response to polysaccharide antigens. Immunoglobulin G_3 antibody is responsible for the primary antibody response to many viruses.

Immunoglobulin M concentrations at birth usually are low because IgM does not cross the placenta; however, IgM synthesis can be increased in utero in response to intrauterine infection. In the initial immune response, the first antibody to be produced is IgM antibody, which is of relatively low affinity. Subsequently, after activation of B cells, there is isotype switching to higher affinity antibodies such as IgG and IgA. Immunoglobulins G and M, but not IgA, can bind complement. Immunoglobulin M antibody remains confined to the intravascular space in contrast to IgG antibody, which is in the intravascular and interstitial spaces. Immunoglobulin A antibody is found primarily in secretions such as saliva, nasal secretions, sweat, and breast milk. It provides local immunity and prevents systemic access of foreign antigens. Secretory IgA, primarily IgA subtype 1, is found in very high concentrations in breast milk and provides an important protective function against infection for breast-feeding infants. Normal plasma levels of IgG, IgA, and IgM at different ages are shown in Table 7–9.

Clinical Disorders

The more common forms of antibody-mediated immunodeficiency are discussed in this section. By far the most common form of B-cell–mediated immunodeficiency is **IgA deficiency,** which occurs at a frequency of as high as 1 in 500, compared with **agammaglobulinemia,** which occurs at a frequency of approximately 1 in 50,000. Diagnosis of **hypogammaglobulinemia** is suggested by low concentrations of immunoglobulins (usually <250 mg/dL) and an inability to make specific antibody. Not all patients presenting with low immunoglobulin concentrations in infancy have hypogammaglobulinemia. Those with THI can make specific antibodies to diphtheria and tetanus toxoids by age 6 to 10 months. Treatment involves replacement therapy with intravenous globulin. An approach to the evaluation of disorders of antibody-mediated immunity is shown in Figure 7–2.

X-LINKED AGAMMAGLOBULINEMIA

X-linked agammaglobulinemia (XLA) is the prototype form of hypogammaglobulinemia. Male infants typically present with recurrent infections within their first year. The primary defect is caused by a developmental arrest

Table 7–4. Clinical Signs and Symptoms in Primary Immunodeficiency Disorders

Clinical Signs/Symptoms	Deficiency of Antibody-Mediated Immunity	Deficiency of Cell-Mediated Immunity	Pediatric HIV Infection
Increased sinopulmonary disease	Common	Common	Common
Increased infection with encapsulated organisms	Common	Common	Common
Increased infection with opportunistic organisms	Rare	Common	Common
Oral candidiasis	Rare	Common	Common
Systemic fungal infections	Rare	Unusual	Common
Pneumocystis carinii pneumonia	Rare	Common	Common
Tonsil/lymphoid tissue	Decreased or absent	Frequently absent	Frequently enlarged
Liver and spleen	Normal	Usually normal	Frequently enlarged

HIV = human immunodeficiency virus.

Table 7–5. Initial Workup for Suspected Immunodeficiency

Complete blood count with differential (absolute lymphocyte count)

HIV antibody (if positive in child <15 mo; HIV polymerase chain reaction to confirm)

Quantitative immunoglobulin levels (IgG, IgA, IgM, and IgE)

Isohemagglutinin levels (>2 y)

Diphtheria, tetanus, and *Haemophilus influenzae,* antibody titers

T-cell–surface marker subsets (CD3, CD4, CD8)

Skin testing for *Candida,* mumps, and tetanus (>2 y)

CH50 (quantitates complement component activity)

in B-lymphocyte differentiation as a result of a mutation in the gene for Bruton tyrosine kinase, which belongs to the src family of tyrosine kinases.

Affected male infants usually are well during the first few months, when they are protected by maternal IgG. When maternal IgG is catabolized and infants cannot synthesize their own IgG, recurrent infections, frequently sinopulmonary infections, develop. If treatment is prompt or if exposure to infections is minimal, individual infections may be no more severe than those in the general population. The infections usually are chronic or recurrent, with symptoms recurring shortly after antibiotic treatment is discontinued. The most frequent infectious agents are common pyogenic bacteria, including *S. aureus, S. pneumoniae,* and *H. influenzae;* later in the course, mycoplasma might be an important pathogen in patients with chronic lung disease. Septicemia, bacterial meningitis, and osteomyelitis occur in as many as 10% of male infants who do not receive treatment. Affected infants usually are not susceptible to opportunistic infections, although they may have sensitivity to enteroviruses, including vaccine-related complications or severe echovirus meningoencephalitis, despite normal T-cell function. Findings on physical examination include absence of adenoids, tonsils, and lymph nodes.

Laboratory studies in patients with XLA show total immunoglobulin concentrations of less than 250 mg/dL, without B cells in the peripheral blood. Patients cannot make a specific antibody response, although they have normal T-cell function. Early diagnosis and initiation of replacement immunoglobulin (IVIG) are essential to prevent complications, including the development of chronic pulmonary disease. Despite the use of IVIG, some patients can have chronic sinusitis and otitis media. Risks of IVIG are discussed in the section on treatment. Prophylactic antibiotics are now generally discouraged because of the emergence of antibiotic-resistant bacteria. Patients with XLA frequently require more aggressive treatment to clear

(*text continues on page 260*)

Table 7–6. Evaluation of Immune System

	Quantity	Function
B cell	IgG, IgM, IgA, IgE IgG subclasses (IgG$_{1-4}$) B-cell numbers (CD19)	Isohemagglutinins Specific antibody response to tetanus (protein) and Pneumovax In vitro proliferation to PWM
T cell	Absolute lymphocyte count Chest radiograph (thymus) T-cell numbers (CD3$^+$) T-cell subsets (CD4, CD8)	Delayed hypersensitivity skin testing (candida, mumps, tetanus) T-cell in vitro proliferation to mitogens (PHA, concanavalin A) T-cell in vitro proliferation to antigens (candida, tetanus) ADA/PNP concentrations Cytokine production
Complement	C3, C4 Concentration of specific components (C7–9)	CH50 Hemolytic activity of other complement components
Phagocytic	Absolute neutrophil count	NBT reduction Enzyme assays (MPO, G-6PD) Bacterial killing Chemotaxis assays

ADA/PNP = adenosine deaminase/purine nucleoside phosphorylase; G-6PD = Glucose-6-phosphatase; IgA, -E, -G, -M = immunoglobulins A, E, G, M; MPO = myeloperoxidase; NBT = nitroblue tetrazolium; PHA = phytohemagglutinin; PWM = pokeweed mitogen.

Table 7–7. Clinical and Laboratory Features of Disorders of Immunity

Clinical Disease	History	Physical Examination	Humoral Immunity
Disorders of antibody-mediated immunity			
X-linked agammaglobulinemia	Male infants with recurrent infection with common pyogenic bacteria in their 1st year	Absence of adenoids, tonsils, and lymph nodes	Total Ig <250 mg/dL; no B cells in the peripheral blood
Common variable immunodeficiency	Recurrent infections in 1–2 decades of life, sinopulmonary infections from pyogenic bacteria; GI disorders; autoimmune diseases, malignancy	Presence of tonsils and adenoids, splenomegaly	Hypogammaglobulinemia; B cells in the peripheral blood
Hyper-IgM syndrome	Recurrent infections with common pyogenic bacteria in the 1st year; distinctive clinical features include presence of opportunistic infections such as *Pneumocystis carinii*	Presence of lymphoid tissue; may have lymphoid hyperplasia	Hypogammaglobulinemia; with normal or elevated IgM
IgA deficiency	Most patients are healthy; symptoms can include recurrent sinopulmonary infections and autoimmune disorders	Generally normal	Normal IgG and IgM with decreased IgA
Disorders of cell-mediated immunity			
Ataxia–telangiectasia	Typically at 3–6 y of age; progressive ataxia and then recurrent sinopulmonary infection	Cerebellar ataxia, oculocutaneous telangiectasia	IgA deficiency, low IgG$_2$ subclass level, variable defect to make specific Ig
Severe combined immunodeficiency syndrome	Heterogeneous disorder characterized by onset of recurrent infections by 3–6 mo; infections may be bacterial or opportunistic infections including PCP	Failure to thrive/absence of lymphoid tissue; oral thrush is common	Total Ig <250 mg/dL
DiGeorge syndrome	Variable presentation including recurrent infection, congenital heart defect, congenital tetany, abnormal facies	Abnormal facies, failure to thrive	Variable findings; Igs are usually normal
Wiskott–Aldrich syndrome	Eczema and bleeding in infancy; recurrent infections by 1–2 y; increased incidence of lymphoreticular malignancy	Eczema, failure to thrive	Normal IgG and may have elevated IgA and IgE; no production of antibody to polysaccharide antigens
Hyper-IgE syndrome	Present in childhood with recurrent staphylococcal infections of the skin and lung	Eczema-like skin rash, coarse facial features	Elevated IgE with normal IgG, IgM and IgA; eosinophilia is common
Disorders of phagacytic function			
Chronic granulomatous disease	Recurrent infections with catalase positive organisms	Lymphadenopathy is common	Normal
Leukocyte adhesion deficiency	Delayed separation of umbilical cord; recurrent infections include skin abscesses, pneumonia		
Disorders of complement			
Deficiency of complement components; C2 deficiency	Recurrent infections with encapsulated organisms; increase in autoimmune disorders such as lupus		

ADA = adenosine deaminase; GI = gastrointestinal; Ig = immunoglobulin; NBT = nitroblue tetrazolium dye test; NOI = neutrophil oxidative index; PCP = *Pneumocystis carinii* pneumonia; PNP = purine nucleoside phosphorylase.

Cellular Immunity	Complement System	Phagocytic System	Other Tests
Normal T-cell function			
Normal T-cell function			
Partial T-cell defect			Most patients have mutations in the gene for CD40 ligand
Normal T-cell function			
Cutaneous anergy, depressed T-cell function			Elevated serum α-feto protein level
Lymphopenia (<1200); reduced T cell proliferation to mitogens and antigens			Screen for ADA or PNP deficiency; Mutations may be defined, ie, ZAP 70 etc
Variable findings; generally, thymic hypoplasia results in decreased T cells; T-cell proliferative studies vary			Thymic hypoplasia Chromosomal deletions in 22q11
T-cell responses to mitogens are variable			Thrombocytopenia and small platelets Defect in WASP
Generally, normal T-cell proliferation to mitogens but decreased responses to specific antigens			Eosinophilia
Normal		Abnormal respiratory burst (NBT or NOI) Abnormal phagocyte adhesion and migration	
	Decreased CH50		

Table 7–8. Immunoglobulin Classes (Isotypes)

	IgG	IgM	IgA
%-total immunoglobulin	70–80	5–10	10–15
Mean adult value	1200 mg/dL	150 mg/dL	300 mg/dL
Distribution	Intravascular/interstitial spaces	Intravascular	Secretions/intravascular
Transplacental passage	Yes: after 30–32 wk	No	No
Synthesized in utero	No	Yes	Yes (late)
Activates complement	Yes	Yes	No
Subclasses	4	0	2

infections. For example, the treatment of pneumonia may require prolonged administration of intravenous antibiotics. With early diagnosis and appropriate treatment, children with XLA can survive into adulthood without significant morbidity.

COMMON VARIABLE IMMUNODEFICIENCY

Common variable immunodeficiency (CVI) is a primary immunodeficiency with hypogammaglobulinemia that is distinct from XLA. Distinguishing features are B cells in the peripheral blood, autoimmune disease, and later age of onset. CVI is a heterogeneous group of disorders without a unifying pathogenesis. The disease frequently is caused by an intrinsic B-cell defect, although abnormalities of cytokines or interactions between T and B cells have been implicated. In addition, there is no clear mode of inheritance, although CVI can cluster in families.

Most patients with CVI are well in early childhood, but recurrent infections develop during the second and third decades of life. The most common manifestations of CVI are chronic sinopulmonary infections from pyogenic bacteria and chronic diarrhea frequently due to

Table 7–9. Normal Plasma Values for Immunoglobulins at Various Ages

Age	IgG (mg/dL)	IgA mg/dL	IgM mg/dL
Newborn	600–1670	0–5	6–15
1–3 mo	218–610	20–53	11–51
4–6 mo	228–636	27–72	25–60
7–9 mo	292–816	27–73	12–124
10–18 mo	383–1070	27–169	28–113
2 y	423–1184	35–222	21–131
3 y	477–1334	40–251	28–113
4–5 y	540–1500	48–336	20–106
6–8 y	571–1700	52–535	28–112
14 y	570–1570	86–544	33–135
Adult	635–1775	106–668	37–154

Giardia lamblia. Malabsorption also is commonly seen; small bowel biopsy specimens show flattened villi. Additional features are autoimmune hemolytic anemia and thrombocytopenia, inflammatory bowel disease, gluten-sensitive enteropathy, and nodular lymphoid hyperplasia. Malignant neoplasms, including non-Hodgkin's lymphoma, thymoma, and gastric adenocarcinoma, occur in approximately 10% of patients and increase in frequency with age. In contrast with the physical examination of patients with hypogammaglobulinemia and XLA, who do not have lymph nodes and tonsils, patients with CVI show presence of lymph nodes and tonsils. Splenomegaly is present in approximately 25% of patients with CVI. Laboratory evaluation shows hypogammaglobulinemia with typically normal T-cell function. The mainstay of treatment is IVIG and aggressive management of infections.

HYPER-IGM SYNDROME

Hyper-IgM syndrome is a complex clinical syndrome characterized by low levels of IgG but normal to increased levels of IgM. It is typically X-linked but may be autosomal recessive. Patients with X-linked hyper-IgM syndrome have mutations in the gene for the CD40 ligand on T cells. Absence of T-cell CD40 ligand results in abnormal interactions between T and B cells and an inability of B cells to undergo isotype switching from IgM- to IgG- or IgA-producing cells. In addition, deficiency of CD40 ligand on T cells results in a partial T-cell defect and susceptibility of patients with hyper-IgM to infections with intracellular pathogens. Like patients with XLA, patients with hyper-IgM syndrome usually become symptomatic within the first 2 years of life. Sinopulmonary disease develops from common encapsulated bacteria. Distinctive clinical features are infections with intracellular pathogens such as *P. carinii* and *Cryptosporidium parvum*. Chronic diarrhea, sclerosing cholangitis, and chronic hepatitis can occur. In addition, patients with hyper-IgM syndrome frequently have chronic neutropenia, lymphoid hyperplasia, and autoimmune diseases such as hemolytic anemia and thrombocytopenia.

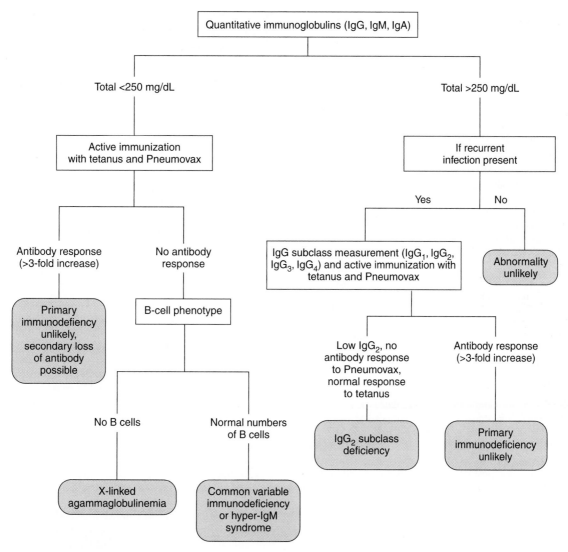

Figure 7–2. Algorithm showing an approach to the evaluation of clinical disorders of antibody-mediated immunity.

Patients with hyper-IgM syndrome have increased risk of neoplasms such as lymphoma and tumors of the liver and biliary tract. The results of laboratory studies show a deficiency in IgG and IgA but normal to increased levels of IgM. B cells are present in the peripheral blood, and patients usually have normal T-cell numbers and function. Treatment requires replacement therapy with IVIG and PCP prophylaxis with trimethoprim–sulfamethoxazole. Consideration should be given to the use of recombinant granulocyte colony stimulatory factor (G-CSF) for chronic neutropenia and flucytosine for long-term treatment of *Cryptosporidium*. Bone marrow and stem cell

transplantation have been used successfully to treat this disorder.

SELECTIVE IgA DEFICIENCY

Selective IgA deficiency, the most prevalent primary immunodeficiency, occurs in approximately 1 in 500 individuals. Most cases occur sporadically, although risk is increased among family members. Most patients with IgA deficiency are healthy. Symptomatic patients present with recurrent sinopulmonary infections, allergy, gastrointestinal diseases, and autoimmune disorders. The age of onset of symptoms is variable. Laboratory study results include normal IgG and IgM with decreased IgA (<10 mg/dL). Patients with IgA deficiency may have a coexisting IgG$_2$ subclass deficiency. Treatment with IVIG is not indicated; in fact, commercial γ-globulin preparations contain small amounts of IgA capable of sensitizing patients with IgA deficiency. On rare occasions, this sensitization results in an anaphylactic response to IVIG or blood transfusions.

IgG Subclass Deficiencies

Deficiencies in IgG subclasses can occur despite normal total IgG levels. The most common one is **IgG$_2$ deficiency.** Patients typically present with recurrent infections, including sinopulmonary infections and otitis media caused by pyogenic organisms. Laboratory evaluation usually shows decreased IgG$_2$ levels and no specific antibody response to immunization with unconjugated polysaccharide vaccines such as Pneumovax. Pre- and postimmunization titers are obtained at the time of and 3 weeks after immunization with Pneumovax. Normal response to immunization is a greater than threefold increase in antibody titer to three or more serotypes of *S. pneumoniae* contained within the Pneumovax vaccine. Use of IVIG to treat IgG$_2$ subclass deficiency is controversial and recommended only in patients with severe recurrent infections.

Treatment

Replacement therapy with IVIG remains the mainstay of therapy for disorders of antibody-mediated immunity. Risks of IVIG include those associated with the infusion of blood and blood products. Although there were numerous reported cases of the transmission of hepatitis C during the early 1990s, IVIG preparations currently are acid treated, making the transmission of hepatitis C unlikely. There have been no reported cases of HIV transmission with IVIG. Additional treatment approaches for patients with hypogammaglobulinemia are aggressive treatment of infections with antibiotics. Patients with hypogammaglobulinemia should not receive live-virus vaccines such as OPV or the combination of mumps, measles, and rubella vaccine.

■ DISORDERS OF CELL-MEDIATED IMMUNITY

Development of Cell-Mediated Immunity

Differentiation of stem cells into a mature population of T lymphocytes occurs in the thymus. Prothymocytes colonize the fetal thymus at 8 to 9 weeks of gestation, initially entering the subcapsular region of the thymus. As the T cells move through the cortex to the medulla, they differentiate into mature T cells. Cell surface markers change as the T cell matures, with early T-cell precursors co-expressing CD4 and CD8. As T cells differentiate, they acquire a mature T-cell receptor and the cell-surface antigens CD3 and CD11. The presence of CD4 on mature T cells correlates with T-helper activity, whereas the presence of CD8 correlates with T-suppressor and T-cytotoxic activities. By 12 weeks of gestation, functioning T cells are present in the human fetus; by 40 weeks, the T-cell population generally is mature. This process of generating a mature T-cell population requires positive and negative selections in the thymus, with most T-cell precursors dying before maturity. At birth, the full-term newborn frequently has an elevated total lymphocyte count (mean of 4500/μL) with normal total T-cell numbers in the peripheral blood. In addition, CD4 cells make up 60% of peripheral T cells, and the ratio of CD4 to CD8 exceeds 3:1. The numbers of CD4 cells slowly decrease with age; by 6 years, 40% of the peripheral blood cells are CD4 cells, and the ratio of CD4 to CD8 reaches the adult value of 2:1. The changes in lymphocytes, T cells, and T-cell subpopulations are shown in Table 7–10.

The two main populations of T cells, CD4 and CD8 cells, have distinct functions. T-helper cells, or CD4 cells, play an important role in helping B cells produce antibody by generating stimulating cytokines such as interleukin-2 (IL-2; Figure 7–1). The CD4-positive cells are stimulated by interacting with antigen in the context of class II molecules in the major histocompatibility complex on antigen-presenting cells such as dendritic cells

Table 7–10. Peripheral Blood Lymphocytes, T Cells, T-Cell Subpopulation by Age

	Lymphocyte Count (per μL)	CD2 (%lymphs)	CD4 (%CD3)	CD8 (%CD3)	CD4:CD8 Ratio
Third trimester early	—	—	80	15	5:1
Third trimester term/newborn	>3000	55	60	20	3:1
Newborn to 2 y	>2000	65	50	20	2:1
2–4 y	>1500	65	40	20	2:1
4–6 y	>1200	65	40	20	2:1
Adult	>1200	65	40	20	2:1

and macrophages. In contrast, CD8-positive cytotoxic T cells play an essential role in fighting infection that involves targeting and killing cells infected with viruses. This recognition process involves the direct interaction of CD8-positive T cells with viral antigen presented on cells in the context of class I molecules in the major histocompatibility complex.

Clinical Disorders

Although the clinical spectrum depends on the severity of disease, patients with disorders of cell-mediated immunity tend to present earlier during infancy and usually require more aggressive treatment and intervention for survival than do those with isolated B-cell disorders. T cells play an important role in the organization and activation of other components of the immune response such as the B-cell and macrophage responses (Figure 7–1). Abnormal antibody-mediated immunity is an important component of T-cell disorders.

SEVERE COMBINED IMMUNODEFICIENCY SYNDROME

Severe combined immunodeficiency syndrome (SCID) is a heterogeneous disorder characterized by the absence of functional T cells and abnormal antibody-mediated immunity. Progress has been made recently in defining the molecular defects underlying several forms of SCID. The defect in X-linked SCID, the most common form, has been identified as a mutation in the gene for the IL-2 receptor γ-chain. Other recently defined forms of SCID are a T-cell–receptor signaling defect with mutations in the *ZAP70* gene, deficiency of Jak3 kinase, IL-7 receptor α-chain deficiency, mutations in CD25 (IL-2 receptor α-chain), and defective IL-2 production. Approximately half the patients with the autosomal-recessive form of SCID have a deficiency in the enzyme adenosine deaminase (ADA), which results in the accumulation of metabolites toxic to the lymphocyte.

Infants with SCID usually present with serious or recurrent infections by 3 to 6 months of age. Other manifestations are failure to thrive and chronic respiratory, gastrointestinal, or cutaneous infections. However, the first indication of SCID frequently is pneumonia with an opportunistic organism such as *P. carinii* or cytomegalovirus. In addition, oral ulcers, oral esophageal candidiasis, severe varicella, and secretory diarrhea are seen commonly in infants with SCID. Laboratory evaluation shows lymphopenia (<1200/μL) in most patients, although a normal lymphocyte count does not exclude the diagnosis of SCID. Further evaluation for SCID should include quantitation of T-cell subpopulations and determination of T-cell function. Classification of T-cell subpopulations by flow cytometry contribute to the identification of the type of SCID (Table 7–11). Studies of T-cell function include T-cell proliferative responses to mitogens (phytohemag-

Table 7–11. Classification of T-Cell Immunodeficiencies by Flow Cyotmetry

T⁺B⁺NK⁺
Hyper-IgM
MHC deficiency
ZAP70 CD8-SCID
Wiskott–Aldrich syndrome
Omenn syndrome
T⁻B⁺NK⁺
DiGeorge syndrome
IL-7 receptor α-chain deficiency SCID
T⁻B⁺NK⁻
X-linked SCID
Jak3-kinase–deficient SCID
T⁻B⁻NK⁺
RAG1 and RAG2 defects
T⁻B⁻NK⁻
ADA deficiency
PNP deficiency
Reticular dysgenesis

ADA = adenosine deaminase; Ig = immunoglobulin; IL-7 = interleukin-7; MHC = major histocompatibility complex; NK = natural killer cell; PNP = purine nucleoside phosphorylase; SCID = severe combined immunodeficiency syndrome.

glutinin and concanavalin A), antigens (tetanus, *Candida*), and alloantigens (mixed lymphocyte culture). Patients with SCID also have reduced serum immunoglobulin levels and an inability to form specific antibody.

Treatment of SCID depends on the pathogenesis of the disorder. The optimal treatment for most patients with SCID is histocompatible bone-marrow transplantation from a sibling. Success with bone-marrow transplantation, if performed early and before the onset of severe infections, has been seen in as many as 90% of patients. However, most patients do not have matched donors for bone-marrow transplantation. Alternative therapeutic options are stem cell transplantation or haploidentical bone-marrow transplantation, eg, from a parent, after depleting the bone marrow of mature T cells. Infants with enzyme deficiencies such as ADA may receive enzyme replacement therapy as an alternative. In some recent clinical trials, some patients with ADA deficiency received stem cell gene therapy with some early promising results. Two patients with X-linked SCID were treated successfully with gene therapy. Gene therapy might become a more common therapeutic approach as the technology improves and additional molecular mechanisms are defined.

Infants with SCID should not receive live-virus vaccines because dissemination can occur, as in vaccine-induced poliomyelitis after OPV. Close contacts of the patient also should receive killed poliovirus vaccine. All blood products should be irradiated to avoid graft-versus-host reaction and screened for cytomegalovirus. IVIG and prophylaxis against PCP should be administered until bone marrow engraftment is complete.

DiGeorge Syndrome

DiGeorge syndrome is characterized by thymic hypoplasia, tetany from hypoparathyroidism and hypocalcemia, abnormal facies, increased susceptibility to infection, and congenital heart disease. Chromosomal microdeletions in 22q11 have been found the majority of patients, although the molecular defect has not been determined. Most cases are sporadic, and male and female infants can be affected. DiGeorge syndrome results from a developmental defect that affects third and fourth pharyngeal pouch evaginations at 6 to 8 weeks of gestation. Thus, this syndrome is a multisystem developmental disorder affecting the thymus and parathyroid glands and certain aortic arch structures, resulting in congenital heart defects.

The spectrum of immunodeficiency differs, with some patients having "partial DiGeorge syndrome" and essentially normal immune function. In the other extreme, some patients have severe immunodeficiency with a clinical presentation similar to SCID. Infants with DiGeorge syndrome usually are identified because of their congenital heart disease and hypocalcemia. In general, the thymic hypoplasia results in decreased but not absent T cells (30–40% CD3 cells). Serum immunoglobulin levels usually are near normal for age, and T-cell proliferative studies depend on the severity of the immunodeficiency. Patients with severe immunodeficiency have benefited from thymic transplants and human leukocyte antigen (HLA)–identical bone marrow transplantation. The bone marrow transplant cannot be depleted of T cells; its success requires the presence of mature T cells from the donor because of the thymic hypoplasia seen in DiGeorge syndrome. Children with this syndrome require comprehensive management that includes genetics, cardiology, immunology, developmental neuropsychology, craniofacial surgery, and endocrinology.

Wiskott–Aldrich Syndrome

Wiskott–Aldrich syndrome (WAS) is an X-linked disorder characterized by thrombocytopenia, eczema, and recurrent infections. Cellular and antibody-mediated immunity are abnormal. The defective gene in WAS has been cloned and is known as *WASP; WASP* is important for normal immune cell function and is thought to involve cycloskeletal reorganization after the activation of T-cells or platelets.

Patients typically present with eczema and bleeding during early infancy. Recurrent infections frequently develop later, often during the first 1 to 2 years. The infections usually are secondary to encapsulated organisms, such as *S. pneumoniae,* although patients also are susceptible to opportunistic infections, including PCP. Patients with WAS also have an increased incidence of lymphoreticular malignant disease, autoimmune hemolytic anemia, and arthritis. Laboratory studies usually show no production of antibody to polysaccharide antigens, elevated IgA and IgE, normal IgG, and low IgM concentrations. Isohemagglutinins are absent, and T-cell responses to mitogens are variable. The diagnosis is suggested by thrombocytopenia and small platelets.

Survival into adulthood is rare, and the cause of death is commonly related to bleeding, infection, or malignant disease. Treatment is, at minimum, supportive with IVIG and aggressive management of acute infections. Patients may benefit from an HLA-mixed lymphocyte culture–identical bone marrow transplant. Successful bone marrow transplantation normalizes the platelet count, reconstitutes the immune system, and relieves eczema.

Ataxia–Telangiectasia

Ataxia–telangiectasia (AT) is an autosomal recessive disorder characterized by cerebellar ataxia, oculocutaneous telangiectasia, recurrent sinopulmonary tract infections, and variable immunodeficiency. The immunodeficiency can involve antibody- and cell-mediated immunities. Patients with AT have defective mechanisms of DNA repair and increased susceptibility to chromosomal breaks and translocations after irradiation. The defect in AT has been discovered in a gene on chromosome 11q22-23, which encodes a phosphatidylinositol-3-kinase–like protein that is believed to be important in DNA repair.

Patients typically present at 3 to 6 years of age with progressive cerebellar ataxia and telangiectasia. The immune dysfunction usually develops later and is accompanied by recurrent sinopulmonary infections. Older patients with AT might have insulin-resistant diabetes mellitus and increased incidence of malignant disorders such as lymphosarcoma, leukemia, adenocarcinoma, dysgerminoma, and medulloblastoma. Diagnosis of AT is confirmed by an elevated serum α-fetoprotein level. The immunologic abnormalities are variable and usually progressive. Patients commonly have IgA deficiency and low IgG$_2$ subclass levels, with variable defects in the ability to make antibodies to specific antigens. Most patients have abnormal cell-mediated immunity characterized by cutaneous anergy and depressed, but not absent, T-cell function.

There is no specific treatment to limit progression of AT. Intravenous immunoglobulin might be indicated if there is IgG subclass deficiency and significant infections. Progression of the disease is variable, and many patients survive into adulthood.

Chronic Mucocutaneous Candidiasis

Chronic mucocutaneous candidiasis (CMC) is a rare disorder in which patients have persistent *Candida* infection of the skin, mucous membranes, and nails. The pathogenesis of CMC is unknown, although family history has been present in as many as 20% of patients.

Approximately half the patients have an associated endocrinopathy, such as Addison's disease, hypoparathyroidism, hypothyroidism, or diabetes mellitus. Patients with CMC are anergic on delayed hypersensitivity skin testing to *Candida* despite normal responses to mumps and tetanus. These results are supported by absent T-cell proliferative responses to *Candida* despite normal responses to mitogens and other specific antigens such as tetanus. Patients with CMC have normal antibody-mediated immunity. Patients usually require systemic treatment with antifungal agents such as fluconazole. They typically survive into adulthood with the primary complication of an endocrinopathy such as unsuspected adrenal insufficiency.

HYPER-IGE SYNDROME

Hyper-IgE syndrome is a rare multisystem disorder characterized by abnormalities of dentition, bones, and connective tissue, recurrent staphylococcal pulmonary and skin infections, dermatitis, and a markedly elevated serum IgE level. Although the underlying cause of hyper-IgE syndrome is unknown, the proximal region of chromosome 4 is thought to contain a disease locus for the disorder. Patients typically present in childhood with coarse facies and recurrent staphylococcal infections of the skin and lung; complications include abscess formation and the development of pneumatoceles. Allergic bronchopulmonary aspergillosis frequently complicates the underlying pulmonary disease. Patients often have a chronic inflammatory skin condition similar to eczema. Recurrent bone fractures, scoliosis, and delayed shedding of primary teeth with noneruption of secondary teeth are seen in over half of the patients. Laboratory studies show eosinophilia and elevated IgE levels with normal IgG, IgA, and IgM levels. T-cell function is variable, with generally normal T-cell proliferative responses to mitogens but decreased responses to specific antigens. Some patients have abnormal phagocytic chemotactic responses, although this finding is not universal. Treatment is supportive, with prophylactic antibiotics against staphylococcal infections and aggressive treatment of acute infections. Some patients have benefited from treatment with IVIG and γ-interferon.

Treatment

The ideal treatment for severe T-cell–mediated immunodeficiency is bone marrow transplantation using an HLA-identical donor. Alternative treatments are stem cell transplantation or bone marrow transplantation from a haploidentical donor, usually the child's parents, after depletion of mature T cells to prevent graft-versus-host disease. Less severe forms of T-cell–mediated immunodeficiency can be managed with intravenous antibiotics,

PCP prophylaxis, and supportive care as indicated. Most patients require IVIG. The patients should not receive live-virus vaccines, and blood transfusions should be negative for cytomegalovirus and irradiated. ADA deficiency is a unique form of SCID in which patients can receive enzyme replacement therapy. Early clinical trials using gene therapy to treat ADA deficiency and X-linked SCID currently are in progress, with some evidence of potential therapeutic benefit.

■ DISORDERS OF THE COMPLEMENT SYSTEM

The complement system has more than 20 components, and deficiencies in many of these components have been reported. Most of these are inherited as autosomal recessive traits, although C1 esterase inhibitor deficiency is autosomal dominant. The most common defect in the complement system is C2 deficiency, which occurs in 1 of 10,000 individuals.

The complement system plays an important role in host defense by (1) causing lysis of cells and bacteria, (2) mediating opsonization by coating foreign antigens with complement and thereby promoting phagocytosis, and (3) producing peptide fragments that generate inflammatory responses, including chemotactic and vasodilatory factors. The two major pathways of the complement system are the classic and alternative. The classic pathway is activated by antibody and involves complement components C1, C4, and C2, which activate C3 and the terminal components of the complement cascade. The alternative pathway may function independently of antibody and includes factors B, D, and properdin, which subsequently activate C3 and the terminal components of the cascade.

DEFICIENCY OF COMPLEMENT COMPONENTS

Patients with complement deficiency have variable clinical presentations depending on the component that is deficient. Patients deficient in C1, C2, C3, or C4 have increased susceptibility to encapsulated bacteria and autoimmune disorders such as systemic lupus erythematosus. In contrast, patients with deficiencies of the terminal complement components C5 through C9 have selected susceptibilities to meningococcal and gonococcal infections. Screening laboratory evaluation is done best by quantitation of the hemolytic complement. This is a functional assay and requires the presence of functional complement components C1 through C9. If hemolytic complement is decreased or absent, the quantity and function of each complement component should be determined.

There is no specific therapy for complement deficiencies. Treatment includes immunizations against *H. influenzae*, *S. pneumoniae*, and *Neisseria meningitidis*. Prophylactic antibiotics using trimethoprim–sulfamethoxazole might benefit some patients. Children with deficiencies in early complement components should be observed carefully for the development of autoimmune diseases.

DEFICIENCY OF MANNOSE BINDING PROTEIN

Mannose binding protein (MBP) plays an important role in the immune response by acting as an opsonin and activating the classic complement pathway. Recent studies suggest that low serum levels of MBP are associated with recurrent infections in childhood. As many as 25% of children with unexplained recurrent infections may have deficiencies in MBP. Children typically present at 6 to 18 months of age with recurrent otitis media, sinopulmonary infections, skin infections, and diarrhea. Reports have indicated that the spectrum of clinical involvement is variable, with some patients having more severe infections, including chronic cryptosporidial diarrhea and meningococcal meningitis. Treatment usually is supportive and similar to the approach used with patients deficient in components of the complement cascade.

■ DISORDERS OF THE PHAGOCYTIC SYSTEM

Infants with defects in phagocyte function frequently present with recurrent infections during their first year of life. The clinical disorders of phagocytes can be divided into those with decreased neutrophil counts and those with normal or increased neutrophil counts but abnormal neutrophil function.

The phagocytic system is made up of a number of different cell types, including neutrophils and macrophages, which play an important role in host defense. Phagocytes play a role in the immune response by accumulating in areas of inflammation and participating in the local inflammatory response. They also play an important role in host defense through phagocytosis and, subsequently, by killing certain types of pathogens.

LEUKOCYTE ADHESION DEFICIENCY

Leukocyte adhesion deficiency (LAD) is a rare disorder characterized by abnormal phagocyte adhesion and migration. The more common form of the disease, LAD type I, is caused by a deficiency in the cell-surface β_2 integrin CD11/CD18. As a result of this autosomal recessive disorder, immune cells cannot attach to, and subsequently migrate through, the endothelial surface and accumulate in sites of inflammation. Patients present with delayed separation of the umbilical cord (>3 weeks), poor wound healing, and recurrent infections. The more common infections are skin abscesses, otitis media, perirectal abscesses, bacteremia, and pneumonia. The organisms typically seen

are *S. aureus, Escherichia coli,* and *Pseudomonas aeruginosa.* Severity of disease depends on the levels of integrin present on the cell surface. Patients without CD11/CD18 usually present with severe recurrent infections and die within the first few years of life. Patients with LAD also may have normal β2 integrin expression but a mutation in the gene that disrupts its adhesive function. Another type of LAD is LADII, a defect in the surface expression of the Sialyl Lewis epitype. Bone marrow transplantation has been successful in some of these patients.

CHÉDIAK–HIGASHI SYNDROME

Chédiak–Higashi syndrome is a rare autosomal recessive disorder characterized by recurrent pyogenic infections, partial albinism, platelet storage pool defect, and giant cytoplasmic granules in granulocytes. The pathogenesis of this disorder is not well understood. Patients have a lysosomal storage defect and abnormal phagocyte chemotaxis. Children present with recurrent pyogenic sinopulmonary infections, skin infections, and subcutaneous abscesses. They have increased susceptibility to *S. aureus,* streptococci, gram-negative organisms, and fungi. The diagnosis is made by identifying the giant granules in myeloid cells on the peripheral smear. Treatment is supportive, with aggressive treatment of acute infections. Some patients have responded successfully to bone marrow transplantation.

CHRONIC GRANULOMATOUS DISEASE

Chronic granulomatous disease (CGD) is an inherited disorder caused by an abnormal respiratory burst in phagocytes. The phagocytes cannot generate oxygen radicals such as superoxide anion and, as a result, have defective intracellular killing. There is an X-linked form of CGD, which is the more common, and an autosomal recessive form. The X-linked form is caused by a defect in one of the membrane-associated nicotinamide adenine dinucliotide phosphate subunits. The autosomal recessive form is caused by a defect in one of the cytosolic components, which is also required for a normal oxidative burst.

Patients present with recurrent infections caused by catalase-positive microorganisms. The most common organisms are *S. aureus, Serratia marcescens,* and *Aspergillus* species. Patients frequently present with cutaneous abscesses, lymphadenitis, dermatitis, pneumonia complicated by empyema or lung abscess, perirectal abscess, and recurrent osteomyelitis. Patients also may have a chronic inflammatory disease that might manifest as chronic lymphadenopathy and intermittent fevers with no identifiable microorganisms. Treatment usually is supportive, with aggressive diagnosis, treatment of infections, and prophylaxis with trimethoprim-sulfamethoxazole. Many patients have benefited from γ-interferon; a significant reduction in recurrent infections in those patients receiving γ-interferon was noted in placebo-controlled clinical trials. The mechanism of action of γ-interferon in this disease is unknown, although it has been postulated to increase respiratory burst activity.

■ PEDIATRIC ACQUIRED IMMUNODEFICIENCY SYNDROME (AIDS): APPROACHES TO DIAGNOSIS & TREATMENT

Pediatric AIDS is a leading cause of death in children throughout the world. At the end of 2000; global estimates included 2.0 million children living with HIV/AIDS. The majority of these children live in the developing world, and the majority of new infections (estimated 600,000 in the year 2000) occur in neonates in the developing world. Chemoprophylaxis of HIV-infected pregnant women and their newborns and obstetric procedures that decrease transmission from mother to infant have decreased new cases of perinatal HIV in the United States to fewer than 500 per year. However, in those children infected with HIV, the clinical signs and symptoms are indistinguishable from those seen in children with inherited primary immunodeficiency disease (Table 7–4). Therefore, it is important to examine all children with too many infections or unusual infections for HIV-1.

Transmission

Most children infected with HIV acquired the virus by transmission from their infected mothers. The risk of transmission without chemoprophylaxis varies throughout the world, from as low as 14.4% in Europe to more than 30% in coastal cities in the United States. Rates of transmission are dramatically decreased by the administration of zidovudine with or without other antiretroviral agents during pregnancy. Results of a randomized, placebo-controlled trial indicate that giving zidovudine to the mother orally during pregnancy (after 14 weeks of gestation), intravenously during labor, and to the infant for 6 weeks after delivery reduced transmission from 25% (placebo group) to 8% (zidovudine group). Decreasing the HIV-1 viral burden during pregnancy by the use of combination antiretroviral therapy and careful obstetric practice to ensure the delivery of a term infant with minimal exposure to maternal blood have further decreased the transmission rate to approximately 2%. The use of zidovudine chemoprophylaxis to mother and infant and the treatment of pregnant women with combination antiretroviral therapy to decrease their viral burdens is now recommended throughout the United States. Risk factors for the transmission of HIV from mother to infant are multifactorial. Factors contributing to such transmission are high viral load during pregnancy, advanced maternal disease, primary infection during pregnancy, and low maternal CD4 count. Obstetric factors contributing to transmission are rupture of membranes for longer than 4 hours, prematurity (<32 weeks of gestation), and chorioamniocentesis and "skin breaks" and bloody gastric aspirates in newborns. In the United States most (two thirds) of infants with HIV-1 infection acquire their infection peripartum, as the infant passes through the mother's birth canal and is exposed to HIV-1 in the mother's blood and cervical vaginal secretions. Transmission also can occur in utero or postpartum in breast-fed infants.

An important strategy to prevent transmission is a universal approach that offers HIV testing with the right of refusal to all pregnant women, regardless of the prevalence of HIV infection in their communities or their perceived risk for infection. This uniform policy should reach HIV-infected pregnant women in all populations and geographic areas of the United States and has been recommended by the Institute of Medicine. Although this universal approach will necessitate increased resources, the effect of implementation of HIV-1 counseling and testing services for pregnant women will result in medical interventions that have been documented to reduce HIV-related morbidity in women and their infants and should ultimately reduce medical costs.

Diagnosis of HIV Infection in Children

The diagnosis of HIV-1 infection in infants and children is based on (1) epidemiologic risk factors, (2) clinical presentation, and (3) confirmation by serologic test or documentation of the virus and/or genome in the peripheral blood. The "gold standard" for the documentation of genome in the peripheral blood is DNA polymerase chain reaction (PCR), which detects the integration of viral genetic material into the human chromosome. The standard test for the diagnosis of HIV infection in adults is enzyme-linked immunosorbent assay IgG anti-HIV with confirmation using western blot analysis. Immunoglobulin G antibody in infants born after 32 weeks of gestation and until age 18 months may reflect maternal antibody because of the active transport of IgG across the placenta at 32 weeks of gestation. Therefore, the documentation of HIV-1 infection in infants younger than 18 months is based on the identification of HIV-1 in peripheral blood mononuclear cells by culture or the identification of the genome by DNA-PCR. The finding must be confirmed with a second test performed on separate blood samples. With the use of DNA-PCR, it is now possible to diagnose 96% of infants who have HIV-1 infection by age 28 days. The recommended schedule for testing infants at risk is as close to birth as possible (within 72 hours); if there is no evidence of virus, tests should be repeated at age 1 month and again at age 2 to 4 months. If an infant has no evidence of virus or genome by culture or DNA-PCR on two occasions with both tests performed after age 1 month and one after age 4 months, there is greater than 96% certainty that the infant is not infected with HIV-1.

After HIV-1 infection is documented, baseline immunologic studies should be obtained. Those studies are total T-cell count, percentage and total numbers of CD4 and CD8 cells, and quantitative immunoglobulin levels. In addition, the HIV-1 viral load should be quantitated by plasma RNA-PCR, which measures the circulating plasma virus not yet incorporated into the human genome.

Clinical Manifestations

The clinical features of AIDS in children and the differences between children and adults are shown in Table 7–12. However, the natural history of HIV-1 in children in the United States is changing. With the increased identification of HIV-1–infected women during pregnancy, the prompt diagnosis of the 2% to 8% of infants who prove infected within the first few months of life, and the rapid initiation of combination antiretroviral therapy in those infected infants, fewer clinical manifestations are seen with HIV-1 infection. The rapid initiation of combination antiretroviral therapy controls viral burden and prevents the destruction of CD4 cells. Thus, increasing numbers of HIV-1–infected children are living to their

Table 7–12. Clinical Features of AIDS in Children and Adults

Common in children and adults
Opportunistic infections (not CNS)
Chronic mucocutaneous *Candida*
Neurologic abnormalities
Chronic diarrhea
Chronic fevers
Diffuse adenopathy
Hepatosplenomegaly
Chronic eczema
Renal disease
Cardiomyopathy
More common in children
Recurrent bacterial infections
Chronic interstitial pneumonitis
Parotitis
Failure to thrive
Early onset developmental delay
More common in adults
Neoplasms
Opportunistic infections of CNS

AIDS = acquired immunodeficiency syndrome; CNS = central nervous system.

second decade of life and beyond relatively asymptomatic. Without early diagnosis and treatment, common clinical features are failure to thrive, developmental delay, oral candidiasis, diarrhea, chronic eczema, and intermittent fevers of unknown origin. Abnormal antibody-mediated immunity in HIV-infected children predisposes them to overwhelming infections with encapsulated organisms. Chronic sinopulmonary disease and skin and soft tissue infections are common. Physical examination findings can include splenomegaly and lymphadenopathy.

Children with HIV are susceptible to opportunistic infections with *P. carinii, Mycobacterium avium intracellulare, Candida, Cryptosporidiosis,* and *Mycobacterium tuberculosis*. Chronic herpes simplex infection is common in HIV-1–infected children, and chronic varicella frequently follows a primary infection. Pulmonary disease is common in children with AIDS. In a child with HIV-1 and pulmonary infiltrates, the differential diagnosis is broad and ranges from lymphocytic interstitial pneumonitis to acute bacterial pneumonia, viral pneumonia, fungal pneumonitis, and PCP.

HIV-1 infection of the central nervous system and developmental delay are among the most devastating complications of pediatric AIDS. Without early diagnosis and treatment, encephalopathy may be the first manifestation of HIV-1 infection; the rate of progression varies, and children may remain stable for several years or deteriorate rapidly over a few weeks. Developmental delay and intellectual deterioration usually are accompanied by neurologic abnormalities such as increased muscle tone, paresis, or Bells palsy. Acquired microcephaly may be the first sign of neurologic disease. Computed tomographic scans show atrophy of the brain with ventricular enlargement; calcifications and contrast enhancement in the basal ganglia and frontal lobes plus attenuation of white matter may be present.

Most children currently infected with HIV-1 likely will live for extended periods. Before the institution of antiretroviral therapy, the median life expectancy after diagnosis of HIV-1 infection was approximately 35 months; the current median life expectancy with the use of three antiretroviral agents is unknown but is greatly improved.

Management

HIV-1 infection in children is a multisystem disorder and a chronic illness with acute exacerbations. Management includes providing prompt antiretroviral treatment and supportive care within a multidisciplinary setting. Children infected with HIV-1 should be referred to a pediatric HIV specialist for consultation because the guidelines for antiretroviral therapy continue to change.

HIV-1 viral burden, quantitated by RNA-PCR copy per milliliter, is substantially greater in children than in adults at the time of diagnosis; remains elevated for up to 2 to 3 years in children compared with 2 months in adults; and subsequently declines to 100,000 copies rather than 10,000 copies as in adults if antiretroviral therapy is not initiated. Therefore, the early initiation of antiretroviral therapy to control the high viral load is particularly important in children. Most specialists recommend the initiation of combination antiretroviral therapy at the time of diagnosis and as early as age 28 days.

Zidovudine, a thymidine analogue and reverse transcriptase inhibitor, is safe in children. As a single agent, however, it reduces viral load modestly and only temporarily. When accompanied by a second nonthymidine analogue–reverse transcriptase inhibitor, such as dideoxyinosine or Epivir, the impact on viral load is greater and sustained for longer periods. The addition of a protease inhibitor to the regimen further improves the treatment efficacy of HIV-1 in children. However, the number of antiretroviral agents available as suspensions for the treatment of young children is limited. If a child fails one combination regimen and develops increased viral burden, decreased CD4 cells, and/or progressive clinical disease, a change in regimen requires at least two new antiretroviral agents. Failure to change more than one drug almost always results in an increasingly resistant virus. Therefore, initiation and change of antiretroviral regimens must be done with caution. Regardless of the therapy selected, it is important to monitor decreases of viral load by RNA-PCR and increases in CD4 counts to assess the effect of therapy and adjust treatment appropriately.

Prompt diagnosis and specific treatment of all bacterial, viral, and fungal infections are essential. Nutrition should be followed carefully, and nighttime enteral feedings or hyperalimentation should be used when failure to thrive is a major problem. Although there is no specific management for the central nervous system disease, treatment is directed at its neurologic manifestations. For example, as lower extremity neurologic signs develop, providing leg braces may allow for longer periods of normal ambulation.

Because PCP is the most common opportunistic infection in HIV-1–infected children, prophylaxis with trimethoprim–sulfamethoxazole is recommended for all HIV-exposed infants between age 6 weeks and 4 months. Prophylaxis should be continued between 4 and 12 months if HIV infection is indeterminate. However, if HIV infection has been reasonably excluded, prophylaxis should be discontinued. For those children in whom HIV-1 infection is documented between 1 and 5 years of age, prophylaxis should be initiated or continued if the absolute CD4 count is less than 500 cells/mL or the CD4 percentage is less than 15%. Between 6 and 12 years, prophylaxis should be continued if the CD4 count is less than 200 cells/mL or the CD4 percentage is less than 15%.

Childhood immunizations, including hepatitis B, should be provided. Inactivated poliovirus vaccine must be substituted for OPV in the patient and all household contacts. HIV-1–infected children should receive the conjugated polyvalent pneumococcal vaccine (Prevnar) and, if exposed to measles, immunoglobulin. Likewise, zoster immunoglobulin should be administered after exposure to varicella.

There has been significant progress recently in the prevention and treatment of pediatric AIDS, which has greatly improved prognosis. It is likely that many children with HIV-1 infection will live through adolescence and that new manifestations of this increasingly chronic illness will be identified during the next few years.

■ MOLECULAR MECHANISMS IN PRIMARY IMMUNODEFICIENCY DISORDERS

Remarkable progress has been made in our understanding of the molecular defects causing primary immunodeficiency disorders (Table 7–13). This information has improved our understanding of how the normal immune system functions and guided our approach to treatment of primary immunodeficiency disorders.

Understanding molecular mechanisms has lead to new diagnostic approaches and aided the development of new therapeutic interventions. Characterization of these defects at a molecular level has opened the door to sophisticated techniques to identify the precise genetic mutation and family members at risk for passing the disorder onto their offspring. Involvement of genetic counselors may be very important for these families.

The recent progress in understanding molecular mechanisms also has led to the development of new therapeutic approaches. Newer treatments include the use of recombinant enzyme replacement therapies, such as polyethylene glycol-modified bovine adenosine deaminase for ADA deficiency and the use of recombinant cytokines such as γ-interferon for CGD and hyper-IgE syndrome. Identification of the precise genetic defect is allowing the definition of genotype–phenotype associations for specific diseases. For example, definition of the precise abnormality in the *WASP* gene in a child with WAS allows prediction of the relative risk of severe thrombocytopenia versus the development of malignant disease. This knowledge can be used to guide therapy.

The ultimate treatment for many of these diseases would be to cure the illness with gene therapy. Because many of the primary immunodeficiencies currently are treatable by bone marrow transplantation, a potential therapeutic approach is placement of the functional gene in bone marrow stem cells. Gene therapy in autologous peripheral blood lymphocytes has been used successfully to treat ADA deficiency in patients whose conditions were unresponsive to enzyme replacement. Some of those chil-

Table 7–13. Molecular Defects Found in Some of the Primary Immunodeficiencies

Disorder	Classification	Molecular Defect
Ataxia–telangiectasia	Combined T/B cell	*ATM* gene (phosphatidylinositol-3 kinase-like gene)
Agammaglobulinemia	B cell	Bruton tyrosine kinase
Hyper-IgM	B/T cell	CD40 ligand (on T cells)
SCID X-linked	Combined T/B cell	IL-2 γ-chain
SCID-AR	Combined T/B cell	ADA/PNP
SCID-AR	CD8 lymphopenia	ZAP70
Wiskott–Aldrich syndrome	T/B cell	WASP protein, proline rich
SCID X-linked		Jak3 tyrosine kinase
LAD		β2 integrin
Lymphoproliferative syndrome		IL-2 receptor α-chain
SCID-AR		IL-7 receptor α-chain
SCID-AR		RAG1 and RAG2 deficiencies

ADA/PNP = adenosine deaminase/purine nucleoside phosphorylase; AR = autosomal recessive; IL-2 = interleukin-2; LAD = leukocyte adhesion deficiency; SCID = severe combined immunodeficiency.

dren have had good clinical responses to peripheral lymphocyte gene therapy, although frequent treatments are required because peripheral lymphocytes have limited life spans. Clinical studies using stem cell gene therapy currently are under way, with the hope of providing a cure for patients with ADA deficiency. Preliminary results show that retroviral gene therapy might successfully transfer a gene into stem cells and that this gene might remain expressed several years after initial treatment. It is not yet known whether the patients have substantial therapeutic benefit from these treatments. Further studies are needed to develop efficient gene delivery systems, including viral vectors and liposomes, that are safe and allow for long-term expression of the desired gene in vivo.

REFERENCES

Antiretroviral therapy and medical management of pediatric HIV infection and 1997 USPHS/IDSA report on the prevention of opportunistic infections in persons infected with human immunodeficiency virus. Pediatrics 1998;102(suppl).

Auger I et al: Incubation periods for Paediatric AIDS patients. Nature 1988;336:575.

Bryson Y et al: Establishment of a definition of the timing of vertical HIV-1 infection. N Engl J Med 1992;327:1246.

Buckley RH: Breakthroughs in the understanding and therapy of primary immunodeficiency. Pediatr Clin North Am 1994; 41:665.

Buckley RH et al: Hematopoietic stem-cell transplantation for the treatment of severe combined immunodeficiency. N Engl J Med 1999;340:508.

Cavazzana-Calvo M et al: Gene therapy of human severe combined immunodeficiency (SCID)-X1 disease. Science 2000;288:669.

Conley ME et al: Diagnostic criteria for primary immunodeficiencies. Clin Immunol 1999;93:190.

Connor E et al: Reduction of maternal-infant transmission of human immunodeficiency virus type 1 with zidovudine treatment. N Engl J Med 1994;331:1173.

el Habbal MH, Strobel S: Leukocyte adhesion deficiency. Arch Dis Child 1993;69:463.

Guidelines of antiretroviral agents in pediatric HIV infection on the Internet (The Living Document: January 7, 2000). Available at: www.hivatis.org.

Levy J et al: The clinical spectrum of X-linked hyper IgM syndrome. J Pediatr 1997;131:47.

Markert ML et al: Transplantation of thymus tissue in complete DiGeorge syndrome. NEJM 1999;341:1180.

Nachman SA et al: Nucleoside analogs plus Ritonavir in stable antiretroviral therapy-experienced HIV-infected children, a randomized controlled trial. JAMA 2000;283:492.

Nelson D, Kurman CC: Molecular genetic analysis of the primary immunodeficiency disorders. Pediatr Clin North Am 1994; 41:657.

Ochs HD et al: *Primary Immunodeficiency Diseases. A Molecular and Genetic Approach. 1999.* Oxford University Press, 1999.

Pacheco SE, Shearer WT: Laboratory aspects of immunology. Pediatr Clin North Am 1994;41:623.

Rogers M: HIV/AIDS in infants, children and adolescents. Pediatr Clin North America 2000;47.

Savitsky K et al: A single ataxia-telangiectasia gene with a product similar to PI-3 kinase. Science 1995;268:1749.

Shearer W et al: Viral load and disease progression in infants infected with human immunodeficiency virus type 1. N Engl J Med 1997;336:1337.

Shyur SD, Hill HR: Recent advances in the genetics of primary immunodeficiency syndromes. J Pediatr 1996;129:8.

Smart BA, Ochs HD: The molecular basis and treatment of primary immunodeficiency disorders. Curr Opin Pediatr 1997;9:570.

Summerfield J et al: Mannose binding protein gene mutations associated with unusual and severe infections in adults. Lancet 1995;345:886.

Wahn U: Evaluation of the child with suspected primary immunodeficiency. Pediatr Allergy Immunol 1995;6:71.

Wood RA, Sampson HA: The child with frequent infections. Curr Probl Pediatr 1989;19:229.

Rheumatic Diseases

Mary Denise Moore, MD

Rheumatic diseases refer to a diverse group of chronic and complex inflammatory conditions, with peak onset in early adult life. The hallmark is arthritis of the peripheral joints and axial skeleton, but the inflammatory process also can affect other organ systems such as skin, eye, kidneys, lungs, heart, and central nervous system. There is considerable overlap in the clinical features of the rheumatic disorders. Often the characteristic clinical feature are not evident for months or even years after onset of symptoms, making it difficult to establish an accurate diagnosis. The causes of most rheumatic diseases remain unknown, but there has been an explosion in information on the role of the immune response in chronic inflammation and the development of new immunotherapies that specifically target pathologic aspects. The morbidity and mortality of the rheumatic diseases have improved markedly over the past decade, and future advances are anticipated. Patients with these conditions represent many challenges in terms of diagnosis and treatment and in the prevention of secondary complications such as opportunistic infections and adverse effects from medications (e.g., growth failure in children requiring prolonged systemic corticosteroids). Decreased bone mineral content can occur from immobility from the disease or as a complication of corticosteroid use.

In children, the most common forms of chronic arthritis are juvenile rheumatoid arthritis (JRA) and the spondyloarthropathies. Systemic lupus erythematosus (SLE) and dermatomyositis occur less commonly in children. The systemic vasculitides are distinctly uncommon in childhood, with the exception of Kawasaki disease and Henoch–Schonlein purpura (HSP), conditions that have a much more favorable outcome than the other vasculitides.

In evaluating children with rheumatic complaints, the importance of a detailed history and physical examination, including a comprehensive family history, cannot be overemphasized. The working impression from the history and examination will assist greatly in the development of a thoughtful, logical, and appropriate diagnostic and treatment plan. General goals of management are determination of the patient's diagnosis, control of pain, prevention of disability, adequate rest, and appropriate exercise. The family and child need education on the disease process, its treatment, and a realistic assessment of disease outcome. The child presenting with nonorganic musculoskeletal pain is a therapeutic challenge. It is important to identify these children early to avoid putting the child through an extensive and unnecessary evaluation and focus on symptom control, return to school, and normal function.

■ APPROACH TO THE CHILD WITH MUSCULOSKELETAL COMPLAINTS

Musculoskeletal symptoms are the third most common reason for children to see a health care provider. Only visits for routine well-child care and acute infections are more common. Most children will have a transient cause of their symptoms, usually minor trauma, overuse syndromes, joint hypermobility, or a reactive process from an intercurrent infection. Evaluation begins with careful history taking, thorough physical examination, and a few simple laboratory investigations. A more comprehensive investigation should be reserved for those children with more serious or persistent symptoms or in whom the screening studies suggest an underlying inflammatory or systemic condition (Figure 8–1). A list of some of the more prevalent causes of musculoskeletal pain is presented in Table 8–1. Orthopedic causes are common and discussed in more detail in Chapter 22.

History and Physical Examination

A comprehensive history is essential. A checklist for the patient to fill out can be useful in a busy outpatient setting. Details should be obtained on the timing and progression of symptoms, pain characteristics, and conditions that relieve symptoms because they will guide the diagnostic evaluation. Relief of joint symptoms with one of the ubiquitous nonsteroidal anti-inflammatory drugs (NSAIDs) does not necessarily indicate the presence of a rheumatic disease because the NSAIDs are also analgesic and antipyretic. **Arthralgia** refers to pain in the joints and is due more often to a less serious process. **Arthritis,** also called synovitis, involves clinical signs of inflammation such as palpable joint swelling, as described below. Inflammatory pain tends to be chronic and relatively indolent, with a vague progressive onset and course. **Migratory arthritis**

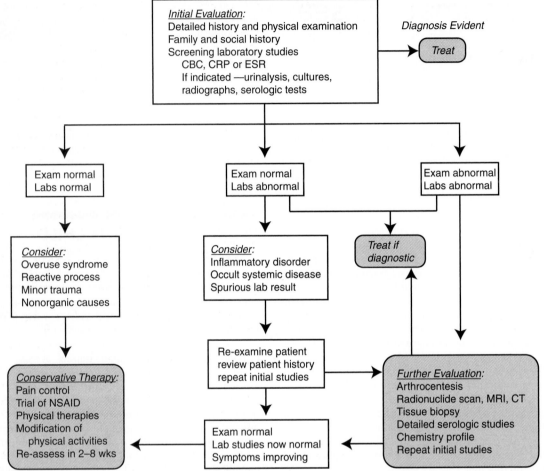

Figure 8–1. Algorithm for the evaluation of a child with a musculoskeletal complaint. CBC = complete blood count; CRP = C-reactive protein; ESR = erythrocyte sedimentation rate; NSAIDs = nonsteroidal anti-inflammatory drugs.

refers to inflammation that resolves in one joint as it appears in the next joint; this is classically seen in acute rheumatic fever and gonococcal arthritis but can occur in a number of other conditions. The arthritis of JRA tends not to migrate but to take on an additive pattern, and the child may present with joint pain first and note obvious joint swelling weeks later. Inflammatory pain typically is worse in the morning, often associated with morning stiffness (which may be marked), and improves with exercise. In contrast, mechanical pain is relieved by rest and tends to be worse at the end of the day and after strenuous activity. The patient should be asked about prior episodes of musculoskeletal disease and precipitating factors such as trauma, sports activities, recent immunizations, travel, exposures, and intercurrent illnesses.

A history of trauma may be misleading, especially in young children, as most toddlers experience daily incidents

of minor trauma. The presence or absence of systemic symptoms should be determined. Symptoms of possibly serious or chronic underlying inflammatory conditions include weight loss, progressive weakness or immobility, growth failure, fever, chills, bruising, pallor, and chest pain. The child should be asked specifically about signs and symptoms typical for rheumatic diseases such as mouth ulcers, Raynaud's phenomenon, morning stiffness, and photosensitivity. With the exception of growing pains, nighttime pain, in particular pain that awakens the child from sleep, is unusual and suggests a more serious condition such as musculoskeletal infection, malignancies, or fractures. A tactful inquiry into social factors and school absences is vital because this can provide clues to establishing nonorganic causes of symptoms. However, it may be difficult in the initial visit to establish sufficient rapport to elicit sensitive information. The child might not

Table 8–1. Common Causes of Musculoskeletal Pain in Childhood

Noninflammatory
  Trauma
    Contusions
    Sprains, strains
    Fractures, subluxation
    Overuse syndromes (e.g., Little League shoulder)
    Child abuse
  Structural
    Slipped capital femoral epiphysis
    Avascular necrosis (idiopathic or secondary to underlying disorder)
    Patellofemoral disorders
    Joint hypermobility
  Other
    Growing pains
    Nonorganic (fibromyalgia, myofascial, psychogenic)
    Reflex sympathetic dystrophy
Inflammatory
  Infectious
    Osteomyelitis
    Septic arthritis
    Postinfectious (reactive) arthritis
    Viral arthritis
    Cellulitis
    Diskitis
    Lyme disease
  Rheumatic diseases
    Juvenile rheumatoid arthritis
    Spondyloarthropathies
    Systemic vasculitis
      Systemic lupus erythematosus
      Kawasaki disease
      Henoch–Schonlein purpura
  Systemic diseases
    Hematologic/oncologic disorders (leukemia, sickle cell, local tumor, hemophilia)
    Metabolic disorders
    Inflammatory bowel disease

feel comfortable enough with the practitioner or might consider the problem (e.g., bullying at school, family discord) to be unrelated to the musculoskeletal symptoms. The child should be asked about sleep quality, depressive symptoms, and social functioning. The family history is often overlooked and this omission can delay the establishment of the correct diagnosis, as in the case of the older boy with intermittent episodes of inflammatory arthritis and a family history of spondyloarthropathy.

The physical examination begins with obtaining growth parameters and, if indicated, body temperature and blood pressure. It is useful to watch the patient and family before they are aware of being observed because this can provide clues about family functioning or suggest symptom exaggeration if the child is more ambulatory before the examination. The entire musculoskeletal system should be examined because occult sites of involvement can be uncovered that can redirect the clinical evaluations (e.g., a stiff, tender back in an adolescent with a swollen knee, or multiple swollen joints in a child with monoarticular complaints). Similarly, referred pain must be considered, particularly in children with knee pain. The joints should be examined for swelling, warmth, tenderness, restriction of motion, and pain on motion because these signs usually indicate inflammatory arthritis. The degree of discomfort should be determined. The articular examination usually will be normal in children with overuse syndromes, nonorganic diseases, and simple arthralgia. In inflammatory arthritis, the joints are not usually red; pain and tenderness will be mild to moderate, and joint contracture and muscle atrophy may be prominent. It would be uncommon for a child with a rheumatic disease to have extreme pain or be unable to bear weight, and other conditions such as malingering, infection, fracture, neurologic disorders, or malignancy should be investigated.

Laboratory Investigation

The choice of diagnostic testing is guided by the information provided in the history and physical examination. A complete blood count (CBC) and an erythrocyte sedimentation rate (ESR) or C-reactive protein (CRP) should be obtained in virtually all children when a rheumatic disease is suspected. A normal physical examination and normal laboratory studies are quite helpful in ruling out serious underlying inflammatory conditions in the vast majority of patients. Other initial studies to consider are urinalysis, appropriate cultures (blood, synovial, urogenital, stool), serologic tests for infectious agents (i.e., Lyme or parvovirus titers), and studies of renal and hepatic function. The CRP and ESR are nonspecific indicators of inflammation and can be completely normal in children with inflammatory arthritis, in particular those with involvement of only a few joints. On serologic testing, many JRA patients, especially those with pauciarticular JRA, will have low titers of antinuclear antibody (ANA). Similarly, low titers of ANA are seen in most rheumatic diseases and the titer does not correlate with disease severity. In contrast to adult rheumatoid arthritis (RA), rheumatoid factor (RF) is present in only 10% of JRA cases, overall. Antinuclear antibody and RF occasionally can be present in healthy individuals or in other systemic conditions and are helpful only in distinguishing the type of JRA after the diagnosis is established. More detailed serologic evaluation (complement levels, anti–double-stranded DNA, antinuclear cytoplasmic antibodies) should be obtained in children suspected of having SLE or one of the less common systemic vasculitidies. Histocompatility locus antigen (HLA) testing is not a useful clinical tool, except for testing for HLA B27 in a youngster suspected of having a spondyloarthropathy. However, approximately 10–30% of patients with a spondyloarthropathy are negative for this antigen. Arthrocentesis is mandatory in any child with a swollen joint who is suspected of having an infectious arthritis. Results of synovial fluid test can be helpful in establishing noninflammatory arthritis, such as trauma. Synovial fluid should be examined for cell count, differential, Gram stain, glucose, and culture. Serologic studies and determination of total protein concentration of the synovial fluid are not helpful. In most types of inflammatory arthritis, the synovial fluid will have cell counts ranging from 1000 to 50,000 cells/mm³ and a predominance of polymophonuclear leukocytes. In infectious arthritis, the synovial glucose is usually lower and the cell count often is greater than 50,000 cell/mm³. However, there is considerable overlap, and the diagnosis of infectious arthritis usually is confirmed by culture. With the exception of infectious arthritis, synovial fluid examination is not helpful in distinguishing the type of inflammatory arthritis.

Radiographs of the involved area will be normal in children with new onset of inflammatory arthritis and are most useful in excluding other causes of symptoms, such as infections, tumors, and orthopedic conditions. Referred pain, such as hip problems presenting with knee complaints, should be considered when ordering radiographs. Similarly, obtaining radiographs of the uninvolved side is useful for comparison. Radionuclide scans, computed tomography, and magnetic resonance imaging can be considered in children with severe or more chronic symptoms, where a more detailed investigation is necessary.

Noninflammatory Musculoskeletal Conditions

GROWING PAINS

Growing pains have nothing to do with growth and can affect up to 15% of school-aged children. Growing pains are common in preschool age boys, are associated with physical activity, and generally occur late in the day and early evening. These pains often awaken the child from sleep and respond to analgesics and massage. The patient typically has difficulty localizing the pain, which may involve the thighs, knees, calves, and pretibial surfaces. Physical examination and laboratory studies must be normal. Growing pain is never unilateral and does not cause persistent limp. Management consists of careful observation for development of other symptoms, NSAIDs or analgesics given just before bed, and a balance of rest and physical activity. Most cases improve spontaneously.

JOINT HYPERMOBILITY SYNDROME

Up to 12% of school-aged children have been found to have hyperextensible joints; it is more common in younger children and girls. Joint laxity is also more prevalent among dancers, gymnasts, and instrumental musicians. Joint laxity leads to an increased incidence of arthralgia, transient joint effusions, dislocations, and diffuse pain syndromes such as fibromyalgia. Half of youngsters with joint hypermobility will consult a health care provider because of symptoms. Children with hypermobility also may have mitral valve prolapse. The criteria for hypermobility are listed in Table 8–2. These children do not have skin laxity or other physical signs of the hereditary connective tissue disorders such as Marfan or Ehler–Danlos syndromes. However, joint laxity and increased pain do occur in those disorders. Similar to growing pains, the management of hypermobility syndrome is conservative and includes curtailment of offending physical activities, physical therapy (strengthening, bracing, pain control), and NSAIDs or analgesics as required. Hypermobility will improve or resolve with time.

REFLEX SYMPATHETIC DYSTROPHY

Reflex sympathetic dystrophy is an infrequent condition in adolescents. Terms previously used for this entity include reflex neurovascular dystrophy, causalgia, and Sudeck atrophy. The adolescent will present with an extremely painful, swollen, mottled, cool extremity, often after minor trauma. The involved limb can be very dry or have increased sweating. Pain is extreme, with a burning or "pins and needle" sensation, and the individual will not use the extremity or tolerate even light touch. Diagnosis is made most often clinically but can be confirmed by bone scan, thermography, and plain radiographs (regional osteopenia) in long-standing cases. In adults, the condition is usually secondary to underlying conditions such as diabetes and degenerative cervical spine dis-

Table 8–2. Criteria for Joint Hypermobility[1]

1. Passive dorsiflexion of the fifth finger beyond 90 degrees with the forearm flat on a table
2. Passive apposition of the thumb to the flexor aspect of the forearm
3. Hyperextension of the elbow beyond 10 degrees
4. Hyperextension of the knee beyond 10 degree
5. Forward flexion of the trunk so that the palms of the hands rest easily on the floor

[1] Presence of any three criteria establishes joint hypermobility.

Reproduced, with permission, from Beighton P: The Ehlers–Danlos syndromes. In: Beighton P (editor): *Heritable Disorders of Connective Tissue.* Mosby-Year Book, 1993:200.

ease. In children, an underlying cause is not usually found, but occasionally a stress fracture or other orthopedic condition can trigger reflex sympathetic dystrophy. Treatment is focused on pain control, prompt mobilization of the involved extremity, and education of the patient as to the pathophysiology of the symptoms. Physical therapy, counseling, and biofeedback have been shown to be effective. There is a high incidence of psychosocial discord in the families of these children, which also must be addressed. Most episodes will remit spontaneously but can recur. Persistent and chronic disease can result in contractures and disability.

OSTEOPOROSIS

The past two decades have seen an explosion of research and new information in osteoporosis and in the prevention and treatment of established bone loss. Approximately half of adult bone mass is acquired during adolescence, with bone mass increasing 8% each year during the adolescent growth spurt. Achievement of normal peak bone mass during childhood is quite important because it may not be possible to correct this deficiency later in life. All children should be counseled about adequate calcium and vitamin D intake and the importance of sufficient regular physical exercise to maintain bone density. Conditions associated with decreased bone mass include amenorrhea, eating disorders, metabolic diseases, prolonged administration of corticosteroids and any disorder limiting physical mobility. Patients with JRA, RA, and spondyloarthropathy have diminished bone mass, even without corticosteroid use. Corticosteroids are used frequently in the treatment of the rheumatic diseases. The risk and severity of corticosteroid-induced osteoporosis is related to the cumulative dose and the duration of treatment. A careful balance between disease control and use of the lowest dose of corticosteroids is necessary. If the steroid dose cannot be reduced, other anti-inflammatory agents should be added for disease control to allow a reduction in the daily steroid dose (steroid-sparing effect). Children identified with significant osteopenia should be referred for evaluation and treatment, which can include estrogen, vitamin D, and treatment with one of the bisphosphonates, such as alendronate or etidronate. Although the bisphosphonates have been studied and are effective in postmenopausal osteoporosis and steroid-induced osteoporosis in adults, there are few studies on the use of these agents in children or young adults. Treatment recommendations for osteoporosis are in transition: several large-scale trials are underway to determine optimal doses, duration of therapy, and indications for use of medications in younger patients. Unless severe, decreased bone density per se does not lead to musculoskeletal pain. Children with significant osteoporosis are at high risk for extremity fractures and vertebral fractures after relatively minor trauma. Children with osteoporotic vertebral stress fractures usually complain of chronic low-grade back pain and progressive kyphosis but can present occasionally with more acute severe pain.

FIBROMYALGIA

Fibromyalgia is quite common, particularly in older adolescent females. These patients have diffuse long-standing chronic pain. Review of systems usually will reveal multiple complaints, including sleep disturbance, fatigue, mood disorders, generalized joint and muscle aching, back ache, abdominal pain, and chronic headaches. Often, there will be a lifelong history of vague chronic symptoms, sometimes starting with infantile colic. A positive family history of fibromyalgia or irritable bowel syndrome is also common. Physical examination will be completely normal, except for tender points across the back and anterior chest wall. The patient occasionally may have pain on joint examination but should have no clinical signs of inflammation. Laboratory studies are normal, including serologic studies, acute phase reactants, radiographs, and routine blood tests. There is significant overlap of this condition with chronic fatigue syndrome and with the mood and somatization disorders. School problems and other stresses are often present. Management of these adolescents can be extremely challenging and at times frustrating. The diagnosis of fibromyalgia is based on the typical history of chronic, stable diffuse pain, normal laboratory investigations, and the presence of specific tender points on physical examination. The focus is on pain control, patient education, normalization of sleep habits, stress reduction, and the use of non-narcotic analgesics and physical therapy to control symptoms. An aerobic exercise program can be particularly effective. Low doses of amitriptyline or nortriptyline given at night can improve sleep quality, because these agents have a mild sedative effect, without disturbing sleep rhythm. Treatment of concomitant mood disturbance is also quite important. In the evaluation of these patients, an appropriate and limited workup is indicated, followed by a trial of conservative therapies. The parent, practitioner, and child must come to an agreement as to what types of symptoms warrant further diagnostic evaluation and what therapies will be tried. Careful and consistent follow-up with a supportive health care provider can prevent a prolonged and unnecessary evaluation and has been shown to reduce the long-term cost of treatment. In general, adolescents have a better prognosis than adults with fibromyalgia. In community-based studies, most fibromyalgia patients have remained stable or improved over time.

NONORGANIC MUSCULOSKELETAL PAIN

Unexplained musculoskeletal pain is extremely common and increases markedly with advancing age. Disorders include chronic fatigue syndrome, myofascial pain, fibromyalgia, nonspecific low back pain, "psychogenic rheumatism," and, less commonly, conversion disorders. Most of these conditions have considerable overlap. Chronic back pain is also common in children: half of all children will experience episodes of back pain and 8–30% will have chronic back pain. Most of these children will not seek medical attention. Of those who do, a specific cause for the back pain will be found in only about half. Nonorganic musculoskeletal pain can be one of the more challenging conditions to evaluate because patients can have severe pain, prolonged symptoms, and will seek evaluation from many health care providers. Parents may become upset when no organic etiology can be determined as the cause of their child's pain. The term "psychogenic" is probably best avoided because it can be perceived as pejorative. However, it is important to discuss the role of psychological factors in pain expression when planning the diagnostic and therapeutic evaluation. Warning flags suggesting an organic etiology include age younger than 10 years, the presence of systemic symptoms, inflammatory or nocturnal pain, neurologic signs or symptoms, and constant pain. Further evaluation is warranted in the presence of one or more of these factors. Malingering and/or factitious causes are not common in children and usually can be ascertained by careful investigation. Symptom extension, where a child has persistent symptoms weeks after resolution of an acute infection and normalization of laboratory studies, is quite common. Nonorganic musculoskeletal pain should be considered in the older child presenting with frequent school absences, psychosocial stresses, or bizarre, diffuse, and/or vague symptoms with a normal laboratory and physical examination. Often the child's reported disability and dysfunction are out of proportion to the physical examination. For these children, a limited diagnostic evaluation, careful observation, and symptom control may be indicated as the first line of management. A trial of physical therapy, analgesics, and/or NSAIDs is recommended and the child should be scheduled for a reexamination in 4–8 weeks. The child can be advised to keep a diary of symptoms, reassured in a sympathetic tone, and transitioned back to school and normal physical activity.

Inflammatory Musculoskeletal Conditions

REACTIVE ARTHRITIS AND TOXIC SYNOVITIS

Toxic (or transient) synovitis of the hip is the most common nontraumatic cause of childhood arthritis and is considered a form of reactive arthritis. Another name for this condition is "observation hip." It more commonly affects boys aged 3–6 years, usually after an upper respiratory infection. The child limps or refuses to bear weight and complains of pain in the groin, anterior thigh, or knee. The results of laboratory investigations are normal or show mild increases in ESR and white blood cell count. Aspiration of the hip will show inflammatory fluid and sterile cultures. The condition is self-limiting and rarely lasts more than 10 days; management involves rest and analgesics. Recurrence with subsequent upper respiratory infections is not uncommon, but care should be taken to rule out other causes such as avascular necrosis of the femoral head (Perthé disease) when the limp persists. Similarly, the child with recurrent episodes of hip disease ultimately might be diagnosed with a spondyloarthropathy.

Reactive or postinfectious arthritis refers to a transient inflammation of synovial tissue in association with infection in another part of the body. By definition, no organism will be recovered from the joint. Common etiologies associated with reactive arthritis include enteric pathogens (*Salmonella, Shigella, Yersinia,* or *Campylobacter*), parvovirus, rubella, viral hepatitis, mononucleosis, and cytomegalovirus. A short-lived arthritis can occur after streptococcal infections and has been called "poststreptococcal reactive arthritis." This entity originally was believed to be distinct from rheumatic fever because these children did not meet clinical criteria for rheumatic fever. However, there have been case reports of children diagnosed with poststreptococcal reactive arthritis who were later found to have carditis or who subsequently developed rheumatic fever. The issue as to whether or not these children should also receive rheumatic fever prophylaxis is not settled. **Reiter syndrome,** a type of reactive arthritis associated with spondyloarthropathy, should be considered in the older patient presenting with reactive arthritis, ocular symptoms, enthesitis (inflammation of tendons), and/or urethritis. Reactive arthritis can involve only one joint or several joints, as in rubella infection, or it can be polyarticular, as in acute rheumatic fever or hepatitis B infection. Reactive arthritis also can be seen after exposure to medications.

The diagnosis of reactive arthritis is established after a careful history and, if possible, by confirmatory serologies and exclusion of other causes of the arthritis. Reactive arthritis typically lasts less than 6 weeks and often is invoked as the etiology of short-lived arthritis of undetermined etiology. Treatment is with NSAIDs, pain control, and limited weight bearing on affected joints (crutches or cane). Most children recover completely and do not experience recurrences.

ACUTE RHEUMATIC FEVER

Rheumatic fever was once a common cause of polyarthritis. Although its incidence has declined in the United States, the disease still occurs in epidemics, with peak ages of onset from 5 to 15 years. This condition is the prototypic reactive arthritis: symptoms usually occur a few weeks after a streptococcal infection with group A streptococci as a host immune response is mounted against the infection.

The pathogenesis is felt to be due to the process of molecular mimicry in which antibodies to bacterial products cross-react with host antigens in various tissues, resulting in inflammation. Diagnosis is made on clinical grounds by using the modified Jones criteria (Table 8–3). These criteria are only guidelines and must be interpreted carefully, especially in patients who present only with arthritis (see below). Children with other causes of arthritis can have serologic evidence of a preceding streptococcal infection and meet Jones criteria but have another disease.

The onset of rheumatic fever typically follows streptococcal pharyngitis after 1–3 weeks and is characterized by nonspecific malaise and fever. Polyarthritis is the most common major manifestation, occurring in up to 75% of patients. Articular pain often is severe and out of proportion to objective findings. The arthritis is frequently migratory, resolving in one joint after 3–10 days before going on to involve another. Large joints of the lower extremities tend to be affected more frequently. The arthritis is exquisitely sensitive to even low doses of aspirin; failure to respond to salicylates should suggest another diagnosis.

Carditis, present in 40% of patients, is suspected in children with resting tachycardia but is diagnosed with certainty in those with new heart murmurs. A systolic murmur suggesting mitral insufficiency is heard most commonly. The next most common murmurs are a mid-diastolic rumble at the apex (Carey–Coombs murmur) and an early diastolic murmur of aortic regurgitation. Right-sided lesions are uncommon. Myocarditis (e.g., resting tachycardia, cardiomegaly, and congestive heart failure) and pericarditis may accompany valvular involvement but rarely occur in isolation.

Less common manifestations of rheumatic fever include Sydenham chorea, erythema marginatum, and subcutaneous nodules. Sydenham chorea, seen in fewer than 15% of patients, may occur in isolation weeks after the inciting infection or other signs of the disease. These children may present with emotional lability and develop involuntary movements of the face and upper extremities. These disappear during sleep and are exacerbated by emotional factors that may wrongly suggest a conversion reaction. Erythema marginatum is an evanescent, macular eruption with serpiginous borders and central clearing. It is virtually always associated with carditis but is uncommon, occurring in fewer than 10% of patients. Subcutaneous nodules, which are even rarer, are painless swellings smaller than 1 cm in diameter. They are found over bony prominences and extensor tendons.

Establishing evidence of an antecedent streptococcal pharyngitis is a sine qua non for the diagnosis of rheumatic fever. Streptococci may be detected by rapid antigen tests, pharyngeal culture, or elevated serum levels of antistreptococcal antibodies. Antistreptolysin O titers are elevated in 80% of patients when first measured. In those with normal antistreptolysin O titers, antibodies to the streptococcal proteins hyaluronidase and deoxyribonuclease B will increase the yield to 90%. With the exception of isolated chorea, rheumatic fever is always associated with an acute phase response, so the ESR or CRP level will be elevated.

A diagnosis of rheumatic fever is established clinically through the application of the Jones criteria (Table 8–3). A few caveats are in order. Arthralgia cannot be considered a minor criterion if arthritis is the major one. The arthritis of rheumatic fever is not always migratory and can be monoarticular. Echocardiographically documented but clinically inaudible valvular insufficiency is not sufficient evidence of carditis. Similarly, PR prolongation on electrocardiography is not diagnostic of cardiac involvement.

Once a diagnosis is established, all patients should receive a full treatment course of penicillin to eradicate an ongoing streptococcal infection, even without a positive throat culture. This is followed by continuous antistreptococcal prophylaxis administered as 1.2 million U of benzathine penicillin every 3–4 weeks. Oral prophylaxis with twice-daily penicillin is effective, but compliance can be a problem. Children with rheumatic heart disease also should receive prophylaxis for bacterial endocarditis. Relief of joint symptoms and fever typically is achieved rapidly with salicylates administered as aspirin, 60–100 mg/kg/day in four divided doses. Corticosteroids (prednisone, 2 mg/kg/day) are indicated for congestive heart failure. Children without carditis fare well, although they are at risk for heart involvement with subsequent

Table 8–3. Criteria for the Diagnosis of Rheumatic Fever[1,2]

Major Manifestations	Minor Manifestations
Carditis	Clinical findings
Polyarthritis	Arthralgia
Chorea	Fever
Erythema marginatum	Laboratory findings
Subcutaneous nodules	Elevated acute phase reactants (erythrocyte sedimentation rate, C-reactive protein)
	Prolonged P–R interval

[1] The presence of two major criteria, or of one major and two minor criteria, indicates a high probability of acute rheumatic fever if supported by evidence of Group A streptococcal infection.
[2] Supporting evidence of antecedent group A streptococcal infection: positive throat culture or rapid streptococcal antigen test; elevated or increasing streptococcal antibody titer.

Reproduced, with permission, from Dajani AS et al: Guideline for the diagnosis of rheumatic fever; Jones criteria, updated 1992. Circulation 1993;87:302.

attacks; therefore, continuous antibiotic prophylaxis is crucial and should be maintained at least into adult life. Although up to 70% of those with heart involvement have no major sequelae, those with severe carditis are likely to have permanent valvular lesions.

Rheumatic Disorders

JUVENILE RHEUMATOID ARTHRITIS

Juvenile RA encompasses a heterogeneous group of idiopathic disorders, the hallmark of which is chronic synovitis predominantly afflicting peripheral joints, although the cervical spine is often involved. Juvenile RA refers to persistent arthritis lasting more than 6 weeks in children younger than 16 years. This age distinction is somewhat arbitrary as adult RA can present in children, particularly in older adolescent females. Like most rheumatic diseases, JRA is more common in females. The American College of Rheumatology subdivides JRA into three main subtypes: systemic onset, polyarticular, and pauciarticular. Juvenile RA subtypes are based on the clinical course 6 months after onset. Some centers divide the subtypes further based on the results of serologic studies and the presence or absence of HLA B27 or RF. Outside the United States, many rheumatologists reserve the term rheumatoid for children with positive serum RF.

Juvenile RA occurs with a prevalence of approximately 1 in 1000. At any one time, half of the cases are inactive. Epidemiologic studies of JRA have been mainly descriptive and are complicated further by the differences in diagnostic criteria, the marked heterogeneity in disease expression, and the inability to identify specific etiologic agents. Despite major advances in the understanding of the inflammatory response, the etiology of JRA remains unknown. Stress, infection, and trauma can play a role in triggering the onset of arthritis and causing exacerbations of existing disease. The actual contribution of each factor is not known. Genetic factors also contribute to the development of JRA, but the association is much less consistent than the strong association of HLA B27 in the spondyloarthropathies. Juvenile RA probably encompasses several diseases of differing etiologies. In addition, other types of inflammatory arthritis, such as reactive arthritis and Lyme arthritis can be difficult to distinguish from pauciarticular JRA. Another difficulty is that inflammatory conditions evolve over time, and it might be decades later that another rheumatic disease becomes evident. The classic example is a young boy with pauciarticular JRA who develops typical spinal involvement, intestinal disease, or psoriasis in adult life and is then rediagnosed as having a spondyloarthropathy.

Pauciarticular JRA. Pauciarticular JRA is the most common subtype, representing about half of all JRA cases, and can be subdivided further into two groups: young girls (often with +ANA) and older boys. In pauciarticular JRA, four or fewer joints are involved. The typical child presents with an asymmetric arthritis in a large weight-bearing joint. Knee and ankle are most common, but virtually any joint can be involved. However, isolated hip involvement is distinctly uncommon and suggests a spondyloarthropathy. The pain will be mild and the child will present with persistent swelling, limp, and/or contracture of peripheral joints. Morning stiffness may be prominent and joint symptoms typically improve later in the day. Occasionally, children will present with abrupt onset of inflammatory arthritis and fever, but the initial presentation is usually more indolent. Levels of CBC, ESR, and CRP may be elevated and the child may have a mild anemia. However, these blood tests often are completely normal. Antinuclear antibody is positive in a low titer in more than 75% of cases and the presence of ANA correlates strongly with the development of chronic uveitis. The inflammatory eye disease of JRA historically had a 10% risk of severe vision loss or even blindness. However, the risk of severe visual sequelae has dropped significantly due to early diagnosis, better treatment, and identification of milder cases. All children with JRA need regular examinations to detect eye disease, which is asymptomatic early on and apparent only on slit-lamp examination.

Polyarticular JRA. Polyarticular JRA accounts for 40% of JRA and refers to chronic arthritis affecting five or more joints. This condition also is subdivided into two subgroups depending on the presence or absence of RF. Low titer ANA also occurs frequently in the polyarticular type. The RF-negative children tend to be younger, with a more variable course and better prognosis, although some may develop a positive RF and progressive arthritis later on in the disease process. The RF-positive JRA represents early-onset adult RA. As such, it also has a female predominance and has features common in adult RA, including rheumatoid nodules, Raynaud phenomenon, and early progression to erosive disease and joint damage. Eye inflammation is less common but can in polyarticular disease.

Systemic-onset JRA. Systemic-onset JRA, or Still disease, accounts for 10% of JRA cases, occurs with equal frequency in girls and boys, and tends to present with a much more abrupt onset. Children are often quite ill at presentation, and this subtype is the one associated most often with fatalities. Systemic signs and symptoms include a characteristic rash (rheumatoid rash) in 75% of cases, fever, lymphadenopathy, serositis, leukocytosis, and marked increases in acute phase reactants. High fever typically occurs once or twice daily, at which time the child is extremely irritable and may complain of arthralgia and myalgia. The rash is a transient, salmon colored, macular, or slightly papular, blanching eruption occurring at the time of the temperature spike. In systemic JRA, the arthritis may not be apparent for weeks or even months to years after the onset of systemic symptoms, making this condition extremely difficult to differentiate from other causes of fever of unknown origin. The arthritis that subsequently develops is usually polyarticular, and significant joint damage develops in approximately 25% of patients. In general, the systemic features regress within 6 months of onset and the arthritis remits or progresses to joint destruction. Uveitis is quite rare in systemic JRA.

An unusual complication of systemic JRA is called **macrophage activation syndrome,** which can occur at any point in the clinical course but is seen most frequently after exposure to new medications. It is important to recognize this complication and start prompt treatment because there is considerable morbidity and even mortality. This disorder is similar to other hematophagocytic syndromes and is caused by excessive activation and proliferation of macrophages, with marked increases in T-cell and macrophage-derived cytokines. The child develops an acute overwhelming dramatic illness, secondary to severe multisystemic inflammation, and marked derangement in hematologic studies (disseminated intravascular coagulation). Diagnosis can be confirmed by biopsy, and treatment is with high doses of parenteral corticosteroids. Cyclosporine A may be useful in those children not responding to corticosteroids.

Radiographic features of JRA. Radiographs at the onset of JRA will be normal or show only soft tissue swelling. Typical destructive changes may take years to develop, if ever. Radiographs are useful for baseline studies and, more importantly, to rule out other causes of the articular symptoms. The first evident radiographic changes are soft tissue swelling and juxta-articular osteoporosis, followed by bone erosion, loss of articular cartilage, decreased joint space, and bone destruction. A distinctive feature in the developing child is regional overgrowth or undergrowth in joints with persistent disease. The most common example of this is leg length discrepancy in a child with pauciarticular JRA of one knee. The chronic inflammatory process and increased blood flow in synovial tissue lead to advanced bone maturation, resulting in the involved leg being longer than the uninvolved extremity.

Treatment of JRA. All children with JRA need individualized treatment plans and should be managed by a practitioner experienced in the treatment of these disorders, especially if agents more potent than NSAIDs are required (Table 8–4). Pain should be controlled, using appropriate non-narcotic analgesics, with narcotics reserved for severe pain. Conservative therapies should not be overlooked and include topical agents, moist heat, splinting or casting for comfort, crutches or canes, sufficient rest, and an appropriate exercise program.

Virtually all patients require an NSAID for control of symptoms. The NSAIDs reduce joint swelling, relieve pain, and have a modest effect on the overall inflammatory process. There are several NSAIDs to chose from, and several newer agents are being tested in clinical trials in children. In general, an NSAID that needs to be taken only once or twice daily is preferred, especially for the school-age child. The younger child may need a liquid preparation. Several selective inhibitors of cyclooxygenase-2 have

Table 8–4. Drug Therapy of Juvenile Rheumatoid Arthritis[1]

Drug	Dose
Aspirin	80–100 mg/kg/day orally divided 4 × per day (max 4000 mg/day)
Ibuprofen	40 mg/kg/day orally divided 3 × per day (max 3600 mg/day)
Naproxen	10–20 mg/kg/day orally divided 2 × per day (max 1500 mg/day)
Tolmetin sodium	20–30 mg/kg/day orally divided 3 × per day (max 2000 mg/day)
Indomethacin	2–3 mg/kg/day orally divided 3 × per day (max 150 mg/day)
Celcoxib	
Relcoxib	
Disease-modifying antirheumatic drugs	
Hydroxychloroquine	6.5 mg/kg/day orally (max 400 mg/day)
Sulfasalazine	40–50 mg/kg/day (orally divided 2 × per day) (max 3000 mg/day)
Intramuscular gold salts	1 mg/kg/week (max 50 mg/week) intramuscularly
Auranofin (oral gold)	0.15 mg/kg/day initially orally, 0.2 mg/kg/day if not effective after 6 mo (max 9 mg/day)
Methotrexate	10–15 mg/(mg/m^2/wk) (max 20–30 mg/wk)–oral or subcutaneously
Etanercept	0.4 mg/kg (max 25 mg) subcutaneously twice a week
Infliximab	5 mg/kg intravenous infusion, repeated at 2 and 6 wk

[1] Nonsteroidal anti-inflammatory drugs approved by the Food and Drug Administration for use in children.

been marketed recently in the United States and abroad and can be useful in the child who cannot tolerate the usual NSAIDs. These agents (celecoxib, rofecoxib, among others) have less gastrointestinal toxicity but are more expensive and do not have the cardiovascular protective effect of the earlier NSAIDs. Salicylates are used less frequently in children because of increased risk of gastrointestinal toxicity, the rare risk of Reyes syndrome, and the need for more frequent laboratory studies, including salicylate levels. Serum levels of the other NSAIDs are not useful clinically. In general, patients on chronic NSAIDs should have laboratory studies every 3–4 months, including a CBC, measurement of liver enzymes, and a urinalysis to monitor for drug toxicity.

Short courses and/or low doses of corticosteroids can be useful for rapid and sustained control of inflammation. However, corticosteroids can have significant long-term side effects. Thus, long-term use and high doses are reserved for children with severe systemic disease or incapacitating polyarthritis. Because malignancies such as leukemia and neuroblastoma can mimic systemic JRA, it is important to consider an oncology consultation before starting systemic corticosteroids in systemic JRA to avoid masking the diagnosis of malignancy. Intraarticular injection of corticosteroids is safe and can be very helpful, especially in the child with significant pain or loss of function in only a few joints.

The past decade has seen major advances in the understanding and treatment of chronic inflammatory arthritis. There is increasing emphasis on early identification of patients at risk of severe disease and aggressive control of inflammation, often with the simultaneous use of several pharmacologic agents. A detailed discussion of the use of agents individually and in combination is beyond the scope of this chapter. Medications include methotrexate, leufludomide, hydroxychloroquine, sulfasalazine, gold salts, and novel biologic agents that specifically inhibit inflammatory mediators, specifically interleukin-1 (IL-1) and tumor necrosis factor (TNF; Table 8–4). Two injectable anti-TNF inhibitors, etanercept and infliximab, have been recently approved by the U.S. Food and Drug Administration and are marketed for the treatment of RA and JRA. Both agents have a good safety profile and usually are used in combination with another agent, such as methotrexate or leflunomide. Clinical trials are underway for other biologic agents, including an anti-IL-1 inhibitor. Gold salts are used less frequently because of the high incidence of toxicity and added costs for weekly laboratory monitoring. For unknown reasons, systemic JRA patients are unusually susceptible to adverse reactions to salicylates, gold salts, and azulfadine; these agents should be used with caution in this subtype. Mild cases of JRA refractory to a trial of NSAIDs can be managed with hydroxychloroquine or sulfasalazine, which have very good safety profiles. For moderate to severe cases, low

dose methotrexate should be used early in the disease and can be given weekly as an oral dose or subcutaneously. Methotrexate has been approved by the U.S. Food and Drug Administration for use in JRA and is effective in the treatment of uveitis, which has not responded to corticosteroid therapy.

Prognosis of JRA. The hallmark of the rheumatic diseases is inflammation of synovial tissue. There is a marked increase in macrophages and T lymphocytes, local production of inflammatory mediators, and recruitment of neutrophils into the joint space leading to synovial hypertrophy, increased vascularity, and joint fluid secretion. Over time, the inflammatory process extends from the synovium, with local invasion of cartilage, and then erosion of bone. If inflammation does not remit or cannot be controlled by treatment, the final result may be end-stage joint damage and ankylosis. The natural course of JRA is extremely variable. However, most children do quite well with early recognition and management. Remission rates vary from 26% to 65% and historically, severe disability occurs in 20–45%. This marked variation in outcome is due to differences in clinical criteria, length of follow-up, and types of treatment. With the recent advances in treatment, the long-term outcome is expected to improve markedly. Children with pauciarticular JRA do the best, although this subtype is at highest risk for inflammatory eye disease and its ocular complications (vision loss, glaucoma, and cataracts). The children with the highest incidence of more severe articular outcome are RF+ polyarticular and systemic JRA patients with persistent polyarthritis. Chronic inflammatory arthritis for longer than 5 years is also predictive of more severe disability. An important consideration is that children initially diagnosed with JRA may be rediagnosed years later with a different rheumatic disease. This was seen in one series in 22% of JRA patients followed for decades, and most of those children were ultimately diagnosed with a spondyloarthropathy.

SPONDYLOARTHROPATHIES

The spondyloarthropathies encompass a group of diseases, with considerable overlap in clinical features. The majority of these conditions have in common the presence of HLA B27 (overall about 75–90%), male predominance, enthesitis, and inflammatory arthritis in the peripheral and axial skeleton. The spondyloarthropathies are divided into six subtypes. Classic ankylosing spondylitis (which represents about half of all cases of spondyloarthropathy) does not occur in young children. The child may present with an asymmetric pauciarthritis that, only decades later, is correctly diagnosed. Children presenting with isolated hip arthritis are particularly likely to develop ankylosing spondylitis or another subtype.

The spondyloarthropathies are ancient disorders. Ankylosing spondylitis has been described in skeletal remains dating to the 30th century B.C. In contrast, adult RA appeared during the Renaissance. The incidence of ankylosing spondylitis is about 2 in 1000. In children, the spondyloarthropathies account for one third of cases of chronic arthritis and children also may fulfill JRA criteria. The etiology of the spondyloarthropathies is still unknown. There have been tremendous advances in the past two decades in the understanding of the immune response, identification of microbial triggers of inflammation, and delineation of the contributions of HLAs and enteric infections in these diseases. Theories of the role of HLA B27 include molecular mimicry (where a bacterial antigen is similar in structure to B27), posttranslational modification of the B27 molecule (resulting in an altered structure and subsequent autoimmune response), and the association of the B27 molecule with a deficient or altered host response to various infectious agents, resulting in the triggering of a chronic immune response. A transgenic HLA B27 rat model has contributed to our understanding of these disorders.

Clinical features of the spondyloarthropathies. The hallmark of the spondyloarthropathies is enthesitis, which refers to inflammation at the sites of attachment of connective tissue (tendons, fascia, ligaments) to bone. Typical sites of involvement include the lower extremities (e.g., heel, plantar fascia) and the sacroiliac joints. In addition to enthesitis, these conditions can be associated with synovitis, tendonitis, spinal disease (especially the sacroiliac joint), and mucocutaneous features.

The importance of a careful history and physical examination cannot be overstated. The patient or parents should be asked specifically about a family history of spondyloarthropathies, psoriasis, and inflammatory bowel disease. Enthesitis, especially of the lower extremities, often is misdiagnosed as an overuse syndrome. Clinical features useful to distinguish spondyloarthropathy from JRA are the presence of enthesitis and tarsal disease. The discriminative value of either sign approaches that of axial disease in making the diagnosis of spondyloarthropathy. Back involvement in children usually originates from inflammation of the sacroiliac joints. Symptoms may be bilateral. Pain is inflammatory in nature, of mild to moderate intensity, and persists for months. A careful and thorough physical examination should be done. The mouth should be inspected for lesions and the skin examined for psoriasis (especially the nape of the neck, elbows, knees, and umbilicus). Shoes should be removed and the feet examined carefully for nail pits, sausage toes (dactylitis), and signs of enthesitis.

Histocompatibility locus antigen B27 is not a useful screening tool in asymptomatic individuals. Its main use is to support a clinical diagnosis of a spondyloarthropathy. Patients with significant inflammation may have low-grade anemia and elevated levels of CRP and ESR. Routine radiographs will be normal early on, except for soft tissue changes. The most common early radiographic changes in the spondyloarthropathies are from enthesitis and sacroiliitis and characterized by bony erosion and then sclerosis and ankylosis of the adjacent bone. Magnetic resonance imaging will show profound alterations in involved bone and attached connective tissues years before standard radiographs will. Other useful imaging procedures are ultrasound and radionuclide scanning, particularly for evaluation of enthesitis. Computed tomography is not useful for enthesitis but can be quite useful for evaluation of sacroiliac disease.

Ankylosing spondylitis is quite uncommon in children and is diagnosed by characteristic changes in the spine or by presence of bilateral sacroiliitis. Onset is usually in young adulthood, primarily in males. Most patients will present with insidious, persistent chronic low back pain. Other features are enthesitis, peripheral arthritis, and, less commonly, extraarticular manifestations.

Reiter syndrome refers to an acute reactive arthritis occurring after an enteric infection or, less commonly, after a genitourinary infection. Young white males predominantly are affected. The original description of Reiter syndrome included the triad of peripheral arthritis, conjunctivitis, and urethritis, but most patients first present with peripheral arthritis alone. The arthritis will be abrupt and self-limited, lasting weeks to months. Patients can experience recurrences. Enthesitis is also quite common. Similarly, most patients will develop conjunctivitis, low back pain, and mucocutaneous manifestations (mouth ulcers, rashes, nail changes) at some point in their clinical course. Back pain is most often from sacroiliac involvement, is often unilateral, and will progress to ankylosing spondylitis in about 10% of cases.

Psoriatic arthropathy is an arthropathy associated with psoriasis that can manifest in extremely different ways, from peripheral asymmetric arthritis, a polyarthritis resembling RA, spinal or sacroiliac disease, or a combination. Most patients will have typical psoriatic skin lesions before developing arthritis, but the psoriasis may appear years later. Psoriatic arthropathy is more common in adults, with a male predominance, but can occur in children.

Enteropathic arthropathy occurs in about one third of patients with inflammatory bowel disease and may be the initial manifestation of their illness. Acute arthritis in peripheral joints usually coincides with active bowel inflammation and will subside once the gastrointestinal disease is controlled. Ten percent of patients eventually will develop spinal disease, usually sacroiliitis and occasionally ankylosing spondylitis. Other features are mouth ulcers, skin lesions (erythema nodosum, pyoderma gangrenosa), and uveitis. Interestingly, a high frequency of patients with other arthropathies have occult gastrointestinal inflammation demonstrated by endoscopic examination and biopsy.

Undifferentiated spondyloarthropathy is a term used for suspected spondyloarthropathy without the symptoms characteristic of the other subtypes. This situation is fairly common in childhood-onset cases because the classic radiographic findings of sacroilitis or spondylitis may not be evident for several years. This group of patients will be predominantly male and HLA B27 positive and will not have RF or other autoantibodies. The previous term for the spondyloarthropathies was *seronegative arthritis.* However, RA and JRA patients can be seronegative. Thus, this designation is now used infrequently. A subgroup of undifferentiated spondyloarthropathy was once called *seronegative enthesopathy,* or *SEA syndrome,* and these patients primarily were young males with chronic enthesitis. Most of these cases, followed over time, will evolve into one of the spondyloarthropathies discussed above.

Prognosis and treatment of the spondyloarthropathies. Similar to the treatment of the child with JRA, the initial focus of treatment for the spondyloarthropathies is on pain control, appropriate balance of rest and exercise, use of analgesics, and a trial of NSAIDs. Exercises to preserve back flexibility, an appropriate overall exercise program, and inserts to protect heels or plantar fascia can be useful. For reactive arthritis, this is usually sufficient to control disease. Many rheumatologists also will treat an acute exacerbation of reactive arthritis with a course of doxycycline because this has been shown to reduce its duration. For more recalcitrant and persistent peripheral arthritis, other agents can be added. The doses and types of agents are similar to those used to treat RA and JRA, including sulfasalazine, methotrexate, doxycycline, chronic NSAIDs, and low dose prednisone. Some of the newer biologic agents also might control spondyloarthropathy. Injection of corticosteroids into involved joints and bursae also may provide considerable and long-standing relief of symptoms.

The prognosis of the spondyloarthropathies is generally favorable, with permanent disability less common than in systemic and polyarticular JRA or adult RA. Long-term studies have shown marked variations in progression to classic ankylosing spondylitis (9–92%), mainly due to differences in classification criteria and length of follow-up. In a recent series of patients with childhood-onset spondyloarthropathy of more than 10 years' disease duration, those with enteropathic or psoriatic arthropathy had remission rates of 50–70%, whereas no patient with ankylosing spondylitis was in remission. Severe outcome is more likely with hip or spine involvement and prolonged elevation of ESR.

SYSTEMIC LUPUS ERYTHEMATOSUS

Systemic lupus erythematosus (SLE) is an inflammatory disorder of unknown etiology, occurring predominantly in young women, with an increased incidence in Asian, Hispanic, and African American ethnic groups. In the United States, the overall incidence is about 1 in 2000 individuals. The hallmark features of SLE are the production of multiple autoantibodies, vasculitis, and inflammation of multiple organ systems. The etiology is multifactoral. Disease expression and long-term prognosis are also quite variable and unpredictable.

Diagnosis is based on exclusion of other rheumatic diseases and the presence of 4 of 11 specific classification criteria including rashes, presence of certain serologic markers, arthritis, nephritis, serositis, and neurologic or hematologic abnormalities (Table 8–5). The SLE classification criteria are 96% specific and sensitive. As in many other rheumatic diseases (including JRA), most patients will have a positive ANA. Antibodies to double-stranded DNA (anti-dsDNA) and various cytoplasmic antigens are much more sensitive and specific for a diagnosis of lupus. Up to 12% of first-degree relatives of patients with SLE have the disease and up to 40% will have positive ANAs or other laboratory abnormalities without associated symptoms.

Clinical features. Systemic lupus erythematosus is characterized by the inappropriate production of autoantibodies to nuclear constituents that, with complement and other mediators, can trigger an immune reaction in virtually any organ. Thus, patients with this disease can present to virtually any subspecialty, from the psychiatrist to the orthopedic surgeon. The disorder should be considered in any patient with unusual symptoms and evidence of inflammation, especially if the patient is a young female. It is not uncommon for SLE to present within the first few years after menarche, after institution of estrogen-containing oral contraceptives, or around pregnancy and delivery.

Among the most common symptoms of SLE are arthralgia, arthritis, fatigue, fever, headache, and weight loss. Cutaneous manifestations are frequent and include the classic butterfly malar eruption, generalized photosensitivity, alopecia, Raynaud's phenomenon, and cutaneous vasculitis (palpable purpura, livedo reticularis). Renal involvement occurs in 50–70% of patients, ranging from minimal mesangial proliferation to diffuse proliferative glomerulonephritis on biopsy specimens. Inflammatory lesions can occur throughout the central nervous system, resulting in seizures, psychosis, stroke, and coma.

Laboratory features. Antinuclear antibodies are found in 97% of patients with SLE. As such, the ANA is a good screening test for SLE but lacks specificity. It is possible to confirm a clinical diagnosis of SLE in the laboratory in most cases by demonstrating the presence of anti-dsDNA or the extractable nuclear antigen Sm (Smith). Active SLE most often is accompanied by low levels of the complement components C3 and C4. The combination of a depressed complement level and elevated anti-dsDNA is 100% specific for SLE. Similarly, anti-dsDNA titers and complement levels can be used to monitor disease activ-

Table 8–5. American College of Rheumatology Classification Criteria for Systemic Lupus Erythematosus[1]

Criterion	Definition
Malar rash	Fixed erythema, flat or raised over malar eminences, sparing nasolabial folds
Discoid rash	Erythematous raised lesions with hyperkeratosis and follicular plugging; atrophic scarring
Photosensitivity	Cutaneous reaction to sunlight
Oral ulcers	Usually painless
Arthritis	Nonerosive involvement of ≥2 joints
Serositis	Pleuritis or pericarditis
Renal disorder	Proteinuria >0.5 g/d or persistently greater than 3+ on dipstick *or* Cellular casts
Neurologic disorder	Seizures or psychosis
Hematologic disorder	Hemolytic anemia with reticulocytosis *or* Leukopenia <4000/mm³ on ≥2 occasions *or* Lymphopenia <1500/mm³ on ≥2 occasions *or* Thrombocytopenia <100,000/mm³
Immunologic disorder	Positive lupus erythematosus preparation *or* Antibody to native DNA in abnormal titer *or* Antibody to Smith nuclear antigen *or* Chronic false-positive serologic test result for syphilis for at least 6 mo with negative treponemal testing
Antinuclear antibody	Abnormal titer of antinuclear antibody by immunofluorescence in the absence of drugs known to be associated with "drug-induced lupus erythematosus"

[1] Diagnosis based on exclusion of other rheumatic diseases and the presence of at least 4 of 11 criteria.

Reproduced, with permission, from Tan EM et al: The 1982 revised criteria for the classification of systemic lupus erythematosus. *Arthritis Rheum* 1982;25:1271.

ity and often can predict a disease flare. Deficiencies of early complement components leading to a lupuslike disease are suspected if the total hemolytic complement is quite low or persistently depressed. Hematologic features of SLE include leukopenia, lymphopenia, thrombocytopenia, and Coombs-positive hemolytic anemia. Patients with SLE and antiphospholipid antibodies or the lupus anticoagulant are prone to recurrent arterial and venous thromboses (stroke, thrombophlebitis) and miscarriage.

Treatment. Treatment for SLE is based on the organ systems involved. Arthritis and mucocutaneous disease are manageable with nonsteroidal drugs and hydroxychloroquine. All children with SLE must wear sunscreens to avoid cutaneous and systemic flares. Estrogen-containing oral contraceptives should be avoided. Corticosteroids are indicated for any visceral involvement or severe hematologic disease and typically are begun at a dose of 2 mg/kg/day of prednisone (maximum 60–80 mg/day). The dosage of medication is titrated on the basis of the patient's symptoms and objective measures of disease activity (phys-

ical examination, urinary sediment, and levels of C3, C4, and DNA antibodies). Whenever possible, steroids should be converted to alternate-day dosing to minimize side effects. Severe symptomatic flares (e.g., onset of renal insufficiency, seizures, and coma) are best managed with intravenous pulse methylprednisolone (30 mg/kg, up to 1000 mg). Immunosuppressive therapy is added in children with severe uncontrolled disease or in whom the steroid dose cannot be reduced. Significant renal involvement, such as diffuse proliferative glomerulonephritis, requires monthly intravenous cyclophosphamide because corticosteroids alone are not sufficient to prevent end-stage renal failure. Methotrexate and azathioprine are effective in managing nonrenal manifestations and can allow reduction of the corticosteroid dose. Autologous bone marrow transplantation has been used to control disease in severe SLE unresponsive to other therapies.

Prognosis. The prognosis for patients with lupus has improved dramatically in the past 50 years. The 10-year survival rate is now greater than 90%. Nevertheless, this disease results in considerable morbidity because of the disease and the complications of treatment, such as accelerated atherosclerosis, increased susceptibility from infection, and musculoskeletal complications of prolonged corticosteroid use. The overall risk of corticosteroid induced avascular necrosis of the hips can exceed 25%. Death in SLE patients occurs primarily from infection but can be a result of renal failure, pulmonary hemorrhage, severe central nervous system disease, and early myocardial infarction.

OTHER LUPUS SYNDROMES

Drug-induced lupus is seen in individuals taking any number of prescription drugs, most commonly antihypertensives (hydralazine, procainemide, α-methyldopa), making this disorder more common in adults. Drug-induced lupus can be seen in children taking anticonvulsants, usually dilantin and occasionally phenobarbital. The child will develop vague constitutional symptoms, joint disease, rashes, mouth ulcers, and a positive ANA. The child also might manifest pleuritis or pericarditis. Renal disease and positive anti-dsDNA are very unusual in drug-induced lupus. Patients usually have antihistone antibodies, but these antibodies also can occur in SLE. The condition is self-limited and resolves when the medication is stopped. A short course of corticosteroids may be needed to control symptoms.

Most infants born to mothers with SLE will be healthy, although there is an increased incidence of maternal complications such as miscarriage and preterm labor. Transplacental passage of maternal autoantibodies may result in **neonatal lupus syndrome,** which presents with distinct cardiac, cutaneous, and hematologic manifestations that can occur independently or in combination. Complete congenital heart block occurs when maternal anti-Ro antibody (also called anti-SS-A) crosses the placenta and binds to the fetal conduction system, resulting in permanent injury. In addition to heart block, half of these babies also will have structural heart lesions. Infants may present with photosensitive skin eruptions a few weeks after birth. The skin eruptions resemble discoid lupus or may consist of serpiginous flat or slightly raised erythematous linear lesions, similar to those of subacute cutaneous lupus. Some infants can develop thrombocytopenia, hemolytic anemia, or leukopenia from other maternal autoantibodies acquired transplacentally. The heart block is permanent, but the other features will resolve within months as the acquired maternal antibody declines. The rash may scar.

All infants born to women with lupus should be examined carefully for these manifestations and a screening electrocardiogram and chest radiograph should be considered. Treatment is sun avoidance and directed therapy for any hematologic manifestations. Other than heart pacing, there is no treatment for the heart block. If a baby is born with congenital heart block to a healthy mother, the mother should be screened for autoimmune diseases (including testing for anti-Ro) and counseled about the subsequent risk to future children.

Systemic Vasculitis

Vasculitis is inflammation and damage to vessel wall endothelium and has a multitude of causes. Vasculitis can occur in virtually any organ; thus, the clinical signs and symptoms can be extremely variable. In contrast to adults, the two most common vasculitis syndromes of childhood are Kawasaki disease and Henoch-Schonlein purpura (HSP). Both conditions have an acute onset, a self-limited course, and overall good prognosis.

Systemic vasculitis is uncommon in young children but should be considered in the older adolescent, particularly if other conditions have been ruled out and the youngster is systemically ill with multisystem organ involvement, constitutional symptoms, and laboratory evidence of inflammation. Prompt diagnosis and early treatment are crucial to limiting disease progression and preventing severe sequelae. Histologic examination of involved organs is essential to making an accurate diagnosis. Equally important is the recognition of other diseases that can mimic vasculitis because the clinical course and treatment will depend significantly on the patient's diagnosis. Mimics of vasculitis include drug reactions, infections (parvovirus, hepatitis, Epstein–Barr virus), endocrine disorders, and gastrointestinal diseases. Although malignancies and cholesterol emboli are relatively common vasculitis mimics in adults, they are seldom the etiology of vasculitis mimics in children.

HENOCH–SCHONLEIN PURPURA

Henoch-Schonlein purpura is the most common vasculitis of childhood, with an incidence of about 15/100,000 children. Seventy-five percent of cases occur in children age 2–11 years. Henoch–Schonlein purpura was described first in the 19th century. Other names are anaphylactoid purpura and allergic vasculitis. Histologic lesions show leukocytoclastic vasculitis and immunoglobulin A deposition. Small vessels (capillaries, arterioles, and venules) are involved. The etiology of HSP is still unknown, but documented cases have occured after infection with several agents including Epstein–Barr virus, adenovirus, enteric bacteria, and streptococcus. Henoch–Schonlein purpura is more common in the spring and fall months, and 75% of patients will report a preceding upper respiratory infection.

Clinically, HSP typically presents with a purpuric rash, abdominal pain, arthritis, and nephritis. Other manifestations are intussusception (2–3%), scrotal swelling, and renal involvement (20–50%). Long-term outcome depends on the extent of kidney involvement. In general, renal involvement will be present within 2–3 months of onset. Progression to end-stage renal impairment is rare (<1%) and more common in older children.

Treatment for HSP is primarily supportive. Intravenous fluids may be necessary for children with severe gastrointestinal symptoms. The role of corticosteroids is controversial. Corticosteroids will improve the rash, arthritis, and abdominal symptoms and shorten the duration of hospitalization, but it is unclear if they reduce the progression of renal disease. There are anecdotal reports of improvement in clinical symptoms after administration of intravenous immunoglobulin (IVIG).

KAWASAKI DISEASE

In 1967, a Japanese allergist, Professor T. Kawasaki, first described an outbreak of a peculiar illness in very young children. A few years after this outbreak in Japan, there was an outbreak in Hawaii (predominantly in children of Asian ancestry) and then an outbreak in the United States in the late 1970s, strongly suggesting a transmissible agent. At first, the illness was thought to be relatively benign, but a few years after Dr. Kawasaki's initial description, the association of this disease with fatalities and the development of coronary vasculitis was reported.

Kawasaki disease is an acute vasculitis occurring almost exclusively in very young children. Eighty percent of cases occur in children younger than 5 years. It is diagnosed very rarely in children 8 years or older. Approximately 6000 cases occur annually in the United States and Japan. For unknown reasons, children of Asian ancestry have a 5–10-fold increased incidence of the disease.

Despite intense research effort since this disease was first recognized over 30 years ago, the etiology of Kawasaki disease is unknown. An infectious cause is likely in view of the epidemic nature and clustering of outbreaks, the self-limited course, and the occurrence in young children. There is considerable overlap in the clinical and laboratory features of Kawasaki disease and diseases from bacterial toxins such as staphylococcal and streptococcal toxic shock syndromes.

Clinical features. The clinical features of Kawasaki disease can be divided into three phases. The first, or acute, phase lasts about 10 days, if untreated, and is marked by a temperature as high as 40°C accompanied by a polymorphous exanthem. The rash can resemble scarlatina, measles, erythema multiforme, urticaria, and Rocky Mountain spotted fever (illnesses for which Kawasaki disease may be mistaken). Other findings in the acute phase are conjunctival suffusion without discharge (sparing the limbus), marked erythema of the lips and oral mucous membranes, strawberry tongue, and indurative edema of the hands and feet. Cervical lymphadenitis (about 40% of children) may be mistaken for bacterial adenitis. Cardiac manifestations during this phase include tachycardia, gallop rhythm, congestive heart failure, pericardial effusion, and arrhythmias. Other organ systems may be involved in the first days to weeks. Nonspecific

gastrointestinal symptoms include abdominal pain, diarrhea, vomiting, and evidence of hepatic dysfunction. An enlarged, tender liver in a child with Kawasaki disease should raise the possibility of hydrops of the gallbladder (acalculous cholecystis), which can be confirmed sonographically. Children with Kawasaki disease are commonly very irritable. Lumbar puncture often shows a lymphocytic pleocytosis (aseptic meningitis). Urethritis, manifested as sterile pyuria, is the most frequent genitourinary finding. This will be missed if the sample is obtained by catheterization or bladder puncture. Arthritis and arthralgia occur during the second, or subacute, phase, which is signaled by gradual subsiding of fever, marked thrombocytosis, and desquamation of the palms and soles beginning at the fingertips. Up to 40% of untreated patients have echocardiographically documented coronary artery dilatation and aneurysms in the third, or convalescent, phase, typically 3–6 weeks after the onset of symptoms. Coronary aneurysms have been reported in infants with prolonged febrile illnesses without rashes or conjunctivitis, a condition previously called infantile polyarteritis nodosa.

Diagnosis. The diagnosis of Kawasaki disease is based initially on clinical criteria alone (Table 8–6). However, atypical or incomplete cases not meeting the criteria but demonstrating coronary aneurysms also occur. Only 20–25% of children with Kawasaki disease will have aneurysms. Coronary aneurysms are extremely rare in children but can be seen in Wegener's granulomatosis, polyarteritis nodosa, and Behçet disease; conditions that are virtually never seen in young children. Difficulties arise in patients who do not meet criteria, do not have aneurysms, or meet the criteria, but actually have another cause of their disease. Similar to the situation with acute rheumatic fever, the diagnostic criteria should be used

Table 8–6. Criteria for the Diagnosis of Kawasaki Disease

Fever of at least 5 d duration, unresponsive to antibiotics (generally ≥40°C) and four of the following:
  Extremity changes: palmar and plantar erythema, indurative edema, desquamation of hands and feet, Beau lines (transverse ridges across nails months after resolution of illness)
  Polymorphous exanthem: earliest changes often seen in perineum, urticaria, morbilliform papules, scarletiniform erythroderma
  Lymphadenopathy: unilateral cervical, >1.5 cm; firm, nonfluctuant
  Mucosal changes; erythema; dry, cracked, fissured lips; strawberry tongue; marked erythema of oropharyngeal mucosa
  Conjunctival injection; bilateral bulbar, limbal sparing; nonexudative; painless

as guidelines only. The differential diagnosis in a child suspected of having Kawasaki disease includes staphylococcal and streptococcal disease, leptospirosis, Rocky Mountain spotted fever, and a variety of viral infections (Epstein–Barr virus, adenovirus, influenza, measles). Noninfectious conditions to consider include drug reactions, Steven–Johnson syndrome, and systemic juvenile rheumatoid arthritis.

Laboratory evaluation. Laboratory studies demonstrate a significant inflammatory reaction with leukocytosis, anemia, elevation of acute phase reactants, and marked thrombocytosis (platelet counts of 650,000 to up to 2 million/cc^3). These findings peak in the second week of illness and gradually resolve over several weeks in untreated patients. Patients also demonstrate increased serum levels of several cytokines (IL-1, IL-6, soluble IL-2 receptor, TNF), expansion of B and T cells in the peripheral blood, and evidence of lymphocyte and macrophage activation. All patients should have an echocardiogram 3–6 weeks after onset of fever. In a large series of 800 patients, none of the patients who had normal echocardiograms at 3–4 weeks had abnormal echocardiograms later.

Treatment. High dose aspirin (80–100 mg/kg/day given orally) plus IVIG 2 g/kg over 10–12 hours should be given as soon as the diagnosis is clear and other etiologies have been ruled out. When IVIG and aspirin are administered within 7–10 days of onset, defervescence occurs promptly and clinical manifestations associated with the later stages of illness may not occur. High dose aspirin is continued until signs of acute inflammation subside (usually 7–10 days) but should be reduced to 5–10 mg/kg/d when the platelet count begins to increase. Salicylates are discontinued once the platelet count normalizes but are continued indefinitely in those with coronary involvement. Corticosteroids increased the incidence of aneurysms in the pre-IVIG era and should be reserved for refractory myocarditis.

Other Rheumatic Disorders

SERUM SICKNESS

Serum sickness occurs when a foreign protein (classically horse serum) is administered, resulting in circulating antigen–antibody complexes that fix to the walls of blood vessels and initiate an immune reaction and subsequent vasculitis. Serum sickness can occur after exposure to several drugs. Clinically, this is manifested as urticarial skin lesions and polyarthritis, often in association with fever. Commonly implicated drugs are antibiotics (e.g., cefaclor, sulfonamides, and penicillins) and anticonvulsants (e.g., phenytoin). Treatment is removal of the drug and supportive therapy. A short course of oral or parenteral corticosteroids can help ameliorate symptoms.

MIXED CONNECTIVE TISSUE DISEASE (MCTD)

Mixed connective tissue disease is one of the "overlap" syndromes with features of SLE, systemic sclerosis, myositis, and arthritis. It is defined by the presence of antibody to the extractable nuclear antigen ribonucleoprotein. Classically, children with mixed connective tissue disease present with Raynaud phenomenon, puffy hands, and arthritis. They are less likely to have significant renal involvement than children with SLE. Mixed connective tissue disease initially was thought to have a benign course and prognosis. However, over time, many cases ultimately will evolve into a diagnosable rheumatic disorder, usually scleroderma or SLE. Mixed connective tissue disease most likely is a subset of conditions referred to as **undifferentiated connective tissue disease.** This term refers to patients with nonspecific rheumatic symptoms (e.g., Raynaud phenomenon, polyarthritis, positive ANA) who do not yet meet classification criteria for a definable rheumatic disease. Patients with rheumatic diseases also can have overlap syndromes where rheumatic and nonrheumatic disorders coexist.

DERMATOMYOSITIS

Dermatomyositis is characterized by chronic inflammation in skin and muscle. The etiology is not known. Cases occasionally occur in clusters, suggesting an infectious trigger.

Clinical features. The child usually will present with progressive proximal weakness and a distinctive rash on sun-exposed areas. Joint symptoms, fatigue, vague abdominal pain, mild dysphagia, and low-grade fever are also common. Some patients also may have mild to moderate muscle pain. Significant weight loss is not common.

On physical examination, the child will have the characteristic rash, which consists of Gottron papules (reddish nodules on the knuckles), a psoriasiform eruption over the extensor surfaces of the elbows and knees, and a purplish discoloration of the eyelids (heliotrope rash). Photosensitive eruptions also occur on the face and can extend down the upper trunk in a V or shawl distribution. The facial rashes can be mistaken for the malar rash of SLE, but Gottron papules are not seen in SLE. Other signs of vasculitis are nail-fold telangiectasias and ulcerative lesions of the skin and gastrointestinal tract. On muscle testing the child will have a positive Gowers maneuver, diminished proximal muscle strength, and normal reflexes.

On laboratory testing, patients usually have normal levels of ESR, CRP, and CBC. Occasionally, the platelet count can be mildly low. Muscle enzymes will be moderately high and more than 70% of patients will have a positive ANA. Muscle biopsy will show inflammation and changes in capillaries.

The diagnosis of dermatomyositis is made on the basis of the criteria of Bohan and Peter (Table 8–7). If

Table 8–7. Criteria for the Diagnosis
of Dermatomyositis

Diagnosis requires the classic skin eruption and three of
four other findings:
Rash
   Purplish, edematous discoloration of eyelids
   Scaly eruption over metacarpal and proximal
      interphalangeal joints, knees, elbows, malleoli
      (Gottron papules)
Muscular weakness
   Progressive symmetric involvement of proximal limb
      girdle, anterior neck flexors, and abdominal
      musculature
   Gowers sign, difficulty climbing stairs, arising from
      chair, combing hair
Muscle enzyme elevations
   Creatine kinase
   Aldolase
   Aspartate aminotransferase
   Lactate dehydrogenase
Electromyographic abnormalities
   Insertional irritability
   Spontaneous activity at rest
   Short, small polyphasic motor units
   Positive sharp waves
Muscle biopsy
   Vascular compromise and capillary dropout
   Perifascicular atrophy of type I and II fibers

Reproduced, with permission, from Bohan A, Peter J: Polymyositis and dermatomyositis. *N Engl J Med* 1975;292–344, 403.

weakness is documented, the rash is classic, and serum muscle enzyme concentrations are elevated, a diagnosis may be confirmed through characteristic changes in muscle seen on magnetic resonance imaging. This may obviate muscle biopsy or electrophysiologic testing. One third of adult patients with dermatomyositis will have an occult malignancy. However, malignancy is not seen in childhood dermatomyositis. Similarly, polymyositis is very uncommon in children.

Treatment. Due to the seriousness of sequelae in untreated or inadequately treated patients, all children with dermatomyositis should be referred to a specialist with experience in treating this condition. High dose corticosteroid therapy is the mainstay of therapy, given orally or as pulse methylprednisolone to control inflammation rapidly. Corticosteroids are continued in high doses until muscle strength improves and serum muscle enzyme levels normalize and then are gradually tapered. Usually it is not possible to convert to alternate-day dosing during periods of disease activity. For unclear reasons, dermatomyositis can cause flares after a minute drop in the prednisone dose. Failure to respond to corticosteroids or the development of significant corticosteroid side effects calls

for the addition of immunosuppressive therapy, usually methotrexate, given orally or subcutaneously. Intravenous immunoglobulin has been shown in a randomized, placebo controlled trial to be efficacious as well. In refractory cases, cyclophosphamide, cyclosporine, and other agents in combination with corticosteroids have been tried. Hydroxychloroquine can be useful in treating the cutaneous disease but has little effect on the muscle inflammation.

Prognosis. Untreated, the mortality rate for childhood dermatomyositis approaches 33% and over two thirds of survivors have severe long-term disability. Death is now uncommon (<1%), occurring primarily in children with fulminant disease and/or severe gastrointestinal manifestations with perforation. Children also can die from infectious complications. More than 75% of children can be expected to have a monocyclic course lasting 2 years or less. Delay in diagnosis and effective therapy is correlated with the late development of dystrophic calcification of muscle and soft tissues. Rarely, children may develop features of another rheumatic disease such as scleroderma or, occasionally, SLE.

SCLERODERMA

Diffuse scleroderma (systemic sclerosis) is rare in children. Most children with scleroderma have one of the localized forms, linear scleroderma or morphea (isolated patches of sclerotic skin). Like other rheumatic diseases, the etiology of scleroderma is unknown. This disorder also has a female predominance. Scleroderma is characterized by the increased deposition of collagen in skin (which manifests as progressive tightening) and, on occasion, other organ systems. The most severe form, systemic sclerosis, involves multiple organs.

Skin changes begin with edema and are followed by induration, sclerosis, and eventually atrophy. The skin of the digits, hands, face, or arm usually is affected first. The disease then progresses proximally. Dysphagia results from thickening of the lower third of the esophagus. Hypertension, renal failure, pulmonary fibrosis, and cardiac involvement also may occur. This disease is commonly associated with the Raynaud phenomenon and tends to be relentlessly progressive.

The diagnosis is based on clinical suspicion and may be confirmed by a biopsy specimen of affected tissue. No single laboratory test is useful for the diagnosis. The ANA and RF may be positive but usually have lower titers than those found in patients with SLE.

Treatment is aimed at decreasing deposition of collagen and controlling associated phenomena such as hypertension and digital necrosis. The long-term prognosis for children with systemic scleroderma is not well established but is probably similar to that of adult cases and depends greatly on the extent of renal, cardiac, and pulmonary involvement. The CREST variant of systemic sclerosis is not common in children. CREST refers to calcinosis,

Raynaud phenomenon, esophageal dysmotility, sclerodactyly, and telangiectasias; CREST tends to be more indolent than classic systemic sclerosis.

The localized forms of scleroderma usually are not associated with systemic involvement, but some patients may have a positive ANA. Local involvement causes flexion contractures and growth abnormalities. The natural history varies from total spontaneous remission to progression of lesions over several years. Treatment emphasizes good physical therapy to soften the skin and maintain range and function. Drugs occasionally are indicated for more severe or rapidly progressive disease. In several small series of patients with linear scleroderma, low dose methotrexate was particularly useful in controlling extension and softening the involved skin.

REFERENCES

Ayoub, E, Majeed HA: Poststreptococcal reactive arthritis. Curr Opin Rheumatol 2000;12:306.

Brooks P: Use and benefits of nonsteroidal anti-inflammatory drugs. Am J Med 1998;104:9S.

Cabral DA et al: Spondyloarthropathies of childhood. Pediatr Clin North Am 1995;42:1051.

Cassidy JT, Petty RE: *Textbook of Pediatric Rheumatology,* 3rd ed. Saunders, 1995.

Conn DL: When should you consider vasculitis? Bull Rheum Dis 1998;47:1.

Dajani AS et al: Guideline for the diagnosis of rheumatic fever: Jones criteria, updated 1992. Circulation 1993;87:302.

Drugs for Rheumatoid Arthritis. Med Let 2000;42:57.

Flatø B et al: Outcome and predictive factors in juvenile rheumatoid arthritis and juvenile spondyloarthropathy. J Rheumatol 1998;25:366.

Goldenberg DL: Fibromyalgia syndrome a decade later; what have we learned? Arch Intern Med 1999;159:777.

Jennette JC, Falk RJ: Small vessel vasculitis. N Engl J Med 1997; 337:1512.

Klippel JH (editor): *Primer on the Rheumatic Diseases.* Atlanta: Arthritis Foundation, 1997.

Koopman W: *Arthritis and Allied Conditions,* 13th ed. Williams & Wilkins, 1997.

Lanzkowsky S et al: Henoch–Schoenlein purpura. Pediatr Rev 1992; 13:130.

Leung D et al: The immunopathogenesis and management of Kawasaki syndrome. Arthritis Rheum 1998;41:1538.

Melish ME: Kawasaki syndrome. Pediatr Rev 1996;17:158.

Moore MD: Rheumatic diseases. In: Weinstein SL (editor). *The Pediatric Spine: Principles and Practice.* New York: Raven Press, 2000.

Olivieri I et al: Enthesiopathy: clinical manifestations, imaging and treatment. Baillieres Clin Rheumatol 1998;12:665.

Petty RE: Classification of childhood arthritis: a work in progress. Baillieres Clin Rheumatol 1998;12:181.

Roberts NW: Keys to managing systemic lupus erythematosus. Hosp Pract 1997;1997:113.

Schaller JG: Juvenile rheumatoid arthritis. Pediatr Rev 1997;18:337.

Siegel DM et al: Fibromyalgia syndrome in children and adolescents: clinical features at presentation and status at follow-up. Pediatrics 1998;101:377.

Szer IS: Chronic arthritis in children. Compr Ther 1997;23:124.

Tizard EJ: Henoch–Schoenlein purpura. Arch Dis Child 1999;80:380.

Van Solingen RM et al: When it's not a rheumatic disease. Bull Rheum Dis 1998;47:2.

Wallace DJ: Lupus for the non-rheumatologist. Bull Rheum Dis 1999;48:1.

Yanagawa H et al: Results of the nationwide epidemiologic survey of Kawasaki disease in 1995 and 1996 in Japan. Pediatrics 1998; 102:1469.

Infectious Diseases

Allan S. Lau, MD, FRCP(C), Alan Uba, MD, & Deborah Lehman, MD

9

This chapter begins with a discussion of important general concepts in the diagnosis and management of pediatric infectious diseases. Key aspects of the clinical assessment including history taking, physical examination, and use of laboratory services are addressed, followed by a discussion of existing classes of antimicrobials and basic principles of their use. Because of the rapid pace of change in this area, detailed information regarding specific drugs and their dosing is generally avoided. A discussion of the approach to the child with fever follows. Fever is a common presenting complaint, associated with many infectious and noninfectious etiologies, and it is important that providers use an evidence-based, age-appropriate approach to its evaluation. In the subsequent section, individual infectious diseases are grouped and discussed according to the organ system most involved. Finally, several special topics, including infectious disease concerns in group day-care settings and the immune compromised host, are addressed.

■ LABORATORY APPROACH TO THE CHILD WITH A POSSIBLE INFECTION: HISTORY & PHYSICAL EXAMINATION

A detailed history and physical examination are the cornerstones of the evaluation of a child with a suspected infection. The information obtained allows the clinician to develop and narrow the differential diagnosis and formulate a subsequent diagnostic and therapeutic plan.

Although a thorough medical history is important to all areas of pediatric medicine, nowhere is it more essential than in the approach to an ill child with a possible infectious disease. Historical points unique to infectious diseases include questions regarding immunization history, previous antibiotic use, and recent contacts and exposures to infectious diseases. Knowledge of exposures, whether they involve household contacts, food, domestic pets or other animals, personal travels, or visitors from overseas, frequently hold the clues to an accurate and timely diagnosis.

The medical history begins with an inquiry into the nature of the present illness, including the duration and severity of each symptom. The progression and sequence of complaints also can provide essential clues to the diagnosis. For example, children with Kawasaki syndrome present with prolonged fevers and several signs and symptoms, such as conjunctivitis and rash, that may resolve before presentation and thus would not be identified unless specifically elicited by the history taker.

Specific symptoms should direct the examiner through a series of additional historical questions. For example, the child presenting with diarrhea should be questioned about food exposures to raw meats and eggs, recent travel, animal contacts, day-care attendance, and recent antibiotic use. Hemolytic uremic syndrome has been associated with patients who consume meat contaminated with specific strains of *Escherichia coli. Salmonella* is commonly found in poultry and dairy products. The travel history may suggest exposure to intestinal parasites such as *Entamoeba histolytica* in Mexico or *Cryptosporidium,* reported in municipal water supplies in several U.S. cities during 1995. History of animal contacts may indicate exposure to reptiles likely to carry *Salmonella.* The family should be questioned about day-care attendance because *Giardia* and *Cryptosporidium* can be transmitted in day-care settings. Recent antibiotic use should prompt the clinician to consider *Clostridium difficile* colitis.

Although most pediatric pneumonia is caused by common viral and bacterial pathogens, a careful history is critical to identifying less common pathogens that often present with symptoms that are persistent and unresponsive to conventional therapy. Tuberculosis is one of the most frequently overlooked causes of persistent pneumonia: families should be questioned extensively about potential exposures including contact with high-risk individuals such as immigrants from tuberculosis-endemic areas and homeless or incarcerated individuals. Questions should extend beyond immediate family members to include unrelated child care providers, such as nannies and caretakers in day-care centers. Children with risk factors or pneumonia that is unresponsive to a standard course of antibiotics should have a purified protein derivative (PPD) placed. *Legionella* is associated with known outbreaks in hospitals, hotels, and cruise ships via exposure to contaminated water and air-conditioning systems. *Chlamydia psittaci* causes pulmonary infiltrates and high fever after exposure to infected domestic birds. Coccidioidomycosis is a common cause of lymphadenopathy and pneumonia and is contracted by inhalation of spores in the San Joaquin

Valley, California. Similarly, histoplasmosis and blasto-mycosis may cause pneumonia in individuals exposed to the fungal spores in parts of the Midwest and Mississippi valley, respectively.

Patients with fever of unknown origin (FUO) should be questioned extensively regarding potential exposures. Brucellosis may be contracted by drinking unpasteurized milk. Exposure to malaria and other parasitic infections can occur during travel to endemic areas. Cat-scratch disease, now known to be caused by *Bartonella henselae,* is transmitted to humans by exposure to cats, most frequently kittens. This usually causes painless lymphadenopathy, but several reports have found serologic evidence of acute *B. henselae* infection in children with FUO and liver or spleen lesions.

No medical history is complete without a thorough investigation of animal exposures. The examiner should ask specifically about pets, including dogs, cats, reptiles, rats, and birds. Other animals, such as bats, squirrels, and raccoons, can transmit serious infectious diseases; possible exposures always should be investigated when confronted with a seriously ill child.

Every child with a persistent infectious disease or an infection with an unusual organism should be evaluated for an underlying immunodeficiency. The most common immunodeficiency is infection with human immunodeficiency virus (HIV). Transmission of HIV to children is now almost exclusively perinatal, making exploration of relevant aspects of the parents' medical and social histories also important.

A detailed medical history should be followed by a comprehensive physical examination. The examiner should be especially attentive to the presence of lymphadenopathy, swollen joints, and skin lesions. A child with endocarditis may have nothing more than a persistent fever and splinter hemorrhages or an abnormal urinalysis. A thorough musculoskeletal examination is a mandatory part of every physical examination. Osteomyelitis frequently presents with refusal to ambulate and point tenderness over the affected bone.

By taking the time to obtain a complete history and physical examination, the clinician can narrow the differential diagnosis and formulate a rational diagnostic and therapeutic plan that minimizes unnecessary anxiety, laboratory testing, and hospitalization.

■ LABORATORY MEDICINE IN INFECTIOUS DISEASES

The laboratory provides supportive and definitive evidence for the diagnosis of an infectious pathogen: A strong understanding of the general principles involved in modern laboratory medicine will aid the clinician greatly.

Basic Principles in Using Laboratory Services

Because of the rapid pace of change in this area, practitioners need to keep abreast of new testing procedures and technologies as they become available. Many cultures can now be completed much more quickly than in the past: With modern techniques, blood cultures are reportable within 48 hours, urine and throat within 1–2 days, and herpes simplex virus (HSV) and cytomegalovirus (CMV) cultures within 3 days. Cultures for anaerobes, mycobacteria, and fungi still require longer incubation times.

When seeing patients with fever or suspected infections, physicians should focus on the subset of patients whose diagnosis or management would be influenced by the results of microbiologic testing. If there is no clinical relevance for performing cultures and other diagnostic tests, these procedures are seldom indicated. Excessive and unnecessary investigations are a common problem. For example, if an infection (such as upper respiratory tract infection [URI] of nonspecific etiology) is trivial or self-limiting, little effort should be made to prove a specific etiology. Other examples are the performance of six or eight blood cultures when one or two would have been sufficient or ordering three stool examinations for parasites without waiting for the results of the first test.

Once a decision is made to perform a test, the physician is responsible for careful specimen collection under optimal conditions. Cultures from normally sterile sites, such as cerebrospinal fluid (CSF), blood, and joint fluid, must be collected using aseptic techniques. When samples are collected from skin or mucosal surfaces (e.g., expectorated sputum or urine specimens), efforts should be made to minimize contamination. Urine specimens for bacterial culture are most reliable if collected by midstream void, catheter, or suprapubic puncture rather than by a plastic bag attached to the perineal skin. In general, body fluids and tissue are preferred over swab specimens; stool specimens are preferred over rectal swabs. Whenever possible, bacterial cultures should be obtained before beginning antimicrobial therapy.

After collection, specimens should be transported promptly to the laboratory or held at the proper temperature to avoid bacterial overgrowth or death of fastidious organisms. When in doubt, specimens should be stored at refrigerator temperature. In some situations, especially for viral cultures, inoculation of specimens at the bedside or into special transport media may enhance isolation.

To enhance the recovery of pathogens, clinicians should fully complete test request forms including information regarding the type of specimen, site and time of collection, patient's age, symptoms, clinical diagnosis, prior antibiotic treatment, and suspected agents. This information will guide the choice of laboratory media and procedures. If an unusual infection is suspected, the laboratory should be alerted and the clinical microbiologist or an infectious disease specialist consulted.

When results are reported to the clinician, they should be interpreted carefully on the basis of the nature of the specimen and the clinical history. All skin and exposed mucosal surfaces have their own normal bacterial and fungal flora, creating potential difficulties in interpreting the results of cultures. Without knowledge of the patient's clinical history and the method of specimen collection, it is difficult to distinguish contamination from infection. Correct interpretation is easy when a single pathogen is recovered from a usually sterile site. Likewise, contamination should be suspected when multiple organisms of low virulence are found in urine or respiratory tract specimens. When a common contaminant is isolated in pure culture from a normally sterile site (e.g., *Staphylococcus epidermidis* in CSF and blood cultures), proper interpretation of the results requires knowledge of the clinical setting and the medical history of the host. For example, the presence of a ventriculoperitoneal shunt (in the case of CSF culture) or cardiac disease with foreign graft materials (in the case of blood culture) increases the likelihood of a true *S. epidermidis* infection. Likewise, if the patient is an immunocompromised host, isolation of a bacterial species of usual low virulence must be interpreted with care. In summary, judicious use of laboratory tests to aid diagnosis and management must be coupled with proper interpretation of the significance of the microbe identified.

Laboratory Methods for Detection of Pathogens

Laboratory studies can facilitate diagnosis by providing direct and indirect evidence of specific pathogens. Table 9–1 lists specific laboratory techniques currently available to clinicians. These are discussed in the following sections.

DIRECT DEMONSTRATION OF A PATHOGEN

Direct detection methods are of great value to the clinician because they are usually quick and relatively inexpensive. Staining of clinical specimens is the most direct method to demonstrate the presence of a pathogen. Specimens also may be cultured with subsequent staining and identification of resultant growth. Newer direct techniques involve the identification of specific bacterial antigens or sequences of bacterial DNA.

Staining and microscopy. Gram staining is a time-tested method of staining bacteria that aids in the initial general identification of the organism. The result of the Gram stain often guides the initial choice of antibiotic; with anaerobic or extremely fastidious bacterial infections, it may provide the only clue that a pathogen is present.

Other stains commonly used in the clinical laboratory are Wright or Giemsa to identify malaria parasites from thick blood smears, silver stains to identify fungal elements, and Ziehl–Neelsen to identify acid fast organisms such as mycobacterium. Recently, aramine orange, a fluorescent dye that stains acid fast bacilli, has been used in addition to the Ziehl–Neelsen stain. The bright fluorescence of this dye enhances identification of the bacteria.

Fluorescent antibody staining is used widely to identify pathogens from specimens and cultures. A smear of the infected material is placed on a glass slide, which is then coated with an antibody (typically a mouse monoclonal antibody) directed against a specific antigenic determinant of the pathogen. Unbound antibody is washed from the slide. If the monoclonal antibody is fluorescein tagged, the slide can be examined directly for antigen-expressing cells; this technique is called *direct immunofluorescence.* If the monoclonal antibody is not tagged, the slide can be stained with a fluorescein-tagged antibody directed against the species of the monoclonal antibody. The preparation then can be examined for fluorescence in a technique called *indirect immunofluorescence.* This approach offers the advantage of versatility without the need for different individual specific antibodies tagged with fluorescein. The major limitation of this technique is the subjectivity of slide interpretation; positive and negative control slides should be included for each determination. Laboratory personnel must be skilled in the interpretation of these slides. Antibody kits for immunofluorescent staining are currently available for the diagnosis of respiratory syncytial virus (RSV), *Bordetella pertussis,* HSV, varicella-zoster virus (VZV), and *Chlamydia trachomatis* infections. Special tests for Rocky Mountain spotted fever (*Rickettsia rickettsii*) and typhus (*Rickettsia typhi*) can be obtained from regional reference laboratories.

Direct identification of pathogens also can be made without staining techniques. Samples are examined under a standard light microscope as a "wet preparation." These preparations can be used to look for yeast or trichomonas in vaginal secretions and mycelial forms of fungus in skin scrapings. Potassium hydroxide is often added to dissolve unwanted cellular material. Unspun urine samples can be used to identify bacteria and white blood cells in the setting of urinary tract infections (UTIs) and Trichomonas. Dark field examination of suspected syphilitic lesions allows the examiner to visualize *Treponema pallidum.*

Major obstacles complicate the identification of viruses as etiologic agents. Viruses are not easily cultured, and some are impossible to grow in vitro. Polymerase chain reaction (PCR) assays and copy DNA probes are not routinely available for most viruses because of prohibitive costs and technical problems. To date, many regional laboratories have used PCR assays for HSV-1 and -2 and

Table 9–1. Identification of Pathogens in Laboratory Medicine

Method	Pathogens
Direct demonstration techniques	
Staining & microscopy	
Direct microscopic identification	
Potassium hydroxide	Fungus: yeast or mycelia
Dark field examination	*Treponema pallidum*
Electron microscopy	Viruses
Standard stains	
Gram	Gram-positive or negative bacteria
Giemsa or Wright	Malaria in thick blood smear
Ziehl–Nieelsen	Acid fast bacteria, mycobacteria
Aramine orange	Acid fast bacteria
Fluorescent antibody staining (on specimen or cell culture)	
Direct immunofluorescence (DFA)	Bacteria, viruses
Indirect immunofluorescence (IFA)	Bacteria, viruses
Identification by culture	
Standard bacteriology/mycology protocols	Bacteria, fungus
Selective media	
Colony morphology & odor	
Biochemical tests	
Different environmental conditions	
Antibiotic sensitivities	
Viral cultures in cell lines	Viruses
Cytopathic effects	
Immunofluorescence	
Detection of microbial antigens & antibodies	
Latex agglutination	Bacteria, fungus
ELISA	Bacteria, viruses
Western blot	E.g., HIV
Detection of nucleotide sequences by molecular biology techniques	
PCR assay	Bacteria (e.g., mycobacteria), viruses
Branched DNA assay	E.g., HCV
Nucleic acid hybridization (Northern or Southern blot)	E.g., HIV
Indirect demonstration techniques[1]	
Tzank smear	HSV, VZV
Skin tests	Mycobacteria, coccidiomycosis
Antibody testing	
Direct (acute & convalescent sera)	Bacteria, viruses
ELISA	Bacteria, viruses
Western blot	E.g., HIV

[1] Based on the host's immune response to pathogen.
ELISA = enzyme-linked immunosorbent assay; HCV = hepatitis C virus; HIV = human immunodeficiency virus; HSV = herpes simplex virus; PCR = polymerase chain reaction; VZV = varicella zoster virus.

Varicella zoster in routine diagnostics. Examination of potentially infected materials (e.g., stool) by electron microscopy is convenient for identifying viruses as pathogens. In an extension of that technique, gold-labeled antibodies specific for viral antigens permit identification of some viruses through visualization of antibody-viral binding (immuno-electron microscopy).

Identification of pathogens by culture. Identification by culture is traditionally considered the "gold standard" by which one establishes a diagnosis of a known pathogen from a usually sterile body site. Unfortunately, growth of a pathogen in culture is influenced by many factors including use of the correct growth media, the patient's history of antibiotic use, and the nature of specimen collection. Laboratories use numerous protocols and algorithms to identify specific bacterial pathogens. These include the use of selective media, biochemical tests, morphologic distinctions, and different environmental conditions. For instance, CSF cultures are usually plated onto 5% sheep blood agar and chocolate agar and grown in a carbon dioxide–enriched environment. Genitourinary cultures for *Neisseria gonorrhoeae* are plated onto antibiotic-containing agar (Thayer–Martin medium) for selective isolation. *Yersinia* species require incubation at colder temperature (4°C) for growth and also favor iron supplementation. Culture of unusual or fastidious organisms including *Mycobacterium tuberculosis, Legionella,* or *B. pertussis* requires special media; laboratory personnel should be alerted so that the appropriate medium is used. To identify the specific species of bacterial pathogen, Gram staining and morphologic characteristics of isolated colonies are identified and various biochemical tests are performed. Antibiotic sensitivity also can be tested to help guide therapeutic management.

Many yeasts, especially *Candida* species, can be cultured on standard bacteria media. However, most mycelial organisms require the use of fungal medium (e.g., Sabouraud medium). The diagnostic laboratory should be informed when a fungal infection is suspected, and the sample should be handled appropriately using the proper culture medium.

Viral cultures are often more labor intensive and take longer to grow because viruses must be grown in active cell cultures. Specific cell lines are needed for specific viruses. Therefore, the laboratory must be aware of which viruses are suspected in a particular patient. Usually, the diagnosis of a viral infection is made by identification of specific change in the morphology of the host cells in culture. This cytopathic effect (CPE) provides evidence that the virus was present in the inoculated sample. Demonstration of CPE can take days to weeks for most viruses. However, recent use of monoclonal antibody tagged with fluorescein has enhanced the identification of the virus (e.g., HSV and CMV) in the cultured cells, without the need to wait for the onset of a CPE. The fluorescein-labeled, virus-containing cells are identified with the use of a simple light microscope.

Detection of microbial antigens & antibodies. Detection of pathogen-specific antigen is a useful and fairly rapid method to support a suspected diagnosis. These techniques identify specific epitopes of a pathogen with the use of antibodies to the epitope.

Latex agglutination tests are used fairly commonly in pediatrics to help identify infections caused by *Hemophilus influenzae* type b (HIB), group B *Streptococcus* (GBS), *Streptococcus pneumoniae, Neisseria meningitides,* and *E. coli.* These tests work by coating a tiny latex particle with the antibody to the pathogen-specific epitope.

When these particles are mixed with the body fluid in question, they agglutinate by antigen–antibody bridging between the latex particles. This agglutination reaction is visible to the eye or by light microscopy. A drawback to this technique is that false-positive results are common, often necessitating more definitive tests for diagnostic confirmation.

The enzyme-linked immunosorbent assay (ELISA) is another antigen-antibody–based test that is performed easily and rapidly on clinical specimens. It is inexpensive, sensitive, readily available, and easily quantifiable for measuring either a pathogen-specific antigen or antibody. Antigen detection is accomplished by immobilizing a specific antibody into the wells of a tissue culture plate. The sample to be tested is then added, and the antigen immobilized and subsequently recognized by a second pathogen-specific antibody. After washings, a third antibody (which is covalently linked to a chromophore or enzyme) is added to develop the color. The intensity of the color development in the reaction is directly proportional to the amount of antigen in the clinical sample. Similarly, ELISA can be used to detect antibodies specific for the pathogen in question. In this scenario, antigens are used for immobilization on the plastic plate instead. As an alternative to the plastic well technique, the primary antibody is immobilized onto a membrane and the sample, second, and third antibodies are added sequentially. This membrane ELISA forms the basis for most commercially available rapid group A streptococcal tests.

Detection of pathogen-specific nucleotide sequences by molecular biology techniques. Polymerase chain reaction is a new and increasingly available method for the direct detection of pathogens. It involves identification of sequences of DNA that are specific to a certain pathogen and can be used with viral, fungal, bacterial, and parasitic pathogens. Briefly, two specific oligodeoxynucleotides that define the 59 and 39 ends of the DNA sequence of interest are added to total DNA extracted from the clinical sample. A special polymerase, Taq (from *Thermus aquaticus*), is added; Taq has polymerase activity only at high temperatures. The mixture is repeatedly heated and cooled. This allows for a logarithmic amplification of the sequence of interest, if it is present in the sample. This amplified DNA sequence can then be identified by gel electrophoresis followed by nucleic acid hybridization assays as described below. In theory, this technique can detect a single copy of the sequence of interest. Because of the enormous sensitivity of the technique, inadvertent contamination with very minute amounts of DNA can produce false-positive results. Thus, strict quality assurance measures must be undertaken by any laboratory performing these assays. Currently, PCR techniques are available for detection of HSV, parvovirus, HIV, and other pathogens by many reference laboratories.

An alternative to this approach is nucleic acid hybridization (Northern analysis for RNA and Southern analysis for DNA), which is more cumbersome and far less sensitive than PCR. This technique may produce false-negative results because relatively high concentrations of nucleic acids from the pathogen in question must be present.

INDIRECT DEMONSTRATION OF AN INFECTIOUS AGENT

These techniques use identification of an immune response as indirect evidence that a specific pathogen was (or is) present in a patient. They presume that the patient is able to mount an immune response and that enough time has elapsed from initial infection for this to have occurred.

Tzanck smear. This technique involves identification of multinucleated giant cells from skin lesions. The presence of these cells is suggestive of a HSV or VZV infection. To perform this test correctly, one must scrape the base of a cutaneous vesicle and place the epithelial cells onto a glass slide. The dried slide is then stained with Wright, Giemsa, Papanicolaou, or other stain and examined under a light microscope.

Skin test. Intradermal injection of an antigen preparation to look for a delayed hypersensitivity response (erythema, induration) was once a widely used immunodiagnostic test in clinical medicine. Infectious concerns, problems with standardization of preparations, and improvement in other types of testing have led to a general decrease in the use of these tests, with several exceptions.

The Mantoux tuberculin skin test is still widely used as a screening test for mycobacterial infections. Recommendations regarding pediatric screening and definitions of a positive responder are based on population risk groups and are addressed in Chapter 1. These guidelines are also thoroughly reviewed in the *Red Book* of the American Academy of Pediatrics. In the Mantoux test, 5 U of PPD is injected intradermally, and the site is checked for induration 48–72 hours later. Children with tuberculous and those with nontuberculous mycobacterial infections may have positive reactions, although nontuberculous (atypical) mycobacterial infections classically demonstrate a smaller area of induration. The clinician should be aware that early in the disease a child's test result may be negative and later, if repeated, may be positive. In addition, with active disease, generalized anergy to skin testing may exist, and a positive control to rule this out also should be performed.

Skin testing for coccidiomycosis occasionally can be helpful in a child whose clinical picture and history fit this diagnosis. Unfortunately, a positive skin test result may merely reflect past exposure or self-limited previous disease rather than current active disease.

Antibody testing. Quantification of serum antibody titers to a pathogen-specific antigen provides indirect evidence of a specific infection. As a general rule, paired serum samples are assayed with an "acute" serum sample obtained at the time of clinical presentation and a "convalescent" serum sample obtained 4–6 weeks later. A fourfold increase in antibody titer between the two samples indicates a recent infection. Antibody against pathogen-specific antigens also can be assessed with the ELISA method. Some of these assays measure immunoglobulin M (IgM) production, therby making the test more specific for acute disease. Examples of pathogens detected by this method are *Epstein-Barr virus* (EBV), *Cytomegalovirus* (CMV), HIV, and *Mycoplasma*.

Western blots, or immunoblots, are qualitative tests used to detect antibody against pathogen-specific protein antigens. A mixture of these antigens is separated electrophoretically by molecular weight. The antigens are immobilized on a membrane, and the membrane is blocked to prevent nonspecific binding. The serum sample is then applied to the membrane, incubated, and washed. The blot is processed in a manner similar to ELISA. Positive blots produce darkly colored bands that correspond to the molecular weight of the desired antigen. This technique currently is used to confirm positive ELISA results for the diagnosis of HIV.

Use of Laboratory Tests to Guide Therapy

There are two general types of laboratory tests to guide the therapeutic use of antibiotics: (1) in vitro tests that assess the susceptibility of the infecting organisms to different antimicrobials and (2) measurement of antibiotic levels or bactericidal activity in the serum. The most commonly used method for testing the susceptibility of an infecting organism to different antimicrobials is the disc diffusion method, in which antibiotic impregnated discs are used to inhibit the growth of bacterial colonies. Different concentrations of the antibiotic are often used and, based on the surrounding growth, a particular bacterium is reported as sensitive, intermediately sensitive, or resistant to the antibiotic being tested. To further characterize the susceptibility of the bacteria, the laboratory may elect to perform dilution susceptibility tests including the minimal inhibitory concentration (MIC) and minimum bactericidal concentration (MBC) of an antibiotic for an infecting organism. The MIC of the drug is defined as the lowest concentration that prevents visible growth of the test organism under a standardized set of conditions. The MBC of the drug is the lowest concentration that results in complete killing of the test organism or that permits no more than a 0.1% survival of the initial inoculum under standardized conditions. Both MIC and MBC are expressed quantitatively in micrograms, international units, or micromoles of antibiotic per milliliter.

To measure the effectiveness of antimicrobial therapy, there are two general types of in vitro tests: measurement of blood or body fluid antibiotic activity against the responsible organism and assay of actual antibiotic concentrations in blood or other body fluids. In the former, the serum bactericidal test determines the killing power of patient's serum against the infecting organism. The result is expressed as the highest dilution of the patient's serum that will produce the desired effects. This test is cumbersome and labor intensive. It is not commonly used except under unusual conditions with difficult management problems. In the latter, antibiotic levels may be measured to assess the adequacy of the chosen dose and route of administration and to prevent overdose, which may lead to toxicity (e.g., aminoglycoside).

An indirect way to assess the adequacy of treatment is to monitor the patient's erythrocyte sedimentation rate (ESR) or C-reactive protein (CRP). Both are nonspecific indicators of the presence of inflammation and may be elevated in a variety of infectious and noninfectious conditions. The ESR depends on the size and shape of the red blood cells and the plasma level of fibrinogen and globulins. Although an elevated ESR is supportive evidence for an inflammatory state, a normal ESR does not preclude the presence of underlying disease. A suddenly falling sedimentation rate in an acutely ill patient may mean the development of dissemination intravascular coagulation. Other circumstances that can produce a falsely low ESR include liver failure, congestive heart disease, sickle hemoglobinopathies, and extreme elevation of leukocytes as in the leukemias.

C-reactive protein is a serum protein produced by the hepatocytes that can be precipitated by the C-polysaccharide of certain pneumococcal strains. Its synthesis is induced by inflammatory signaling factors including interleukin-6. Because of its rapid degradation, CRP often is used to monitor acute treatment response.

■ ANTIMICROBIAL THERAPY

In the second half of the 19th century, Louis Pasteur formulated the germ theory and postulated that severe infections are caused by microbial agents. This theory led to the introduction of the pasteurization process for dairy and other food products. In addition, these early works resulted in the introduction of vaccination against bacterial and viral pathogens. These advances in microbiology and disease pathogenesis laid the foundation for modern medicine. The control and management of infectious diseases are among the greatest achievements of medical science.

Using the historical work on germ theory as a basis, therapy directed against microbes was developed in the 20th century. The first antibiotic to be discovered was penicillin, a natural product of *Penicillium* mold. Since then, innumerable microbial products have been investigated and chemically modified, leading to the generation of a great variety of antibiotics. These modified products, termed *semisynthetic antibiotics,* represent most of the antibiotics in clinical use today. Beneficial effects of these semi-synthetic products include increased antimicrobial activity, increased stability and solubility, and improved pharmacokinetics and bioavailability (i.e., wider distribution and tissue penetration and longer half-life). However, along with the vast array of new antibiotics have come enormous concerns regarding their overuse and misuse, which can result in increased microbial resistance, iatrogenic complications, and unnecessary costs to the health care system. Antibiotics are one of the most frequently prescribed classes of drugs, accounting for approximately 11% of all drug costs, or more than $80 billion in the United States. It has been estimated that two thirds of antibiotic prescriptions in hospitals are of questionable value. For example, clinical research data have determined that 50% of physicians prescribe antibiotics for the common cold. It is a common belief among the public that antibiotics are useful in treating and preventing complications of viral diseases. Thus, pediatricians frequently face enormous parental pressure to relieve symptoms by prescribing antibiotics. Indiscriminate use of antibiotics can lead to iatrogenic complications arising from adverse side effects and drug toxicity, emergence of resistant bacteria, and the masking of more serious infections.

The decision to prescribe an antibiotic is based on proof or strong suspicion that the patient has a bacterial infection. If the patient has a noninfectious process or an infection of probable viral etiology, withholding an antibacterial agent is rational. However, if the patient appears to be septic and critically ill, empiric use of antibiotics is essential. The specific antibiotic chosen is based on knowledge of the pathogens most likely to cause infection at a specific site in a specific host. Table 9–2 provides a list of clinical infections, their most likely etiologies, and recommendations regarding antibiotic therapy. Many of these conditions are discussed further in the subsequent organ-based sections.

Principles of Antibiotic Therapy

To prescribe antibiotics appropriately, the clinician must know the likely antibiotic sensitivities of the suspected pathogens. In addition, the achievable tissue concentration of various antibiotics at the site of the infection must be considered in selecting an appropriate agent. If more than one antibiotic is active against the likely pathogen, the specific agent should be chosen on the basis of relative toxicity, convenience of administration, and cost. Further, preference should be given to the drug with the narrowest spectrum against the presumed pathogen. If the site of infection is readily accessible for sampling (e.g., blood, urine, CSF), bacterial cultures should be performed to guide therapy. Once the infectious agent is definitively identified, therapy should be directed specifically against the organism, and the spectrum of the antibiotics narrowed to avoid toxicity and the emergence of resistance.

(text continues on page 298)

Table 9–2. Empiric Antibiotics of Choice: A Prescribing Guide for Infectious Diseases

Diagnosis	Probable Pathogen(s)	Recommended Antibiotic(s)	
		Either	Or
Ears and sinuses	Streptococcus pneumoniae	Amoxicillin[1]	Trimethoprim-sulfamethoxazole, azithromycin, erythromycin/sulfa
Acute otitis media	Haemophilus influenzae (most strains not typable) Moraxella catarrhalis	For recurrences, or failure	PO amoxicillin/clavulanate, cefuroxime PO ceftriaxone IM Cephalexin, erythromycin, clindamycin
Acute sinusitis Upper airway Pharyngitis	As above	Same as in otitis media	Same as in otitis media
Exudative	S. pyogenes (group A Streptococcus)	Penicillin V	
Membranous	Corynebacterium diphtheriae	Erythromycin + Antitoxin	Penicillin
Epiglottitis	HIB	Cefotaxime, cefuroxime	Ampicillin + chloramphenicol
Eyes Cellulitis Preseptal			
Spontaneous	HIB	Cefotaxime, cefuroxime	Ampicillin + chloramphenicol
After trauma (especially penetrating trauma near the eye, eg, insect bites, scratches)	HIB S. aureus, streptococci	Cefotaxime ± nafcillin	Cefuroxime
Orbital	HIB Staphylococcus aureus S. pneumoniae	Cefotaxime + nafcillin + surgery	Ceftriaxone + vancomycin
Conjunctivitis			
Neonate <5 d	Neisseria gonorrhoeae	Penicillin	Cefotaxime
Neonate >5 d	Chlamydia trachomatis	Erythromycin	Sulfonamide
Central nervous system Meningitis			
Neonate	Group B Streptococcus Escherichia coli Listeria monocytogenes	Ampicillin + cefotaxime	Ampicillin + gentamicin
Infant or child	HIB S. pneumoniae Neisseria meningitidis	Ceftriaxone + vancomycin	Vancomycin + cefotaxime
Abscess with or without trauma (trauma refers to penetrating trauma, including postneuro-surgery)	Microserophilic streptococci Anaerobes Microserophilic streptococci S. aureus	Vancomycin + cefotaxime + metronidzole	Vancomycin + chloramphenicol Add anti-pseudomonas drug for chronic otitis/mastoiditis

(continued)

Table 9–2. (Continued)

Diagnosis	Probable Pathogen(s)	Recommended Antibiotic(s) Either	Or
Abdomen			
Peritonitis			
Primary	S. pneumoniae E. coli	Ampicillin + gentamicin	Cefotaxime
After perforation	Enterobacteriaceae Anaerobes, gram negative rods	Clindamycin + gentamicin	Cefoxitin, meropenen
Secondary to continuous ambulatory peritoneal dialysis (CAPD)	Coagulase negative staphylococci Enterobacteriaceae Anaerobes	Vancomycin + cefotaxime	Cefazolin + gentamicin Vancomycin + gentamicin
Necrotizing enterocolitis in neonates (NEC)	Coagulase negative staphylococci	Vancomycin + cefotaxime ± clindamycin	Clindamycin + gentamicin
Kidneys			
Pyelonephritis	Enterobacteriaceae (most frequently E. coli)	Ampicillin + gentamicin	Cefotaxime or septra
Cystitis and asymptomatic bacteriuria	Enterobacteriaceae (most frequently E. coli)	Trimethoprim/sulfa	Amoxicillin or cefixime
Perinephric abscess	Enterobacteriaceae S. aureus	Nafcillin + cefotaxime	Nafcillin + gentamicin
Skin and soft tissues			
Cellulitis			
Extremity	S. aureus S. pyogenes	Nafcillin + penicillin (to prevent treatment failure when S. pyogenes is infective agent)	Clindamycin
Face (buccal cellulitis)	HIB	Cefotaxime	Ampicillin + chloramphenicol
Impetigo	S. pyogenes S. aureus	Cephalexin	Erythromycin or cloxacillin
Fasciitis	S. pyogenes	Penicillin + surgery	Clindamycin, meropenen
Myositis	S. aureus	Nafcillin + surgery	Vancomycin
Bones (osteomyelitis)			
In neonates	Group B Streptococcus S. aureus Enterobacteriaceae	Nafcillin + gentamicin	Nafcillin + cefotaxime
Acute hematogenous	S. aureus Streptococci	Nafcillin + consider appropriate coverage for HIB in children <24 mo	Clindamycin
In children with sickle cell anemia	S. aureus Salmonella sp.	Nafcillin + ampicillin	Cefotaxime + vancomycin
After puncture wound to the foot	Pseudomonas aeruginosa	Ticarcillin + tobramycin	Ceftazidime + tobramycin
Joints			
Infections in neonates	Group B Streptococcus S. aureus Enterobacteriaceae	Nafcillin + gentamicin	Nafcillin + cefotaxime
Infections in infants and children	HIB S. aureus S. pneumoniae	Cefotaxime ± nafcillin	Cefuroxime

(continued)

Table 9–2. (Continued)

Diagnosis	Probable Pathogen(s)	Recommended Antibiotic(s)	
		Either	Or
Infections in adolescents	S. aureus N. gonorrhoeae S. pneumoniae	Nafcillin + penicillin	Ceftriaxone + nafcillin
Postoperative infections	S. aureus Coagulase negative staphy- lococci Enterobacteriaceae	Vancomycin + cefotaxime	Vancomycin + gentamicin
Blood (septicemia/ bacteremia)			
Neonates <7 d	Group B Streptococcus E. coli L. monocytogenes	Ampicillin + gentamicin	Ampicillin + cefotaxime
Nosocomial	Coagulase negative staphylococci S. aureus Enterobacteriaceae	Vancomycin + cefotaxime	Vancomycin + tobramycin
In children	HIB S. pneumoniae N. meningitidis	Cefotaxime	Ampicillin + chloramphenicol
In adolescents	N. meningitidis N. gonorrhoeae S. aureus	Penicillin + nafcillin	Cefotaxime

[1] High dose amoxicillin should be used in patients at high risk for drug-resistant streptococcus pneumoniae: age <2 y, abx therapy within proceeding 1–3 mo; day-care attendance.
HIB = H. influenzae type b.

ROUTE OF ADMINISTRATION AND RELATED CONSIDERATIONS

Systemic antibiotics can be given orally or parenterally through the intravenous (IV) or intramuscular routes. Several factors should be considered when choosing the specific route of administration. To ensure direct delivery and enhance bioavailability, the IV route is commonly used with hospitalized patients. Antibiotics can be administered intramuscularly in patients who do not have an IV device in place, unless they have a bleeding disorder or are in shock. For outpatients, antibiotics usually are given orally. An exception would be a single intramuscular administration of an antibiotic in a child when family compliance is questionable or pending outcome of culture results. Another exception would be long-term IV antibiotics administered as part of a home therapy program. In recent years it is becoming increasingly popular to initiate antibiotic therapy parenterally during an initial hospital-based phase of treatment and then to complete the course of antibiotics using the oral route when the patient has improved and is stable enough to be discharged. This practice is used most commonly in treating osteomyelitis and septic arthritis. Although this innovative treatment pro-

tocol saves hospital costs and serves the patient well for early discharge, the patient must be monitored carefully to ensure compliance and avoid potential complications.

Although IV administration of an antibiotic would appear to ensure drug delivery, this is not always true. Stability within delivery solutions varies with different antibiotics. Further, interactions between injected drugs may interfere with drug activity. For example, aminoglycosides are inactivated by penicillins when they are allowed to mix before an infusion. Intravenous drugs always should be given separately. If this is not possible, the compatibility of the mixed agents must be verified. Because pediatric doses involve relatively small volumes, the total volume of the infusion system itself must be taken into account when delivering antibiotics intravenously.

In pediatrics, the smell and taste of an antibiotic has a significant impact on compliance with oral therapy. Success also is influenced by the concomitant ingestion of food and drink. Food may reduce the gastrointestinal discomfort generated by certain antibiotics and therefore indirectly enhance compliance. For certain antibiotics, however, the benefit of reduced gastrointestinal upset is outweighed by the decrease in bioavailability that results from the presence of food. Table 9–3 provides a list of

Table 9–3. Antibiotic Administration and Food Consumption

Antibiotics that should be taken on an empty stomach
Clindamycin
Erythromycin base and stearate
Penicillins (except those listed below)
Rifampin
Tetracyclines (except those listed below)
Antibiotics that should be taken with food
Amoxicillin
Amoxicillin-clavulanic acid
Doxycycline
Erythromycin
Metronidazole
Minocycline
Penicillin V
Nalidixic acid
Nitrofurantoin
Sulfonamides

Table 9–4. Classification of Antibiotics by Mechanism of Action

Inhibition of cell wall synthesis	Inhibition of protein synthesis
Penicillins	Aminoglycosides
Cephalosporins	Chloramphenicol
Vancomycin	Clindamycin
Aztreonam	Erythromycin
Imipenem	Spectinomycin
	Tetracyclines
Inhibition of nucleic acid synthesis	Inhibition of folate synthesis
Metronidazole	Sulfonamides
Quinolones	Trimethoprim
Rifampin	

Adapted, with permission, from Prober CG: Antibacterial therapy. In: Rudolph AM et al (editors): *Rudolph's Pediatrics*, 20th ed. Appleton & Lange, 1996:499.

antibiotics that should be taken on an empty stomach and those that should be taken with food.

DURATION OF THERAPY

For many infectious diseases, the recommended duration of antibiotic treatment is based on empiric historical experience rather than controlled trials. In general, however, therapy should be guided by the patient's clinical response rather than adherence to an arbitrary duration of therapy. Guidelines for the treatment of specific infectious disease are discussed later in the chapter.

RESPONSE TO THERAPY

The response of the patient to antibiotic therapy is monitored by clinical assessment and laboratory testing. Clinical monitoring involves sequential physical examinations, with special attention to vital signs such as body temperature and the site of original infection. Fever and signs of inflammation should resolve within several days of initiating appropriate antibiotic treatment. Laboratory monitoring may include repeating bacterial cultures to ensure sterilization and serial measurement of nonspecific indicators of inflammation. For severe infections, the peripheral white blood cell count (WBC) and acute phase reactants (ESR or CRP) should be followed until they are normal. Sometimes it may be necessary to determine that adequate concentrations of the antibiotic are achieved in vivo. This can be done by measuring the antibiotic concentration in the serum or, alternatively, assaying for the serum bactericidal test, which is reflective of antibiotic killing effects on the organism (see above, Laboratory Tests to Guide Therapy). In general,

a lack of clinical or laboratory response to treatment mandates a change in therapy (e.g., change in antibiotic, surgical drainage).

MECHANISMS OF ACTION

Antibiotics work by attacking targets present in bacteria that are absent or less vulnerable in human cells. This directed attack is referred to as *selective toxicity*. Antibiotics can be grouped according to their site of action (Table 9–4). These sites include inhibition of the synthesis of bacterial cell wall, nucleic acids, proteins, and folate.

BACTERIOSTATIC VERSUS BACTERICIDAL

Antibiotics also can be categorized as bacteriostatic or bactericidal (Table 9–5). Bacteriostatic agents inhibit

Table 9–5. Classification of Antimicrobials: Based on Bactericidal Versus Bacteriostatic Effect

Bactericidal	Bacteriostatic[1]
Penicillins	Clindamycin
Cephalosporins	Macrolides (e.g., erythromycin)
Aminoglycosides	Sulfonamides
Vancomycin	Tetracycline, minocycline
Quinolones	Chloramphenicol[2]

[1] At high concentrations, bacteriostatic drugs can be bactericidal.
[2] Chloramphenicol usually is classified as bacteriostatic against many microbes (e.g., *S. aureus* or *Gram-negative rods*), but it has been shown to be bactericidal against *S. pneumoniae*, *N. meningitides*, and *H. influenzae*.

bacterial cell replication but do not kill the organism. In this case, they halt bacterial growth and allow the host's immune mechanisms to clear the infection. Theoretically, if host immunity is suppressed or the infection is in an area of poor immunologic surveillance (e.g., CSF or vitreous humor), bacteriostatic agents may not be effective. Chloramphenicol and erythromycin are bacteriostatic against most bacteria, although chloramphenicol is bactericidal against the most common and important pediatric pathogens including HIB, *S. pneumoniae,* and *Neisseria meningitidis.* Examples of bactericidal antibiotics are penicillins, cephalosporins, vancomycin, and aminoglycosides. They cause microbial death by cell lysis. Some antibiotics have dual properties and may be bacteriostatic or bactericidal depending on the specific bacteria, concentration of the drug, and nature of the tissue environment. These antibiotics include the sulfonamides and tetracyclines.

EMERGENCE OF ANTIBIOTIC RESISTANCE

The development of microbial drug resistance results from widespread excessive and indiscriminate use of antimicrobial agents, coupled with the ability of bacteria to acquire and spread resistance and the capacity of humans to spread bacteria. Antimicrobial drug resistance is a major driving force behind the incessant search for newer drugs. Few antibiotics can escape the ability of bacteria to develop resistance. Development of resistance has resulted in major changes in the therapy of important pathogens for children, including *Staphylococcus aureus,* HIB, and *S. pneumoniae.* For instance, infections caused by *S. aureus* no longer can be treated with penicillin, and some strains are not even sensitive to methicillin and cloxacillin, prompting the excessive use of vancomycin as the standard of therapy for *S. aureus.* In the hospital setting, this is a very serious issue: the frequent use of vancomycin has led to the emergence of vancomycin-resistant enterococci, which pose a difficult management problem for the treatment of immunocompromised patients. Another example is the emergence of penicillin- and cephalosporin-resistant pneumococci in many parts of the world. Emergence of resistant organisms in the community and the hospital results in longer hospital stays, frequent use of newer generations of expensive drugs, increased morbidity from those infections, and about a twofold increase in mortality rate. Resistance can result from a mutation or the insertion of foreign DNA by recombination. More often, resistance results from the transfer of genes carried on extrachromosomal resistance plasmids. Transfer of the plasmids is mediated most commonly by conjugation and followed by transformation, transduction, or transposon transfer. During the emergence of antibiotic resistance, it is quite common for clinical bacterial isolates to develop resistance to a number of antimicrobial agents, i.e., multiresistance.

Mechanisms of resistance include the production of enzymes that inactivate or modify the antibiotic, decreased antibiotic uptake or an active efflux transport system, and alteration in the antibiotic's bacterial target. β-Lactamase is probably the best known enzyme produced by resistant bacteria to inactivate penicillins and cephalosporins. By altering specific outer membrane proteins, certain bacteria can decrease the uptake or penetration of an antibiotic (e.g., imipenem). An example of resistance secondary to alteration of the antibiotic's target is the development of penicillin-binding proteins with markedly reduced antibiotic affinity, resulting in strains of *S. pneumoniae* that are poorly killed by penicillin. Bacteria may develop resistance by more than one mechanism.

COMBINATION THERAPY WITH ANTIBIOTICS

In general, single antibiotic therapy should be used to treat an uncomplicated infection. The drug chosen should have the narrowest spectrum of activity necessary to eradicate the targeted organism so that the emergence of resistance can be minimized. For certain clinical conditions, however, combination antibiotic therapy is indicated. The most common reason for combining two or more antibiotics is to provide broad empiric therapy in an ill or septic patient until the infecting pathogen has been identified. Other indications for combination therapy are infections caused by relatively resistant organisms, infections involving multiple bacteria, sepsis or febrile neutropenic episodes in an immunocompromised host, and infections where the risk of antibiotic resistance to single agent therapy is great. Combination therapy is often necessary to effectively treat infections involving resistant organisms: management of most *Pseudomonas aeruginosa* infections requires the use of two drugs, such as tobramycin and piperacillin, for synergistic effects. Although extensive in vitro data demonstrate synergism between various antibiotics, definitive proof of the clinical relevance of these interactions is generally lacking. Combination therapy also is indicated for infections involving more than one bacterium that cannot be adequately treated with a single agent. Examples are intrapelvic and intraabdominal infections, which usually are caused by a mixture of aerobic and anaerobic organisms. In addition, antibiotics are prescribed in combination to provide greater inhibition or killing of the pathogenic bacteria than would occur with single-drug therapy. This is particularly important for the management of immunocompromised hosts with sepsis or episodes of fever and neutropenia (see below). Combining two agents at times also can prevent or delay the emergence of resistance. For instance, multiple drugs are used to treat mycobacterial infections. It is also known that some gram-negative rods including *Enterbacter, Klebsiella,* and *Serratia* species can develop resistance to cefotaxime during the course of treatment with one drug alone, despite being sensitive to the antibiotic initially. This has prompted the use of double coverage with the addition of lower dose aminoglycoside to the third-generation cephalosporin regimen for optimal treatment. In summary, the possible beneficial effects of combination antibiotic therapy should be weighed against possible harmful outcomes, including an increased incidence of superinfection and toxicity, increased cost, and potential antagonism.

PROPHYLACTIC USES OF ANTIBIOTICS

Prophylactic antibiotics are used routinely in several clinical situations including prevention of infections in immunodeficient individuals, bacterial endocarditis in patients with abnormal cardiac valves, certain recurrent infections (e.g., urinary tract infections in patients with vesicoureteral reflux), and to prevent the spread of certain diseases (e.g., meningococcal infections) in the contacts of patients. Specific situations where antibiotic prophylaxis has been proven to be effective are summarized in Table 9–6. A single pathogen is involved in most of the situations in which efficacy has been documented.

It is often assumed that the antibiotic used to treat an infection effectively should be able to prevent the infection. Although logical, this may not necessarily be the case. For example, patients with meningococcal infections can be treated effectively with penicillin or cefotaxime. However, these antibiotics are not secreted in the nasopharyngeal mucosa and therefore not useful in the prophylaxis of

Table 9–6. Prophylactic Uses of Antibiotics

Disease/Infection	Medication of First Choice
Proven	
Haemophilus influenzae type b	Rifampin
Leprosy	Dapsone
Neisseria meningitidis infections	Rifampin
Pneumocystis carinii pneumonia	Trimethoprim-sulfamethoxazole
Rheumatic fever	Penicillin
Syphilis	Penicillin
Vibrio cholerae	Tetracycline
Recurrent urinary tract infection	Trimethoprim-sulfamethoxazole
Recurrent otitis media	Sulfisoxazole
Possibly useful	
Asplenia	Trimethoprim-sulfamethoxazole
Bacterial endocarditis	Penicillin
Pertussis	Erythromycin
Postoperative infections	Choice depends on the surgery

Reprinted, with permission, from Rudolph AM et al (editors): *Rudolph's Pediatrics*, 20 ed. Appleton & Lange, 1996.

close contacts of patients with these infections. Rifampin is the drug of choice in this situation.

When administering antibiotics prophylactically, it is important that the duration of their use is appropriate. For example, most perioperative prophylactic regimens need be given for only 24–48 hours or less. Unfortunately, antibiotics are often continued for more than 7–10 days postoperatively. This unrestricted practice only serves to increase antibiotic side effects and encourages the emergence of resistant bacteria. In contrast, contaminated or infected operative sites should be treated with a full course of antibiotics.

ANTIBIOTICS IN NEONATES

Newborn infants, in particular low-birth-weight premature neonates, are more susceptible to the deleterious effects of many medications. As a result of immature hepatic and renal function, a relatively large extracellular fluid volume, and the presence of substances that can compete for protein binding with antibiotics (e.g., bilirubin vs. ceftriaxone), the absorption, distribution, metabolism, and excretion of antibiotics in the neonate differ from those in the older child or adult.

Immaturity of hepatic enzyme systems can cause transient deficiencies of specific enzymes required for drug metabolism or elimination. For example, deficiency of hepatic glucuronyl transferase in the neonate leads to the diminished conjugation of chloramphenicol to its inactive form, thus increasing the active drug level to a potentially toxic range that can cause cardiovascular collapse and death. This presentation, known as *gray baby syndrome,* can be avoided by using an alternative drug or monitoring serum drug levels. Similarly, some drugs can cause deleterious effects by competitively displacing bilirubin from albumin, resulting in potentially dangerous bilirubin levels. Those drugs include the sulfonamides, moxalactam, cefoperazone, and ceftriaxone. The latter two drugs are excreted in the bile, unlike most of their cephalosporin counterparts, which are excreted by the kidney.

Renal function in the immediate newborn period also is diminished with a glomerular filtration rate of approximately 30–60% that of an adult. Thus, the dosing intervals for many antibiotics need to be prolonged (e.g., ampicillin and cephalosporins) in the neonatal period. However, during the first 2 weeks of life, renal function increases, so that doses and dosing intervals must be readjusted by 7–28 days of life. Due to increased immaturity of multiple systems, premature infants require even greater attention to avoid overdosing and toxicity.

ANTIBIOTIC TOXICITIES

In addition to their beneficial effects, all antibiotics have potential toxicities. Side effects attributed to each agent are addressed in the following section on specific antimicrobials.

It is also well recognized that certain antibiotics cross the placenta and can be potentially toxic or teratogenic to the fetus (Table 9–7). In addition, many antibiotics are excreted in breast milk (Table 9–8). The potential for transplacental transfer and breast milk excretion always should be considered before prescribing antibiotics to pregnant women and lactating mothers.

At all ages, special attention should be paid to antibiotics that have a narrow toxic-to-therapeutic ratio (e.g., aminoglycosides, vancomycin, and chloramphenicol). In patients with renal or hepatic impairment, the clinician must be aware of the pharmacologic properties of the drug and its route of excretion. For example, in patients with significant renal impairment, antibiotics that are excreted by the kidney must be administered carefully.

The dosage of the drug should be adjusted appropriately to accommodate the residual function of the respective organ (Tables 9–9 and 9–10).

Pharmacology of Antimicrobial Agents

The following discussion is an abbreviated review of antimicrobial agents, including antibacterial, antiviral, antifungal, and antiparasitic drugs. Readers are encouraged to consult additional resources for more in-depth information regarding specific agents.

ANTIBACTERIAL AGENTS

Antibacterial agents can be divided into four major groups based on their mechanism of action (Table 9–4). These

Table 9–7. Transplacental Passage of Antibiotics and Their Potential Adverse Effects

Antimicrobial Agent	Trimester	Adverse Effects to Fetus or Infant
Amikacin	1, 2, 3	Potential ototoxicity
Amoxicillin	3	None
Ampicillin	1, 2, 3	None
Azlocillin	3	Unknown
Carbenicillin	2, 3	None
Cefazolin	1, 2, 3	None
Cefoperazone	3	None
Cefotaxime	2	None
Cefoxitin	3	None
Ceftizoxime	3	None
Ceftriaxone	3	None
Cefuroxime	3	None
Cephalexin	3	None
Cephalotin	3	None
Chloramphenicol	3	Potential circulatory collapse
Clindamycin	2, 3	None
Cloxacillin	3	None
Dicloxacillin	3	None
Erythromycin	2, 3	None
Gentamicin	2, 3	Potential ototoxicity; neuromuscular weakness
Imipenem	3	Potential seizure activity
Kanamycin	3	Ototoxicity
Lincomycin	3	None
Methicillin	3	None
Nafcillin	3	None
Nitrofurantoin	3	Hemolysis in G6PD deficiency
Penicillin G	1, 2, 3	None
Streptomycin	3	Ototoxicity
Sulfonamides	3	Hemolysis in G6PD deficiency; jaundice and potential kernicterus
Tetracyclines	3	Depressed bone growth; abnormal teeth; possible inguinal hernia
Tobramycin	1, 2	Potential ototoxicity
Trimethoprim	1, 2	Teratogenic in animals

G6PD = glucose-6-phosphate dehydrogenase.

Modified and reproduced with permission from Remington JS, Klein JO: *Infectious Diseases of the Fetus and Newborn Infant.* Saunders, 1995.

Table 9–8. Antibiotics Excreted Into Breast Milk

Antibiotics excreted in substantial amounts	Aminoglycosides, chloramphenicol, erythromycin, metronidazole, sulfonamides, tetracycline, trimethoprim-sulfamethoxazole
Antibiotics excreted in only trace amounts	Acyclovir, cephalosporins, clindamycin, nitrofurantoin, penicillins

Table 9–10. Antibiotics in Patients With Hepatic Failure

Dose reduction required
Chloramphenicol
Clindamycin
Doxycycline
Erythromycin
Antibiotics to be used with caution
Rifampin
Tetracyclines

include agents that disrupt the synthesis of bacterial cell wall, proteins, nucleic acids, and folate. Major classes of antibiotics and commonly used agents in each of these groups are discussed in this section.

Cell wall synthesis inhibitors

β-Lactam agents. Many different antibacterial agents contain a β-lactam, or monobactam, ring (Table 9–11). This is the site of covalent binding to penicillin-binding proteins (PBPs) as well as action of bacterial β-lactamases. With the exception of the monobactams, all agents in this class have a five-membered (penicillins) or a six-membered (cephalosporins) ring adjacent to the β-lactam structure.

Mechanism of action. The cell walls of bacteria consist of peptidoglycans, protein receptors, enzymes, and lipopolysaccharides. The peptidoglycan, the major structural framework of the cell wall, is a network of alternating polysaccharide chains (glycans) that are cross-linked with short polypeptides unique for different species of bacteria. Peptidoglycans are synthesized by enzymes located on the inner membrane of the bacteria. β-Lactam antibiotics exert their action by binding to PBPs located on the inner membrane, causing inhibition of cross-linking of the polysaccharide chains, thereby leading to bacterial killing. Different types of PBPs exist in different bacteria with different sensitivities to different antibiotics.

Spectrum of activity & clinical uses. Because of the relatively few toxicities associated with these drugs, β-lactams are used widely in many clinical infections. The penicillins are active against a variety of aerobic and anaerobic gram-positive and gram-negative organisms. Penicillin G and its oral equivalent (penicillin VK) are active against gram-positive organisms, including the hemolytic streptococci, many isolates of *S. pneumoniae,* non–β-lactamase-producing strains of *S. aureus,* and most oral streptococci. Of the gram-negative aerobes, only *N. meningitidis* and non–penicillinase-producing isolates of *N. gonorrhoeae* are susceptible to this agent. Nafcillin and oxacillin have a spectrum of activity similar to penicillin G, with additional activity against β-lactamase–producing strains of *S. aureus.* The aminopenicillins, such as amoxicillin and ampicillin, are among the most commonly prescribed antibiotics in pediatrics. These agents have a spectrum of

Table 9–9. Antibiotics in Patients With Renal Failure

Major decrease in dose	No dose adjustments
Aminoglycosides	Clindamycin
Vancomycin	Chloramphenicol
Trimethoprim-sulfamethoxazole	Metronidazole
	Rifampin
Minor decrease in dose	Avoid
Penicillins	Methenamine
Cephalosporins	Nalidixic acid
Tetracyclines	Nitrofurantoin
Erythromycins	Polymyxin B
	Spectinomycin

Table 9–11. β-Lactam Antibiotics

Penicillin derivatives
Penicillin VK, penicillin G
Aminopenicillins: ampicillin, amoxicillin
Penicillinase-resistant penicillins: e.g., cloxacillin, methicillin, nafcillin
Antipseudomonal penicillins: e.g., carbenicillin, piperacillin, ticarcillin
Penicillin + β-lactamase inhibitor: e.g., piperacillin/tazobactam, amoxicillin/clavulanic acid, amoxicillin/sulbactam
Monobactams
Aztreonam
Carbapenems
Imipenem, meropenem
Cephalosporins
First generation: e.g., cefazolin, cephalexin, cephradine
Second generation: e.g., cefoxitin, cefotetan, cefuroxime, cefuroxime axetil
Third generation: e.g., cefotaxime, ceftriaxone, ceftizoxime, ceftazidime, cefoperazone, cefpodoxime
Fourth generation: cefepime, cefpirome

activity similar to that of penicillin G but are also active against non–β-lactamase-producing strains of *H. influenzae, Listeria monocytogenes,* many strains of *E. coli,* and *Moraxella catarrhalis.* Amoxicillin has been the initial drug of choice in the pediatric age group for outpatient management of otitis media, uncomplicated UTIs, and sinusitis. Because of its effects on *E. coli,* group B streptococcus, and *Listeria,* ampicillin is used commonly in neonatal antiinfective therapy. Amoxicillin combined with the β-lactamase inhibitor clavulanic acid (Augmentin) provides an oral agent with all of the activity of ampicillin and coverage of β-lactamase–producing strains of *H. influenzae, M. catarrhalis,* and *S. aureus.*

The extended-spectrum penicillins, such as carbenicillin and piperacillin, have expanded activity against gram-negative aerobes but are susceptible to β-lactamases. They are active against many isolates of *P. aeruginosa* and members of the Enterobacteriaceae family. These antibiotics often are used in combination with aminoglycosides for synergistic effects.

The cephalosporin derivatives often are divided into "generations." In general, antibiotics in the higher generations are more active against gram-negative bacteria, with concomitant loss of activity against gram-positive organisms. For instance, the first-generation agents are active against most aerobic gram-positive cocci including β-lactamase–producing strains of *S. aureus.* An important exception is group D streptococci (enterococci), which is not covered by any of the cephalosporins. First-generation cephalosporins are also active against many strains of *E. coli* and *Klebsiella* species. Second-generation agents, such as cefuroxime, have expanded gram-negative activity against *H. influenzae* and *M. catarrhalis.* However, cefuroxime should not be used alone in septic shock or nosocomial-acquired sepsis: Neither first- nor second-generation cephalosporins can achieve adequate CSF concentrations for the treatment of meningitis or are active against organisms including *Listeria,* enterococci, *Pseudomonas,* or anaerobes (with the exception of reasonable coverage of anaerobes by cefotetan or cefoxitin). As compared with the earlier generation of agents, the properties of third-generation cephalosporins include improved penetration into the CSF, diminished gram-positive activity, and expanded gram-negative activity. In contrast to other cephalosporins, ceftazidime has expanded activity against *P. aeruginosa* and *Pseudomonas cepacia.* Because of their increased activity against gram-negative pathogens such as *H. influenzae* and *E. coli,* cefotaxime and ceftriaxone usually are recommended for the treatment of meningitis and sepsis in children. Cephalosporins in general are not active against anaerobes (with the exception of cefoxitin and cefotetan) and have no activity against *Listeria* and enterococci. Thus, the combination of ampicillin and cefotaxime or cetizoxime, or ampicillin and an aminoglycoside, is used in the treatment of neonatal meningitis. Recently, fourth-

generation cephalosporins have been introduced. Cefepime is a new broad-spectrum cephalosporin with in vitro activity similar to that of cefotaxime or ceftriaxone. It has excellent activity against the common pediatric meningeal pathogens *S. pneumoniae* and *N. meningitides.* It is also active against *P. aeruginosa* and *Enterobacter* species and methicillin-susceptible *S. aureus.* Because of its broad spectrum of activity, use of cefepime has been reserved for more complex situations such as empiric treatment in immunocompromised hosts.

Side effects. In general, β-lactam agents have few side effects: Type I hypersensitivity, manifested by urticaria and wheezing, is the most serious. Extremely high doses or intraventricular administration of β-lactam agents can precipitate seizures. Prolonged high dosage administration of any of these agents can result in a type-specific neutropenia, which is reversible after cessation of drug therapy. Many of these agents, in particular oxacillin and nafcillin, have been associated with dose-dependent elevations in serum hepatic transaminase activity and thrombophlebitis.

Vancomycin

Mechanism of action. Vancomycin inhibits cell wall synthesis by binding to the polypeptide side chain of the peptidoglycan in the cell wall, thereby inhibiting polymerization. After intravenous injection, vancomycin diffuses throughout the body, although it is not absorbed from the gastrointestinal tract. During meningeal inflammation, the CSF concentration is approximately 10–20% that of the serum. The drug is excreted unmetabolized in the urine. Thus, the dosage should be reduced in patients with renal impairment.

Spectrum of activity & clinical uses. The primary activity of this antibiotic is against gram-positive bacteria. Although there have been several recent reports of resistant strains, essentially all *S. aureus,* coagulase-negative staphylococci, streptococcal species, and most enterococci are sensitive to this antibiotic. Gram-positive bacilli, including *Clostridium* species, are also very sensitive. However, gram-negative bacteria are resistant. Widespread use of vancomycin in the tertiary care setting has led to the recent emergence of vancomycin-resistant enterococci.

The clinical uses of vancomycin include treatment of infections due to methicillin-resistant *S. aureus,* coagulase-negative staphylococci, multiply resistant pneumococci, and enterotoxin-producing *C. difficile.* The first three organisms are treated intravenously. Antibiotic-associated enterocolitis due to *C. difficile* is treated with oral vancomycin.

Side effects. Historically, vancomycin was thought to be notoriously toxic, with adverse reactions including ototoxicity and nephrotoxicity due to impurities in the preparations. With newer formulations, these adverse reactions are uncommon and usually related to serum concentrations above 50 mg/L. Serum concentration therefore should be monitored and the dosage adjusted if it exceeds 25–40 mg/L. Nephrotoxicity has been reported when vancomycin is used in combination with an aminoglycoside. One of the more common side effects of vancomycin is the "red man" syndrome, which is characterized by fever, chills, erythema, and paresthesia. These symptoms appear to be mediated by histamine and are related primarily to the rate of drug infusion.

Aztreonam

Aztreonam is a member of a new and unique class of antibiotics referred to as the *monobactams.*

Spectrum of activity & clinical uses. Aztreonam is resistant to a broad range of β-lactamases and thus is active against most gram-negative organisms. Activity against gram-positive bacteria is very limited. Although monobactams are β-lactam antibiotics, their structure is so different that cross immunogenicity with other β-lactam does not appear to be a problem. Therefore, they can be used with caution in patients with penicillin or cephalosporin allergies. Clinical experience with aztreonam in children is limited. It should be reserved for unusual cases that cannot be treated with other drugs active against gram-negative rods.

Side effects. In comparison with aminoglycosides, aztreonam appears to be less nephrotoxic and ototoxic.

Imipenem

Imipenem is the first of a new class of β-lactam antibiotics called *carbapenems.* Because imipenem is metabolized rapidly by renal brush border enzymes, it is administered with cilastatin, a drug that inhibits renal metabolism.

Spectrum of activity & clinical uses. Imipenem has the broadest antimicrobial spectrum of any currently available antibiotic, with activity against gram-negative and gram-positive aerobes and anaerobes. However, it is not active against methicillin-resistant *S. aureus* and *S. epidermidis* or *Mycoplasma* and *Legionella.* Due to its broad spectrum of activity, the use of Imipenem is reserved for the management of difficult cases that cannot be treated optimally with other antibiotics. Meropenem is an analog that can be considered as an alternative.

Side effects. Imipenem appears to have a toxicity profile similar to that of other β-lactam agents. Imipemem, but not Meropenem, has been associated with an increased tendency to cause seizures at high doses, especially in children with meningeal infections.

Protein synthesis inhibitors
Aminoglycosides

Commonly used antibiotics in this class include gentamicin, tobramycin, and amikacin. Others such as neomycin, kanamycin, and streptomycin are used for unusual infections or resistant organisms. However, the toxicity of the latter three compared with that of newer agents, precludes their generalized use.

Mechanism of action. The cellular uptake of aminoglycosides in gram-negative bacteria involves several phases. In the first stage, the cationic aminoglycoside binds to the anionic sites of lipopolysaccharide, phospholipids, and outer membrane proteins. This disrupts the outer membrane integrity and provides a molecular explanation for the synergy observed between certain β-lactam antibiotics and aminoglycosides. Once the aminoglycoside has entered the bacterial cell, it binds to the bacterial ribosomes (30S subunit), which leads to inhibition of protein synthesis, further destruction of the integrity of the outer membrane, and inhibition of DNA replication. These events culminate in the bacteria's ultimate death.

Spectrum of activity & clinical uses. The activity spectrum of aminoglycosides is limited to the treatment of gram-negative aerobic infections such as *E. coli, Pseudomonas, Enterobacter, Serratia, Klebsiella,* and *Proteus* species. Tobramycin appears to have the most activity against *Pseudomonas* species. Although not active against *Listeria monocytogenes* or *Enterococcus fecalis* by itself, aminoglycosides may be used with vancomycin or a broad-spectrum β-lactam to achieve synergistic coverage of these microbes.

Side effects. These agents must be prescribed and monitored with caution because their narrow therapeutic index. An irreversible deafness may occur, usually at high drug concentrations (e.g., 10–15 μg/mL of gentamicin). Nephrotoxicity is reversible but can create major problems in the management of seriously ill patients. As a rare complication, these agents can produce paralysis in patients with preexisting neuromuscular disease (notably myasthenia gravis). The use of these agents is usually reserved for UTIs and empiric coverage of short duration.

Chloramphenicol

This lipophilic drug provides high CSF concentrations even without meningeal inflammation. However, because of the availability of third-generation cephalosporins, this drug is no longer in common use for the treatment of meningitis.

Mechanism of action. Because it is highly hydrophobic, chloramphenicol appears to enter the bacterial cell by passive diffusion across the outer membrane. It inhibits protein synthesis by binding to the 50S subunit of the 70S ribosome. However, many gram-negative aerobes "tolerate" this action by ceasing to grow without dying.

Clinical uses & spectrum of activity. Until recently, chloramphenicol was used extensively for the treatment of suspected *H. influenzae* infections including sepsis, meningitis, pneumonia, and septic arthritis. The drug is also bactericidal against other typical childhood pathogens, including *S. pneumoniae* and *N. meningitidis,* and active against most anaerobic bacteria. The potentially serious toxicity of this drug has led to decreased use in recent years. Current indications include typhoid fever, rickettsial diseases, brain abscesses, and a variety of other infections in which anaerobes predominate. Chloramphenicol should be considered an alternative drug in the treatment of penicillin-allergic patients.

Side effects. Because of cross-reactivity and binding of the drug to 70S ribosomes in human mitochondria, prolonged administration of this agent results in bone marrow toxicity and potential pancytopenia. For certain individuals, irreversible aplastic anemia develops after brief exposure to this drug. The incidence of this idiosyncratic complication is approximately 1 in 50,000. In addition, significant poisoning of mitochondria in the myocardium can produce a generalized shock presentation (gray baby syndrome).

Miscellaneous protein synthesis inhibitors

Although chemically dissimilar, the tetracyclines, macrolides (e.g., erythromycin), and clindamycin have similar sites of action. Tetracycline prevents binding of transfer RNA to the 30S ribosome, whereas both erythromycin and clindamycin block protein synthesis by binding to the 50S ribosomal subunit. Each agent has a slightly different spectrum of activity.

Tetracycline is used in the treatment of a variety of infections including rickettsial diseases, Lyme disease, nongonococcal arthritis, and *Propionibacterium acnes* infections, the organism most often associated with inflammatory acne. A common side effect of tetracycline is yellow discoloration of the teeth seen in some children after treatment. Thus, this drug should not be used in children younger than 8–10 years unless there are no alternatives.

Macrolides. Erythromycin is an effective alternative to penicillin for the treatment of streptococcal and pneumococcal infections and is often used as an alternative to oral penicillins in allergic patients. Erythromycin is also indicated for the treatment of respiratory and genital mycoplasma, pertussis, diphtheria, chlamydia, legionella, gastroenteritis due to *Campylobacter,* and gonorrhea or syphilis during pregnancy. In combination with a sulfonamide, erythromycin can be used to treat acute otitis media. Oral erythromycin formulations often result in gastrointestinal disturbances such as nausea, vomiting, diarrhea, and abdominal cramps. A more serious but rare side effect is cholestatic hepatitis. Intravenous erythromycin frequently is associated with thrombophlebitis. Two newer macrolide antibiotics, Azithromycin and Clarithromycin, have a spectrum of activity similar to that of the older macrolides but fewer gastrointestinal side effects. In addition to improved tolerance, the newer macrolides have improved activity against atypical mycobacterial infections. They are also active against non–*C. difficile* species and *Prevotella melanogenicus* (formerly known as *Bacteroides melanogenicus*). Azithromycin has an exceptionally long half-life, allowing for once-daily dosing and reduced duration of therapy for many common infections. Because of their extended spectrum of activity, Azithromycin and Clarithromycin should not be used as first-line therapy for otitis media or pharyngitis caused by *S. pyogenes.*

Clindamycin is active against most aerobic and anerobic gram-positive bacteria and most anaerobic (but not aerobic) gram-negative rods. The most important uses of clindamycin are in treating severe anaerobic infections, including those caused by *Bacteroides fragilis.* Clindamycin often is used in combination with an aminoglycoside for the treatment of intraabdominal and pelvic infections and for aspiration pneumonia. It should not be used for the treatment of central nervous system infections (CNS; e.g., brain abscess) due to its poor penetration into the CSF. Clindamycin also can be used to treat a variety of staphylococcal and streptococcal infections as an alternative to penicillin and is used extensively in treating acne vulgaris (*P. acnes*). Adverse reactions to clindamycin include gastrointestinal disturbances such as diarrhea and mild hepatotoxicity. In severe case of toxicity, patients may develop pseudomembranous colitis due to overgrowth of toxin-producing *C. difficile.* This complication can be treated with oral vancomycin or metronidazole.

Alterations of nucleic acid synthesis
Rifampin (Rifamycin)

Mechanism of action. Rifampin binds bacterial DNA-dependent RNA polymerase, which effectively inhibits transcription.

Clinical uses. Rifampin is an important antituberculous drug and active against some nontuberculous mycobacteria. Because it achieves high mucosal concentrations, rifampin is used frequently to eliminate carriage of *N. meningitidis, H. influenzae, S. pyogenes,* and *S. aureus.* Except as a prophylactic agent, rifampin is not used alone.

Side effects. All patients receiving this antibiotic should be advised that their body secretions, including urine, saliva, sweat, and tears, will develop an orange discoloration. Other adverse effects include dermatitis and a flu-like syndrome. Rare complications can include thrombocytopenia, hemolytic anemia, acute renal failure, and cholestatic hepatitis.

Because rifampin induces hepatic microsomal P-450, patients receiving rifampin have altered liver metabolism of several other drugs using this system. Examples are anticonvulsants (e.g., phenobarbital), antibiotics (e.g., chloramphenicol), oral contraceptives, warfarin, and propranolol. Adjustments should be made to the dosage of these drugs to maintain therapeutic concentrations.

Quinolones

Nalidixic acid was the first member of this drug class to be used clinically. However, because of its poor bioavailability and the rapid development of bacterial drug resistance, its use was limited to the treatment of UTIs. Recently, norfloxacin, ciprofloxacin, and other 6-fluorinated piperazinyl quinolones have been developed.

Mechanism of action. Bacterial topoisomerase II, which introduces negative superhelical twists into double-stranded bacterial DNA, is a requirement for DNA replication. These antibiotics inhibit the formation of a DNA–topoisomerase complex, resulting in inhibition of DNA synthesis.

Clinical uses & spectrum of activity. Nalidixic acid, as the prototype, is active against gram-negative enteric isolates but has no useful activity against gram-positive bacteria or pseudomonas. It is only partly absorbed from the gastrointestinal tract; thus, large doses are necessary to attain therapeutic urinary concentrations.

The fluorinated quinolone derivatives have a much broader spectrum of activity including most gram-positive bacteria (including methicillin-resistant *S. aureus*) and most gram-negative rods (including many *Pseudomonas* species). These antibiotics are available in oral and intravenous forms. As such, they represent the first agents available for the oral treatment of systemic infections caused by resistant gram-negative enteric isolates (including *Pseudomonas* species) and have been used successfully as alternatives to IV antibiotics for non–life-threatening gram-negative infections (e.g., osteomyelitis and UTIs).

Side effects. High doses of nalidixic acid have been associated with visual disturbances. The observation that drugs of this class inhibit cartilage formation in young animals currently precludes their general use in children.

Metronidazole

Mechanism of action. Metronidazole is a hydroxy-aliphatic derivative of nitroimidazole. It is active only against anaerobes and some protozoa that produce nitrore-ductase, a unique enzyme necessary for conversion of the drug to its active components. The resultant hydroxy-lamino and nitroso intermediates subsequently interfere with synthesis of nucleic acids.

Clinical uses & spectrum of activity. This agent has been used extensively to treat life-threatening anaerobic infections, including intrapelvic and intraabdominal sepsis and brain abscesses. It is also a suitable and less expensive alternative to vancomycin in the treatment of pseudomembranous colitis caused by *C. difficile*. In addition, it is used for the treatment of vaginal *Trichomonas* and some protozoal infections.

Side effects. Metronidazole therapy often is associated with nausea and a metallic taste. More serious but less frequent adverse reactions include a reversible peripheral neuropathy, seizures, encephalopathy, and neutropenia. Several studies conducted in laboratory animals have indicated that prolonged use of high dose metronidazole can be carcinogenic. However, supporting evidence among humans is currently lacking. Due to potential mutagenic effects, metronidazole probably should not be used in pregnant women.

Antimetabolites (folate synthesis inhibitors)
Sulfonamides

Mechanism of action. The sulfa agents are analogs of para-aminobenzoic acid, a necessary precursor for bacterial folate synthesis. Because humans cannot synthesize folate, these antibiotics specifically target bacteria and have a rel-

atively high therapeutic index. In addition, trimethoprim and pyrimethamine selectively inhibit dihydrofolate reductase, another enzyme necessary in the bacterial synthesis of folates. The combination of trimethoprim with sulfamethoxazole has synergistic effects and is marketed commercially as Bactrim or Septra.

Clinical uses & spectrum of activity. Sulfa drugs alone or in combination with trimethoprim are used for the outpatient treatment of a variety of non–life-threatening infections (e.g., otitis media and UTIs). The combination of a dihydrofolate reductase inhibitor with sulfa has been used extensively for the treatment of a variety of parasitic infections, most notably malaria and *Pneumocystis carinii*, a common infection in acquired immunodeficiency syndrome (AIDS).

Side effects. Sulfonamides can cause a spectrum of hypersensitivity reactions, ranging from mild rashes to a life-threatening Stevens–Johnson syndrome. Hematologic toxicity includes agranulocytosis and hemolytic anemia in patients with deficiency of glucose-6-phosphate dehydrogenase. Sulfonamides are contraindicated in the neonate and during the latter part of pregnancy because they can displace bilirubin from protein-binding sites, possibly leading to jaundice or even kernicterus. At high dosages trimethoprim can cause nausea and vomiting, anemia (secondary to folate deficiency), and other blood dyscrasias. The anemia is reversible with folate treatment.

ANTIVIRAL AGENTS

Although most viral infections are self-limited, they are a frequent cause of significant morbidity and mortality in immunocompromised hosts. Despite many recent advances, antiviral therapy is in its infancy. Most antiviral agents have a spectrum of activity that is limited to one or, at most, two viral genera and often cause irreversible toxicity to the host cell and the target virus. Recent advances in biochemistry and molecular medicine have increasingly allowed the development of antiviral agents that target specific aspects of viral replication. In general, antiviral agents can be divided into four categories (Table 9–12): (1) antimetabolites in nucleic acid synthesis, (2) specific antiviral antiserum, (3) natural immunomodulators such as interferons, and (4) neuraminidase inhibitors. Several additional agents fall outside of those groupings.

Effective antiviral therapy is available for infections caused by HSV, VZV, CMV, HIV, hepatitis B (HBV), hepatitis C (HCV), and respiratory viruses including RSV and influenza viruses (Table 9–13). Due to potential toxicity associated with many of these agents, the use of antiviral therapy should be based on the definitive identification of a specific viral pathogen. For maximum therapeutic effectiveness, treatment should be started early in the course of the disease. In some infections (e.g., HIV), the virus may mutate or acquire other mechanisms to evade the action of the drugs. In these scenarios, combination therapy should

Table 9–12. Antiviral Agents

Antimetabolites
  Vidarabine
  Acyclovir
  Ganciclovir
  Zidovudine (azidothymidine [AZT])
  Dideoxyinosine
  Ribavirin

Human antisera preparations
  Hepatitis B immunoglobulin
  Varicella zoster immunoglobulin
  Human rabies immunoglobulin

Immunomodulators
  Human interferon: α, β, γ

Neuraminidase inhibitors
  Zanamivir oseltamivir

Other drugs
  Amantadine, rimantadine

be considered. Different strains of the same virus can change in geographic distribution and sensitivity to specific therapies. For instance, there are six genotypes of HCV, with type 1 being most prevalent in the United States. This strain is not as sensitive to interferon-α treatment as other genotypes prevalent in some European countries.

Acyclovir

Acyclovir is a guanine derivative effective against HSV and VZV. Acyclovir is activated by viral thymidine kinase, which ensures its specificity against virus-infected but not normal host cells. After initial activation, the acyclovir monophosphate is converted by the host's cellular machinery into several triphosphate forms that compete with deoxyguanosine triphosphate for incorporation into the viral genome (via viral DNA polymerase). Viral DNA elongation is terminated because acyclovir triphosphate lacks a 3-hydroxyl group. The incomplete DNA polymer effectively inhibits further activity of the viral DNA polymerase and thus further viral replication.

Acyclovir is the drug of choice for the treatment of all serious infections caused by HSV and VZV. In particular, acyclovir reduces the morbidity and mortality of herpes encephalitis and neonatal herpes infection. It also is effective for primary and reactivated VZV infections in the immunocompromised host. Orally administered acyclovir is effective for the treatment of initial or recurrent episodes of genital herpes infections. The use of oral acyclovir for primary VZV infections in normal children is controversial because of the marginal benefits observed and the high cost of the drug. Acyclovir is not active against other *Herpes* group viruses including EBV and CMV infections. Because of the specificity of its activation, acyclovir is considered a relatively nontoxic agent. Although its use has

been associated with a number of CNS symptoms including hallucinations and cortical dysfunction, it is not clear whether the acyclovir or other factors have been causal. Patients receiving acyclovir always should be well hydrated to prevent the rare complication of nephrotoxicity caused by crystallization of drug in the renal cortex.

Zidovudine

Zidovudine was the first agent licensed and approved for the treatment of HIV infections. Unlike acyclovir, zidovudine is triphosphorylated by cellular kinases. The 5-triphosphate derivative inhibits retroviral reverse transcriptase by prematurely terminating chain elongation of the viral DNA. Zidovudine often is used in the treatment of HIV-infected children and children with AIDS. Because of its mechanism of activation, the drug is associated with significant side effects including bone marrow suppression. This is manifested as neutropenia or megaloblastic anemia. Recent studies have demonstrated the gradual development of significant drug resistance to this agent among many clinical isolates of HIV. New classes of anti-HIV drugs, including protease inhibitors and new reverse transcriptase inhibitors, have been developed to help fight this infection. Protease inhibitors interfere with the processing of viral proteins during replication, resulting in inhibition of HIV replication.

Ribavirin

Ribavirin is a nucleoside analog with relatively broad activity in vitro and in vivo against RNA viruses. Ribavirin has several potential modes of action, including inhibition of viral RNA polymerases and reduction of cellular pools of guanosine triphosphate, by competitively inhibiting cellular inosine monophosphate dehydrogenase activity. In the United States, ribavirin is used mainly for treating RSV infections with aerosol administration in hospitalized, critically ill infants. Two recent studies have demonstrated a beneficial effect of combination therapy with oral ribavirin and parenteral interferon-α in the treatment of chronic HCV infection. The sustained response rate (as defined by undetectable HCV RNA serum levels 24 weeks after treatment) increased to 38% in new patients and 49% in relapsed patients with chronic HCV. The responders also had improvements in liver histology and hepatic function tests. Other potential uses of ribavirin are under investigation.

Rimantadine & amantadine

Rimantadine and amantadine are tricyclic aminohydrocarbons with antiviral activity directed uniquely against influenza A virus. Both compounds have a similar mechanism of action: inhibiting the early phases of viral replication by preventing uncoating of the viral genome and virus-mediated membrane fusion. Both are used in the prevention and treatment of influenza A infections. Recommendations regarding the preventive use of amantadine or rimantadine are based on individual clinical factors and the local prevalence of

Table 9–13. Antiviral Therapy: Current Recommendations for Specific Diseases

Clinical Indication (Disease/Virus)	Antiviral Agent
HSV encephalitis	Acyclovir IV
Neonatal herpes simplex	Acyclovir IV or ARA-A IV
Mucocutaneous HSV Immunocompromised host	Acyclovir IV
Prophylaxis for HSV recurrence	Acyclovir PO
Primary HSV in normal host HSV stomatitis, genital HSV	Acyclovir PO or IV
Recurrent genital HSV in normal host Prophylaxis for HSV recurrence	Acyclovir PO Acyclovir PO

Varicella (chickenpox)
  Pneumonia or pregnancy
  Immunocompromised host
	Acyclovir IV
	Acyclovir IV

Herpes zoster
  Normal host
  Immunocompromised host
	Consider Acyclovir PO
	Acyclovir IV

Cytomegalovirus
  Normal host
  Immunocompromised host
  Retinitis
	No Rx
	Ganciclovir & consider IVIG
	Induction & suppression Rx
	Ganciclovir, Foscarnet, or Cidofovir

Epstein–Barr virus	No Rx for infectious mono, steroid for airway obstruction
Human herpes virus-8	Anti-HIV Rx and interferon-α
Enteroviral meningitis	No Rx or Pleconaril
Hepatitis A	No Rx within 2 wk of exposure, γ-globulin

Hepatitis B
  Acute
  Chronic
	No Rx
	Interferon-α; Lamivudine

Hepatitis C	Interferon-α; interferon-α & ribavirin
Influenza A & B	Zanamivir inhaled or oseltamivir PO
Influenza A	Rimantadine or Amantadine
Human papilloma virus (condyloma acuminata)	Cryotherapy or interferon-α

Parvovirus B19
  Mild case in normal host
  Severe anemia
	No Rx
	IVIG

Respiratory syncytial virus
  RSV disease
  RSV prevention
	Consider Ribavrin in high risk patients (e.g., heart disease, cystic fibrosis,
	    premature infants & severely ill)
	RSV IVIG or Palivizumab

HSV = Herpes simplex virus; IV = intravenous; IVIG = intravenous immunoglobulin; PO = per os (oral treatment) or (per mouth); RSV = respiratory syncytial virus; Rx = treatment.

Table adapted from information in *Nelson's Pocket Book 2000, Sanford Guide to Antimicrobial Therapy,* 2000.

influenza A. For a therapeutic benefit, treatment should be initiated within 48 hours of the onset of influenza symptoms. Side effects of these agents most commonly involve the gastrointestinal tract and CNS.

Two new drugs have been approved recently for the treatment of influenza A and B. They are neuraminidase inhibitors and act by inhibiting the release of influenza virions from the host cell surface. Zanamivir (by inhalation therapy) and oseltamivir (by oral route) have been shown to be effective against influenza A and B when used within 36–48 hours of the onset of symptoms. They have been shown to reduce symptoms and speed recovery.

ANTIFUNGAL AGENTS

Three classes of compounds are useful for the treatment of fungal diseases in children: polyenes (e.g., amphotericin B), antimetabolites (e.g., flucytosine), and imidazole derivatives (e.g., ketoconazol).

Polyene agents

Amphotericin B

Mechanism of action. Amphotericin B binds to sterols on the fungal cell membrane, which results in the loss of membrane integrity, leakage of intracellular constituents, and osmotic lysis of the fungal cell. Amphotericin B recently has been shown to lyse cells by oxidant injury. Toxicity is caused by cross-over binding of the drug to cholesterol on human cells.

Clinical uses & side effects. Amphotericin B is administered parenterally and is the drug of choice for most systemic fungal infections in children, including *Aspergillus, Candida, Cryptococcus, Histoplasma, Blastomyces,* and *Coccidioides.* Amphotericin is used in combination with flucytosine for its synergistic effect on cryptococcal infections, especially those involving the CNS. The toxicity of amphotericin B is significant; hypokalemia and oliguria are the most common complications and result from the binding of amphotericin B to the renal tubules. A syndrome of fever, chills, and rigors that frequently accompanies drug infusion often can be modified or eliminated by pretreatment with meperidine and antihistamines. However, these side effects do not seem to be as common in young children as in adults. Phlebitis can be minimized by simultaneous infusion of hydrocortisone. Coadministration of blood leukocytes with amphotericin B is contraindicated because of the potential for the development of severe pulmonary injury.

Nystatin. Nystatin is a polyene antifungal agent with presumed mechanisms of action similar to those of amphotericin B. Nystatin is currently available only for nonsystemic use in the treatment of superficial mucosal *Candida* infections (e.g., thrush).

Antimetabolites

Flucytosine. Flucytosine (5-fluorocytosine) is an antimetabolite with limited activity against human fungal infections. After entry into fungal cells, flucytosine is deaminated to form 5-fluorouracil, an inhibitor of DNA synthesis. Because of the rapid development of drug resistance to this agent, flucytosine is rarely used alone. Most studies have examined the use of flucytosine in combination with amphotericin B. This combination is recommended for the treatment of cryptococcal meningitis and candidal meningitis in the newborn. The major toxicity of flucytosine is myelosuppression. Because the drug is excreted by the kidney, changes in dosage are required for individuals with renal impairment.

Imidazoles

Ketoconazole, **miconazole**, **fluconazole**, and **itraconazole** are imidazoles with different activities against *Candida* species, *Histoplasma capsulatum, Coccidioides immitis, Blastomyces dermatitidis,* and *Cryptococcus neoformans.* They affect membrane permeability by competitive inhibition of cytochrome P-450 enzymes. Ketoconazole has been used successfully for the treatment of many dermatomycoses and mucocutaneous candidiasis. Miconazole is available in over-the-counter (OTC) preparations for the treatment of tinea pedis and tinea cruris. Fluconazole has been shown to be effective in the treatment of systemic candidiasis, coccidioidomycosis, and cryptococcosis. Intraconazole has been used to treat aspergillosis, blastomycosis, coccidioidomycosis, and histoplasmosis. Itraconazole and fluconazole are available in IV and oral formulations. To difference degrees, all of these agents have gastrointestinal and hepatic toxicities. Nausea and vomiting occur commonly with ketoconazole. This agent has also been known to downregulate ergosterol synthesis and therefore should not be used in conjunction with amphotericin B. Changes in liver function tests can occur with use of all of these agents.

ANTIPARASITIC AGENTS

A comprehensive review of the many antiparasitic agents available is beyond the scope of this chapter. Readers are advised to consult other references for more detailed information. Only a brief overview of several of the more commonly used agents is provided.

Antimalarials

Chloroquine phosphate is the main antimalarial drug in use today. Chloroquine, a weak base, is actively taken up by the malarial parasites. Alkalinization of the food vacuoles presumably prevents subsequent hemoglobin hydrolysis by inhibiting the parasites' acid proteases and intracellular transport of macromolecules. Chloroquine is used for the prevention and treatment of most forms of malaria, except for infections caused by *Plasmodium falciparum.* Gastrointestinal and CNS side effects, although common, are dose dependent. **Primaquine** is used for eradication of the extraerythrocytic phase of malarial infections caused by *Plasmodium vivax* and *Plasmodium ovale.* This agent should be used cautiously as it can precipitate hemolysis in patients with glucose-6-phosphate dehydrogenase deficiency. The combination of **pyrimethamine** and **sulfadoxine** (Fansidar) is used for the treatment of chloroquine-resistant falciparum malaria. Alternatively, pyrimethamine can be used in combination with sulfadiazine. Pyrimethamine is potentially hepatotoxic and can cause bone marrow suppression. This side effect can be prevented by the coadministration of folinic acid. Other antimalarial agents include **quinine sulfate, mefloquine,** and **atovaquone.** Mefloquine recently became the drug of choice for chloroquin-resistant *P. falciparum.*

Antihelminthics

Mebendazole, pyrantel pamoate, and **niclosamide** are orally administered agents used for the treatment of most intestinal parasites encountered in the United States. However, they have different mechanisms of action. **Mebendazole** is used for the treatment of pinworms (*Enterobius vermicularis*), ascariasis (*Ascaris lumbricoides*), *Ancylostoma duodenale,* and *Necator americanus* infections. **Thiabendazole** is recommended for the treatment of *Strongyloides stercoralis* infection and some infections caused by *Toxocara* species. **Niclosamide** and **praziquantel** are used for the treatment of *Taenia* infections, including neurocysticercosis.

Other agents

Pentamidine is used as an alternative drug for the treatment of *P. carinii* infections in individuals who are intolerant of, or nonresponsive to, trimethoprim-sulfamethoxazole therapy. Furazolidone is used for the treatment of *Giardia lamblia* infections in young children because this compound is available in liquid form and is well tolerated. **Praziquantel** is used for the treatment of a variety of fluke and schistosoma infections.

Natural Immunomodulators

Cytokines

Cytokines are naturally occurring proteins that function as short-range signaling molecules to enhance cell-to-cell interactions. They are important in the regulation of immune responses, growth and development, and homeostasis. The ability to mass produce several of these compounds has made it possible to use them as therapeutic agents in the modulation of the immune system. Several prototypes of this class of molecules are discussed below.

Hematopoietic growth factors. Granulocyte-macrophage colony stimulating factors (GM-CSF) and granulocyte colony stimulating factors (G-CSF) are growth factors that exert their major biological effects on the hematopoietic system.

Granulocyte colony stimulating factor is a late-acting hematopoietin whose effects are restricted mainly to the neutrophil lineage. In contrast, GM-CSF is a multilineage

hematopoietin that acts on multiple steps in myeloid differentiation, from the early stem cell to the mature macrophage. Human GM-CSF and G-CSF are used therapeutically in recipients of bone marrow transplantation and cancer chemotherapy and patients with dysfunctional hematopoiesis. Both GM-CSF and G-CSF have clearly reduced the incidence of neutropenia and infection after conventional cytotoxic chemotherapy and high dose chemotherapy preceding bone marrow transplantation. Similar results have been described in aplastic anemia, myelodysplasia, drug-induced agranulocytosis, and chronic neutropenia. In general, recipients show increases in peripheral blood granulocyte counts and fewer opportunistic infections and require a shorter period of hospitalization. Treatment appears to be well tolerated, despite the common occurrence of mild to moderate flu-like symptoms and occasional fluid retention problems. The bedside use of these growth factors represents a major contribution of biotechnology to a difficult management area.

Interferon. Interferons have antitumor, immunomodulatory, and antiviral effects and can be divided into three major types: α, β, and γ. The U.S. Food and Drug Administration has approved the use of interferons for the treatment of a variety of clinical conditions including hepatitis B and C infections, human papilloma virus infection (condyloma acuminata), multiple sclerosis, and malignant neoplasms including hairy cell leukemia, chronic myelogenous leukemia, malignant melanoma, and Kaposi's sarcoma. Interferon-γ is approved for prophylactic use in patients with chronic granulomatous disease to prevent recurrence of bacterial infections.

Specific immunoglobulins

Passive immunization using specific high-titer human IgG preparations is recommended for a variety of viral illnesses. For example, immunoglobulin preparations containing high titers of antibodies against respiratory syncytial virus have been approved recently for use in high-risk premature neonates. Most of these preparations are available through the Red Cross. The risk of infection, including HIV and hepatitis C, from these products is very low. However, anaphylaxis can occur with administration. Caution must be used when administering any of these products to patients with IgA deficiency because minute quantities of IgA in each preparation might prompt the development of endogenous anti-IgA antibody and result in subsequent hypersensitivity reactions to transfusion of blood products.

■ LABORATORY APPROACH TO THE CHILD WITH FEVER

In response to infection, chemical mediators (e.g., endogenous pyrogen and interleukin-6) are elaborated, which produce an elevation of body temperature. The resultant fever is presumed to have beneficial effects in mobilizing the host's immune system. Specifically, experimental evidence has shown improvement in neutrophil function and migration, T-lymphocyte proliferation, and interferon production in response to fever.

Fever is one of the most frequent concerns prompting a telephone call or visit to the pediatrician. Parents often worry that the fever itself, especially if it is high, can result in injury (e.g., brain damage) or death. Physicians consider fever a sign of illness caused most often by infection and are concerned primarily with identifying the source of illness and excluding serious bacterial infections. The vast majority of febrile children seen in the primary care setting will have an infectious etiology. Most of these infections will be relatively benign and self-limited (e.g., viral upper respiratory infections) or responsive to straightforward therapies (e.g., otitis media). However, among the febrile children seen in an office setting, a few will have a more serious and/or life-threatening illness. The differential diagnosis for the febrile child is long and must include infectious and noninfectious etiologies (e.g., neoplastic and rheumatologic diseases). Consideration of less common and noninfectious causes is especially important in children who present with persistent fever. It is also important to remember that young infants, in particular neonates, may not mount a febrile response to serious or overwhelming infections. Hypothermia can be a marker of infection in the very young (e.g., neonates) or the very ill in whom normal homeostatic mechanisms are compromised.

Of utmost importance when evaluating a child with fever is the individualized care of each patient. Clinical guidelines can be extremely useful in outlining general principles and providing expert opinion; however, they also must be tailored to the specific clinical situation. Diagnostic investigations and therapy should not supplant the importance of good follow-up (in the inpatient or outpatient setting), education, and support for family members.

Acute Fever

An important goal of the evaluation of febrile infants and children is to identify those at highest and lowest risk for having a serious bacterial infection. High-risk patients need to be treated more aggressively and may be candidates for empiric antibiotic therapy. Similarly, physicians hope to identify very low-risk patients in whom no further workup or treatment is necessary.

CLINICAL APPROACH

One approach to the ill child with a history of fever is for the provider to ask himself or herself a series of questions: Is fever present? Does the child appear "toxic"? Is there a source for the fever on physical examination? What is the risk of serious bacterial infection? Are laboratory tests indicated? Is treatment necessary?

Is fever present? Different factors influence normal body temperature, which should be defined by a range rather than by an absolute number. There is a normal diurnal variation in body temperature, with lowest values occurring in the morning and highest values occurring in the evening. Small differences in temperature also have been observed based on the patient's age, sex, and ethnicity. Further, the method by which the temperature is taken influences the value obtained. Different techniques (e.g., tactile, axillary, oral, tympanic, and rectal) have been used by parents and physicians to report body temperatures in infants and children. Virtually all of these have received some criticism over their accuracy and/or relative ease of use. For example, axillary temperatures can be affected by skin perfusion, thickness, and environmental temperature. Overbundling in young infants has been reported to elevate body temperature into the febrile range. Oral temperatures can be affected by respiratory rate and the consumption of hot or cold liquids. Likewise, tympanic temperatures can be influenced by the presence of a middle ear infection. In infants and young children, a rectal temperature with a glass–mercury or digital–electronic thermometer is considered the gold standard for taking temperatures.

Normal variations in body temperature and different measurement techniques have caused some confusion regarding a uniform definition for what constitutes fever. In a survey of residency directors in pediatrics and emergency medicine, physicians agreed on the definition of fever only a little over one third of the time. The survey produced a range of temperatures (from 37.4°C to 38.6°C) that were accepted as fever. For practical purposes, a rectal temperature of 38.0°C is a commonly accepted definition of fever. There is some evidence in the pediatric literature that the risk of a serious bacterial infection increases with the height of fever. The Baraff guidelines (see below) use a temperature of 39.0°C in older infants and children with fever to enter the diagnostic algorithm.

Does the child appear "toxic"? *Toxicity* refers to the apparent severity of a child's illness based on observation and physical examination.

To identify objective observational items that might help clinicians assess the risk of serious illness in a febrile child, McCarthy and his colleagues at Yale designed the Yale Observation Scale (Table 9–14). This tool consists of six observational items: an evaluation of the child's cry, reaction to parents, state variation, response to social overtures (e.g., smile), color, and hydration status.

Each item is given a score of 1 (normal), 3 (moderate impairment), or 5 (severe impairment). In a prospective study utilizing this scale with 312 febrile children 2 years of age or younger, 92.3% with scores of 16 or greater versus 2.7% with scores of 10 or less points were diagnosed with a serious illness as defined by a bacterial pathogen in the CSF, blood, stool, deep soft tissue, or pleura; an infil-

Table 9–14. The Yale Observation Scale

Observation Item	Normal (1)	Moderate Impairment (3)	Severe Impairment (5)
Quality of cry	Strong cry and normal tone *or* content and not crying	Whimpering *or* sobbing	Weak *or* moaning *or* high-pitched
Reaction to parent stimulation	Cries briefly then stops *or* content and not crying	Cries off and on	Continual cry *or* hardly responds
State variation	If awake → stays awake *or* is asleep and stimulated → wakes up quickly	Eyes close briefly → awake *or* awakes with prolonged stimulation	Falls to sleep *or* will not rouse
Color	Pink	Pale extremities *or* acro-cyanosis	Pale *or* cyanotic *or* mottled *or* ashen
Hydration	Skin normal, eyes normal, *and* mucous membranes moist	Skin normal, eyes normal, *and* mouth slightly dry	Skin doughy *or* tented *and* dry mucous membranes *and/or* sunken eyes
Response (talk, smile), anxiety to social overtures	Smiles *or* alerts (≤2 mo)	Brief smile *or* alerts briefly (≤2 mo)	No smile, face dull, expressionless *or* no alerting (≤2 mo)

Each item is scored 1, 3, or 5 (as indicated in parentheses). See text for interpretation of scoring.

trate on chest x-ray; aseptic meningitis; or a significant abnormality in the electrolytes or blood gas. The Yale Observation Score in combination with the medical history and physical examination produced a sensitivity of 92% for serious illness.

Is there a source for the fever on physical examination? After the fever is documented and the history reviewed, a thorough physical examination must be performed to identify any detectable source of infection. Rashes (exanthems and enanthems), lymphadenopathy, organomegaly, and bone or joint abnormalities (e.g., septic arthritis or osteomyelitis) should not be overlooked. It must be remembered, especially in young infants, that the identification of a minor source of infection (e.g., viral upper respiratory infections and otitis media) in a febrile child does not preclude the presence of a more serious disorder (e.g., UTI, meningitis, sepsis). Diagnostic algorithms differ with respect to the significance they place on the finding of a minor viral illness or otitis.

If no source is detected in the initial evaluation, further workup, including laboratory data and radiologic studies, must be considered. These children fall into a category that has variously been called fever without a source, fever of unclear etiology, and fever without localizing signs. The term fever of unknown origin generally refers to a persistent fever that has not been identified by initial diagnostic investigation. It is discussed in a subsequent section.

Are laboratory tests indicated? The laboratory is an essential tool for localizing sites of serious bacterial infection in patients for whom no source of infection has been iden-

tified by history and physical examination. Diagnostic tests are directed at identifying potential infections in the blood (e.g., bacteremia or sepsis), CSF (e.g., meningitis), lungs (e.g., pneumonia), urinary tract (e.g., cystitis, pylonephritis), and stool (e.g., gastroenteritis) Table 9–15.

When making decisions regarding the diagnostic workup, the clinician must weigh the risk of complications, cost, and patient discomfort associated with performing specific tests against the potential benefit of detecting a specific disease based on its likelihood, severity, and risk of morbidity and mortality, if undetected or untreated.

For example, efforts to identify infections in the CSF, blood, and urine are influenced by the potential severity and sequellae associated with those infections. Undetected or inadequately treated meningitis can result in permanent disability or death. Undetected bacteremia can go on to cause septic shock and multisystem organ failure. Likewise, undetected UTIs can lead to renal scarring.

Table 9–15. Initial Laboratory Investigations for Possible Sepsis

Complete blood count, with white blood cell count and differential
Urinalysis
Blood culture
Urine culture
Stool culture and microscopic examination
Cerebrospinal fluid studies: cell count, glucose, total protein
Cerebrospinal fluid culture
Chest radiograph

What is the risk of serious bacterial infection? Various clinical protocols have been developed to assist clinicians in determining whether the afebrile infant or child is at high or low risk for serious bacterial infection. One of the most widely accepted is the Rochester Criteria, which is designed to help clinicians identify infants younger than 3 months of age who are at low risk for serious bacterial infection and uses a combination of findings from the medical history, physical examination, and laboratory evaluation (Table 9–16). Research has shown that infants with normal Rochester Criteria have significantly lower rates of serious bacterial infection than those with positive findings. One study of the Rochester Criteria in 931 febrile infants no older than 2 months of age demonstrated a negative predictive value of 98% (95% confidence interval: 97.2–99.6) for serious bacterial infection (Jaskiewicz et al). Low-risk infants may be managed with careful observation and follow-up, but without antibiotics, in the outpatient setting. In contrast, high-risk infants require parenteral antibiotics and hospitalization.

Is treatment necessary? Once the initial evaluation is completed, the clinician must decide when and if antibiotic treatment should be initiated. Information from laboratory testing may come back in minutes (e.g., urinalysis, complete blood count [CBC], Gram stains) or hours to days (e.g., cultures). Abnormalities in the urinalysis, CSF analysis, or chest radiograph can point to specific sites of infection and specific organisms. In many situations, decisions regarding antibiotic therapy will need to be made empirically based on the child's appearance and predictions of the most likely bacterial pathogens. Such predictions are in turn influenced by factors such as patient age, gender, history of contacts or exposures (including travel, household contacts, and child care), and suspected organ involvement.

In infants and children who appear "toxic," antibiotic therapy is often begun immediately after cultures are obtained. In other cases, an abnormal WBC (too high or too low) may be used to make decisions regarding the initiation of empiric antibiotic coverage. In addition to antibiotics, the patient must be managed properly with attention to fluid and electrolyte status, cardiovascular and respiratory function, renal output, and neurologic function. Readers are referred to Chapter 10 (Injuries and Emergencies) for a comprehensive discussion of the management of the acutely sick and septic child.

Once the decision is made to begin antibiotic therapy, other choices must be made: What is the most appropriate agent? By what route should the antibiotic be administered (e.g., topical, oral, IV)? and Does the patient require hospitalization?

Ceftriaxone, a third-generation cephalosporin, has become an increasingly popular choice for empiric antibiotic coverage of febrile infants and young children. It has a broad spectrum of activity that covers most of the common pediatric bacterial pathogens. It also has the relatively unique advantage of a very long half-life, which allows for once-a-day dosing. In selected cases, patients can receive an intramuscular injection of ceftriaxone and be followed up in the office the following day. However, this option should not be used as a substitute for IV therapy in patients who otherwise require hospitalization. Also, overuse of ceftriaxone in the outpatient setting will lead to increased antibiotic resistance to this effective antibiotic.

Clinicians should consider several medical and nonmedical factors when making a decision regarding whether to treat a child as an inpatient or an outpatient:

Medical aspects

1. Is the patient "toxic"? Any severely ill or "toxic"-appearing child requires close observation and monitoring in an inpatient setting.

2. What is the suspected site of infection? Patients with suspected serious illness (e.g., meningitis, osteomyelitis) should be hospitalized.

3. Are there other medical indications outside of the suspected infection? Children may need to be admitted for IV fluids in the treatment of dehydration or oxygen in the treatment of pneumonia.

Table 9–16. The Rochester Criteria (Modified)[1]

Goal	Defines febrile infant at low risk of serious bacterial infection if following criteria are met
History	
Previously healthy	Term infant, normal perinatal course, no antibiotics, no medical conditions, no hospitalizations
Physical examination	
Well appearing	
No focal bacterial infections	
Laboratory	
WBC	5000–15,000 cells/mm³
Band count (immature neutrophils)	<1500 cells/mm³
Urinalysis	Normal (≤10 WBC/high-power field on spun urine sediment)
Stool WBC (if diarrhea is present)	<5 WBC/high-power field

[1] Examination of the stool was not a part of the initial Rochester Criteria.
WBC = white blood cell count.

Reproduced, with permission, from McCarthy PL et al: Observation scales to identify serious illness in febrile children. Pediatrics 1982;70:802.

4. Does the patient require intravenous antibiotics? Is the suspected infection amenable only to intravenous antibiotics, or is the patient unable to take oral antibiotics?

Nonmedical aspects

1. Does the patient have ready access to medical care? Does the family have transportation back to the hospital?
2. Can the family be contacted for follow-up? Does the family have a telephone?
3. Are the parents or caretakers able to observe for worsening of the patient's status?
4. Is compliance with outpatient management (e.g., administration of oral antibiotics) a concern?

Although those steps may seem straightforward, the application of management strategies in febrile infants and children continues to be controversial. Several factors contribute to this controversy: (1) Most febrile infants and children will have benign, self-limited infections. (2) The signs and symptoms of serious illness in infants and young children can be nonspecific, and judging the "toxicity" of infants and very young children may be difficult even for the best of clinicians. (3) Physicians disagree on the amount of laboratory testing necessary to exclude serious illness. Performing laboratory tests (e.g., blood draws, catheterization, lumbar puncture) on every febrile infant and child risks potential complications and involves time, expense, and at least discomfort to the patient. (4) Even the use of screening laboratory tests will not entirely eliminate risk of serious infection. (5) Inappropriate empiric antibiotic use results in therapy-related complications (e.g., side effects, allergic reactions), unnecessary costs, and rising bacterial antibiotic resistance. (6) The use of empiric antibiotics without proper cultures and/or follow-up may result in partly treated infections, which may delay definitive diagnosis and treatment.

Practice guidelines recently were published on the management of febrile illness in children. Although they continue to be a matter of debate, these guidelines were developed by an expert panel to outline an evidence-based approach to this common clinical problem (Figure 9–1). Similar guidelines are currently being developed by the American Academy of Pediatrics.

SPECIAL CONSIDERATIONS IN THE MANAGEMENT OF ACUTE FEVER

The febrile infant younger than 3 months of age. The management of young infants is complicated by the following issues.

1. The medical history is provided by parents or caretakers and not directly from the patient.
2. The physical examination is more difficult because of limited cooperation and fewer signs for assessment.

3. The relative immaturity of the young infant's immune system often is associated with a decreased or delayed host response.
4. Young febrile infants may have a higher risk of serious bacterial infections than older children with fever.

On the basis of these limitations, until recently, all febrile infants younger than 3 months of age were recommended to undergo a "rule-out sepsis" evaluation. This included examination and culture of the blood, urine, and CSF and a chest radiograph. These infants were admitted to the hospital and given empiric parenteral antibiotics until the results of the cultures were known. Over the past 15 years, however, the optimal management of young febrile infants has undergone a reexamination. In part, this is the result of a better understanding of the epidemiology of bacterial infections in this age group and a decreasing incidence of certain infections. For example, immunization in infancy against HIB has reduced the incidence of invasive disease due to this organism by over 90%. Another factor producing this change has been a greater appreciation of the costs, inconvenience, and nosocomial complications that are incurred during hospitalization of these infants. New outpatient treatments (e.g., ceftriaxone) have contributed to a decrease in the pressure to hospitalize patients. Current management guidelines provide clinicians with more opportunities for decision making based on specific clinical factors and their assessment of the severity of illness. Several unique aspects of the approach to the young infant with fever are addressed below.

Does the infant appear "toxic"? At times, the only manifestation of serious illness in a young infant is a change in activity, increased irritability, or lethargy. Physicians use a combination of subtle and semiobjective signs, such as those included in the Yale Observation Scale (Table 9–14) to assess toxicity and the need for further diagnostic evaluation. Unfortunately, some studies have shown that the Yale Observation Scale is less sensitive in detecting serious illness in this age group than in older infants and children.

Is there a source for the fever on physical examination? A careful physical examination must be performed, with special attention to clues that may point to the source of fever: Tachypnea may signal a pneumonia that cannot be detected by auscultation. Decreased movement of an extremity may be an indication of an osteomyelitis or septic arthritis. A bulging fontanelle and nuchal rigidity are excellent indicators of CNS infection, but the absence of these signs does not exclude the possibility of meningitis.

Are laboratory tests indicated? The infant with fever without localizing signs can have occult infection in the blood, urine, CSF, or lungs. A CBC (including WBC and differential) and a blood culture can be obtained by venopuncture. A high (>15,000) or low (<5000) WBC suggests increased risk of serious bacterial infection (see below) and may prompt further laboratory testing. Urine

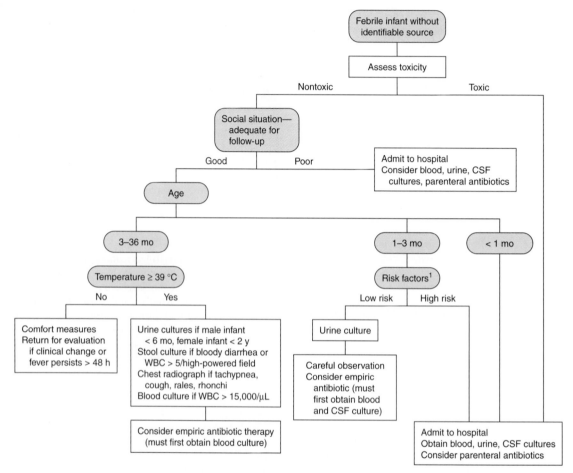

Figure 9–1. Algorithm demonstrating the approach to the febrile infant and young child.[1] See Table 9–16. CSF = cerebrospinal fluid; WBC = white blood cell count. (Reproduced, with permission, from Baraff LJ et al: Practice guidelines for the management of infants and children 0 to 36 months of age with fever without source. Agency for Health Care Policy and Research. *Ann Emerg Med* 1993;22:1198.)

and CSF specimens can be examined for the presence of white blood cells and bacteria and samples of both sent for culture. In infants with tachypnea or respiratory distress, a chest radiograph can confirm the suspicion of pneumonia. Chest radiographs are unlikely to show respiratory disease in a child without signs of respiratory illness.

What is the risk of serious bacterial infection? The incidence of serious bacterial infection in febrile infants younger than 3 months of age has been estimated to be 3–10%. The Rochester Criteria protocol has been used successfully to assign infants to high- and low-risk categories (Table 9–16). However, in one study of "low-risk" infants age 2–3 months with febrile episodes, 5.4% had a serious bacterial infection: the diagnoses were roughly

evenly distributed between bacteremia, UTIs, and bacterial gastroenteritis. The risk of serious bacterial disease increases significantly, to more than 10%, in toxic-appearing infants. Recently, a large collaborative trial by the Pediatric Research in the Office Setting network collected data on more than 3000 febrile infants younger than 3 months of age. As expected, infections associated with the upper respiratory tract accounted for the majority of the cases: upper respiratory infection, 35%; otitis media, 16%; and bronchiolitis, 8.4%. The other commonly found diagnoses were gastroenteritis (7.8%), UTI (4.7%), bacteremia (1.5%), and bacterial meningitis (0.4%).

Is treatment necessary? Any toxic-appearing infant or child should undergo a full evaluation for sepsis and meningitis and be hospitalized for treatment. Most clinicians agree that all infants younger than 1 month of age, well appearing or otherwise, should be hospitalized and treated with parenteral antibiotics pending initial laboratory and culture results. There has been growing support for the outpatient management of infants 1–3 months of age who meet standard low-risk criteria (e.g., Rochester Criteria). The outpatient administration of Ceftriaxone, a third-generation cephalosporin, has been studied in this context because of its activity against the common bacterial agents seen in infancy (including *S. pneumoniae, N. meningitides,* and *H. influenzae*), its excellent penetration into the CSF, and its longer half-life, which permits once-daily dosing. If this management plan is selected, blood, urine, and CSF cultures should be obtained before antibiotic administration to avoid potential future confusion in distinguishing a viral from a partly treated bacterial infection. In selecting outpatient management, close follow-up by the primary health care provider is essential and must be ensured before discharging the patient from the outpatient setting.

Approach to the older febrile infant (3–36 months of age). Febrile illnesses occur frequently in this age group, and temperatures as high as 39–40°C may be encountered routinely by primary care providers. The same questions can be asked after fever is documented.

Does the child appear "toxic"? Any severely ill child with signs and symptoms of meningitis (e.g., extreme irritability or lethargy) or cardiovascular instability suggestive of septic shock should be admitted to the hospital. Nontoxic-appearing children from 3 to 36 months of age may be considered for outpatient management.

Is there a source for the fever on physical examination? The concept of occult bacteremia refers to infants and children who appear well and have no identified source of fever detected by history or on physical examination, but whose blood culture taken at the time of initial presentation subsequently grow bacteria. The most commonly reported pathogen is *S. pneumoniae,* followed by HIB and *N. meningitidis.* With the introduction of HIB vaccine in the late 1980s, disease due to this organism is waning.

Are laboratory tests indicated? If no source of the fever is identified after the initial history and physical examination, the clinician must consider the role of further diagnostic testing. Blood, urine, and CSF are potential occult sites of infection, in addition to the lungs (e.g., pneumonia) and the musculoskeletal system (e.g., osteomyelitis). Although not all agree, many experts have recommended further testing in children whose temperature is 39.0°C or higher (Figure 9–1). In addition to blood cultures, urine cultures should be obtained in boys younger than 6 months of age and girls younger than

2 years of age. Stool cultures and chest radiographs should be performed if there are any suggestive signs or symptoms such as diarrhea with blood or mucous or tachypnea and respiratory distress.

What is the risk? Much of the research on febrile infants and children has focused on the risk, significance, and prevention of occult bacteremia. Previously, rates of bacteremia in children 3–36 months old were similar to the overall incidence of serious bacterial infections in the younger infants, between 3% and 11%. The risk of bacteremia has been shown to increase with increasing fever (39°C) and elevation of WBCs (>15,000/mm³). Recent studies, however, have shown a lower rate of bacteremia, including *S. pneumoniae,* since the introduction of immunization against *H. influenzae.* A 1998 study from Children's Hospital in Boston reported a prevalence of occult bacteremia of 1.6% in this age group.

Complications of persistent bacteremia, especially HIB, can include otitis media, cellulitis (e.g., periorbital, buccal), meningitis, arthritis, pericarditis, and epiglottitis. Although much of the interest in occult infections in this age group focuses on bacteremia, the prevalence of UTIs in febrile children 2–24 months of age is substantially greater—approximately 5%. Girls have over a twofold higher risk than boys.

Is treatment necessary? The empiric antibiotic treatment of febrile children without an identifiable source remains controversial. Some discourage the use of antibiotics without a discernible focus of infection because of cost, potential for allergic or other adverse reactions, and contribution to increasing bacterial antibiotic resistance. Others believe that empiric antibiotic use, oral or intramuscular, can prevent serious infectious complications.

In patients who are subsequently found to have bacteremia, follow-up and clinical reassessment are essential. The child with *S. pneumoniae* bacteremia, the most commonly isolated pathogen, who is afebrile and appears well can be managed as an outpatient with continued close follow-up. The child who is persistently febrile requires close re-evaluation for complications of bacteremia. Any child who appears ill on reevaluation, or in whom *H. influenzae* or *N. meningitidis* is isolated from the blood culture, should be hospitalized for parenteral antibiotics.

Fever of Unknown Origin

In the broadest sense, FUO (unspecified, undetermined) can include fevers occurring for any duration of time. Traditionally, however, the term has been applied to illnesses of a longer duration in which the initial diagnostic evaluation has been unrevealing. It is the prolonged nature of the fever that differentiates FUO from the fevers without localizing signs.

Children attending schools or day-care centers are exposed to a large number of community-acquired infections and, as a result, may present with what appears to parents to be excessively frequent or continuous fever. These intermittent fevers may occur with irregular or regular patterns lasting several days to several weeks but typically are due to a series of unrelated, self-limited viral infections. These benign infections must be differentiated from more ominous pathogens. Additional differential diagnoses of intermittent fever include malaria, relapsing fever, rat bite fevers, and cyclic neutropenia.

DIFFERENTIAL DIAGNOSIS

In 1961, Petersdorf and Beeson published their classic paper detailing the results of an evaluation of 100 adults with FUO. They defined an FUO as (1) an "illness of more than 3 weeks duration," associated with a (2) "fever higher than 100°F on several occasions," and in which the (3) "diagnosis remained uncertain after 1 week of hospitalization." In that study, infections, neoplasms, and collagen disorders made up, respectively, 36%, 19%, and 15% of final diagnoses. Of additional significance was a reported mortality rate of 32%.

In the almost four decades since that report was issued, a number of studies have been published on FUO in the pediatric population. Data from seven pediatric case series, consisting of 786 patients, are summarized in Table 9–17. Although the definition of FUO differed from study to study, diagnoses differed significantly from those found in an adult population. Most cases of FUO in children represented atypical presentations of common diseases. Infectious diseases accounted for more than half (52.3%) of pediatric cases, followed by collagen–vascular and inflammatory causes (11.5%) and malignancy (5.0%). Overall, 21.8% of cases remained undiagnosed. In one report, 67% of cases were undiagnosed. Of interest, HIV infection was reported in just one instance, but most of those studies predated clinical and serologic diagnosis of HIV.

CLINICAL APPROACH TO THE CHILD WITH PROLONGED FEVER

An approach similar to that used for the child with an acute febrile illness can be used in the evaluation of children with prolonged fever. Consideration of a series of clinical questions is helpful.

Is fever present? The diagnostic evaluation of prolonged fever begins with documentation of the fever and fever patterns. The definition of fever was addressed earlier. A description of the fever should include the duration, timing (continuous or intermittent, day or night, daily or weekly), and temperature elevation. Fevers can be continuous or sustained, intermittent or spiking, or relapsing. In some conditions, temperature may return to normal or even subnormal levels between fever spikes. In many cases,

Table 9–17. Final Diagnosis in Children With Fever of Unknown Origin[1]

Diagnoses	No.	%
Total	786	100
Infection	411	52.3
Respiratory infections	114	14.5
Urinary tract infections	31	3.9
Bacterial meningitis	14	1.8
Tuberculosis[2]	15	1.9
Collagen–vascular/inflammatory	90	11.5
Juvenile rheumatoid arthritis	40	5.1
Systemic lupus erythematosus	11	1.4
Crohn disease	12	1.5
Malignancy	39	5.0
Leukemia	19	2.4
Lymphoma	8	1.0
Undiagnosed	171	21.8

[1] A composite summary based on published literature on fever of unknown origin, including Gartner 1992, Steele 1991, Feigin & Shearer 1976.
[2] Includes pulmonary, meningitis, disseminated, and site unspecified.

the pattern of fever or response to antipyretics does not correlate with the severity of illness or ultimate diagnosis. Documentation and description of the fever has become more difficult recently because the evaluation of many of these patients has moved from inpatient to outpatient settings. Optimally, multiple daily temperature measurements should be obtained and recorded by an objective, trained individual. Parental reports may be complicated by unintentional (e.g., misunderstanding of normal temperature) or intentional (e.g., factitious fever, Münchausen syndrome by proxy) errors. In many situations it is unrealistic for the temperature to be measured by someone other than the parent. In those cases, the parent should be instructed carefully on how to take a temperature and keep a fever diary by measuring the temperature three to four times per day. In addition to a description of the fever and its pattern, a thorough history is the cornerstone of the evaluation of FUO. Examples of how historical factors may lead to specific diagnoses are listed in Table 9–18. A detailed travel history should include all previous travel experiences (recent and distant past, domestic and foreign). Exposures should be explored, including ill contacts, animals (domestic and wild), potential water or food sources, and medications. A family's ethnicity and medical history also may be relevant.

Does the child appear toxic? Does the patient appear acutely or chronically ill? A toxic-appearing patient requires

Table 9–18. Historical Considerations in Diagnosis of Fever of Unknown Origin

History	Diagnoses	Test
Medications	Drug fever	Stop medication
Foods		
Unpasteurized milk or cheese	Brucellosis	Serology, culture
Animal exposure (wild and domestic)		
Rodent	Tularemia	Serology, culture
Rodent	Rat-bite fever	Serology, culture
Many species	Leptospirosis	Serology, culture
Dog	Visceral larva migrans	Stool for parasites: *Toxocara canis*
Travel history (endemic area)		
Foreign travel	Malaria	Thick blood smear examination
Southwestern United States	Coccidioidomycosis	Serology, culture
Central river valleys, United States	Histoplasmosis	Serology, culture, stains
Mississippi and Ohio river basins	Blastomycosis	Serology, culture, stains
Family history	Familial Mediterranean fever	Clinical diagnosis

immediate, thorough evaluation in the hospital setting. Patients who otherwise appear well are candidates for initial outpatient evaluation.

Is there a source for the fever on physical examination? By definition, preliminary examination has not identified a source for the fever. However, it is essential that careful physical examinations be repeated to observe for subtle or fleeting signs that can help lead to a specific diagnosis. Table 9–19 lists some of these physical examination findings.

Which laboratory tests are indicated? Consultation with infectious disease, hematology–oncology, and/or rheumatology specialists can be useful in directing further workups. Usually, several screening laboratory tests have been performed as part of the initial diagnostic evaluation. Typically, these have included a CBC with complete differential count and markers of inflammation (e.g., ESR or CRP). The CBC can demonstrate abnormalities (increases or decreases) in white blood cell, red blood cell, or platelet count. A low hemoglobin concentration may reflect anemia of chronic disease or nutritional deficiencies. A decrease in multiple hematopoietic cell lines (anemia, leukopenia, and thrombocytopenia) may indicate primary marrow failure, leukemic infiltrate, or a malignant neoplasm that has invaded the bone marrow space. Rarely, an etiologic agent may be visualized directly on a peripheral blood smear, as may be the case in infections with *Borellia, Plasmodia,* or *Erlichia.* An elevation in ESR or CRP suggests an ongoing inflammatory process such as infection, collage vascular disease, or occult malignancy.

The clinical laboratory provides a large variety of tests that can be used to identify or exclude specific diseases. However, because of the wide range of conditions associ-ated with fever, it is impractical to order tests to exclude all possibilities. Further diagnostic evaluation should be guided by clues obtained in the history and physical examination and by pursuing the most common or most urgent causes of FUO (Table 9–20). Bacteremia, UTI, and meningitis can be detected through appropriate sample analysis and culture, as previously discussed. Skin testing with PPD should be performed during every evaluation for FUO to rule out infection with tuberculosis. A wide range of serologic tests is available. Elevations in antinuclear antibody can support the diagnosis of systemic lupus erythematosus. Serologic titers can be obtained for many specific infectious diseases such as EBV, tularemia, brucellosis, toxoplasmosis, salmonellosis, coccidiomycosis, and Lyme disease, to name a few. However, a directed workup based on a detailed history and physical examination is usually a more fruitful and cost-effective approach. Wide range testing without historical evidence of exposure can lead to false-positive results.

Radiologic examinations are frequently part of the evaluation of patients with FUO. In particular, chest and sinus radiographs are important because of the frequency with which respiratory tract infections are identified. Although more sophisticated imaging studies (e.g., ultrasonography, computed tomography [CT], magnetic resonance imaging [MRI], and nuclear medicine scans) are widely available, their usefulness as routine screening procedures in the evaluation of FUO is less certain. More invasive procedures such as biopsies (e.g., bone marrow, skin, lymph node, liver) and exploratory laparotomy may be indicated in certain settings where patients remain febrile and are sick.

What is the risk? Children with FUO are less likely than adults to have a life-threatening illness. Most children with

Table 9–19. Physical Examination Considerations in Diagnosis of Fever of Unknown Origin

Physical Examination	Diseases	Diagnostic Studies
Ocular		
Conjunctivitis	Kawasaki's disease	Clinical diagnosis
	Tularemia (oculoglandular type)	Serology, culture
	Leptospirosis	Serology, culture
	Histoplasmosis	Serology, culture
	Cat-scratch fever	Special stain, serology
	SLE	Clinical diagnosis, serology (ANA)
Fundoscopic	Toxoplasmosis, cytomegalovirus (congenital infections)	Chorioretinitis
Roth spots	Bacterial endocarditis	Blood culture, echocardiogram
Uveitis	Autoimmune disorders	Slit lamp
Hepatomegaly	Visceral larva migrans (toxocariasis)	Clinical diagnosis, histology, ELISA
	Hepatitis A, B, C	Serology
Jaundice	Hepatitis A, B, C	Serology
	Leptospirosis	Serology, culture
Lymphadenopathy	Cat-scratch	Skin test, serology
	Tularemia	Serology, culture
	Kawasaki	Clinical diagnosis
Arthritis	Autoimmune	Clinical diagnosis, serology (ANA)
	Septic arthritis	Culture
Bone pain or tenderness	Osteomyelitis	Culture
	Leukemia	Complete blood count, bone marrow aspiration
Skin		
Erythematous maculopapular rash	Kawasaki disease	Clinical diagnosis
Salmon-colored rash	Autoimmune (JRA, SLE)	Clinical diagnosis, serology (ANA)
Osler, Janeway lesions	Bacterial endocarditis	Blood culture, echocardiogram

ANA = antinuclear antibody; ELISA = enzyme-linked immunosorbent assay; JRA = juvenile rheumatoid arthritis; SLE = systemic lupus erythematosus.

FUO represent atypical presentations of common diseases. Infectious and collagen-vascular/inflammatory conditions are the two most commonly identified categories of disease. The risk of adverse outcomes differs from diagnosis to diagnosis. The mortality rate reported in two studies was 9–18%.

Is treatment necessary? Treatment must be disease directed. Because numerous infectious and noninfectious causes can produce prolonged fever, thorough investigation must precede attempts at empiric therapy. Undirected treatment with broad-spectrum antibiotics can potentially mask infections and delay the diagnosis of meningitis, osteomyelitis, and endocarditis. When a diagnosis cannot be made, close follow-up, serial examinations, and reevaluations are essential. In a significant number of cases, the etiology of FUO is never determined, and the fever resolves spontaneously without obvious sequelae.

■ LABORATORY COMMON INFECTIOUS DISEASES & PRESENTATIONS BY ORGAN SYSTEM

Eye, Mouth, & Neck Infections

EYE INFECTIONS

Eye swelling and inflammation of the conjunctiva can be a manifestation of a variety of different clinical conditions in the pediatric age group. The loose connective tissue of the eyelid predisposes this area to swelling in response to a variety of disease states. When the swelling and redness is of acute onset, the principal diagnoses are allergic reactions, trauma, insect bites, and infection.

Table 9–20. Laboratory Considerations in Diagnosis of Fever of Unknown Origin

Screening laboratory
    Complete blood count
    Erythrocyte sedimentation rate or C-reactive protein
    Urinalysis and urine culture
    Blood culture
    Cerebrospinal fluid analysis and culture[1]
    Tuberculosis skin test

Serology
    Antinuclear antibodies
    Rheumatoid factor
    Febrile agglutinins
    Antibodies for specific pathogens, e.g., Lyme titers

Radiology
    Chest radiograph, sinus radiograph
    Others: ultrasonography, computed tomographic scan, magnetic resonance imaging, nuclear scan[1]

[1] When indicated.

The history and initial physical examination may provide important information regarding the etiology of eye swelling and inflammation. A history of allergy (e.g., allergic rhinitis) or injury should be elicited. Physical examination may reveal an insect bite mark in the center of the swelling or signs of atopic disease (e.g., allergic shiners, infraorbital folds or "Dennie lines," horizontal nasal crease). Even when other causes are suspected, it is always important to consider the possibility of periorbital and orbital infections. In some cases, an insect bite or trauma may be the precipitating event in periorbital cellulitis. In addition, conjunctivitis can be caused by local infectious processes(e.g., viral and bacterial infections) or systemic inflammatory conditions such as Kawasaki disease.

Acute infectious conjunctivitis. A variety of conditions can cause inflammation of the conjunctiva, including allergic reactions, trauma, and infection. Infectious etiologies and their prevalence differ by age. A more extensive discussion of neonatal conjunctivitis and the diagnostic approach to the pediatric red eye can be found in Chapter 21.

Acute conjunctivitis in the neonate. In contrast to the preantibiotic era, the most common cause of conjunctivitis in the neonate is the ophthalmic medication applied at birth to prevent gonococcal ocular infection. Medications such as silver nitrate are responsible for a chemical irritation that occurs after application, lasts for several days, and resolves spontaneously. Infectious causes of neonatal conjunctivitis often involve pathogens acquired during passage through the birth canal including *Chlamydia trachomatis, Neisseria gonorrhea,* and HSV.

Conjunctivitis due to *C. trachomatis* appears after an incubation period of 1–2 weeks. Diagnosis can be made by tissue culture, Giemsa stain, and antigen assays (e.g., fluorescent antibody stain, enzyme immunoassays). Over half of newborns with *C. trachomatis* conjunctivitis will develop pulmonary symptoms including pneumonia. For that reason, *C. trachomatis* conjunctivitis is treated with systemic antibiotics (e.g., erythromycin).

Neisseria gonorrhea is an important cause of neonatal conjunctivitis because of the significant associated risk of permanent damage to the eye, which can lead to blindness. Ocular prophylaxis (silver nitrate or erythromycin) administered shortly after birth has dramatically reduced the incidence of *N. gonorrhea* conjunctivitis. The incubation period for gonococcal infection is 3–5 days. Diagnosis can be made by Gram stain and culture. Because gonoccal conjunctivitis may be accompanied by disseminated infection, therapy involves the use of parenteral antibiotics (e.g., third-generation cephalosporins).

Conjunctivitis due to HSV (HSV-2 more commonly than HSV-1) usually occurs with other signs of systemic infection, including cutaneous lesions, and nervous system involvement. The incubation period is 3 days to 3 weeks. Diagnosis can be made by Tzanck smear or viral culture. Treatment involves a combination of topical (e.g., vidaribine) and systemic (e.g., acyclovir) antiviral agents.

The reader is referred to Chapter 21 (Ophthalmology) for additional information on neonatal conjunctivitis.

Acute conjunctivitis in the older infant and child. Clinical studies in the past two decades have delineated the infectious causes of conjunctivitis in children. In 1981, Gigliotti and associates performed diagnostic tests for routine bacteria, *Chlamydia, Mycoplasma,* and viruses on 99 children with acute conjunctivitis and 102 age-matched healthy controls. Their results showed that pediatric conjunctivitis is caused primarily by pathogens commonly associated with other upper respiratory infections. *Hemophilus influenzae* is the most frequent bacteria identified (42–68% of cases in a recent review by Boder), with *S. pneumoniae* the next most common (7–21% of cases). Other bacteria less frequently isolated are *M. catarrhalis, N. gonorrhea,* and *N. meningitidis.* It should be noted that *S. aureus* and *S. epidermidis* are cultured with almost equal frequency from the eyes of children with and without conjunctivitis. Adenovirus is the most common viral cause of conjunctivitis, accounting for 20% of cases. Enterovirus also has been isolated during epidemics of hemorrhagic conjunctivitis. Infection with measles virus causes conjunctivitis in association with fever, cough, coryza, and a distinctive (morbilliform) rash.

It can be difficult to distinguish clinically between the most common bacterial and viral causes of conjunctivitis. In the study by Gigliotti and colleagues, bilateral disease was seen most often with *H. influenza* conjunctivitis (71%). However, *S. pneumoniae* (50%) and adenovirus

(35%) also frequently caused bilateral involvement. Likewise, purulent conjunctivitis occurred most often with bacterial infections (*H. influenzae* and *S. pneumoniae*) but occurred in almost half of the cases caused by adenovirus. Although preauricular lymphadenopathy is more suggestive of a viral rather than a bacterial etiology, its presence is relatively uncommon in viral (17%) and bacterial (7%) conjunctivitis.

The presence of associated infections, such as otitis media and pharyngitis, can provide clues to the specific etiology. Several "conjunctivitis syndromes" have been reported. The most common is the conjunctivitis–otitis syndrome first described by Bodor in 1982. In the original study, three fourths of purulent conjunctivitis cases were associated with otitis media, and in those cases, the most common infectious organism isolated was *H. influenzae*. The otitis media typically occurred within 3–4 days after the onset of eye symptoms. Purulent conjunctivitis and/or otitis media developed in siblings of index cases almost half the time. Systemic antibiotic therapy (e.g., oral amoxicillin and clavulanate) without topical antibiotics has been shown to successfully treat the otitis and conjunctivitis. The combination of pharyngitis and conjunctivitis (pharyngoconjunctival fever) is seen most often in association with adenovirus infection. As the name implies, the infection is accompanied by conjunctivitis, sore throat, and fever. Kawasaki disease causes a nonexudative, bilateral conjunctivitis, persistent fever, rash, lymphadenopathy, and mucus membrane changes. This disease is described in Chapter 8 (Rheumatic Diseases).

If trauma or conditions predisposing to corneal ulceration (e.g., HSV, some strains of adenovirus) are suspected, fluorescein staining should be performed. Any significant trauma or corneal ulceration on initial examination should prompt a complete ophthalmologic evaluation and consultation. The laboratory can be used to differentiate viral from bacterial conjunctivitis with a variety of stains, cultures, and antigen assays.

Practically speaking, however, many clinicians treat acute conjunctivitis almost uniformly with antibiotics. In part, this is due to the known predominance of bacteria as the cause of acute conjunctivitis in young children. Other factors influencing the frequent use of antibiotic treatment may include concern over bacterial superinfection of viral conjunctivitis and the requirement for treatment in children returning to some child care centers. A wide range of topical solutions and ointments are available. Systemic therapy may be indicated in some cases (e.g., intolerance of topical application, conjunctivitis associated with otitis media). Because of the high prevalence of β-lactamase producing *H. influenzae,* antibiotics used should be resistant to those enzymes.

Periorbital & orbital cellulitis

Pathogenesis. The orbit is a bony cavity surrounded by the paranasal sinuses: medially by the ethmoid sinus, infe-

riorly by the maxillary sinus, and superiorly (in older children) by the frontal sinus. In some areas, only a very thin bony wall separates the adjoining spaces (e.g., the lamina papyracea separating the ethmoid sinus and orbit). These close anatomic relationships are a factor in the development of many orbital and periorbital infections. The area around the eye can be divided into two clinically important areas by a coronal fascial plane that runs from the bony orbital rim to the tarsal plate of the eyelid. The periorbital and orbital spaces are separated by the fibrous orbital septum, which serves as a barrier to edema and infection. Infections anterior to the orbital septum are classified as periorbital or preseptal cellulitis.

Several routes of entry have been hypothesized for periorbital and orbital infections:

1. direct inoculation (e.g., trauma)
2. extension of infection from an adjacent site (e.g., sinusitis, conjunctivitis, hordeolum)
3. deposition of organisms during bacteremia

Etiology. The most frequently reported bacterial isolates in periorbital and orbital infections are HIB, *S aureus, S epidermidis,* and *Streptococcus* species (e.g., *S. pneumoniae*). Before universal immunization against HIB, *H. influenzae* represented half of all isolates in periorbital cellulitis. Many of these infections are presumed to have resulted from the hematogenous spread of HIB. In contrast, cases of periorbital cellulitis secondary to insect bites or trauma are caused more commonly by *S. aureus* and *Streptococcus* species. On the basis of the anatomic proximity to the sinuses, the bacteria responsible for orbital cellulitis are the same as those responsible for acute sinusitis. A relatively even distribution between typeable and nontypeable *H. influenzae, S. aureus,* and *Streptococcus* species has been reported. Anaerobic and mixed infections may play a more frequent role in orbital than in periorbital infections.

Clinical manifestations. Periorbital erythema and edema are the presenting signs in periorbital (preseptal) and orbital cellulitis. Most patients with either infection present with fever. Table 9–21 compares some of the clinical features of periorbital and orbital cellulitis.

Diagnosis. Whenever a child presents with a red and swollen eye, it is critical that the clinician be able to identify a periorbital and/or orbital infection. A history of viral URI, trauma, insect bites, and allergy should be elicited. The child should be asked about the presence of eye pain (including foreign body sensation), photophobia, and any visual changes (blurry vision or double vision). A history of ill contacts with conjunctivitis should suggest the diagnosis of adenovirus infection, which may mimic periorbital cellulitis in younger children.

The physical examination can be especially useful in distinguishing periorbital from orbital infection (Table 9–21).

Table 9–21. Comparison of Periorbital and Orbital Cellulitis

	Periorbital Cellulitis	Orbital Cellulitis
History		
Incidence	More common	Less common
Age	Toddler to preschool-age	School-age
Physical examination		
Fever	Usually present	Usually present
Periorbital swelling and redness	Present	Present
Chemosis	Present	Present
Conjunctival infection	Present	Present
Proptosis	Absent	Present[1]
Ophthalmoplegia	Absent	Present[1]
Visual acuity	Normal	Normal or impaired[1]
Pathogenetic mechanism		
Sinusitis	Common	Common
Trauma/skin infections	Common	Uncommon

[1] Features distinguishing orbital involvement.

Proptosis, ophthalmoplegia, and decreased visual acuity are the hallmarks of orbital infection. These findings are absent in periorbital infection. Physical examination also should identify skin injury and possible entry points. Palpation of the face can be performed for sinus tenderness, although this is an infrequent finding in pediatric sinusitis. The mouth should be examined for evidence of dental abscess, including pain on palpation of the teeth. The presence of preauricular lymphadenopathy, bilateral disease, and a conjunctival pseudomembrane suggests infection due to adenovirus.

Radiologic imaging of the orbits are indicated when the clinical examination is equivocal or whenever suspicion of orbital infection exists. Computed tomography and MRI can show an abscess and thickening of the extraocular muscles consistent with orbital involvement. Other laboratory tests are of limited benefit in making the diagnosis of periorbital and orbital cellulitis. The WBC and ESR may be elevated, but these findings are nonspecific. Cultures of the blood or CSF are more likely to be positive in cases due to HIB.

Treatment & complications. Treatment of periorbital and orbital cellulitis consists of antibiotics aimed at the most common etiologic organisms. All patients who appear toxic or have evidence of orbital involvement should be hospitalized. Outpatient therapy for periorbital cellulitis is possible for selected patients, including those with mild infections whose compliance with medications and close follow-up can be ensured. Antibiotic regimens may include an antistaphylococcal penicillin (e.g., nafcillin) and an aminoglycoside or third-generation cephalosporin. Surgery is indicated for abscess formation, sinus drainage, or lack of clinical response to medical therapy. Prevention of a significant number of these infections is now possible through the use of the HIB conjugate vaccines.

The most frequent complications of periorbital cellulitis are meningitis and lid abscess. Orbital cellulitis, although rare, can be complicated by periosteal abscess, meningitis, and cavernous sinus thrombosis.

SORE MOUTH OR THROAT

Sore throat is a frequent complaint encountered by pediatric health providers. It has been reported that pharyngitis brings almost 1% of the population to a physician each year, making it one of the most common infectious diseases encountered in the office setting.

A large variety of infectious agents can produce inflammation in and around the oropharynx. In older children, this results in complaints of sore throat or dysphagia. In younger children, irritability, increased drooling, or decreased appetite may be the only symptoms of sore throat.

Sore throat due to the common respiratory viruses (e.g., rhinovirus, coronavirus) is typically accompanied by fever, rhinorrhea, and cough. Several other infectious agents associated with pharyngitis produce relatively distinctive skin (exanthem) and mucous membrane (enanthem) eruptions. Examples are adenoviruses (pharyngoconjunctival fever), coxsackievirus (hand, foot, and mouth disease), and HSV (gingivostomatitis).

Stomatitis & gingivostomatitis. In young infants, *Candida albicans* can produce whitish plaques on the tongue, palate, and buccal mucosa. Infection of the oral cavity with *C. albicans* is referred to as oral candidiasis or thrush. Gentle brushing of the involved areas with a tongue blade can be used to distinguish thrush from residual milk particles. Thrush will be more adherent to the underlying mucosa, and removal of the whitish plaques will reveal inflamed mucosal surfaces. Laboratory tests (wet mounts, Gram stains, and culture) usually are unnecessary to make the diagnosis. Oral candidiasis typically responds to the application of the topical antifungal agent nystatin. Alternatively, topical application of clotrimazole and oral administration of fluconazole have been used for persistent infections.

In infants and young children, infection with coxsackievirus or HSV (primarily HSV-1) can produce vesicular or ulcerative oral lesions. These conditions may be classified as pharyngitis, stomatitis, gingivitis, or gingivo-stomatitis depending on the site(s) of involvement.

Herpes simplex virus typically results in a cluster of vesicles around the lips, gingiva (i.e., gingivostomatitis), and the anterior portion of the tongue. Primary infections with HSV can range from asymptomatic to severe. Symptomatic cases are associated with fever, irritability, dysphagia, and cervical lymphadenopathy. The vesicles eventually break and form ulcers. The diagnosis is usually a clinical one, although Tzanck smears (multinucleated giant cells and intranuclear inclusions), antigen assays, and viral cultures can be used to confirm the diagnosis. Treatment is aimed primarily at pain relief during the acute infection. Analgesia may be accomplished through the use of topical preparations containing viscous lidocaine or systemic analgesics (e.g., acetaminophen, ibuprofen, codeine). Patients must be monitored for signs of dehydration, which may result from decreased oral intake. Antiviral agents, such as acyclovir, may be useful in specialized settings (e.g., immunodeficiency states or severe disease). A recent study showed that oral Acyclovir given to children with primary HSV gingivostomatitis shortened the time to healing and prevented hospitalization for dehydration. Recurrences have been attributed to a variety of physiologic stresses (e.g., sun, febrile illness, emotional duress).

In contrast to HSV infection, the lesions of coxsackievirus have been characteristically described in the posterior aspect of the mouth, including tonsils and soft palate. Transmission of the virus occurs by the fecal-to-oral route. When lesions are limited to the mouth, infection with coxsackievirus is referred to as **herpangina.** Some serotypes of coxsackievirus (e.g., coxsackievirus A16) are associated with other cutaneous manifestations: Oral lesions in combination with similar vesicular lesions on the palmar aspect of the hands and feet describe the clinical syndrome known as **hand, foot, and mouth disease.** The maculopapular lesions on the hands, feet, and buttocks often become vesicular. The progression from vesicles to ulcers is similar to that seen in HSV infection. The diagnosis of coxsackievirus infection is made on clinical grounds and additional laboratory tests usually are not indicated. Like HSV, the disease is often self-limited and requires only symptomatic treatment in normal hosts.

Pharyngitis & tonsillitis

Etiology. In children, the etiology of pharyngitis (tonsillopharyngitis) can be divided into viral, bacterial, and idiopathic causes. The viruses responsible for pharyngitis include adenovirus, parainfluenza virus, enterovirus, influenza virus, HSV, and EBV. Rhinovirus and coronavirus may produce sore throat in conjunction with other upper respiratory symptoms (e.g., common cold). Of the bacterial agents, group A *Streptococcus* (GAS) is the most frequently isolated. Overall, GAS has been responsible for somewhere between 15% and 30% of all cases of pharyngitis. Other bacteria responsible for pharyngitis are non–group A streptococci (groups C, F, and G), *Arcanobacterium haemolyticum,* and *Neisseria* species (*gonorrhoeae* and *meningitidis*). *Mycoplasma pneumoniae* and *Chlamydia pneumoniae* are among the less common causes of pharyngitis.

The frequency with which various etiologies are identified differs with the age of the child and the time of year. Overall, viruses are the most common cause. This is especially true in children younger than 2 years, in whom viruses may be responsible for half of all episodes of pharyngitis. Viral infections are more common during the colder months of the year. School-aged children (5–15 years of age) represent the group most frequently infected with GAS. Infections typically occur during the winter and spring. Outbreaks of groups C, G, and F streptococci have been reported in adolescents (e.g., college students).

Diagnosis. The traditional approach to pharyngitis (tonsillopharyngitis) focuses on distinguishing GAS infections from all other causes. The importance given to GAS infection relates primarily to its association with rheumatic fever. Studies from the 1950s found that early treatment of GAS infection reduced the incidence of rheumatic fever. A resurgence of rheumatic fever occurred in certain geographic areas of the United States in the 1980s.

In approaching the patient with pharyngitis, the clinician should investigate aspects of the history and physical examination that increase or decrease the likelihood of GAS infection (Table 9–22). Classic manifestations of GAS tonsillopharyngitis include the acute onset of sore throat, dysphagia, fever, headache, nausea, vomiting, and abdominal pain. A history of exposure to someone with documented GAS infection also may be elicited. On physical examination, the throat, tonsils, and uvula are bright red and edematous. The tonsils may be covered with exudate. Petechiae on the palate, although infrequently present, suggest GAS infection. A scarlatiniform rash also may be present, although such a rash is reported in more than 50% of cases of *A. haemolyticum.* The anterior cervical nodes typically are swollen and tender.

Signs and symptoms that diminish the likelihood of GAS include viral URI symptoms (e.g., rhinorrhea, cough), hoarseness, conjunctivitis, viral exanthems or enanthems, myalgia, and diarrhea. The presence of generalized lymphadenopathy and hepatosplenomegaly suggests EBV infection. The absence of fever, lymphadenitis, or tonsillar exudate decreases the likelihood of GAS.

Scoring systems have been devised to differentiate GAS infection from other (primarily viral) causes based on clinical and epidemiologic factors. Unfortunately, only a small minority of patients may present with the classic manifestations of GAS pharyngitis. Likewise, there is significant overlap in clinical and epidemiologic

Table 9–22. Comparison of Group A Streptococcal (GAS) and Viral Pharyngitis

	GAS Infection	Viral Infection
History		
Sore throat	Yes	Yes
Rhinorrhea	No	Yes
Cough	No	Yes
Hoarseness	No	Yes
Headache	Yes	Yes or no
Stridor	No	Yes or no
Conjunctivitis	No	Yes or no
Stomachache	Yes	Yes or no
Exposures to GAS	Yes	No
Physical examination		
Fever	Yes	Yes or no
Tonsillar exudates	Yes	Yes
Tender cervical adenopathy	Yes	Yes or no
Palatal petechiae	Yes[1]	No
Scarlatiniform rash	Yes[1]	No
Laboratory		
White blood cell count	Yes[2]	No

[1] Probably has the greatest specificity for GAS infection. However, the low frequency of this finding makes it insensitive for diagnosing GAS.

[2] Risk of GAS infection may be higher with higher elevations of white blood cell count (especially ≥20,500) and neutrophil predominance.

features between GAS and other infectious causes. Overall, the ability of these scoring systems to predict positive laboratory tests (culture or rapid antigen) has been in the range of 50–80%. Therefore, due to the difficulty of making the diagnosis of GAS infection clinically, the laboratory plays a central role in confirming the diagnosis. The clinical laboratory provides several methods for establishing the diagnosis of GAS pharyngitis. Culture, rapid antigen assays, and serologic tests are widely available (Table 9–23). In the clinic, a single throat culture is the standard for making the diagnosis of GAS pharyngitis. Modifications of the single-culture technique (e.g., use of multiple cultures, culturing of surgical specimens) or documentation of an increase in antistreptolysin O antibody titer can increase the detection rate of GAS. However, these techniques are often impractical and not available in the usual clinic setting. Isolation of GAS by throat culture usually occurs within 24–48 hours. A useful adjunct to the culture has been the development of antigen detection techniques. Several antigen assays are available, including latex agglutination, enzyme and optical immunoassays, and chemiluminescent probes. Historically, rapid antigen tests for GAS have had a lower sensitivity (<80–90%) than culture. However, the high specificity (95%) of these rapid antigen techniques allows treatment of children who test positive without having to perform a culture. The newer assays have sensitivities more closely approaching culture. Antigen studies are popular because of their ease of use and the availability of immediate results. The results of an antigen assay performed in the office can be available immediately, and, if positive, antibiotic therapy can be initiated at the same visit. A positive antigen test result precludes the need for a culture; however, when a negative result is obtained, due to the lower sensitivity, a standard culture should be performed (Figure 9–2).

Treatment. The goals of treatment for GAS pharyngitis include:

1. bacteriologic cure
2. prevention of nonsuppurative sequelae (e.g., acute rheumatic fever)
3. prevention of suppurative complications
4. hastening of clinical recovery
5. reduction of transmission

Bacteriologic cure is, for the most part, readily achieved with the administration of any number of antibiotics. Prevention of acute rheumatic fever was demonstrated in the

Table 9–23. Diagnostic Tests for Group A Streptococcal Pharyngitis[1]

	Sensitivity	Specificity	Time for Result	Advantage	Disadvantage
Culture	Good	Good	24–48 h	Early diagnosis	Role of carrier
Rapid antigen assay	Fair	Good	Minutes	Earliest diagnosis	Less sensitive, ? more recurrence with early treatment
ASO titers[2]	Good	Good	Weeks	? Gold standard	Too late for therapy to prevent rheumatic fever

[1] Many diagnostic algorithms use a combination of rapid antigen and culture (see Figure 9–2).

[2] Acute and convalescent sera.

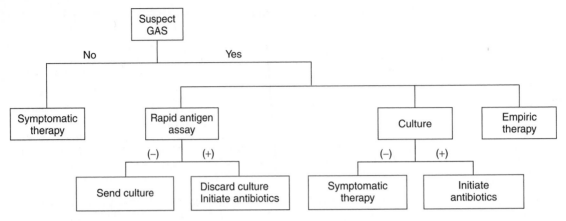

Figure 9–2. Management strategies in pharyngitis. GAS = group A *Streptococcus*.

1950s through treatment of GAS pharyngitis with benzathine penicillin. The incidence of suppurative complications, such as peritonsillar abscess or severe invasive infection (e.g., sepsis), is also likely to be reduced with antibiotic therapy.

The duration of symptoms of pharyngitis is shortened by 1–2 days in patients who receive treatment. It should be noted that symptoms related to GAS pharyngitis will typically resolve in 3–4 days even without treatment. Since the early studies, penicillin has remained the treatment of choice for GAS pharyngitis. The use of alternative antibiotics, including other penicillins (e.g., amoxicillin, ampicillin, amoxicillin-clavulanate), cephalosporins, clindamycin, and erythromycin, have been demonstrated to achieve bacteriologic cure. Erythromycin is standardly recommended for patients with penicillin allergy, although resistance to erythromycin by GAS does occur. The duration of antibiotic therapy is typically a 10-day course of oral antibiotics or a single dose of intramuscular benzathine penicillin G. Symptomatic treatment involves the use of oral analgesic agents such as acetaminophen and ibuprofen.

Treatment failures & carriers. Recurrent symptoms or repeated throat cultures positive for GAS can represent treatment failure, recurrent disease, or the GAS carrier state. Antibiotic failure is believed to occur in 10–30% of cases.

Treatment failure can result from poor compliance (the most common cause), copathogens (other β-lactamase-producing bacteria in the oropharynx), antibiotic resistance or penicillin tolerance, and biologic properties of the bacteria. Penicillin tolerance exists when there is a large difference between the MICs and MBCs. In recent years, erythromycin-resistant GAS has been reported in 5% of cases in the United States and almost 50% in Finland and Japan.

Recurrent disease may represent up to half of all "treatment failures." However, it is difficult to distinguish treatment failure from recurrent disease without knowledge of the serotypes of the organisms responsible for the initial and subsequent episodes. Recurrence may result from reexposure and the high background prevalence of the carrier rate. In addition, early treatment may suppress the development of protective antibodies, thus allowing reinfection.

The existence of the GAS carrier state has been known since 1947. Carriers of GAS are defined as individuals with positive throat culture results who demonstrate no increase in antistreptolysin O titers. Carriers may be detected during episodes of pharyngitis from other causes (symptomatic) or during screening (asymptomatic). The symptomatic carrier cannot be differentiated from the carrier of acute infection without the results of acute and convalescent titers. The carrier state is especially common in pediatric patients (an estimated 10% of school-aged children) and may last for weeks to months. The etiology of the carrier state is unknown, and neither host- nor organism-specific factors (e.g., serotype) have been identified that predispose to this condition. After adequate treatment for the acute infection, no further antibiotic therapy is indicated for the chronic carrier state.

The management of treatment failures depends on the presumed cause. When compliance is a problem, a single intramuscular injection of benzathine penicillin is an effective choice. The therapy for compliant patients with recurrent or persistent disease and for the GAS carrier state is less easily defined. Usually, alternative antibiotics, such as erythromycin, amoxicillin-clavulanate, cephalosporins, or clindamycin, are used.

Complications. Pharyngitis caused by gas can result in suppurative and nonsuppurative complications. Suppurative complications include peritonsillar abscess, retropharyngeal abscess, septicemia, and toxin-mediated shock.

Peritonsillar abscess (or quinsy) is characterized by trismus and a muffled or "hot-potato" voice. Physical examination reveals unilateral tonsillar enlargement and erythema. The uvula and soft palate are deviated away from the infected side due to inflammation and accumulation of purulent material. Cultures of abscess fluid usually show a combination of aerobic (GAS, *S. aureus, H. influenzae*) and anaerobic (*Fusobacterium, Peptostreptococci, Bacteroides*) organisms. Radiologic imaging such as intraoral ultrasound and CT may differentiate peritonsillar abscess from peritonsillitis or parapharyngeal space abscess. Medical management includes antibiotics (usually penicillin), hydration, and pain control. Surgical treatment may be necessary, including needle aspiration, incision and drainage, and immediate or delayed tonsillectomy. **Retropharyngeal abscess** follows infection of the lymph nodes occupying a potential space in the retropharynx. These lymph nodes drain the sinuses and nasopharynx. Direct trauma (e.g., foreign body, airway instrumentation) or extension of infection from an adjacent site (e.g., vertebral tuberculosis) also can lead to abscess formation in this area. Symptoms of upper respiratory infection precede the development of stridor, muffled voice, and stiff neck. In a study from the Children's Hospital of Pittsburg, one third of the children diagnosed with retrophayngeal abscess also had torticollis. Physical examination may reveal a unilateral swelling of the posterior pharynx. Fluctuance may be felt on palpation of the involved area. Microbiology of the abscess fluid is similar to that seen with peritonsillar abscess, i.e., aerobic and anaerobic bacteria. Lateral neck radiographs, CT, and, less commonly, MRI and ultrasound have been used to aid in diagnosis. Management of retropharyngeal abscess includes antibiotics, hydration, pain control, and surgical drainage.

Group A *Streptococcus* also can cause invasive disease including sepsis and necrotizing fasciitis. A specific **toxic shock syndrome** caused by GAS was first described in 1987. The development of streptococcal toxic shock syndrome is believed to be related to the production of streptococcal pyrogenic exotoxins (e.g., mitogenic factor and streptococcal superantigen). The clinical criteria used to define streptococcal toxic shock syndrome are listed in Table 9–24.

Nonsuppurative complications of GAS pharyngitis include **acute rheumatic fever** and **acute poststreptococcal glomerulonephritis.** Acute rheumatic fever is the principal reason that so much time and effort are directed toward identifying individuals with GAS pharyngitis. This entity is discussed in Chapter 8 (Rheumatic Diseases). The incidence of rheumatic fever has been shown to be significantly diminished by antibiotic therapy for GAS pharyngitis if initiated within 9 days of the onset of illness. Acute

Table 9–24. Case Definition for Streptococcal Toxic Shock Syndrome[1]

I. Isolation of group A β-hemolytic streptococci
  A. From a normally sterile site (e.g., blood, cerebrospinal fluid, peritoneal fluid, tissue biopsy specimen)
  B. From a nonsterile site (e.g., throat, sputum, vagina)

II. Clinical signs of severity
  A. Hypotension: systolic blood pressure <90 mm Hg in adults *or* <5 percentile for age in children

and

  B. Two of the following signs
    1. Renal impairment, creatinine >2 mg/dL for adults, or twice the upper limit of normal for age
    2. Coagulopathy: platelets <100,000/μL or signs of disseminated intravascular coagulation
    3. Hepatic involvement: alanine aminotransferase (SGPT) aspartate aminotransferase (SGOT) or total bilirubin levels twice the upper limit of normal for age
    4. Adult respiratory distress syndrome
    5. A generalized erythematous macular rash that may desquamate
    6. Soft tissue necrosis, including necrotizing fasciitis or myositis, or gangrene

[1] An illness fulfilling criteria IA and II (A and B) can be defined as a definite case. An illness fulfilling criteria IB and II (A and B) can be defined as a probable case if no other cause for the illness is identified.

From Committee on Infectious Disease, American Academy of Pediatrics: Severe Invasive group A streptococcal infections: a subject review. Pediatrics 1998;101:13–70.

rheumatic fever is associated with M types 3 and 18 serotypes. Unlike acute rheumatic fever, the incidence of glomerulonephritis does not appear to be reduced by treatment of GAS pharyngitis. Acute glomerulonephritis is associated with the M type 12 serotype and is discussed further in Chapter 16 (Kidneys and Electrolytes).

INFECTIONS IN THE NECK

Parotitis. Parotitis is an inflammation of the parotid salivary glands and must be distinguished from anterior cervical lymphadenopathy (see below). On physical examination, parotid swelling is usually identifiable by its location as a swelling centered above or at the angle of the jaw, often displacing the lobe of the ear. The two main causes are viral parotitis (e.g., mumps) and acute suppurative parotitis.

Viral parotitis is usually caused by the mumps virus (a paramyxovirus) but also can be due to infection with coxsackievirus group A, EBV, influenza A, lymphocytic-choriomeningitis, parainfluenza virus, and, in the case of the immunocompromised patient, CMV. With mumps, the incubation period is about 2–3 weeks after exposure. The child presents with pain and swelling of one or both parotid glands, which may develop within a few hours. The affected parotids are usually tender to palpation, and the child experiences pain with the ingestion of sour-tasting substances. On examination, the Stensen duct is erythematous, and tonsils may be displaced medially from ipsilateral swelling of the affected salivary glands. The submandibular glands also may be involved, resulting in erythema of the Wharton duct. A mild to moderate fever may be present. The swelling resolves gradually over the course of a week. Complications of mumps include meningoencephalitis, pancreatitis, oophoritis, and orchitis and epididymitis (in up to one third of adolescent and adult males). Treatment is symptomatic. Analgesics may be helpful, and diet should be adjusted to accommodate the patient's ability to chew. The worldwide vaccination program, in which a live attenuated mumps virus is used, has markedly decreased the incidence of this disease.

Although considered in the differential diagnosis of parotid swelling, acute suppurative parotitis is a far less common cause in children. Predisposing factors include conditions that decrease salivary flow such as dehydration, sialolithiasis, and certain medications. Bacterial seeding usually takes place from bacteremia or a local infection in the oral cavity. The most common organism is *S. aureus*. Other common agents include *Streptococcus pyogenes* and α-hemolytic streptococci. Patients with the infection are often toxic and febrile. The swelling is unilateral and very tender. The opening of the Stensen duct is inflamed, and pus can be expressed from the duct on gentle palpation. Complications include rupture of the parotid, with local spread of infection to the face, ear, or temporomandibular joint, and development of osteomyelitis of the mandible. If pus can be expressed from the duct, Gram-stain results may be useful to direct initial therapy. In the absence of pus, needle aspiration of the gland may be necessary for cultures. Cultures should be sent for aerobes, anaerobes, fungi, and mycobacteria. Laboratory evaluation may show an increased ESR, WBC, and serum amylase level. Therapy consists of parenteral antimicrobial agents: Initial empiric therapy should include coverage of *S. aureus,* streptococcal species, and anaerobes. Surgical drainage is sometimes required.

Enlarged lymph nodes. "Bumps in the neck," or enlarged cervical lymph nodes, are common complaints that bring children and adolescents to the pediatrician. Fortunately, most of these are self-limited or easily treatable. It is the task of the physician to determine when such complaints suggest a more serious etiology and warrant further investigation. The most common causes of neck swelling in children are listed in Table 9–25. In addition to a variety of infectious and infiltrative etiologies, certain congenital lesions may present as an acutely enlarged neck mass.

Table 9–25. Most Common Causes of Neck Swelling

Infectious etiologies
Regional lymphadenopathy
Bacteria
Reactive lymphadenopathy
Staphylococcus aureus
Group A β-hemolytic *Streptococcus*
Bartonella henselae (cat scratch disease)
Mycobacterium tuberculosis
Mycobacterium avium-intracellulare
Viruses
EBV
CMV
HSV
Adenovirus
Parasitic/fungal/other
Toxoplasma gondi
Kawasaki syndrome
Coccidiomycosis
Kikuchi disease
Generalized lymphadenopathy
HIV
EBV
CMV
Rubeola
Noninfectious etiologies
Tumors: e.g., lymphoma, other malignancies, cystic hygroma
Congenital cysts: e.g., branchial cleft cyst, thyroglossal duct cyst
Parotid swelling
Storage disorders

CMV = cytomegalovirus; EBV = Epstein–Barr virus; HIV = human immunodeficiency virus; HSV = herpes simplex virus.

Such lesions include branchial cleft cyst, cystic hygroma, thyroglossal duct cyst, and dermoid cyst.

Clinical approach: history & physical examination. To identify abnormalities, physicians first must have an understanding of the characteristics of normal lymph nodes in children. Compared with adults, children have larger, more easily palpable, lymph nodes. Further, children's lymph nodes typically mount a more exaggerated response to infection and other inflammatory stimuli. Normally palpated lymph nodes occur in the cervical, inguinal, and, occasionally, axillary regions: They usually are smaller than 1–2 cm in diameter. Lymph nodes found in the occipital, pre- or postauricular, supraclavicular, epitrochlear, and popliteal areas are usually abnormal and indicate some intrinsic or adjacent inflammatory process. Further, lymph nodes larger than 2 cm are generally indicative of a pathologic process.

When evaluating a patient with lymphadenopathy, it is important to consider whether the lymph node is isolated or part of generalized lymphadenopathy. Generalized lymphadenopathy, enlarged lymph nodes in multiple locations, is usually a response to a systemic process involving the reticuloendothelial system and may be associated with liver and spleen enlargement. Enlargement of an isolated lymph node is frequently a local response to a nearby infection (e.g., *M. tuberculosis*) or due to an infiltrative process such as lymphoma.

A detailed and complete medical and social history is an essential part of the workup of a child presenting with enlarged lymph nodes. Historical clues are often critical to making the diagnosis in cases of lymphadenopathy caused by *M. tuberculosis, B. melitensis, B. henselae, Toxoplasma gondii, Francisella tularensis,* and HIV. The review of systems should focus on overall health, fever, night sweats, weight loss, upper respiratory symptoms, cough, sore throat, rashes, and bone pain. Recent dental work or a history of dental pain may implicate an occult dental abscess with lymphatic drainage.

A history of potentially relevant exposures also should be pursued, including ill contacts, pets, unpasteurized milk, and farm animals (Table 9–26). A detailed travel history may hold important clues to the diagnosis (e.g., coccidiomycosis, histoplasmosis, or tuberculosis).

The physical examination can help to narrow the differential diagnosis When the adenopathy is associated with prolonged fever, conjunctivitis, mucous membrane erythema, and rash, Kawasaki disease should be considered. When exudative pharyngitis is present, reactive lymphadenopathy secondary to infection with EBV, CMV, adenovirus, or *S. pyogenes* is likely. Isolated conjunctival injection associated with cervical adenopathy has been described in the oculoglandular form of tularemia and the Parinaud oculoglandular syndrome. The presence of a rash suggests the diagnosis of a generalized viral process such as measles, varicella, or rubella. When abdominal examination reveals hepatosplenomegaly, the lymphadenopathy may be due to a systemic process such as EBV, CMV, HIV, or malignant neoplasm. If the history is consistent, more unusual etiologies, such as brucellosis, should be considered.

Involvement of specific lymph nodes may help guide the diagnosis. Occipital and posterior auricular nodes are enlarged in rubella; occipital nodes may be enlarged in an infection with tinea capitis. Axillary and cervical lymphadenopathy are commonly involved in cat-scratch disease. Knowledge of the body's lymphatic drainage can be helpful in identifying a source for lymph node enlargement. Epitrochlear nodes drain the ulnar side of the hand and forearm. Inguinal nodes drain the lower extremities and the genital regions.

Specific etiologies. The most common cause of enlarged lymph nodes is **reactive lymphadenopathy,** which is secondary to a systemic or local infection. Lymphadenopathy in the anterior cervical region most frequently is a reaction to pharyngitis, otitis media, or a viral URI. These lymph nodes can be quite enlarged and tender but usually have no overlying erythema and are not fluctuant. If cultured, these lymph nodes would be sterile, histologically showing an infiltration of benign lymphocytes. The lymph nodes are usually multiple and will shrink over the course of the illness. In general, the nodes themselves require no diagnostic intervention.

Occasionally, one of these lymph nodes may become more tender and develop overlying erythema with or without fluctuance. In these cases, the involved node has become superinfected and is termed **cervical adenitis.** The most common pathogens are *S. pyogenes* and *S aureus.* These usually respond to warm soaks and oral antibiotics. The antibiotic chosen should cover the pathogens (e.g., a first-generation cephalosporin or an antistaphylococcal penicillin). Occasionally, oral antibiotics are unsuccessful and IV antibiotics are needed. This is usually indicative of the formation of an abscess. The choice of IV antibiotics should mirror the oral antibiotics mentioned. If there is no response in 48 hours to the administration of parenteral therapy, a surgeon should be consulted for incision and drainage.

Although gram-positive bacteria are the most commonly encountered organisms in cervical adenitis, others pathogens should be considered. Cervical adenitis caused by *M. tuberculosis* is referred to as *scrofula.* It frequently presents as a nontender, mobile, unilateral cervical lymph node. Placement of a PPD is mandatory in any workup of cervical lymphadenitis. If scrofula is diagnosed, treatment involves antituberculous chemotherapy and surgical excision. A diligent search for the source case should be undertaken. Compared to *M. tuberculosis,* nontuberculous mycobacterial infection of cervical lymph nodes is by far the more common cause of lymphadenopathy. This usually occurs in younger children (generally younger than 5 years). The enlarged nodes usually are unilateral and can be of significant size. The overlying skin is frequently erythematous, with a bluish hue. As

Table 9–26. Historical Clues to Diagnosis of Infectious Lymphadenopathy

Exposure	Etiologic Organisms
Kitten	*Bartonella henselae*
	Toxoplasma gondii
Raw milk	*Brucella* species
Rabbits	*Francisella tularensis*
Rats/mice	*Streptobacillus moniliformis, Spirillum minus*
	Leptospirosis

with tuberculous adenitis, these nodes are nontender. A minimally reactive PPD may be present. Definitive diagnosis is made surgically, and treatment ideally involves complete surgical excision, not chemotherapy.

Cat-scratch disease is a very common cause of chronic lymphadenitis in children. The organism responsible is *Bartonella henselae,* a small pleomorphic gram-negative bacillus. Cat-scratch disease typically presents as an enlarging nontender lymph node, frequently located in the cervical, axillary, or inguinal regions. After the scratch of a kitten, a papule develops at the site, followed by enlargement of the lymph node draining the involved area within 2–3 weeks. Needle biopsy has been reported to create sinus tracts that are difficult to treat and thus should be avoided. If the node is removed surgically, a Warthin–Starry stain will reveal the bacillus. Diagnosis is best made by serology, which is now commercially available. The disease is self-limited and requires no intervention. The enlarged nodes usually resolve within a few months. However, the node may eventually suppurate. Although antibiotics are generally not effective and not needed, some previous reports have reported that trimethoprim-sulfamethoxazole may be useful.

Kikuchi disease, or histiocytic necrotizing lymphadenitis, should be considered in patients with chronic lymphadenitis. This syndrome is characterized by cervical lymph node swelling, tenderness, fever, and night sweats. It occurs more commonly in females and is diagnosed on the basis of an excisional biopsy. The etiology is idiopathic, but the disease is generally self-limited.

Laboratory evaluation. The workup of a child or adolescent presenting with an enlarged lymph node or group of lymph nodes should proceed in a stepwise fashion and be directed by pertinent findings in the history and physical examination. Empiric therapy with antibiotics is appropriate if the node appears to be superinfected. If, after antibiotic treatment, the node persists or continues to enlarge, a more thorough workup should be done to rule out less common causes of lymphadenopathy. Serologic testing for cat-scratch disease, EBV, HIV, and toxoplasmosis should be performed if the history is compatible. A chest radiograph is frequently indicated to evaluate for mediastinal adenopathy and pulmonary nodules. Regardless of exposure history, a PPD should be placed to identify mycobacterial infection. Other unusual etiologies need to be considered, such as fungal pathogens (e.g., *H. capsulatum, Aspergillus* species, and *C. neoformans*) and less commonly encountered bacteria (e.g., *Yersinia, Actinomyces,* and oral anaerobes such as *Peptostreptococcus*). The possibility of a noninfectious etiology such as lymphoma, Langerhans cell histiocytosis, and metastatic tumor should be explored, especially if the enlarged node is accompanied by systemic symptoms such as fever and weight loss. Diagnosis of these entities generally requires

tissue. Indications for lymph node biopsy are presented in Table 9–27.

Respiratory Infections

Respiratory infections can be classified according to their area of primary involvement, in the upper, middle, and lower airway, each of which is associated with a characteristic set of symptoms. In early childhood, infections of the respiratory tract are due most often to viruses, followed by bacteria. These common complaints usually begin after the first few months of life, when the protective immunoglobulin acquired transplacentally from the mother begins to wane. Thereafter, the child undergoes natural immunization with each new respiratory infection. It is not uncommon for a young child to have six to eight upper respiratory infections per year. The most common infections are associated with nasal congestion and rhinorrhea. These include simple URIs, sinusitis, and otitis media.

UPPER RESPIRATORY TRACT INFECTIONS

The common cold. The common cold is a minor illness that is a major nuisance to children, parents, daycare providers, health care workers, and much of society. Colds are important not so much for their severity as for their frequency. The Public Health Service has reported that half the population experiences a cold during a single winter season. Children, especially preschool-aged children, are prone to developing recurrent colds. Attendance in day care contributes to this high frequency through increased exposure to potential pathogens. The high prevalence of the common cold generates enormous health care and non–health care expenditures. Colds are responsible for more missed school and work than any other illness in the United States, with estimates near 50 million days per year. In addition to absenteeism, colds generate health care costs related to physician visits and the use of prescription and nonprescription medications.

Pathogenesis & etiology. Transmission of viruses that cause URIs is believed to occur primarily through direct (sneezing, hand-to-nose) or indirect (fomites) con-

Table 9–27. Indications for Biopsy of a Lymph Node

Persistent enlargement despite empiric therapy
Persistent enlargement or no improvement with negative workup results
Solid fixed mass
Mass located in supraclavicular area
Accompanying constitutional signs of persistent fever, weight loss

tact with nasal secretions. Children literally pick up cold viruses from school or day care and bring them home to other family members. Inoculation with a virus is followed by invasion of the respiratory epithelium lining the nasopharynx, sinuses, and upper respiratory tract. The typical incubation period is 2–5 days. Viral replication results in cholinergic stimulation, direct cellular damage, and the release of inflammatory mediators and cytokines. These events produce changes in vascular permeability, mucosal edema, and mucus production. Numerous viruses are responsible for producing symptoms of the common cold. Rhinovirus and its many serotypes are the most commonly identified agent, representing approximately one third of all cases. Other viral causes are parainfluenza, RSV, coronavirus, adenovirus, and influenza virus.

Clinical manifestations. The principal symptoms associated with a URI are nasal congestion and rhinorrhea. Fever, sore throat, sneezing, cough, and hoarseness may be associated. The symptoms usually last for approximately 1 week, although there is considerable variation in duration. The diagnosis of the common cold is made by history and physical examination. Because of the generally mild and self-limited nature of the disease, specific diagnostic evaluations are rarely warranted. A variety of viral culture and antigen techniques are available in specialized circumstances (e.g., RSV). Medical complications of the common cold include otitis media, sinusitis, and exacerbation of reactive airway diseases (asthma).

Treatment. Currently, the most effective management for URIs is education. Parents should be given information regarding the natural course of the infection, including the expected duration of illness, and the signs and symptoms that would require physician evaluation or reevaluation. Families also should be instructed on methods to limit transmission (e.g., hand-washing) of cold viruses. Many therapies have been advocated to prevent or treat the common cold. Humidification, hydration, saline nose drops, and bulb suctioning of the nostrils may loosen nasal secretions and provide temporary relief in some patients. In addition, many families use a range of traditional OTC preparations and alternative and folk medicines for treating colds. Alternative therapies include herbs and teas, chicken noodle soup, vitamin C, and homeopathic medicines. In the United States, the market for OTC cold preparations produces $2 billion in annual sales. The frequent use of these products necessitates that physicians familiarize themselves with their ingredients. Despite the hundreds of preparations available, there are only four types of active ingredients in typical OTC cold medications: antihistamines, decongestants, expectorants, and cough suppressants.

The mechanisms of action of these compounds are often theoretical, and their clinical effects in children are primarily speculative and anecdotal. Many OTC preparations contain combinations of these four ingredients, and some contain additional active ingredients such as antipyretics and analgesics (e.g., acetaminophen, ibuprofen). Antihistamines (e.g., diphenhydramine, brompheniramine, chlorpheniramine) block H-1 receptors and may produce some anticholinergic effects. Although histamine has no demonstrated role in the pathophysiology of the common cold, anticholinergic effects of the antihistamines theoretically may reduce mucous secretion. Decongestants (e.g., phenylephrine, phenylpropanolamine, pseudoephedrine) are sympathomimetics that can produce vasoconstriction through α-adrenergic stimulation. Vasoconstriction may reduce mucous-membrane swelling and mucous secretion. Expectorants (e.g., guaifenesin) have been suggested to act by thinning respiratory tract secretions. Cough suppressants (e.g., codeine, dextromethorphan) may act on the medullary cough center to reduce cough.

Despite their widespread use, it is unclear whether any of the cold or cough medication ingredients, individually or in combination, is effective in providing relief from common cold symptoms in children. There is little, if any, scientific data in the pediatric literature to support their use. In addition, cough and cold preparations have the risk of adverse effects (e.g., sedation, respiratory depression, sleeplessness, agitation, hypertension, tachycardia, mucus plugging). Prolonged use of topical nasal decongestants can produce rebound congestion secondary to local irritation or ischemia. Because of the frequency with which these compounds are found in homes, they are commonly involved in intentional and unintentional drug poisonings. Families should be educated on the use and misuse of these preparations. Attention should be paid to appropriate indications, dosing (age and weight dependent), and potential adverse effects. Currently, antibiotics, antiviral, and antiinflammatory agents have no role in the therapy of the common cold in children. Despite a flurry of interest in vitamin C for the prevention and therapy of the common cold, little scientific evidence supports its use. Researchers have reported some success with intranasal α_2-interferon in preventing colds due to rhinovirus; however, general use of the cytokine for the common cold is not indicated at present. Other agents under investigation are anticholinergic agents and antiinflammatory agents (e.g., corticosteroids and nonsteroidal antiinflammatory medications).

Ear pain. Ear aches are one of the most frequent presenting complaints to the primary care physician. Although infectious causes predominate, other conditions can produce direct or referred pain in this area. Among those are foreign bodies, local trauma, and temporomandibular joint pain. A host of infectious processes of the ear and nearby structures can present with ear ache: otitis media, otitis externa, myringitis, mastoiditis, cervical lymphadenitis, folliculitis, furunculosis, and cellulitis of the outer ear structures. The following discussion focuses on two of the most common of these conditions: otitis externa and acute otitis media.

Otitis externa. Otitis externa refers to an inflammatory process involving the external ear structures including the external auditory canal and auricle. An intact epithelial lining and acid pH normally contribute to the local defense of the external auditory canal. The pathophysiology of otitis externa centers primarily on alterations in those local defenses and in some cases on systemic host immunity. High humidity, frequent or prolonged water immersion ("swimmer's ear"), local trauma, or underlying dermatitis can compromise local defenses and lead to infection and inflammation of the external ear. *Pseudomonas aeruginosa* and *S. aureus* are common bacterial isolates associated with otitis externa. Streptococci, mycoplasma, and fungi (e.g., *Candida* species) are found less commonly. The primary symptom of otitis externa is ear pain. Ear discharge (otorrhea) might occur. Systemic signs such as fever are uncommon. The history and physical examination usually are sufficient to make the diagnosis of otitis externa. The hallmark of this condition is pain with manipulation of the external auricle or pressure on the tragus. This pain results from stretching of the inflamed auditory canal. Otoscopy reveals erythema, edema, and exudate in the auditory canal. Laboratory evaluation, such as cultures, may be indicated in unusually severe cases or treatment failures. Otitis media with perforation of the tympanic membrane also can produce ear pain and otorrhea.

Treatment of otitis externa consists of topical drops containing a combination of antibiotic and steroid ingredients (e.g., Cortisporin otic suspension, which contains neomycin, polymyxin B, and hydrocortisone). Prevention of recurrent episodes of otitis externa involves avoidance of precipitating factors (e.g., swimming, local trauma from cotton swabs) and/or prophylaxis therapy. Prophylaxis with topical solutions containing alcohol or preparations of boric or acetic acid have been used. These compounds act by sterilizing the auditory canal and restoring the normally acid pH.

Acute otitis media. Otitis media refers to inflammation of the middle ear. In fact, otitis media represents a spectrum of acute and chronic diseases (Table 9–28). Otitis media is one of the most frequent diagnoses made in children younger than 15 years. The National Center for Health Statistics reported 24.5 million office visits for otitis media in the United States in 1990. In a large study from Boston (Teele, 1989), more than 80% of children had episodes of otitis media by age 3 years. Nearly half of the same group (46%) had three or more ear infections. Otitis media produces short-term costs related to physician visits, antibiotic prescriptions, school absenteeism, and work loss by parents. It is the most common reason that antibiotics are prescribed to children. Long-term costs associated with otitis media include the need for placement of myringotomy tubes, hearing evaluations, and therapy for secondary speech and language problems. In addition, the development of bacterial antibiotic resistance caused by the routine administration of antibiotics is of increasing concern throughout the world.

Certain factors are associated with increased risk of recurrent otitis media. These are young age at first ear infection, male sex, family history of recurrent ear infections, participation in day care, and exposure to cigarette smoke. Individuals of Native American or Eskimo ancestry and individuals with cleft palate or Down syndrome may be particularly susceptible to severe or persistent otitis media. In contrast, there are data showing

Table 9–28. Spectrum of Middle Ear Infections

	Description	Otoscopy	Tympanometry Compliance	Pressure[1]
Otitis media without effusion	E.g., myringitis	Erythematous, opaque TM; bullae may be present	Normal	+
Acute otitis media (suppurative otitis media, purulent otitis media)	Implies rapid onset of local and/or systemic illness	Erythematous, opaque, bulging TM	Decreased	+
Otitis media with effusion (secretory, serous, or non-suppurative otitis media)	Implies presence of effusion in an asymptomatic patient	Translucent or opaque TM; bubbles or air fluid levels may be seen	Decreased	+ or −

[1] Implies positive or negative pressure within the middle ear space relative to atmospheric pressure.
TM = tympanic membrane.

that breast feeding protects against the development of ear infections.

Pathogenesis. The middle ear is an air-filled cavity lined by respiratory mucosa and connected to the nasopharynx via the eustachian tube. The intact eustachian tube maintains aeration and allows drainage of the middle ear. Conditions that produce inflammation and swelling in the nasopharynx (e.g., common cold, allergies) cause dysfunction and obstruction of the eustachian tube. Obstruction and the development of negative pressure within the middle ear allow fluid to accumulate. In infants and young children, the narrower, shorter, and more horizontal orientation of the eustachian tube contributes to more frequent obstruction. Bacteria colonizing the nasopharynx can reflux into the fluid-filled middle ear space. The proliferation of bacteria and the resultant host inflammatory response produce the signs and symptoms of acute otitis media.

The most common organism isolated in otitis media is *S. pneumoniae,* followed by *H. influenzae* and *M. catarrhalis* (Table 9–29). Most of the *H. influenzae* are nontypable strains. Although a respiratory virus (e.g., RSV, rhinovirus, adenovirus, parainfluenza virus) may be a frequent inciting event in otitis media, isolation of virus without bacterial coinfection has been reported in fewer than 10% of cases.

Clinical manifestations. Classically, the child with acute otitis media presents with the history of a prodromal viral URI followed by the development of ear pain (otalgia) or pulling on the ear. Fever, increased irritability, and anorexia are common and may be the only indicators of acute otitis media in infants. Parents often bring their children to the pediatrician with concerns over worsening cold symptoms (e.g., new onset fever), increased night–awakening, or fussiness. Otorrhea can occur from perforation of the tympanic membrane after the buildup of inflammatory material within the middle ear.

Diagnosis. The diagnosis of acute otitis media can be strongly suspected based on the clinical history (e.g., ear ache, worsening common cold symptoms). Direct visualization of the tympanic membrane with otoscopy can confirm the diagnosis. It is crucial for students of pediatrics to be familiar with the normal landmarks (e.g., color, location of the malleus, cone of light, and neutral position of the tympanic membrane) to recognize pathologic changes. In acute otitis media, the tympanic membrane may appear erythematous, opaque, and bulging or retracted. The light reflex or normal cone of light may be diminished or absent. Yellowish white fluid and air–fluid levels may be visualized. If perforation of the tympanic membrane has occurred, purulent exudate can be seen in the external auditory canal.

Pneumatic otoscopy and tympanometry are techniques that can be used to detect changes in compliance of the tympanic membrane (Table 9–28). Compliance of the tympanic membrane is reduced by the presence of fluid in the middle ear space or significant retraction (increased or decreased pressure in the middle ear). Medical instruments that can perform tympanometry are available in many pediatric offices. In addition to measuring compliance, the tympanogram can measure volume of the external auditory canal. The external canal volume is increased dramatically by a perforated tympanic membrane or patent ventilating tube. This result reflects the combined measurement of canal and middle ear spaces.

Treatment. At present, antibiotics are the treatment of choice for acute otitis media in the United States. In most cases, treatment is empiric, and the selection of antibiotics is based on coverage of the typical upper respiratory pathogens. Recently, there has been renewed interest in tympanocentesis, a technique used to remove fluid from the middle ear by puncturing the tympanic membrane. Tympanocentesis can provide symptomatic relief by reducing pressure buildup in the middle ear and allow fluid to be collected for culture and antibiotic sensitivities. Tympanocentesis has been recommended in treatment failures to help in appropriate selection of antibiotics.

Additional factors that influence antibiotic selection are cost, availability of an oral suspension for younger children, palatability (i.e., taste), and dosing frequency. Amoxicillin has long been the initial drug of choice. The factor that determines whether amoxicillin will continue to be first-line therapy is bacterial antibiotic resistance. A high proportion of bacteria such as *H. influenzae* and *M. catarrhalis* produce β-lactamase, an enzyme capable of degrading penicillins. Also, in recent years, the prevalence of penicillin-resistant *S. pneumoniae* (through alterations in penicillin-binding sites) has increased significantly. As a result, a panel from the Centers for Disease Control has recommended using high dose amoxicillin (80–90 mg/kg) rather than the usual dosage (40–50 mg/kg) in individuals at high risk for acquiring penicillin-resistant *S. pneumoniae.* High dose amoxicillin can overcome intermediate-resistant *S. pneumoniae.* Risk

Table 9–29. Etiology of Acute Otitis Media

Organisms	% Infections[1]	β-Lactamase Producing (%)
Streptococcus pneumoniae	38	None[2]
Haemophilus influenzae (nontypable)	27	20–40[3]
Moraxella catarrhalis	10	>90[3]

[1] Barnett 1995.
[2] Resistance of *S. pneumoniae* mediated by alterations in penicillin-binding proteins.
[3] Bluestone and Klein 1995.

groups for resistant *S. pneumoniae* include children attending day care, children with recurrent otitis media, and recent antibiotic use. With the emergence of resistant *S. pneumoniae,* recommendations regarding the prophylactic use of antibiotics to decrease the incidence of acute otitis media have been tempered to minimize selection pressure favoring resistant organisms.

Second-line antibiotics include a variety of penicillin, erythromycin/sulfa, and cephalosporin-type antibiotics. The possibility of β-lactamase-producing bacteria should be considered after failure of first-line therapy. Clinicians should select antibiotics with an awareness of the common agents and antibiotic resistance patterns seen in their local communities. Duration of therapy for acute otitis media is generally 7–10 days of an oral antibiotic. Shorter courses of antibiotics (5 days) have been effective in some studies. Intramuscular ceftriaxone, as a single dose or in multiple doses, also has been used successfully in treating otitis media.

It is of interest that antibiotics are not universally prescribed for acute otitis media. In the United States, antibiotics have been the standard therapy since they first became available. The introduction of antibiotic therapy has coincided with a dramatic decrease in complications of otitis media, most noticeably mastoiditis. However, other countries, such as the Netherlands, have reported low rates of mastoiditis despite not routinely treating acute otitis media with antibiotics. Although the explanation for these differences are not known, the facts are intriguing. The widespread use of antibiotics for acute otitis media is no doubt contributing to the alarming increase in the frequency of bacterial antibiotic resistance. This concern, as well as the costs and side effects of antibiotic therapy, have generated interest in the possibility of a "no-treatment" option for acute otitis media. Further clinical studies are needed to document the outcome of such an approach.

Recurrent and persistent otitis media are common problems encountered by primary care physicians. Recurrent infections typically are treated with separate courses of antibiotics. The choice of antibiotic may be the same or different depending on the interval of time separating the most recent infections. Persistent infections are managed with a change in antibiotics. Differentiation between closely spaced recurrences and persistent infections can be difficult. Diagnosing recurrent infections in this setting requires that the patient has had documented normal ear examinations between infections.

Medical management of recurrent infections primarily depends on the use of antibiotic prophylaxis. Daily administration of low dose antibiotics (commonly amoxicillin or sulfisoxazole) has been used to reduce the incidence of recurrences. Selection of appropriate patients for prophylaxis is based on the number of infections experienced in a given time frame (e.g., three to four infec-

tions within 6 months). Recommendations regarding the use of prophylaxis are currently being reevaluated because of concerns for the potential to select out resistant organisms. Systemic corticosteroids (e.g., oral prednisone) have been advocated by some in the treatment of persistent effusion. Currently, this use is controversial and these drugs should not be prescribed routinely.

Myringotomy tubes (e.g., ventilating or "pressure-equalizing" tubes) provide a surgical approach to the treatment of recurrent and persistent ear infections. Myringotomy tubes create a hole in the tympanic membrane, which prevents the accumulation of fluid in the middle ear space. These tubes essentially bypass the obstructed eustachian tube. Most myringotomy tubes spontaneously fall out in approximately 6 months. Some children need permanent myringotomy tubes, which require a second surgical procedure to be removed. National guidelines exist concerning the management of persistent middle ear effusions.

Follow-up & complications. In otitis media, pain and fever should improve within 2–3 days of appropriate therapy. If this does not occur and the patient has been compliant with the initial therapy, a treatment failure should be suspected and a change in antibiotic considered. No additional medical follow-up may be necessary in uncomplicated infections in which symptoms resolve quickly. However, it is not uncommon for primary care providers to see patients 2–6 weeks later to document clearing of the infection. Patients at risk for persistent or recurrent otitis media require more frequent follow-up to monitor resolution of infections. In addition to perforation of the tympanic membrane and mastoiditis, rare acute complications of otitis media include lateral sinus thrombosis, meningitis, and abscess formation. The long-term effects of persistent middle ear effusion include conductive hearing loss and language delay.

Acute sinusitis. The paranasal sinuses (maxillary, ethmoid, sphenoid, and frontal) are air-filled cavities lined by ciliated columnar epithelium and mucus-producing goblet cells. The coordinated action of cilia allows drainage of these spaces into the nasopharynx through a series of ostia. Developmentally, the maxillary and ethmoid sinuses are present at birth, whereas the sphenoid and frontal sinuses appear later in childhood. The actual incidence of sinusitis in the pediatric age group is unknown. However, some estimates can be made based on the frequency of viral URIs. Sinusitis is suspected to complicate URIs in 0.5–10.0% of cases, a 20-fold range. Because preschool-aged children have an average of five to eight colds per year, this could translate into almost one episode of sinusitis per child per year when using the highest estimates of 10%.

Pathogenesis & etiology. Inflammation and edema of the nasopharynx due to viral URIs or allergic rhinitis impair drainage of the sinuses. Obstruction of the sinus ostia allows the accumulation of fluid in the sinus cavity.

As in otitis media, bacteria can enter and multiply within the enclosed space of the sinuses, resulting in infection. Other conditions can impair drainage of the ostia—such as alterations in the character of mucus (e.g., cystic fibrosis), and decreases in ciliary activity (e.g., immotile cilia syndromes). The common respiratory pathogens are the typical pathogens associated with acute sinusitis: *S. pneumoniae,* nontypable *H. influenzae,* and *M. catarrhalis.* As in acute otitis media, respiratory viruses (adenovirus, parainfluenza virus, influenza virus, and rhinovirus) are believed to be responsible for a minority of the episodes of acute sinusitis.

Clinical manifestations. In children, sinusitis produces persistent symptoms of nasal congestion, nasal discharge, and cough. Wald and others defined persistent respiratory symptoms as lack of improvement by 10 days. Cough can occur day and night. The nasal discharge can be clear and colorless or appear purulent. Patients or family members may report malodorous breath and painless, periorbital edema occurring in the morning. The facial pain and frontal headache commonly described by adults are uncommon complaints in children with sinusitis. Sinusitis also may produce more severe symptoms marked by high fever (temperature >39°C) and purulent nasal discharge. In cases with severe symptoms, it may be appropriate to initiate treatment before symptoms have persisted for 10 days.

Diagnosis. The diagnosis of sinusitis in children often is made primarily on the basis of history and physical examination. The differential diagnosis of sinusitis includes recurrent viral upper respiratory infections, nasal allergies (allergic rhinitis), and, rarely, nasal foreign bodies. In contrast to bacterial sinusitis, the common cold is expected to show significant improvement over 7–10 days. Unfortunately, some children, especially those in day care, experience frequent viral URIs—one cold may be resolving just as another is beginning. To parents, the symptoms may seem persistent. In these cases, a history of waxing and waning symptoms is helpful but may be difficult to elicit. Children with allergic rhinitis may have a history of atopic disease (e.g., eczema, asthma), nasal itching, sneezing, and a seasonal occurrence. A history of drainage from one nostril suggests a mechanical cause such as a foreign body.

On physical examination, the nasal mucosa appears erythematous and swollen, although this may be seen in viral URI and sinusitis. There also may be copious nasal discharge and halitosis. In contrast, the mucosa may be pale and boggy in allergic rhinitis. The presence of allergic shiners, allergic nasal crease, and Dennie lines also can support the diagnosis of atopic disease. Palpation over the sinuses (ethmoid, maxillary, and, in older children, the frontal sinuses) may produce tenderness, although this is an unusual finding in pediatric sinusitis. As a diagnostic test, some experts have recommended transillumination of the maxillary sinuses in older children (>10 years). In

this technique, the room is darkened and a light source is placed on one of the patient's inferior orbital rims. The patient is asked to open his/her mouth and the amount of light transmitted through the palate is assessed. The procedure is repeated over the contralateral sinus. If the light transmitted is markedly diminished on one side, it suggests opacification of the maxillary sinus on that side.

Traditional plain film sinus series (three views: anteroposterior, lateral, and occipitomental) or CT have been used in the radiologic diagnosis of sinusitis. Both studies demonstrate opacification, mucosal thickening (>4 mm), and the presence of air–fluid levels within the sinuses. Unfortunately, the specificity and sensitivity of these findings in diagnosing bacterial sinusitis have been questioned. Healthy individuals and those with common cold symptoms can have mucosal thickening and air–fluid levels. In practice, radiologic imaging (preferably CT) may be indicated in more severe or persistent cases. Aspiration of the maxillary sinuses is the gold standard for diagnosing acute bacterial sinusitis. This procedure allows documentation of infected sinus fluid with cultures and sensitivities. However, it is an invasive procedure, requiring referral to an otolaryngologist. It is usually reserved for severe or atypical cases and treatment failures.

Treatment. The treatment of sinusitis centers on antibiotic therapy. The agents chosen are similar to those used to treat other respiratory infections, including otitis media. The prevalence of resistant organisms should be considered. As in otitis media, amoxicillin often is considered the initial antibiotic of choice. Second-line agents, including amoxicillin-clavulanate (Augmentin), erythromycin ethylsuccinate-sulfisoxazole (Pediazole), and cephalosporins may be indicated in areas with high rates of β-lactamase-producing organisms or in patients with complicated disease or treatment failures. Symptoms should improve within 2–3 days of appropriate antibiotic therapy. The duration of therapy depends in part on the individual patient's rate of clinical response. Children who respond rapidly to antibiotics may need shorter courses, whereas slow responders may benefit from a longer duration of therapy. Typical regimens vary from 10 to 21 days. Antibiotics are often continued for 7 days after the resolution of symptoms in patients who have had a slow response to antibiotics. Additional medical therapies such as decongestants, antihistamines, and nasal corticosteroids have not been proven to be effective in children with sinusitis.

MIDDLE RESPIRATORY TRACT INFECTIONS: FEVER & STRIDOR

Because of the potentially life-threatening nature of stridor, patients presenting with this complaint warrant careful evaluation and follow-up.

Differential diagnosis. The causes of stridor are listed in Table 9–30. Although these etiologies are quite diverse, all lead to a fixed or functional obstruction and

Table 9–30. Causes of Respiratory Stridor

Extrinsic airway compression and narrowing
  Malformations/syndromes
    Macroglossia (Beckwith syndrome)
    Craniofacial anomalies (e.g., Pierre–Robin syndrome)
    Neurologic disorders with poor tongue and oromotor tone
    Aberrant vascular structures (e.g., double aortic arch, aberrant right subclavian artery, pulmonary sling)
  Masses
    Enlarged lymph nodes
    Enlarged tonsils
    Hemangiomas
    Cysts: e.g., thyroglossal duct cyst
    Tumors: e.g., thyroid, thymus, cystic hygroma
    Hematoma
  Trauma
    Neck and chest injury
  Infection
    Tonsillitis
    Peritonsilar abscess
    Retropharyngeal abscess
    Diphtheria

Intrinsic airway narrowing and/or collapse
  Malformations
    Laryngotracheomalacia
    Tracheoesophageal fistula
    Subglottic webs, cysts, laryngocele, stenosis
  Masses
    Foreign body in the airway
    Laryngeal polyps or papillomatosis
  Trauma
    Intubation
    Burns
    Neck injury
  Infection
    Tracheitis, bacterial
    Epiglottitis
    Croup
    Diphtheria
  Other
    Allergic reaction: e.g., anaphylaxis, angioneurotic edema
    Vocal cord paralysis
    Laryngospasm

narrowing and/or compression of the airway in the regions of the pharynx, larynx, and trachea. Infectious etiologies include croup (or laryngotracheitis), epiglottitis, bacterial tracheitis, diphtheria, peritonsillar abscess, and retropharyngeal cellulitis or abscess. The following discussion focuses on viral croup, bacterial tracheitis, epiglottitis, and diphtheria. Table 9–31 presents clinical features that characterize and distinguish the most common of these infectious disorders. Peritonsillar and retropharyngeal abscess are discussed under the section on Sore Throat or Mouth.

Viral croup (acute laryngotracheitis). Croup occurs as the result of inflammation in the subglottic area. Inflammatory edema and swelling reduce the caliber of the trachea. Croup is a relatively common childhood illness and is diagnosed most frequently in children aged 1–2 years. Boys are affected more frequently than girls (ratio of 3:2). The seasonal occurrence of croup mirrors the appearance of respiratory viral infections during fall and winter. Parainfluenza virus types 1, 2, and 3 account for up to 75% of all documented cases of croup. Respiratory syncytial virus and influenza virus (types A and B) are the next most frequent causes. Other viruses, including measles, can cause croup. The typical case begins with symptoms of a viral upper respiratory infection (e.g., rhinorrhea and fever). Hours to days later, symptoms of upper airway obstruction develop. The hallmarks of croup are hoarseness, a "barking" or "croupy" cough, and inspiratory stridor. The amount of respiratory distress can range from mild to severe, depending on the degree of airway narrowing. Although most patients with croup are probably managed at home, croup can cause life-threatening respiratory obstruction. Of note, attempts have been made to distinguish between viral croup and **spasmodic croup.** Spasmodic croup probably lies along a spectrum of illness with viral croup. In addition to viral infection, allergy and muscle spasm have been postulated to cause spasmodic croup. Unlike viral croup, episodes of spasmodic croup are not accompanied by fever or viral URI symptoms. Barking cough and stridor occur primarily at night and recur for several nights. Repeated episodes of spasmodic croup are not uncommon and may represent an element of upper airway hypersensitivity.

The diagnosis of viral croup is based primarily on findings in the history and physical examination. Viral studies (e.g., cultures, antigen detection, serology) do not aid in the management of typical cases and are generally not indicated. An anteroposterior radiograph of the neck will demonstrate a tapering subglottic narrowing that resembles a church steeple ("steeple sign"). However, like viral studies, a radiograph usually is not necessary to diagnose typical cases of viral croup.

The therapy for croup depends on the severity of clinical findings. Standard treatments include humidified air, corticosteroids, and inhaled racemic epinephrine. Humidified air (e.g., by baths, showers, croup kettles, and croup tents) has long been the mainstay of therapy despite only anecdotal evidence supporting its use. The loosening of secretions, reduction of irritation, and effect on laryngeal receptors have been proposed as mechanisms of action. Mist therapy is often considered reasonable if it does not interfere with observation of the patient or result in increased agitation. Corticosteroids have been used in

Table 9–31. Comparison of Infectious Causes of Stridor

	Croup	Bacterial Tracheitis	Epiglottitis
Age	Infant to preschool	Infant to preschool	Older infant to preschool
Prodrome	Viral URI	Viral URI	Usually none
Toxicity	Variable mild to severe	Severe	Severe
Drooling	No	Yes or no	Yes
Microbiology	Viral, ? role of allergy in spasmodic croup	*Staphylococcus aureus*	*Haemophilus influenzae* type b
Radiographic findings	Subglottic narrowing ("steeple sign" on AP), dilated hypopharynx, air trapping	Subglottic narrowing, irregular tracheal margin, intratracheal membranes	"Thumb" sign, thickened aryepiglottic folds
Treatment	Variable depending on severity (see text)	Artificial airway, antibiotics	Artificial airway, antibiotics

AP = anteroposterior view; URI = upper respiratory infection.

the treatment of viral croup for more than 40 years. A meta-analysis of nine randomized studies has reported fewer intubations and greater clinical improvement at 12 and 24 hours after treatment with corticosteroids when compared with controls. The mechanism of action may be through effects on local inflammation, capillary permeability, and host allergic responses. The choice of corticosteroid and the dose, route (oral, parenteral, or inhaled), and duration of therapy have varied from study to study. Traditionally, corticosteroids had been reserved for patients ill enough to be hospitalized. In recent years, there has been increasing evidence for its use as an outpatient therapy.

Inhaled racemic epinephrine (via nebulizer or intermittent positive pressure breathing) has been used in the treatment of croup for more than 30 years. Although racemic epinephrine (equal quantities of levorotatory and dextrorotatory isomers) is the compound that has been used primarily, there is evidence to suggest that L-epinephrine may be equally effective. The α-adrenergic action of epinephrine is believed to result in vasoconstriction and the reduction of edema in the subglottic area. Onset of action is rapid (10–30 minutes), and duration of activity is short (2 hours). In the past, it had been recommended that all patients who received racemic epinephrine should be hospitalized because of the short duration of activity and the risk of rebound swelling. Recently, combination therapy with racemic epinephrine and corticosteroids has been used successfully in the outpatient treatment of croup.

Epiglottitis (supraglottitis). Epiglottitis (or supraglottitis) is characterized by inflammation of the epiglottis and adjacent structures including the aryepiglottic folds. The incidence of epiglottitis has decreased dramatically since the early 1990s, when universal immunization of infants against HIB infection was instituted. Before the

availability of *Hemophilus* flu vaccines (HIB), most cases of epiglotitis were due to this organism. Most cases occurred in children 1–5 years old, with a slight preponderance in boys. In a significant percentage of cases, primary infection of the epiglottis is followed by bacteremia. Other etiologic organisms identified less commonly are *S. pneumoniae, H. parainfluenza,* and *S. aureus.* Epiglottitis presents with the acute onset of fever, toxicity, and respiratory distress. Typically, patients are brought to the hospital within hours of becoming ill. Although viral URI symptoms may precede some cases, the progression of illness is more rapid than that seen in viral croup or bacterial tracheitis. Cough is usually absent. Apprehension, dysphagia, drooling, respiratory distress, and toxicity are the prominent signs. Children with epiglottitis typically resist lying down. In the classic "tripoding" posture of epiglottis, the child prefers to sit upright with arms back and neck extended to maximize airway caliber.

When the diagnosis of epiglottitis is suspected, care must be taken not to agitate the patient and precipitate airway obstruction. Procedures that are uncomfortable or that will delay therapy should be withheld. These procedures include examination of the pharynx with a tongue depressor, laboratory testing (e.g., WBC, blood culture, antigen assays), and radiographs. Patients should be allowed to sit in a position of comfort. Lateral radiographs of the neck demonstrate a swollen epiglottis (the thumb sign) and thickened aryepiglottic folds. The management of epiglottitis is directed at stabilizing and maintaining the airway through intubation or tracheostomy. Epiglottitis often progresses quickly to complete airway obstruction. Anesthesia and otolaryngology services should be consulted, and emergency procedures such as intubation or tracheostomy should be readily available, if the need arises.

Antimicrobial therapy must include coverage for *H. influenzae,* usually a third-generation cephalosporin or ampicillin plus chloramphenicol. In patients fully immunized against HIB, antibiotic coverage may be expanded to cover *S. aureus* (β-lactamase-resistant penicillin or vancomycin).

Bacterial tracheitis. Infection of the upper respiratory tract (URT) by bacteria other than diphtheria was common through the early 1900s. For reasons that are unclear, reports and literature on nondiphtheritic infections of the URT disappeared over the next half-century. Then, in 1979, two separate series of children with upper airway obstruction caused by an exudative tracheitis were reported. This condition has been called bacterial tracheitis, or membranous or pseudomembranous laryngotracheobronchitis. Bacterial tracheitis is an infection of the trachea that results in narrowing of the airway by inflammatory edema and exudates. The incidence of bacterial tracheitis is much lower than that of viral croup and higher than that of epiglottis. Cases occur most frequently in preschool-aged children; boys are more commonly affected than girls. Most evidence suggests that an initial insult to the airway predisposes to bacterial infection. The most common inciting event is viral croup, although other airway injuries (e.g., endotracheal intubation) have been associated with bacterial tracheitis. Patients with Down syndrome also may be at higher risk for this condition, possibly through alterations in immunity or airway anatomy. *Staphylococcus aureus* is the major isolate from these patients. Other common respiratory pathogens (e.g., streptococcal species, *Hemophilus species,* and *M. catarrhalis*) also have been isolated. In a number of patients with bacterial tracheitis, viruses responsible for croup (e.g., parainfluenza, influenza, RSV, and measles) have been identified.

Bacterial tracheitis shares features of viral croup and epiglottitis. As the pathogenesis suggests, illness often begins with symptoms of URI and viral croup. Patients with bacterial tracheitis often have higher fever and appear more ill than in typical croup. Like epiglottitis, upper airway obstruction is severe and may develop rapidly. Bacterial tracheitis should be suspected in patients with severe or worsening croup symptoms. Little in the way of diagnostic testing is indicated. White blood cell count and blood cultures are unlikely to be of help in the acute setting. Lateral neck radiographs may show a narrowed subglottic airway, with irregular margins secondary to the inflammatory pseudomembrane. Unlike viral croup, treatment with nebulized racemic epinephrine produces no benefit in bacterial tracheitis. The definitive diagnosis of bacterial tracheitis is made during direct visualization by an otolaryngologist or anesthesiologist. Laryngoscopy can be diagnostic and therapeutic by documenting the location and severity of airway injury and allowing removal of purulent secretions.

Most patients with bacterial tracheitis require the placement of an artificial airway (e.g., endotracheal tube). Antibiotic therapy should be directed toward *S. aureus* and other respiratory pathogens.

Diphtheria. Early in the 1900s, the term *croup* was synonymous with laryngeal diphtheria. At that time, diphtheria was the leading serious infection of the larynx and infraglottic airway. Since the 1950s, immunization programs have dramatically reduced the number of cases of diphtheria. Currently, only a few cases are reported annually in the United States. Infection with *Corynebacterium diphtheriae* is characterized by a localized infection in the URT. The hallmark of the infection is a pseudomembranous lesion identified most frequently in the URT including pharynx, tonsils, uvula, and, less frequently, in the nose, larynx, and lower respiratory tract. Clinically, laryngeal diphtheria is similar to bacterial tracheitis and is notable for producing a fibrinous tracheal exudate. In most cases of diphtheria, the onset of symptoms is gradual. Patients present with a low-grade fever and sore throat, followed by dysphagia and drooling. Over 1–2 days, an exudate appears and forms a shiny, sharply outlined pseudomembrane. In fewer than 5% of patients, diphtheria of the laryngotracheal area occurs with tonsillopharyngeal involvement. Different degrees of hoarseness, stridor, and respiratory distress occur, depending on the extent and thickness of the membrane in relation to the caliber of the airway. *Corynebacterum diphtheriae* also may damage other organ systems by elaboration of a cytotoxic protein, diphtheria toxin, that interferes with protein synthesis by the host cells. Diphtheria toxin produces degenerative changes in the heart (myocarditis), liver, spleen, kidney, adrenal gland, and brain. The diagnosis can be accomplished by culturing the bacteria from lesions in the throat, nostrils, and skin using a special media. Direct staining and immunofluorescence antibody staining are not reliable. Management of the patient is targeted at neutralizing the diphtheria toxin and reducing transmission of the bacteria. Intravenous diphtheria antitoxin neutralizes circulating toxin but has no effect on the toxin that is bound to tissue. It should be administered as soon as possible after onset of disease and before the availability of culture results. Antibiotics, including penicillin or erythromycin, are indicated to render the patient noncontagious. Adjunctive treatment, including airway and cardiovascular supports, should be initiated as needed.

Clinical approach to the child with stridor & fever. An algorithm outlining an approach to the child who presents with stridor and fever is shown in Figure 9–3. Initial management should focus on identifying those patients who are in need of immediate airway assistance (e.g., intubation), regardless of etiology. Many of the infectious and noninfectious causes of acute stridor can produce complete obstruction of the upper airway. Therefore, assessment of the general state of the patient and patency

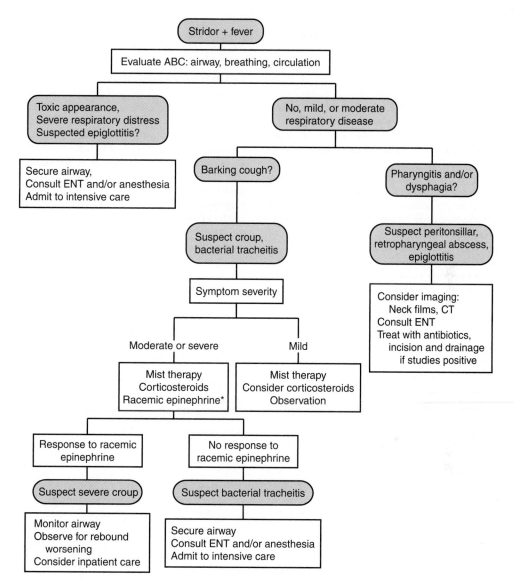

Figure 9–3. Approach to the child with fever and stridor. *Patients receiving racemic epinephrine should be treated with corticosteroids, especially if outpatient management is being considered. CT = computed tomography; ENT = ear, nose, and throat specialist; RX = treatment.

of the airway is essential. In doing so, clinicians should ask themselves several questions: Does the child appear toxic (severely ill, obtunded)? What is the work of breathing? Is there evidence of respiratory fatigue? These questions can be addressed by observing and monitoring the patient's level of consciousness, degree of stridor, respiratory distress (e.g., retractions, accessory muscle use, nasal flaring), air movement, and color. Patients who appear toxic or at risk of complete airway obstruction should be treated immediately without delaying to per-

form diagnostic procedures. The need for serial reexaminations cannot be overestimated. The patient's clinical and airway status may change rapidly. Selection of initial therapy and requirement for additional therapy and/or hospitalization will be determined by changes in the patient status.

Once the child has been assessed and stabilized with regard to airway and cardiovascular status, the most important aspect of the subsequent evaluation is the performance of a thorough history and physical examination.

The history should include questions that explore key features of the infectious diseases described previously (Table 9–31) and noninfectious etiologies such as allergic reactions, foreign body aspiration, trauma, and chronic predisposing conditions (Table 9–30).

The immunization record also should be reviewed, with special attention paid to HIB and diphtheria vaccines. A diagnosis of viral croup is suggested by the presence of URI symptoms, barking cough, and hoarseness. Sore throat and dysphagia are prominent features in epiglottitis and peritonsillar and retropharyngeal abscesses. High fever and toxicity suggest one of the bacterial causes of stridor. When performing the physical examination, it is important to defer any procedures that are likely to cause increased agitation and deterioration in the child's respiratory status (e.g., examination of the oropharynx) until appropriate personnel are present (e.g., otorinolaryngologist, anesthesiologist) and airway support can be assured. In general, the laboratory plays a limited role in the evaluation of patients with stridor and fever. Marked elevations in WBC, CRP, or ESR suggest bacterial infection. However, these tests are nonspecific and usually add little to the diagnostic evaluation. Microbiologic studies for viral or bacterial pathogens (e.g., Gram stains, cultures, antigen detection, serology) are useful in cases of severe disease but usually are obtained only after the airway has been secured.

Radiologic studies, although helpful, are indicated infrequently in the evaluation of upper airway obstruction. In viral croup, the diagnosis is primarily clinical. In suspected bacterial tracheitis and epiglottitis, the importance of securing the airway outweighs any benefit of radiologic imaging.

The diagnosis of bacterial tracheitis or epiglottitis is confirmed by direct visualization of the airway under controlled conditions. Initial therapy is directed to assessing and optimizing the child's respiratory status. Because most patients presenting to a physician's office or emergency room with fever and stridor will have viral croup, mist therapy is often initiated and corticosteroids and racemic epinephrine administered based on the severity of the stridor. In patients who fail to respond to racemic epinephrine, other diagnoses, such as bacterial tracheitis, should be strongly considered. Subsequent therapy should be directed to the specific etiology identified.

LOWER RESPIRATORY TRACT INFECTIONS

Lower respiratory tract infections are common causes of morbidity and mortality in children. The child often presents with symptoms of cough and fever, in association with wheezing and crackles (rales), the cardinal signs of bronchial and lung parenchymal involvement. In children, inflammation of the bronchi and parenchyma often is associated with upper airway infection.

Viral infections, including RSV, parainfluenza, and influenza, are the most common causes of lower respiratory tract infection. Frequent community-acquired bacterial pathogens are *S. pneumoniae, S. aureus,* and *S. pyogenes. Hemophilus influenzae* is no longer a common cause of pneumonia in the United States because of the widespread use of the HIB conjugate vaccine. Bacterial infections such as *B. pertussis, C. diphtheriae, M. tuberculosis,* and *M. mycoplasma* are also found in the pediatric age group. Nosocomially acquired pneumonia in chronically ill children usually is caused by gram-negative bacilli, including *E. coli, Enterobacter, Klebsiella,* and *Pseudomonas* species. Aspiration also should be considered in a chronically debilitated child. In those cases, pneumonia often is due to gram-positive and -negative organisms and anaerobes including anaerobic streptococci and *Bacteroides.* In newborns, bacterial causes of pneumonia are related to pathogens commonly associated with neonatal sepsis, including GBS and *E. coli. Staphylococcus aureus* also can cause devastating disease in this age group. In addition, young infants may present with afebrile pneumonitis, a relatively benign infectious syndrome caused by different organisms, including *C. trachomatis, P. carinii,* and CMV.

Common pediatric lower respiratory tract infections are discussed in more depth below. For a broader discussion of the differential diagnosis of wheezing and its management, the reader is referred to Chapter 18 (Respiratory Diseases). Unique aspects of respiratory infections occurring during the perinatal period are discussed in Chapter 4 (The Perinatal Period).

Pertussis syndrome. Pertussis syndrome is caused most frequently by *B. pertussis* and *Bordetella parapertussis.* Viruses such as adenovirus can cause a similar clinical presentation.

The syndrome usually is divided into the catarrhal, paroxysmal cough, and convalescent phases. The prodromal catarrhal phase lasts approximately 2 weeks. This is followed by 2–4 weeks of paroxysmal coughing and then 4–12 weeks of a convalescent period; hence, its name the "hundred day cough" in ancient Chinese literature. Mild fever with URI symptoms is typical of the catarrhal stage. The characteristic coughing that occurs during the second phase usually brings the patient to the attention of the physician. This cough is of increasing severity and staccato in nature. It can be followed by a whoop-like, high-pitched inspiratory noise (hence the name "whooping cough") that is caused by deep inspiration through partly obstructed airways. Post-tussive emesis is another common finding in this syndrome.

The incidence of pertussis has declined steadily in the United States over the past four decades due to national efforts to immunize all children against this disease. However, recurrent peaks of the *B. pertussis* and *B. parapertussis* diseases occur every 4 years. *Bordetella pertussis,* the cause of classic pertussis, is highly contagious, especially during the catarrhal prodrome. When exposed to a patient in this phase, as many as 90% of susceptible children will acquire the disease. *Bordetella parapertussis* causes a less severe and more protracted course that is frequently diagnosed as bronchitis or URI unless paroxysmal symptoms develop. Adults and children can serve as vectors for disease.

Common complications of pertussis include pneumonia and, in the case of infants, apnea and hypoxia. Other complications include seizures, atelectasis, intracerebral bleeding from tearing of small blood vessels during coughing, hypoglycemia, and neurologic deficits from hypoxia. Younger infants seem to be more susceptible to those complications. Long-term outcomes in a large British study noted learning disabilities three times as often in children who had pertussis when compared with vaccinated children with no clinical history of the disease.

Laboratory findings often include peripheral leukocytosis with lymphocytosis (often up to 80% of the total WBC). Diagnosis usually is made by culture and/or immunofluorescent antibody staining. Immunofluorescent antibody often is more sensitive than culture, with good specificity in experienced laboratories. Serologic tests are also available, which are useful for epidemiologic studies but of limited value in clinical management.

Due to the potential for significant hypoxia and other complications, young infants and other children with severe disease should be hospitalized for monitoring and supportive care (e.g., oxygen, IV fluids). Antimicrobial therapy is used to reduce infectivity but does not alter the severity or duration of the disease in the affected patient. Erythromycin is the drug of choice and should be administered for 14 days to prevent relapse. Trimethoprim-sulfamethoxazole is the alternative drug. Close contacts, regardless of age of immunization history, should be treated with erythromycin prophylactically to reduce secondary transmission.

Bronchiolitis. Bronchiolitis is a clinical syndrome defined by inflammation of the bronchioles and is usually due to a viral infection. It is characterized by rapid respirations, chest retractions, and wheezing, all signs of bronchiolar obstruction due to inflammatory changes, thick, tenacious secretions, and bronchiolar constriction. In infants aged 2–6 months, bronchiolitis is a major cause of hospitalization. Epidemics, typically related to RSV, occur in late fall and winter.

Respiratory syncitial virus is the most common etiologic agent, accounting for at least three-fourths of all cases. Other viruses have been associated with bronchiolitis, including parainfluenza viruses 1 and 3, adenovirus, enterovirus, and influenza viruses. The infection is highly contagious; RSV infection develops in nearly half of the infants in any given community during the first epidemic. These infections decrease in severity with age, suggesting that certain age-dependent anatomic factors are important in the pathogenesis. In addition, there is a progressive reduction in severity after repeated infections, which suggests that immunity plays a role in mitigating the clinical course.

Clinically, the infant presents with rhinorrhea, cough, and a low-grade fever, followed (within 1–2 days) by the onset of rapid respirations, intercostal and subcostal retractions, and wheezing. The infant may be irritable, feed poorly, and vomit. Infants younger than 6 months may present with central apnea before other signs of airway inflammation are present.

On physical examination, the hallmark is an elevated respiratory rate, often greater than 50–60 breaths/minute, associated with an increased pulse rate, with or without fever. Other signs of URT infection may be present, including conjunctivitis, otitis media, and pharyngitis. Chest retractions and a prolonged expiratory phase are often noted. Wheezing and/or rales are typically heard throughout the lungs. The respiratory distress may prevent adequate intake of fluids and lead to dehydration. Cyanosis develops in a minority of patients, but severe gas-exchange abnormalities may be present without cyanosis. An increase in respiratory rate is a more sensitive indicator of impaired oxygenation: Respiratory rates of 60 or higher frequently are associated with reduction of partial pressure of arterial oxygen (PaO_2) and elevation of partial pressure of arterial carbon dioxide ($PaCO_2$).

The radiographic appearance of bronchiolitis is nonspecific and includes diffuse hyperinflation of the lungs with flattening of the diaphragms, prominence of the retrosternal space, and bulging of the intercostal spaces. In most infants, patchy or peribronchial infiltrates are also seen, suggesting an interstitial pneumonitis. Rarely, a small pleural effusion may be observed.

Diagnosis of acute viral bronchiolitis is made based on the clinical presentation, time of year, age of the child, and known presence of RSV in the community. Viral identification can be performed rapidly on nasal secretions using immunofluorescent techniques now available for RSV and most other respiratory viruses including parainfluenza, influenzas A and B, and adenovirus. These results can be confirmed by viral culture of nasopharyngeal washings, but immunofluorescent techniques remain the diagnostic method of choice.

The treatment of bronchiolitis involves general supportive measures such as IV hydration and administration of oxygen by air tent or cephalic hood. Aerosolized bronchodilators may provide transient improvement of the airway obstruction in some patients who have a reactive component to their symptoms. Specific RSV antiviral therapy is available, but its use is controversial and usually limited to the treatment of the most severe cases and RSV-infected patients with increased risk for serious infection, such as those with complex congenital heart disease, chronic lung disease (e.g., cystic fibrosis), or multiple congenital anomalies. In these situations, aerosolized ribavirin is delivered by a specialized small particle generator. Its use has been associated with a small but significant shortening of the clinical course of the disease. An additional concern regarding the use of ribavirin relates to possible toxic effects via environmental exposure by health care workers caring for patients receiving the medication. New delivery systems appear to be fairly effective in minimizing exposure to others. Two types of immunoglobulin therapy, including RSV immunoglobulin and monoclonal antibody (palivizumab), have been shown to be efficacious for prevention of RSV infection in high-risk infants and young children.

Alveolar infections: pneumonia & pneumonitis. Infections of the alveoli are termed pneumonitis and pneumonia. Although most alveolar respiratory infections are mild or moderate in severity, some pathogens may be life-threatening. For example, *S. aureus* infection is aggressive and carries a high mortality rate in infants who are not treated promptly and properly.

Most bacterial pneumonias arise from invasion of the pathogen after an initial host infection with a respiratory virus. Consequent to the initial viral infection, the following factors enhance the risk of bacterial pneumonia development:

1. increases in the production of mucosal secretions, which are laden with bacteria
2. aspiration of the fluid into the respiratory tract and lung
3. a decrease in ciliary activity, resulting in diminished capacity to clear bacteria from the respiratory tract
4. a transient decrease in phagocytosis and bactericidal activity of alveolar macrophages

Other predisposing factors are congenital anatomic defects such as sequestration of a pulmonary lobe and tracheo-esophageal fistula, aspiration of fluid or a foreign body, congenital or acquired immune defects, cystic fibrosis, and congestive heart failure.

Age is probably the single most important variable in determining the probable microorganisms involved. Because the URT often is colonized by human pathogens and normal flora, bacterial cultures obtained through the upper airway may not be conclusive. Detection of bacterial antigen in urine, serum, or nasopharyngeal secretions or of viral antigen in nasopharyngeal secretions may offer additional diagnostic information. Usually, a specific etiologic diagnosis can be made only if the bacterial pathogen is recovered from the blood.

Several of the more common organisms associated with alveolar infection in children, their clinical presentation, and treatment are discussed below.

Viral pneumonia. Influenza viruses cause disease predominantly in winter, and their incidence may vary yearly depending on the dominant strain. Severe disease

and death occur primarily in infants with underlying cardiorespiratory disease or those with superimposed bacterial pneumonia. A protective role for passively acquired maternal antibody has been suggested but not proved.

Parainfluenza viruses also cause lower respiratory disease in young children. However, this infection more frequently presents as croup. Parainfluenza infection is not common in infants younger than 3 months of age. When it occurs, it is more prone to be associated with pneumonitis. Reinfections are less severe and often confined to the URT.

Bacterial pneumonia. Pneumonia due to *S. pneumoniae* occurs most commonly in late winter and early spring, during the peak of viral respiratory infections. It typically presents with the abrupt onset of fever, restlessness, and respiratory distress after an upper respiratory viral infection.

Auscultation of the chest may show diminished breath sounds and fine crackles (rales) on the affected side, but those findings are less common in infants than in older children. Dullness on percussion may be caused by consolidation or the presence of pleural effusion or empyema. Nuchal rigidity without meningeal infection may occur with involvement of the right upper lobe.

Laboratory studies usually show leukocytosis (15,000–40,000 WBC/μm); a WBC of less than 5,000/μm has been associated with a poor prognosis. A positive blood culture for *S. pneumoniae* is diagnostic; however, bacteremia is found in fewer than 30% of cases. Lobar consolidation on chest radiograph is less common in infants than in older children. Parapneumonic effusion is relatively common.

Penicillin is the treatment of choice for pneumococcal pneumonia. Even with strains determined to have intermediate susceptibility to penicillin, drug levels in the lung usually are adequate to eradicate the organism. Erythromycin is an alternative choice if the patient is allergic to penicillin. With the recent emergence of penicillin- and cephalosporin-resistant strains, vancomycin should be considered in a toxic child until the antibiotic sensitivities of the specific pathogen are determined.

Before the introduction of the HIB vaccine, HIB accounted for most cases of bacterial pneumonia in children younger than 5 years of age. Clinical and radiographic findings are similar to those found in other cases of bacterial pneumonia. *Hemophilus influenzae* tends to produce a lobar pattern of consolidation, but disseminated pulmonary disease and bronchopneumonia have been described. Empyema often is present in the young infant. Although it may be difficult to distinguish from pneumococcal pneumonia, it is more insidious in onset, and the course usually is prolonged over several weeks.

A diagnosis of *H. influenzae* pneumonia is established by isolation of the organism from blood, pleural fluid, lung aspirate, or bronchoscopic washings. Latex agglutination tests for *H. influenzae* antigens on tracheal secretions, blood, urine, and pleural fluid may be helpful in making an early diagnosis.

Suspected *H. influenzae* pneumonia should be treated with an IV second- or third-generation cephalosporin (e.g., cefuroxime). The third-generation cephalosporins (e.g., cefotaxime) have the added advantage of excellent meningeal penetration if meningitis is a possible complication.

Streptococcus aureus infections are common in children. This organism can cause a wide spectrum of clinical disorders, ranging from mild furuncles to disseminated sepsis and toxic shock syndrome. *Streptococcus aureus* infections are often difficult to treat because of antibiotic resistance patterns, the invasive nature of the organism, and its ability to form sequestered sites of infection.

Because *S. aureus* can colonize the respiratory tract, it sometimes can cause a primary pneumonia with a presentation similar to that with *S. pneumoniae*. Alternatively, staphylococcal pneumonia can be a complication of bacteremia or septicemia arising from another site. Several characteristic and often ominous signs that distinguish staphylococci from other causes of pneumonia include: (1) rapid progression of respiratory distress, (2) frequent formation of pneumatoceles, (3) empyema and pyopneumothorax due to rupture of pneumatoceles, and, most important of all, (4) the toxic appearance of the patient with impending septic shock. Other sites of infection often associated with staphylococcal pneumonia are otitis media, sinusitis, lymphadenitis, and periorbital cellulitis. Additional complications can include endocarditis, septic arthritis, and osteomyelitis. Thus, staphylococcal pneumonia is a serious infection that may evolve to a medical emergency.

Diagnosis is established by isolation of the organism from blood, pleural fluid, lung aspirate, or bronchoscopic washings. Radiologic examination may show the various stages of the formation of pneumatoceles, empyema, and pyopneumothorax. In the presence of empyema, pleurocentesis should be performed, as should the fluid sent for Gram stain and culture and measurement of total protein, glucose, and pH. A pH of less than 7.2 usually suggests a pyogenic process.

In the past, the treatment of choice for staphylococcal pneumonia was IV administration of a β-lactamase–resistant penicillin such as nafcillin or cloxacillin. However, in recent years, it has been shown that many strains adapt mutations that alter their penicillin-binding proteins, rendering them resistant to all penicillin and cephalosporin products. Fortunately, these strains remain sensitive to vancomycin. These organisms are known as methicillin-resistant *S. aureus.* Thus, the first-line empiric therapy for staphylococcal pneumonia in a toxic child should be vancomycin. In the case of severe infections, combination therapy with nafcillin or vancomycin and

an aminoglycoside or rifampin may be considered to provide synergistic effects. In the child who is less severely ill or when a less resistant strain has been identified, first- and second-generation cephalosporins such as cefazolin and cefuroxime can be used. Cefixime, cefotaxime, and ceftriaxone are not recommended for treating staphylococcal infections. Other drugs, including clindamycin, erythromycin, and trimethoprim-sulfamethoxazole, may be useful to complete the course of treatment but probably should not be used during the acute treatment phase. With empyema, it is important to drain the purulent material because an acidic and enclosed environment will inactivate β-lactam antibiotics, making them unable to optimally exert their killing effects. If indicated, a chest tube should be placed for continuous drainage.

Other organisms causing pneumonia. As the incidence of bacterial and viral lower respiratory tract infections decreases with age, infections with other organisms, such as *C. pneumoniae* and *M. pneumoniae,* increases in older children.

Chlamydia pneumoniae is more common in late childhood and in young adults and appears to exist worldwide. It is a distinct strain of *Chlamydia* that causes severe pharyngitis without exudate, laryngitis, fever, lymphadenopathy, and pneumonia. The pneumonia, when present, is usually unilobar. The WBC is generally normal, and the ESR is elevated.

Mycoplasma pneumoniae is a major cause of respiratory infections in school-aged children and young adults. This organism accounts for 33% and 70% of all pneumonia in children aged 5–9 years and 9–15 years, respectively. It is unusual before the age of 3–4 years, with the peak incidence of disease occurring between the ages of 10 and 15 years. Previous infections, as demonstrated by the presence of circulating antibodies, prevent or ameliorate subsequent ones. Patients with immunodeficiency states or sickle cell anemia have more severe mycoplasma infections than do normal hosts. *Mycoplasma pneumoniae* is the most common infectious cause of acute chest syndrome in patients with sickle cell anemia. *Mycoplasma pneumoniae* is spread through the respiratory tract by inoculation with infected respiratory droplets. The incubation period is thought to be 2–3 weeks.

In *M. pneumoniae* infections, pneumonia, tracheobronchitis, and bronchopneumonia are the most commonly recognized clinical syndromes. Undifferentiated URT infections, pharyngitis, croup, bronchiolitis, otitis media, and bullous myringitis also have been described. Occasionally, patients with respiratory infections may present with multisystemic manifestations involving the skin, CNS (meningitis, encephalitis), heart (myocarditis or pericarditis), joints (arthritis), and blood. Hematologic manifestations include mild degrees of hemolysis, as shown by a positive reaction to Coombs testing and minor reticulocytosis occurring 2–3 weeks after the onset of illness. Symptoms typically begin gradually and are characterized by headache, malaise, and fever. Sore throat is a frequent complaint. Cough is prominent and usually worsens during the first 2 weeks of the illness. All symptoms resolve gradually within 3–4 weeks. On physical examination, fine rales in the lung fields are the most prominent finding.

Roentgenographic features are nonspecific and usually described as interstitial or bronchopneumonic; lower lobe involvement is the most common. Unilateral, centrally dense infiltrates are described in 75% of patients. Hilar lymphadenopathy may be seen in one third of patients. Pleural effusion is unusual but has been described. White blood cell count and differential counts are usually normal.

A variety of serologic responses occur after *M. pneumoniae* infection. Cold hemagglutinins develop late in the first or second week, appearing with titers of at least 1:32 in approximately 50% of patients. These increase fourfold or more by the third week and last about 6 weeks. Specific IgG levels against *M. pneumoniae* also can be measured: The diagnosis can be confirmed by a fourfold increase or decrease in the antibody level over 2–3 weeks (i.e., acute and convalescent titers). Rapid diagnostic testing has not yet proved reliable, although a DNA probe assay is available that has shown good sensitivity and specificity. Cultures of the throat or sputum may demonstrate *M. pneumoniae,* but these studies are not widely available.

Macrolides (e.g., erythromycin, azithromycin and clarithromycin) and the tetracyclines are effective in shortening the course of mycoplasma illnesses. Macrolides are the drug of choice in small children because of the risk of tetracycline toxicity in this age group. It should be given in full therapeutic doses until several days (usually 7–10) after defervescence. For patients older than 9 years, tetracycline is an alternate choice. Despite the efficacy of these drugs in ameliorating the clinical course, the organism may not be eradicated.

Legionella is an entity that has been found increasingly to be a cause of pneumonia in children over the past few years. The increased incidence is probably reflective, in part, of improved methods for detection. Nosocomial cases often are linked to hospital water supplies. Children with underlying pulmonary disease and those who are immunosuppressed seem to be at greatest risk. Culture, direct fluorescent antibody testing, and urinary antigen detection systems are currently available and highly sensitive and specific. Clinical disease typically presents with cough, fever, and chest pain. Diarrhea and neurologic symptoms also can be seen. Therapy involves antibiotic treatment with erythromycin or other macrolide such as azithromycin. Alternative agents include flouroquinolones or Septra. In the immunocompromised

patient, the addition of a second drug, such as rifampin, may be beneficial. Nosocomial infections deserve careful investigation of water supplies and appropriate measures to decrease environmental reservoirs of the organism.

Chlamydia trachomatis may cause up to one third of all cases of pneumonia in infants aged 2–6 months. The illness is characterized by persistent cough, tachypnea, nonspecific abnormalities on chest radiograph, eosinophilia in the blood, and elevated specific immunoglobulin level. The infant is usually afebrile. Clinical findings often are preceded by purulent conjunctivitis in the first 2 months after birth. Pneumonia is usually mild but on occasion can be severe. The diagnosis can be made by staining a smear of nasopharyngeal material with fluorescein-conjugated monoclonal antibody against *C. trachomatis,* which is available commercially. Infants with chlamydial pneumonia often have specific IgM antibodies, which are also diagnostic. Because of placental–fetal transfer, specific IgG is significant only if found in levels at least fourfold greater than that of the mother. Macrolides are the treatment drugs of choice. Alternatives include ampicillin or sulfonamide. For children who receive outpatient treatment, the combination of erythromycin and sulfisoxazole offers activity against *Chlamydia* and other common bacterial pathogens.

Pneumocystis carinii infection can occur in infants younger than 1 year of age as an afebrile pneumonia similar to *C. trachomatis* or in isolated patients with underlying immunodeficiencies. Infection is common and acquired in early life, but most cases are subclinical. Onset of symptoms in otherwise normal infants is slow and insidious. Nonspecific signs of restlessness, poor feeding, and diarrhea are common. Characteristically, fever is absent or low grade. Cough, although not prominent, may appear later over 1–4 weeks. Eventually, patients exhibit increasingly severe tachypnea, dyspnea, intercostal retractions, and flaring of the nasal alae. Pulmonary physical findings consist primarily of fine rales. Roentgenographic evidence of pulmonary infiltrates can be documented early in the course of the disease.

In most infants and older children with AIDS, *P. carinii* pneumonia presents abruptly. High fever and nonproductive cough appear initially, followed by tachypnea and coryza. The course quickly progresses to full-blown disease, with cyanosis and respiratory failure. Death may supervene if no treatment is given. The treatments of choice includes trimethoprim/sulfamethoxazole or pentamidine isethionate. Alternatives are trimethoprim/dapsone, primaquine/clindamycin, and trimetrexate/folinic acid.

Tuberculosis. *Mycobacterium tuberculosis* was once thought to be declining in incidence, with the hope of eradication a real possibility. The past decade, however, has shown it to be a persistent and devious survivor. Especially in the developing world, tuberculosis remains an important cause of morbidity and mortality in children. In the United

States, tuberculosis is much less common. However, in certain populations, the disease is increasing in incidence and the organism is becoming increasingly drug resistant. Most cases occur in children younger than 1 year of age, with a median age of 3 years. The reservoir for infection of these children is adults with newly acquired or reactivated disease. As with many infectious diseases, tuberculosis is closely associated with socioeconomic status and found most frequently in areas of poverty and crowding.

Tuberculosis is transmitted by respiratory droplets from the cough or sneeze of an infected individual. This individual is usually an adult with numerous bacilli in a lung cavity. After inhalation by the host, the bacilli travel to the pulmonary alveoli and multiply. An inflammatory response is induced that involves mobilization of polymorphonuclear leukocytes and macrophages to surround the bacilli, forming the typical epithelioid cell tubercle. During the early stage of infection, some tubercle bacilli may enter the bloodstream and disseminate (this is especially true for younger infants). Most bacilli are killed without establishing disease. Others may progress or become quiescent. The first 12 months after primary infection is the time of greatest risk for dissemination. Children are particularly susceptible to disseminated disease. Infected children younger than 5 years of age have a 4% chance of having meningitis or miliary tuberculosis; this risk then decreases but increases again at puberty. Bone infection with tuberculosis usually occurs 2–3 years after primary infection, with renal involvement following 2–3 years after that.

Four to 6 weeks after infection, delayed hypersensitivity to tuberculin develops and skin testing with the PPD produces a positive reaction. Symptoms at this time are usually minimal or nonexistent. Respiratory symptoms may be absent. The primary lesion becomes centrally necrotic (i.e., the process of caseation), and the immune response walls off the area with collagen to form a capsule. At this point, the lesion resolves completely, becomes fibrotic, or calcifies. On occasion, the course of this primary complex is more acute, with progression to bronchopneumonia or lobar pneumonia. These patients frequently are febrile and have respiratory symptoms and night sweats.

Despite caseation or calcification of the parenchymal focus, viable tubercle bacilli may exist for years. The lymph nodes draining the primary lesion continue to enlarge, sometimes encroaching on adjacent structures such as bronchi (5–20% in primary tuberculosis) or blood vessels. If the lymph node breaks though the wall of the bronchi or blood vessel, exuded infectious caseous material is then free to disseminate to other parts of the lungs or body. The infection may spread to involve the meninges, bones, superficial lymph nodes, and urinary tract.

Skin testing with five tuberculin units of PPD administered by intradermal injection (Mantoux method) is helpful in establishing the presence of an infection but does not distinguish between past infection and active disease. The results of skin testing should be read by trained medical personnel after 48–72 hours by measuring the extent of induration (not erythema) at the test site. Interpretation of the skin test relies on knowledge of the individual's risk factors. An induration of 10 mm or more usually is considered to be a positive reaction. With a history of exposure, suggestive symptoms, and positive physical signs, even a reaction of 5 mm or greater can be regarded as positive. These interpretation criteria were revised recently to reduce the high percentage of false-positive test results in populations with low disease prevalence. Children who have been previously vaccinated with bacillus Calmette–Guérin (BCG), an attenuated strain of *Mycobacterium bovis* (see below), frequently react to subsequent tuberculosis skin testing. However, the current recommendation is to ignore prior BCG administration and treat the individual on the basis of his or her risk group: Children who have received BCG are in a high-risk group because they or their family members come from an area with a high prevalence of tuberculosis. In symptomatic and asymptomatic PPD-positive children, a chest radiograph should be obtained to determine whether pulmonary disease is present.

It must be emphasized that the Mantoux test is a screening test, and a negative reaction does not rule out the diagnosis of tuberculosis, especially in infants and the immunocompromised host. Annual screening for tuberculosis is recommended in areas of high disease prevalence and high-risk populations. Testing of low-risk individuals is dictated by local health departments. The reader is referred to Chapter 1 for a more in-depth discussion regarding tuberculosis screening.

The diagnosis of tuberculosis is often difficult. Empiric therapy is started frequently on the basis of a reactive PPD or demonstration of acid fast bacilli from clinical specimens. *Mycobacterium tuberculosis* can be cultured from sputum, gastric aspirates, and other tissues. Cultures always should be performed to establish antimicrobial sensitivity patterns. *Mycobacterium tuberculosis* is a slow-growing organism, frequently requiring up to 6 weeks to grow in culture. Newer molecular biologic techniques such as DNA probes and PCR assays have allowed more rapid identification of *M. tuberculosis* from clinical specimens such as sputum and CSF.

Treatment strategies for tuberculosis take into account the potential for the development of drug resistance within the heterogeneous population of bacilli that are present in a given host. Traditional treatment protocols combine the use of three or four different antituberculosis medications for extended periods. Characteristic properties of selected antimycobacterial drugs and the various therapeutic regimens are summarized in Tables 9–32 and 9–33. Individuals likely to be infected with

Table 9–32. Antituberculosis Chemotherapy

Drug	Unique Features	Toxicity	Dose (mg/kg)
Isoniazid (INH)	CSF penetration	Hepatic, rare peripheral neuritis	10–15
Rifampicin (RIF)	CSF penetration	Hepatic, gastrointestinal tract	10–20
Pyrazinamide (PZA)	Intracellularly active; CSF penetration	Hepatic, gastrointestinal tract, rash	20–40
Streptomycin	Penetrates inflamed meninges; resistance develops rapidly; used in combination therapy; IM administration	Ototoxicity, rare nephrotoxicity	20–40
Ethambutol (EMB)	Bacteriostatic	Optic nerve toxicity	25

CSF = cerebrospinal fluid; IM = intramuscular.

drug-resistant strains initially should be treated with four antituberculosis medications. Immunocompromised individuals require longer and frequently lifetime treatment for tuberculosis.

The most commonly encountered clinical scenario is that of the immunocompetent child with a reactive Mantoux test result but no known exposure. Frequently, such a child is the marker for an index case within the family, and contacts should be investigated aggressively. If a complete physical examination and chest radiograph do not show active tuberculosis, the child should begin a 9-month course of isoniazid. Isoniazid prophylaxis in this setting has decreased the complication rate by 88% over a 10-year period and has completely prevented tuberculous meningitis and miliary tuberculosis.

Effective prevention of tuberculosis relies on rapid identification and therapy of infected individuals. Currently, vaccination with BCG is used in Europe and many developing countries with high endemic rates of disease. Immunization with BCG does not prevent primary infection with *M. tuberculosis,* but it has been shown to reduce the incidence of hematogenous spread and severe pulmonary disease by 20–80%, thereby providing significant protection against disseminated forms of the disease (e.g., tuberculous meningitis, miliary tuberculosis, and bone and joint infections). In the United States, BCG has been used for PPD-negative children who have continued and unavoidable exposure to adults with active tuberculosis. Use of the vaccine is contraindicated in children and adults with underlying immunodeficiencies, including infection with HIV.

Central Nervous System Infections

Infections of the CNS are more common in children than in adults. However, because of the nonspecific nature of the signs and symptoms associated with these disorders, especially in infants, and a general reluctance to perform invasive procedures in infants and children, their diagnosis can be challenging. The following section discusses common types of CNS infections seen in children and is organized by clinical syndrome and etiologic agent.

MENINGITIS

Meningitis refers to inflammation of the meninges, which results in the clinical presentation of neck stiffness,

Table 9–33. Recommended Therapy for Tuberculosis Infection and Exposure

PPD (+) without disease	INH × 9 months
TB exposure	
PPD (−)	INH × 3 months; repeat PPD; if negative discontinue
PPD (+)	INH × 9 months if disease workup negative
PPD (+) INH resistance	RIF or RIF + EMB × 6–12 mo
PPD (+) INH & RIF resistance	PZA + EMB × 6–12 mo
Pulmonary TB	
Sensitive organism	INH, RIF, PZA × 2 mo, followed by INH, RIF × 4 mo
Suspect resistant organism	INH, RIF, EMB, PZA × 2 mo followed by INH, RIF, EMB × 6 mo until sensitivities available
Known INH resistance	RIF + EMB + PZA × 18 m
TB meningitis, bone/joint disease	INH, RIF, PZA, streptomycin × 2 mo, followed by INH, RIF × 10 mo (Dexamethasone when indicated × 1 m)
TB during pregnancy	INH + RIF + EMB × 9 mo

INH = isoniazid; PPD = purified protein derivative; PZA = pyrazinamide; RIF = rifampin; TB = tuberculosis; EMB = ethambutol.

fever, headache, and irritability. Cerebrospinal fluid findings include abnormal numbers of leukocytes and, often, abnormalities in protein and glucose concentrations. Based on the clinical presentation and CSF results, meningitis often is categorized as septic or aseptic based on whether a bacterial or nonbacterial etiology is suspected. However, this preliminary categorization does not always accurately predict the actual pathogen.

Bacterial meningitis

Clinical presentation. A child or infant with bacterial meningitis usually is acutely ill. This diagnosis is one of the most feared in pediatrics because of its potential for mortality. Even with prompt, appropriate diagnosis and treatment, morbidity can be quite high. The risk for long-term CNS sequelae is related to many factors, including the specific pathogen, the host's age and immune status, and the timeliness and appropriateness of treatment.

In the neonate, signs of meningitis can be quite variable and nonspecific. Such signs include irritability, poor feeding, hyper- or hypothermia, lethargy, vomiting, seizures, bulging fontanelle, and poor tone. Because neonatal meningitis often is associated with generalized sepsis, other signs not related to the CNS, such as hypotension, jaundice, and respiratory distress, may be seen. Neonates are at risk for the development of meningitis, in part because of intrinsic defects in their immune system, such as alterations in cytokine synthesis and impaired immune-cell function (e.g., T and natural killer cells). These factors and perinatal exposure to bacteria in the maternal gastrointestinal and genitourinary tracts explain why the highest incidence of meningitis is seen in the neonatal period.

Older children with meningitis typically present with fever, headache, vomiting, and photophobia. The Kernig and Brudzinski signs may be present, reflecting meningeal irritation and neck rigidity. The Kernig sign is performed by flexing the hip and knee and then extending the knee with the hip still flexed. Pain in the back and neck regions with this maneuver represents a positive test result. The Brudzinski maneuver is considered positive if the hips flex when the neck is passively flexed. Presence of these signs indicates meningeal irritation in this age group. In young infants (younger than 2 years of age), absence of these signs does not preclude the diagnosis of meningitis. Seizures, altered mental status, and focal neurologic deficits are additional presenting signs of meningitis that can occur in a child of any age. Progression of the disease can be quite variable, depending on such factors as the age of the patient, the specific organism involved, and the therapy instituted. Focal neurologic signs may develop with time. Paresis, cranial nerve palsies, papilledema, and papillary abnormalities can occur as a result of increased intracranial pressure or vascular thrombosis.

Mechanisms of bacterial invasion of the meninges remain similar for all age groups. The disease usually begins with a viral infection of the URT with subsequent bacterial attachment to the mucosa and invasion of the bloodstream. Through hematogenous seeding of the meninges and CSF, the bacteria encounter a rich nutrient environment relatively deficient in host defense antibodies, phagocytes, and complement, where they multiply rapidly. Bacterial components, such as the lipopolysaccharides of gram-negative bacteria, lead to production of inflammatory cytokines and chemokines. These substances, notably interleukin-1 and interleukin-8, platelet-activating factor, and tumor necrosis factor α (TNF-α or cachectin), lead to chemotaxis and activation of granulocytes, stimulation of phagocytosis, activation of the complement cascade, and permeability changes in the blood–brain barrier. These developments result in brain edema, increased intracranial pressure, and decreased blood flow to the brain. Decreased transport of glucose across the blood–CSF barrier due to inflammation and increased use results in hypoglycorrhachia. Purulent exudate may cover the surface of the brain, spinal cord, and ventricles, resulting in the clinical symptoms and signs of meningeal irritation.

Etiology & epidemiology. Specific bacterial pathogens are associated with certain age groups and underlying conditions (Table 9–34). The most common pathogens in the neonatal period include GBS, *E. coli,* and *L. monocytogenes.* Other, less frequently seen bacteria include *Klebsiella, Enterobacter, Serratia,* and *Hemophilus* species. Occasionally, *S. pneumoniae* and *Enterococcus* species are seen as pathogens in neonatal meningitis.

In infants aged 1–3 months, the primary pathogens are GBS and *S. pneumoniae.* Infection with GBS at this time is termed "late onset" and is somewhat different in its presentation than its neonatal counterpart; HIB, *N. meningitides,* and *Salmonella* also are seen less commonly.

From 3 months to 3 years of age, HIB, *N. meningitides,* and *S. pneumoniae* are the most common agents of bacterial meningitis. The advent of *H. influenzae* vaccines during the past decade has markedly decreased the incidence of invasive HIB disease, including meningitis and epiglottitis.

From 3 to 12 years of age, the incidence of septic meningitis decreases significantly, with the most common bacterial pathogens being *S. pneumoniae, N. meningitides,* and, occasionally, *H. influenzae.* In older children and adults, *S. pneumoniae* and *N. meningitides* predominate.

Certain conditions, congenital and traumatically acquired, predispose children to specific types of bacterial meningitis. For example, children with galactosemia have an increased susceptibility to *E. coli* infection and meningitis. Patients with asplenia, sickle cell disease, nephrotic syndrome, and deficiencies of IgG2 and IgG4 have an increased incidence of septicemia and meningitis

Table 9–34. Bacterial Pathogens in Meningitis and Empiric Therapy by Age Group[1]

Age Group	Likely Organisms	Empiric Therapy
Neonate	Group B *Streptococcus, Escherichia coli* and other gram-negative organisms, *Listeria monocytogenes*	Ampicillin + cefotaxime
1–3 mo	Group B *Streptococcus* (late onset), *Streptococcus pneumoniae*, and rarely, *L. monocytogenes*	Vancomycin + ampicillin + cefotaxime
3 mo–3 y	*S. pneumoniae, Haemophilus influenzae,*[2] and *Neisseria meningitidis*	Vancomycin with either cefotaxime or ceftriaxone
3–12 y	*S. pneumoniae, N. meningitidis,* and occasionally, *H. influenzae*[2]	Vancomycin with either cefotaxime or ceftriaxone
12 y–adult	*S. pneumoniae* and *N. meningitidis*	Vancomycin with either cefotaxime or ceftriaxone

[1] Empiric use of vancomycin must be customized depending on the incidence of *S. pneumoniae* resistance to penicillin and cephalosporins in the community.
[2] *Haemophilus influenzae* is uncommon in the United States because of the *H. influenzae* type b vaccine.

associated with encapsulated organisms such as *S. pneumoniae* and HIB. Recurrent *N. meningitidis* infections are seen in children with C5–C8 complement system defects. Children with anatomic defects, such as a congenital dermal sinus or traumatic CSF leak, are at risk for meningitis from a variety of gram-positive and gram-negative organisms. Staphylococcal meningitis is rare except in patients with ventriculoperitoneal shunts for the treatment of hydrocephalus. In most cases, the predominant organism is coagulase-negative *Staphylococcus.*

Specific organisms. Several types of bacterial meningitis deserve a more detailed description of their pathophysiology and clinical presentations. Meningitis caused by GBS, *S. pneumoniae, H. influenzae, N. meningitidis,* and *L. monocytogenes* will be discussed.

Group B *Streptococcus* is the most common cause of neonatal meningitis in the United States. Gastrointestinal and genitourinary tract colonization occurs in up to one third of pregnant women. Screening pregnant women during the third trimester of pregnancy and administering intrapartum prophylactic IV antibiotics for GBS carriers and all high-risk women has significantly decreased the incidence of early onset neonatal disease and is currently the standard of care. Despite these efforts, GBS infection continues to be a major cause of neonatal morbidity and mortality in developed countries.

Group B *Streptococcus* is responsible for several distinct clinical syndromes characterized by early and late onsets of disease. Early onset disease classically occurs within the first 72 hours postnatally. Presentation involves respiratory distress with pneumonia, sepsis, and meningitis in approximately 30% of cases. The profound shock and respiratory insufficiency are usually the most problematic aspects of this disease for the clinician. Late onset GBS infections usually occur around 2–4 weeks of age and are less severe than early onset disease. Presentation

can occur up to age 4 months. Meningitis is seen more often in late onset disease, occurring in more than three fourths of infants with this clinical syndrome.

The incidence of **H. influenzae** meningitis has decreased steadily in developed countries with efforts to universally immunize infants with HIB vaccines. *Hemophilus influenzae* type b is an encapsulated form that is associated with more invasive disease than any other strains. This type also is commonly associated with many other childhood diseases such as otitis media, sinusitis, epiglottis, pneumonia, and bacteremia. By age 5 years, most children will have natural immunity to this organism and rarely manifest invasive HIB disease.

Hemophilus influenzae meningitis is seen more frequently from October to November and from February to April. The incidence is increased in day-care centers and is greater among African Americans, Alaskan Eskimos, Apaches, and Navajos. The increased incidence in African Americans may be due to socioeconomic factors. The suboptimal living conditions and greater exposure of Navajos and Alaskan Eskimos and decreased natural antibody titers and responsiveness to HIB vaccines may be important factors in their higher rates of infection. Unvaccinated children in close contact with a household member in whom invasive disease has developed are at increased risk for infection. Prophylactic treatment with antibiotics (usually rifampin because of its nasopharyngeal mucosal penetration) is recommended for all members of households, including the patient, in which there is a child younger than 4 years of age. Alternatively, ceftriaxone can be used for prophylaxis. Children younger than 1 year of age who have had invasive disease are still at risk for recurrence and should be vaccinated.

Neisseria meningitidis is a frequent cause of meningitis in children younger than 5 years, although it can be seen in any age group. There are at least 13 serogroups; A, B,

C, and W135 are most prevalent in the United States. Disease can follow colonization of the URT after exposure to another colonized or infected person. This gram-negative diplococcus can produce two distinct clinical entities, meningococcemia and meningitis, which can exist separately or together. The disseminated disease associated with meningococcemia often is a fulminant, devastating process, even with prompt and appropriate therapy. The onset is typically abrupt, with the sudden appearance of fever, chills, and prostration. Rash is common, usually beginning as a pink maculopapular exanthem and progressing rapidly to the more classic petechial or purpuric rash, leading to the ecchymosis notoriously associated with this disease. Other foci of infection are pericarditis, endocarditis, and pneumonia. In meningococcal meningitis without sepsis, the usual presenting signs and symptoms are fever, headache, malaise, meningismus, and altered mental status. Household and close contacts of patients with meningococcal meningitis should receive antibiotic prophylaxis (rifampin is the recommended agent).

A quadrivalent meningicoccal vaccine is available that covers serotypes A, C, Y, and W-135. It is administered as a single dose and can be given concomitantly with other vaccines. Because it is a polysaccharide vaccine, it is not immunogenic for children younger than 2 years of age. It is currently recommended for high-risk individuals such as those with asplenia and persons with defects in the terminal complement pathway. Travelers to the "meningitis belt," which extends from Senegal to Ethiopia, also should receive the meningococcal vaccine if their visits occur between December and June. Military recruits receive annual meningococcal vaccinations. The Centers for Disease Control has recently broadened their recommendations to include the consideration of vaccination for college students who will be living in dormitories.

Streptococcus pneumoniae is a gram-positive diplococcus that is responsible for a variety of diseases in pediatrics, including otitis media, pneumonia, sinusitis, and bacteremia. Meningitis caused by this pathogen can be quite severe, with a relatively high degree of associated morbidity and mortality. Predisposing host factors include hemoglobinopathy, status post splenectomy, suppurative otitis media or sinusitis, and a CSF leak. Transmission is via contact with respiratory secretions, and the incubation period ranges from 1 to 30 days. Presentation is similar to that of other types of nonneonatal septic meningitis. A new 7-valent conjugate pneumococcal vaccine recently has been licensed and is recommended for routine use in infancy. With its universal administration, the incidence of invasive pneumococcal infections, including meningitis, is expected to decline.

Listeria monocytogenes is a β-hemolytic gram-positive rod that can cause neonatal sepsis and meningitis.

Early onset disease usually presents with pneumonia or sepsis and is acquired through transplacental or ascending intrauterine infection. Late onset disease occurs after the first postnatal week and may result in meningitis. It is acquired during or after birth. Maternal infection may occur from ingestion of contaminated meat or dairy products.

Diagnosis. The diagnosis of meningitis usually centers on evidence of inflammation in the CSF. A lumbar puncture must be performed when there is clinical suspicion of meningitis unless contraindicated by factors such as intracranial hypertension, an overlying infectious skin lesion, or severe clinical instability, making technical performance of spinal tap impossible. Because infants are at increased risk for meningitis associated with sepsis and the signs and symptoms of meningitis are so nonspecific and variable in this age group, the clinician should maintain a very low threshold for performing a lumbar puncture in an infant.

The CSF findings for a child with bacterial meningitis usually include leukocytosis, increased protein concentration, and hypoglycorrhachia (low CSF glucose relative to serum glucose; see Table 9–37). It is important to remember that normal values for these parameters differ with age (Table 9–35). Other factors need to be considered when evaluating CSF findings, such as a history of previous antibiotic administration or traumatic lumbar puncture. It has been shown that oral antibiotics before lumbar puncture, even for a few doses, will affect the CSF cultures and make the diagnosis more difficult. A maternal history of antibiotic administration before delivery also will affect the clinical course and laboratory findings in the newborn. In these cases, the physician will have to rely on the interpretation of CSF counts and glucose levels to guide therapy. No hard and fast rules exist regarding how these factors influence the CSF. Various formulas have attempted to correct for red blood cell contamination of the CSF from a previous traumatic tap but have not proved very useful. Gram stain of the CSF may provide invaluable and immediate information that can aid the clinician in selecting an antibiotic before culture results are known. Occasionally, the Gram stain will show bacteria even before pleocytosis

Table 9–35. Normal Values of Cerebrospinal Fluid in Children

	Neonates (<1 mo)	Infants (>1 mo)
White blood cell count	<30	<10
Percent neutrophils	60	0
Protein levels (mg/dL)	<90	<40
Glucose levels (mg/dL)	70–80	50–60

develops, especially in the case of pneumococcal or meningococcal meningitis.

Another diagnostic aid is latex agglutination testing, which detects bacterial antigen in the CSF. The use of these tests are most helpful in the setting of prior antibiotic therapy, which may interfere with culture results. Unfortunately, they are neither very sensitive nor specific.

Blood culture always should be obtained in the setting of suspected meningitis. Results may be positive in up to 90% of cases of *H. influenzae* and meningococcal meningitis and 80% of pneumococcal meningitis cases. In neonates, there is a high correlation between positive blood cultures and CSF cultures in meningitis due to *H. influenzae* and *S pneumoniae* and a lower correlation in meningitis due to GBS and *N. meningitidis*. Initial investigations also should include a peripheral CBC with a WBC and differential. Normal-appearing CSF does not completely rule out the possibility of meningitis. If cultures are sterile, causes of aseptic meningitis syndrome must be considered.

Management. Empiric treatment for presumed bacterial meningitis includes intravenous antibiotics, fluid and electrolyte management, and, in specific cases, steroid therapy. In the setting of concurrent sepsis and/or significant neurologic compromise, other supportive measures may be necessary. These may include the use of anticonvulsants, means to decrease cerebral hypertension or hydrocephalus, and ventilatory support.

Antibiotic therapy should be initiated promptly (Table 9–34). In the neonate, coverage should include GBS, coliforms, and *Listeria*. The combination of cefotaxime and ampicillin is an appropriate choice. Ampicillin with gentamicin is less desirable but may be used as alternative coverage in some centers. Cefotaxime is a better choice than other third-generation cephalosporins because it does not displace bilirubin from serum proteins. *Listeria* is less of a concern in infants older than 3 months of age, and most clinicians would discontinue using ampicillin in empiric therapy after this age.

Because of increasing resistance to penicillin and cephalosporins among *S. pneumoniae* isolates, empiric therapy for infants and children with streptococcal meningitis who are older than 1 month of age should include vancomycin in addition to cefotaxime or ceftriaxone. Ampicillin should be added if the patient is at risk for *Listeria*. Once the organism is identified and sensitivities determined, antibiotic therapy can be tailored appropriately.

Traditionally, the use of steroids in the management of meningitis has been considered controversial. More recently, several studies have demonstrated some benefit from the use of steroids in *H. influenzae* meningitis. This benefit was demonstrated when steroids were given before or concomitantly with antibiotics. The rationale behind administration of steroids involves potential attenuation of the bacteriolytic inflammatory response associated with antibiotic administration. The benefit probably is most pronounced in infants and children with profound alterations in consciousness or cerebral hypertension. Different studies have shown different degrees of benefit. In a study from Costa Rica, a statistically significant decrease in the incidence of one or more neurologic sequelae and a trend toward reduction of audiologic impairment in infants and children treated with dexamethasone before the initiation of antibiotic therapy (vs. antibiotic therapy alone) were reported. Of note, in most studies on the use of steroids, no differences were observed between mortality rates with or without adjunctive steroid therapy. On occasion, upper gastrointestinal bleeding has been reported as a complication of adjunctive steroid use in the management of patients with meningitis. Although the issues regarding the use of steroids are not completely settled, many experts recommend their use under specific circumstances, namely that IV dexamethasone (0.15 mg/kg) be given at the beginning of antimicrobial therapy and every 6 hours for 16 doses in suspected cases of bacterial meningitis and for proven *H. influenzae* meningitis.

The patient with meningitis must be monitored closely for the development of complications. Frequent physical and neurologic examinations, including daily measurement of head circumference in infants, should be performed. The status of electrolytes, body weight, and urine specific gravity should be followed to look for evidence of the syndrome of inappropriate secretion of antidiuretic hormone (STADH). This syndrome is usually transient and managed by fluid restriction if the patient is not hypovolemic or does not have decreased blood pressure. Other acute complications include toxic encephalopathy, cerebral edema, transtentorial herniation, cranial nerve palsies, deafness, seizures, subdural effusion, cerebral infarction, and cortical vein thrombosis. Subdural effusion is common and rarely lasts more than 3 months. Invasive therapy for subdural effusion usually is not required unless there are associated focal neurologic changes.

Long-term sequelae of meningitis may include hearing deficits, seizures, language disorders, mental retardation, motor abnormalities, visual impairment, behavior disorders, learning disorders, attention deficits, and decreased intelligence quotients (Table 9–36). Hearing loss is the most frequent long-term complication and is seen most often after meningitis due to *S. pneumoniae*, followed by *N. meningitidis* and *H. influenzae*. Age of onset and duration of illness before treatment do not appear to affect the occurrence of subsequent hearing loss. All children should undergo hearing evaluation after meningitis on an annual basis for several years.

Aseptic meningitis. Aseptic meningitisis is characterized mostly by a lymphocytic CSF pleocytosis, evidence of meningeal irritation on clinical examination, and a history consistent with meningitis. However, there are no

Table 9–36. Potential Long-term Complications of Bacterial Meningitis and Recommended Follow-up Evaluations

Complications
  Hearing loss—most common
  Visual impairment
  Neurologic deficits: hemiparesis, hypertonia, motor deficits, seizures, hydrocephalus
  Mental retardation, learning and behavioral disorders, attention deficits, language disorder

Follow-up evaluations
  Hearing tests
  Vision examinations
  Neurologic assessment: physical examination, electroencephalogram; when indicated, radiologic imaging including computed tomography and magnetic resonance imaging scans
  Psychological tests
  Language and learning assessment

significant changes in level of consciousness, no growth on routine bacterial cultures, and no obvious etiologic agent on routine stains. Table 9–37 provides a list of clinical and CSF characteristics that help differentiate aseptic from septic meningitis. A wide variety of pathologic processes can cause this syndrome (Table 9–38).

Table 9–37. Characteristics of "Septic" Versus "Aseptic" Meningitis

	"Septic"— Typically Bacterial	"Aseptic"— Usually Viral
Presentation	Usually acutely ill; no seasonal pattern	May be more insidious or chronic; often seasonal
CSF WBC	Pleocytosis usually >1000 cells/mm^3	Pleocytosis usually hundreds to a few thousand cells/mm^3
CSF glucose concentration	Typically low, i.e., <40 mg/dL	May range from low to normal
CSF protein concentration	Elevated, usually 100–500 mg/dL	May range from normal to mildly elevated

CSF = cerebrospinal fluid; WBC = white blood cell count.

Table 9–38. Aseptic Meningitis: Etiology

Infection	
Viral	Enterovirus (most common): Coxackievirus, echovirus, poliovirus
	Arbovirus: St. Louis encephalitis, Eastern equine encephalitis, Western equine encephalitis, Venezuelan equine encephalitis, Powassan and California encephalitis
	Mumps, measles, rubella
	Herpes simplex virus
	Adenovirus
	Varicella, Epstein–Barr virus, cytomegalovirus
	Influenza, parainfluenza
Bacterial	*Mycobacterium tuberculosis*
	Leptospira
	Syphilis
	Borrelia (Lyme disease)
	Nocardia
	Partially treated bacterial meningitis
Rickettsial	Rocky Mountain spotted fever
Mycoplasmal	*Mycoplasma pneumoniae, Mycoplasma hominis*
Fungal	Coccidioides, Blastomyces, Histoplasma, Cryptococcus
Protozoan	Toxoplasma, Malaria, Amebiasis, Cysticercosis
Post-vaccination	Influenza, rabies
Drugs	Trimethoprim-sulfamethoxazole, intrathecal drugs
Toxins	Heavy metals (eg, lead, mercury, and arsenic compounds)
Vascular	Collagen vascular diseases, hemorrhage, thrombosis
Neoplastic	Metastatic tumors, primary meningioma
Foreign bodies	Ventriculoperitoneal shunts, pressure monitors
Other	Kawasaki disease

Viral causes of aseptic meningitis. Viral causes for aseptic meningitis are very common (Table 9–38). However, the presentations and outcomes can be quite variable depending on the specific virus involved.

Enteroviruses are RNA viruses that belong to the picornavirus family and can cause a variety of illnesses including gastroenteritis, URIs, conjunctivitis, rashes, hepatitis, myositis, myocarditis, and pericarditis. Enteroviruses are a common cause of aseptic meningitis. Encephalitis also can occur, although this is uncommon. In neonates with X-linked hypogammaglobulinemia, enterovirus can cause a chronic form of meningoencephalitis, which can be fatal. Otherwise, most enteroviral diseases, including meningitis, resolve spontaneously, leaving minimal, if any, sequelae.

Transmission is by the fecal–oral route and is most prevalent during the summer and fall.

Poliovirus is a specific enterovirus that usually causes asymptomatic infection but may present as aseptic meningitis with paralytic lower neuron disease. Given widespread immunization practices, poliomyelitis is exceedingly rare in the United States, with most cases representing vaccine-related or imported disease. Current vaccine schedules in the United States advocate the use of an inactivated injectable vaccine. This is a recent change reflecting a shift in the risk:benefit ratio regarding continued use of the live oral vaccine. Because polio has been eradicated from the western hemisphere, the risk of polio is in fact greater with the vaccine than with wild-type disease.

Infection with the **mumps virus** is a known cause of aseptic meningitis and encephalitis. It can also be associated with neuritis or myelitis. Central nervous system involvement may occur 1 week before or up to 3 weeks after the onset of parotitis. Lethargy, nuchal rigidity, photophobia, and vomiting are common manifestations. This form of meningitis usually is self-limiting and has an excellent prognosis.

In viral meningitis, the typical CSF WBC count is lower than that seen in bacterial meningitis (i.e., $100–1000/mm^3$). Although a polymorphonuclear cell pleocytosis can be seen early in the disease, this usually changes to a lymphocytic predominance within 12–48 hours. The hypoglycorrhachia is usually absent or much milder, and the elevation in CSF protein concentration is usually much lower in patients with aseptic meningitis than in patients with bacterial disease. Thus, due to the nonspecific nature of the findings, studies on the CSF are often inconclusive. The diagnosis of viral meningitis is aided by negative routine bacterial cultures in the context of appropriate physical signs, season, and CSF findings. Cerebrospinal fluid viral cultures can be helpful, but their sensitivity is often quite variable (50–75% for enteroviral CSF cultures). Stool and nasopharyngeal viral cultures by themselves may provide additional evidence of enteroviral infection, but the result is not diagnostic of enteroviral meningitis. Some centers have used immunofluorescence antibody assays on nasopharyngeal samples to identify certain subtypes of enteroviruses. An enteroviral PCR test with excellent specificity recently has become available in major laboratories.

Nonviral infectious causes of aseptic meningitis. *Mycobacterium tuberculosis* was once a very common cause of meningitis in young children. During the latter half of the 20th century, screening, effective therapy, and general improvement in public health had drastically decreased the incidence of mycobacterial disease in the United States. During the past 15 years, however, tuberculosis and mycobacterial disease have experienced a resurgence, particularly in patients with AIDS. Tubercular meningitis usually occurs within the first 12 months after a primary infection and is seen most commonly in children younger than 5 years of age. The onset is subacute, and symptoms are classically quite nonspecific. Fever, listlessness, headache, and anorexia are common during the first 1–2 weeks. These symptoms can progress to involve more significant changes in the level of consciousness, cranial nerve deficits, evidence of meningismus, peripheral tremor, and deep tendon reflex abnormalities. Without treatment, opisthotonos, hemiplegia or paraplegia, and coma can develop, and the patient ultimately will die. Cerebrospinal fluid findings in tubercular meningitis typically include a WBC of 10–8500 cells/mm³ with a lymphocyte predominance, although early in the disease one may see a large number of neutrophils. Cerebrospinal fluid glucose concentrations are initially normal but then decrease. Protein concentrations are characteristically elevated, becoming extremely high in advanced disease. Presumptive diagnosis is made usually on the basis of CSF findings and symptomatology. Computed tomography or MRI may show a basilar exudate. Definitive diagnosis involves CSF cultures, which traditionally are positive in 45–90% of cases and can take up to 8 weeks to grow. Acid fast stains of CSF are rarely positive, although use of large volumes and multiple lumbar taps can increase positivity. Reactivity of PPD or positive chest radiographs are seen in only about half the cases, although PPD results usually become positive later in the course of the disease. Therapy involves a combination of antimycobacterials, usually including isoniazid, rifampin, streptomycin, and pyrazinamide for a duration of 12 months (Table 9–33). Adjunctive use of corticosteroids in the first month of treatment is recommended in the case of advanced disease. Mortality remains high, at 20%, in children younger than 5 years of age.

Three spirochetes that can infect the CNS are *Leptospira, Borrelia burgdorferi,* and *T. pallidum.* **Leptospirosis** is an uncommon zoonosis seen in the United States that is transmitted by contact with urine from infected animals such as dogs, livestock, or rodents. Clinical disease can range from mild to fulminant (Weil syndrome) and usually is biphasic in nature. Leptospiremia, fever, and headache are the most common findings during the first 4–7 days of the illness. The second phase occurs after 1–3 days of improvement and marks the beginning of the immunologic response to this disease, during which rash, uveitis, and meningitis are seen. The meningitis usually lasts for 2–3 days. The CSF findings typically reveal fewer than 500 white blood cells/mm³, with a mononuclear cell predominance. The glucose concentration is usually normal, with the protein concentration usually normal to elevated. Leptospira generally cannot be cultured from the CSF during the period when the patient exhibits clinical meningitis, but rather only during the initial phase of the disease. A more severe form of leptospirosis infection (Weil syndrome) occurs in 10% of patients and is characterized by fever, jaundice, hemorrhage, altered state of consciousness, and renal insufficiency. The diagnosis usually is made by isolation of the leptospires from body fluid or tissues. Antibody testing may be helpful in the second stage of the disease, when CSF and blood cultures are likely to be sterile. Polymerase chain reaction techniques for the detection of leptospire DNA are currently under development for clinical use. Penicillin G is the drug of choice for the treatment of these infections. Tetracycline can be used as an alternative in older children.

Borrelia burgdorferi can cause a form of meningitis in Lyme disease. The diagnosis often is made clinically on the basis of the presence of the characteristic rash and the history of a tick bite. Meningitis is just one of several neurologic manifestations that can occur with Lyme disease. Others are facial palsy, encephalitis, chorea, and radiculoneuropathy. Diagnosis is also supported by positive serology for *B. burgdorferi.* Treatment depends on the stage of the disease: IV ceftriaxone or cefotaxime is given for late stage disease including CNS involvement. Amoxicillin with probenecid is used in early stage infections.

Syphilis, caused by the spirochete ***T. pallidum,*** is a disease that can involve many organ systems. It can affect the CNS in congenital and acquired infections, causing an aseptic meningitislike syndrome. In acquired neurosyphilis, symptoms appear decades after the initial infection. The CSF may show increased protein concentration, increased WBCs, and a positive Venereal Disease Research Laboratory (VDRL) test result. A negative VDRL result does not exclude neurosyphilis. The fluorescent treponemal antibody absorption test (FTA-ABS) can be positive in the newborn because of passively transferred immunoglobulins from the mother. Patients with congenital neurosyphilis should have repeated evaluations of the CSF every 6 months for 3 years or until the CSF has returned to normal. Treatment for congenital neurosyphilis consists of penicillin for 14 days. The VDRL follow-up titers must be performed at 3, 6, and 12 months. If the CSF VDRL result is reactive after 6 months, treatment should be repeated.

Fungal infections of the CNS are not common in children. The organisms seen most frequently are *C. neoformans, C. immitis,* and *H. capsulatum.* **Cryptococcus neoformans** infections of the CNS occur most commonly in patients with immunologic defects involving T-cell–mediated functions. *Cryptococcus neoformans* is a frequent CNS pathogen in adult patients with AIDS but is much less common in the pediatric AIDS population. This encapsulated yeast is found in bird droppings and soil. It can cause a wide spectrum of disease involving lungs, myocardium, bone, and skin in addition to the CNS. Meningitis caused by *C. neoformans* may be acute or chronic, with the course often depending on the degree of immunosuppression seen in the host. The diagnosis can be made by identification of the organism in CSF sediment using an India ink preparation; however, this process is associated with a fairly low sensitivity (50%). Culture is more sensitive but can take 4–8 weeks to grow. Cryptococcal antigen assays are very sensitive (up to 90%) for CNS disease and probably are the initial diagnostic test of choice. Treatment of CNS cryptococcal infection includes use of amphotericin B in combination with flucytosine for synergistic effects. For less severely ill patients, oral fluconazole can be used as an alternative. Patients with AIDS usually require life-long suppressive therapy.

Coccidioides immitis is another fungus found in the soil, primarily in the southwestern United States and northern Mexico. After the organism is inhaled, it invades the respiratory tract. Rarely, disseminated disease occurs, affecting many organs including the CNS. Diagnosis can be made by serologic testing early in the illness (i.e., within 1–3 weeks) or skin testing later in the disease course. Cultures of the CSF are often sterile despite active disease. Bronchoalveolar lavage specimens may be more revealing, with appropriate culture. The treatment of choice consists of oral fluconazole with amphotericin B. Intravenous amphotericin B is a possible alternative. Relapse of the infection in the CNS is common, and some experts recommend continuation of fluconazole indefinitely.

Histoplasma capsulatum can cause an aseptic meningitislike syndrome of chronic duration. This mycosis is acquired by inhalation of the conidia from contaminated soil. Usually, the primary pulmonary infection is asymptomatic and self-limited. If meningitis develops, it is associated with disseminated disease and seen most often in the context of compromised cell-mediated immunity. Definitive diagnosis is by culture, but the CSF is positive in only 30–60% of cases. Serologic diagnosis (complement fixation) and staining techniques are probably the most practical and widely used methods of diagnosis given the 4–6-week incubation period needed for cultures. A recently introduced ELISA for urinary histoplasma antigen is believed to be very sensitive. Treatment of histoplasmal meningitis involves the use of amphotericin B. Whereas itraconazole has been used for non-CNS infection, it is not recommended for CNS histoplasmosis. Even with prompt and appropriate care, long-term cure rates are poor for this disease.

Amebic meningitis, parasites, & rickettsia. **Naegleria fowleri** and **Acanthamoeba** species are free-living amoebas that can cause CSF disease in humans. These species exist in cyst forms and the invasive trophozoitic forms. *Naegleria fowleri* also occurs in a flagellate form. Infections with *N. fowleri* usually follow fresh-water exposure; organisms enter the CNS through the cribriform plate to the subarachnoid space. *Acanthamoeba* infections are seen usually in immunocompromised individuals; these organisms usually reach the brain via hematogenous spread. Fatality is common with both infections.

Toxoplasma gondii is a protozoan parasite that can cause congenital infection and reactivated disease in patients with AIDS. Humans become infected from eating incompletely cooked meat and from exposure to oocysts in cat feces. Congenital disease can result in intrauterine meningoencephalitis: Sequelae include chorioretinitis and mental retardation. Cerebral calcifications are seen often on CT or MRI. If acquired in adulthood, the disease usually is asymptomatic. Pyrimethamine combined with sulfonamides (e.g., sulfadiazine) is used for treatment.

Cysticercosis is an infection caused by the larval stage of the pork tapeworm, *Taenia solium.* Cysticercosis, although uncommon in the United States, is frequent in South America, Central America, and Southeast Asia. Humans are hosts for the adult tapeworm; swine are the tapeworm's intermediate host. Infection occurs after the ingestion of eggs in undercooked meat. Oncospheres are liberated and penetrate the intestine to enter the lymphatic system, where they are carried to other sites. The oncospheres develop into fluid-filled cysticerci that may be present in any area of the brain. The inflammatory response causes their death and an area of calcification. The cysts can appear individually or in clumps. Seizures are common, and obstruction of CSF may lead to hydrocephalus. Spinal cysticerci also can cause arachnoiditis or symptoms of a mass lesion. The CSF may contain eosinophils. The diagnosis is made by CT findings, serologic ELISA, and hemagglutination tests. Serum antibodies are 80–95% sensitive and specific. No treatment is necessary for asymptomatic disease. Active or progressive disease can be treated with praziquantel, but death of the parasite can cause increased inflammatory response, leading to headache, nausea, and seizures. Thus, corticosteroids should be given before the first dose of treatment. Surgery is not indicated except to relieve hydrocephalus or a mass effect.

Trichinosis results from eating undercooked meat that contains larvae of the nematode *Trichinella spiralis.* Larvae can migrate into the brain and meninges, producing encephalitis and meningitis. Delirium, seizures, paresis, and coma can occur. Electroencephalography may show findings consistent with diffuse encephalopathy. Larvae are found in the CSF in 25% of patients. The peripheral WBC typically is increased, with a marked eosinophilia. No treatment is available for cerebral trichinosis. Thiabendazole can be given within 24 hours after a patient has been known to ingest infected meat. Corticosteroids may be of some benefit for treating the cerebral inflammatory reaction.

Rickettsia and rickettsialike organisms are obligate intracellular pleomorphic bacteria. *Rickettsia rickettsii* (Rocky Mountain spotted fever), *Coxiella burnetii* (Q fever), *Rickettsia prowazekii* (typhus), *R. typhi, Rickettsia tsutsugamushi,* and *Ehrlichia* species have been reported to cause aseptic meningitis.

Partially treated bacterial meningitis can cause a clinical and laboratory picture consistent with aseptic meningitis. The clinical presentation may be less acute and symptoms nonspecific. The CSF may show close to normal findings. Diagnosis can be difficult in these cases because cultures are often sterile. Latex agglutination studies on CSF may be helpful in this scenario, aiding in diagnosis and treatment. If partially treated bacterial meningitis is suspected, the patient should receive a full course of antibacterial therapy.

Noninfectious causes of aseptic meningitis. Many noninfectious etiologies can cause aseptic meningitis and should be kept in mind when constructing a differential diagnosis. An abbreviated list includes toxins (lead, mercury, arsenic), trauma, medications (trimethoprim-sulfa, IV immunoglobulin), malignant neoplasms, and collagen vascular diseases.

Approach to the evaluation of aseptic meningitis syndrome.

As with other infectious diseases, evaluation of the patient begins with a thorough history. In addition to obtaining detailed information regarding the present illness, the history should note the child's immunization status, travel history, previous infections, and possible animal and tuberculosis exposures. The time of year is also important because enteroviral infections are more common during the summer. The clinical presentation usually is acute, with fever, nuchal rigidity, headache, photophobia, and vomiting. To assess for viral etiologies, stool and nasopharyngeal cultures are useful and reliable. In contrast, etiologic viruses are less likely to grow from culture of the CSF. Because many different processes are responsible for the aseptic meningitis syndrome, a careful evaluation must be performed before the diagnosis of viral meningitis is made. In particular, it is important not to ascribe partially treated bacterial or mycobacterial meningitis to viral causes.

Because it is difficult to distinguish viral from bacterial illness by clinical and CSF findings in young children and infants, these individuals should be treated presumptively for bacterial illness, until culture results and other tests are available. However, older patients who are not seriously ill, who have not been pretreated with antibiotics before lumbar puncture, and who can be observed closely do not necessarily need to be treated immediately with antibiotics. Sometimes, a second lumbar puncture 8–12 hours later can help clarify the diagnosis when the first lumbar puncture shows a few polymorphonuclear leukocytes: If the infection is viral, the follow-up CSF findings should show a lymphocytic predominance.

In summary, patients should be evaluated carefully for the possibility of bacterial causes of sepsis and meningitis. Aseptic meningitis syndrome often is a diagnosis of exclusion.

ENCEPHALITIS & MENINGOENCEPHALITIS

Infections of the CNS that involve the parenchyma of the brain are termed encephalitis. Sometimes, both meninges and parenchyma are involved, leading to the clinical designation of meningoencephalitis. Specific etiologies for these two entities are discussed below.

Viral etiologies

Herpes simplex virus. Herpes simplex virus is a DNA virus that is responsible for localized and systemic diseases. In children and infants, HSV can cause an extremely devastating form of encephalitis. Neonatal infection usually is acquired during or just before delivery from a maternal genital source. Primary maternal HSV-2 infection during delivery presents a greater risk for transmission to the infant than does recurrent maternal infection. Many pregnant mothers are unaware of their HSV status because primary and recurrent infections can be asymptomatic.

Neonatal HSV encephalitis presents with temperature instability, poor feeding, changes in the level of consciousness, seizures, and/or focal neurologic deficits. Unlike HSV encephalitis in older children and adults, neonatal HSV CNS infections often are not localized and therefore are less commonly associated with focal neurologic signs. The CSF findings may be normal in infants with HSV encephalitis, especially early in the disease. Usually, there is a mild to moderate pleocytosis, with a mononuclear predominance and the presence of erythrocytes. Viral CSF cultures are well known to be sterile. Serum HSV titers may demonstrate a fourfold or greater increase between acute and convalescent serum specimens. Currently, PCR assay of CSF samples is available in many reference laboratories and is the test of choice for the diagnosis of HSV encephalitis.

Computed tomographic or MRI findings may show evidence of temporal or frontal lobe hemorrhage. Electroencephalography and brain scans are less helpful. Treatment consists of IV acyclovir, which has less risk of neurologic and renal toxicity than does vidarabine. Both drugs have been shown to reduce morbidity and mortality in HSV encephalitis.

Other viral causes. Cytomegalovirus can cause encephalitis in the setting of congenital infection. About half the infants with symptomatic, congenital infections may have evidence of brain damage. Microcephaly, periventricular calcification, seizures, and focal neurologic deficits, including sensory neural hearing loss, can be seen. Infection also may be acquired perinatally from contact with infected maternal secretions during delivery or from breast milk, but this type of postnatal acquisition rarely causes CNS involvement. The CSF evaluation shows a pleocytosis with increased protein concentration. Diag-

nosis is often made by culture. The "shell vial" culture technique, in which cytospin and monoclonal antibody staining are used, is a sensitive and rapid test for CMV in body fluids. Cytomegalovirus-specific IgM from serum is diagnostic in the neonate. Another useful test is CMV antigen assay, which recently has become available for rapid diagnosis. At this time, treatment is primarily supportive. A few clinical trials have investigated the use of ganciclovir for congenital CMV infections, but to date no consensus has emerged regarding its use.

Varicella zoster virus is a rare cause of encephalitis. Cerebellar involvement is typical and usually resolves spontaneously. Cerebral involvement is less common and often associated with more significant neurologic impairment and higher mortality rates, depending on the host.

Arboviruses are arthropod-borne viruses that include the Bunyaviridae, Togaviridae, Flaviviridae, Reoviridae, and Rhabdoviridae families. The prognosis for patients with these infections differs with the specific virus implicated in the infection.

Eastern equine encephalitis usually is severe, with a high mortality rate. It is caused by an RNA togavirus and occurs throughout the central and eastern seaboard and Gulf states in North America. It is also seen in Central and South America. The virus is spread by mosquitoes from avian reservoirs. Outbreaks in humans often are preceded by an increased incidence of disease in pheasants and horses. Patients present with symptoms that are similar to other types of viral encephalitis but may be more severe. Seizures and coma are common. The CSF often has an increased WBC, with a predominance of polymorphonuclear leukocytes. The diagnosis is made by serologic testing or brain biopsy. Mortality rates are high, and survivors often are left with significant neurologic and other morbidities.

Saint Louis encephalitis, the most common arbovirus in the United States, occurs most frequently along states bordering the Ohio and Mississippi rivers. The virus is spread by mosquitoes that breed in irrigated farmland in rural areas and in stagnant sewage in cities. Birds serve as reservoirs. Morbidity and mortality rates are higher in the elderly. Death and sequelae in children are rare.

California encephalitis (La Crosse encephalitis) is caused by several California serogroup viruses and has a widespread distribution in the United States and Canada. The disease is most common in the upper Midwest. The virus is spread by mosquitoes living in hardwood forests. Animals such as squirrels serve as reservoirs. Encephalitis occurs mainly in children aged 5–10 years of age. The initial illness may be accompanied by seizures and stupor. Sequelae may include behavioral changes and learning disabilities. There is no specific treatment.

Western equine encephalitis is a togavirus transmitted by mosquitoes from avian reservoirs. Equine outbreaks often precede human disease. The disease occurs in the central and western United States and Canada and in South America. Infants are at greatest risk for neurologic sequelae. There is no treatment.

Rabies is caused by an RNA virus classified as a rhabdovirus. Transmission usually occurs as a result of an animal bite, with the virus present in saliva. Airborne infection has been reported in bat caves. The disease also has been transmitted after corneal transplantation, when it was unknown that the donor died of rabies. Reservoirs of the disease in the United States are mainly wild animals.

After a bite from an infected animal, the virus is inoculated into subcutaneous tissue and muscle. There it replicates slowly with symptoms usually appearing 1–3 months after the bite. Areas with greater nerve supply (fingers, genitalia, face) have shorter incubation periods than arm or leg bites. Children also have shorter incubation periods.

The virus ascends the infected peripheral nerves to the spinal cord, where it selectively infects the limbic system and then the rest of the brain. Patients initially may have pain and numbness at the inoculation site, with a prodrome of anxiety, malaise, and headache. This progresses to an encephalomyelitis with apprehension, delirium, meningismus, and mildly convulsive movements. Attempts to swallow or even the sight of water can result in painful laryngospasm (hydrophobia). A smaller percentage of patients may present with an ascending paralysis similar to the Guillain–Barré syndrome. Patients usually die of aspiration secondary to laryngospasm or of arrhythmias due to viral myocarditis.

Fluorescent antibody staining can detect virus in corneal epithelium and skin samples. Antibodies to rabies can be detected in nonimmunized individuals about 1 week after the onset of symptoms. Diagnosis of rabies in the biting animal can be made by fluorescent antibody staining of brain tissue. After a bite injury to a child, domestic animals should be observed for 10 days because dogs and cats can shed the virus in saliva up to 12 days before they demonstrate symptoms. If no symptoms appear in the biting animal, immunotherapy for the child is not indicated.

Exposed individuals are treated by immunoprophylaxis. In the United States, skunks, raccoons, and bats are most likely to be infected, followed by foxes, coyotes, cattle, dogs, and cats. Rabies is rare in rodents and rabbits. When the decision to treat is made, the individual must receive passive and active immunizations. Passive immunity is achieved with rabies immunoglobulin; one half the dose is infiltrated into the wound, and the other half given intramuscularly. Active immunization is achieved by giving human diploid cell vaccine intramuscularly.

Other nonviral causes. Cerebral malaria is the most severe complication of *P. falciparum* infections. It affects children, usually younger than 6 years of age, almost exclusively and is a major cause of mortality in patients with malaria. In these patients, the plasmodia invade red blood cells, causing them to be "sticky" with respect to endothelial cells. Proinflammatory cytokines, including TNF-α, are produced, leading to upregulation of adhesion molecules on immune cells and other inflammatory processes and the induction of fever. This adds to the tendency toward microvasculature sludging and thrombosis, ultimately resulting in CNS damage. Consequently, the patient presents with fever, mental status changes, seizure, focal neurologic deficits, and even coma. Of these, mental status changes are the most common CNS presentation. A travel history can be crucial in making the diagnosis of this extremely serious but treatable disease. Diagnosis of cerebral malaria is made by the combination of travel history, CNS presentation, and microscopic examination of thick and thin blood smears from these patients. The Giemsa or Wright stain can be used on the smears for parasite visualization. A fluorescent antibody test is available in some centers as a specific diagnostic test. DNA probes have been developed recently as additional diagnostic tools. Treatment of cerebral malaria involves the use of IV quinidine gluconate in an intensive care setting. The patient must be monitored for arrhythmias and hypoglycemia during therapy. Once the clinical condition has improved and parasitemia is reduced, oral quinine therapy can replace IV quinidine. Steroids are contraindicated in cerebral malaria because their use is associated with increased morbidity and mortality.

Postinfectious encephalitis is a relatively common cause of encephalitis in which a current infectious agent cannot be isolated from the brain tissue but probably results from the immunologic response to a previous infection. Agents known to trigger this response include measles, rubella, mumps, VZV, and *M. pneumoniae* infections. It also has been observed in patients after immunization with these vaccines.

Gastrointestinal Infections

INFECTIOUS DIARRHEA

Diarrhea is the second most common acute infection in pediatrics after URI. Worldwide, it is a leading cause of illness and death for millions of children. The most serious complications of diarrhea are severe dehydration, electrolyte disturbances, and hypovolemic shock. Children younger than 4 years and those living in socioeconomically disadvantaged areas are at greatest risk.

Diarrhea is defined as an increase in water content of the stool associated with an increase in frequency. Infectious agents lead to diarrhea in the host by several different pathogenic mechanisms. After adherence to intestinal mucosa cells by the use of projections such as flagella, pili, or fimbria, bacteria release mucinases and proteases. These enzymes result in gastrointestinal mucosal cell death, with loss of digestive enzymes in the mucosal villi. Loss of these enzymes leads to malabsorption of specific substances including lactose, resulting in the clinical appearance of an osmotic diarrhea. With bacterial invasion into the cells, direct enterocyte destruction ensues. Secretory diarrhea is the result of bacterial toxin production (e.g., cholera toxin), which leads to huge losses of electrolytes and water.

Endemic diarrhea is the most common type of gastroenteritis encountered. By definition, it is spread in children through close contact, as in families, day-care centers, and residential institutions. Viral causes predominate with rotavirus and Norwalk agent, the principal etiologic organisms. However, bacterial pathogens such as *Salmonella, Shigella,* and *Campylobacter* species are important causes of endemic diarrhea. *Food and waterborne epidemic diarrhea* refers to outbreaks occurring in many individuals at the same time after the ingestion of contaminated substances. Inadequate storage and preparation of food leads to the contamination. The most common organisms causing this type of outbreak are *Salmonella, Clostridia,* and enterotoxin-producing *S. aureus.* Certain food sources are more likely to harbor specific organisms. For example, poultry, eggs, and unpasteurized milk are common sources of *Salmonella* outbreaks.

Evaluation of patients presenting with acute diarrhea requires a detailed history and physical examination. Important aspects of the history to elicit are shown in Table 9–39. The ordering of diagnostic tests should be tailored to the likely etiologies. Table 9–40 provides a summary of the characteristic features of infectious agents commonly associated with childhood diarrhea. The stool should be tested for blood and fecal leukocytes: The presence of erythrocytes and leukocytes indicates an invasive diarrhea from organisms such as *Campylobacter, Shigella, Salmonella, Yersinia,* and hemorrhagic *E. coli.* Stool cultures and examination for ova and parasites should be reserved for patients with suggestive histories such as day-care outbreaks, foreign travel, prolonged and/or severe diarrhea, and stools that are positive for blood and leukocytes. Acid fast staining may aid in the detection of *Cryptosporidium* oocysts and *Mycobacterium* strains. Most laboratories routinely test stools for *Salmonella,*

Table 9–39. Important Questions for Evaluating the Patient With Diarrhea

Stool: frequency, color/consistency, odor, presence of blood or mucus
Travel
Antibiotic use
Contact with ill patients
Day-care attendance
Camping and exposure to wild animals
Pet and domestic animal exposure

Shigella, and *Campylobacter.* If less common organisms, such as *Yersinia* or *E. coli,* are suspected, the laboratory should be notified and specific requests for pathogen identification made.

The mainstay of therapy for all patients with acute diarrhea is appropriate management of fluid and electrolyte abnormalities. Treatment with antimicrobial agents is rarely indicated and frequently results in prolonged shedding of the offending organism. Likewise, the use of antiperistaltic agents has not been shown to be of benefit in the treatment of children with infectious diarrhea.

The following section focuses on several of the more common causes of infectious diarrhea in children. For a discussion of the broader differential diagnosis and clinical approach to acute and chronic diarrhea, the reader is referred to Chapter 13 (The Gastrointestinal Tract and Liver).

Bacterial diarrhea. *Salmonella* is a non–lactose-fermenting, motile, gram-negative rod with three pathogenic species: *Salmonella enteritidis, Salmonella choleraesuis,* and *Salmonella typhi. Salmonella enteritidis* and *S. choleraesuis* cause acute gastroenteritis by enterocyte invasion into the small bowel. Leukocytes and blood may be found in the stools of an acutely infected patient who may or may not have systemic symptoms. *Salmonella* also can cause bacteremia, with subsequent seeding of focal infections such as osteomyelitis. These complications appear to be more common in young infants and neonates. This organism also is associated with an asymptomatic carrier state. Transmission of *Salmonella* occurs through the fecal–oral route and requires a large inocula of contaminated food or water. Reptiles, such as domestic turtles, have long been known to be carriers of *Salmonella.* Recently, other domestic reptiles, such as iguanas and snakes, have been implicated in *Salmonella* outbreaks. Eggs, poultry, and other meat products have high *Salmonella* infection rates and frequently are the source in reported outbreaks. The highest incidence of infection occurs in infants and children younger than 5 years of age.

Treatment of gastroenteritis without bacteremia usually is contraindicated in *Salmonella* infections because it can prolong the carrier state. In some cases, azithromycin, ciprofloxacin, or trimethoprim/sulfa can be used. Immunocompromised patients, patients with hemoglobinopathies, and infants younger than 3 months should be treated because these groups have a high incidence of *Salmonella* bacteremia. In severe cases, IV therapy with ceftriaxone is indicated.

Salmonella typhi is the cause of typhoid or enteric fever. It is transmitted by the fecal–oral route due to contaminated food or water. Humans are the only known carriers. Fewer than 500 cases are reported annually in the United States, with most cases occurring in individuals younger than 20 years. Bacteremia is universal, with invasion of the reticuloendothelial system. The bacterial cell wall contains

Table 9–40. Childhood Diarrhea: Characteristic Features of Each Causative Agent

Pathogen	Site of Action	Season	Stool	Clinical	Laboratory Results
Bacterial (10–20%)					
Salmonella enteritidis, choleraesuis typhi	Small and large bowel, bacteremia	Late summer, early fall	Foul smelling, ±blood, soft, mucus	Gradual onset, extra-intestinal, with cramps, chronic carrier	Neutrophil "left shift," no fever
Shigella sonnei flexneri boydil dysenteriae	Large bowel (low inoculum)	Fall	Fruity smell (vinegar) Watery, mucus, bloody	High temperature, toxic Seizures (infants)	Low WBC, neutrophil "left shift"
Campylobacter jejuni fetus abortus	Large bowel	Summer	Foul smell, soft, mucus, ±blood	Most common; low-grade temperature, cramps; self-limited	
Yersinia enter-colitica	Ileum	Winter	±Diarrhea, ±blood	Fever, abdominal pain, arthritis (Reiter syndrome), mesenteric lymphadenopathy (pseudoappendicitis; in older children)	
Vibrio cholerae	Small bowel	Epidemic	Large volume watery	Dehydration, cramps	
Aeromonas hydrophilia		Late summer–early fall	Chronic diarrhea (adults more than children) Acute diarrhea (children <2 y)		
Escherichia coli					
ETEC ("turista")	Small bowel	Summer	Watery, no blood, large volume	Abrupt onset, no fever, cramps	Not helpful
EPEC	Small bowel	Fall	Musty odor; (–) blood, mucus; ±fever	Gradual onset, chronic infection, FTT in infants <3 mo	
EIEC	Large bowel	Any	Small volume	Dysentery, (+) fever	
EHEC	Large bowel	Any	Bloody, no fever	Hemolytic uremic syndrome (0157:H7)	High WBC
Viral (70–90%)					
Rotavirus	Small bowel (upper)	Winter (October–May)	Large volume, foul smelling; (–) blood, mucus	Dehydration, ±fever, (+) vomiting, mostly children 6–24 mo	
Adenovirus (types 40, 41)	Small bowel	Any	Watery	<2 y, abdominal pain, fever, emesis	
Norwalk	Small bowel	Winter	Explosive	Abrupt onset: vomiting, no fever, adults/school-aged children	

EIEC = enteroinvasive *Escherichia coli*; EHEC = enterohemorrhagic *Escherichia coli*; EPEC = enteropathogenic *Escherichia coli*; ETEC = enterotoxigenic *Escherichia coli*; WBC = white blood cell count; FTT = failure to thrive.

a potent pyrogenic endotoxin, resulting in high fevers and a paradoxical bradycardia. Emesis and constipation are followed by diarrhea, hepatosplenomegaly, cholestatic jaundice, and the characteristic maculopapular rash called "rose spots." Complications include small bowel perforation, glomerulonephritis, and numerous neurologic symptoms such as encephalopathy, acute cerebellar ataxia, optic neuritis, aphasia, deafness, and cerebral thrombosis. The organism has become increasingly resistant to antibiotics, and many strains in the developing world have shown multiple resistance patterns. Empiric treatment with a third-generation cephalosporin should be initiated until the susceptibility pattern is available. Other choices are oral ciprofloxacin and azithromycin in less severe cases. A vaccine is available and recommended for intimate carrier contact, community outbreaks, or travel to an endemic area.

Shigella is a non–lactose-fermenting, nonmotile, gram-negative rod transmitted through fecal–oral contamination. Although most cases of shigellosis in the United States are caused by *Shigella sonnei* and *Shigella flexneri, Shigella dysenteriae* is more important in underdeveloped countries. Outbreaks are common in day-care centers and may follow ingestion of contaminated food and water. Only very small inocula are required for transmission. The incubation period is approximately 2–4 days. Symptoms include fever, upper abdominal pain associated with tenesmus, headache, and profuse watery, mucoid stools containing blood and leukocytes. Additional features are seizures and the occasional finding of lax anal sphincter tone, presumably due to release of a neurotoxin. Bacteremia is rare. The WBC remains normal, but a marked increase in immature forms of granulocytes or leukopenia may occur. Complications are frequent and include toxic megacolon, cholestatic hepatitis, hemolytic uremic syndrome, and Reiter syndrome (arthritis, conjunctivitis, urethritis, and dermatitis). Treatment previously consisted of trimethoprim-sulfamethoxazole or ampicillin; however, the organism has shown increasing resistance to these traditional antibiotics. Most strains remain susceptible to parenteral third-generation cephalosporins (e.g., Ceftriaxone or Cefixime), and these should be the empiric treatment of choice pending identification of the specific susceptibility pattern. In milder cases, azithromycin or ciprofloxacin can be used.

Campylobacter jejuni is the most commonly isolated bacterial fecal pathogen. It is a curved, gram-negative organism causing grossly bloody diarrhea, fever, and abdominal pain that may mimic appendicitis. Bacteremia occurs with *Campylobacter fetus* and *Campylobacter abortus* but rarely with *C. jejuni*. Animals, including poultry, dogs, cats, and wild birds, serve as important reservoirs. The incubation period is 1–7 days, and the diarrhea and abdominal pain continue for an average of 1 week. Erythromycin shortens the fecal excretion but does little to alleviate symptoms. Other medications that can be used include azithromycin or oral ciprofloxacin.

Yersinia enterocolitica is an aerobic, motile, non–lactose-fermenting, gram-negative coccobacillus. Rodents and swine serve as important reservoirs. Ingestion of large inocula from contaminated meat, dairy products, and seafood is required. An incubation period of 4–6 days precedes the onset of symptoms. Symptomatic patients typically present with fever, abdominal pain, and mucoid, bloody diarrhea in which leukocytes are demonstrated. Complications are frequent and include erythema nodosum, reactive arthritis, terminal ileitis, mesenteric adenitis, meningitis, myocarditis, hepatitis, and glomerulonephritis. In severe cases, *Yersinia* infection is treated with IV ceftriaxone or chloramphenicol. Trimethoprim-sulfamethoxazole may be used for patients who are less ill. Ciprofloxacin and norfloxacin are newer antibiotics that have been used successfully to treat this infection. In general, only infections outside the gastrointestinal tract are treated.

Escherichia coli has four different subclasses, each named for its distinct mechanism of action on the intestinal mucosa. Enterotoxigenic *E. coli* (ETEC) secretes one or more heat-labile or heat-stable toxins and can resemble infections with cholera. It is the only subclass that is not associated with fecal blood or leukocytes on stool examination. Enteropathogenic *E. coli* (EPEC) can lead to chronic infection, malabsorption, and failure to thrive by a mechanism that is not well understood. In contrast, enteroinvasive *E. coli* (EIEC) produces an acute illness that mimics shigellosis. In general, gastroenteritis due to *E. coli* has an incubation period of less than 24 hours and rarely requires antimicrobial treatment. Because enteropathogenic *E. coli* has a chronic presentation, it may need to be treated in infants younger than 3 months of age; oral neomycin has been used successfully.

Enterohemorrhagic *E. coli* (EHEC) is easily transmitted through the fecal–oral route. Strains of EHEC produce cytotoxins. Among them, subclass 0157:H7 has been responsible for outbreaks in many day-care centers and epidemic hemolytic uremic syndrome. Epidemics have been traced to undercooked, contaminated meat. Treatment of EHEC is controversial; some studies have indicated that antimicrobial therapy increases the incidence of hemolytic uremic syndrome.

Vibrio infections are important causes of diarrhea worldwide. Infection with these aerobic, motile, curved, gram-negative organisms result in crampy abdominal pain and explosive, watery diarrhea. Noncholera strains are common in seawater, especially in summer. A large inoculum is required, and incubation is less than 24 hours. Uncooked crustaceans and mollusks (e.g., oysters, crabs, and shrimp) are well-known carriers. Once the flagella attach to intestinal enterocytes, enterotoxin produced by cholera bacteria alters production of cellular cyclic adenosine monophosphate. Rapid and severe fluid loss resulting in death from hypovolemia is common. Cholera itself is more common in Asia, the Middle East, and southern Europe. Management includes meticulous fluid and electrolyte replacement and antimicrobial therapy, including tetracycline or trimethoprim-sulfamethoxazole. Newer agents such as oral ciprofloxacin and norfloxacin are used also.

Although antibiotics can cause diarrhea by several mechanisms (e.g., alteration in normal bowel flora leading to overgrowth of other organisms, decreased carbohydrate transport and intestinal lactase levels), antibiotic-associated colitis (its most severe form is known as pseudomembranous colitis) usually is the result of a toxin produced by **C. difficile.** The use of broad-spectrum antibiotics allows for increased growth of this organism and subsequent toxin production. Ampicillin, clindamycin, and the cephalosporins are commonly implicated antimicrobials. Symptoms may not appear for weeks after discontinuation of the antibiotic. Blood, mucus, and leukorrhea are commonly found in the stool. On colonoscopy, the mucosa typically is lined with grayish plaque-like lesions. *Clostridium difficile* (without the toxin) may be found in the stool of normal, healthy infants without diarrhea. Thus, the identification of this organism, without the toxin or suggestive clinical symptoms, is not an indication for treatment. Severe cases may require treatment with oral vancomycin or metronidazole. In the very ill patient with pseudomembranous colitis who cannot tolerate oral medications, IV metronidazole can be used.

Staphylococcal enterotoxin–mediated disease typically produces vomiting, retching, and diarrhea. The diarrhea usually is less prominent than the upper gastrointestinal symptoms. The incubation period is brief, usually 3–5 hours. Antimicrobials are of no help because the symptoms are due to heat-stable enterotoxins and not the organism itself.

Parasitic diarrhea. *Giardia lamblia* is a flagellated protozoan, with the cyst form being the infectious agent. After infestation, the trophozoites are found in the duodenum and shed intermittently in the stools. The protozoa are transmitted through the fecal–oral route; day-care outbreaks are common. Many patients remain asymptomatic, and symptoms can differ greatly among patients. Flatulence and abdominal pain with diarrhea are most common, but malabsorption and failure to thrive are also seen, especially in children. Those with IgA deficiency and cystic fibrosis are at highest risk for severe disease from *G. lamblia.* The diagnosis can be made by examination of fresh stool specimens by direct inspection or ELISA. In adults, the preferred treatment is with quinacrine. In children, however, furazolidone is recommended; metronidazole can be used as an alternative.

Entamoeba histolytica results in loose, bloody, mucoid stools after ingestion of infectious cysts. Hepatic abscesses result from metastasis to the liver through the portal veins. Stool examinations and immunoassays can aid in the diagnosis. Treatment consists of furazolidone, albendazole, or metronidazole.

Cryptosporidium may cause outbreaks of frequent, watery stools in day-care settings. Although infection is self-limited in the normal host, significant chronic diarrhea occurs in the immunocompromised host, resulting in dehydration and malnutrition. There is no effective therapy.

Isospora belli is another protozoan that causes severe diarrhea in AIDS patients but can be treated with trimethoprim-sulfamethoxazole or by combining pyrimethamine and sulfadiazine.

Viral diarrhea. Viral diarrhea is the most common type of infectious diarrhea encountered and spread in children through close contact in families, day-care centers, hospitals, and residential institutions. Infections usually are self-limited, and the agents do not need to be routinely identified. Most can be identified by electron microscopic examination of the stool, if specific diagnosis is necessary. In addition, enzyme immunoassays are available to test for rotavirus and adenovirus.

Rotavirus is an RNA virus with five known antigenic subtypes. Of all the gastrointestinal pathogens, rotavirus is the leading cause of infantile diarrhea and dehydration. Transmission is by the fecal–oral route, with a 1–3-day incubation period. It is highly contagious, and outbreaks in day-care centers are common. Seasonal peaks occur in winter. Infection is characterized by the abrupt onset of vomiting, fever, and diarrhea. Blood, mucus, and leukocytes are not commonly seen in the stool. Premature infants are at increased risk for severe disease. Treatment consists of supportive therapy to maintain fluid and electrolyte balance. Strict enteric precautions also are essential to prevent further spread of the disease.

Adenovirus, especially subtypes 40 and 41, also is responsible for endemic diarrhea. It causes symptoms similar to those from rotavirus infection and spreads easily in close contact environments. Adenovirus typically affects older children, is associated more often with significant abdominal pain, and may have a more protracted course.

Norwalk agent is another RNA virus that causes diarrhea and usually is accompanied by fever, abdominal cramps, and emesis. Fecal–oral transmission is common. Outbreaks also can follow ingestion of contaminated shellfish and salads. The incubation period is 1–2 days.

VIRAL HEPATITIS

Hepatitis, or inflammation of the liver, is caused by a variety of etiologies. However, it is most frequently due to infection. A viral pathogen is most commonly responsible, but bacterial, fungal, and parasitic infections also occur (Table 9–41). It should be noted that systemic infections such as influenza, herpes viruses, and measles also can cause transient hepatic inflammation resulting in abnormal liver function. In neonatal hepatitis, the microbial agents usually are acquired in utero or at birth and include hepatitis A, B, and C viruses, CMV, rubella, syphilis, and toxoplasmosis. Among the cases in which an etiology is proved, hepatitis B is the most common etiology.

Similar clinical features are seen with various viral hepatidities, but there are several unique differences (Table 9–42). Clinical presentations can range from a mild, asymptomatic, anicteric illness to fulminant disease associated with liver failure leading to death. Alternatively, the patient may recover symptomatically and become a chronic carrier with persistent hepatitis leading to the development of liver cirrhosis and, ultimately, hepatocarcinoma.

Chronic hepatitis refers to an ongoing inflammation of the liver that persists after the patient has recovered symptomatically from an acute infection. Causes of chronic hepatitis include infectious agents and autoimmune or metabolic diseases. Infection with viral hepatitis B, C, and D, all of which are parenterally transmitted, can result in chronic disease. In contrast, the enterally transmitted forms (A and E) do not lead to chronic hepatitis. Historically, chronic hepatitis can be divided into two forms: chronic active and chronic persistent. Chronic active hepatitis features portal triad infiltration by immune cells, including lymphocytes and plasma cells, resulting in encroachment of the hepatocytes. This often leads to fibrosis, necrosis, and cirrhosis because of a chronic inflammatory process. With chronicity over a few decades, the patient eventually develops hepatocellular carcinoma. This

Table 9–41. Etiologic Organisms for Infectious Hepatitis

Viruses	Fungi
Hepatitis A, B, C, D, E	*Candida albicans*
Herpes family	*Blastomyces dermatitidis*
CMV, EBV, HSV, VZV	*Histoplasma capsulatum*
Adenovirus	
Enterovirus	Parasites
Parvovirus B19	*Toxoplasma gondii*
Influenza	*Entameba histolytica*
Measles	*Schistosoma* species
	Toxocara canis
Bacteria	
Neisseria gonorrhoeae	
Leptospira	
Mycobacterium tuberculosis	
Treponema pallidum	

CMV = cytomegalovirus; EBV = Epstein–Barr virus; HSV = herpes simplex virus; VZV = varicella zoster virus.

is especially common in hepatitis C infections. In chronic persistent hepatitis, the infiltrating immune cells are less extensive and limited to the portal triad. Consequently, it carries a better prognosis and is not associated with cirrhosis. Whether chronic active and chronic persistent hepatitis are two distinct forms of chronic hepatitis remains uncertain. Most likely, both represent a continuous spectrum of chronic hepatitis.

Several key points that relate to the diagnosis of the viral hepatidities should be kept in mind. As always, a thorough history is essential. A history of exposure to a jaundiced individual or ingestion of contaminated food or water may provide the initial clue leading to the diagnosis of hepatitis A. Potential parenteral exposures to hepatitis B also should be explored. These include tattoos, transfusions or use of other blood products, IV drug use, or inadvertent needle-stick injuries, and exposures through sexual transmission. The definitive differentiation between hepatitis viruses cannot be made clinically and relies on serologic testing, as described below.

The viral etiologies of hepatitis are discussed in more depth below. The broader differential diagnosis for jaundice and the approach to the infant or child who presents with jaundice are addressed in Chapter 13 (The Gastrointestinal Tract and Liver).

Hepatitis A. The hepatitis A virus is a common cause of hepatitis in developing and developed countries. This virus is a member of the picornavirus family. It is a nonenveloped, single-stranded RNA virus and is transmitted through the fecal–oral route. Ingestion of contaminated food or water is a major source of infection. The incubation period is 15–40 days; 90% of children are asymptomatic. The virus is shed in feces 14–21 days before the onset of jaundice and continues until approximately 1 week after its appearance. Therefore, most individuals are infectious for a long time before they realize that they have the disease. Because of this silent infectious period and the frequency of asymptomatic cases, this disease is notoriously difficult to control. Large outbreaks often are associated with day-care centers. The diagnosis is best made by the determination of IgM levels against the virus. Prophylaxis is recommended for household and other close contacts; intramuscular immunoglobulin (0.02 mL/kg for one dose) should be given within 2 weeks of exposure. Strict hand washing is the best prophylactic measure. Preexposure prophylaxis is recommended for travel to developing countries. A recently available killed virus vaccine provides excellent immunity when given in two doses 6–12 months apart.

Hepatitis B. Hepatitis B virus is a DNA virus belonging to the hepadnavirus family. It is double shelled and has several antigenically distinct parts. The outer lipoprotein envelope is the surface antigen (HBsAg). The inner core (HBcAg) contains three distinct parts: the genome of the

Table 9–42. Viral Hepatitis: Types A, B, C, D, and E

	Hepatitis A	Hepatitis B	Hepatitis C	Hepatitis D[1]	Hepatitis E[2]
Incubation period	15–40 d	50–180 d	1–5 mo	21–90 d	15–60 d
Transmission	Fecal-oral	Parenteral, sexual, mucosal, or perinatal	Parenteral, sexual, or perinatal (including breast feeding)	Parenteral (same as HBV)	Fecal-oral
Chronic infection	No	~5% of infected adults; if perinatally acquired, can approach 90%	50% of posttransfusion acquired cases	Yes	No
Treatment or postexposure prophylaxis	Can give immunoglobulin if within 2 wk of exposure	Interferon-α, lamivudine, immunoglobulin postexposure	Interferon-α, interferon-α + ribavirin	Interferon-α	No
Vaccine available	Yes	Yes	No	No	No
Associated sequelae of chronic disease		Cirrhosis, hepatocellular carcinoma, immune complex manifestations	Cirrhosis, hepatocellular carcinoma common	Cirrhosis	

[1] Coinfection with HBV (requires presence of HBV for replication). The most common cause is fulminant hepatitis.
[2] Usually self-limited infection but significant risk of fulminant hepatitis in pregnant women. HBV = hepatitis B virus.

partially stranded DNA, the DNA-dependent DNA polymerase, and the hepatitis B "e" antigen (HBeAg). Viral shedding occurs into blood, semen, and saliva, so transmission can be parenteral, sexual, mucosal, or perinatal. The incubation period is 50–180 days.

A radioimmunoassay is available to measure serum concentrations of HBsAg. Antibodies to HBsAg and HBcAg also can be measured. Response to the hepatitis B virus can be documented, and asymptomatic patients can be screened by determining the presence of antibody against HBsAg. The immunologic response to hepatitis B infection is outlined in Figure 9–4. A period of several weeks, called the "window phase," often elapses between the disappearance of HBsAg and the appearance of IgG anti-HBsAg antibody. Immunoglobulin M and anti-HBcAg antibody can be detected during the window phase; measurements of this antibody also can help differentiate recent from previous hepatitis B infection. The HBeAg correlates with active viral replication and infectivity, and the presence of antibody against HBeAg implies less viral replication and chance of infecting others. The carrier state results when there is an ineffective immune response; these patients remain infectious to others. In adults, the carrier state occurs in about 5% of those infected, whereas in newborns, it may run as high as 90%.

Hepatitis B is the most common cause of infectious hepatitis in the neonatal period. Transmission to the newborn is most frequent if the mother is positive for HBeAg. In such cases, transmission is as high as 90%. In contrast, if the mother is HBsAg positive but HBeAg negative, transmission is less than 20%. Routes of transmission include viral invasion across the placenta during late pregnancy or labor (prenatal), ingestion of maternal blood or amniotic fluid (natal), and breast feeding with cracked and bleeding nipples (postnatal). To prevent perinatal infection, hepatitis B immunoglobulin and recombinant hepatitis B vaccine should be given to all newborns of infected mothers soon after birth. This should be followed by completion of hepatitis B vaccination during infancy.

Although the mortality rate associated with acute hepatitis B infection is less than 1%, complications and morbidity are very significant. Complications include fulminant hepatitis, cirrhosis, and hepatocellular carcinoma, especially after decades of the chronic carrier state. Other extrahepatic manifestations are the result of immune complex vasculitis and manifest as glomerulonephritis, arthritis, serum sickness, polyarteritis nodosa, and urticaria. Therapies for chronic hepatitis B infection are now available. One example is interferon-α, which has been licensed in the United States for this indication. Response rates of 35% have been seen in controlled trials after 4–6 months of therapy, as documented by normalization of liver enzyme levels and improved histologic appearance of the liver on biopsy. In addition, there was a delayed response to interferon therapy in another 10–15% of treated patients. Different patient groups have different response rates. Patients infected at or shortly after birth appear to have more recalcitrant disease and are less responsive to interferon therapy. Other promising antiviral therapies currently under investigation include lamivudine and thymosin as well as ribavirin in combination with interferon-α (see following section on hepatitis C).

Hepatitis C. Hepatitis C virus is a single-stranded RNA virus and a member of the flavivirus family. This virus is the most common cause of non-A, non-B posttransfusion hepatitis. The incubation period is long, 1–5 months, and transmission usually occurs through parenteral, sexual, or perinatal exposure. It has been estimated that 3 to 4 million patients, mostly adults, are infected with HCV in the United States alone. Clinical disease is usually mild; most acute infections are anicteric but demonstrate mild and fluctuating elevations in alanine aminotransferase, aspartate aminotransferase, and bilirubin levels. Chronic carriage occurs in 50% of posttransfusion acquired infections. Of the patients with chronic HCV infection, at least 20% will develop cirrhosis and final progression to hepatocellular carcinoma over 20–30 years. Hepatitis C virus can be found in breast milk of infected mothers, but reliable data on risk of transmission from breast milk are not currently available. Transfusion-acquired HCV is uncommon nowadays since the introduction of screening tests including HCV antibody assays for blood products during the past decade.

In chronic hepatitis C, 40–50% of patients may initially respond to interferon-α (given as 3 million units three times a week for 6 months), with resolution of abnormal liver function tests and loss of detectable serum

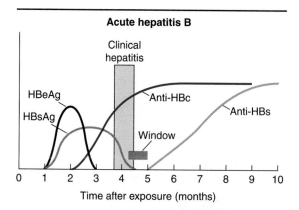

Acute hepatitis B

Clinical hepatitis

HBeAg

HBsAg

Anti-HBc

Anti-HBs

Window

Time after exposure (months)

Figure 9–4. Schematic representation of viral markers in the blood throughout the course of self-limited, hepatitis B surface antigen (HBsAg)–positive primary hepatitis B virus infection. (Reproduced, with permission, from Mandell GL et al [editors]: *Principles and Practice of Infectious Diseases*, 3rd ed. Churchill Livingstone, 1990:1209.)

HCV RNA in 75%. Unfortunately, the therapeutic effects are not sustained, and more than 50% of patients relapse after cessation of interferon therapy. Subsequent treatment involves using interferon-α at higher doses for at least 12 months. Two recent studies in 1998 indicated that, with parenteral interferon-α therapy in combination with oral ribavirin, the sustained response rate (as defined by better hepatic functions and undetectable HCV RNA serum levels 24 weeks after treatment) increased to 38% in new patients and 49% in relapsed patients. During acute HCV infection, interferon-α treatment alone was shown to reduce the risk of chronicity. In addition, in patients with HCV-related cirrhosis, interferon-α therapy appears to reduce the risk of hepatocarcinoma. Combined interferon-α and ribavirin treatment is necessary to reduce the risk of recurrent HCV infection post–liver transplant. Taken together, these studies demonstrate the superiority of the combination use of interferon-α with other antiviral drugs. α-Interferons are currently approved for use as monotherapy and combination therapy with ribavirin for the treatment of hepatitis C.

Hepatitis D. This defective virus is really a coinfection or superinfection because it requires the presence of the HBV for replication. Also known as the delta virus, this small, circular, single-stranded RNA virus has an incubation period of 21–90 days. Transmission can be parenteral, sexual, or perinatal. Disease tends to be quite severe, with the highest mortality of all viral hepatidities (about 20%). Cirrhosis and portal hypertension often develop in those who survive the acute illness. Individuals who abuse IV drugs are at particularly high risk for this infection.

Hepatitis E. Hepatitis E is seen more commonly in adolescents and young adults and is similar to hepatitis A. This single-stranded RNA member of the calicivirus family was first identified in 1990. It has been called enterically transmitted non-A, non-B hepatitis. Transmission is by the fecal–oral route, and the incubation period is 2–9 weeks. The mortality rate is less than 1%. In pregnant women, however, this rate reaches 20%.

Cardiac Infections

For a comprehensive review of cardiac infections including endocarditis and pericarditis, the reader is referred to Chapter 17 (Circulation).

Bone & Joint Infections

Bacterial infections of the skeletal system can occur at any age but are most common in young children, in whom bone growth is rapid. Damage to the growth plate (epiphysis) of the bone can have disastrous consequences to the skeletal system of a growing child. In the preantibiotic era, osteomyelitis and septic arthritis were crippling diseases. Now, with proper management, compliance and follow-up, most children with these infections recover completely.

OSTEOMYELITIS

The pathogenesis, etiology, signs and symptoms, and management of osteomyelitis differ as a function of age and site of infection.

Pathogenesis. Bony infections in neonates, older infants, and children represent suppurative sequelae of bacteremia, penetrating trauma, or extension of infection from an adjacent foci. In the vast majority of immunologically normal children younger than 10 years of age, osteomyelitis develops as a late complication of bacteremia or septicemia. In children beyond the neonatal age group and without hemoglobinopathies, bony infections of hematogenous origin occur almost exclusively in the metaphyses of the long bones. It has been suggested that the explanation for this observation lies in the unique vascular anatomy of immature bone at these sites. The terminal arterial ramifications of the nutrient artery form loops immediately adjacent to the epiphyseal plates and drain into a large venous sinusoidal system that occupies the intramedullary portion of the metaphyses. Consequently, decreased rates of blood flow through this region of bone predispose to osseous colonization and subsequent infection during bacteremia. Once the infection is established, it extends to the cortex (causing periosteal elevation), through the intramedullary cavity or subperiosteum, and into the adjacent capsule of the joint beyond the epiphyseal growth plate. In children with sickle cell disease, the diaphyseal portions of long bones typically are involved, most likely the result of prior bone infarctions associated with red blood cell sludging and vasocclusion. In addition to a hematogenous origin, osteomyelitis can arise from direct bacterial inoculation of bone. Penetrating injuries of the foot, such as stepping on a nail or repeated heel sticks for blood sampling in a neonate, may introduce bacteria directly into bone. Premature infants often require venous or arterial catheters and repeated instrumentation and are at increased risk for bone infections. Osteomyelitis of the bones of the hand as a result of human or animal bites may represent direct inoculation or spread from an adjacent site of infection. Osteomyelitis of the facial bones typically follows extension from an infected sinus or from dental abscesses.

Clinical presentation. Neonatal osteomyelitis typically presents 2–8 weeks after birth. Bone infections in this age group usually represent late suppurative complications of bacteremia or direct inoculation of bone. Any bone may be involved. Systemic signs and symptoms of infection, such as fever, irritability, and poor oral intake, are often absent. Unlike bony infections in older infants and children, osteomyelitis in the neonate usually is multifocal, with involvement of joints and bones. Lack of spontaneous movement of an extremity (pseudoparalysis) or evidence of joint space involvement (see below) are the usual clinical signs. Beyond the neonatal period, infections of the femur, tibia, or humerus account for approximately two thirds of all cases of osteomyelitis; involvement of the hands and feet accounts for another 15%. Infection in the skull, vertebrae, or pelvis is rare in childhood. Concomitant joint infection and multiple foci of involvement are rare in children older than 3 years of age. However, osteomyelitis is a common complication of septic arthritis in children younger than 3 years of age, and up to 25% of these cases may be multifocal.

Focal pain, tenderness, and limp or decreased use of an extremity are characteristics of bone infections regardless of age. Most infants and children present with the constellation of fever, focal tenderness to palpation of the affected bone, and pain on passive motion of the affected extremity. Soft tissue swelling, local erythema, and drainage might not be present early in osteomyelitis of hematogenous origin but may accompany infections caused by penetrating trauma. In older children, osteomyelitis arising from penetrating injury is insidious at onset and lacks systemic signs of infection. Individuals with puncture wounds of the feet or bite injuries of the hands may experience persistent or episodic pain for several weeks to months before seeking medical attention. In these patients, focal tenderness, erythema, and drainage often are discovered on examination.

Etiology. The bacterial pathogens associated with neonatal osteomyelitis are similar to the etiologies of neonatal sepsis. Group B *Streptococcus*, *E. coli*, and *S. aureus* are the most common organisms identified. Under some circumstances, *N. gonorrheae* also should be considered. Most neonatal skeletal infections appear to accompany late onset sepsis and represent vertical rather than horizontal acquisition of pathogens.

Beyond the newborn period, *S. aureus* is the most common bacterial pathogen of bone in children. *Hemophilus influenza* type b and *S. pneumoniae* also cause a significant number of hematogenously acquired skeletal infections in children younger than 3 years of age. *Hemophilus influenza* type b and *S. pneumoniae* osteomyelitis usually are encountered as a complication of a joint infection. With the success of early *H. influenzae* vaccination, the incidence of skeletal infection due to this pathogen has decreased dramatically.

In several special circumstances, nonconventional organisms may be implicated. These include bone infections in patients with hemoglobinopathies and those arising from penetrating injuries to the foot, human or animal bites, and sinusitis or dental infections. Although *S. aureus* is still a significant bone pathogen among children with hemoglobinopathies, an increased percentage of these infections are due to *Salmonella* species and other gram-negative rods. *Pseudomonas aeruginosa* and *S. aureus*

are the most common causes of osteomyelitis after penetrating injury to the foot. Oral streptococci, *Eikenella corrodens,* and facultative anaerobes may cause osteomyelitis after human bites. Osteomyelitis due to *Pasteurella multocida* can follow dog or cat bites. Anaerobic bacteria, *M. catarrhalis,* and aerobic streptococci and staphylococci may cause osteomyelitis accompanying sinusitis or dental infections.

Diagnosis. A number of infectious and noninfectious processes can present with bone and joint swelling (Table 9–43). However, osteomyelitis should be considered in any child with:

1. nonuse or decreased use of an extremity
2. a limp or refusal to bear weight; focal, bony pain; and unexplained musculoskeletal swelling

A thorough history and physical examination are essential to identify any recent direct trauma, open wounds, or infections associated with bacteremia. It is also important to inquire about the presence of relevant underlying diseases such as hemoglobinopathies or metabolic and immune disorders. Neonatal osseous infections must be differentiated from birth trauma and congenital neurologic defects. Beyond the neonatal age group, osteomyelitis complicating penetrating trauma, sinusitis, or dental infections must be distinguished from soft tissue infections, bone cysts, malignant neoplasms, and chronic multifocal osteomyelitis (a syndrome of recurrent symptoms and signs of osteomyelitis without positive cultures). In older children with suspected osteomyelitis, the differential diagnosis includes septic arthritis, bacterial sepsis, leukemia, tumor (including osteosarcoma), collagen vascular diseases trauma, bone infarcts, and metabolic bone disorder.

The diagnosis of osteomyelitis may be especially difficult in several situations. Pelvic osteomyelitis frequently is confused with an acute abdomen or other intrapelvic processes. In patients with sickle cell disease, aseptic bone infarctions may present with signs and symptoms that are

Table 9–43. Differential Diagnosis for Bone and Joint Swellings

Bacterial osteomyelitis
Septic arthritis
Other infections: viral (e.g., rubella, hepatitis B), fungal, parasitic, rickettsial
Tumors: benign or malignant; bone cyst, histiocytosis, metastatic bone tumors
Collagen vascular diseases; juvenile rheumatoid arthritis
Acute rheumatic fever
Trauma, hemarthosis
Bone infarctions; sickle cell crisis
Metabolic bone disorder; scurvy, rickets

very similar to those of bone infections. In these cases, even a technetium scan may not differentiate the two entities reliably.

Laboratory and radiographic testing can assist in diagnosis and pathogen identification (Table 9–44). Children with osteomyelitis secondary to bacteremia usually have elevated peripheral WBCs and acute phase reactants (e.g., ESR and serum CRP levels). Results of blood cultures are positive in one half to two thirds of cases. Needle aspirates from infected bone yield pathogens in at least 70–80% of cases.

Plain radiographs of the affected bone often do not show any changes for up to 2 weeks after symptoms first appear. Although the earliest radiographic finding is the loss of the periosteal fat line, focal bony destruction is the most commonly identified abnormality. Periosteal elevation and destruction are later findings. The identification of a sequestrum (avascular, dead bone separated from adjacent bone) and involucrum (the thickened sheath around a sequestrum) on radiography indicates a chronic, long-standing infection.

Technetium-99m bone scans demonstrate increased bony uptake early in the course of osteomyelitis and can identify silent foci of infection, especially in multifocal disease. Results of these scans may be falsely negative in individuals with long-standing infections. Gallium or indium scans also may be useful. These tests are indicative of inflammation with migration of white blood cells to the site of infection; thus, they are positive in soft tissue infection and septic arthritis. Computed tomography and MRI also are useful modalities for demonstrating osteomyelitis.

Table 9–44. Laboratory Investigations for Evaluating Osteomyelitis and Septic Arthritis

Hematologic tests		
White blood cell counts, elevated		
C-reactive proteins		
Erythrocyte sedimentation rate, elevated in >95%		
Bacterial cultures		
Sources	*Yield (%)*	
Blood	50–60	
Bone aspiration	70–80	
Pus culture at surgery	80	
Joint fluid	<50	
Radiologic imaging		
Bone plain films		
Technetium-99m scan[1]		
Gallium or indium scan[1]		
Computed tomographic scan		
Magnetic resonance imaging		

[1] Commonly used radiologic tests.

Treatment. Successful management of bony infections in neonates and children requires close cooperation between the pediatrician and the orthopedic surgeon. For proper treatment, bacterial culture of blood and closed bone aspirate should precede empiric antimicrobial therapy because it is crucial for establishing the diagnosis and specific etiology. In borderline cases and in cases of chronic osteomyelitis, open surgical biopsy or debridement may be required to obtain the cultures.

Empiric antibiotic therapy is based on the likelihood of specific pathogens given specific clinical situations. In neonates, because of the prevalence of GBS, *E. coli,* and *Staphylococcus,* a broad-spectrum, parenteral cephalosporin, such as ceftriaxone or cefotaxime, combined with an anti-staphylococcal penicillin is recommended. Once the organism and its sensitivity are identified, antibiotic therapy can be adjusted accordingly.

For children younger than 5 years of age, initial antibiotic coverage should include gram-positive cocci and *H. influenzae.* Thus, cefuroxime, a second-generation cephalosporin, can be used. An alternative regimen might be ceftriaxone or cefotaxime in combination with an anti-staphylococcal penicillin.

Children older than 5 years of age with systemic signs and symptoms of infection should have therapy directed against *S. aureus.* Cloxacillin and nafcillin are the drugs of choice in this setting. Parenterally administered clindamycin is recommended for patients who are allergic to penicillin. For children with hemoglobinopathies and other immunocompromising conditions, a broader spectrum of coverage is essential, including gram-negative organisms. To provide anaerobic coverage, clindamycin is included in combination regimens for the empiric treatment of osteomyelitis due to bites or dental abscesses.

Therapy for the treatment of osteomyelitis secondary to puncture wounds of the foot may be delayed until culture results are known because this type of infection is indolent and rarely life threatening. If *P. aeruginosa* is isolated from the wound, combination therapy with an antipseudomonal penicillin or cephalosporin plus an aminoglycoside is suggested (especially in the case of immunocompromised hosts). Once the pathogen and its sensitivities have been identified, therapy can be narrowed and directed against the specific organism.

Parenteral therapy should be continued until most of the initial clinical symptoms have resolved. In the past, serum bactericidal titers, using the patient's own serum against the organism isolated or a reference strain of *S. aureus,* were used to monitor oral therapy. Alternatively, serum antibiotic levels can be measured directly.

Nowadays, some experts advocate at least one week of IV antibiotic therapy followed by consideration of oral antibiotic therapy to complete the treatment course *only* if the following criteria are met:

- The organism has been identified or the patient has shown improvement with antistaphylococcal therapy alone.
- An effective oral agent is available and tolerated by the child.
- Compliance with oral therapy is ensured.
- Adequate follow-up will be provided for clinical monitoring of progress.
- The patient is not a neonate.

For neonates, or in cases in which the criteria for oral therapy have not been met, the antibiotic course should be completed by the parenteral route. Parenteral therapy may be completed outside the hospital under the supervision of a home IV therapy team.

The optimal total duration of antimicrobial therapy (parenteral plus oral) remains controversial. In general, for uncomplicated cases due to staphylococci in a previously well patient, a minimum of 3–4 weeks of therapy is probably adequate. Clinical findings should resolve rapidly, and the ESR and WBC should return to normal 1 week before cessation of therapy. For *Pseudomonas* osteomyelitis from puncture wounds in patients without joint involvement, the infection can be treated with a short course of 10–14 days, especially when combined with adequate curettage. Chronic staphylococcal osteomyelitis, especially in the presence of foreign bodies such as orthopedic pins, usually is treated with at least 1 month of parenteral therapy followed by at least 8–10 months of oral therapy. Open drainage and debridement of necrotic bone are rarely required but recommended in: cases of chronic osteomyelitis or neonatal osteomyelitis, instances in which a closed aspirate yields grossly purulent material, patients with associated joint infection, patients who have nonfocal pain along the shaft of the infected bone or have persistent bacteremia despite adequate antimicrobial therapy, instances of failure of systemic symptoms and laboratory markers to normalize in a reasonable amount of time, and cases of *Pseudomonas* osteomyelitis.

Complications. Complications of osteomyelitis are rare, and, in general, most children recover without significant sequelae. The most common complications are the development of chronic infection and impaired function of the affected extremity. Symptoms of chronic infection, characterized by constant or episodic pain at the site of the original infection, may not manifest themselves until 8 weeks or more after completion of therapy. In some patients, a sinus tract with drainage may develop. In approximately 25% of these patients, the infection does not respond to extensive surgical debridement and prolonged antimicrobial therapy. These patients may require extended antimicrobial therapy in addition to extensive surgical reconstruction and bone grafting.

Because the metaphyseal growth plate is the most common site of bony infection in children, a small percentage of patients, in particular neonates, may experience loss of longitudinal bone growth. Without adequate treatment, this limb shortening is a well-known complication of childhood osteomyelitis.

INFECTIOUS ARTHRITIS

Infectious arthritis can be divided into three major syndromes: (1) acute pyogenic, (2) neonatal, and (3) reactive arthritis. Although these syndromes share many clinical characteristics, the etiologic agents and management are different.

Clinical presentation. Infectious arthritis in infants and children is characterized by fever and joint pain. The onset of illness usually is abrupt, with complaints of joint pain with passive and active motion. When lower extremities are involved, the child may limp or refuse to bear weight. When the hip joint is involved, the affected limb usually is held in the position of greatest comfort, i.e., flexed and externally rotated (the "frog-leg" position). On occasion, pain may be perceived at a site distal to the actual infection. For example, the child with a septic hip joint may point to the knee as the source of pain.

Examination of the affected joint shows pain on motion and overlying warmth, erythema, and swelling. Large joints such as the knees, hips, and elbows are affected most commonly in children, accounting for almost two thirds of cases. The small joints of the hands often are involved in posttraumatic infections, particularly after human or animal bites.

Diagnosis. The differential diagnosis for arthritis in children is broad and includes infectious diseases, malignant neoplasms, rheumatologic disorders, trauma, osteomyelitis, septic bursitis, fasciitis, myositis, cellulitis, and occult abscesses (Table 9–43). Occult abscesses may mimic the clinical presentation of infectious arthritis. For instance, a psoas muscle abscess may present with fever and pain on hip movement. Antecedent events such as gastroenteritis, urethritis, tick bite, pharyngitis, or sexually transmitted diseases (STDs) may precede the development of a reactive arthritis. A history of injury, penetrating trauma, or bleeding dyscrasia usually is present in cases of hemarthrosis.

In the neonate, prolonged ventilation, use of indwelling venous catheters, and hyperalimentation are risk factors for infectious arthritis. Because of the relative immaturity of the immune system, pyogenic arthritis in the neonate frequently is multifocal and associated with concomitant osteomyelitis. Bacterial arthritis in older children typically is monoarticular, unlike some forms of reactive and rheumatologic arthritis. Juvenile rheumatoid arthritis, Kawasaki syndrome, Henoch–Schönlein purpura, Crohn disease, and other rheumatologic disorders must be considered in children when multiple, hot, swollen joints are present. In general, symmetric multiple joint involvement usually excludes infectious causes. However, Reiter syndrome must be considered in these cases, particularly with involvement of the eyes, skin, and mucous membranes (see below). Commonly available laboratory studies usually are nonspecific in patients with infectious arthritis (Table 9–44). Elevations in peripheral WBC, ESR, and CRP are typical in children with joint space infections. Arthrocentesis with synovial fluid analysis is the most useful study for establishing the presumptive diagnosis of infectious arthritis. The recovery of grossly purulent fluid with a high protein content and low glucose concentration is characteristic of infectious arthritis.

The definitive diagnosis of pyogenic arthritis requires the recovery of a bacterial pathogen from purulent synovial fluid or blood cultures. The bacterial recovery rate from infected synovial fluid is less than 50%; blood culture results are positive in approximately one third of cases.

Plain radiographs are not helpful in the early diagnosis of infectious arthritis. Radionuclide scans are useful in making the diagnosis, and technetium-99m bone scans may identify a coexisting osseous infection. Gallium scans are helpful for identifying the infected joints but are not specific. Ultrasound studies can confirm joint effusions and are particularly helpful when used to guide diagnostic arthrocentesis in suspected hip infections. Magnetic resonance imaging can distinguish joint infections from cellulitis or suspected deep abscesses.

Specific clinical syndromes

Acute pyogenic arthritis. In children, acute infectious arthritis usually is the result of hematogenous seeding of a large joint after an occult or overt episode of bacteremia. Systemic signs and symptoms of infection usually are present. Less commonly, a penetrating injury to the joint may lead to bacterial infection. Beyond the newborn period and up to 2 years of age, HIB, *S. aureus,* and *S. pneumoniae* are the usual bacterial pathogens. Recent efforts to vaccinate young children against HIB has reduced the incidence of acute pyogenic arthritis caused by this organism. In older children and young adolescents, *S. aureus, N. gonorrhoeae,* and *S. pyogenes* are the most common bacterial pathogens identified. *Salmonella* and other aerobic gram-negative bacteria are seen usually in patients with diarrheal illnesses or immunodeficiencies. Oral streptococci, *Fusobacterium* species, and *Eikenella corrodens* may cause pyogenic arthritis in children after a human bite. *Pasteurella multocida* may be implicated with dog or cat bites. The diagnosis of acute pyogenic arthritis is confirmed by recovering bacteria from purulent joint fluid or blood.

Treatment of acute bacterial arthritis consists of antimicrobial therapy and judicious surgical intervention. In cases of suspected hematogenous origin, an antistaphylococcal penicillin or cefuroxime would provide appropriate coverage. If gram-negative rods or gonococcus are suspected, cefotaxime, ceftriaxone, or penicillin can be used. In patients with hypersensitivity to penicillins, clindamycin and aztreonam provide appropriate alternative coverage. Clindamycin or an antistaphylococcal penicillin can be used for the initial management of pyogenic arthritis after trauma or bites. Recent studies have suggested that pneumococcal or *H. influenzae* arthritis can be treated successfully with 10–14 days of therapy, whereas 21 days are required for staphylococcal infections. These shorter periods of therapy are contingent on observing prompt resolution of the initial signs and symptoms of infection. Joint infections caused by *N. gonorrhoeae* are readily treated by a 7-day course of parenteral ceftriaxone. The role of surgery in the management of acute pyogenic arthritis is focused primarily on the need for drainage of local purulent materials. All patients should undergo an initial closed arthrocentesis for diagnostic purposes. Repeated arthrocentesis or closed drainage is recommended in cases in which the effusions reaccumulate rapidly. Open drainage and debridement are suggested in cases that do not respond rapidly to conservative therapy and those with concomitant osteomyelitis. However, hip involvement requires emergent open drainage of the joint. This recommendation is based on the relatively high incidence of long-term sequelae after hip infections; necrosis of the femoral head is a significant concern because the blood supply to this area of the bone is tenuous and can be compromised by an actively inflamed joint.

Neonatal arthritis. Pyogenic arthritis and osteomyelitis often are associated infections in the neonate, and the bacterial pathogens are similar. Group B *Streptococcus, Enterobacteriaceae, N. gonorrhoeae,* and *S. aureus* are the most common organisms identified. Most infants with neonatal arthritis have a preceding episode of bacteremia. Typically, the infection presents 2–8 weeks after birth. As with osteomyelitis, the first clinical sign of a neonatal skeletal infection may be pseudoparalysis, the absence of spontaneous movement of an affected extremity. Detailed examination often shows an effusion and pain on passive motion of the joint involved.

Definitive diagnosis is made by recovery of purulent materials from the affected joint. The duration of treatment for neonatal joint infections is largely empiric. Initial antimicrobial therapy is based on the pathogens typically encountered in these infections. Antistaphylococcal penicillin (oxacillin or nafcillin) combined with a broad-spectrum cephalosporin (cefotaxime, ceftazidime) is appropriate coverage for most bacterial pathogens. Amphotericin B should be used in cases of suspected fungal arthritis. Once the pathogen is identified, focused parenteral therapy should be continued for at least 3 weeks. Isolated neonatal infectious arthritis may be treated successfully with repeated arthrocenteses or closed drainage. However, if the underlying bone becomes involved, open drainage and bony debridement are usually necessary.

Reactive arthritis syndrome. Reactive arthritis is defined as a sterile arthritis that occurs in the absence of bacteremia or sepsis and often accompanies or immediately follows an infectious illness. In general, the arthritis in these conditions is thought to be immune mediated, but the inflammatory process is less aggressive than that seen in pyogenic conditions. Reactive arthritides are discussed in more depth in Chapter 8 (Rheumatic Diseases).

Gastrointestinal infections, particularly with **Shigella** and **Yersinia** species, must be considered in the differential diagnosis of arthritis. The knees are most commonly involved in both cases. The organism usually is recovered from the stool but not from the synovial fluid. In addition to using antimicrobial therapy for the elimination of pathogens from the gastrointestinal tract, nonsteroidal antiinflammatory agents are required for treatment of the arthritis.

Reiter's syndrome is a constellation of conjunctivitis, urethritis, reactive arthritis, rash, diarrhea, and stomatitis that may follow a number of infections, including bacterial gastroenteritis, chlamydiosis, or group A streptococcal infections.

The **gonococcal arthritis–dermatitis** syndrome is considered a complication of untreated primary infection caused by *N. gonorrhoeae*. The syndrome represents a continuum of symptoms that include dermatitis and arthritis caused by disseminated gonococcal infection.

After an untreated primary infection, patients present with a febrile, toxic illness characterized by a petechial rash, especially on the dorsum of the hands and feet, and periarthritis typically involving the tendon sheaths of the hands and feet. Cultures of joint fluid are almost always sterile, whereas cultures from the primary source of infection (genitourinary tract, throat, or rectum) and the blood are often positive. If left untreated, these symptoms initially resolve, only to return weeks later with arthritis of a large weight-bearing joint, usually the knee. At this later stage, the cultures of synovial fluid and primary infection sites are often positive. The arthritis-dermatitis syndrome may be readily treated with 7 days of parenteral ceftriaxone or oral amoxicillin. As with any gonococcal infection, these patients should be screened for other STDs.

Lyme disease is an arthropod-borne illness that is caused by *B. burgdorferi. Ixodes dammini,* the eastern deer tick, is the vector responsible for disease in most parts of the northeastern and midwestern United States. *Ixodes pacificus* is the vector in the western United States, and other *Ixodes* species have been implicated in the southeast. All *Ixodes* vectors have multiple hosts. The white-footed mouse in the United States and the black mouse in Europe are the typical reservoirs of infection because these species tolerate intense spirochetemia. The tick larvae feed on infected mice and then leave their hosts to

develop into nymphs that infect new hosts the following year. The nymphs become adult ticks and seek larger mammals, such as deer and humans, in the late summer or early fall of the second year.

Human disease caused by *B. burgdorferi* follows the bite of an infected tick. The spectrum of disease is broad, with most cases being asymptomatic. When present, symptoms appear after an incubation period of 3–31 days. The classic early feature of infection is a characteristic rash called *erythema chronicum migrans* that appears in 50–75% of patients. It begins at the site of the bite and then develops into an erythematous plaque that expands circularly and clears centrally. Subsequently, the rash may progress into variable colors and forms, such as purpura or vesicles. Altogether, the primary and secondary forms typically last several weeks and may recur. The appearance of the rash may be accompanied by constitutional symptoms including fatigue, fever, arthralgia, and arthritis, all of which resolve spontaneously.

Major concerns for Lyme disease are late manifestations, including joint, CNS, and cardiac complications that occur several months after the primary infection. Approximately one half of children with untreated primary infections will have episodes of arthritis, usually involving large joints such as the knees. Without treatment, these patients can develop chronic synovitis and permanent joint disability. Central nervous system disease can affect up to 15% of patients who do not receive treatment and has a variety of manifestations including meningitis, encephalitis, cranial nerve palsies, radiculitis, and transverse myelitis. Cardiac disease is not a common complication of Lyme disease: Atrioventricular block of different degrees is the most common manifestation. Myocarditis and pericarditis occur rarely.

Lyme disease is best diagnosed clinically. A history of travel to an endemic region and tick bite in an individual with erythema chronicum migrans is highly suggestive of the diagnosis. Although recovery of *B. burgdorferi* from the skin lesion is diagnostic, this test is not widely available. Serologic testing is of limited value because the IgM response to a mixture of *Borrelia* antigens occurs as late as 4 weeks after the initial infection. In addition, the available ELISA for detection of antibody is nonspecific. In fact, the Centers for Disease Control and the Food and Drug Administration support a two-step testing procedure, in which ELISA is performed first and, if positive, is followed by Western blot analysis. Serologic testing is only of value in patients with a suggestive history or with clinical findings that are suggestive of early or late infection.

The recommended treatment regimens for Lyme disease are shown in Table 9–45. A short course of oral therapy is effective treatment for children with erythema chronicum migrans and no systemic symptoms. Prophylactic antibiotics for children with tick bites is unproved

Table 9–45. Recommended Treatment of Lyme Disease in Children

Disease Category	Drug(s) and Dose
Early localized disease[1]	
≥8 y	Doxycycline, oral regimen, 100 mg twice a day for 14–21 days
All ages	Amoxicillin, oral regimen, 25–50 mg/kg/day divided into 2 doses (maximum, 2 g/day) for 14–21 days
Early disseminated and late disease	
Multiple erythema migrans	Same oral regimen as for early disease but for 21 days
Isolated facial palsy	Same oral regimen as for early disease but for 21–28 days[2]
Arthritis	Same oral regimen as for early disease but for 28 days
Persistent or recurrent arthritis[3]	Ceftriaxone, 75–100 mg/kg, IV or IM, once a day (maximum, 2 g/day) for 14–21 day; or penicillin, 300 000 U/kg/day, IV, given in divided doses every 4 h (maximum, 20 million U/day) for 14–21 days
Carditis	Ceftriaxone or penicillin: see persistent or recurrent arthritis
Meningitis or encephalitis	Ceftriaxone or penicillin: see persistent or recurrent arthritis

[1] For patients who are allergic to penicillin, cefuroxime axetil and erythromycin are alternative drugs. IV = intravenously; IM = intramuscularly.

[2] Corticosteroids should not be given. Treatment has no effect on the resolution of the nerve palsy; its purpose is to prevent late disease.

[3] Arthritis is not considered persistent or recurrent unless objective evidence of synovitis exists at least 2 months after treatment is initiated. Some experts administer a second course of an oral agent before using an IV-administered antimicrobial agent.

Reproduced with permission from the American Academy of Pediatrics: *Report of the Committee on Infectious Diseases (Red Book),* 25th ed. Author, 2000:377.

but has been used in highly endemic regions, such as New England. However, recent guidelines do not recommend this approach routinely. In fact, transmission of *B. burgdorferi* occurs in only approximately 10% of patients with bites by infected ticks. Use of measures to reduce the risk of tick bite (e.g., protective clothing, insect repellents), frequent tick checks, and prompt tick removal when found (within 24–48 hours of attachment) are among the most effective methods to prevent infection. Parenteral therapy is recommended for established complications of late disease. In contrast, the efficacy of prolonged courses of antimicrobial therapy for chronic fatigue syndrome or other nonspecific CNS symptoms in seropositive individuals without recognized manifestations of early or late Lyme disease is unknown.

Acute rheumatic fever is a late, nonsuppurative sequela of group A streptococcal pharyngitis. This syndrome is the result of an immune response against specific streptococcal strains that cross-react with cardiac and other tissues. Migratory polyarthritis is one of the unique features of this disease. Patients present with frank arthritis (joint effusion, pain, warmth, and tenderness), typically of the large joints (knees, ankles, wrists, and elbows), in a sequential pattern. Arthritic presentations of the joints flare and resolve spontaneously, with each episode lasting several days. Cardiac valvular and myocardial involvement frequently are observed. Acute

rheumatic fever is discussed in more depth in Chapter 8 (Rheumatic Diseases).

Urinary Tract Infections

The term urinary tract infection encompasses a variety of conditions that have in common the presence of an infectious agent somewhere in the urinary system. Infections are separated primarily into those that involve the renal parenchyma (upper tract) and those that are limited to the bladder (lower tract). Some terms used to describe specific urinary tract infections are listed in Table 9–46. Pediatric UTIs can present a number of challenges to the clinician in the areas of detection, diagnosis, treatment, and follow-up. The goals of UTI management include symptomatic relief, microbiological cure, identification of predisposing conditions, and the prevention of complications.

EPIDEMIOLOGY

Pediatric health providers encounter UTIs on a regular basis in the primary care setting. Epidemiologic information regarding UTIs in children generally has been derived from school-based screening studies and those of febrile infants and children. These sources have shown that the incidence of UTI is influenced by age, sex, and presence of the penile foreskin in boys.

Table 9–46. Urinary Tract Infection (UTI): Terms and Definitions

Bacteriuria	Isolation of bacteria from the urine; symptomatic or asymptomatic bacertiuria (see text)
Cystitis[1]	Commonly implies an infection limited to the bladder (lower tract UTI)
Pyelonephritis	Involvement of the renal parenchyma (upper tract UTI)
Pyuria	Presence of white blood cells in the urine; ≥5 white blood cell count/high-power field
Sterile pyuria	Presence of white blood cells in the urine with no identifiable infectious agent

[1] Noninfectious causes of bladder inflammation, also occur (e.g., hemorrhagic cystitis secondary to certain antineoplastic chemotherapy agents).

In neonates, UTIs are more common in boys than in girls, although studies vary widely. Premature newborns may have an even higher rate of infection than term newborns. In infants and older children, the incidence of UTIs is clearly greater in girls. Bacteriuria has been detected in 0.03% of boys and 1–2% of girls in school-aged children. In febrile infants and children with no localizing signs, UTIs represent the most commonly identified serious bacterial infection (see section on Approach to the Child With Fever). Overall, the frequency of UTI in febrile children between 2 months and 2 years of age is approximately 5%. When cases are separated by sex, UTIs are more than twice as common in girls as in boys. In boys, the presence of the foreskin has been shown to increase the risk of UTI. In a study of almost 4000 infants by Wiswell and colleagues, uncircumcised boys had a 10-fold greater incidence of UTI than did circumcised boys. Subsequent studies have confirmed an increased risk of 5–20-fold.

CLINICAL MANIFESTATIONS

Bacteria in the urinary tract may result in asymptomatic or symptomatic infection. In older children, the occurrence of asymptomatic bacteriuria has been well documented in large, school-based, screening studies. The occurrence of asymptomatic bacteriuria in infants and younger children is less clearly defined.

In symptomatic disease, the manifestations of UTI change with age. Infants and younger children may present with fever alone or in combination with nonspecific symptoms such as irritability, anorexia, abdominal pain, and vomiting. Older children and adolescents are more likely to exhibit signs and symptoms suggesting UTI. These include the classic manifestations of dysuria, urinary frequency, urinary urgency, and cloudy or malodor-

ous urine. In the previously continent school-aged child, the development of enuresis (secondary enuresis) should prompt the clinician to consider the possibility of a UTI.

Severe symptoms and constitutional signs (e.g., fever and back pain) suggest upper urinary tract involvement. It is generally assumed that bacteria isolated from the urine of a febrile infant or young child is an indicator of pyelonephritis. Costovertebral angle tenderness is a useful indicator of pyelonephritis in adolescents and adults but is infrequently elicited in infants and young children.

PATHOGENESIS

The urinary tract represents a normally sterile environment lined by uroepithelial cells. Infection may occur by (1) ascent of periurethral organisms through the urethra or (2) deposition of blood-borne organisms into the urinary tract. Ascending infection is the principal route of infection beyond the neonatal period. In neonates, isolation of bacteria from blood and urine cultures provides evidence for hematogenous spread.

Bacterial virulence factors and host susceptibility factors play a role in developing a UTI. Some bacteria (e.g., *E. coli*) exhibit fimbriae or pili, which allow them to adhere to uroepithelial cells. Children also may possess certain physiologic and anatomic characteristics that influence their likelihood of having a UTI. Factors that increase their risk include residual urine in the bladder, uroepithelial cell adhesiveness, presence of the penile foreskin, and congenital urogenital anomalies. Residual urine in the bladder can be secondary to a neurogenic bladder, infrequent or dysfunctional voiding, obstructive lesions, and vesicoureteral reflux (VUR). Other medical conditions, such as diabetes mellitus, renal calculi, constipation, and immunodeficiency, are associated with increased risk for UTIs.

MICROBIOLOGY

Escherichia coli is responsible for the vast majority of acute UTIs in children (80% or more). *Klebsiella–Enterobacter, Proteus mirabilis,* and viridans streptococci are other, less frequently isolated organisms. *Escherichia coli* may be a less important cause of UTI after instrumentation of the urinary tract (e.g. catheterization) or in patients with an underlying anatomic abnormality (e.g., obstructive lesions).

DIAGNOSIS

The pediatric health provider must have a low threshold for suspecting a UTI. As already discussed, UTIs should be considered in febrile infants with no localizing signs, children with nonspecific abdominal complaints, and children with urinary complaints (e.g., enuresis, frequency, dysuria).

When a UTI is suspected based on the history and physical examination, a number of indirect and direct laboratory tests are available to document the presence of infection. The initial laboratory procedure is to perform a urinalysis (UA) with or without microscopy. The dipstick UA can indirectly detect the presence of bacteria and white blood cells by using reagents that change color in the presence of nitrite or leukocyte esterase. (Bacteria such as *E. coli* can convert nitrate into nitrites, and white blood cells, if present, can release leukocyte esterase.) Urine microscopy and Gram stain of the urine can be used to directly visualize bacteria and white blood cells. The principal advantages of the UA, microscopy, and Gram stain are that the results are obtained rapidly. This allows clinicians to start treatment immediately if the findings are consistent with a UTI. The disadvantages of the conventional UA and microscopy are that they are less sensitive and less specific than the urine culture. An enhanced UA has been developed that has been reported to approach the sensitivity of culture.

Culture of the urine remains the gold standard for diagnosing a UTI. Because of the lower sensitivity and specificity of the conventional UA, urine culture should be performed regardless of the UA results. Urine culture allows specific identification of the organisms involved and the determination of their antibiotic sensitivities. However, interpretation of a positive urine culture is influenced by (1) the method of urine collection, (2) the specific organism or organisms isolated, and (3) the bacterial colony count.

Urine specimens can be collected for laboratory evaluation in several different ways:

1. midstream, "clean-catch" in children who are toilet trained and can void on demand
2. bag specimens (a sterile plastic bag taped to the perineal region)
3. transurethral bladder catheterization
4. suprapubic aspiration (a sterile needle is inserted directly across the abdominal wall into the bladder)

Each technique has advantages and disadvantages. For example, bag specimens are noninvasive but much more likely to become contaminated by perineal bacteria, whereas suprapubic aspiration is more invasive but the least likely method to become contaminated.

Quantitative urine cultures provide results in terms of bacterial colony counts. Bacterial colony counts of 100,000 or more of a single organism are consistent with UTI regardless of the method of collection. Colony counts less than 100,000 require additional interpretation but may be acceptable from suprapubic aspiration or catheterization specimens, or if multiple clean-catch samples yield the same results. Unusual organisms or multiple organisms suggest improper collection and a contaminated specimen. Urine cultures also provide information regarding the antibiotic sensitivities of the identified

pathogens. The principal disadvantage of the culture technique is the delay required (usually 1–2 days) before results are obtained.

Adjunctive tests have been used to differentiate upper from lower tract disease. Elevation of the ESR and CRP suggests a more systemic infection such as pyelonephritis. Nuclear medicine imaging with technetium-99m or a gallium renal scan can be performed in the acute setting to demonstrate abnormal uptake in the renal parenchyma. Other urine tests, such as documentation of antibody-coated bacteria and increased urine concentrations of lactate dehydrogenase isoenzyme 5 and *N*-acetyl β-D-glucosaminidase, have limited usefulness in the clinical setting. Likewise, bilateral ureteral catheterization and kidney biopsy are not commonly used to verify upper tract involvement.

TREATMENT

In the office or emergency department, the clinician's initial treatment plan will be based on the history, physical examination, and results of the urinalysis and any other immediate laboratory work. In formulating a therapeutic plan, the clinician must answer the following questions:

1. Should treatment be initiated immediately? (empiric therapy vs. waiting for culture results)
2. What is the most appropriate antibiotic? (drug of choice, route of administration, and duration of therapy)
3. What is the most appropriate setting for therapy? (inpatient vs. outpatient)

When the diagnosis of a UTI is supported by the initial evaluation, empiric therapy usually can be initiated. This is especially true if symptoms are severe, or upper tract disease is suspected (e.g., febrile infant with UTI). The choice of antibiotic should be based on the likely organism, usually *E. coli,* and the patterns of antibiotic resistance in the local area. In particular, *E. coli* has demonstrated an increasing frequency of ampicillin resistance. Adjustments to therapy can be made once the identity of the bacteria and its antibiotic sensitivities are known.

In determining the setting and route of therapy, pediatric health providers must consider the age of the patient, the severity of infection, and the patient's hydration status or ability to maintain hydration. Well-appearing patients with uncomplicated lower tract infections (cystitis) can be treated with a variety of oral antibiotics including amoxicillin, trimethoprim/sulfamethoxazole, and cephalosporins. Sick patients with upper tract infections (pyelonephritis) should be managed in the hospital with intravenous antibiotics including ceftriaxone, trimethoprim-sulfa, or gentamicin. Recent studies have supported the use of antibiotics (oral or intramuscular) in an outpatient setting in select patients. Inpatient therapy is still appropriate in neonates and very young infants who are at higher risk for bacteremia and sepsis. Ill or toxic-appearing patients and patients who are dehydrated may need admission for monitoring, IV fluids, and antibiotic therapy.

The duration of antibiotic therapy for UTIs is typically 7–14 days, with the longer course used in cases of upper tract disease. In most cases, a repeat urine culture (to document clearing of the infection) is not necessary if the patient is clinically responding and the organism has known sensitivities. However, for complicated patients with pyelonephritis, a repeat urine culture is indicated to monitor the progress of treatment.

FOLLOW-UP INVESTIGATIONS

The most controversial aspect of UTI management is the need for follow-up radiologic imaging of the urinary tract. The goals of radiologic imaging are (1) to identify host factors that may predispose to or increase the risk of recurrent infection and (2) to detect or prevent possible sequelae of infection (e.g., renal scarring). Many experts consider a UTI, especially in a male infant, to be a marker for anatomic malformation or dysfunction. Some of these abnormalities can predispose children to recurrent UTIs and subsequent renal scarring. Unfortunately, it is not known how often these abnormalities exist in children without UTI. Also, the optimal management for some of these conditions, once identified, remains unclear. Radi-

ologic testing can be invasive (i.e., require procedures that are uncomfortable to the patient), expensive, and require exposure to radiation. Therefore, the primary care provider must weigh the risks and benefits in deciding whether additional investigation is indicated after a documented UTI. A recent American Academy of Pediatrics Practice Parameter on UTI recommends diagnostic imaging in every febrile infant and young child with a first documented UTI. Of note, these guidelines refer to infants and children between 2 months and 2 years of age. The management of older children and children with uncomplicated cystitis is less clear.

A description of some of the radiographic studies used to evaluate the urinary tract is provided in Table 9–47. Currently, ultrasound and voiding cystourethrograms (VCUGs) are the procedures used most frequently to evaluate the upper and lower urinary tracts. Ultrasound can evaluate the kidney (hydronephrosis, congenital anomalies), ureters (duplication, dilatation, ureteroceles), and bladder (bladder thickening, diverticula). During the acute infection, ultrasound also can demonstrate perirenal or renal parenchymal diseases (e.g., abscess). The VCUG requires injecting radio-opaque contrast into the bladder by transurethral catheterization. Fluoroscopy is performed throughout the procedure. The VCUG can demonstrate obstructive lesions (e.g., posterior urethral valves) and is most sensitive for detecting and grading degrees of VUR.

Table 9–47. Imaging Studies in Urinary Tract Infection

	Detects	Advantages	Disadvantages
Renal ultrasound	Renal size, shape, position Echogenicity Hydronephrosis, hydroureter, ureteroceles, bladder thickening	Little discomfort No radiation No IV contrast	Low sensitivity for renal scars No functional assessment Dependent on skill of sonographer
IV pyelogram	Renal scarring Abnormal urinary tracts		Radiation Requires IV contrast (risk of contrast allergy)
VCUG[1]	Vesiculoureteral reflux (grading) Posterior ureteral valves Ureteroceles, bladder diverticula Bladder functions, emptying		Requires bladder catheterization Radiation
Radioisotope renal scans	Acute pyelonephritis Renal scars	Low radiation No contrast	
Nuclear VCUG	Vesicoureteral reflux	Low radiation	Requires bladder catheterization Difficult to grade reflux Less anatomic detail than VCUG

[1] The retrograde voiding cystourethrogram (VCUG) consists of instilling contrast material directly into the bladder via a small catheter inserted through the urethra.
IV = intravenous.

The most common urinary tract abnormality identified with radiographic evaluation is VUR, occurring in over half of children with UTI younger than 1 year of age. *Vesicouloureteral reflux* refers to the reflux of urine from bladder to ureter that may predispose to the development of UTIs and renal scarring by allowing the reflux of sterile or infected urine up to the kidneys. Medical (e.g., prophylactic antibiotics) and surgical (e.g., surgical reimplantation of the ureters) options exist for the treatment of reflux. Other abnormalities that can be detected by imaging are congenital renal abnormalities (e.g., dysplastic, horseshoe kidneys), duplicated collecting systems, bladder diverticula, obstructive lesions (e.g., posterior urethral valves), and urolithiasis.

Sexually Transmitted Diseases

Sexually transmitted diseases are an important cause of morbidity in the neonatal and adolescent age groups. Although adolescents and young adults are at greatest risk, newborns of infected mothers also can acquire many of these same infections. More than two dozen infectious agents are known to be transmitted by genital, anal, and oral sexual contact. Patients often are infected with more than one STD at a time; the identification of one infection should prompt an investigation for the presence of others. Only the more common STDs are discussed below. Additional information regarding STDs during adolescence is provided in Chapter 2 (Adolescence). Infection with HIV is discussed in Chapter 7 (Immunologic Disorders).

CHLAMYDIA TRACHOMATIS

Chlamydiae are some of the most common bacterial pathogens found in the human host. However, chlamydia lacks the capability to produce its own adenosine triphosphate and therefore is an obligate intracellular parasite, similar to viruses. Properties of chlamydiae that resemble those of bacteria include possession of both DNA and RNA, replication through binary fission, the presence of a cell wall, and their susceptibility to antimicrobials. The genus *Chlamydia* is divided into three species: *C. psittaci*, which causes psittacosis and ornithosis; *C. pneumoniae*, which causes pneumonia and bronchiolitis; and *C. trachomatis*, which is the leading cause of nonspecific urethritis and the most common nonviral STD in the United States (Table 9–48).

Chlamydia trachomatis has many different serotypes: types A–C are the leading cause of blindness worldwide. The types responsible for the common STDs include types D–K; types L1–L3 are the cause of lymphogranuloma venereum. The life cycle of chlamydiae is complex and involves attachment and then phagocytosis of the infectious elementary body by a host epithelial cell. The elementary bodies then reorganize into reticulate bodies,

Table 9–48. Chlamydial Infections

Species	Serotypes	Clinical Manifestations
Chlamydia trachomatis	A, B, C	Trachoma
	D–K	Urethritis, epididymitis, cervicitis, pelvic inflammatory disease, conjunctivitis, infantile pneumonia
	L1–L3	Lymphogranuloma venereum
Chlamydia psittaci		Psittacosis, ornithosis
Chlamydia pneumoniae		Pharyngitis, pneumonia

which take over the cellular machinery for reproduction while arresting cellular DNA and RNA replication. Once abundant in the cytoplasm, reticulate bodies condense and reorganize back into elementary bodies. Multiplication of *C. trachomatis* deprives the host cell of its own cellular adenosine triphosphate, resulting in host cell death, lysis, and release of elementary bodies. Epithelial cell phagocytosis of the newly released chlamydial particles spreads the infection and perpetuates the cycle.

Chlamydial urethritis presents with dysuria, sterile pyuria, and urethral inflammation and discharge. It is estimated that 10–25% of infected men and 35–50% of infected women are asymptomatic despite being infectious to others. The disease may localize to the initial point of contact with the organism, resulting in urethritis, cervicitis, conjunctivitis, pharyngitis, or proctitis. It also may ascend the genitourinary tract, resulting in epididymitis and prostatitis in male patients and salpingitis in female patients. Secondary scarring of the fallopian tubes increases the risk of subsequent ectopic pregnancy and infertility.

This infection may also result in Reiter syndrome and a perihepatitis (Fitz–Hugh–Curtis) syndrome. Features of Reiter syndrome include arthritis, ocular inflammation, and urethritis. Although usually associated with *C. trachomatis*, it also may be seen with other infections, most notably several organisms responsible for gasteroenteritis. The perihepatitis syndrome associated with *C. trachomatis* may present with right upper quadrant pain, referred shoulder pain, pleuritic pain, and elevated liver transaminases. The liver may be tender to palpation with an audible hepatic friction rub.

Newborns of mothers infected with *C. trachomatis* have a 30–50% chance of acquiring the infection with passage through the birth canal. Ocular and nasal mucosa are the areas most likely to be infected. The resulting conjunctival erythema and purulent ocular discharge cannot be distinguished clinically from other causes of conjunctivitis, including gonococcus and viruses. Spread from the upper to lower respiratory tract may result in interstitial pneumonitis by 1–6 months of age. These infants usually present with a pertussislike cough, hyperinflated chest, fever, and peripheral eosinophilia. The conjunctivitis and pneumonitis frequently occur sequentially rather than simultaneously.

Testing for chlamydial disease remains difficult. A urethral Gram stain revealing granulocytes without intracellular gram-negative diplococci (*N. gonorrhea*) is suggestive. Other tests require proper collection of infected epithelial cells. In newborns, samples should be collected from nasal respiratory mucosa or the conjunctiva. Culture remains the gold standard but takes time and is labor intensive. Rapid testing is available with an ELISA-identifying antigen and immunofluorescent antibody staining to identify intracellular elementary bodies. More recently, PCR and ligase chain reaction tests have become available.

In older children and teenagers, doxycycline or azithromycin is the drug of choice for treatment of chlamydial infections. Alternatives include tetracycline and erythromycin. In newborns, systemic therapy with erythromycin is recommended for conjunctivitis and pneumonitis. In addition, the newborn's mother and her partner should be treated.

NEISSERIA GONORRHOEAE

After *Chlamydia, N. gonorrhoeae*, a gram-negative diplococcus, is the most commonly reported bacterial STD in the United States and is responsible for more than 1 million reported cases per year. The organism's virulence is associated largely with its ability to use pili from its cell wall to adhere to mucoepithelial surfaces. Columnar epithelium is most susceptible to infection.

Asymptomatic infection is less frequent than with chlamydial infection; however, it does occur and is most common in women and in pharyngeal infections. Most infections are symptomatic and localized to the site of contact with the organism. Symptoms are similar to those seen with chlamydial infection, such as urethritis, cervicitis, conjunctivitis, pharyngitis, and proctitis. Ascending infections of the genitourinary tract include prostatitis in male patients and salpingitis in female patients. Disseminated disease occurs in fewer than 2% of patients. Hematogenous spread most frequently results in septic arthritis, tenosynovitis, and dermatitis (see section on Reactive Arthritis Syndrome). Skin lesions may be maculopapular, vesicular, or purpuric in appearance. Less frequent manifestations of disseminated disease include endocarditis and meningitis.

In newborns of infected mothers, gonococcal ophthalmia neonatorum may develop after a variable incubation period of several days to weeks. This usually presents with copious purulent discharge from the infant's eyes. Without proper diagnosis and treatment, rapid progression of the infection results in corneal ulceration, opacification, and blindness. The use of prophylactic ocular erythromycin ointment or 1% silver nitrate administered shortly after birth greatly reduces the rate of neonatal infection.

Diagnosis of gonococcal disease is confirmed by Gram stain and culture of purulent body fluids from the suspected site of infection. Cultures require the use of Thayer–Martin medium, with an increased carbon dioxide environment to enhance bacterial growth. Antimicrobial sensitivity testing is essential to guide therapy because of the rapid increase in numbers of penicillinase-producing organisms. Accepted treatments are outlined in Table 9–49. Third-generation cephalosporins are used to treat disseminated disease in older children and adolescents. In milder infections, oral amoxicillin, cefixime, or azithromycin may be used. In neonates, IV cefotaxime is preferred due to the effects of ceftriaxone on bilirubin binding. Concurrent therapy for chlamydial infection is recommended in all patients in whom gonorrhea is diagnosed.

SYPHILIS

Syphilis is caused by *T. pallidum,* a prototypic spirochete bacterium. The organism is a thin, delicate spirochete, 5–20 mm long, with an appearance of a helical coil. It can be visualized with dark field microscopy or immunofluorescence. Humans are the only hosts. Transmission is almost totally through sexual contact, with the exception of congenital infections and very close physical contact between mucous membranes of the hosts. The treponemal organism attacks the human cells and multiplies actively during the initial phase. The fetus and neonate are good targets because of the relative immaturity of the mucosal barrier and immune system of these hosts.

The incidence of syphilis in the United States had been decreasing over the past few decades; however, there has been a recent resurgence in the incidences of acquired and congenital syphilis, especially in major inner cities. The number of cases of congenital syphilis increased from fewer than 200 in the early 1980s to approximately 3000 in 1991. This has become a major problem for pediatric practitioners in many metropolitan centers. Particularly challenging is the approach to the well-appearing infant born to a serologically positive mother. For children newly diagnosed outside of the neonatal period, sexual abuse must be presumed, and a report must be made to children's protection services.

Acquired syphilis (i.e., beyond the perinatal period) has three stages. The primary stage is characterized by chancre, which is a single, painless, ulcerated lesion with a raised border at the site of entry of the organism (e.g.,

Table 9–49. Treatment for Gonococcal Infections[1]

Type of Infection	Drug of Choice	Alternatives[2]
Urethritis, vulvuvaginitis, cervicitis, proctitis	Ceftriaxone IM	Spectinomycin IM Cefixime PO Ciprofloxacin PO Ofloxacin PO
Pharyngitis	Ceftriaxone IM	Cefixime PO Ciprofloxacin PO Ofloxacin PO Trimethprim-sulfamethoxazole PO
Disseminated disease	Ceftriaxone IV	Cefotaxime IV Ciprofloxacin IV Ofloxacin IV Spectinomycin IM q 12 hrs
Neonatal GC conjunctivitis	Ceftriaxone IV or IM × 1 dose	Cefotaxime IV or IM × 1 dose

GC = gonococcal; IM = intramuscular; IV = intravenous; PO = per oral.
[1] For specific information regarding dosing and treatment variations, see the *Report of the Committee on Infectious Diseases (Red Book),* 25th ed (American Academy of Pediatrics, 2000). Concomitant treatment for chlamydia trachomatis is recommended due to the high prevalence of coinfection.
[2] Quinolones (Ciprofloxacin, Ofloxacin) are not currently licensed for routine use in children <18 y.

on the glans penis or labia or within the vagina). It often is accompanied by regional lymphadenopathy. The primary lesion heals spontaneously in 1–2 months. The secondary stage begins several months later with the onset of fever, sore throat, headache, rhinitis, arthralgia, malaise, and anorexia. Signs include generalized lymphadenopathy, hepatosplenomegaly, and a copper-colored maculopapular rash that begins on the trunk and spreads rapidly to involve the extremities, including the palms and soles. Mucous patches are common. Other dermatologic manifestations are alopecia and condyloma. In some patients, complications, including meningitis, hepatitis, and glomerulonephritis, may develop. At this stage, patients are very infectious, and the lesions often are positive for *Treponema* by immunofluorescence. Serologic tests are invariably positive. If undiagnosed, symptoms resolve spontaneously after approximately 2 weeks. Tertiary or latent syphilis occurs months to years after untreated secondary syphilis. The lesions are gummatous in appearance and probably the result of hypersensitivity reactions. Tertiary syphilis is primarily a disease of adults and can affect any organ. During this phase of the disease, the patient is no longer infectious to others. Gradual destruction of the nervous and cardiovascular systems predominates in the third stage as a result of long-standing vascular disease and endarteritis.

Serologic testing is the cornerstone of diagnosis. There are two general categories of tests. Nontreponemal antigen tests use a component of normal tissue (e.g., beef heart cardiolipin) as an antigen to assay for reagin, a nonspecific antibody formed by patients with syphilis. The most commonly used nontreponemal tests are VDRL and rapid plasma reagin (RPR). Older tests that use complement fixation are seldom used today. Results of these surrogate markers become positive by 4 weeks after the initial infection and remain so through the second stage of disease, with high titers of more than 1 : 32. During the latent phase and after therapy, the VDRL and RPR titers often decrease gradually. False-positive test results are encountered frequently in a number of other disorders, such as collagen vascular diseases, malaria, EBV infections, and other nonvenereal treponemal infections as well as drug reactions. The RPR test is simpler than the traditional VDRL.

If VDRL or RPR results are positive, the serum should be tested specifically for treponemal antibody with the FTA-ABS to confirm the diagnosis. This test is sensitive and specific for treponemal antibody. It is positive in most patients with primary syphilis and in virtually all secondary cases. In general, it remains permanently positive despite treatment. False-positive FTA-ABS results occur infrequently in systemic lupus and other rare diseases with abnormal globulins. Diagnosis also can be made by identifying motile spirochetes on material from the primary chancre using dark field microscopy. Current treatment recommendations are given in Table 9–50.

Congenital syphilis develops by two different routes: (1) transplacental transmission of the spirochete, mostly

Table 9–50. Recommended Therapy for Syphilis[1]

	Children	Adults
Neonatal (≤4 wk of age) proven or highly probable disease	Aqueous crystalline penicillin G 100,000–150,000 U/kg/day, administered as 50,000 U/kg per dose IV every 12 h during the first 7 days of life, and every 8 h thereafter for a total of 10 days *or* Procaine penicillin G 50,000 U/kg per dose IM a day in a single dose for 10 days	—
Primary, secondary, and early latent syphilis[2]	Benzathine penicillin G 50,000 U/kg IM, up to the adult dose of 2.4 million U in a single dose	Benzathine penicillin G 2.4 million U IM in a single dose *or* *If allergic to penicillin and not pregnant* Doxycycline 100 mg orally twice a day for 14 days *or* Tetracycline 500 mg orally 4 times a day for 14 days
Late latent syphilis or latent syphilis of unknown duration	Benzathine penicillin G 50,000 U/kg IM, up to the adult dose of 2.4 million U, administered as 3 doses at 1-wk intervals (total 150,000 U/kg up to the adult dose of 7.2 million U)	Benzathine penicillin G 7.2 million U total, administered as 3 doses of 2.4 million U IM each at 1-wk intervals *or* *If allergic to penicillin and not pregnant* Doxycycline 100 mg orally twice a day for 4 wk *or* Tetracycline 500 mg orally 4 times a day for 4 wk
Tertiary	—	Benzathine penicillin G 7.2 million U total, administered as 3 doses of 2.4 million U IM at 1-wk intervals
Neurosyphilis[3]	Aqueous crystalline penicillin G 200,000–300,000 U/kg/day given every 4–6 h for 10–14 days in doses not to exceed the adult dose	Aqueous crystalline penicillin G 18–24 million U a day, administered as 3–4 million U IV every 4 h for 10–14 days *or* Procaine penicillin 2.4 million U IM daily PLUS probenecid 500 mg orally 4 times a day, both for 10–14 days

[1] IM = intramuscularly; IV = intravenously.
[2] Early latent syphilis is defined as being acquired within the preceding year.
[3] Patients allergic to penicillin should be desensitized.

Reproduced, with permission, from American Academy of Pediatrics: *Report of the Committee on Infections Diseases (Red Book),* 25th ed. 2000:555–556.

in the first half of gestation, and (2) perinatal acquisition by direct contact with the organism through the vaginal canal. Many infants who are infected by the former route are stillborn. Manifestations of the congenital infection in the survivors vary and may be nonspecific. The skin and bones are the most commonly affected sites. Bullous lesions on the skin, including the palms and soles, develop in most untreated cases. Profuse serous rhinorrhea, called "snuffles," is a characteristic mucous membrane lesion. Consequent to mucosal and cartilage infections in the nasal area, destruction of the nasal cartilage

ensues, resulting in the classic saddle nose deformity. In addition, osteochondritis is diffuse and symmetric with involvement of the metaphyseal plates. Periosteal elevations in the humerus and tibia are most common. Involvement of the reticuloendothelial system results in splenomegaly and generalized lymphadenopathy. Late congenital syphilis is characterized by the Hutchinson triad: Hutchinson teeth (peg shaped, notched upper central incisors), interstitial keratitis, and cranial nerve VIII deafness. Table 9–50 summarizes the treatment alternatives and follow-up for congenital syphilis.

HERPES SIMPLEX VIRUS

Herpes simplex virus is responsible for an increasing number of clinically significant infections each year. Two strains, HSV-1 and HSV-2, are identified by biologic and antigenic differences. They are among the most common infectious pathogens in the pediatric age group. Herpes simplex virus belongs to a family of DNA viruses that also includes CMV, VZV, EBV, and herpes viruses 6–8. It has the capacity to persist, in active or dormant forms, throughout the life of the host. For primary infection, mucocutaneous epithelial cells provide the initial target for viral infection, whereas neural cells in trigeminal and sacral root ganglia constitute the sites of latent infection. In disseminated diseases, HSV-1 and HSV-2 can infect other tissue sites such as brain, liver, and lung.

Because of biologic differences, the two serotypes have different modes of transmission: HSV-1 is transmitted mainly through a nongenital route, whereas HSV-2 most commonly is transmitted venereally or from maternal genitalia to the newborn. As a general rule, HSV-1 infections occur most frequently during childhood and usually affect body mucosal sites above the waist, including mouth, lips, and eyes. In contrast, HSV-2 infections occur most often during adolescence and young adulthood and involve genital sites. HSV-2 produces vesicles similar to those of HSV-1, but these occur most often on the genitals. Men have lesions on the glans, prepuce, or penile shaft. Women usually have lesions on the cervix but may have scattered involvement of the labia.

After a primary infection, the virus becomes latent in the ganglion cells of the nerves innervating the site of inoculation. Recurrence may be frequent and can be precipitated by a number of factors such as stress, trauma, or fever. Recurrent disease presents with painful ulcerating vesicles and can be located on oral, rectal, vaginal mucosa, the penis, or labia. Regional lymphadenitis is common.

In neonates, most herpes infections are caused by HSV-2 due to transmission from the maternal genital tract to the infant during vaginal delivery. The incidence of neonatal herpes infection has been estimated to be in the range of 1:3000 to 1:30,000 deliveries, with a higher incidence reported in premature than in term newborns. Transplacental transmission has been shown to occur in a very small number of infants who present at birth with a congenital syndrome. The affected infants typically have CNS and ocular anomalies, accompanied by vesicular cutaneous lesions and scarring.

Neonatal herpes can manifest itself as localized or severe systemic disease complicated with meningoencephalitis. Without effective antiviral therapy, disseminated HSV disease has a mortality rate greater than 70%. Almost all survivors have serious CNS sequelae. Without treatment, the initially localized disease will progress to the disseminated form after 1–2 weeks.

Disseminated HSV disease affects primarily the liver, adrenal gland, and CNS. The infant may present with hepatosplenomegaly, jaundice, a bleeding diathesis, and seizures. In some cases, pneumonia has been described. Shock and disseminated intravascular coagulation may lead to death. Involvement of the eye may present with conjunctivitis, keratitis, and chorioretinitis and can lead to corneal scarring, cataracts, and blindness.

The diagnosis of an herpetic infection is strongly suggested by the demonstration of multinucleated giant cells in a Wright stained smear of cells scraped from the base of a vesicle. The diagnosis can be confirmed by viral culture of vesicular fluid or by immunofluorescence antibody assays against the HSV.

Patients with overt herpetic lesions should have strict barrier isolation to avoid spread of the infectious fluid. Hospital personnel should wear protective gowns and gloves when caring for these patients. Immunocompromised hosts should avoid contact with individuals with overt HSV disease.

For adolescents and adults, the use of condoms and the practice of "safe sex" cannot be overemphasized. Treatment of primary genital herpes with orally administered acyclovir shortens the clinical course but does not prevent recurrent infections. Small daily doses of the drug may be useful in preventing frequent recurrences after resolution of the acute infection. To minimize perinatal transmission, infants whose mothers are suspected of having active HSV-2 infection should be delivered by cesarean section before rupture of membranes or within 4 hours of membrane rupture. For neonates with HSV infection, systemic administration of acyclovir is indicated. Similarly, antiviral therapy should be instituted for patients with encephalitis and for immunocompromised hosts.

HUMAN PAPILLOMAVIRUS

Human papillomavirus is the most common STD in the United States. The DNA papillomavirus causes a painless, firm, warty lesion at the site of infection. The incubation period may be several months. Diagnosis is made by inspection. The application of 3% acetic acid turns human papillomavirus lesions white and may aid in the diagnosis. Human papillomaviruses 16 and 18 are risk factors for cervical and anal carcinoma. Newborns exposed to human papillomavirus during the birthing process may develop laryngeal papillomatosis, leading to airway obstruction many months after delivery. Treatment options differ and include topical application of podophyllin in tincture of benzoin for nonmucosal lesions, application of trichloroacetic acid, cryosurgery, laser therapy, systemic interferon administration, and surgical excision.

OTHER INFECTIONS

Trichomonas vaginalis is a frequent cause of vaginitis in the female population and urethritis in the male population. The vaginal discharge is often foul smelling, frothy, and yellow-green. The cervix usually is edematous and covered with punctate lesions against a background of diffuse erythema. Wet mounts reveal live, motile organisms and numerous granulocytes. The infection can be treated with metronidazole.

Bacterial vaginosis is a polymicrobial infection associated with decreased numbers of vaginal lactobacilli and overgrowth of vaginal anaerobic organisms including *Gardnerella vaginalis.* Many patients have asymptomatic infections. The most common symptoms are profuse vaginal discharge with an offensive, fishy odor. No associated pelvic pain, dysuria, or dyspareunia is present unless accompanied by another STD. The diagnosis is made on clinical grounds based on the presence of three of the following four criteria: (1) gray-white discharge adherent to vaginal mucosa; (2) vaginal pH greater than 4.5; (3) positive amine test, in which volatile amines are released with the addition of 10% KOH solution to vaginal secretions, thus enhancing the fishy odor; and (4) presence of clue cells (vaginal epithelial cells speckled by the adherence of organisms) in addition to numerous leukocytes on a saline wet mount of vaginal fluids. Treatment is with a single dose of metronidazole.

Haemophilus ducreyi is a nonmotile, gram-negative rod that causes chancroid. At the site of inoculation, a painful ulcer with scalloped and irregular borders develops. Regional lymphadenopathy is also present. The diagnosis is confirmed by bacterial culture of the exudate. Treatment consists of trimethoprim-sulfamethoxazole, erythromycin, or ceftriaxone.

■ INFECTIOUS EXANTHEMS PRESENTING AS RASH & FEVER

Rash and fever are common during childhood. Classically, there are six infectious exanthems (Table 9–51). Although this classification scheme is somewhat antiquated, it is a marker for the progress we have made in

Table 9–51. Historical Nomenclature of Infectious Exanthems

Disease	Infectious Agent
First	Rubeola or measles
Second	Streptococcal scarlet fever
Third	Rubella or German measles
Fourth	Filatov–Dukes disease
Fifth	Erythema infectiosum (parvovirus B19)
Sixth	Human herpes virus 6 (roseola)

identifying the infectious etiologies for a variety of common childhood illnesses.

Although most childhood exanthems accompanied by fever are self-limited and benign, some are life threatening and require immediate medical attention and treatment. For this reason, most ill children with rash should be examined promptly by medical personnel. This section discusses the common early childhood infectious exanthems and several other important causes of rash and fever.

Classic Viral Illnesses of Childhood

MEASLES

Rubeola, commonly referred to as the "10-day measles," is a highly contagious viral illness characterized by three stages: incubation, prodrome, and rash. Although the widespread use of the measles vaccine has significantly decreased the incidence of this infection, recent outbreaks in inadequately vaccinated children and adolescents remind us of the high morbidity and mortality associated with this disease.

Rubeola is an RNA virus of the Paramyxoviridae family. It spreads very efficiently through households with a greater than 90% infection rate in exposed susceptible individuals. Before the vaccine was available, measles occurred in epidemics during the spring every 2–4 years.

The incubation period is typically 8–12 days after exposure. During the prodromal phase, the patient has low-grade fever and "the three Cs": cough, coryza, and conjunctivitis, often with photophobia. This is followed by the appearance of the pathognomonic measles enanthem, Koplik spots. Koplik spots are gray, pinhead-sized dots surrounded by a ring of erythema on the buccal mucosa. They may last as briefly as 12 hours and frequently are missed on physical examination. The symptoms of the prodrome worsen until the fever spikes and the rash erupts. The maculopapular rash usually starts as faint macules around the neck and ears and spreads quickly to cover the face, arms, and chest within 24 hours. During the second day of rash, the lower torso and legs become involved. By the third day, the rash reaches the feet and has areas of confluence that are centripetal in distribution: The most densely confluent areas are located proximally and superiorly. The severity of the disease appears to be related directly to the severity of the rash. In severe cases, the rash may become hemorrhagic with the appearance of petechiae and ecchymosis.

Measles frequently is associated with otitis media and bronchopneumonia. As many as one third of affected children have patchy infiltrates on chest radiograph. Infrequent but potentially serious complications are laryngotracheitis and encephalomyelitis. Subacute sclerosing panencephalitis, a rare complication of persistent measles virus infection, is characterized by behavioral and intellectual deterioration and myoclonic seizures occurring several decades after the initial infection. The disease progresses to bulbar palsy, hyperthermia, and decerebrate posturing. Death occurs 1–2 years after the onset of symptoms.

Measles usually is diagnosed clinically but can be confirmed by serology. Assays measuring IgM and IgG are available commercially. In subacute sclerosing panencephalitis, high titers of measles antibody are found in the serum and CSF.

RUBELLA

Rubella, alternatively known as "German measles" or "3-day measles," continues to be a relatively common communicable disease despite efforts to vaccinate all children. Of major clinical significance is the risk for severe congenital anomalies associated with rubella infections that occur during pregnancy in susceptible hosts.

Rubella is caused by the rubivirus, a pleomorphic RNA virus in the togavirus family. During clinical illness, the virus is present in nasopharyngeal secretions, blood, feces, and urine. The disease is spread by oral droplets or the transplacental route. Before the vaccine was available, the peak incidence of disease was in children aged 5–14 years. Currently, most cases are seen in teenagers and young adults. In close quarters, the virus is highly contagious among susceptible individuals. Maternal antibody provides passive immunization for the first 6 months postnatally in infants. Active infection with rubella virus confers permanent immunity.

Several characteristic clinical features can help distinguish rubella from other childhood infections associated with exanthems. After an incubation period of 14–21 days, the disease typically begins with a prodrome of mild catarrhal symptoms, which often go unnoticed. A characteristic finding in rubella is the markedly tender lymphadenopathy that appears at least 24 hours before the rash and may last for several days. Usually, the postauricular, posterior cervical, and postoccipital nodes are most involved. The exanthem that subsequently develops is maculopapular and confluent, beginning on the face and spreading quickly to the trunk and extremities within the first 24 hours. The rash is nonpruritic and typically lacy in appearance. On the second day, the appearance becomes more pinpoint, resembling scarlet fever. The eruption usually clears by the third day. Occasionally, mild desquamation ensues. The oropharynx and conjunctiva usually are inflamed, but there is no photophobia as occurs in rubeola. A slight fever may accompany the rash for up to 3 days. Polyarthritis also may be seen, especially in older girls and women, and lasts several days to 2 weeks. With primary maternal infection during pregnancy, 25–90% of the fetuses may become infected depending on when during gestation the infection occurred. The highest rate of transmission occurs during the first trimester. Congenital anomalies can be seen in up to 30% of congenital rubella infections

acquired before 12 weeks of gestation. With infection beyond 20 weeks' gestation, congenital anomalies are rare. The most common anomalies are congenital cataracts, patent ductus arteriosus, sensorineural hearing loss, and meningoencephalitis. In addition, infants with congenital rubella syndrome may have growth retardation, radiolucent bone disease, hepatosplenomegaly, thrombocytopenia, jaundice, and purpura. The appearance of the skin lesions gives the name "blueberry muffin syndrome." The clinical diagnosis of rubella can be confirmed by acute and convalescent IgG titers or by direct measurement of rubella IgM antibody. Viral culture of the urine is diagnostic in congenital infections. Except for cases of congenitally acquired disease, rubella is a self-limited illness. The vaccine is important to improve herd immunity and reduce the risk of infection in pregnant women. Young women should be vaccinated or tested for immunity to rubella before the onset of sexual activity. Routine childhood immunization with the rubella vaccine [as a component of the MMR (measles, mumps, and rubella vaccine)] is recommended at 12–15 months and again at 4–6 years of age.

STREPTOCOCCAL SCARLET FEVER

Scarlet fever is characterized by an erythematous, sandpaperlike rash, with fever caused by one of the erythrogenic exotoxins produced by GAS, *S. pyogenes*. It is associated most often with pharyngeal infection (see section on Sore Mouth or Throat), but can be seen with pyoderma and impetigo. Transmission occurs by contact with respiratory secretions from a person with active streptococcal infection, especially in overcrowded environments such as schools, military camps, and the living quarters of the underprivileged. Infection can occur at any age but is most frequent in children older than 3 years of age.

The incubation period is 1–7 days, with an average of 3 days. Initially there is a rapid onset of fever and chills, vomiting, headache, and a toxic appearance. Examination of the posterior pharynx reveals erythematous tonsils, which frequently are covered with a white exudate. The tongue may initially appear white with prominent edematous papillae ("white strawberry tongue"). After several days, the white coat desquamates, leaving the erythematous papillae ("red strawberry tongue"). The exanthem usually appears at the same time as the fever and is characterized by fine, mildly erythematous papules that are seen first in the axilla, groin, and neck. Within 24 hours, the rash generalizes but spares the face. The cheeks and forehead are flushed, and there is circumoral pallor. The rash is most intense at pressure sites, and there may be some petechiae. Pastia lines are areas of linear hyperpigmentation in the deep creases, particularly the antecubital fossae. Miliary sudamina are small vesicular lesions that appear on the abdomen, hands, and feet in severe cases. The rash desquamates after approximately 1 week.

The diagnosis of scarlet fever is made clinically, and GAS can be cultured readily from the pharynx or wound. Patients with suspected scarlet fever should receive penicillin or erythromycin.

ERYTHEMA INFECTIOSUM (FIFTH DISEASE)

Erythema infectiosum is a common childhood illness caused by parvovirus B19, a single-stranded DNA virus. It is a relatively benign disease in the normal host but can cause aplastic anemia in patients with hemolytic anemia and HIV infection. Fetal hydrops may occur rarely when pregnant women experience a primary parvovirus B19 infection.

The disease is seen commonly in school-aged children, and community epidemics have been described. Approximately 50% of adults show serologic evidence of past infection. Outbreaks occur most frequently in the spring. Infection is spread by contact with respiratory secretions or blood.

The clinical presentation most frequently seen with parvovirus B19 infection is erythema infectiosum. This is a mild systemic illness, with low-grade fever and a distinctive rash. The cheeks show red flushing, with circumoral pallor, giving the appearance of "slapped cheeks." The rash on the torso and extremities is a pale maculopapular eruption, frequently lacy in appearance. This rash intensifies with fever and exposure to sunlight. The rash is frequently pruritic. The illness lasts approximately 3–5 days, and there are no sequelae. A child is usually noninfectious once the rash appears. In older children and adults, especially women, there may be associated arthralgia and arthritis. Rarely, the rash will be limited to hands and feet, giving a "glove and stocking" appearance.

Parvovirus B19 affects the red cell precursors in the bone marrow and reduces the number of circulating reticulocytes. This does not cause a significant anemia in healthy children, but severe anemia, termed *transient aplastic crisis,* can develop in children with conditions that are associated with a shortened red blood cell life span. This is seen most commonly in children with hemoglobinopathies and has been reported in patients infected with HIV. These patients have prolonged excretion of the virus and, if hospitalized, should be kept in respiratory isolation. The aplastic crises may be quite prolonged but have been successfully treated with IV immunoglobulin.

The diagnosis of erythema infectiosum is made clinically, but serologic tests measuring IgM and IgG are available. In addition, parvovirus B19 DNA can be detected by PCR assays or Southern hybridization in bone marrow from patients experiencing aplastic crises.

HUMAN HERPES VIRUS 6 (ROSEOLA)

Roseola infantum is a common acute viral illness seen in infants and toddlers. The child with roseola typically presents with 3–4 days of high fever, followed by a diffuse erythematous maculopapular eruption that emerges as the fever subsides.

The etiology of roseola has recently been found to be human herpes virus 6. Epidemiologic studies also have implicated this virus in children who present with febrile seizures, leading to the expression "roseola without the rash."

Although patients may have mild pharyngeal inflammation or coryza, the first symptom noted usually is the sudden onset of high fever. Temperatures as high as 39.5–41.0°C are common. Within the first 24–36 hours of fever, the WBC is elevated, often with increased neutrophil counts. Over the second to third day of fever, the WBC decreases, sometimes resulting in neutropenia. With resolution of the fever on the third or fourth day, a diffuse maculopapular rash erupts, beginning over the trunk. The rash quickly spreads to the arms, neck, face, and legs. This eruption usually lasts less than 24 hours.

Roseola infantum is a self-limited illness and requires no treatment. Antipyretics may be helpful in relieving the discomfort of the fever and reducing the risk of febrile seizure.

VARICELLA

Varicella zoster and herpes zoster are two clinical manifestations of the same virus. Varicella, or "chickenpox," is the primary infection that presents with diffuse vesicular skin lesions. It is a disease of early childhood; 90% of individuals contract the disease and develop immunity during the first decade of life. In contrast, herpes zoster is a localized reactivation of the infection characterized by distribution of lesions limited by dermatomes. A primary infection with varicella usually confers lifelong immunity against the systemic disease, but second episodes have been reported, particularly during periods of stress and in immunocompromised hosts. The viral agent that causes varicella and herpes zoster is *Herpesvirus varicellae,* a DNA virus. It is indistinguishable by electron microscopy from *Herpesvirus hominis.* The skin lesions of both species also are identical histologically.

The virus is highly contagious and can be transmitted through direct contact and large and small airborne droplets. Chickenpox is seen usually during the winter and spring months. Herpes zoster has no seasonal preference. The incubation period for varicella infection is 11–21 days. Viremia usually occurs 2 days before the onset of the exanthem. A mild prodrome of fever, malaise, and anorexia precedes the rash, usually by 24 hours. The rash consists of generalized, pruritic vesicular lesions that begin on the trunk and spread to the face and proximal extremities. A pertinent feature useful in distinguishing chickenpox from other vesicular exanthems is that the lesions can always be seen at different stages of healing. At any time during the infection, one should find erythematous papules, "tear drop" vesicles on an erythematous base, ruptured vesicles, and crusted vesicles with scabs. In primary infections, the vesicular lesions are limited to the skin. Rarely, lesions may spread to the mouth, esophagus, trachea, and intestines. Varicella pneumonia and hepatitis are rare complications.

After the primary infection, the virus remains dormant in a dorsal root ganglion in the normal host. Herpes zoster develops during periods of stress and in immunocompromised hosts. Reactivation of virus replication causes pain in the corresponding dermatome. Within a few days, an eruption of vesicular lesions on an erythematous base occurs in the same dermatome. The lesions last 5–10 days, and regional lymphadenopathy may be seen. The dermatomes of the second thoracic to the second lumbar nerves are the most commonly involved. In severe cases and in immunocompromised hosts, more than one dermatome may be involved. Rarely, herpes zoster may involve the ophthalmic branch of the trigeminal nerve, leading to a potentially serious ocular infection.

The fetus can be infected if primary varicella develops in a pregnant woman. Infection in the first half of pregnancy may result in the congenital varicella syndrome, which is a constellation of malformations characterized by abnormalities in epidermal tissue development. These include limb atrophy, cicatrized skin with severe scarring, CNS injury with cortical atrophy and microcephaly, and eye anomalies including chorioretinitis and cataracts. Affected infants usually die in the first year after birth. The few survivors have profound neurologic abnormalities. In contrast, no malformations were observed in the offspring of 48 women who experienced zoster during pregnancy, suggesting that the risk of viremia and maternal–fetal transmission is low in women with prior chickenpox infection.

Severe perinatal varicella may occur when a woman experiences a primary infection (as shown by the appearance of the viral exanthem between 5 days before and up to 2 days after delivery) at the very end of her pregnancy. This is due to the fact that it takes at least 5 days for maternal antibodies to develop and be transferred to the fetus before delivery. In primary infections, the infected mother is viremic 2 days before the onset of rash. Thus, maternal infection with primary varicella during this period can lead to life-threatening disease in the neonate (30–50% mortality rate). Diagnosis of varicella infections is usually clinical, but ELISA titers can confirm an acute infection. Varicella and herpes zoster infections are almost always self-limited in the otherwise healthy child. However, patients with eczema can have an especially severe course of varicella (eczema herpeticum).

Immunocompromised patients, newborns younger than 10 days, or children with varicella pneumonia, vari-

cella encephalitis, or hemorrhagic chickenpox (black pox) should receive high dose parenteral acyclovir for 7–10 days. Topical therapy is required for eye involvement. Oral acyclovir has been shown to decrease the duration of symptoms and the number of pox lesions when given to otherwise healthy children with chickenpox. However, the use of acyclovir in this setting is controversial.

A live-attenuated varicella vaccine, first developed and tested in Japan, is now available in the United States. Studies have shown a 90% rate of antibody production and 80% efficacy in children who are subsequently exposed to varicella. Passive immunity can be induced by using varicella-zoster immunoglobulin in exposed, high-risk patients, including immunocompromised hosts and cancer patients, and neonates at risk for severe perinatal infections.

Other Infectious Diseases Presenting With Rash & Fever

RICKETTSIAL INFECTIONS

Rocky Mountain spotted fever is a rickettsial disease associated with fever and a characteristic rash. It is caused by *R. rickettsii*, an obligate intracellular pathogen. The disease is transmitted to humans by a tick bite (*Dermacentor americanus*). Ticks are the reservoir and vector for *R. rickettsii*. The infection is widespread in the United States and most common in the southeastern states. Of interest, sporadic cases have been reported in the northeast, including New York City. Most cases occur in the spring and summer months.

The incubation period for Rocky Mountain spotted fever is 1–14 days, depending on the size of inoculum. Patients appear toxic and present with fever, headache, delirium, myalgia, nausea, vomiting, and rash. The erythematous macular rash first appears on the wrists and ankles and then quickly becomes maculopapular or petechial as it spreads proximally to the trunk. The infection can be severe, lasting as long as 3 weeks, and involve the CNS, heart, lungs, kidneys, and gastrointestinal system. In the most severe cases, disseminated intravascular coagulation, shock, and death can occur.

The clinical diagnosis of Rocky Mountain spotted fever must be suspected early to benefit from treatment. The diagnosis often is confirmed retrospectively by demonstrating a fourfold increase in serum antibody titer to *R. rickettsii* or immunohistology of biopsy specimens obtained from skin lesions and is suspected in patients with proteus OX-2 agglutinating antibodies. Chloramphenicol, fluoroquinolone, and tetracycline are the most effective antibiotics and should be administered until the patient is afebrile for at least 2 days. Side effects of tetracycline limit its use in children.

Epidemic typhus is a rickettsial disease transmitted by the body louse *Pediculus humanus*, which carries the infectious agent *R. prowazekii* from human to human. The disease is seen most commonly in areas of overcrowding and unsanitary conditions where lice spread quickly. Epidemic typhus is not transmitted between humans without the presence of the vector. The incubation period is 1–2 weeks. High fever, myalgia, headache, and malaise are the first symptoms and often mistaken for influenza or other viral infections. Four to seven days later, a rash appears on the trunk and spreads to the limbs, leaving a concentrated eruption in the axillae. Initially, the rash is maculopapular but later becomes petechial or hemorrhagic. Mental changes are common, sometimes progressing to delirium or coma. Myocardial or renal failure may supervene. The illness is rarely fatal in children who do not receive treatment, but it is severe and usually lasts 2 weeks. In adults, however, the mortality rate is 10–41%.

The diagnosis is based on a high level of clinical suspicion, especially in endemic areas. A fourfold increase in antibody titers against *R. prowazekii* confirms the diagnosis. The disease can also be suspected in patients with positive proteus OX-2 agglutinins. To be effective, treatment should be instituted early, with chloramphenicol or tetracycline given parenterally or orally. Topical insecticides containing pyrethrins are most effective in controlling the spread of lice.

Endemic typhus resembles epidemic typhus clinically but runs a much milder course. Endemic typhus is caused by *R. typhi,* which is transmitted to humans by the rat flea. The incubation period is 1–2 weeks. The patient has mild fever, headache, and myalgia, followed by a discrete maculopapular rash on days 3–5 of the illness. The symptoms last about 1 week. Because visceral involvement is unusual, the disease is rarely fatal. The diagnosis is confirmed by a fourfold increase in antibody to *R. typhi.* Because of the benign nature of the infection, a single dose of tetracycline (5 mg/kg; maximum, 200 mg) is effective in eradicating the organism.

TOXIN-RELATED EXANTHEMS

Toxic shock syndrome is caused by an exotoxin of *S. aureus* or, less commonly, *S. pyogenes*. These toxins serve as superantigens that activate most T cells through direct binding to the β chain of T-cell receptors. Among the various homeostasis disturbances, dysregulation of the immune system results in uncontrolled expression of proinflammatory cytokines. Most notably, these cytokines include interleukins and TNF. Some of these factors are directly cytotoxic and induce a process similar to disseminated intracellular coagulation, with massive fluid loss from the intravascular space.

The patient presents with rapid onset of high fever, myalgia, abdominal pain, vomiting, diarrhea, pharyngitis, and headache. Most notably, a diffuse, intense sunburnlike rash appears within 24 hours, along with hyperemia of the pharynx, conjunctiva, and vaginal mucosal membranes. Petechiae may develop several days later. Severe cases can be complicated by hypotension, renal failure, hepatitis, thrombocytopenia, and encephalopathy with altered mental status. The disease can be fatal especially during episodes of cardiovascular instability. Recovery occurs after 7–10 days and is heralded by desquamation of the rash, particularly of the palm and the sole.

The diagnosis of toxic shock syndrome is made by fulfilling six major clinical criteria: (1) temperature above 39°C, (2) diffuse macular erythroderma, (3) subsequent desquamation of the rash, (4) hypotension, (5) three or more organs involved (gastrointestinal system, muscle, mucous membrane, kidney, liver, hematologic, and CNS), and (6) negative findings on blood and CSF cultures (except for *S. aureus*).

In the past, most cases were diagnosed in women aged 15 to 25 years who used hyperabsorbent tampons in the presence of vaginal colonization with *S. aureus*. With recognition of this syndrome and proper avoidance of those tampons, the syndrome has become rather uncommon in this age group. Recently, colonization or infection with toxin-producing staphylococcal strains have occurred postoperatively as a complication of primary surgical infections. In the management of patients with toxic shock syndrome, cardiovascular support and vigorous fluid resuscitation are essential. Multiorgan failure or dysfunction should be identified and managed conservatively. Tampons should be removed, and infected wounds should be explored and properly drained. In women with menstrual-related toxic shock syndrome, further use of tampons must be avoided. Antimicrobial agents including nafcillin or cephazolin are used to eradicate the toxin-producing *S. aureus.* However, this may not affect the course of the acute disease because of the pathogenic mechanisms involved. Treatment, however, may reduce the risk of recurrence. In addition, the use of IV immunoglobulin has been met with an uneven but significant degree of success. This modality of therapy should be considered carefully in severe cases.

Staphylococcal scalded skin syndrome is characterized in children by the acute onset of fever, irritably, malaise, and a generalized fine erythematous rash. This is followed by exudative and crusty lesions around the mouth and eyes. Subsequently, the skin develops wrinkles and desquamates spontaneously, demonstrating the characteristic Nikolsky sign (exfoliation of the skin caused by gentle rubbing). The disease is caused by toxin secreting coagulase-positive *S. aureus* bacteria. In its early phase, the clinical presentation may resemble toxic shock syndrome, scarlet fever, drug-induced toxic epidermal necrolysis, or Kawasaki disease.

■ INFECTIOUS DISEASE ISSUES IN DAY-CARE CENTERS

In the United States, the number of children in out-of-home or nonparental child care has increased dramatically over the past several decades. Two factors contributing to this increase are the number of working mothers and the geographic mobility of young families. There are more working mothers in two-parent and single-parent households. Between 1970 and 1994, the percentage of married mothers with children younger than 6 years who worked outside of the home more than doubled, rising from 30% to 62%. The increased likelihood that parents will live far away from their place of birth means that families are less likely to have relatives nearby who can help with child care. By 1995, the number of children younger than 6 years in day care or preschool reached 13 million.

Infants and children who attend group day care are at increased risk of acquiring many of the typical childhood infections. A number of factors are responsible. Group day care places children in close physical contact. Larger groups raise the risk of infectious exposures. Further, the mixing of younger infants with older children allows the exchange of pathogens that are typically age specific (e.g., enteric infections in pre—toilet-trained children and *H. influenzae* colonization in older children). Normal infant behaviors (e.g., mouthing objects) and decreased hygienic behaviors in younger children (e.g., hand washing, toilet training) also contribute to the increased risk for infection in these settings.

Respiratory tract infections followed by gastrointestinal infections are the most common infectious diseases seen in day-care centers. In a prospective study by Wald and colleagues, respiratory tract infections represented 89% of all disease episodes. The risk of otitis media and diarrheal illness has been reported to be two to three times greater in children attending day care than in those who do not. Besides more frequent acute otitis media, children in day care have been shown to experience higher rates of middle ear effusions and tympanostomy tube placement.

Table 9–52 provides a list of infections that have been documented in children and staff of day-care centers.

In addition to the obvious direct health effects on the child, the increased frequency of infections can lead to other consequences, financial and social. Families need more frequent physician contacts, including office visits, emergency room visits, and hospitalizations. Increased episodes of illness lead to the use of more OTC and prescription med-

Table 9–52. Infectious Agents Documented to Have Occurred Among Children or Adult Providers Attending Day Care

Respiratory tract
  Viruses
    Respiratory syncytial virus
    Influenza, parainfluenza
    Adenoviruses, rhinoviruses
    Enteroviruses
    Parvovirus B19
    Measles, mumps, rubella
  Bacteria
    Streptococcus pneumoniae
    Haemophilus influenzae
    Moraxella catarrhalis
    Group A *Streptococcus*
    Mycobacterium tuberculosis
    Bordetella pertussis
    Corynebacterium diphtheriae

Gastrointestinal tract (GI) and liver
  Viruses
    Rotavirus, Norwalk
    Astrovirus, calcivirus
    Enteric adenovirus
    Hepatitis A and B

GI tract (*cont.*)
  Bacteria
    Shigella, Salmonella
    Escherichia coli (0157:H7; 0114:NM; 0111:K58)
    Clostridium difficile
    Campylobacter
  Parasites
    Giardia lamblia
    Cryptosporidium

Skin
    Streptococcus pyogenes
    Staphylococcus aureus
    Scabies (*Carcoptes scabiei var hominis*)
    Lice (*Pediculus humanis var corporis and capitis*)
    Herpes simplex

Multiple organ systems
    Cytomegalovirus, varicella zoster
    Human immunodeficiency virus

Invasive bacterial disease
    Haemophilus influenzae type b
    Neisseria meningitidis
    Streptococcus pneumoniae

Reproduced, with permission, from MT Osterholm: Infectious disease in child day care: An overview. Pediatrics 1994;94(6, suppl):997–998.

ications. The sick child who cannot attend day care also causes parental work loss or school absenteeism.

More frequent antibiotic usage contributes to increasing bacterial antibiotic resistance. Otitis media is the most frequent childhood illness resulting in an antibiotic prescription. A two- to threefold increase in otitis media due to day-care attendance adds pressure on bacteria to develop antibiotic resistance. Children in day care have been shown to be at increased risk for harboring penicillin-resistant *S. pneumoniae.* This in turn has resulted in recent changes in the treatment recommendations for otitis media in children attending day care, specifically the use of high doses (80–90 mg/kg/day) rather than regular doses (40–50 mg/kg/day) of amoxicillin (see Acute Otitis Media section). Day-care centers have attempted to implement a variety of measures aimed at decreasing the potential for spread of infectious diseases. Ensuring that all children are up to date with immunizations is one such effort. Universal immunization against HIB disease in infancy has dramatically reduced the number of cases occurring in the first 2 years of life. Laws that require age-appropriate immunization in children attending licensed day-care centers are present in almost all states. Additional measures include implementation of hygienic behaviors such as frequent hand washing of children and day-care center staff and the daily cleaning of toys, sinks, eating areas, and diapering/toilet areas. Centers should have separate areas for diaper changes and food handling and preparation.

When certain infections, such as invasive HIB or *N. meningitides,* are diagnosed at a child care center, the children and staff should be treated with prophylactic antibiotics (rifampin in the case of *H. influenza* and *N. meningitides*) to prevent further spread of the infectious disease. Immune globulin can be administered to children and caregivers after a hepatitis A outbreak at a day-care center.

In summary, more and more children are being cared for in group child care settings, which increase their risk for common and some not so common childhood infections. Age-appropriate immunizations, an emphasis on personal hygiene, and the separation of toileting from food preparation areas can reduce the risk of infection.

■ INFECTIOUS DISEASE ISSUES IN INTERNATIONALLY ADOPTED CHILDREN

Approximately 10,000 foreign-born children are adopted into homes in the United States each year. These children come from many different countries, including China, Korea, Vietnam, Central and South America, India, and Eastern Europe. Comprehensive medical evaluations are not required for entry into the United States, and these children commonly arrive with acute and sometimes chronic infectious diseases. Among the conditions diagnosed are HIV infection, hepatitis B and C, syphilis, intestinal parasitic infections, tuberculosis, and, more commonly, scabies and lice.

The medical evaluation often begins before a child's arrival into the United States, with the review of medical documents, photographs, and, more recently, videotapes of the child in its native country. Medical records can be inaccurate and difficult to interpret. Birth history, growth parameters, and immunization history usually are available but may be unreliable. Specifically, screening tests and immunization records frequently are incorrect.

After his/her arrival into the United States, the newly adopted child should be evaluated by a specialist within the first week or sooner, if any acute illness or unstable medical condition is present. During the initial visit, a review of medical records and a thorough medical examination should be performed. This can be done by an adoption specialist, infectious diseases specialist, or a pediatrician or family practitioner with experience in the area of internationally adopted children.

Recommended screening tests and examinations for all internationally adopted children include an evaluation for anemia, a UA, stool examination for ova and parasites, serologies for hepatitis B and C, syphilis, HIV, and the placement of a PPD. A complete list of recommended screening tests is included in Table 9–53.

Table 9–53. Recommended Screening Tests for Internationally Adopted Children

Complete blood count and differential
Urinalysis
Lead level
Stool examination for ova and parasites and culture
Stool for Giardia EIA
Hepatitis B panel: HBsAg, HBsAb, HBcAb
Hepatitis C antibody
HIV ELISA
RPR or VDRL
PPD (Mantoux skin test)

ELISA = enzyme-linked immunosorbent assay; HBsAg = hepatitis B virus surface antigen; HBcAg = hepatitis B virus inner core; HBeAg = hepatitis B "e" antigen; HIV = human immunodeficiency virus; PPD = purified protein derivative; RPR = rapid plasma reagin; VDRL = Venereal Disease Research Laboratory.

Adapted from Aronson J: Pediatr Annals 2000;29:218–223.

Infection with HIV is uncommon in children adopted from abroad. In infants younger than 18 months, a reactive HIV ELISA should be confirmed with HIV PCR because transplacentally acquired HIV antibody may persist for up to 18 months in children born to HIV-infected women.

Infection with HCV recently has been identified as a problem in internationally adopted children, especially those children adopted from China and Eastern Europe. Children may be infected with HCV perinatally or from the use of contaminated needles during medical procedures. Hepatitis B is especially prevalent in children adopted from Asia, Africa, and Eastern Europe. Perinatal transmission of HBV is much more common than that of HCV. The use of nonsterile needles also places children at risk for HBV infection.

There is a high prevalence of tuberculosis in many of the countries where children are frequently adopted from, and it is estimated that 1–2% of internationally adopted children are infected with *M. tuberculosis*. All children should have a PPD placed and interpreted in 48–72 hours by a medical professional. A measurement of at least 10 mm should be considered evidence of infection in an otherwise asymptomatic child. It is not uncommon for a foreign born child to have received BCG. These children also should be screened with a PPD. A recent report of a young adoptee from the Marshall Islands with undiagnosed cavitary tuberculosis highlights the importance of timely screening of internationally adopted children. The young boy transmitted tuberculosis to 20% of his contacts before his eventual diagnosis.

Evaluation of vaccine status is a complex issue and requires knowledge of the vaccine practices of specific countries. In general, vaccine records from most countries of origin should be disregarded: The vaccines frequently are not administered at the correct intervals, are often stored improperly, which may reduce efficacy, and are sometimes simply not provided despite documentation. An exception to this rule are the immunization records of children adopted from Korea, where vaccine documentation and administration are generally reliable. For all other countries, the vaccine series should be repeated in full for young children. If an older child has a record of having received multiple vaccines, serologic evaluation for immunity to diptheria, tetanus, measles, mumps, rubella, and varicella is reasonable to guide further booster immunization.

Common parasitic infections include giardiasis and scabies. These are especially prevalent in children adopted from orphanages abroad. After treatment for *Giardia,* follow-up stool examinations may reveal other parasitic pathogens that were masked by the giardia infection. Other common infections are *Entamoeba histolytica, Dientamoeba fragilis, Blastocystis hominis,* and *Ascaris lumbricoides.*

It is estimated that up to 50% of all internationally adopted children have some underlying medical condition requiring intervention. These infections are frequently contagious, thereby putting the adoptive family and community at risk. Fortunately, most of these infections are treatable, especially if diagnosed early. Other, noninfectious issues such as nutritional disorders, lead toxicity, prenatal exposure to illicit drugs and alcohol, and emotional neglect also need to be addressed in a timely manner by an experienced practitioner.

■ INFECTION OF THE IMMUNOCOMPROMISED HOST

The spectrum of infectious diseases prevalent in immunocompromised hosts is quite different from that of the normal child. In the normal host, invasion of infectious pathogens causes activation of different branches of the immune system, including cellular- and humoral-mediated responses. In the immunocompromised host, however, deficiency in different branches of the immune system results in defective responses and failure to protect the host from dissemination of the microbial agents. By studying these compromised patients, we can appreciate the importance of intact host defense mechanisms to maintain homeostasis.

The vast majority of organisms that are readily available to invade the immunocompromised host are the commensal or saprophytic microbes of the exogenous or endogenous flora. These opportunistic organisms account for most of the serious infections in these patients. In patients with specific immune defects, certain infectious organisms may predominate. These diseases include sickle cell anemia, cystic fibrosis, diabetes mellitus, and congenital, functional, or surgical asplenia.

Causative Agents

The organisms that account for more than 95% of serious infections in the immunosuppressed host are listed in Table 9–54. These originate predominantly from normal microbial flora of the intestinal tract, oral cavity, and skin. In the immunocompromised host, no organism isolated from sites including blood, bone marrow, CSF, or from biopsy specimens can be discounted as a contaminant without careful clinical evaluation, even if these can be treated as insignificant or nonpathogenic in a normal host.

Clinical Manifestations

Serious infection rarely occurs without any sign or symptom. Fever usually is the hallmark of infection and

Table 9–54. Some Common Causative Agents of Serious Infections in Immunosuppressed Patients

Bacteria	Viruses
Pseudomonas aeruginosa	Varicella zoster
Escherichia coli	Cytomegalovirus
Klebsiella-Enterobacter species	Herpes simplex
	Epstein–Barr
Staphylococcus aureus	Hepatitis A, B, and C
Staphylococcus, coagulase-negative	
	Protozoa
Mycobacterium avium-intracellulare	*Toxoplasma gondii*
Vancomycin-resistant enterococci	*Pneumocystis carinii*
	Cryptosporidium species
Legionella	*Microsporida* species
	Isospora species
Fungi	
Candida albicans	
Candida non-*albicans* species	
Aspergillus species	
Cryptococcus neoformans	
Mucor species	

is seldom abated by immunosuppressive drugs. In these patients, fever always must be considered to be of infectious etiology until proved otherwise. Because of deficient immune responses, the patient usually cannot localize infection at the portal of entry. Thus, the expected signs and symptoms of a specific infection may not occur. For example, the neutropenic patient may have perianal abscess without signs of significant inflammation. Likewise, the patient with bacterial meningitis may not have obvious signs of meningeal irritation or neutrophils in the spinal fluid. As in normal hosts, bacterial sepsis in these immunocompromised hosts presents with fever, but jaundice, abdominal pain, lethargy, petechiae, and erythematous macules also may occur. Careful physical examination must search for oral or anal lesions, infected IV sites, ulcerative skin lesions, and subtle mucositis. Whereas *S. epidermidis* is considered a contaminant in the blood culture of a normal host, it should be treated seriously in an immunocompromised patient with central venous lines. In fact, *S. epidermidis* is the most frequent cause of bacteremia in the febrile neutropenic host with an indwelling central catheter (e.g., Hickman–Broviac).

General Principles of Management

Key principles in the management of infections in the immunosuppressed host are listed below:

- Fever should be considered a sign of infection unless proved otherwise.
- Granulocytopenia with an absolute neutrophil count of 500/mm^3 or less renders the host highly susceptible to bacterial infection.
- Any organism should be considered a potential pathogen.
- When the causative agent for an infection is identified, surveillance should be continued for mixed or sequential infections.
- Immunosuppressive therapy should be withheld or modified during infection, if the status of the primary disease permits.
- Broad-spectrum antibiotics, preferably bactericidal, should be administered when indicated with monitoring for toxicity.
- GM-CSF or G-CSF should be used when indicated for the prevention and treatment of certain conditions associated with granulocytopenia.
- Systemic fungal infection should be considered when the febrile granulocytopenic patient continues to be unresponsive to a course of broad-spectrum antibiotic treatment.

Preventing Infection

Immunodeficient children and their caregivers should be instructed about their increased susceptibility to infection. They should be asked to report early signs and symptoms of infection, follow basic principles of good hygiene, and avoid contact with individuals with even minor contagious diseases. These patients should receive vaccinations according to the guidelines of the Centers for Disease Control and Prevention for the immunization of immunosuppressed infants and children. Diphtheria, tetanus, pertussis, *H. influenzae,* and hepatitis B vaccines are recommended as routine immunizations. Live oral polio vaccine is contraindicated in the severely immunocompromised patient, and close contacts of such patients should not receive the vaccine. The enhanced inactivated polio vaccine should be given instead. The live mumps, measles, and rubella vaccine is contraindicated in most severely immunocompromised patients, although it can be given to HIV-infected patients. Influenza and pneumococcal vaccines are suggested for those immunosuppressed patients who might have an immune response to the antigen. Prophylactic antibiotics, such as trimethoprim-sulfamethoxazole, should be used to prevent *P. carinii* pneumonitis and certain bacterial infections. Alternatively, aerosolized pentamidine given once a month is equally effective in preventing the infection in children who do not tolerate trimethoprim-sulfamethoxazole. Unfortunately, there is no generally accepted regimen for fungal prophylaxis.

REFERENCES

Laboratory Medicine in Infectious Diseases

Murray PR et al: *Manual of Clinical Microbiology,* 6th ed. Washington, DC: American Society for Microbiology, 1995.

Rogers WO et al: Microbiology testing and the pediatrician's office. Pediatr Infect Dis J 1997;16:33.

Antimicrobial Therapy

American Academy of Pediatrics: *Report of the Committee on Infectious Diseases (Red Book).* Author, 2000.

Gilbert DN et al: *The Sanford Guide to Antimicrobial Therapy,* 30th ed. Antimicrobial Therapy Inc., 2000.

Grossman M: Bacterial and viral infections. In: Rudolph AM et al (editors): *Rudolph's Pediatrics,* 20th ed. Appleton & Lange, 1996:499.

Lau AS: *Advances in Biotherapeutics: Interferons, Myeloid Hematopoietic Growth Factors and Chemokines.* Biotechnology International, Universal Medical Press, 2000.

Long SS et al: Section on anti-infective therapy. In: Long SS et al (editors): *Principles and Practice of Pediatric Infectious Diseases.* Churchill and Livingstone, 1997:1570.

Nelson JD: *Pocketbook of Pediatric Antimicrobial Therapy,* 14th ed. Williams & Wilkins, 2000–2001.

Approach to the Child with Fever

Baraff LJ et al: Practice guideline for the management of infants and children 0 to 36 months of age with fever without source. Agency for Health Care Policy and Research. Ann Emerg Med 1993; 22:1198.

Gartner JC Jr: Fever of unknown origin. Adv Pediatr Infect Dis 1992;7:1.

Jaskiewicz JA et al: Febrile infants at low risk for serious bacterial infection: An appraisal of the Rochester criteria and implications for management. Febrile Infant Collaborative Study Group. Pediatrics 1994;94:390.

Klassen TP, Rowe PC: (The Rochester Criteria) Selecting diagnostic tests to identify febrile infants less than 3 months of age as being at low risk for serious bacterial infection: A scientific overview. J Pediatr 1992;121(5, pt 1):671.

McCarthy PL et al: (Yale Observation Scale) Observation scales to identify serious illness in febrile children. Pediatrics 1982; 70:802.

Steele RW et al: Usefulness of scanning procedures for diagnosis of fever of unknown origin in children. J Pediatr 1991;119:526.

Eye, Mouth, & Neck Infections

Barnett ED, Klein JO: The problem of resistant bacteria for the management of acute otitis media. Pediatr Clin North Am 1995; 42:509.

Bluestone CD, Klein JO: *Otitis Media in Infants and Children,* 2nd ed. Saunders, 1995.

Bodor FF: Conjunctivitis–otitis syndrome. Pediatrics 1982;69:695.

Bodor FF: Diagnosis and management of acute conjunctivitis. Semin Pediatr Infect Dis 1998;9:27.

Cohen R et al: A multicenter, randomized double blind trial of 5 versus 10 days of antibiotic therapy for acute otitis media in young children. J Pediatr 1998;133:634.

Drugs for treatment of acute otitis media in children. Med Lett. 1994;36:19.

Gigliotti F et al: Etiology of acute conjunctivitis in children. J Pediatr 1981;98:531.

Weiss A et al: Acute conjunctivitis in childhood. J Pediatr 1993; 122:10.

Respiratory Infections

American Academy of Pediatrics Committee on Infectious Disease: Severe invasive group A streptococcal infections: A subject review. Pediatrics 1998;101:136.

Dworsky ME, Stagnio S: Newer agents causing pneumonitis in early infancy. Pediatr Infect Dis J 1982;1:188.

Schwartz B et al: Pharyngitis: Principles of judicious use of antimicrobial agents. Pediatrics. 1998;101(suppl):171.

Stark JM: Lung infections in children. Curr Opin Pediatr 1993;5:273.

Turner RB et al: Pneumonia in pediatric outpatients: Cause and clinical manifestations. J Pediatr 1987;111:194.

Central Nervous System Infections

Bonadio WA: The cerebrospinal fluid: Physiologic aspects and alterations associated with bacterial meningitis. Pediatr Infect Dis J 1992;11:423.

Feigin RD et al: Diagnosis and management of meningitis. Pediatr Infect Dis J. 1992;11:785.

Leggiardo RI: Penicillin and cephalosporin-resistant Streptococcus pneumoniae: An emerging microbial threat. Pediatrics 1994; 93:500.

Saez-Llorens X, McCracken GH Jr: Bacterial meningitis in neonates and children. Infect Dis Clin North Am 1990;4:623.

Toltzis P: Viral encephalitis. Adv Pediatr Infect Dis 1991;6:111.

Wald ER et al: Dexamethasone therapy for children with bacterial meningitis. Pediatrics 1995;95:21.

Approach to the Child with Diarrhea

American Academy of Pediatrics: Provisional Committee on Quality Improvement. Subcommittee on Acute Gastroenteritis. The management of acute gastroenteritis in young children. Pediatrics. 1996;97:424.

Guerrant RL, Bobak DA: Bacterial and protozoal gastroenteritis. N Engl J Med 1991;325:327.

Pickering LK: Therapy for acute infectious diarrhea in children. J Pediatr 1991;118:S118.

Hepatitis

Davis GL et al: Interferon alpha-2b alone or in combination with ribavirin for the treatment of relapse of chronic hepatitis C. N Engl J Med 1998;339:1493.

Hepatitis B virus: A comprehensive strategy for eliminating transmission in the United States through universal childhood vaccination. Recommendations of the Immunization Practices Advisory Committee (ACIP). MMWR 1991;40:1.

Hoofnagle JH, Di Bisceglie AM: Serologic diagnosis of acute and chronic viral hepatitis. Semin Liver Dis 1991;11:73.

McHutchison JG et al: Interferon alfa-2b alone or in combination with ribavirin as an initial treatment for chronic hepatitis C. N Engl J Med 1998;339:1485.

Tabor E: Etiology, diagnosis, and treatment of viral hepatitis in children. Adv Pediatr Infect Dis 1988;3:19.

Osteomyelitis

Faden H, Grossi M: Acute osteomyelitis in children. Reassessment of etiologic agents and their clinical characteristics. Am J Dis Child 1991;145:65.

Mader JT et al: Antimicrobial treatment of osteomyelitis. Clin Orthoped 1993;295:87.

Welkon CJ et al: Pyogenic arthritis in infants and children: A review of 95 cases. Pediatr Infect Dis 1986;5:669.

Urinary Tract Infections

The American Academy of Pediatrics Practice parameter: The diagnosis, treatment, and evaluation of the initial urinary tract infection in febrile infants and young children. Pediatrics 1999;103:843.

Andrich MP, Majd M: Diagnostic imaging in the evaluation of first UTI in infants and children. Pediatrics 1992;3:436.

Feld LG et al: Urinary tract infections in infants and children. Pediatr Rev 1989;11:71.

Sexually Transmitted Diseases

American Academy of Pediatrics, Committee on Adolescence. Sexually transmitted diseases. Pediatrics 1994;94:568.

Centers for Disease Control and Prevention: 1998 Guidelines for treatment of sexually transmitted diseases. MMWR 1998;47:1.

Ikeda MK, Jenson HB: Evaluation and treatment of congenital syphilis. J Pediatr 1990;117:843.

Pelvic inflammatory disease: Guidelines for prevention and management. MMWR 1991;40:1.

Shafer MA, Sweet RL: Pelvic inflammatory disease in adolescent females. Epidemiology, pathogenesis, diagnosis, treatment, and sequelae. Pediatr Clin North Am 1989;36:513.

Rash & Fever

Irving WL et al: Roseola infantum and other syndromes associated with acute HHV6 infection. Arch Dis Child 1990;65:1297.

Kirk JL et al: Rocky Mountain spotted fever. A clinical review based on 48 confirmed cases, 1943–1986. Medicine 1990;69:35.

Ware R: Human parvovirus infection. J Pediatr 1989;114:343.

Williams CL et al: Lyme disease in childhood: Clinical and epidemiologic features of ninety cases. Pediatr Infect Dis J 1990;9:10.

Adoption & Day-care Infections

Aronson J: Medical evaluation of an internationally adopted child. Pediatr Ann. 2000;29:218.

Goodman R et al: Proceedings of the International Conference on Child Day Care Health: Science, prevention, and practice. Pediatrics 1994;94(suppl 6):987.

Holmes SJ et al: Child-care practices: Effects of social change on the epidemiology of infectious diseases and antibiotic resistance. Epidemiol Rev 1996;18:10.

Osterholm MT: Infectious disease in child day care: an overview. Pediatrics 1994;94(6, suppl):997.

Injuries & Emergencies 10

Joel A. Fein, MD, Dennis R. Durbin, MD, & Steven M. Selbst, MD

Each year, approximately 100 million individuals are treated in emergency departments in the United States, and 25–30% of them are children. An estimated 10% of ambulance runs in this country involve individuals younger than 19 years. The emergency department has become the safety net for health care by treating those with life-threatening illness and injury and those with minor problems who are uninsured or poorly insured. Most children are treated in general emergency departments rather than in specialized pediatric emergency departments. Most are brought to the hospital because the caretaker or the patient perceives the problem to be serious and requiring urgent treatment. Only a small percentage of visits involve life-threatening emergencies, but most pediatric deaths are preventable or treatable if the problem is recognized early and managed appropriately.

The three leading causes of death in pediatric patients are injury, infection, and sequelae of prematurity and congenital malformations. Automobile-related injuries, including occupants involved in crashes and pedestrians hit by cars, are the most common causes of death due to trauma. Other traumatic deaths involve drownings, poisonings, falls, fires, and smoke inhalation. Unfortunately, the number of deaths associated with firearms (used intentionally or unintentionally), homicide, and suicide has increased rapidly over the past few years. Deaths from infectious diseases usually involve the respiratory tract or the central nervous system (CNS).

Children require special attention because they are so different from adults. Children are less tolerant of blood loss, more likely to sustain serious respiratory problems, and more at risk for head injury. Therefore, the care of ill and injured children requires special training, special equipment of variable sizes, different medications, and unique diagnostic and procedural skills.

This chapter focuses on several important emergencies in pediatrics. We first discuss cardiopulmonary resuscitation (CPR). We then discuss sudden infant death syndrome (SIDS); shock; the injured child, including head injury; near-drowning; and burns and smoke inhalation. These discussions are followed by sections on child abuse, poisonings, and status epilepticus. A discussion on asthma, an important pediatric emergency, can be found in Chapter 17.

■ CARDIOPULMONARY RESUSCITATION IN INFANTS & CHILDREN

Cardiopulmonary arrest (the absence of a pulse and spontaneous respirations), fortunately, is rare in the pediatric age group. In children, cardiopulmonary arrest commonly results from a prolonged period of hypoxia secondary to a respiratory arrest. Hypoxia plays a central role in many events leading to cardiopulmonary arrest in children. The hypoxia may be acute or chronic and result from an acquired or a congenital illness. The primary goal of CPR is to reestablish cardiac output and tissue oxygen delivery through the use of artificial ventilation and chest compressions and the administration of pharmacologic agents.

The etiology of cardiopulmonary arrest in children differs greatly from that in adults. Adult arrests typically are sudden in onset and primarily cardiac in origin. In contrast, children typically go through a series of physiologic changes after respiratory arrest, leading to cardiopulmonary arrest. Table 10–1 lists the most common identifiable causes of cardiopulmonary arrest in children. Resuscitation from respiratory arrest is successful in more than 50% of cases. Once cardiac arrest occurs, success rates for resuscitation are consistently less than 10%. Because respiratory arrest frequently precedes cardiac arrest in children, recognition of the child at risk of deterioration and intervention before full cardiopulmonary arrest occurs are of paramount importance.

Most pediatric cardiopulmonary arrests occur in children younger than 1 year. This is due to the higher occurrence of congenital anomalies that predispose some children to cardiopulmonary arrest and the unique differences in the anatomy and physiology of infants. The airway of a child differs from that of an adult: The trachea is more flexible, the tongue relatively larger, the glottic opening higher and more anteriorly placed in the neck, and the airway itself proportionately smaller, rendering infants more susceptible to airway compromise. Although the use of pediatric CPR is based on the adult model of resuscitation, important differences exist on the basis of these and other unique qualities of children.

Table 10–1. Most Common Identifiable Causes of Cardiopulmonary Arrest in Children

Respiratory
  Pneumonia
  Aspiration
  Airway obstruction
Sudden infant death syndrome
Congenital heart disease
Central nervous system disease
  Infection
  Trauma (including child abuse)
  Status epilepticus
Drowning
Smoke inhalation
Poisoning
Anaphylaxis

Management

Cardiopulmonary resuscitation in the pediatric age group should be part of a community-wide effort that integrates basic life support (BLS), advanced life support (ALS), and postresuscitation care. Basic life support is the phase of emergency care that supports ventilation and circulation in the arrest victim without the use of adjuncts. It is used typically in the prehospital setting. Advanced life support begins with BLS and adds adjunctive equipment, medications, and special techniques for establishing and maintaining effective ventilation and circulation.

The basic approach to pediatric CPR is the same as in adults with respect to the initial priorities: establishment of *A*irway, *B*reathing, and *C*irculation (the ABCs).

Establish unresponsiveness. The first step in the sequence of CPR is to establish the unresponsiveness of patients by gently shaking, tapping, or shouting at them. Once unresponsiveness is established, help should be summoned (by shouting), and the patient placed in a supine position on a firm, flat surface. If the rescuer is alone, provide BLS to the child for approximately 1 minute before activating the Emergency Medical Services system. Care should be taken in positioning the child at risk for head or neck injury. The child should be turned as a unit, with firm support of the head and neck so that the head does not twist or tilt forward or backward.

Airway. Once the patient is positioned properly, the first priority in management is evaluation and treatment of the airway. Most airway obstruction is related to the tongue and the mandibular block of soft tissues lying against the posterior wall of the hypopharynx. This obstruction can be relieved by manual maneuvers, including the head tilt and chin lift or jaw thrust to pull the tissues forward physically. Because of the lack of firm cartilaginous sup-

port in the trachea of an infant or small child, hyperextension of the neck can lead to collapse of the trachea. Therefore, the head should be placed in a "sniffing position," with the occiput slightly higher than the shoulders.

If manual manipulation of the airway cannot maintain airway patency, artificial airways, such as oropharyngeal and nasopharyngeal airways, can be used. These function to stent or support the mandibular block of tissue off the posterior pharyngeal wall.

Breathing. Once a clear airway has been established, the patient should be reassessed for the presence and adequacy of spontaneous breathing. Movement of the chest and abdomen should be seen; movement of air during exhalation should be felt and heard. If no spontaneous breathing is detected, mouth-to-mouth or, in infants younger than 1 year, mouth-to-mouth and nose breathing is begun. Two slow breaths are given, with a pause between for the rescuer to take a breath. The volume should be sufficient to cause the chest to rise. If a mask with one-way valve or other infection control barrier is readily available, rescue breathing should be provided with such a device.

Once available, supplemental oxygen always should be administered to patients requiring resuscitation. If the patient has adequate spontaneous breathing, a variety of oxygen delivery devices can be used, including nasal cannulas, hoods, tents, and masks. If assisted ventilation is required, oxygen should be delivered through a bag-valve-mask or bag-valve-endotracheal tube system.

Endotracheal intubation during CPR might be performed for a variety of reasons. The endotracheal tube can maintain further patency of the airway, protect the airway from aspiration of gastric contents, and facilitate mechanical ventilation and delivery of high concentrations of oxygen to the lungs. For children older than 2 years, the correct endotracheal tube size can be approximated by using a simple formula based on the patient's age:

$$\frac{\text{age (years)} + 16}{4} = \text{endotracheal tube size}$$

Because this is an estimate, the next smaller and larger size endotracheal tubes also should be available. Only personnel skilled in the technique of endotracheal intubation of children should perform the procedure.

Circulation. Once a patent airway is established and adequate oxygenation and ventilation are ensured, many children reestablish cardiac output. Assessment of the adequacy of circulation includes palpating the brachial or femoral artery in children younger than 1 year or the carotid artery in older children. One also should assess the color of the skin and mucous membranes for cyanosis or pallor and capillary refill.

If no effective pulse is present, external chest compressions must begin. Adequate ventilation must be continued

Table 10–2. Recommendations for External Cardiac Compressions in Pediatric Cardiopulmonary Resuscitation

Age	Site	Procedure	Depth	Rate/Min
Infant	One finger below internipple line	2–3 fingers	0.5–1 in	At least 100
Child	One finger above xiphoid notch	Heel of one hand	1–1.5 in	100
Adult	Same as for child	Both hands	1.5–2 in	60–80

Adapted and reproduced, with permission, from Bardossi K: Newest guidelines on pediatric CPR and first aid. *Contemp Pediatr* 1987;4:47.

during chest compressions. A chest compression:ventilation ratio of 5 : 1 is considered optimal for infants and children, except newborns, in whom a ratio of 3 : 1 is used. The position of the hands for chest compressions depends on the age of the child. The depth and rate of compressions likewise are based on the child's age (Table 10–2). In general, the chest should be compressed to approximately one third to one half its total depth, for all ages. The compressions should be smooth, not jerky, and the hand should not be lifted off the chest between compressions.

Drugs

If mechanical means do not reestablish effective circulation, pharmacologic intervention is essential. The primary drugs used in pediatric CPR are oxygen, epinephrine, sodium bicarbonate, atropine, and glucose. Table 10–3 lists the doses and indications of the drugs commonly used during a pediatric resuscitation.

Placement of an intravenous (IV) line during CPR often is the most difficult and time-consuming aspect of resuscitation. During CPR, the preferred access site is the largest, most accessible vein that does not require interruption of resuscitation. Whenever possible, a central IV site should be obtained. Peripheral sites (antecubital, dorsum of the hand, saphenous vein) are a second choice and may be difficult to obtain owing to circulatory collapse. Frequently, the most rapid means of obtaining circulatory access is via intraosseous (into the bone) infusion into the anterior tibial bone marrow. Specific intraosseous needles are available, or a large spinal needle may be used. If IV access proves difficult, the endotracheal tube provides an effective route for administration of some drugs into the systemic circulation (Table 10–4). Doses of the resuscitation drugs given through an endotracheal tube probably should be greater than the IV doses; however, optimal doses of drugs for endotracheal administration have not been determined because drug absorption may vary widely.

OXYGEN

The most important agent delivered during CPR is oxygen. Because hypoxia plays such an important role in the development of cardiopulmonary arrest and irreversible organ injury, all children requiring CPR should receive 100% oxygen until resuscitation is achieved.

Table 10–3. Drugs and Procedures Commonly Used in Pediatric Cardiopulmonary Resuscitation

Drug	Dose	Indication
Oxygen	100%	Hypoxia (assumed in every resuscitation)
Fluids (0.9% NaCl solution)	20 mL/kg	Inadequate peripheral circulation
Epinephrine (1:10,000)	Initial: 0.01 mg/kg (0.1 mL/kg) Subsequent: 0.1 mg/kg (0.1 mL/kg of 1:1000)	Asystole, hypotension, electromechanical dissociation, to convert from fine to coarse ventricular fibrillation, symptomatic bradycardia
Atropine	0.02 mg/kg Minimum: 0.1 mg Maximum: 2 mg	Bradycardia with inadequate perfusion Second- or third-degree atrioventricular block
Bicarbonate	1 meq/kg	Metabolic acidosis
Glucose (D10W)	0.5–1 g/kg (5–10 mL/kg)	Hypoglycemia
Defibrillation	2 J/kg	Ventricular fibrillation or ventricular tachycardia without a pulse
Synchronized cardioversion	0.2–1 J/kg	Symptomatic supraventricular or ventricular tachycardias

Table 10–4. Drugs That Can Be Given via an
Endotracheal Tube During Resuscitation

Lidocaine
Atropine
Naloxone (Narcan)
Epinephrine

EPINEPHRINE

Catecholamines are the primary class of drugs used to stimulate the cardiovascular system during resuscitation. Epinephrine, the primary agent used, has α- and β-adrenergic stimulating effects. The α-adrenergic stimulation results in vasoconstriction with resultant elevation in systolic and diastolic blood pressures. This in turn improves coronary perfusion pressure, resulting in improved oxygen delivery to the heart. The β-adrenergic stimulation enhances spontaneous contractions and increases the contractile force of the heart. Controversy has arisen recently over the proper dose of epinephrine to be used during CPR. Clinical studies in animals and humans have demonstrated that a higher dose than traditionally recommended may improve the ability to obtain return of spontaneous circulation. Therefore, the currently recommended initial dose of epinephrine remains 0.01 mg/kg (0.1 mL/kg of a 1:10,000 solution) intravenously. Second and subsequent doses for unresponsive asystolic and pulseless arrest may be 10 times higher, or 0.1 mg/kg (0.1 mL/kg of a 1:1000 solution) given every 3–5 minutes. Indications for the use of epinephrine include asystole, electromechanical dissociation, hypotension, symptomatic bradycardia, and conversion of a fine ventricular fibrillation to a coarse pattern, which is believed to be converted more easily to a sinus rhythm with electrical defibrillation.

SODIUM BICARBONATE

Sodium bicarbonate is indicated for significant metabolic acidosis. It is important to recognize that, with the onset of respiratory failure, respiratory acidosis can develop. The treatment for this type of acidosis is to provide adequate ventilation. With the onset of circulatory failure, lactic acid is produced and a concomitant metabolic acidosis develops. Sodium bicarbonate combines with hydrogen ions in the blood to produce carbon dioxide and water. This additional production of carbon dioxide must be eliminated through ventilation. Thus, sodium bicarbonate should not be used until after 10 minutes of conventional CPR. Providing effective ventilation and chest compressions to generate adequate coronary perfusion pressures during CPR are most important. If arterial blood gases are known, sodium bicarbonate should be given according to the formula:

$$\text{meq NaHCO}_3 = \frac{\text{base deficit} \times \text{weight (kg)} \times 0.4}{2}$$

If blood gases are not available, the initial dose is 1 meq/kg given intravenously. Potential side effects of bicarbonate administration include hypernatremia, hyperosmolarity, impairment of oxygen delivery to the peripheral tissues due to a shift in the oxyhemoglobin dissociation curve to the left, and inactivation of catecholamines if given through the same IV line without interposed flushing of the line.

ATROPINE

Atropine is a parasympatholytic agent. It increases heart rate by increasing the rate of discharge from the sinus node, increases conduction through the atrioventricular node, and reverses vagally mediated hypotension. Indications for atropine are bradycardia associated with hypotension, ventricular ectopy, or symptoms of myocardial ischemia and the treatment of second- or third-degree heart block. A minimum dose of atropine (0.1 mg) is recommended to prevent a paradoxic bradycardia caused by the CNS action of atropine at low doses of the drug.

GLUCOSE

Rapid assessment of blood glucose is a priority in the evaluation of any patient in need of resuscitation. If hypoglycemia is present, the initial dose of glucose is 0.5–1 g/kg given as 5–10 mL/kg of 10% dextrose in water (D10W) or 2–4 mL/kg of D25W. The blood glucose level should then be monitored to determine the need for subsequent doses.

Intravenous Fluids

During CPR, IV fluids usually are used to keep an IV line patent for drug administration. Ringer's lactate or 5% dextrose in normal saline may be used for this purpose. Volume expansion in the patient with circulatory collapse usually is achieved with colloid solutions such as 5% albumin, crystalloid solutions such as Ringer's lactate or normal saline, or blood products such as packed red blood cells or fresh-frozen plasma. The initial amount of volume is typically 20 mL/kg given as a bolus infusion. Subsequent fluid administration is determined by reassessment of the adequacy of cardiac output, as detailed above.

Defibrillation

Defibrillation is a relatively uncommon intervention in pediatric resuscitation. The most common arrhythmia seen in children presenting in cardiopulmonary arrest is asystole. Because it is unusual for a child's heart to fibrillate, the rhythm should be confirmed before defibrillation is attempted. Defibrillation produces a mass depolarization of the myocardium followed by the spontaneous return of sinus rhythm.

The larger adult defibrillator paddles are recommended for children weighing more than 10 kg. The smaller pediatric paddles should be used for infants weighing less than 10 kg. The paddles should rest firmly on the chest wall; one is placed over the right side of the upper chest and the other over the apex of the heart. The recommended dose of energy for ventricular fibrillation is 2 J/kg. If the first defibrillatory attempt is unsuccessful, second and third attempts are made with a dose of 4 J/kg. If these also are unsuccessful, lidocaine should be given and attention turned to correcting acidosis, hypoxemia, or hypothermia before proceeding with further attempts at defibrillation.

Synchronized cardioversion is distinguished from defibrillation. It is the timed depolarization of myocardial cells used when a patient is symptomatic with hypotension or poor perfusion from a rapid supraventricular or ventricular tachycardia. The depolarization must be synchronized with the existing rhythm. The energy dose is usually one tenth to one half the usual defibrillation dose (0.2–1 J/kg).

Summary

Pediatric CPR requires effective integration of mechanical skills and pharmacotherapy used in BLS and ALS paradigms. The immediate goal of CPR in children is to reestablish substrate delivery to preserve vital organ function and reverse ongoing tissue injury.

■ SUDDEN INFANT DEATH SYNDROME

Sudden infant death syndrome is defined as the sudden death of an infant younger than 1 year that remains unexplained after a complete postmortem examination. It should be emphasized that SIDS is a diagnosis of exclusion. The differential diagnosis of SIDS includes overwhelming infection (sepsis), congenital heart disease, cardiac arrhythmia, seizure, trauma (child abuse), poisoning, gastroesophageal reflux associated with apnea, infantile botulism, congenital CNS lesions associated with apnea, brain tumor, hypoglycemia, and inborn errors of metabolism. Sudden infant death syndrome is the leading cause of death in infants between 1 month and 1 year of age. In the United States, the overall incidence of SIDS is approximately 1–2 of 1000 live births. The peak incidence is at 2–3 months after birth; it is rare before 1 month and after 9 months.

Several epidemiologic studies have demonstrated a number of factors significantly related to the risk of SIDS. Rates of SIDS are highest in poor and nonwhite infants, children of mothers who smoke or who have a history of substance abuse, preterm or small-for-gestational age infants, siblings of prior SIDS victims, and infants recovering from mild upper respiratory tract symptoms.

Infants who have experienced an **acute life-threatening event,** such as prolonged apnea requiring resuscitation, may be at a higher risk for recurrence of such events. These and other infants determined to be at a higher risk of SIDS (such as siblings of SIDS victims) may be offered home monitoring with an electronic cardiorespiratory monitor, and their caretakers should be instructed in BLS. Considerable controversy exists regarding the guidelines for instituting and terminating home monitoring.

Many theories have been offered to explain the mechanism of SIDS. One of the most actively studied areas is the **apnea hypothesis,** which speculates that apnea is the main mechanism and terminal event in SIDS. The apnea may be central, in which there is no respiratory effort; obstructive, in which there is an effort to breathe, but there is anatomic or functional obstruction to airflow; or a combination of the two. Although the apnea hypothesis has been one of the most active areas of SIDS research, it has not proved convincing. Most infants with prolonged apnea do not die of SIDS, and most SIDS victims did not have a known apnea event before death.

Other theories that have received attention include abnormal respiratory control response to hypoxia and hypercarbia; upper airway obstruction due to abnormal neuromuscular control; abnormalities in sleep patterns; cardiac arrhythmias, particularly the prolonged QT syndrome; and an imbalance of sympathetic innervation to the heart, rendering the heart more susceptible to life-threatening arrhythmias. Infantile botulism has been considered the cause in some infants. Recently, it has been reported that positioning infants in the prone position for sleeping is associated with an increased risk of SIDS. The mechanism responsible for this relation between SIDS and sleep position has not been defined. Several studies have demonstrated a drastic reduction in the incidence of SIDS in regions where infants predominantly sleep on their sides or backs. The American Academy of Pediatrics now recommends that healthy infants be placed to sleep on their sides or backs.

Although no consensus exists as to the major determinant of SIDS, a single pathologic mechanism is clearly unlikely. Further research is needed to explore the interaction between sleep and other physiologic control systems in the developing infant.

■ SHOCK

Shock is a complex pathophysiologic state of circulatory dysfunction that results in the inability of the body to deliver adequate oxygen, glucose, and other nutrients to tissue beds. In **early or compensated shock,** blood flow is maintained by compensatory mechanisms but is uneven in the microcirculation. Cardiac output and most vital signs may be normal. However, if untreated, compensated shock progresses to **late or uncompensated shock.** Unless this process is corrected, **irreversible shock occurs,** with permanent damage to important organs such as the brain and heart.

The etiology of shock can be divided into three categories: hypovolemic, distributive, and cardiogenic. Table 10–5 summarizes the etiology of shock in children. Hypovolemic shock is the most common category. When the circulating blood volume is reduced, cardiac output falls. The body compensates for the decrease in cardiac output by increasing heart rate, systemic vascular resistance, and myocardial contractility. This response maintains the child's blood pressure until almost 40% of blood volume is lost. However, the systemic vasoconstriction leads to ischemia in many tissues; thus, cell metabolism and function suffer. As cells die, they release enzymes that can cause vasodilation and pooling of blood in capillary beds. "Toxic" substances are released, which depress myocardial function and affect the coagulation system, resulting in disseminated intravascular coagulopathy.

In distributive shock, peripheral vascular resistance is severely reduced. Although this is triggered most often by gram-negative infection (septic shock), it can be due to gram-positive organisms or viruses. Distributive shock also can result from anaphylaxis due to an allergic reaction to medications, insect bite, or snake bite. Transection of the spinal cord is rare in children but may lead to vasodilation and shock. However, this should not be considered the source of shock in the initial evaluation of the trauma patient because hypovolemic shock is much more common. Toxic shock syndrome is another example of distributive shock; it is triggered by toxin-producing

Staphylococcus aureus colonizing the vagina after the use of heavy-absorbency tampons or invading injured skin. Diarrhea, vomiting, and diffuse erythematous rash frequently are the first symptoms, followed by shock. Overdoses of some medications also can cause hypotension and shock. Distributive shock results in increased venous capacitance by shunting past some capillary beds and ischemia in many underperfused tissues. The result is release of other vasoactive substances such as serotonin, endorphins, prostaglandins, leukotrienes, and histamine, which cause further capillary leakage and inadequate tissue oxygenation. Cardiac function is affected by poor perfusion and release of toxic myocardial depressant factors.

In cardiogenic shock, abnormal heart function results in failure to meet the metabolic demands of the body. Although this is the least common cause of shock in children, it can result from arrhythmias (such as supraventricular tachycardia), cardiomyopathies (such as viral myocarditis), drug intoxication, or tension pneumothorax and pericardial tamponade, which inhibit the heart's ability to fill and pump adequately. The body compensates for decreased stroke volume by increasing systemic vascular resistance to maintain blood pressure and increasing sodium and water retention to increase central blood volume. However, this increased afterload and preload only further increase the metabolic demands on the heart and may result in myocardial ischemia and decreased ventricular function. Figure 10–1 summarizes the pathophysiology of shock in children.

Diagnosis & Clinical Manifestations

The diagnosis of shock is made by an abbreviated physical examination (Table 10–6). When evaluating a child who may be in shock, complete vital signs should be obtained. Initially the child is anxious or irritable, with cool extremities and tachycardia, and may appear gray or ashen due to poor perfusion. Pulses may be weak and thready, and capillary refill may be delayed beyond 2–3 seconds. (Capillary refill cannot be determined accurately in hypothermic patients.) At this point, blood pressure may be normal due to compensatory mechanisms; hypotension is a late finding with shock in the pediatric patient. Later, as shock progresses and decompensation occurs, tachypnea, somnolence, and oliguria may develop. Eventually, obtundation, periodic breathing, apnea, and hypotension ensue. Cardiopulmonary arrest may result.

Additional **physical findings** may be present, depending on the cause of the shock. For instance, there may be evidence of trauma or burns. Fever or hypothermia may occur in patients with septic shock. Petechiae may be noticed if a coagulopathy has developed, or a fine, erythematous, sandpaperlike rash may be present in toxic shock syndrome. Hepatomegaly may be present, with muffled heart sounds or a gallop rhythm, if cardiac failure is the

Table 10–5. Differential Diagnosis of Shock

Hypovolemic shock	Cardiogenic shock
Hemorrhage	Cardiomyopathy
Internal bleeding	Congenital heart disease
External bleeding	Congestive heart failure
Gastroenteritis	Arrhythmia
Diabetes mellitus or	Tension pneumothorax
insipidus	Pericardial effusion
Severe burns	or tamponade
	Hypoxia (near-drowning,
Distributive shock	smoke inhalation)
Septic shock	
Toxic shock syndrome	
Anaphylaxis	
Drug intoxication	
Neurogenic shock	
(spinal cord transection)	

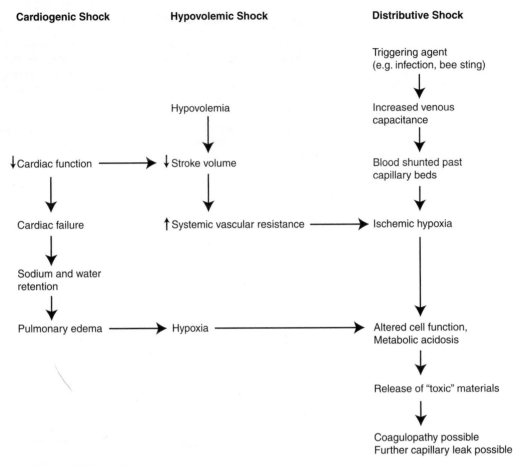

Figure 10–1. Algorithm showing simplified pathophysiology of shock.

cause of shock. However, distended neck veins may be absent when shock is present.

A brief, relevant **history** should be obtained while the child is being examined to help determine the etiology. It is important to learn whether there has been trauma or burns, whether the child has had fever or other signs of infection, whether allergies are present, and whether the child could have taken any medications or has had evi-

Table 10–6. Recognition of Shock

Gray, ashen color	Decreased urine output
Tachycardia	Cool, clammy skin
Delayed capillary refill	Weak pulses
Altered mental status— irritable, lethargic	Hypotension

dence of diabetes. If the patient in shock is a teenage girl, it should be noted whether she is menstruating and using tampons.

The diagnosis of shock is made clinically before any laboratory tests are obtained. However, several **laboratory studies** may help to determine the cause or guide management. Because of poor perfusion, an arterial or venous blood gas will always show some degree of metabolic acidosis. Hypoxia and hypercarbia also may be noted. A complete blood count may show leukocytosis with a left shift as a nonspecific response to stress or a sign of infection. A blood glucose level should be determined, including a bedside rapid dextrose strip to rule out hypoglycemia. Hepatic enzyme and blood urea nitrogen (BUN) and creatinine concentrations may be elevated because liver and renal functions are impaired owing to poor perfusion. A coagulopathy may be present. A chest radiograph may show evidence of pulmonary venous congestion (shock lung), and the heart size may be normal or enlarged. This radiographic picture is seen often after fluid resuscitation has begun. A blood culture should be obtained if sepsis is suspected; a vaginal culture also should be obtained, and a tampon, if present, should be removed if toxic shock is suspected.

Management

Shock must be recognized and treated immediately; the initial management is the same regardless of the cause. Figure 10–2 summarizes the management of shock in pediatric patients. The first intervention is to assess the

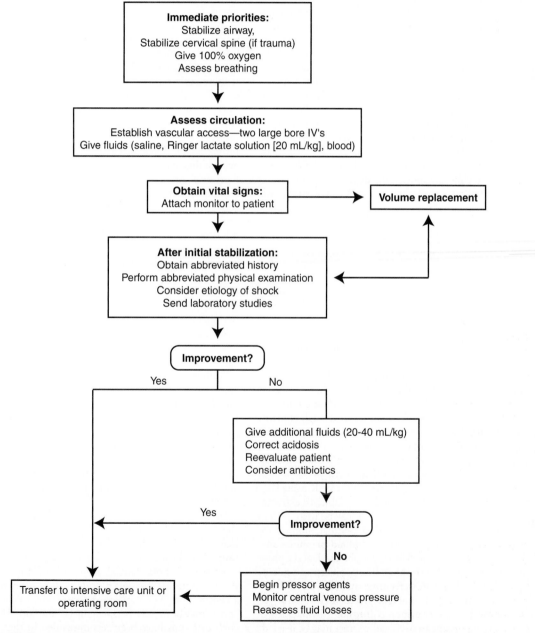

Figure 10–2. Algorithm showing the initial management of shock in the pediatric patient.

child's airway and ensure that it is not obstructed. The child's breathing effort should be assessed by looking at the chest wall and auscultating the lungs.

Oxygen (fractional inspired oxygen [FiO_2], 100%) should be delivered even if the child is not obviously cyanotic. It is desirable to maintain a partial pressure of oxygen (PaO_2) of at least 100 mm Hg. Once the airway and breathing have been assessed, the circulation should be evaluated. Vascular access must be obtained quickly. It is preferable to place two large-bore, short catheters into peripheral veins. Hand veins and those in the antecubital fossae may offer the best opportunities for success. However, even those may be difficult to cannulate in a child who is in shock. If unsuccessful after a brief search for peripheral access, the physician should consider alternative routes. The femoral vein may be cannulated by passing a guidewire through a needle and then inserting a catheter over the wire (Seldinger technique). When venous access is accomplished, blood can be sent for laboratory studies, including type and cross-match. Besides the femoral vein, the internal jugular and subclavian veins can be accessed in a similar manner. These are technically more difficult to reach and have a higher complication rate; thus, access should be attempted only by those with experience. If venous access is not possible, the intraosseous route should be attempted in children younger than 6 years. Specific intraosseous needles, an 18- or 20-gauge spinal needle with a stylet, or a bone marrow needle may be used. Using aseptic technique, the needle is inserted into the flat medial surface of the proximal tibia 2 cm below the tibial tuberosity; this provides an effective route for delivery of fluids and medications during resuscitation. In addition, a saphenous vein cutdown can be used as an alternative means of securing vascular access, but this procedure may require additional time and surgical skills.

Once vascular access is achieved, fluid resuscitation must begin promptly. Saline (0.9%) or Ringers lactate solution is the initial fluid, given in a dose of 20 mL/kg very quickly, over about 10 minutes. Although controversy persists, there is no evidence that colloid solutions (albumin, plasma) are more valuable than crystalloid solutions in the initial management. Packed red blood cells should be given to maintain a hematocrit of 33%, at a rate of 10 mL/kg over 1–2 hours. Saline or Ringers lactate solution is given until blood is available. In extreme emergencies, type O-negative blood may be used.

The child should be attached to a cardiac monitor to record heart rate, respirations, and blood pressure continuously. An abbreviated history is obtained, and a physical examination is performed. If hypoglycemia is noted by rapid blood glucose screening, an infusion of 25% dextrose (2–4 mL/kg) should be given quickly, followed by a 10% dextrose continuous infusion. Temperature control is important; an overhead warmer may be needed to prevent hypothermia.

A urinary catheter should be placed to monitor the child's response to fluid resuscitation. The child must be reevaluated constantly. If the patient remains poorly perfused (i.e., with persistent metabolic acidosis, prolonged capillary refill, tachycardia, weak pulses, oliguria, or hypotension), additional fluids are indicated. Another bolus of saline or Ringers lactate solution (20 mL/kg) should be infused rapidly. Most children in shock require at least 40–60 mL/kg in the first hour before improvement is noted; more is needed if ongoing losses occur.

If the circulation remains poor despite adequate fluid resuscitation, pressor agents may be needed. Dopamine is usually the preferred drug. It has different effects depending on the dosage. When infused at 2–5 µg/kg/min, it increases renal, splanchnic, and cerebral blood flow with little direct cardiac action. When infused at 5–10 µg/kg/min, dopamine may increase the blood pressure and usually increases cardiac output. These changes may result in warmer extremities with improved capillary refill. At higher doses, more severe vasoconstriction often occurs; this may be undesirable because it interferes with perfusion. Another useful agent for circulatory failure is dobutamine; it is an effective inotropic agent that improves cardiac output and blood pressure and is purported to have less effect on heart rate or rhythm than other catecholamines. Therefore, it is a useful agent for cardiogenic shock. Other catecholamines include epinephrine infusions, which are used to treat endotoxemia and anaphylaxis, and norepinephrine infusions, which may be helpful when there is low diastolic blood pressure and coronary perfusion is threatened. Both agents cause peripheral vasoconstriction. Amrinone is a newer nonadrenergic inotropic agent that may be useful when there is severe myocardial failure that is resistant to adrenergic agents.

Other agents used in the management of shock include sodium bicarbonate, given intravenously for severe metabolic acidosis (pH < 7.25) that does not respond to fluid therapy alone. Adequate ventilation should be ensured if bicarbonate is used. Further doses are guided by the child's acid–base status as determined by blood gas analysis. Half-strength sodium bicarbonate should be used for infants in the first few months after birth. Bicarbonate therapy is not a substitute for attempts to improve blood flow and ventilation.

Broad-spectrum antibiotics should be given if septic shock is suspected. Calcium chloride is used rarely but may be of value if the ionized serum calcium concentration is low; in addition, it sometimes is given empirically if massive amounts of blood, albumin, or plasma are used in resuscitation. Calcium chloride must be given through a central line (5–7 mg/kg). Alternatively, calcium gluconate may be infused peripherally (10 mg/kg). Although corticosteroids have been recommended in the past by some centers in the management of shock, studies with

Table 10–7. Medications Useful in Treating Shock

Drug	Recommendation Dose	Actions/Remarks
Dopamine	2–5 µg/kg/min	Increases renal, splanchnic, coronary, cerebral blood flow
	5–10 µg/kg/min	Cardiac output ↑, BP ↑
	>10 µg/kg/min	Peripheral vasoconstriction
Dobutamine	7–10 µg/kg/min	Potent inotropic agent, cardiac output ↑, BP ↑, minimal change heart rate or rhythm
Epinephrine	0.05–2 µg/kg/min	Peripheral vasoconstriction, cardiac output ↑, BP ↑
Norepinephrine	2–10 µg/kg/min	Peripheral vasoconstriction, cardiac output ↑, BP ↑
Isoproterenol	0.05–2 µg/kg/min	Heart rate ↑, BP ↑, cardiac output ↑, causes peripheral vasodilation
Sodium bicarbonate	0.5–1 meq/kg	For metabolic acidosis unresponsive to fluids and electrolytes
Antibiotics	Variable	Broad-spectrum drugs if sepsis considered
Calcium chloride	5–7 mg/kg	If ionized calcium is low
Nitroprusside	1–10 µg/kg/min	Peripheral vasodilation, to improve peripheral circulation when BP stable
Amrinone	0.75 mg/kg over 2–3 min Maintenance rate 5–10 µg/kg/min	For low cardiac output states

BP = blood pressure.

adult patients have shown that they have little value in improving the outcome of patients with septic shock.

Diuretic agents occasionally are used with caution to improve pulmonary congestion, which usually is due to capillary leakage and responds best to mechanical ventilation with positive end-expiratory pressure.

Afterload reduction may be helpful when the child is more stable and central venous pressure can be monitored. Nitroprusside and other drugs are used to improve peripheral circulation, but this form of treatment is administered optimally in the setting of the intensive care unit (ICU) rather than of the emergency department. Table 10–7 summarizes the medications useful in managing the child in shock.

Continuous monitoring of pulse, respirations, blood pressure, and pulse oximetry is essential. Frequent reassessment of mental status, skin perfusion, and urine output is also necessary.

Once the child in shock is stabilized, plans should be made to transfer the patient to an ICU. It is very important to maintain constant surveillance of the child's vital signs, urine output, skin perfusion, and mental status.

■ SEIZURE DISORDERS

STATUS EPILEPTICUS

Status epilepticus is a common medical emergency in children. A patient who is experiencing a seizure or series of seizures for 30 minutes or longer without a return to baseline mental state is in status epilepticus (see Chapter 21).

Status epilepticus occurs in 60,000–160,000 persons annually, and the majority of these are in the pediatric age group. The mean age of onset is 5 years, with 64% of the episodes occurring earlier. It is estimated that 1% of the U.S. population will experience an episode of status epilepticus in their lifetimes, with an overall 1% mortality rate. Morbidity and mortality in these patients usually are related to the specific cause of the seizure rather than to the seizure activity itself.

The etiology of status epilepticus is summarized in Table 10–8. In some cases, such as hypoglycemia, hyponatremia, and CNS hemorrhage, treatment of the cause should help considerably in treatment of the seizure. In other cases, seizure activity must be controlled until the cause is discovered. The cause of seizures in children is also age related.

Status epilepticus can be classified as generalized or partial. The most clinically apparent and potentially compromising are the generalized convulsive types of status epilepticus: tonic, clonic, tonic-clonic (**grand mal**), and myoclonic. **Tonic seizures** ("with tone") are manifested as flexion or extension of the extremities. **Clonic seizures**

Table 10–8. Etiology of Status Epilepticus in Children

Mnemonic: "in status"	
Insufficient medications	**A**noxia
Neoplasm/masses	**T**rauma
Spinal infection	**U**nknown/febrile
Toxins	**S**ugar/sodium

manifest as jerking of the extremities, without an initial tonic phase. These movements are usually asymmetric and arrhythmic. **Tonic–clonic** seizures are the most common presentation of status epilepticus; they begin with a short tonic phase and progress to a longer, more dramatic clonic phase of seizure activity. The seizures typically are discontinuous and can begin as a generalized seizure or a partial convulsion that generalizes secondarily.

Seizures can affect ventilation, oxygenation, and perfusion. There is also evidence that prolonged seizure activity can cause irreversible neuronal cell damage despite optimal correction of oxygenation, ventilation, and metabolic derangements. This likely is a result of cellular hypoxia due to increased cellular demand and decreased availability of oxygen. The end-organ dysfunction seen in status epilepticus results initially from sympathetic and parasympathetic activation. Complications include tachycardia, hypertension, diaphoresis, salivary and tracheobronchial hypersecretion, hyperpyrexia, and hyperglycemia. Later in the course of the seizure, metabolic complications result from high energy expenditure and muscular fatigue; these include metabolic acidosis, hyperkalemia, hypoglycemia, hyperazotemia (increased BUN), and hyponatremia (Table 10–9). Respiratory compromise may result from hypoventilation, aspiration or blockage of the aiways by secretions, or glossopharyngeal dystonia. This eventually can lead to cardiopulmonary arrest. In addition to the organ system and cellular dysfunction, trauma to the head and extremities may occur during the severe tonic-clonic movements.

Diagnosis & Clinical Manifestations

In most cases, the diagnosis of generalized convulsive status epilepticus is not subtle. However, recognition of other forms of status epilepticus, such as myoclonic status epilepticus or infantile spasms, can be more difficult. In general, a complete history should be obtained but can wait until the patient is stabilized and the seizure treated. However, some important historical points can be helpful initially in determining the presence and cause of a seizure. A history of prior seizures leads one to question

the inappropriate use of anticonvulsants, whereas a history of diabetes, head trauma, ingestion, or febrile illness suggests other etiologies.

Physical examination begins with vital signs and mental status examination. All generalized convulsive seizures result in the patient's unresponsiveness to voice or command. Most clonic movements are difficult to miss. However, some other motor activity might be difficult to differentiate from spontaneous movements or rigors. In general, one cannot alter or stop the clonic movements of status epilepticus by holding the extremity down. Close observation of mental status and movement patterns may provide diagnosis of very subtle presentations of status epilepticus.

During the postictal period, patients might appear lethargic, confused, and even comatose. The diagnosis of a seizure at this point is based on the history obtained from witnesses. Although this period may still correlate with abnormal CNS neuronal discharges, muscle tone is no longer increased but rather normal or hypotonic. The patient may experience glossopharyngeal hypotonia and increased secretions, which obstruct the airway despite the cessation of seizure activity. Occasionally, the patient may exhibit a gaze preference.

Laboratory values are not as helpful in diagnosing the presence of a seizure. Laboratory evaluation should focus on two issues: guiding management of ABCs and identifying correctable causes of seizures, such as hypoglycemia, hyponatremia, and hypoxia. Rarely, and only if the history is suggestive, is it necessary to evaluate immediately for uremia, hypocalcemia, and hypomagnesemia. Anticonvulsant levels and toxicologic evaluation also may be ordered, but these results are rarely ready in time to alter the initial management.

Management

STABILIZATION

The management of status epilepticus begins as all pediatric emergencies do: with the ABCs (see Cardiopulmonary Resuscitation). However, certain problems associated with status epilepticus deserve special consideration. The establishment of an adequate airway takes priority over all other management issues. The patient's airway may be compromised during the seizure from increased muscular tone in the pharynx and hypopharynx, increased secretions, and decreased level of consciousness with concomitant loss of the gag reflex. An adequate airway must be established, and the quality of air entry and the success of repositioning and jaw thrust should be determined. If these maneuvers are insufficient to provide adequate ventilation, bag-valve-mask manual ventilation or endotracheal intubation should be performed. It should be remembered that, although patients might withstand up to 30 minutes of seizure activity without neurologic sequelae, they can

Table 10–9. Systemic Effects of Status Epilepticus

Early Findings	Late Findings
Tachycardia	Metabolic acidosis
Hypertension	Hyperkalemia
Diaphoresis	Hyperazotemia
Salivary/tracheobronchial hypersecretion	Hypoglycemia
Hyperpyrexia	Hyponatremia
Hyperglycemia	

tolerate only a few minutes of apnea before cardiorespiratory arrest ensues.

Oxygen always should be administered to patients in status epilepticus regardless of the adequacy of ventilation or pulse oximeter reading. In status epilepticus, IV access is helpful for the rapid administration of antiepileptic medications. The need for IV hydration is variable and often determined by the underlying cause of the seizure. Abnormalities of circulation are rarely due to hypovolemia or distributive shock in patients with status epilepticus. Nevertheless, the children in status epilepticus appear to have poor circulation secondary to the increased catecholamine levels and subsequent shunting of blood away from peripheral areas.

A blood sugar concentration should be determined to evaluate the presence of early hyperglycemia or late hypoglycemia seen in status epilepticus. This can be done easily at the bedside. In addition, antipyretics can be administered rectally to counteract the effects of elevated body temperature on the seizure threshold.

ANTIEPILEPTIC MEDICATIONS

Seizures lasting longer than 10–15 minutes are usually treated with anticonvulsant medications. In addition, rapidly reversible causes of seizures, such as metabolic disturbances or expanding cerebral mass lesions, should be addressed. Many anticonvulsant medications can be administered by alternative routes, e.g., endotracheal, intramuscular (IM), or rectal, which should be considered if IV access is not rapidly attained. Medications commonly used for status epilepticus are presented in Table 10–10.

Benzodiazepines. The two most common medications used initially in the management of seizures are lorazepam (Ativan) and diazepam (Valium). Both have a rapid onset of action (within 2–3 minutes) and are effective in stopping seizures 80–85% of the time. Diazepam can be given by the intravenous or rectal route. Its relatively short duration of action, however, necessitates repeated dosages or the use of a second, longer-acting medication such as phenobarbital or phenytoin. The anticonvulsant activity of lorazepam can last 24–48 hours, and it has been shown to be equally as effective in controlling status epilepticus as diazepam. Lorazepam is not well absorbed through the rectal mucosa and thus will not be effective when administered by this route. Midazolam (Versed), a third benzodiazepine, is used infrequently but theoretically effective in controlling status epilepticus. Its main advantage is that it can be given intramuscularly because of its aqueous solubility. When used in conjunction with a barbiturate such

Table 10–10. Anticonvulsant Medications Used in the Acute Management of Status Epilepticus

Drug	Dosage	Route[1]	Onset of Action	Duration of Action	More Common Side Effects[3]
Diazepam (Valium)	0.1–0.2 mg/kg Maximum: 10 mg/dose Repeat q 5 min 0.5 mg/kg	IV PR[2] in saline	2–3 min	10–15 min	1, 2
Lorazepam (Ativan)	0.05–0.10 mg/kg Maximum: 4 mg/dose Repeat q 5 min	IV	2–3 min	24–48 h	1, 2
Midazolam (Versed)	0.05–0.20 mg/kg Maximum: 5 mg/dose	IV, IM	2–5 min	1–5 h	1, 2, 4
Phenytoin (Dilantin)	18–20 mg/kg Maximum: 1 g/dose	IV slowly (0.5–1 mg/ [kg · min] in saline)	20–40 min	24 h	3
Fosphenytoin	15–20 mg PE/kg	IV slowly (3 mg/ [kg · min]) or IM			3
Phenobarbital (Luminal)	20 mg/kg Maximum: 300 mg/dose	IV, IM	20 min (24 h IM)	24–72 h	1 (especially in conjunction with benzodiazepines), 2

[1] All IV medications can be administered by intraosseous route if necessary.
[2] Per rectum (PR) administration, inserted 4–6 cm into rectum with 1 mL syringe or rectal tube.
[3] 1 = respiratory depression; 2 = alters mental status; 3 = hypotension/bradycardia if administered too quickly—monitor electrocardiogram and blood pressure continuously; 4 = amnesia.
ET = endotracheal; IM = intramuscular; IV = intravenous; PE = phenytoin equivalent.

as phenobarbital, the benzodiazepines can potentiate respiratory depression.

Phenytoin. Because of its slower onset of action, phenytoin (Dilantin) is used frequently as a second medication in the management of status epilepticus. The incidence of bradycardia and hypotension resulting from its use can be reduced by administering the drug slowly, at a rate no greater than 0.5–1 mg/kg/min or 50 mg/min maximum. Because of the slow rate of drug administration, phenytoin concentrations might not reach therapeutic levels until 30–50 minutes after onset of infusion. Despite these caveats, phenytoin is used frequently because of its high efficacy and lack of effect on mental status. Therapeutic levels of 10–20 meq/mL are commonly required, and toxic effects include nystagmus and ataxia. An aqueous form of phenytoin, fosphenytoin, recently has become available. Advantages of this formulation include decreased cardiovascular side effects, more rapid administration (3 mg/kg/min), and the potential for IM administration.

Phenobarbital. Phenobarbital also has a relatively delayed onset of action (20 minutes) and an extremely long half-life and duration of action. Its advantages include the potential for IM administration when IV access is difficult and its wide therapeutic range. Many clinicians prefer to use phenobarbital to treat seizures in infants. Disadvantages include a significant risk of respiratory depression, especially when administered in conjunction with a benzodiazepine. Phenobarbital also causes significant depression of mental status. Children who have received phenobarbital may be sedated and appear ataxic for days after the initial dose.

If seizure activity continues for 30–60 minutes after administration of maximum doses of anticonvulsant medications, general anesthesia can be induced to control status epilepticus. This is rarely needed but can be performed intravenously by using barbiturates such as pentobarbital, thiopental, or high dose phenobarbital. General anesthesia can be induced with the use of inhaled anesthetics such as halothane or isoflurane. These medications are titrated until the electroencephalogram shows a "burst-suppression" pattern—a suppression of seizures with occasional flurries of activity. Close cardiorespiratory monitoring must be implemented, and patients are almost always intubated for airway protection and mechanical ventilation.

SUMMARY: GENERAL APPROACH

The decision to administer anticonvulsant medications is based on the child's clinical status, oxygenation, and duration of seizure. If the decision is made to treat the seizure, a benzodiazepine (preferably lorazepam) should be administered after obtaining IV access. This drug can be

repeated two to three times over the subsequent 15 minutes before initiating phenytoin therapy. If IV access cannot be achieved, diazepam (0.5 mg/kg) may be administered rectally, or midazolam (0.2 mg/kg) may be administered intramuscularly. These drugs may be repeated two to three times.

If status epilepticus continues despite benzodiazepine and phenytoin therapy, barbiturate therapy or inhalational general anesthetic should be considered. When these treatments are instituted, the child should have continuous evaluation by physical examination, pulse oximetry, and cardiorespiratory monitoring. Once seizure activity has ceased, clinical assessment should continue to focus on the child's respiratory pattern, mental status, and neurologic examination.

Frequently during the postictal phase, the child will require supplementary ventilatory support in the form of bag-valve-mask positive-pressure ventilation. The duration of this phase may range from a few minutes to a few hours.

FEBRILE CONVULSIONS

Febrile convulsions occur in 3–4% of children younger than 5 years and account for approximately 50% of all seizures in this age group. Because of their relatively benign nature and good prognosis, it is important to be able to differentiate febrile convulsions from seizures secondary to acute CNS infection or epilepsy. The criteria for diagnosis of simple febrile seizures are listed in Table 10–11.

Boys are affected more often than girls, and there is frequently a strong family predisposition to this type of seizure. The typical clinical picture is one in which the child's caretakers had not noticed a fever before the event. The convulsion usually is completed before the child arrives to the emergency department, but the child may be in the lethargic or sleepy postictal state. Postictal electroencephalographic recordings are normal in 85–95% of cases.

Approximately 0.2% of children with febrile convulsions have permanent neurologic sequelae. The benign nature of this entity significantly affects the patient's evaluation in the emergency department. The physician who

Table 10–11. Diagnostic Criteria for Simple Febrile Convulsions

Age 6 mo to 6 y
Fever > 38.4°C
Generalized tonic–clonic seizure
Duration < 15 min
No known underlying cerebral disease
No neurologic sequelae

initially screens the patient should be suspicious of other potential causes for the child's seizure. In infants, many physicians consider performing a lumbar puncture to rule out meningitis. It is unlikely, however, that a pleocytosis will be found on examination of the CNS in a well-appearing child who has no other findings of meningitis. In addition, further episodes of seizure activity within 24 hours of the first episode should raise the suspicion of other diagnoses.

The management of febrile convulsions is similar to the management of seizures. If a febrile child is actively seizing, support of ABCs should be instituted. Antiepileptic medications might be withheld if the total duration of seizure has been short. In many cases, the seizure stops after a few minutes, and the child awakens after a short postictal period. Because most children with this entity are not actively seizing in the emergency department, a detailed history must be undertaken. Physical examination should be directed toward finding a source for the child's fever and ruling out any possibility of cerebral infection. If the child appears well, many physicians do not perform any laboratory analysis. Discharge instructions should include the proper use of antipyretic medications and anticipatory guidance regarding the chances of further seizures. The parents should be instructed to call their physician or return to the emergency department if a second seizure occurs. In the case of "atypical" febrile convulsions, referral to a pediatric neurologist is warranted.

More than 90% of children with febrile convulsions have an excellent prognosis. Approximately one third of these experience another febrile convulsion, and another one third have a third seizure. Only about 2–6% of children in whom febrile convulsions are initially diagnosed go on to have spontaneous afebrile seizures and a diagnosis of epilepsy. This risk increases, however, as the number of febrile convulsion episodes increases and if the initial convulsion is unusually long. A family history of epilepsy also increases this risk.

HYPONATREMIA

A sodium level below 120 meq/L may precipitate epileptic seizures in children. In these cases, the history is usually suggestive of water intoxication. Typically, a small, ill child is given hyposmolar solutions such as weak tea or plain water. Electrolytes such as sodium and potassium are lost in the urine, stool, and sweat and not replaced. The serum concentrations of these electrolytes may decrease and precipitate seizures or cardiac conduction abnormalities. If there is a strong history of water intoxication in a seizing child, it is appropriate to administer enough sodium chloride to increase the serum level by 10 meq/L. This can be accomplished with 15 mL/kg of 0.9% sodium chloride (normal saline) or 2–4 mL/kg of 3% normal saline for children in whom a larger fluid

bolus is not advisable. Seizures due to hyponatremia alone usually stop when a sufficient amount of sodium is administered intravenously. Hyponatremia can be caused by other underlying problems, such as syndrome of inappropriate antidiuretic hormone in a patient with meningitis. In these cases, the cause of the seizure is still unclear, and rapid sodium administration might not be as effective.

■ CHILDHOOD POISONING

Accidental ingestions are common in pediatrics. Children younger than 19 years constituted nearly 70% of the 2.2 million human exposures reported to the American Association of Poison Control Centers in 1998. In pediatrics, two fairly distinct age groups are involved in poisonings. Children younger than 5 years account for the vast majority of pediatric poisonings, virtually all of which (99.7%) are considered accidental. The natural inquisitiveness and impulsivity of toddlers make them vulnerable "hosts" for toxic ingestions. The home environment in which the poisoning typically occurs often is disrupted and under some stress. Factors such as a recent move, new pregnancy, or the absence of one parent have been associated with an increased risk of poisoning in this age group.

Teenagers are the second distinct age group involved in pediatric poisonings. Approximately half the poisonings in this age group are considered intentional, and half, accidental. Drug experimentation and suicidal gestures are commonly associated with poisonings in adolescents.

There are five basic routes of exposure for accidental poisonings. Ingestion accounts for approximately 75% of all poisonings, followed, in decreasing frequency, by dermal exposure, ophthalmic exposure, inhalation, and envenomation (bites and stings).

A wide range of substances is involved in poisonings. Children younger than 6 years are more likely to be poisoned by nonpharmaceutical products. Table 10–12 presents the categories of substances most frequently involved in accidental poisonings in this age group.

Despite the fact that children younger than 12 years account for almost 90% of all pediatric poisonings, the same group accounts for only 40% of all poisoning fatalities in children. In contrast, teenagers account for only 10% of pediatric poisonings but for 60% of deaths due to poisoning in children. The more favorable outcome in the younger group is explained by the less dangerous type and smaller amount of substances ingested, and the fact that the younger children are brought for medical care more promptly after ingestions than are teenagers or adults. Substances causing the largest number of deaths are analgesics and antidepressants, sedatives, hypnotics, stimulants, and cardiovascular drugs, and somewhat less frequently,

Table 10–12. Categories of the Substances Most Frequently Involved in Poisonings for Children Younger than 6 y in 1998

Type of Substance	% All Exposures
Cosmetics/personal care items	13.3
Cleaning substances	11.0
Analgesics	7.6
Plants	7.1
Cough/cold preparations	5.5
Topicals	5.4
Foreign bodies/toys	6.3
Insecticides	3.9
Antimicrobials	3.1
Vitamins	3.3
Gastrointestinal preparations	3.0

Adapted and reproduced, with permission, from Litovitz TL et al: 1998 annual report of the American Association of Poison Control Centers Toxic Exposure Surveillance System. *Am J Emerg Med* 1998;17:435.

alcohol, gases, asthma remedies, hydrocarbons, and other chemicals.

Diagnosis & Clinical Assessment

Most childhood poisonings can be assessed and managed at home by telephone, as demonstrated by the success of Regional Poison Control Centers. These centers are staffed 24 hours a day by specialists highly trained in poison information who have access to computerized information on virtually every potentially poisonous substance available. A child with a potentially serious or an unknown ingestion is referred to a hospital emergency department for medical evaluation.

The approach to the poisoned patient should begin with a brief history of the exposure. Basic historical information to obtain includes confirmation that a poisoning has occurred or is suspected, identification of the potential toxic substance(s), route and dose of the exposure, time of the exposure, any symptoms occurring before arrival at the hospital, any preexisting medical conditions, and the use of therapeutic medications. Although information obtained during the initial history may be inaccurate, it is often possible to make a judgment regarding the potential severity of the exposure and the level of treatment that may be required.

Children frequently present to the emergency department after a poisoning without a specific history of a toxic exposure. For this reason, poisoning is often a diagnosis of exclusion and must be considered in the differential diagnosis of any child in the high-risk age groups (younger than 5 years or teenagers) who presents with an acute unexplained illness or altered consciousness.

As with any potentially critically ill patient, the physical examination of the poisoning victim begins with an evaluation of the patient's ABCs. Specific attention should be paid to the heart rate; respiratory effort and pattern; blood pressure; CNS function, as manifested by the level of consciousness and pupillary size and reactivity; and hemodynamic status of the patient. Assessment of skin temperature, color, and perfusion, the presence or absence of sweating, and bowel and bladder function can provide clues to the type of poison involved. Smelling the patient's breath also can be of value in establishing the type of poisoning because some substances have characteristic odors (Table 10–13).

Many drugs have a characteristic constellation of physical findings because of their effects on the autonomic nervous system. Table 10–14 lists the four most common autonomic toxic syndromes. By performing a directed "toxicologic" physical examination, the physician may be able to make a tentative clinical diagnosis, allowing for the empiric use of specific antidotes or selective toxicologic tests. Because there are frequent exceptions to these guidelines and because ingestion of multiple agents can demonstrate overlapping or divergent effects, the categorization of physical findings into specific syndromes can be very difficult.

One approach to this dilemma is to consider five major acute clinical signs with which poisoned patients may present: coma, cardiac arrhythmias, metabolic acidosis, seizures, and gastrointestinal symptoms.

COMA

A decreased level of consciousness is a common manifestation of poisoning by a variety of drugs and chemicals. Table 10–15 lists several drugs that characteristically cause stupor or coma. The mechanism by which most toxins cause coma is via a diffuse encephalopathy, which results in global depression of the CNS.

Pulmonary aspiration of gastric contents and progressive respiratory failure are constant concerns in the comatose patient. The most common cause of death in

Table 10–13. Substances With Characteristic Odors

Odor	Substances
Sweet	Chloroform
	Acetone
	Ether
Pear	Chloral hydrate
Bitter almond	Cyanide
Garlic	Arsenic
	Phosphorus
Violet	Turpentine
Wintergreen	Methyl salicylate

Table 10–14. Most Common Autonomic Toxic Syndromes

Anticholinergic

Signs	Delirium; tachycardia; dry, flushed skin; dilated pupils; urinary retention; decreased bowel sounds; hyperthermia.
Common causes	Atropine, scopolamine, tricyclic antidepressants, skeletal muscle relaxants, antihistamines, antipsychotics, many plants (e.g., jimson weed and *Amanita muscaria*).

Cholinergic

Signs	Confusion, central nervous system depression, salivation, lacrimation, urinary and fecal incontinence, bradycardia or tachycardia, miosis, diaphoresis, seizures, muscle fasciculations, pulmonary edema, emesis.
Common causes	Organophosphate and carbamate insecticides, physostigmine, edrophonium, and some mushrooms.

Sympathomimetic

Signs	Tachycardia (or reflex bradycardia if agent is a pure α-agonist), hypertension, hyperpyrexia, diaphoresis, mydriasis, delusions, seizures. Hypotension and arrhythmias may also occur.
Common causes	Cocaine, amphetamines, methamphetamines, over-the-counter decongestants (phenylpropanolamine, ephedrine, pseudoephedrine), caffeine, and theophylline.

Opiate or sedative

Signs	Coma, respiratory depression, miosis, hypotension, bradycardia, hypothermia, pulmonary edema, hyporeflexia. Seizures may occur after propoxyphene overdose.
Common causes	Narcotics, barbiturates, benzodiazepines, ethanol, clonidine.

Adapted and reproduced, with permission, from Kulig G: Initial management of ingestion of toxic substances. *N Engl J Med* 1992;326:1677.

Table 10–15. Drugs Associated With Major Symptoms at Presentation

Toxic causes of coma	Toxic causes of anion gap
Antihistamines	Acidosis
Atropine	Carbon monoxide
Barbiturates	Cyanide
Benzodiazepines	Ethanol
Carbon monoxide	Ethylene glycol
Clonidine	Iron
Cyanide	Isoniazid
Ethanol	Methanol
Narcotics	Salicylates
Organophosphates	
Phenothiazines	**Toxic causes of arrhythmia**
Tricyclic antidepressants	β-Blockers
	Calcium channel blockers
Toxic causes of seizures	Digoxin
Anticholinergics	Tricyclic antidepressants
Camphor	Amphetamines
Carbon monoxide	Cocaine
Cocaine	Chloral hydrate
Phencyclidine (PCP)	Phenothiazines
Phenothiazines	Theophylline
Propoxyphene	
Theophylline	**Toxic causes of gastro-**
Tricyclic antidepressants	**intestinal symptoms**
β-Blockers	Arsenic
Type Ia antiarrhythmic	Iron
agents	Lithium
Quinidine	Mercury
Procainamide	Poisonous mushrooms
Phenothiazines	

Adapted and reproduced, with permission, from Olson KR, et al: Physical assessment and differential diagnosis of the poisoned patient. *Med Toxicol* 1987;2:52.

conditions that cause coma, including intracranial trauma, hypoglycemia, hypothermia, meningitis, and encephalitis.

CARDIAC ARRHYTHMIAS

A full 12-lead electrocardiogram (ECG) should be part of the initial evaluation in all patients with suspected toxic ingestion. Sinus tachycardia is a nonspecific finding in a variety of poisonings and usually not helpful in identifying a specific toxin. Drugs with characteristic ECG findings are listed in Table 10–15. Treatment depends on the specific rhythm present and the hemodynamic status of the patient. Sinus bradycardia is characteristic of digoxin, β-blockers, and cyanide, or as a reflex response to hypertension induced by α-adrenergic agonists like phenylpropanolamine. Prolonged QT intervals suggest phenothiazines or type Ia antiarrhythmics (quinidine or procainamide). Widened QRS complexes are seen with tricyclic antidepressants and propoxyphene (a synthetic

comatose patients is respiratory arrest, which may occur abruptly. Therefore, protection of the airway, assisted ventilation, and supplemental oxygen are the most important interventions in comatose patients.

When evaluating a comatose patient for possible poisoning, it is important to look carefully for other serious narcotic). Patients with these findings are at risk for the development of life-threatening ventricular arrhythmias.

METABOLIC ACIDOSIS

Persistent, unexplained metabolic acidosis may be the only initial clue to a toxic ingestion. Evaluation of metabolic acidosis should include measurement of arterial blood gases, serum electrolyte, BUN, glucose concentrations, and serum osmolality. Calculation of the anion gap can be helpful in the differential diagnosis of metabolic acidosis:

$$anion\ gap\ =\ Na\ (meq/L) - Cl\ (meq/L) - HCO_3\ (meq/L)$$
$$(normal\ is\ 8-12\ meq/L)$$

As listed in Table 10–15, poisonings that may lead to an elevated anion gap acidosis include methanol, paraldehyde, iron, ethylene glycol, and salicylates. Likewise, the calculation of the expected serum osmolality with the following formula:

$$\begin{Bmatrix} calculated\ serum \\ osmolality \end{Bmatrix} = 2(Na[meq/L]) + \frac{urea\ (mg/dL)}{2.8}$$
$$+ \frac{glucose\ (mg/dL)}{18}$$

can be compared with the measured serum osmolality for the presence of an osmolal gap. A measured osmolality that is more than 10 mOsm greater than the calculated value suggests the presence of osmotically active substances that are not accounted for by the calculation. The family of alcohols including ethanol, methanol, isopropyl alcohol, ethylene glycol, or glycerol can produce an osmolar gap metabolic acidosis, the presence of which can provide a tentative diagnosis pending results of specific toxicologic testing.

SEIZURES

Like coma, seizures are a feature of many drug and chemical poisonings (Table 10–15). Because poisoning is a relatively uncommon cause of seizures in children, other causes must be considered, including hypoxia, hypoglycemia, hyponatremia, intracranial injury, CNS infections, and febrile seizures. In most cases of drug-induced seizures, immediate identification of the specific toxin is not necessary because the treatment of most toxin-induced seizures is generally similar to that of seizures resulting from other causes. However, seizures caused by toxins are often more difficult to control. Prolonged seizures, with the development of respiratory and metabolic acidosis, also can aggravate the potential effects of a toxin on the cardiovascular system.

GASTROINTESTINAL SYMPTOMS

Gastrointestinal (GI) symptoms of poisoning include emesis, nausea, abdominal cramps, and diarrhea. These might be caused by the direct toxic effects on the intestinal mucosa or systemic toxicity subsequent to absorption. A single, self-limited episode of vomiting may accompany almost any ingestion. However, iron, lithium, mercury, arsenic, or poisonous mushrooms characteristically cause severe vomiting, diarrhea, or both (see Table 10–15). Gastrointestinal hemorrhage also may accompany iron ingestion. Persistent vomiting or diarrhea may result in hypovolemia and shock. Therefore, the adequacy of the patient's circulation must be assessed.

Laboratory Evaluation

Every patient with a potentially significant poisoning should have some routine laboratory evaluation. Studies that should be considered for all patients include a complete blood count, serum electrolyte, BUN and glucose concentrations, arterial blood gas, and serum osmolality. A 12-lead ECG can reveal arrhythmias or conduction delays that may aid in diagnosis or management. A chest radiograph looking for evidence of aspiration or noncardiogenic pulmonary edema may help guide management. A plain radiograph of the abdomen may visualize radiopaque pills (e.g., iron, chloral hydrate, some phenothiazines, and heavy metals).

A differential diagnosis usually can be constructed on the basis of the history, physical examination, and some routine laboratory tests. Even though most drugs and chemicals commonly ingested today can be measured in serum, urine, or gastric aspirates, the routine toxicology screen is of minimal value in the initial care of the poisoned patient in the emergency department. Toxicology screening is expensive, time consuming, and subject to false-positive and false-negative results. However, specific quantitative levels of certain drugs may be useful in determining the need for a specific intervention or antidote. Specific drug levels are most useful when the patient has ingested an overdose of acetaminophen, salicylates, anticonvulsants, digoxin, ethanol, iron, or theophylline. The use of toxicologic screening should be reserved for patients with signs of major toxicity with an unknown substance and for those cases in which there is direct communication with the laboratory about the suspected agents. Many hospitals now use abbreviated qualitative screening of urine for common drugs of abuse as an alternative to comprehensive toxicologic screening.

Management

Initial management of seriously poisoned patients is similar to that of other critically ill patients. An approach to the management of poisoned patients is outlined in Table 10–16. General supportive management accord-

Table 10–16. Initial Approach to the Management of a Poisoned Patient[1]

A	Airway	Positioning Suctioning Consider endotracheal intubation
B	Breathing	Oxygen Assisted ventilation
C	Circulation	Establish intravenous access Fluid boluses (20 mL/kg) as needed
D	1. Dextrose	Check bedside glucose Administer dextrose (0.5 g/kg as needed)
	2. Disability	Assess level of consciousness, consider naloxone Pupillary examination Treat seizures with benzodiazepines and phenytoin if necessary
	3. Decontamination	Irrigation of affected skin or eyes Induced emesis Gastric lavage Activated charcoal Whole-bowel irrigation

[1] See text for specific recommendations regarding poison management.

ing to the principles of BLS and ALS always should be initiated. Priority is given to ensuring a patent airway, adequate ventilation, and the administration of oxygen. If altered mental status or the threat of seizures or life-threatening cardiac arrhythmias is present, endotracheal intubation and mechanical ventilation may be required. Placement of at least one, and preferably two, IV catheters is indicated in all potentially significant poisonings. Hemodynamic instability should be managed promptly with bolus infusions of normal saline as needed to improve peripheral perfusion and to stabilize the vital signs. The evaluation of a bedside test for blood glucose and the administration of dextrose (0.5–1 g/kg IV) for hypoglycemia is the next priority. A rapid assessment of the patient's neurologic examination should be performed, with attention to the level of consciousness and the pupillary light reflexes. Patients with depressed levels of consciousness should receive 2 mg of naloxone (Narcan) regardless of their age or size. Repeated doses may be required to reverse the effects of some synthetic narcotics such as propoxyphene or dextromethorphan.

Toxin-induced seizures can be difficult to control. In general, diazepam or lorazepam can be administered ini-

tially, with consideration for subsequent use of phenytoin (Dilantin) or fosphenytoin if further seizures are noted. Seizures caused by toxin-induced hypoglycemia must be recognized and treated promptly with dextrose.

Decontamination should begin as soon as possible after initial stabilization to limit the systemic absorption of the toxin from the skin or GI tract. For respiratory exposure, removal of the patient from the toxic environment is usually all that is necessary, with careful observation for latent pulmonary effects of the toxin. If a patient's skin or eyes have been exposed to an irritating or corrosive substance, the affected areas should be irrigated with copious amounts of water after contaminated clothing is removed.

Gastrointestinal decontamination of ingested toxins can be accomplished through a variety of means. Considerable controversy exists as to the efficacy and appropriateness of the primary methods of removing a toxin from the GI tract. Options include induced emesis, gastric lavage, the use of activated charcoal, and, most recently, whole-bowel irrigation.

GASTROINTESTINAL DECONTAMINATION

Emesis can occur spontaneously after the ingestion of many substances. If spontaneous emesis has not occurred or has resulted in the evacuation of only a small amount of the ingested agent, the induction of emesis may be considered. Induced emesis can be effective when performed within 30–60 minutes of an ingestion. It is typically used at home by a parent after phone consultation with a physician or Regional Poison Control Center. Syrup of ipecac is the method of choice for inducing emesis. The following doses should be used depending on the child's age: 6–12 months, 10 mL; 1–10 years, 15 mL; older than 10 years, 30 mL. More than 90% of patients vomit within 20–30 minutes after a single dose of ipecac. Emesis is contraindicated in the following situations: if the patient has a decreased level of consciousness; if the toxin may abruptly lead to seizures or coma; after ingestion of a caustic agent; after ingestion of some hydrocarbons; and in children younger than 6 months.

The amount of gastric contents recovered by ipecac-induced emesis is highly variable and generally less than 50%. Because efficacy decreases substantially with longer delays after an ingestion and because protracted emesis delays the institution of further GI decontamination, the use of ipecac in the emergency department has fallen out of favor.

Like induced emesis, the efficacy of **gastric lavage** is highly variable and dependent on its institution within 1–2 hours after the ingestion. Its role may be limited to patients who arrive in the emergency department soon after a potentially life-threatening ingestion. In particular, if the patient is comatose or seizing and tracheal intubation is being considered for airway protection, gastric lavage can be performed after securing the artificial airway. To carry out the most effective lavage, a large-bore orogastric tube should be inserted. After confirming its location in the stomach, aliquots of normal saline are used until the return is clear. Potential complications of gastric lavage include mechanical injury to the airway, esophagus, or stomach and an increased risk of aspiration pneumonia.

Because neither induced emesis nor gastric lavage completely removes an ingested substance, the administration of **activated charcoal,** with or without initial gastric emptying, is recommended in most cases of poisoning. Activated charcoal functions by binding a wide variety of drugs and chemicals, thereby preventing their subsequent absorption from the GI tract. The dose of activated charcoal is 1 g/kg given orally or through a nasogastric tube. Like the gastric-emptying procedures, it is most effective when given as soon as possible after the ingestion. Activated charcoal has been demonstrated to act as a reservoir to adsorb some drugs directly from the blood perfusing the GI tract in a process referred to as GI dialysis. Repeated doses of charcoal may benefit children who have ingested drugs that undergo enterohepatic circulation or active secretion into the intestinal lumen.

Gastric-emptying procedures (emesis or lavage) before the use of activated charcoal have not been demonstrated consistently to provide any additional benefit. Therefore, most authorities recognize activated charcoal as the decontamination procedure of choice in the majority of pediatric poisonings, provided the ingested agent is known to be adsorbed by charcoal. Activated charcoal does not bind well to a few notable substances (Table 10–17).

Several charcoal preparations are packaged in a slurry with 70% sorbitol. Repeated doses of the charcoal–sorbitol combination may result in significant diarrhea with fluid and electrolyte losses. In contrast, activated charcoal alone may cause constipation. If repeated doses of charcoal are to be administered, it is preferable to alternate between preparations with and without sorbitol and titrate the relative amounts of each to achieve the desired effect without unwarranted side effects.

WHOLE-BOWEL IRRIGATION

Whole-bowel irrigation (WBI) describes the technique of administering large volumes of a polyethylene glycol electrolyte lavage solution into the GI tract to produce

Table 10–17. Substances Not Effectively Bound by Activated Charcoal

Acids	Hydrocarbons
Alcohols	Iron
Alkali	Lead
Cyanide	Lithium

diarrhea. It effectively prevents the absorption of potential toxins by mechanically flushing the agent out of the GI tract. Whole-bowel irrigation has been used extensively as a bowel preparation before surgery or colonoscopy. It recently has gained attention in the management of poisonings in the following situations: (1) ingestion of a drug that is not adsorbed by charcoal (e.g., iron); (2) late presentation after ingestion because the drug may have entered the small intestine, rendering it unavailable for charcoal binding; or (3) ingestion of very large amounts of a substance that may result in persistently toxic amounts of drug even after other initial decontamination procedures.

The solution is delivered orally or through a nasogastric tube at a rate of 0.5 L/h for children up to age 5 years and 2 L/h for adolescents and adults. The procedure should be continued until the rectal effluent clears, typically in 6–12 hours. The most common adverse effects of the procedure are nausea or vomiting. Contraindications to the use of WBI include evidence of major GI dysfunction, such as ileus, obstruction, perforation, or severe GI hemorrhage.

Antidotal Therapy

The number of ingestions for which a specific antidote is necessary or available is small. With rare exceptions, stabilization of the patient through general supportive care takes precedence over trying to determine which, if any, antidote should be given. The antidotes most commonly used within the first hour of management are listed in Table 10–18. Some of the antidotes may be harmful if used inappropriately, as when multiple drugs have been ingested, resulting in a confusing clinical picture. Even when available, antidotes do not diminish the need for

Table 10–18. Antidotes Commonly Used in the First Hour of Management After an Overdose

Toxin	Antidote
Opiates	Naloxone
Methanol, ethylene glycol	Ethanol
Anticholinergics	Physostigmine
Organophosphate or carbamate insecticides	Atropine
β-Blockers	Glucagon
Tricyclic antidepressants	Bicarbonate
Digitalis	Digoxin-specific antibody fragments
Benzodiazepines	Flumazenil
Calcium channel blockers	Calcium

Adapted and reproduced, with permission, from Kulig G: Initial management of ingestion of toxic substances. *N Engl J Med* 1992;326:1677.

meticulous supportive care, with primary attention directed to the support of the patient's vital functions.

Prevention

Poison prevention strategies have resulted in lower morbidity and mortality from poisoning in children. Educational activities in the form of anticipatory guidance by the pediatrician can be effective when continually reinforced. These efforts can be aimed at the parents and, in a developmentally appropriate way, the child. "Poison proofing" the environment by storing potentially poisonous household products and medications in proper containers and in places inaccessible to curious toddlers should be expected of every family. One of the most effective methods of prevention from accidental poisoning was the introduction of child-resistant packaging through the Poison Prevention Packaging Act of 1970. Child-resistant closures have significantly reduced the morbidity and mortality from poisoning in children younger than 6 years.

ACETAMINOPHEN

Acetaminophen is one of the most widely used analgesics and antipyretics; it is among the most common medications involved in overdose in children. In therapeutic doses, acetaminophen has few side effects; however, toxic doses may be associated with hepatic necrosis and, rarely, renal failure.

Acetaminophen is absorbed rapidly after an oral dose, reaching a peak plasma level within 30–60 minutes. Absorption may be delayed in an overdose, with peak levels occurring up to 4 hours after ingestion. Acetaminophen is metabolized in the liver predominantly by two mechanisms. The vast majority (up to 94%) of the drug is converted to glucuronide or sulfate conjugates, which are then excreted in the urine. Another 4% is metabolized by the cytochrome P-450 mixed-function oxidase system to a toxic intermediate, which is rapidly inactivated by conjugation with glutathione. This pathway is of primary interest in the overdosed patient. A large dose of acetaminophen may deplete the stores of glutathione available to detoxify the intermediate. This highly reactive intermediate may then bind to hepatic macromolecules, producing a centrilobular hepatic necrosis. The lower incidence of hepatotoxicity in children younger than 6 years may relate to a relatively smaller amount of metabolism via the P-450 pathway. Antidotal therapy for acetaminophen overdose is based on replacement or substitution of glutathione stores to prevent the production of the toxic intermediate.

Diagnosis & Clinical Presentation

Evaluation of a patient after a known or suspected acetaminophen overdose should begin with a determination of the amount ingested. The history is notably unreliable in adolescents who have intentionally ingested acetaminophen. All adolescents should be managed as if they had ingested a potentially toxic amount, with initial evaluation in an emergency department. For children younger than 6 years, if a reliable history indicates ingestion of less than 100 mg/kg, no treatment is required. Most ingestions of 100–150 mg/kg can be managed at home. Ingestions of greater than 150 mg/kg are considered potentially toxic, and all children with this or an unknown amount of ingestion should be evaluated in an emergency department.

The clinical course of an acute acetaminophen overdose follows four stages (Table 10–19). Early symptoms, such as coma, seizures, or cardiac arrhythmias, within the first 24 hours are associated with acetaminophen but are likely related to coingestants. A high index of suspicion of acetaminophen ingestion must be maintained, however, so that an acetaminophen level may be determined to guide possible antidotal therapy.

Management

Management of acetaminophen overdose begins with good supportive care followed by GI decontamination. Activated charcoal should be administered to all patients with an intentional or significant accidental overdose to prevent the occurrence of a potentially toxic acetaminophen level. This is also useful in case there are significant coingestants, which also may be bound to charcoal. A specific serum acetaminophen level should be obtained no sooner than 4 hours after ingestion. This level is then plotted on the Rumack–Matthew nomogram (Figure 10–3)

Table 10–19. Clinical Course of Acetaminophen Overdose

Stage 1	12–24 h after ingestion Nausea, vomiting, diaphoresis, anorexia
Stage 2	24–48 h after ingestion Clinically asymptomatic ALT (SGPT), AST (SGOT), bilirubin, and PT begin to rise
Stage 3	72–96 h after ingestion In patients who are untreated or treated late: peak hepatotoxicity (AST [SGOT] > 1000 IU/L)
Stage 4	7–8 days after ingestion Recovery

ALT (SGPT) = alanine aminotransferase (serum glutamic pyruvic transaminase); AST (SGOT) = aspartate aminotransferase (serum glutamic oxaloacetic transaminase); PT = prothrombin time.

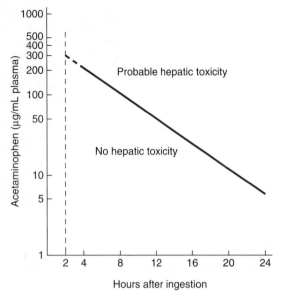

Figure 10–3. Nomogram for interpreting plasma acetaminophen showing semilogarithmic plot of plasma acetaminophen concentrations versus time. (Adapted and reproduced, with permission, from Rumack BH, Matthew H: *Pediatrics* 1975;55:873.)

to predict the likelihood of hepatic injury. Baseline alanine aminotransferase (serum glutamic pyruvic transaminase) and aspartate aminotransferase (serum glutamic oxaloacetic transaminase), bilirubin and glucose concentrations, and prothrombin time are also indicated in significant ingestions.

If the 4-hour acetaminophen level is on or above the nomogram line, indicating possible hepatotoxicity, specific antidotal therapy with oral *N*-acetylcysteine (NAC) is indicated. Because NAC is adsorbed to activated charcoal, its use in patients who have received charcoal has been the subject of recent controversy. Current recommendations are to wait 2 hours after a dose of charcoal before administering NAC or increase the dose of NAC by 40% to account for part of it being bound by the charcoal. *N*-acetylcysteine increases glutathione synthesis and, as a glutathione substitute, inactivates the toxic acetaminophen metabolite. Its efficacy has been proved when given within the first 16 hours after an acute ingestion. *N*-acetylcysteine has maximum efficacy when given within 8 hours of ingestion, when it is protective against hepatotoxicity regardless of the initial plasma acetaminophen level. However, it should be used even up to 24 hours after an ingestion and can be stopped if the acetaminophen level is subsequently found to be nontoxic according to the nomogram.

With prompt recognition of patients at risk of acetaminophen toxicity, good supportive care, and timely institution of antidotal therapy with NAC, outcome should be excellent, with little risk of severe hepatic necrosis.

TRICYCLIC ANTIDEPRESSANTS

Tricyclic antidepressants are among the most widely prescribed drugs in the United States. They are used in the treatment of depression, enuresis, hyperkinesis, sleep disorders, and a number of atypical pain syndromes such as trigeminal neuralgia. Tricyclic antidepressants have the highest case fatality ratio of any class of drugs and consistently are a leading cause of death from poisoning.

Tricyclic antidepressants have a variety of pharmacologic effects, four of which are of primary concern with overdose. These effects are blockage of reuptake of norepinephrine and serotonin at presynaptic sites in the CNS (the primary mechanism for their antidepressant effects), anticholinergic effects, membrane depressant or "quinidinelike" effects on the myocardium, and α-adrenergic receptor blockade. These four effects may result in a characteristic "toxic syndrome" of signs and symptoms, as listed in Table 10–20.

Diagnosis & Clinical Presentation

The tricyclic antidepressants are generally well absorbed from the GI tract. With acute overdose, however, absorption is unpredictable because of the anticholinergic effects

Table 10–20. Signs and Symptoms of Tricyclic Poisoning by Their Mechanism of Action

Blockage of reuptake of norepinephrine and serotonin in the central nervous system	"Quinidine-like" effects
Central nervous system agitation followed by depression	Widened QRS complexes
	Prolonged PR, QT_c intervals
Coma	Second- or third-degree atrioventricular block
	Atrial and ventricular arrhythmias
	Hypotension
Anticholinergic effects	**Peripheral α-adrenergic receptor blockade**
Seizures	Hypotension
Coma	
Tachycardia	
Warm, flushed skin	
Dry skin and mucous membranes	
Dilated pupils	
Decreased or absent bowel sounds	
Urinary retention	

on GI motility. Onset of life-threatening symptoms may be abrupt, usually within 6 hours of the overdose. Tricyclic overdose should be suspected in any patient who presents with seizures, coma, cardiac arrhythmia, or signs of anticholinergic poisoning. Primary attention must be paid to the patient's vital signs and level of consciousness. After this, the physical examination should specifically seek to identify signs of anticholinergic effects, such as dry skin or mucous membranes, dilated pupils, flushing, decreased or absent bowel sounds, and urinary retention. Most of the important effects of tricyclics are on the cardiovascular system and CNS.

The most common causes of death in fatal tricyclic overdoses are hypotension and cardiac arrhythmias. Hypotension can occur secondary to direct myocardial depression, an arrhythmia, or from peripheral α-adrenergic receptor blockade. The "quinidinelike" effects of tricyclics on the cardiac conduction system may result in a widened QRS complex (>100 milliseconds), which is the best clinical predictor of the severity of a tricyclic poisoning. Patients with a widened QRS complex are at increased risk for the development of life-threatening ventricular arrhythmias and sudden death.

Central nervous system effects are usually prominent in tricyclic overdose. An initial phase of agitation or excitement is followed by sedation, which may progress to coma or seizures. Seizures occur in 10–20% of patients, usually after the onset of coma.

Management

As with all critically ill patients, initial priorities in management should focus on the patient's ABCs. Because the onset of coma, seizures, or significant cardiac arrhythmias may be abrupt, a decision to protect the airway with endotracheal intubation must be made early in the assessment of the severity of the ingestion.

Continued monitoring of the patient's respiratory, cardiovascular, and neurologic status is essential. Respiratory failure can occur from CNS depression, seizures, upper airway obstruction, or pulmonary aspiration. Hypoxia and acidosis aggravate the effects of tricyclics on the cardiovascular system and must be treated aggressively.

As soon as the patient's vital functions are stabilized, efforts at GI decontamination are begun. Even in the home setting, induced emesis with syrup of ipecac is contraindicated because of the potential for seizures or an abrupt deterioration in the patient's level of consciousness. Ideally gastric lavage with a large-bore orogastric tube is performed after protection of the airway with an endotracheal tube. Activated charcoal therapy effectively binds tricyclic antidepressants and should be instituted as soon as possible.

Seizures induced by tricyclics are treated with IV diazepam. Recurrent seizures can be managed by loading the patient with a longer acting anticonvulsant such as phenobarbital or phenytoin.

Cardiac conduction abnormalities (prolonged QRS, bradyarrhythmias) are treated by producing an alkalemia (pH 7.4–7.5) with hyperventilation or the use of bicarbonate. When this fails to prevent the onset of malignant ventricular arrhythmias, lidocaine, phenytoin, or ventricular pacing can be tried. Hypotension is managed initially with bolus infusions of isotonic saline (20 mL/kg). If there is no response to repeated fluid boluses, pressor agents should be used.

As soon as possible, all symptomatic patients should be transferred to an ICU for continued monitoring and supportive care. Signs of toxicity usually resolve within 24–36 hours.

IRON

Accidental iron poisoning is among the more common serious ingestions in children younger than 6 years. Factors contributing to the incidence of iron poisoning include its widespread availability and the fact that most people do not consider iron potentially dangerous. A typical scenario of acute iron poisoning involves a toddler who ingests his mother's iron supplement during or just after her new pregnancy.

The toxicity of iron stems from direct corrosive effects on the GI mucosa and systemic effects related to the presence of free iron in the circulation. Systemic toxicity may include cardiovascular, metabolic, and CNS derangements and, infrequently, hepatic failure.

Diagnosis & Clinical Presentation

The severity of acute iron poisoning should be assessed by estimating the amount of elemental iron ingested. Different iron preparations have different concentrations of elemental iron; therefore, the exact name of the preparation and the estimated number of tablets ingested are necessary to make the best determination.

Ingestion of less than 40 mg/kg of elemental iron is considered nontoxic; these children usually can be managed safely at home. Accidental ingestions of more than 40 mg/kg and all intentional ingestions should be evaluated in an emergency department. A proposed strategy for the evaluation and management of iron ingestions is presented in Figure 10–4. As with the evaluation of any potentially ill child, initial emphasis is placed on the overall appearance of the child, the level of consciousness, and the vital signs. Significant vomiting, diarrhea, or GI hemorrhage may result in hypovolemia. Therefore, the adequacy of the patient's circulation should be monitored continuously, with institution of fluid replacement as indicated. Laboratory evaluation after a potentially serious iron ingestion should include a determination of blood

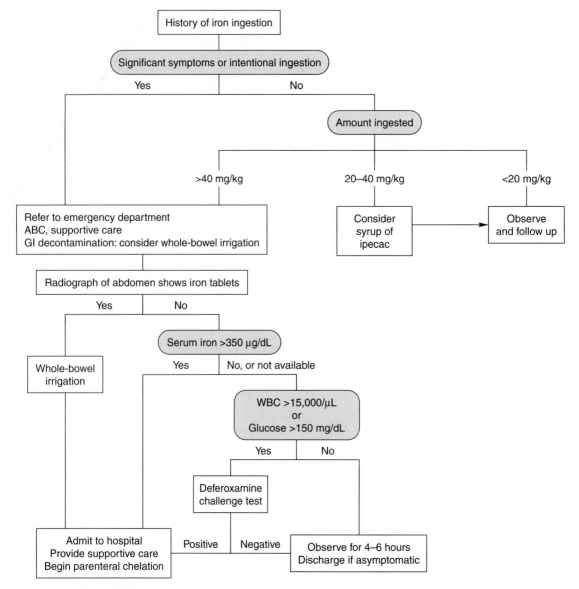

Figure 10–4. Algorithm showing a proposed strategy for the evaluation and management of iron ingestions. ABC = airway, breathing, and circulation; GI = gastrointestinal; WBC = white blood cell count.

glucose and electrolyte concentrations and a complete blood count. An arterial blood gas, blood type, and cross-match may be indicated in patients who manifest signs of serious toxicity. Because many iron preparations are radiopaque, an abdominal roentgenogram is an easy, noninvasive way of estimating the potential for toxicity. The presence of visible iron tablets on an abdominal roentgenogram correlates with more serious symptoms and may guide management decisions about further GI decontamination.

Determination of a serum iron concentration 2–4 hours after an acute iron ingestion provides the most reliable laboratory evidence of the severity of an ingestion. If serum iron levels are not available on an emergency basis, clinical assessment coupled with some simple laboratory tests can be used to assess the severity of an ingestion. Patients with protracted vomiting or diarrhea for 6 hours, a serum glucose level above than 150 mg/dL, or a white blood cell count greater than 15,000/μL, and the presence of radiopaque tablets on a plain roentgenogram of the abdomen correlate highly with toxic serum iron levels. A "challenge" dose of deferoxamine, 50 mg/kg IM, will chelate any free unbound iron in the circulation, thereby producing a characteristic reddish-brown *vin rose* appearance of the patient's urine. This signifies the need for further chelation.

The clinical effects of acute iron poisoning have been divided into four classic phases (Table 10–21). **Phase 1,** which occurs up to 6 hours after an acute ingestion, represents the direct corrosive effects of iron on the GI tract. Most patients with mild to moderate ingestions do not progress beyond this phase. **Phase 2,** classically described as lasting 6–24 hours after ingestion, is characterized by recovery from GI symptoms. This phase may be transient or completely missed in severe iron poisonings that progress rapidly to phase 3. **Phase 3,** which occurs up to 48 hours after ingestion, is characterized by recurrence of GI symptoms and the onset of metabolic acidosis, severe lethargy or coma, and cardiovascular collapse. Circulating free iron is a potent vasodilator and also may increase capillary permeability, resulting in hypovolemia and the development of shock. Iron-induced mitochondrial dysfunction interferes with the normal mechanisms of cellular respiration, resulting in the development of metabolic acidosis. The development of jaundice, hypoglycemia, and coagulopathy secondary to hepatic damage also may occur during this phase. **Phase 4,** which occurs 4–6 weeks after ingestion, is usually seen only after a severe poisoning, with marked early GI corrosive effects, resulting in

Table 10–21. Clinical Phases of Acute Iron Poisoning

Phase 1	0–6 h after ingestion Nausea, vomiting, hematemesis, diarrhea, melena, abdominal pain Lethargy or coma in severe ingestions Tachycardia Hyperglycemia, leukocytosis
Phase 2	6–24 h after ingestion Resolution of gastrointestinal symptoms Intermittent lethargy
Phase 3	12–48 h after ingestion Recurrence of gastrointestinal symptoms Lethargy, coma Cyanosis, tachycardia, cardiovascular collapse Metabolic acidosis, coagulopathy
Phase 4	4–6 wk after ingestion Gastrointestinal scarring and obstruction

the development of pyloric or small bowel strictures. Children typically present with symptoms of GI obstruction.

Management

As outlined in Figure 10–4, management of serious iron ingestions begins with good supportive care. Once vital signs have been stabilized, attention is turned to efforts at GI decontamination. Because iron is not bound to activated charcoal, GI decontamination can be complicated. If the patient is seen soon after the ingestion, an attempt at gastric lavage should be made via a large-bore orogastric or nasogastric tube. If radiopaque material is seen on a postlavage abdominal roentgenogram or if the patient exhibits signs of moderate to severe toxicity, WBI may be attempted. Whole-bowel irrigation has been demonstrated to remove iron tablets safely and effectively from the GI tract, thereby preventing further absorption.

When the patient has been stabilized and GI decontamination has been instituted, a decision must be made concerning the use of the specific chelator, deferoxamine. A serum iron concentration, available within the stabilization phase of management, provides the most reliable method to indicate the need for specific chelation therapy. Serum iron concentrations of 150–350 μg/dL may produce mild phase 1 symptoms but usually do not produce systemic toxicity requiring chelation. Concentrations greater than 350 μg/dL signify the appearance of free iron in the circulation, necessitating a short course of chelation. Concentrations greater than 500 μg/dL are associated with signs of serious systemic toxicity requiring aggressive efforts at GI decontamination, general supportive care, and specific chelation.

Upon chelation with iron, the deferoxamine–iron complex is excreted in the urine. Deferoxamine can be given by intermittent IM injection or continuous IV infusion at a rate of 10–15 mg/kg/h.

The vast majority of children with iron poisoning survive without significant sequelae. Fatality is correlated with the early onset of coma or shock. Good supportive care and specific chelation therapy are required to improve the outcome of seriously poisoned patients.

ETHANOL

Ethanol is widely available in a variety of beverages and many other products, including decongestants, cough medicines, mouthwashes, perfumes, and colognes. The American Association of Poison Control Centers reported more than 7000 cases of ethanol exposure in the pediatric age group in 1994. One fourth of all ethanol exposures in children are from nonbeverage sources, some of which contain ethanol concentrations as high as 80%. Among exposures in all age groups, ethanol, alone or in combination with other substances, was involved in almost 10% of all poisoning fatalities.

Ethanol is absorbed rapidly from the GI tract; peak blood concentrations are reached within 1 hour of ingestion. Ethanol is metabolized primarily in the liver by the hepatic enzyme alcohol dehydrogenase. Despite the fact that this enzyme does not reach adult levels in children until they are 5 years of age, young children metabolize ethanol at a rate twice that of adults. Alcohol dehydrogenase uses nicotinamide adenine dinucleotide as a cofactor, resulting in increased levels of reduced nicotinamide adenine dinucleotide. The increased hepatic cell ratio of reduced to complete nicotinamide adenine dinucleotide inhibits gluconeogenesis. Children younger than 7 years who have limited glycogen stores may become hypoglycemic after an ethanol ingestion because of the inhibition of gluconeogenesis. This hypoglycemia and the global depressant effects of ethanol on the nervous system account for the major mechanisms of ethanol toxicity.

Diagnosis & Clinical Presentation

Ethanol poisoning should be considered in any child presenting with the acute onset of seizures or altered mental status. Information obtained from the history should include not only the availability of alcoholic beverages but also access to mouthwash, perfumes, and over-the-counter liquid cough or cold medications. The physical examination is directed toward a rapid assessment of the patient's ABCs and level of consciousness, as outlined in the section on Diagnosis and Assessment of the poisoned patient. Laboratory evaluation of patients with known or suspected ethanol ingestion should include a rapid evaluation of blood glucose concentration in addition to a blood ethanol level, serum electrolyte and BUN concentrations, and osmolality. Significant ethanol poisoning may result in metabolic acidosis, primarily because of the increased production of lactic acid. A characteristic anion gap and osmolal gap metabolic acidosis is often the first clue to ethanol poisoning in a child with no history of ingestion.

The initial clinical effects of acute ethanol ingestion include nausea and vomiting because of direct gastric irritation. A characteristic odor may be detected on the patient's breath. Early CNS effects include emotional lability, mild ataxia, muscular incoordination, and decreased reaction time. Severe ethanol intoxication may result in coma, hypothermia, respiratory failure, and, rarely, shock. The severity of systemic symptoms and signs correlates with the blood ethanol concentration (Table 10–22). Hypoglycemia, which may be present at blood ethanol concentrations less than 100 mg/dL, may result in lethargy, coma, or convulsions.

Management

The initial priority in management of known or suspected significant ethanol ingestion is the rapid evalua-

Table 10–22. Correlation of Clinical Effects with Blood Ethanol Levels

Ethanol Concentration (mg/dL)	Comon Signs and Symptoms
<25	Usually asymptomatic
25–100	Mild behavioral changes
100–150	Mild incoordination, slowed reactions, visual impairment
150–300	Moderate incoordination, slurred speech
300–500	Severe incoordination, stupor
>500	Coma, depressed respirations, potentially lethal

tion and management of the patient's airway and breathing. As soon as possible, a rapid bedside test of a blood glucose concentration should be performed to determine the presence of hypoglycemia. Patients with documented or symptomatic hypoglycemia should be given 0.5 g/kg of dextrose (2 mL/kg D25W) followed by a dextrose-containing continuous IV infusion, with frequent monitoring of the blood glucose level. If hypoglycemia is not recognized and treated in a timely fashion, significant illness or death may result despite peak ethanol concentrations in a range not typically considered dangerous.

Efforts at GI decontamination are usually of limited value. Because ethanol is absorbed rapidly from the stomach and alters mental status relatively quickly, ipecac-induced emesis and gastric lavage usually are not used if there is a delay in seeking medical attention. Ethanol is not significantly bound to activated charcoal. Unless there is a known or suspected history of coingestion with other substances adsorbed by charcoal, it, too, is of little value.

Any child with hypoglycemia or significant alteration in mental status should be admitted to the hospital for prolonged observation until he or she awake enough to eat and drink. Good general supportive care is usually all that is required in the management of mild to moderate ethanol intoxications. Hemodialysis removes ethanol from the body and may be considered in patients with blood ethanol concentrations greater than 500 mg/dL who are deteriorating despite good supportive care.

CAUSTIC AGENTS

Cleaning products are the second leading category of substances (after cosmetics and personal care items) involved in poisonings in children younger than 6 years. Many of these cleaning products (e.g., bleaches and detergents) contain caustic agents that are available in crystalline and liquid forms. In many households, they are frequently stored in inappropriate containers without child-resistant seals, giving them an attractive appearance for inquisitive toddlers.

Caustic agents include acids and alkalis. Their mechanism of toxicity stems from their potential to produce tissue damage on contact. Acids account for approximately 15% of caustic ingestions in children. They produce tissue damage by coagulation necrosis, a process that usually limits the penetration of the acid into deeper tissue levels. In contrast, alkalis, which are responsible for most significant caustic ingestions in children, produce a liquefaction necrosis. They can penetrate tissues, producing further extensive damage. The extent of injury depends on the pH of the substance (serious damage is seen with pH > 12.5), its concentration, and the amount of time it is in contact with the tissue.

All corrosive acids and alkalis produce inflammation on contact with the skin or mucous membranes. Because acidic solutions taste bitter and cause immediate pain on contact, their exposure is usually limited by the patient unless the ingestion is intentional. In contrast, alkaline solutions are often tasteless and odorless, and large quantities can be ingested before the onset of pain. Granular agents are more likely to cause focal injuries to the oropharynx and proximal esophagus, whereas liquid agents typically can produce extensive, continuous damage throughout the entire length of the esophagus and into the stomach.

Diagnosis & Clinical Presentation

Information obtained from the history should include the specific product name, approximate amount ingested, time of ingestion, and the presence and onset of any symptoms before arrival in the emergency department. Common initial signs and symptoms after a caustic ingestion include drooling, vomiting, stridor, or, in older patients, dysphagia. Nausea, abdominal pain, and abdominal tenderness may also be seen. Physical examination may show erythema of the mucous membranes of the mouth, lips, and perioral skin. Erythema may also be seen in characteristic patterns on the trunk from drooling with contaminated saliva. Oropharyngeal ulcerations, edema, or grayish-white membranes on the mucosa may also be seen. The presence or absence of oropharyngeal findings does not reliably predict the presence or extent of esophageal injury. Up to one third of children with significant esophageal or gastric burns have no oropharyngeal burns.

Management

As with all other potentially serious poisonings, management should begin with an evaluation of the patient's ABCs. Of note, the presence of stridor suggests significant laryngeal edema, and strict attention should be paid to the continued patency of the patient's airway. Efforts at decontamination should include irrigation of the eyes or skin if continued contact with the corrosive substance is suspected. Ipecac-induced emesis is contraindicated with caustic substances so as to limit their contact with the esophagus and oropharynx. Benefits of gastric lavage have not been clearly demonstrated, and the risk of further injury to a damaged esophagus usually precludes its use after caustic ingestions. Patients should be admitted to the hospital for further management. Appropriate supportive care includes withholding oral feedings, judicious use of parenteral nutrition, and careful observation for the development of complications such as hemorrhage, perforation, or sepsis.

Significant esophageal or gastric burns are the most feared complication of caustic ingestions. Therefore, most physicians agree that esophagoscopy is indicated in the evaluation of any patient after a significant caustic ingestion. The absence of oropharyngeal lesions cannot reliably exclude the presence of esophageal burns. The presence of fewer than two serious signs or symptoms (vomiting, drooling, or stridor) has been correlated with the absence of esophageal injury. However, esophagoscopy is still recommended in the evaluation of caustic ingestions.

Of even greater controversy is the management of significant esophageal burns after they are diagnosed. The greatest area of controversy involves the early use of steroids to prevent extensive inflammation with subsequent stricture formation. A recent long-term prospective evaluation of the use of steroids after caustic injury to the esophagus demonstrated no benefit from steroids in the prevention of stricture formation. The severity of the initial burn was highly predictive of the development of strictures, regardless of whether steroids were used.

As soon as the child is able to swallow, liquids should be provided by mouth. Parenteral nutrition may be required if the child cannot eat after an extensive injury. Patients with second-degree (limited to the mucosa) or third-degree (deep ulceration into the muscle) burns of the esophagus should be reevaluated by esophagoscopy 2–3 weeks after the initial injury for the development of strictures. Barium swallow radiographs also can be used to diagnose the presence of strictures. The treatment of strictures includes repeated mechanical dilations, placement of stents to limit the extent of scarring, or, in severe cases, replacement of a segment of esophagus with a colonic or jejunal interposition.

■ CHILD ABUSE & NEGLECT

The syndrome of child abuse was first formally described by radiologist Dr. John Caffey in 1940. He noted a group of children with fractures and subdural hematomas. In 1962, Henry Kemp coined the term **battered** child syndrome to describe children who were beaten by their parents or parental figures. Then, in 1963, Vincent Fontana discussed the **maltreatment syndrome in children,** which introduced the concept that, besides physical abuse, children can be emotionally abused or neglected by depriving them of food, clothing, or medical attention or by leaving them alone and unsupervised.

Child abuse has been defined as any interaction, or lack of interaction, between family members that results in nonaccidental harm to the child's physical or developmental well-being. This includes actions that result in obvious bruises, lacerations, or fractures, in addition to the more unusual forms of abuse, such as intentional poisonings, hypernatremic dehydration because of water deprivation, and subarachnoid hemorrhage from vigorous shaking of infants. Child neglect encompasses a spectrum of parental omissions, including starvation, abandonment, and improper care. A particularly serious form of neglect involves prolonged emotional deprivation of a child by a parent. This may involve failure to meet the emotional needs of a child or constant criticism, and it can result in poor growth of the child, or **failure to thrive.**

Child abuse differs from ordinary punishment; all parents discipline their children, and some use corporal punishment, despite the fact that it may not be the most effective way to change behavior. However, even corporal punishment is not considered child abuse unless significant force is used, resulting in injury to the child. Legally, the child has been abused if discipline results in injury. Unfortunately, many parents believe they can discipline their child by any means they choose.

Child abuse is common in the United States. It is estimated that each year more than 1 million children are physically abused, and 1000 deaths result.

The most severe physical injuries are inflicted on children younger than 6 years because they are less able to flee or defend themselves. Many of these children are more vulnerable or somehow "different" from other siblings; they may be handicapped, chronically ill, or hyperactive or may have had a difficult neonatal course that limited the parents' ability to bond with them. Other high-risk children are twins or siblings of twins, who may be abused because of the stress created by inadequate spacing between children. Likewise, children from unwanted pregnancies may be at risk because a new burden has been placed on the family.

Child abuse occurs in all countries, races, and socioeconomic groups. The abusive parent may have been abused as a child and is depressed and emotionally immature, with poor impulse control. Some of these parents also have unrealistic expectations for their child's growth and development. For example, a child may be abused because a parent is frustrated that the young toddler is not yet toilet trained. Children of young (teenage) mothers are at increased risk of maltreatment. Undoubtedly, many abuse cases in some way involve the use of illicit drugs by caretakers.

Diagnosis & Clinical Manifestations

A witness to the abuse may bring the child for medical attention, in which case the diagnosis of child abuse is obvious. Often, however, the physician is presented with an injured child and must determine whether the injury resulted from intentional harm. Although unintentional injuries do happen, the physician must investigate every injury in a child for evidence of abuse.

The history is important in determining the presence of abuse. A history of significant stress in the family should increase one's suspicion about the injury. One also should be concerned if the cause of the injury is unknown, if the caretakers are reluctant to give information, if they change the story of how the injury occurred, or if they seem inappropriately concerned or tardy in bringing the child for care. Abuse also should be considered if the account of how the injury occurred seems incompatible with the child's developmental abilities. For instance, if the caretakers claim the child climbed and fell from a height, the infant must be old enough or adept enough to accomplish this feat. The history may contribute important information. If the child's records reveal inadequate medical care in the past, e.g., the child was never brought for immunizations or has had frequent "accidents" with injuries, one should have increased concerns about the current injury.

Physical examination should be conducted after completely undressing the child. Child abuse must be considered if the injury does not fit the story. For instance, bruises should not appear on both sides of the head if the story describes the child falling only once; a child cannot get linear bruises from falling down steps. Bruises noted to be in different stages of healing suggest recurrent battering rather than a single episode of trauma; Table 10–23 describes the color of skin bruises at various healing stages. However, "dating" of bruises is not an exact science, and the estimated age of the bruise should not be the sole criterion for a diagnosis of child abuse. Injuries that conform to a particular pattern are usually diagnostic of abuse. For instance, loop-shaped bruises are characteristic of an injury inflicted by a belt or a cord. A circumferential burn

Table 10–23. Estimated Dating of Healing Bruises

Color of Bruise	Days Since Injury
Red	0–1
Bluish-purple	1–4
Greenish-yellow	5–7
Yellowish-brown	>8

of the feet and lower legs or buttocks is characteristic of a child forced or dipped into hot water. Children would not voluntarily put their entire leg into a bathtub if the water were scalding hot, and children never get into a tub with both feet at the same time, or with their buttocks first. Injuries to certain anatomic areas often are caused by abuse. For instance, the hand is commonly injured as a form of punishment, and genitalia may be injured intentionally out of frustration over toilet training. Likewise, frenulum injuries may result from forcibly stuffing an object like a bottle into an infant's mouth.

An injury that otherwise does not seem unusual may take on more importance in the face of signs of general neglect, failure to thrive, malnutrition, poor hygiene, or withdrawn personality. Many serious injuries can occur without obvious bruises; thus, abdominal trauma can result in duodenal hematoma or lacerated liver or spleen without external evidence of injury. Similarly, the "shaken baby syndrome" can present without skin bruising. This syndrome deserves special consideration because it is one of the most common causes of death from child abuse. The typical victim is an infant younger than 1 year who is violently shaken and, in many cases, thrown against a soft surface such as a bed or carpeted floor. The young infant comes to the emergency department because of respiratory distress of sudden onset. The parents usually relate no other history. The baby may be found comatose or may experience seizures. Respiratory arrest may occur in the presence of respiratory distress, yet there is no evidence of upper airway obstruction or lower airway disease. The respiratory distress occurs because of CNS injury, such as a subdural hematoma. Careful physical examination shows a full fontanelle, and retinal hemorrhages occur in 80–90% of cases. Radiographic imaging of the brain will confirm the injury.

Laboratory tests, including radiographs, are often helpful in confirming the diagnosis of child abuse. Fractures are found frequently in abused infants and young children. Half the skeletal injuries in abused children occur in children younger than 1 year, and 90% in children younger than 5 years. Extremities are most commonly fractured, followed by the skull and ribs. Transverse fractures of the diaphysis of long bones are common and caused by direct force against the bone. Spiral or oblique fractures are caused by twisting of the bone. These fractures can occur unintentionally if the foot gets caught between fixed objects and twists as the child falls, but such fractures of the upper extremities are more suspicious. Metaphyseal chip fractures are characteristic of abuse because the forces necessary to produce these are rarely generated by accidental falls in young children. They are caused by vigorous "yanking" or jiggling of extremities left dangling while the child is shaken. Further, skull fractures in young infants should arouse suspicion of abuse; studies have shown that these rarely occur from minor trauma, such as a fall from a bed or down stairs. Also, rib fractures in children younger than 2 years rarely are caused by unintentional trauma. Such fractures are caused by squeezing the infant's thorax rather than by a direct blow, and they cannot occur with chest compressions during resuscitation. Old fractures need an explanation, and multiple fractures, or fractures in various stages of healing, usually are indicative of child abuse.

Because fractures are so common among abused infants, it is recommended that a "skeletal survey" be obtained if abuse is suspected. This survey, which includes radiographs of the chest, skull, and long bones, has the highest yield in infants younger than 2 years; it is rarely worthwhile in children older than 5 years. These radiographs are preferred over a nuclear bone scan, which will not identify metaphyseal fractures or allow determination of the age of the injury. However, a bone scan may help to identify subtle fractures missed by conventional radiography. Computed tomography (CT) is important if head injury is suspected or the shaken baby syndrome is considered. Magnetic resonance imaging may be more useful in identifying small intracranial bleeding.

Other conditions should be considered in the differential diagnosis. For instance, platelet disorders and leukemia can lead to unusual bruising. Further, rickets or osteogenesis imperfecta might lead to unusual or unexplained fractures. The history, physical examination, and some laboratory studies or radiographs should distinguish those conditions from abuse.

Management

Once the diagnosis of child abuse is suspected, the physician is responsible for protecting the child. Ideally, a multidisciplinary team of caregivers, including a pediatrician, nurse, psychologist, and social worker, should be available to participate in the child's care. It is often helpful for members of the caregiving team to interview the child in a quiet, nonthreatening setting. It is important to document the history as thoroughly as possible and record children's exact words if they are old enough to speak. Color photographs of any significant injury are useful, but a good written description of the injury with diagrams will suffice. Hospitalization may be necessary if the injury is serious or if a satisfactory disposition that guarantees the child's safety cannot be arranged. The child should not be sent home to an unsafe environment! Physicians should know how to obtain a court order for custody, if needed, and should know where to refer the child if they cannot provide necessary care for the child and family. Physicians are obligated to report suspected abuse to the local agency that has responsibility for the child's welfare. This reporting must take place regardless of the time of day and regardless of the physician's relationship with the family or desire to avoid court action. The physician need not be certain, but rather only suspicious of abuse, to file a report. If the injury proves to be unintentional, the physician is protected against legal action related to the report. However, failure to report suspected abuse is considered a misdemeanor and may result in fines, civil suits, loss of license, and possible imprisonment. More importantly, there is a 50% chance of repeated abuse and a 10% chance of fatal injury if children are returned to the abusers without proper precautions.

It is best for the examining physician to confront the caretakers with the suspected diagnosis and the need to report it to local authorities. However, the physician must remain nonjudgmental, not accusatory or punitive. It is not the role of the physician to prove that child abuse occurred or to find out who inflicted the injury. The physician can be helpful in arranging for needed follow-up care, counseling, and psychotherapy for the child and family.

Because all but 5–10% of abused children remain with their families, one goal of treatment must be to prevent further child abuse. Ideally, high-risk situations for potential abuse will be noticed before a child is actually harmed. Thus, many centers have set up telephone hotlines for stressed parents to call for advice or crisis nurseries where children can be left temporarily until parents can work out their problems. Primary care physicians can help by scheduling more frequent visits to the office for families at high risk for abuse and by arranging for available community services. The physician can also help by providing information about child rearing and development so that parents can have realistic expectations. The community needs to provide self-help groups, parent education groups, and early intervention programs for high-risk families.

SEXUAL ABUSE

Sexual abuse is defined as any sexual act performed by an adult with a minor younger than 18 years, including indecent exposure, digital manipulation of the genitals, masturbation, fellatio, sodomy, and coitus. Others define sexual abuse as exposure of children to sexual stimulation that is inappropriate for their age, level of psychosocial development, and role in the family.

Because of recent media exposure and parental awareness, reporting of sexual abuse is increasing. It is estimated that more than 300,000, or about 1%, of children are sexually abused each year in the United States.

Girls are six times more likely to be abused than boys. The abuser is usually a family member (35–45%), such as a father, stepfather, uncle, or a trusted friend. Only about 20% are assaulted by strangers, and this usually involves older boys and girls assaulted in the street or other public places.

Sexual abuse is unlike criminal rape in that violence is rarely associated. Usually there is disorganization or stress in the family, such as alcoholism, mental illness, or drug abuse. Abusers usually have weak egos and low self-esteem and are often impotent. They expect failure in adult heterosexual acts and, therefore, seduce children.

The child may become a victim for a variety of reasons. Infants and toddlers cannot verbalize their feelings of fright or confusion and so have no choice but to participate. The young, school-aged child has no concept of real sexuality and does not know to refuse compliance. Also, these young children trust the adult to do nothing wrong. The adult is not hurting the child physically and may instead offer reassurances or bribes. An older child may enjoy the special attention given by the adult, especially if another family member has been physically abusive. Adolescents may pity the adult or feel guilty about reporting the incidents. They also may fear punishment for reporting and are often threatened with harm if they do. When the father is the sexual abuser, the mother may be aware of the abuse but allow it to continue out of fear of breaking up the family or of imprisonment of the father with loss of financial support for the family.

Diagnosis & Clinical Manifestations

The diagnosis of sexual abuse depends primarily on the history from the child or caretaker. Some events are witnessed by the adult who brings the child for care, but more often suspicion exists without definite evidence that abuse has taken place. Some children who are sexually abused have behavioral problems, depression, or anger, but it is difficult to relate these problems to sexual abuse in the emergency department setting. Some may have nonspecific complaints of dysuria, vaginal itch, or discharge. Although some young children can be "coached" to say anything (i.e., in the midst of a custody battle), the physician should be quite concerned about sexual abuse when young children can vividly describe a sexual incident that they experienced. A child's account of the abuse is the most important factor in determining what occurred. A recent review of criminal court cases found that 75% resulted in conviction, yet only 23% had physical evidence of injury, sexually transmitted disease, or seminal fluid.

The physical examination of a child with suspected sexual abuse usually results in normal findings. Signs of trauma are rare, especially as most cases involve fondling or exposure rather than penetration. Even when penetration has occurred, nonspecific or normal findings are noted in about 40% of cases. The size of the hymenal orifice cannot be used reliably to determine whether abuse has occurred because it can change with the degree of relaxation at the time of examination, the position of measurement, presence of estrogenization, and age of the child. Instead, genital findings consistent with sexual abuse (acute cases) include bruising, tears, and lacerations of the hymen, perihymen, and posterior fourchette. In chronic cases, the genitalia may show disruption, scarring, and attenuation or loss of hymenal tissue to indicate prior penetrating trauma. Presence of semen or evidence of sexually transmitted disease indicates sexual abuse until proved otherwise. The perianal area also may show evidence of trauma or infection.

Management

The physician plays a key role in diagnosing sexual abuse. A sensitive interview with the child is of the utmost importance; this should be done in a quiet, nonthreatening environment. If the alleged abuse occurred more than 72 hours before medical attention was sought, it is best to manage the case in a relaxed setting outside the emergency department. The interview questions should be open-ended and nonleading and take into consideration the age and developmental level of the child. Allowing a child to draw or use anatomic dolls may be helpful if the child has difficulty verbalizing. The physician must carefully document the questions asked and the child's responses using the child's exact words and adding a description of the child's affect. Next, a gentle physical examination should be performed; this can be done with the child in the frog-leg position on the mother's lap. The child also can be supine on the examining table in the frog-leg position to allow easy visibility of the genitalia. An alternative is the knee-to-chest position for genital examination. Diagrams and photographs may be helpful to record abnormal findings. Sedation is rarely needed if reassurance is given frequently. An internal pelvic examination is not indicated in prepubertal children. If significant trauma is suspected, examination under general anesthesia may be necessary but is rarely needed.

Some acute infections, such as syphilis or gonorrhea, are almost certainly indicative of sexual abuse; others, such as chlamydiosis, trichomoniasis, herpes simplex virus type 2, and condylomatosis, indicate probable sexual abuse, whereas herpes simplex virus type 1 might be related to sexual abuse. It may not be necessary to collect specimens from all children with alleged sexual abuse, but some children with sexually transmitted diseases because of abuse have no symptoms at the time of evaluation. Thus, it is prudent to obtain cultures for sexually transmitted diseases if there is significant concern that the child was abused. This includes cultures of the oropharynx for gonorrhea and the vagina/urethra and rectum for gonorrhea and *Chlamydia*. Rapid tests for *Chlamydia* should not be used because false-positive results may occur. If a discharge is present, it should be examined for *Trichomonas*. Serology and testing for infection with the human immunodeficiency virus should be considered. A urine pregnancy test should be obtained in the child who is postmenarche. If there was a recent assault, a "rape kit" should be used to collect evidence of the perpetrator's secretions or hair that would likely be found on the victim. This collection includes two saline swabs of the ejaculation site (vagina, rectum, or skin) and two cotton swabs of the throat and gum line if oral–genital contact occurred. Saliva should be obtained from the victim to determine antigen status; the procedure involves placing a sterile gauze pad, 2 inches square, into the victim's mouth and then placing the gauze in a sterile tube. Blood (2–3 mL) also must be obtained from the victim for serologic testing and blood typing. Pubic hairs, if present, should be collected in an envelope, and clothing should be placed in brown paper bags. All evidence must be carefully documented and turned over to police.

Antibiotic therapy for possible sexually transmitted disease can be withheld pending cultures. The alleged abuse must be reported to the local child protective services agency, and the safe disposition of the child must be arranged. The physician should arrange for follow-up evaluation of the child, including counseling for the child and family, if needed.

■ THE INJURED CHILD

Accidents, the leading cause of morbidity and mortality during childhood, account for more than 14 million physician visits, 600,000 hospitalizations, and 22,000 deaths per year. Motor vehicle accidents are the most common cause of death in children. Although the number of deaths caused by motor vehicle accidents in the United States has decreased over the past decade, the incidence of homicide has increased tremendously. Homicide is the second leading cause of death in children younger than 4 years and the most common cause of death for all African-American children.

Although the overall approach to the pediatric trauma patient is the same as that for the adult, the higher incidence of multisystem injury and the relatively limited communication skills in children necessitate an ordered and comprehensive approach to these patients.

The next section addresses the initial evaluation and management of the pediatric trauma patient by following protocols suggested in the Advanced Trauma Life Support course designed by the American College of Surgeons and focusing on the common pediatric entities of head trauma, near-drowning, and fire-related injuries.

Features Unique to Pediatric Trauma Patients

The anatomic differences between children and adults transcend the obvious size discrepancy. Until the age of 11–12 years, children's heads constitute a relatively greater proportion of their total body mass. When they fall, children are more likely to land on their heads. The larger head also contributes to higher level cervical spine injuries (C2–C3) in children. A child's large ratio of body surface area to mass allows more rapid loss of heat and fluids, necessitating close attention to these issues. Because of their small size, children sustain multiple organ system injuries more frequently than adults. Their immature skeletons sustain less frequent bone injuries but more frequent soft tissue and internal organ damage. When bone injury does occur, it may be subtle because of the presence of open growth plates at the epiphyses. These growth plates often are not as strong as the tendons connected to them and therefore can be damaged despite a normal radiographic appearance. Children require age-specific equipment and weight-specific drug dosages during resuscitation. Knowledge of age-specific vital signs and developmentally appropriate examinations of neurologic and mental status also help in assessing pediatric trauma patients.

Optimal care of the most critically injured patients requires a team approach involving personnel trained in surgery, anesthesia, pediatric care, respiratory therapy, and specialty nursing. The identification of one person, usually a trauma surgeon or pediatric surgeon, as the "team leader" helps to ensure proper delegation of duties and facilitates efficient, thorough evaluation and resuscitation.

Management

The assessment and management of the trauma patient begin with the basic principles of CPR: the ABCs (see this chapter, Cardiopulmonary Resuscitation). This is quickly followed by the assessment of neurologic status (disability) and then the exposure of the entire body for evaluation. This approach, known as the **primary survey** of the trauma patient, is summarized in Table 10–24. Although many activities are happening at once during the resuscitation, one must adhere to the order of these priorities. For instance, attention should never be diverted from the airway to correct a circulation problem. Some special considerations in performing the primary survey on children subjected to trauma are presented in Table 10–25.

Even if the child is breathing spontaneously and no supplemental airway maneuvers are deemed necessary, 100% oxygen should be administered to all victims of major trauma. Ensuring cervical spine stabilization while an adequate airway is secured is paramount in all unconscious or head- and neck-injured trauma patients. This is accomplished by putting the patient in a rigid cervical collar with sandbags or placing one's fingers on the mastoid and mandible to impede lateral movement as well as flexion–extension.

Once cervical spine stabilization has been achieved, attention is focused on the adequacy of respiration. Certain traumatic injuries may compromise the child's ability to

Table 10–24. Trauma: Overall Priorities

I. Primary survey
Airway/cervical spine
Breathing
Circulation
Disability (neurologic)
Exposure
II. Resuscitation phase
Control hemorrhage
Supplemental oxygen administration
Fluid administration
Electrocardiogram monitoring
III. Secondary survey
"A finger or tube in every orifice"
Foley/gastric decompression
Blood tests
Head and maxillofacial trauma—check for signs of basilar skull fracture
Cervical spine—continue immobilization until clinically and radiographically cleared
Chest—continuous reevaluation; palpate for fractures
Abdomen—distention; tenderness. Obtain computed tomography scan
Rectum—check prostate in males; bleeding
Pelvis—check stability
Extremities—deformity, tenderness, crepitus
Neurologic—Glasgow Coma Scale; frequent reassessment
Laboratory studies/radiographs
IV. Definitive care phase
History
A—*Allergies*
M—*Medications*
P—*Past illnesses*
L—*Last meal*
E—*Events surrounding the injury*
Determine disposition
Operating suite
Intensive care unit
Regular inpatient care area
Specialized care facility

Adapted and reproduced, with permission, from American College of Surgeons, Committee on Trauma: *Advanced Trauma Life Support Student Manual,* 1993.

expand the lungs. Pneumothorax or hemopneumothorax may need to be evacuated by needle aspiration and subsequent chest-tube catheter placement. In addition, flail chest may occur when two or more adjacent ribs are broken in multiple locations, thereby impeding the development of negative pressure inside of the thoracic cavity. If the patient requires endotracheal intubation, a rapid sequence technique should be used. Pressure should be placed on the

Table 10–25. Special Considerations of the Primary Survey for Pediatric Trauma Patients

Airway	**Circulation**
Cervical spine immobilization	Intraosseous infusion or peripheral vein cutdown if needed
Rapid sequence intubation	Normal vital signs different for children, ie, systolic BP = 80 + (2 × age in years)
Cricoid pressure	
Lidocaine (1 mg/kg) in head trauma	
Ketamine contraindicated as sedative in head trauma	**Disability**
Avoid nasotracheal intubation	Pupillary response
	AVPU (see Table 10–26)
	Treat seizures
Breathing	**Exposure**
Pneumothorax/ hemopneumothorax	Get patient completely exposed
Flail chest not well tolerated	Beware of hypothermia in infants and small children
Pulmonary contusions more common	

BP = blood pressure.

cricoid ring to move it posteriorly, thereby compressing the esophagus and preventing aspiration of gastric contents (Sellick maneuver). In the acute setting, nasotracheal intubation should be avoided because it is difficult to perform in the young child, and the danger exists of entering the cranial vault if there is a cribriform plate fracture.

While the airway and breathing problems are being addressed, vascular access should be obtained. In patients suffering from major trauma (determined by patient condition and mechanism of injury), two large-bore IV catheters should be inserted. If peripheral IV access is not obtained within a few minutes, then a peripheral vein cutdown, central venous access, or an intraosseous infusion should be considered. The techniques for these procedures were discussed previously (see Shock).

Fluid resuscitation is based on the assessment of four organ systems: cardiovascular, renal, CNS, and skin. Tachycardia is often the first sign of hypovolemia. Low blood pressure is a late finding; up to 40% of the blood volume may be lost before hypotension is manifest. More subtle signs, such as weak pulses; confusion; cool, clammy skin; or decreased urine output, may suggest that large amounts of fluids are still needed. Hemoglobin concentrations and hematocrit may not immediately reflect acute blood loss until sufficient time has elapsed for the blood volume to reequilibrate.

It is prudent to begin fluid resuscitation with the administration of 20 mL/kg of lactated Ringer solution and then observe for improvement of the patient's condition. If necessary, this bolus can be repeated several times while waiting to administer 10 mL/kg of packed red blood cells or whole blood. Children requiring further volume support are likely to require operative management of their injuries. The insertion of a Foley catheter to measure urine output will help to determine the adequacy of the fluid resuscitation. However, the presence of blood at the urethral meatus or the presence of a high-riding prostate on rectal examination signify a possible urethral tear and thus are contraindications to this procedure.

During the primary survey, the evaluation of neurologic disability is brief and consists of checking pupillary size and response and assessing mental status (using the AVPU system presented in Table 10–26). The patient is then exposed to complete the initial assessment.

The next part of evaluation is the secondary survey. The goal of the secondary survey is to discover any injuries that were not apparent on initial evaluation (Table 10–24). The catch phrase for this portion of the evaluation used in the Advanced Trauma Life Support protocols is "tubes and fingers in every orifice," which emphasizes its thorough nature. One begins the survey at the head, neck, and face and proceeds caudally to inspect and palpate each and every portion of the body. The patient should be "log-rolled" to permit examination of the back and rectum for injury. The back is palpated for tenderness or step-offs. The Glasgow Coma Scale (GCS) is used at this point to assess neurologic status in more detail (Table 10–27). Intraabdominal or retroperitoneal bleeding may be difficult to assess; suspicion of internal injuries must be high in patients with abdominal tenderness, guarding, or distention. In children, peritoneal lavage is more difficult to perform than in adults, and many trauma centers instead perform abdominal CT in the initial evaluation for intraabdominal pathology.

Fractures suspected because of deformity, crepitus, or tenderness should be immobilized with a splint. Blood loss from femur or pelvic fractures can be extensive, and the patient with isolated orthopedic injuries might require substantial fluid resuscitation. Cervical spine evaluation is best done radiographically with lateral, anteroposterior, and open-mouth (odontoid) views. The immobilization process should continue until the patient is cleared radiographically and clinically. This means that the comatose

Table 10–26. Rapid Neurologic Evaluation

A—*Alert*
V—responds to *Vocal* stimuli
P—responds to *Painful* stimuli
U—*Unresponsive*

Table 10–27. Glasgow Coma Scale for Assessing Neurologic Status

	Adults/Older Children	Numerical Score[1]	Modified Score (infants)
Eye opening	Spontaneous	4	Spontaneous
	To verbal stimuli	3	To speech
	To pain	2	To pain
	None	1	None
Best verbal response	Oriented	5	Coos and babbles
	Confused	4	Irritable cries
	Inappropriate words	3	Cries to pain
	Nonspecific sounds	2	Moans to pain
	None	1	None
Best motor response	Follows command	6	Normal spontaneous movements
	Localizes pain	5	Withdraws to touch
	Withdraws to pain	4	Withdraws to pain
	Flexes to pain	3	Abnormal flexion
	Extends to pain	2	Abnormal extension
	None	1	None

[1] The numerical scores of each of the three categories are added:
A score of 12–15 is found in children who are awake and alert; it is usually considered unnecessary to obtain a computed tomography scan or to hospitalize such children.
A score below 12 is usually considered an indication to admit the child for careful observation, preferably in an intensive care unit.
A score below 8 indicates a severe head injury, usually with considerable cerebral edema and considerable risk of intracranial hypertension.

patient with negative cervical spine radiographs should remain immobilized while in the emergency department. Radiographs of the chest and pelvis are also obtained routinely soon after the secondary survey is complete.

The delineation of the patient's injuries by primary and secondary survey helps to determine that person's eventual disposition: operating suite, ICU, regular inpatient care unit, or specialized care facility (see Table 10–24). Included in this decision is the patient's medical history, present medical illnesses, and the mechanism of injury.

HEAD TRAUMA

One in 10 school-aged children experiences an episode of head trauma with a change in level of consciousness. One third of these children require hospitalization, accounting for almost 250,000 admissions annually. Severe neurologic sequelae occur in 2–5% of head-injured children. In view of these figures, methods of injury prevention and prompt medical management must be emphasized to parents, caretakers, and medical professionals.

Although motor vehicle accidents account for most head injuries in children, falls down staircases (especially in child walkers), falls from standard beds and bunk beds, and violence-related injuries such as child abuse play a role. In addition, penetrating injuries are being encountered more frequently in urban pediatric emergency departments.

Diagnosis & Clinical Manifestations

The primary injury to the CNS is the shearing of the white matter tracts caused by the acceleration and deceleration of the brain within the skull. The neuronal cell death and vascular disruption that occur within the first few milliseconds of impact cannot be reversed. Therefore, management is guided toward prevention of secondary injury to the brain and blood vessels. Head injuries can be divided into focal injuries, such as fractures or hematomas, and diffuse injuries, such as concussion, increased intracranial pressure, and diffuse axonal injury.

FOCAL INJURIES

Scalp lacerations and contusions are common in head injuries. Because of the high degree of vascularity of the scalp, blood loss from a moderately sized laceration can be extensive. Careful exploration of these wounds must include evaluation for retained foreign bodies, such as glass, and assessment of the depth of the wound and underlying skull fractures. The galea aponeurotica, a strong tendinous sheath located just above the periosteal layer of the skull, occasionally is traversed and may need to be sutured separately to control bleeding.

Even after a child sustains minor head trauma, the first change that the parents notice is often a "lump" on the child's head. Because the galea is very loosely attached to the pericranium in toddlers and older children, this finding usually represents a subgaleal hematoma. In infants, however, there is a chance that the collection of blood occurs on a deeper level, between the periosteum and the table of the skull. The cephalhematoma is more common in traumatic newborn deliveries (see Chapter 4).

Collections of blood beneath the limits of the skull can be epidural or subdural in origin. Table 10–28 summarizes the differences between those entities. Subdural hematomas are the result of acceleration/deceleration injuries that cause disruption of the veins that bridge the subarachnoid space to the dural venous sinuses. Subdural hematomas can be acute, subacute, or chronic. **Acute subdural hematomas** become symptomatic within 24 hours of injury. The most common finding in these patients is a change in level of consciousness, ranging from irritability or lethargy to a comatose state. Subacute subdural hematomas present with similar symptoms between 24 hours and 2 weeks after the injury. **Chronic subdural hematomas,** in contrast, present with more subtle neurologic findings 2 weeks or more after injury, when the blood clot slowly expands as it liquefies.

Epidural hematomas are associated less often with underlying brain injury than are subdural hematomas. A blow or penetrating injury to the parietotemporal region results in a skull fracture with underlying disruption of the middle meningeal artery. In children, however, epidural hematomas are commonly venous in origin. Subsequent extravasation of blood between the dura and the inner table of the skull is limited by the dural reflections and results in a convex, lenticular (lens shaped) appearance on CT. Because of the unilateral nature of these lesions, unilateral uncal herniation is seen more commonly in epidural hematomas than in subdural hematomas. Physical examination may show ipsilateral pupillary dilatation secondary to compression of the parasympathetic fibers of the oculomotor nerve and contralateral motor

deficits from disruption of motor tracts. The overall mortality of epidural hematoma is extremely low, and severe neurologic sequelae are rare in survivors.

Cerebral contusions can occur on the area of the brain initially contacting the cranium (coup injury) or on the portion "rebounding" into the opposite side of the cranium (contracoup injury). If disruption of intracerebral vessels results in cerebral hemorrhage and cerebral contusion, uncal herniation may follow. Nevertheless, the most common manifestation of cerebral contusion is posttraumatic epilepsy. Cerebral lacerations usually result from penetrating injury to the brain or a depressed skull fracture.

Skull fractures. Although the concern over skull fractures after minor head trauma often brings children to medical attention, it is usually more important to investigate the underlying pathology and neurologic ramifications of the blow that created the fracture. Controversy exists regarding the appropriateness of obtaining a radiograph of the skull. Many physicians believe that, if sufficient force was generated to create a fracture, a CT scan of the head is necessary to investigate possible intracranial lesions as well. Therefore, the decision to obtain skull radiographs is based on the patient's age, the mechanism of injury, and the need for other radiologic evaluation.

There are several types of skull fractures. **Linear fractures** account for 75–90% of all skull fractures. Although no treatment is usually necessary, the presence of a fracture indicates that a large amount of force was endured during the event. If the fracture is located over a vascular structure, such as the middle meningeal artery, the incidence of epidural hemorrhage increases.

Basilar skull fractures typically occur in the petrous portion of the temporal bone. Although the diagnosis is

Table 10–28. Supratentorial Epidural Versus Subdural Hematoma

	Epidural	Acute Subdural
Etiology	Arterial (middle meningeal)	Venous
		Bridging veins below dura
Incidence	Uncommon	Common
Peak age	Usually >2 y	6 mo (usually <1 y)
Location	Unilateral	Often bilateral
	Usually parietal	Diffuse, over cerebral hemispheres
Skull fracture	Common	Uncommon
Associated seizures	Uncommon	Common
Retinal hemorrhages	Rare	Common
Decreased level of consciousness	Common	Very common
Mortality rate	Low	Moderate
Morbidity in survivors	Low	High
Clinical findings	Dilated ipsilateral pupil	Decreased level of consciousness
	Contralateral hemiparesis	
Radiographic findings (computed tomography)	Convex "lens-shaped" enhancement	Diffuse, concave enhancement surrounding cerebral hemisphere

difficult to make using only a skull radiograph, the clinical picture is helpful. The four potential findings in patients with basilar skull fractures are (1) pooling of blood in the soft tissues below the eyes (**"raccoon eyes"**), (2) ecchymoses located at the mastoid bones behind the ears (**Battle sign**), (3) cerebrospinal fluid (**CSF**) leak from the nose (**rhinorrhea**) or ears (**otorrhea**), and (4) blood behind the eardrum (**hemotympanum**). Computed tomography of the brain might show pneumocephalus (air inside the cranial vault), usually originating from the sinuses. The communication between the paranasal sinuses and the intracranial contents subjects the child to increased risk for bacterial meningitis. In addition, damage to the first, sixth, seventh, and eighth cranial nerves can result in anosmia (loss of the sense of smell), ocular and facial palsy, and sensorineural hearing loss.

Depressed skull fractures sometimes can be diagnosed by palpation of the depression underneath a hematoma or by radiographic evaluation using tangential views of the skull or CT scan. In older children, depression of the skull can be associated with laceration and bruising of the dura, and the fractures require surgical elevation if they extend past the inner table of the skull.

Diffuse Lesions

Concussion syndromes, the most common form of diffuse brain injury, are diagnosed when blunt head injury results in a transient impairment of consciousness with loss of awareness and responsiveness. The duration of the loss of consciousness can range from seconds to hours and is caused by damage to the reticular activating system. The presence of anterograde or retrograde amnesia might help to diagnose concussion if the history of unconsciousness is unclear. Although children with a concussion syndrome may experience a period of lucidity lasting minutes to hours, drowsiness and vomiting may develop over time. Symptoms usually resolve over the next 6–8 hours; however, a few will complain of persistent headaches, dizziness, and subtle differences in memory, anxiety level, and sleep patterns for days to weeks after the injury.

Diffuse axonal injury is characterized by persistent functional or physiologic brain abnormalities unassociated with gross anatomic abnormalities. It is thought to be caused by the shearing of nerve fibers on initial impact. Diffuse axonal injury can result in a prolonged comatose state (>6 hours) and is subsequently associated with a high morbidity and mortality.

The volume of the cranial vault is normally constant and contains three compartments: CSF (10%), blood (10%), and brain tissue (80%). An increase in one component necessitates a decrease in another, or the intracranial pressure (ICP) will increase. If the ICP continues to rise, brain tissue and blood vessels are increasingly compressed, with resulting displacement of brain contents inside and outside the cranial vault (herniation) and disruption of cerebral blood flow.

The exact location of brain herniation depends on the mechanism of ICP. If increased pressure causes displacement of the uncal portion of the temporal lobe through the tentorium, the portion of the brainstem that normally lies below the tentorium is compressed. This can disrupt the parasympathetic fibers of the third cranial nerve and result in an unreactive and dilated pupil on the side ipsilateral to the lesion. Motor deficits are usually contralateral to the lesion. If the uncal herniation is bilateral, as occurs in a diffuse injury, the pupillary and motor deficits will be noted bilaterally as well.

Two less common forms of brain herniation involve the cerebellum and the brainstem. **Cerebellar herniation** usually is a result of a posterior fossa lesion, whereas **brainstem herniation** can occur with almost any severe brain injury. Both entities involve compression of medullary autonomic structures, thereby affecting heart rate, respirations, and level of consciousness. The classic "Cushing triad" is a late finding of increased ICP. The triad consists of hypertension, bradycardia, and irregular respirations. With brainstem compression, decerebrate posturing can also be noted.

Management

The initial priorities in a child with severe head injury involve protection of the airway, maintenance of adequate tissue perfusion, and rapid assessment of neurologic status (Figure 10–5). Although the primary injury to the brain is irreversible, the secondary injury due to hypoxia, hypercarbia, or increased ICP must be minimized in the acute care setting.

The indications for establishing an artificial airway in a child with head trauma are listed in Table 10–29. In view of the 5% incidence of cervical spine fracture in patients with severe head injury, it is prudent to obtain cervical spine radiographs in all but the most minor head trauma patients (see this chapter, Trauma). Hyperventilation using an artificial airway should be instituted in any child with signs of increased ICP. It is most effective when the partial pressure of carbon dioxide ($PaCO_2$) is kept at 25–30 mm Hg, which minimizes cerebral blood flow and reduces cerebral blood volume without causing ischemic damage.

Attention should then be focused on the adequacy of circulation. Neurogenic shock secondary to spinal cord injury is a diagnosis of exclusion and should not be considered until hypovolemic shock has been ruled out. Shock should be dealt with aggressively in the trauma patient, regardless of concern for increased ICP. The perfusion of the brain depends on an adequate mean arterial pressure; lack of perfusion leads to irreversible neuronal cell damage.

After the patient's cardiopulmonary status is stabilized, the secondary survey should be performed. First,

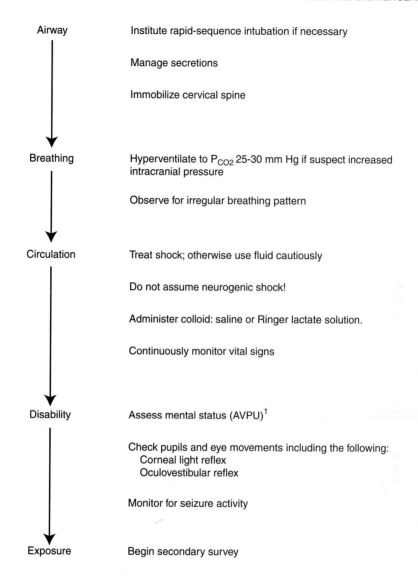

Airway	Institute rapid-sequence intubation if necessary
	Manage secretions
	Immobilize cervical spine
Breathing	Hyperventilate to P_{CO_2} 25-30 mm Hg if suspect increased intracranial pressure
	Observe for irregular breathing pattern
Circulation	Treat shock; otherwise use fluid cautiously
	Do not assume neurogenic shock!
	Administer colloid: saline or Ringer lactate solution.
	Continuously monitor vital signs
Disability	Assess mental status (AVPU)[1]
	Check pupils and eye movements including the following: Corneal light reflex Oculovestibular reflex
	Monitor for seizure activity
Exposure	Begin secondary survey

[1]**AVPU:** Are they **A**lert? Do they respond to **V**oice? Do they respond to **P**ain? Are they **U**nresponsive?

Figure 10–5. Initial management of head trauma. P_{CO_2} = partial pressure of carbon dioxide.

a brief history of the events preceding and subsequent to the trauma episode may be obtained. This history should focus on the time and mechanism of injury, duration of unconsciousness, presence of amnesia, neurologic assessment at the scene, and any preexisting medical conditions. At this point, a more detailed neurologic assessment, including the GCS, should be performed (see Table 10–27). The eyes are examined for abnormal pupillary reflexes or abnormal eye movements that might indicate increased ICP, cranial nerve dysfunction, or seizure activity. The gag reflex should be checked relatively early in the evaluation process to determine the need for intubation. The secondary survey also should include a close inspection of the head for lacerations, depressions, contusions, or signs of basilar skull fracture. Examination of the chest, torso, abdomen, genitalia, and extremities should follow soon after the primary survey.

Table 10–29. Indications for Endotracheal Intubation in the Patient With Head Trauma

Upper airway obstruction
Abnormal respiratory rate or rhythm
Loss of protective airway reflexes
Concomitant trauma
   Chest wall instability
   Pulmonary contusion
Signs of increased intracranial pressure

Evaluation of brainstem function using the oculocephalic ("doll's eye") reflex should be deferred until the cervical spine is evaluated radiographically and clinically. A normal response implies that the cranial nerve pathways most proximal to the brainstem (third, sixth, and eighth cranial nerves) are intact and that, by association, the brainstem is functional. If necessary, the oculovestibular reflexes ("cold caloric") may be implemented if there is no evidence of a perforation of the tympanic membranes. The "normal" reflex is noted as a slow eye deviation toward the cold side and a rapid nystagmus away from the cold side. In general, however, this test can be delayed until after the secondary survey is completed.

SPECIFIC FURTHER MANAGEMENT

If there are signs of increased ICP or of a deteriorating or persistently abnormal neurologic examination, CT of the head is helpful in differentiating focal neurosurgical lesions from more diffuse injury. A head CT scan is also indicated if there is evidence of a skull fracture.

Emergency management of the patient with increased ICP is aimed at reducing the cerebral blood volume to prevent the herniation of brain tissue while maintaining cerebral perfusion pressure. In addition to hyperventilation, other immediate measures can help with this task. The patient's head should be elevated to a 30-degree angle, and adequate arterial blood pressure must be maintained to compensate for the effects of increased ICP. Seizure activity, if present, should be treated. Intravenous mannitol acts as an osmotic diuretic to draw water out of the brain and thereby reduce the "tissue" portion of the intracranial vault. The presence of hypotension or hypovolemia is a relative contraindication to its administration.

Further management of increased ICP may include barbiturate coma, muscle paralysis, and ventriculostomy for CSF drainage. These therapies are usually instituted in an ICU setting.

POST-TRAUMATIC EPILEPSY

The incidence of seizures occurring after head trauma is 5–10%. Most are classified as early post-traumatic seizures, i.e., within 1 week of the initial injury. Twenty percent of these patients go on to experience late seizures more than 1 week after the injury. Post-traumatic seizures are correlated with depressed skull fractures. Early seizures usually are associated with cerebral lacerations and contusions but do not frequently progress to epilepsy. About 50% of patients with late onset seizures will continue to have seizures for the next few years. The drug of choice for such seizures is phenytoin, although in the acute setting a benzodiazepine should be used because of its rapid onset of action.

Disposition of Patients With Head Trauma

The patient who has experienced severe head trauma is almost always admitted to the hospital for aggressive therapy and invasive monitoring. However, patients with less severe injury present a more difficult decision. In general, patients with no history of amnesia and a short duration (<5 minutes) of unconsciousness may be observed without treatment if results of the neurologic examination are normal. This observation usually can occur at home, provided there is a reliable caretaker. Caretakers are instructed to waken the patient every 3–4 hours and allow the patient to walk and talk. In addition, they are instructed to bring the patient back to the emergency department if any signs develop of increased ICP, focal expanding mass, or CNS infection (Table 10–30). In contrast, patients with a prolonged episode of unconsciousness, significant amnesia, posttraumatic seizure, persistent neurologic deficit, or evidence of a depressed or basilar skull fracture should be considered for admission to the hospital and undergo CT of the head. Suspected child abuse victims also should be admitted for evaluation.

Prognosis

There is a 3% mortality rate for all head trauma patients, and a 2–5% incidence of severe handicap. Nevertheless,

Table 10–30. Reasons for Immediate Medical Follow-up of Discharged Head Trauma Patients

Headache worsening or unrelieved by acetaminophen
Frequent vomiting
Change in behavior or gait or difficulty seeing
Fever or stiff neck
Evidence of clear or bloody fluid draining from nose or ear
Difficult to awaken from sleep
Seizure
Bleeding from scalp wound that is unrelieved by 5 min of
   constant pressure

Table 10–31. Factors Associated With a Poor Outcome in Head Trauma

Age < 2 y
Glasgow Coma Scale score < 5
Subdural hematoma
Decerebrate or flaccid posture
Coma > 24 h

complete recovery is the rule for mild to moderate head trauma victims. The GCS is a reliable prognostic indicator in patients with moderate to severe head trauma. Patients with a GCS score of 5 or less and a subdural hematoma have a 75% mortality rate, and surviving children become severely disabled. Factors associated with a worse outcome are listed in Table 10–31. Of all children with severe head trauma, 20% have permanent neurologic deficits, and almost 50% will have some behavioral or emotional problem.

NEAR-DROWNING

Drowning is the third most common cause of death in children aged 1–14 years and a cause of significant neurologic sequelae in near-drowning survivors. **Drowning** is defined as submersion in water resulting in death. **Near-drowning** is defined as survival after asphyxia because of submersion.

Children of all ages are at risk for drowning. However, two age groups are particularly at risk: toddlers and adolescents. Toddlers are most likely to encounter the unknown dangers of ambulating near an open body of water without adequate supervision. Approximately 40% of drowning deaths occur in children younger than 4 years; more than half of these occur in freshwater swimming pools. Adolescent drowning incidents are commonly secondary to unsafe swimming or diving practices or boating accidents; as many as 50% of these deaths are related to alcohol consumption. Most drowning incidents occur during the summer months. An exception is in infants younger than 1 year, in whom bathtub drowning incidents constitute a large percentage. Children with epilepsy have a risk four times greater than that of other children. Child abuse or neglect should be considered in cases of drowning or near-drowning in children who are not ambulatory. Most drowning deaths are preventable; public health measures and legislation are needed to require complete enclosure of all outdoor pools and strict limits on alcohol consumption near boating and swimming areas. In addition, efforts are needed to supply rescue equipment and CPR instruction to responsible individuals at waterside.

Diagnosis & Clinical Manifestations

The initial course of events in submersion injury differs according to the child's age and swimming ability and the mechanism of encounter with the body of water. The common denominator of these events is asphyxia because of respiratory failure, as shown in Figure 10–6. Initially, voluntary breath-holding and voluntary closure of the glottis is accompanied by ingestion of various amounts of water into the GI tract. Ten percent of near-drowning injuries show no evidence of pulmonary aspiration and are termed "dry drowning" injuries. In most cases, however, profound hypercarbia leads to an involuntary gasp and aspiration of water into the airway. The contact of water with the larynx causes reflex laryngospasm and bronchospasm that lead to a marked decrease in ventilation. If water has been aspirated, secondary apnea can occur, thereby adding to the ventilation and oxygenation difficulties. Persistent hypoxemia results from alveolar injury and an intrapulmonary shunt, as the child's airways are perfused but not ventilated. In addition, the denaturation (freshwater) or washout (saltwater) of surfactant adds to the alveolar collapse and hypoxemia. Prolonged hypoxemia results in arrhythmias, pulmonary edema, circulatory failure, and death.

The near-drowning victim's prognosis depends on when the above events were interrupted and the duration of hypoxemia. Neuronal cell damage begins approximately 6 minutes after submersion, becoming irreversible at approximately 9 minutes.

Hypothermia is an invariable sequela of almost all near-drownings. The temperature of the water in which a child is submerged is a double-edged sword. On the one hand, a body temperature below 32°C is likely to result in loss of consciousness and subsequent drowning. The cold heart is more prone to cardiac conduction abnormalities, such as ventricular fibrillation. In addition, the involuntary gasp that leads to fluid aspiration occurs earlier in cold water, and tissue oxygen delivery is impaired in hypothermic states. On the other hand, some evidence indicates that severe hypothermia relates a protective effect to the near-drowning victim by reducing brain metabolism and overall oxygen consumption during a time of severe hypoxemia. Overall, survival has been noted to be better in cases of cold-water submersion than of warm-water submersion. The physical examination of the hypothermic patient may show dilated pupils, increased muscle tone, bradycardia, slow and shallow respirations, and CNS depression. Patients may appear dead. However, the saying, "a patient is not dead until he is warm and dead," reflects the need to continue resuscitation efforts accordingly.

Electrolyte abnormalities are rare in near-drowning victims unless a large amount of water is swallowed, in which case dilutional hyponatremia and hypokalemia may occur.

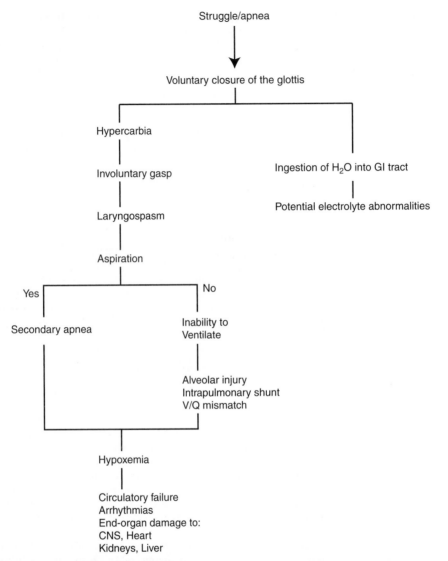

Figure 10–6. Algorithm showing pathophysiology of near-drowning or drowning. CNS = central nervous system; GI = gastrointestinal; V/Q = ventilation-perfusion.

Management

The goals of management of the near-drowning patient are to improve oxygenation and maintain sufficient cardiac output to reverse hypoxic injury to the end organs and prevent further injury to the brain.

ON THE SCENE

Even if the child is still in the water, mouth-to-mouth resuscitation should be initiated immediately. External chest compressions are deferred until the patient is on solid ground and pulses are checked. Once on land, CPR is continued and cricoid pressure is applied to prevent vomiting by compressing the esophagus between the cricoid and the vertebral column. Foreign bodies should be removed from the oropharynx, but the Heimlich maneuver is indicated only if there is a high suspicion of tracheal foreign body. Cervical spine immobilization should be strongly considered if there is any potential mechanism for neck injury. Stabilization for transport to a medical facility should include rewarming by removing wet clothing and covering the child with dry blankets or towels.

HOSPITAL MANAGEMENT

The need for endotracheal intubation is based initially on the presence of apnea or respiratory distress. If the child's trachea was intubated in the prehospital setting, endotracheal tube placement should be evaluated by listening for bilateral and symmetrical breath sounds. Cervical spine immobilization should be considered again unless the history from witnesses absolutely rules out any chance of head trauma or cervical spine injury. If the child is not already intubated, rapid sequence intubation should be performed for the following reasons: apnea, severe respiratory distress, hypoventilation, or decreased level of consciousness. In addition, if further evaluation of breathing shows evidence of pulmonary edema or severe hypoxia, endotracheal intubation should be performed. Severe hypoxia in this scenario is defined as a PaO_2 less than 60 mm Hg despite the administration of an FiO_2 greater than 0.5. Regardless of the condition of the child or need for intubation, 100% oxygen should be provided in the initial resuscitation, and oxygen saturation should be monitored by pulse oximetry. If positive pressure ventilation is required, a high end expiratory pressure and respiratory rate may be required to combat pulmonary edema and hypercarbia. Vigorous suctioning of secretions should be applied in all cases.

After airway and breathing issues are managed, attention must be turned to the circulation to ensure substrate delivery to the tissues. Two competing factors in near-drowning must be considered: hypovolemia and head trauma with increased ICP. Many near-drowning victims are hypovolemic because of capillary leak into the pulmonary parenchyma. Regardless of the ICP considerations, this hypovolemia must be corrected. Intravenous crystalloid fluids should be administered in aliquots of 20 mL/kg to maintain adequate circulation on the basis of heart rate, capillary refill, blood pressure, and urine output. Sodium bicarbonate (1–2 meq/kg) can be administered once adequate ventilation is established.

Most patients with a GCS below 8 require endotracheal intubation and hyperventilation. After an adequate airway has been secured, a nasogastric tube can be inserted to remove any ingested water from the stomach and help prevent dilutional electrolyte disturbances. A Foley catheter can help to assess adequate hydration.

The patient's temperature should be obtained rectally with a thermometer capable of reading temperatures as low as 25°C. Hypothermia should be managed aggressively in the emergency department. If not already done at the scene, the child's wet clothing should be removed, and the child should be dried and wrapped in warm blankets. If the patient's core temperature is 32–35°C, external rewarming methods, such as a radiant warmer and heating blanket, should be used to raise the core temperature. If body temperature is below 32°C, active internal rewarming is accomplished with warmed, humidified oxygen, warmed IV fluids, and warm gastric lavage. Because of the increased incidence of ventricular dysrhythmias in the hypothermic patient, care should be taken not to move the patient too abruptly. In severe cases and when available, extracorporeal blood rewarming can be used for cases of hypothermia with refractory ventricular fibrillation. In patients with severe hypothermia (<32°C) but no apparent cardiac abnormalities, slow rewarming can be accomplished using internal and external rewarming methods. Remember, resuscitation efforts should not be halted in patients with a core temperature below 32°C unless this is considered to be a result of tissue death rather than hypothermic exposure.

Disposition

Transfer to an appropriate inpatient setting should be done quickly to maximize the monitoring status of near-drowning victims. All near-drowning victims require at least 4–6 hours of observation in the emergency department, regardless of how trivial the history or physical examination. Children with a significant history of submersion, a history of apnea or cyanosis, or loss of consciousness, or those who have required CPR must be admitted to the hospital for observation. Patients with abnormal physical findings, abnormal chest x-ray findings, acidosis, or hypoxemia also require admission. In some cases, the respiratory symptoms may not be apparent until 12–24 hours after the incident, when significant pulmonary edema or pneumonitis requires medical intervention. Patients with a change in mental status, respiratory compromise requiring prolonged resuscitation, mechanical ventilation, or high inspired oxygen concentrations should be observed and treated in an intensive care setting (Table 10–32).

Table 10–32. Disposition of Near-Drowning Patients

Observation for 4–6 h	Hospitalization for at Least 24 h	Admission to Intensive Care Unit
All children with history of submersion injury	Apnea/cyanosis Loss of consciousness Required cardiopulmonary resuscitation Findings suggesting anoxia or pulmonary damage	Prolonged cardiopulmonary resuscitation Persistent change in mental status Mechanical ventilation Frequent arterial blood gas monitoring

Table 10–33. Poor Prognostic Factors in Near-Drowning

Prolonged submersion > 10 min
Need for cardiopulmonary resuscitation (CPR)
Delay in necessary CPR efforts in first 10 min
Arrival to emergency department in coma
Initial temperature < 30°C
Initial pH ≤ 7.10

Prognosis

The outcome of the near-drowning victim is related to the amount of irreversible brain injury from hypoxia that occurs during submersion. Poor prognostic factors for survival are listed in Table 10–33. Observation of a stable or improving mental status while in the hospital is a good prognostic sign. A few studies have demonstrated that moderately lower body temperatures may confer some protection against anoxic injury and improve recovery after rewarming and resuscitation. Improvement in mental status within a few hours of injury is an encouraging prognostic indicator.

BURNS

More than 10% of accidental deaths among children between the ages of 1 and 14 years are caused by thermal injury. The nature of these injuries includes scalding, contact with flames or hot solids, and electrical and chemical burns. Although only 3–5% of burn injuries are life-threatening, the pain and psychological ramifications from these injuries argue for efforts to be focused on prevention as well as optimal treatment. Prevention efforts can be helped by informing parents of the benefits of keeping the tap-water temperature below 54.4°C (130°F) and encouraging the use of smoke alarms.

Approximately 80% of burn injuries occur in the home; most injuries in the pediatric population are caused by scalds from hot liquids. However, most deaths in burn patients are caused by direct contact with flames. As children become ambulatory and can gain access to matches or lighters, flame injury becomes the most common form of thermal injury in children 5 to 13 years old. Although a small percentage of thermal injuries is the result of child abuse, 10% of all battered children suffer burns. The typical pattern of these lesions is immersion scald injuries in a stocking-glove appearance or on the buttocks. It is difficult for children to cause a scald burn to the buttocks or symmetric scald burns to extremities on their own bodies. Similarly, few children will intentionally place the full palms of both hands flatly on a hot surface. A high index of suspicion of child abuse needs to be maintained for all cases of burn injury.

Diagnosis & Clinical Manifestations

Burns can be categorized as partial thickness (first- and second-degree burns) or full thickness (third- and fourth-degree burns; Table 10–34).

Partial thickness burns involve some or all of the epidermis or dermis; new skin may be regenerated from this level of burn injury, thereby reducing the need for skin grafting. However, this burn may progress to full thickness if it becomes infected or is subject to further trauma. The appearance depends on the extent of damage to the dermal layer. Shallow lesions result in an exquisitely sensitive blister with underlying erythema. Deeper lesions become white and are painful only to pressure stimulation. This wound is more difficult to distinguish from third-degree burns, especially if a significant amount of edema is present. Second-degree burns usually heal in 10–21 days.

Full thickness burns destroy the entire dermis, including entire hair follicles and sweat glands. The burn usually appears white and is insensitive to painful stimuli. The edges of a full thickness burn are often more shallow and therefore may be painful to touch. Full thickness burns also can be charred or parchmentlike in appearance. It is sometimes possible to see thrombosed superficial vessels through the eschar.

Table 10–34. Degrees of Burn Injury

Type	Degree	Depth	Appearance	Sensitivity
Partial thickness	First	Epidermis	Red	Painful
	Second	Shallow: portion of dermis	Blisters	Exquisitely painful
		Deep	Red/white	May be anesthetic or painful only to pressure
Full thickness	Third	Entire dermis; no remaining adnexal structures	White, parchmentlike, ± blisters, thrombosed veins	Insensitive to stimuli
	Fourth	Muscle, fascia, bone	Black, charred	Insensitive to stimuli

Occasionally the burn injury extends into the subcutaneous tissue, muscle, fascia, or bone. The area is anesthetic and appears charred. There is a danger of systemic toxicity resulting from absorption of toxic products and unrecognized deep infection. Severe scaldings, molten metal burns, and electrical burns result in this type of injury with greater frequency.

Aside from the skin and adnexal structures, other organ systems can be affected by a major burn injury (Table 10–35). In large thermal injuries, circulating blood volume can be diminished because of increased water loss from the external surface and increased capillary permeability in the involved areas. This hypovolemia, in conjunction with direct depression of cardiac output in patients with large burns, may result in "burn shock." These cardiovascular sequelae usually occur only in burn patients with involvement of 30% or more of the body surface area (BSA).

Besides extensive fluid losses, the other most life-threatening complication of thermal injury is infection. Most of these infections originate from the patient's own GI tract rather than those present on the burn unit. Although the bacterium most frequently implicated is *Pseudomonas aeruginosa,* the most serious infections result from invasion by other gram-negative organisms. These organisms are more likely to thrive on wounds that are treated with topical therapy. Conversely, when broad-spectrum antibiotics are used, the incidence of infections with *Candida* increases dramatically.

Management

At the scene, the patient's ABCs, sensorium, and potential for smoke inhalation should be addressed. Smaller burn areas may be doused with cold, wet compresses, whereas larger burns or those encountered more than 10–15 minutes after the injury are covered with clean, dry sheets to minimize heat loss.

Continued assessment of the ABCs should occur in the emergency department. Special attention should be given to the presence of stridor, carbonaceous sputum, edema of the laryngeal structures, or singed nares as evidence of potential burn injury to the upper or lower airways. If these are present, direct laryngoscopy should be performed. Consideration should be given to prophylactic intubation of the trachea if upper airway obstruction appears likely.

The initial approach to the management of fluids in the burn patient begins with a rapid estimation of the wound depth and percentage of BSA involved. The depth of injury should be evaluated, and clinical signs of first-, second-, third-, and fourth-degree burns should be determined (see Table 10–34). The BSA of the injury can be estimated from published diagrams of BSA. Notice that the main difference between infants and older children is the relative surface area of the head. If this type of figure is not available, the size of the child's palm can be used as an estimate of 1% of the BSA. The "rule of 9s" can be applied to adults and children older than 10 years, with BSAs of 9% assigned to the head and each upper extremity and 18% to each side of the torso and each lower extremity.

Patients with burns exceeding 10% of total BSA should have an IV catheter placed for fluid administration. The estimation of the fluid requirements of burn patients should rely on assessing the patient's pulse, capillary refill, mental status, and urine output. Initially, the patient should receive lactated Ringer solution to maintain adequate tissue perfusion. Lactated Ringer solution most closely approximates the extracellular fluid lost through the skin. Therapy begins with administration of 5000 mL/m² per percentage of burn injury, plus maintenance, for the first 24 hours of replacement. One half of the required fluid is administered over the first 8 hours, and the remainder, over the following 16 hours.

After the first 24 hours of burn injury, capillary permeability returns to normal and sodium losses decrease. Therefore, patients are administered D5 one fourth normal saline or D5 one third normal saline with maintenance concentrations of potassium. In addition, serum protein previously lost may be replaced to restore normal plasma oncotic pressure. Children who are able may be allowed to drink hypotonic fluids (Table 10–36). Continued monitoring of serum electrolytes, acid–base status, and urine output cannot be overemphasized.

All persons coming into contact with a burn patient should wear sterile gloves and gowns. Procedures such as IV catheter placement and phlebotomy should be performed with sterile technique. An IV should be placed through an area of burn injury as a last resort. Routine use of parenteral antibiotics is not recommended. The initial

Table 10–35. Common Sequelae of Major Burns

Skin (see text)	Infectious
	Bacterial
Cardiovascular	Pseudomonas
Hypovolemia	Other gram-negative
Myocardial depression	organisms
Renal	Yeast
Acute tubular necrosis	*Candida* species
Acute renal failure	Viral
Hematologic	Nutritional/gastrointestinal
Neutropenia	Increased nutritional
Thrombocytopenia	requirements
Anemia	
Microangiopathic	
hemolytic anemia	
Acute erythrocyte hemolysis	

Table 10–36. Fluid Management of Burn Patients[1]

	Type of Fluid	Amount
First 24 h	Lactated Ringer solution	5000 mL/m² of burned BSA plus maintenance
Second 24 h	Maintenance fluid—dextrose 5% in 0.25% or 0.33% normal saline	3750 mL/m² of burned BSA + 1500 mL/m² of total BSA or to maintain adequate urine output
	Colloid (5% albumin in 0.9% NaCl)	0.5 mL/kg per % burned BSA

[1] Maintain urine output >1 mL/kg/h or 30–60 mL/h; assess tissue perfusion continuously.
BSA = body surface area.

wound management involves cleaning, debriding, and covering the wound with a topical antibiotic agent. If the patient needs to be transferred to another institution, the wound is covered only with sterile, dry gauze or sheets to facilitate reassessment of the wound by the receiving physicians. Because burn injuries are considered "dirty" wounds, tetanus prophylaxis should be considered for all burn patients.

A stepwise approach to burn wound management is presented in Table 10–37. Depending on the severity of the burn and the comfort of the parents, this can be accomplished on an inpatient or outpatient basis. The patient may require analgesia during the initial stage of burn wound healing, especially during dressing changes. Frequent reassessment of the wound is necessary, and systemic antibiotic therapy is indicated only if signs of infection are present. After epithelialization begins to occur, local wound care may be needed less frequently; however, close observation of the wound is still needed.

The decision of whether to admit a patient to the hospital for burn injury depends on many factors, ranging from the presence of associated injuries to the relative safety of the home environment (Table 10–38). If adequate outpatient management cannot be ensured, hospitalization is necessary. Children should also be admitted who require IV fluid resuscitation or who are at risk for infection or neurovascular compromise. Because of the potential for disfigurement or impaired function, children with significant facial or perineal injury are also admitted for care and observation. Transfer to a regional burn center should be considered for children with severe injury or for those who will require long-term management of their injuries.

ELECTRICAL & CHEMICAL BURNS

Two categories of burn injury requiring special consideration are electrical and chemical burns. Injuries from electrical burns are not always immediately recognizable. There may be deep tissue destruction despite the relatively benign appearance of the entry and exit lesions. Electricity tends to travel along blood vessels. Therefore,

Table 10–37. Burns: Wound Management

Procedure	Materials	Comments
Cleaning	Sterile saline + antibacterial soap	Avoid vigorous scrubbing
Debriding	Sterile scissors/forceps	Sterile technique Remove debris and charred epithelium Remove broken blisters
Rinsing	Sterile saline	Copious irrigation

Applying topical cream (lightly over burn area)	Silver sulfadiazine 0.5% (Silvadene)
	Polysporin on face
	Alternatives
	    Silver nitrate 0.5%
	    Mafenide acetate
		Poor penetration of infected burns

Dressing	Nonadherent gauze Loose bulky external gauze	

Table 10–38. Criteria for Hospital Admission of Patients With Burn Injuries

Absolute criteria
  Partial thickness burns >10% BSA, or full thickness
    burn >2% BSA
  Burn of entire hand or foot, or potential for vascular
    compromise of extremity
  Severe burns of face or perineum
  Inadequate patient compliance
  Major electrical burn
  Child abuse or neglect
Relative criteria
  Young age (<2 y)
  Burns crossing a major joint
  Electrical burn of mouth
  Underlying illness or concomitant injury
Consider transfer to a regional burn center
  Partial thickness burns >20% BSA
  Full thickness burns >5% BSA
  Major concomitant injury
  Systemic effects of electrical burn
  Involvement of respiratory tract
  Burn of extremity or chest with neurovascular or respiratory
    compromise

BSA = body surface area.

thrombosis of these blood vessels and injury to muscle, nerves, and bone can occur. This is particularly ominous when the cardiac muscle is involved. Assessment of these patients should include a thorough evaluation of capillary refill, distal sensory and motor neurologic function, and ECG (if there is a chance that the electrical current passed through the heart). Fluid requirements might be higher than originally assumed because of the aforementioned hidden injuries. One type of electrical burn injury that is unique to young children occurs in the corner of the mouth after the child chews through an electrical cord. In these cases, the usual treatment is "masterful observation." The necrotic facial tissue should be left alone until 2–4 weeks later. There is a chance of severe bleeding as the eschar begins to separate after 5–9 days, revealing the underlying labial artery. Parents can be warned about this possibility and should be instructed to apply direct pressure near the point of bleeding and then bring the child to an emergency department.

Chemical injuries in children usually involve household cleaners. Because alkali burns are more severe than acid burns, it is important to determine which agent caused the injury. After removal of all involved clothing, the treatment of these wounds includes copious irrigation with water or saline, generous fluid replacement, and application of a topical antibiotic agent.

SMOKE INHALATION

Inhalational injury is a significant contributor to the morbidity and mortality rates of fire-related injuries.

Diagnosis & Clinical Manifestations

A common result of the derangements caused by smoke inhalation is cellular hypoxia. Patients who are trapped in a closed space during a fire are at highest risk for immediate asphyxia and frequently do not survive the initial resuscitation efforts. Thermal injury due to inhalation of gases hotter than 500°C primarily causes damage to the larynx, supraglottic, and epiglottic regions; thermal injury to the lower airway is rarely seen after inhalation of dry gases, mostly because of the efficient cooling function of the respiratory mucosa, which can exponentially lower the heat of dry inspired gases. The resulting upper airway edema can cause early airway obstruction in these patients. In contrast, steam can cause significant damage to the lung parenchyma. Chemical injury to the lungs is due mostly to the inhalation of the toxic products of combustion, such as plastics, cotton, polyvinyl chloride, and polyurethane. These irritants can facilitate bronchoconstriction, increase mucosal edema, and impair mucociliary transport. In almost all survivors of severe smoke inhalation, bronchopneumonia develops after 2–3 days.

Some of the inhaled products of combustion, e.g., carbon monoxide and cyanide, can severely hinder oxygen transport and delivery.

CARBON MONOXIDE POISONING

Carbon monoxide contributes to cellular hypoxia in three ways: (1) preferential binding to hemoglobin, thereby leaving fewer sites for oxygen binding; (2) shifting the oxygen–hemoglobin dissociation curve to the left, thereby allowing hemoglobin to "hold on" to oxygen more tightly and decreasing the oxygen delivery to the tissues; and (3) binding to cytochrome oxidase, thereby poisoning the intracellular oxygen transport system.

Aside from the cellular anoxia caused by carbon monoxide poisoning, specific organ system damage may also occur. Pulmonary damage because of mucociliary dysfunction, bronchoconstriction, and pulmonary edema can result in severe respiratory distress. The CNS is affected most commonly by carbon monoxide toxicity. The most frequent neurologic findings in patients with carbon monoxide poisoning are memory loss and personality changes. Other early symptoms include slurred speech, dizziness, and headache. Neurologic symptoms, such as seizures, cerebral edema, and hearing or vision loss, may follow later. Cardiac effects, such as focal myocardial necrosis, leukocyte infiltration, and punctate hemorrhages, are manifested as ECG changes ranging from ST segment abnormalities to atrial fibrillation. The muscle, skin, and subcutaneous tissue are particularly susceptible to necrosis, which can lead to myoglobinuria and acute renal failure. Cutaneous findings of carbon monoxide poisoning include blistering, edema, and, infrequently, a "cherry-red" discoloration.

Carbon monoxide poisoning is quantified by measurement of the carboxyhemoglobin (COHb) level, with normal ranges of less than 5% for nonsmokers and less than 10% for smokers. Because of the short half-life of COHb in the presence of oxygen, the levels obtained in the emergency department do not reflect the level at the scene of the fire.

CYANIDE POISONING

The contribution of cyanide toxicity to the morbidity of smoke inhalation has been recently substantiated in the literature. Cyanide is inhaled as a product of the combustion of substances such as polyurethane. The half-life of cyanide is approximately 1 hour. Cyanide causes cellular anoxia by binding to the heme ion in the cytochrome complex A–a3, thereby shutting off the last step of oxidative metabolism. Cellular hypoxia results in CNS effects such as headaches, dizziness, seizures, coma, and death. Cardiac effects include tachycardia and hypertension, followed by bradycardia and hypotension. Determination of cyanide concentrations usually is not helpful in the acute care setting because of the length of time required for values to be returned. However, there is some evidence that serum lactate concentrations can estimate cyanide levels with some accuracy. Antidotes to cyanide toxicity are available and recommended as early adjuncts in the treatment of smoke inhalation.

Management

Before or upon the patient's arrival in the emergency department, certain historical points should be elicited. These include the duration and severity of smoke exposure (open vs. closed space), the types of burning material present, and the presence of unconsciousness at the scene. The physical examination should focus initially on the potential for airway compromise and the presence of respiratory symptoms. For patients exposed to smoke and fire, the initial threats to the airway are from laryngeal or supraglottic burns and edema and from failure to protect the airway from secretions. The indications for endotracheal intubation of these patients are listed in Table 10–39. In cases of unknown mechanism of injury, cervical spine stabilization should be maintained until properly evaluated. Although the presence of respiratory symptoms is a poor prognostic indicator, the absence of such symptoms does not eliminate the possibility of pulmonary injury. Initial assessment also should include the

Table 10–39. Smoke Inhalation: Indications for Endotracheal Intubation

Stridor or hoarseness
Upper airway edema
Profuse tracheal secretions
Severe burns of face, mouth, or nares
Coma
Absent gag reflex
Severe hypoxia or hypercarbia
Carboxyhemoglobin level >50%

extent and severity of burns on the body. The absence of cutaneous burns does not rule out significant inhalational injury.

Oxygen administration is the mainstay of therapy for smoke inhalation. The half-life of carbon monoxide is approximately 5 hours in room air, approximately 1 hour in 100% FiO_2, and less than 0.5 hour in 100% FiO_2 at two atmospheres of pressure (hyperbaric oxygen therapy). Hyperbaric oxygen requires a special hyperbaric chamber, and, despite its potential advantages, the patient must be stabilized before transfer for this type of treatment. In the emergency setting, the highest possible concentration of oxygen should be administered once adequate ventilation has been established. The patient's circulatory status should then be addressed, and symptoms of shock should be treated accordingly. If the patient does not exhibit signs of shock, an estimate of the extent and depth of burn injury helps in arriving at a plan for fluid management. Because of the potential for pulmonary edema, overhydration should be avoided if possible. A Foley catheter for measurement of urine output should be placed to aid in fluid management.

The assessment of neurologic dysfunction follows. As indicated in Table 10–39, the presence of coma or an absent gag reflex are indications for endotracheal intubation. Seizures should be treated expeditiously to prevent further respiratory compromise. PO_2 and COHb concentrations should be measured by arterial blood gas analysis, and a cyanide antidote administered, if available. A cyanide antidote is most helpful when administered early and may require repetitive dosing. The safest and most commonly used antidote is 25% sodium thiosulfate, which binds to cyanide to form an easily excretable sodium thiocyanate. Hyperbaric oxygen therapy should be considered.

Even patients who have not suffered severe sequelae initially from smoke inhalation must be observed carefully for evidence of late injury. Indications for admission of these patients are listed in Table 10–40.

Table 10–40. Indications for Admission of Smoke Inhalation Patients

Closed space exposure
Facial or mucosal burns
Loss of consciousness or change in mental status
Increased secretions or carbonaceous sputum
Abnormal arterial blood gases, chest radiograph, or electrocardiogram
Abnormal respiratory examination
Carboxyhemoglobin level >15%

REFERENCES

Cardiopulmonary Resuscitation in Infants & Children

Goetting MG: Progress in pediatric cardiopulmonary resuscitation. Emerg Med Clin North Am 1995;13:291.

Seidel J: Pediatric cardiopulmonary resuscitation: An update based on the new American Heart Association guidelines. Pediatr Emerg Care 1993;9:98.

Sirbaugh PE et al: A prospective, population-based study of demographics, epidemiology, management, and outcome of out-of-hospital pediatric cardiopulmonary arrest. Ann Emerg Med 1999;33:174.

Young KD, Seidel JS: Pediatric cardiopulmonary resuscitation: A collective review. Ann Emerg Med 1999;33:195.

Zaritsky A: Pediatric resuscitation pharmacology. Ann Emerg Med 1993;22:445.

Sudden Infant Death Syndrome

American Academy of Pediatrics Task Force on Infant Positioning and SIDS: Positioning and SIDS. Pediatrics 1992;89:1120.

Dwyer T et al: The contribution of changes in the prevalence of prone sleeping position to the decline in sudden infant death syndrome in Tasmania. JAMA 1995;273:783.

Klonoff-Cohen HS, Edelstein SL: A case-control study of routine and death scene sleep position and sudden infant death syndrome in southern California. JAMA 1995;273:790.

Perkin RM et al: Apparent life-threatening events: Recognition, differentiation, and management. Pediatr Emerg Med Rep 1998;3:99.

Spiers PS, Guntheroth WG: Recommendations to avoid the prone sleeping position and recent statistics for sudden infant death syndrome in the United States. Arch Pediatr Adolesc Med 1994;148:141.

Shock

Perkin RM, McConnell MS: Unusual causes of pediatric chock: Diagnostic and management pearls to improve patient outcomes. Pediatr Emerg Med Rep 1996;1:53.

Saez-LLorens X, McCracken GH: Sepsis syndrome and septic shock in pediatrics: Current concepts, terminology, pathophysiology, and management. J Pediatr 1993;123:497.

Tobias JD: Shock in children: The first 60 minutes. Pediatr Ann 1996;25:330.

Seizure Disorders

Berg AT et al: Predictors of recurrent febrileseizures: A prospective cohort study. Arch Pediatr Adolesc Med 1997;152:371.

Green SM et al: Can seizures be the sole manifestation of meningitis in children? Pediatrics 1993;92:527.

Mizrahi EM: Seizure disorders in children. Curr Opin Pediatr 1994; 6:642.

Working Group on Status Epilepticus: Treatment of convulsive status epilepticus. JAMA 1993;270:854.

Childhood Poisoning

Gaar GG: Gastrointestinal decontamination for acute poisoning by ingestion: Prevention of absorption of toxic compounds. J Fla Med Assoc 1994;81:747.

Henretig FM et al: Toxicologic emergencies. In: Fleisher G, Ludwig S (editors): *Textbook of Pediatric Emergency Medicine*, 3rd ed. Williams & Wilkins, 1993:745.

Kulig K: Initial management of ingestions of toxic substances. N Engl J Med 1992;326:1677.

Litovitz TL et al: 1998 Annual Report of the American Association of Poison Control Centers. A toxic exposure surveillance system. Am J Emerg Med 1999;17:435.

Lovejoy FH et al: Common etiologies and new approaches to management of poisoning in pediatric practice. Curr Opin Pediatr 1993;5:524.

Acetaminophen

Anker AL, Smilkstein MJ: Acetaminophen: Concepts and controversies. Emerg Med Clin North Am 1994;12:335.

Smilkstein MJ et al: Efficacy of oral N-acetylcysteine in the treatment of acetaminophen overdose. N Engl J Med 1988;319: 1557.

Tricyclic Antidepressants

Berkovitch M et al: Assessment of the terminal 40 millisecond QRS vector in children with a history of tricyclic antidepressant ingestion. Pediatr Emerg Care 1995;11:75.

Goodwin DA et al: Extracorporeal membrane oxygenation support for cardiac dysfunction from tricyclic antidepressant overdose. Crit Care Med 1993;21:625.

Haddad LM: Managing tricyclic antidepressant overdose. Am Fam Phys 1992;46:153.

Iron

Anderson AL: Iron poisoning in children. Curr Opin Pediatr 1994; 6:289.

Mills KC, Curry SC: Acute iron poisoning. Emerg Med Clin North Am 1994;12:397.

Tenenbein M, Rodgers GC: The four A's of decreasing the toll of childhood non-poisoning deaths. Arch Fam Med 1994; 3:754.

Ethanol

Bleich HL, Boro ES: Metabolic and hepatic effects of alcohol. N Engl J Med 1977;296:612.

Leung AKC: Ethyl alcohol ingestion in children, a 15-year review. Clin Pediatr 1986;25:617.

Olson KR, McGuigan MA: Childhood poisoning. In: Rudolph AM (editor): *Rudolph's Pediatrics,* 19th ed. Appleton & Lange, 1991:801.

Caustic Agents

Gorman RL et al: Initial symptoms as predictors of esophageal injury in alkaline corrosive ingestions. Am J Emerg Med 1992;10:189.

Howell JM et al: Steroids for the treatment of corrosive esophageal injury: A statistical analysis of past studies. Am J Emerg Med 1992;10:421.

Lahoti D, Broor SL: Corrosive injury to the upper gastrointestinal tract. Indian J Gastroenterol 1993;12:135.

Child Abuse

AAP Committee on Child Abuse and Neglect: Guidelines for the evaluation of sexual abuse of children: Subject review. Pediatrics 1999;103:186.

Jenny C et al: Analysis of missed cases of abusive head trauma. JAMA 1999;281:621.

Krugman SD et al: Facing facts: child abuse and pediatric practice. Contemp Pediatr 1998;15:131.

Leventhal JM et al: Fractures in young children: Distinguishing child abuse from unintentional injuries. Am J Dis Child 1993;147:87.

Schwartz AJ, Ricci LR: How accurately can bruises be aged in abused children? Literature review and synthesis. Pediatrics 1996;97:254.

The Injured Child

Schwarz DF: Violence. Pediatr Rev 1996;17:197.

Head Trauma

Goldstein B, Powers KS: Head trauma in children. Pediatr Rev 1994;15:213.

Near-Drowning

DeNicola LK et al: Submersion injuries in children and adults. Crit Care Clin 1997;13:477.

Weinstein MD, Krieger BP: Near drowning: epidemiology, pathophysiology, and initial treatment. J Emerg Med 1996;14:461.

Burns

Sheridan RL: The seriously burned child: Resuscitation through reintegration—1. Curr Prob Pediatr 1998;28:105.

Sheridan RL: The seriously burned child: Resuscitation through reintegration—2. Curr Prob Pediatr 1998;28:139.

Smoke Inhalation

Ruddy RM: Smoke inhalation injury. Pediatr Clin North Am 1994;41:317.

Skin

Judith V. Williams, MD, Sheila Fallon Friedlander, MD, & Lawrence F. Eichenfield, MD

■ CLINICAL EVALUATION OF THE SKIN

Skin-related disorders account for approximately 30% of all pediatric visits. The skin is the most accessible body organ and thus provides the first visible clues to many underlying infectious, metabolic, and neurologic disorders. Therefore, understanding the basic terminology and principles of dermatologic diagnosis is important for all pediatric practitioners. Although there are thousands of skin disorders, a much smaller number account for the vast majority of patient visits. This chapter presents the more common entities and reviews an approach to dermatologic diagnosis.

Principles of Diagnosis

Successful evaluation of the patient depends on obtaining an accurate history, performing an appropriate examination, collecting necessary laboratory data, and generating a differential diagnosis. When evaluating patients with skin disorders, it is often appropriate to perform a cursory examination of the skin lesion while simultaneously obtaining a focused history of present illness. Certain basic historical facts must always be elicited: location of the problem; duration of the lesion or rash; associated symptoms, such as itch or pain; and previous treatment. One also must inquire whether the patient has underlying illnesses or any allergies or takes any medications. With this information, one can perform a directed physical examination and then expand history-taking and examination as appropriate. Although focused histories and examinations are often adequate for diagnosis, a complete mucocutaneous examination is appropriate in most patients.

BASIC APPROACH

Evaluation begins with assessment of the characteristics of the individual lesions. The color is noted first, and then the morphology or shape of the lesion. Primary lesions may be macules (flat), papules or nodules (raised, palpable lesions), flat-topped plaques, edematous wheals, or blisters of varying size (vesicles and bullae; see definitions, Table 11–1). Identification of secondary changes is important for diagnosis. Often the primary lesions take on secondary or superimposed changes that can complicate or assist in diagnosis. Scaling or crusting may be late signs of dermatitis. Lichenification is a change secondary to chronic rubbing, and, with excoriations, reveals a pruritic skin disease, such as atopic dermatitis. Erosions, fissures, and ulcerations are skin disruptions of various depths. Table 11–2 lists the most commonly encountered secondary changes of skin lesions.

The examiner should next note the configurations, i.e., how the individual lesions are arranged. Skin lesions in a linear pattern may be from congenital anomalies (epidermal nevus) or skin diseases that localize in areas of trauma or scratching (Koebner phenomenon). Annular lesions may be caused by tinea infection (ringworm) or a variety of other noninfectious disorders (e.g., nummular eczema and granuloma annulare). Table 11–3 lists the most common configurations and examples of each. Identifying the distribution (Table 11–4) usually will limit the diagnostic possibilities. Does the rash involve the entire body or is it limited to the hands and feet? For instance, if a rash presents in a single dermatomal area, it is unlikely to be measles and most probably is herpes zoster.

Two other morphologic descriptions are commonly used to categorize a series of diseases: the papulosquamous and eczematous disorders. **Papulosquamous** (scaling papules) disease refers to the group that shares the common characteristics of discrete scaling papules, usually of an erythematous or violaceous color. **Eczema** refers to less well-defined papules or plaques that usually show some disruption of the epidermis, with oozing, fissuring, or scale crusting present. With time, eczematous lesions often become lichenified, or thickened, because of chronic rubbing.

Patient age, personal and family history, and knowledge of infectious diseases that might be prevalent in the community should be considered in arriving at a diagnosis. Careful clinical inspection of primary and secondary lesion morphology, configuration, and distribution, in addition to patient age and history, will help with diagnosis. The skin conditions presenting in infants and children are listed in Tables 11–5 and 11–6 on the basis of the description of the lesion.

PHYSICAL SIGNS & LABORATORY EVALUATION

Several physical signs and laboratory evaluations are of particular use in the diagnosis of skin disease. **Dermatographism** refers to a change that occurs when the

Table 11–1. Terminology: Primary Skin Lesions and Morphologic Patterns

Macule: Flat area of circumscribed color change; the lesion is not palpable
Patch: Nonspecific term generally referring to larger macules
Papule: Raised palpable lesion <0.5 cm
Nodule: Papule that has enlarged in all three dimensions: length, width, and depth
Plaque: Flat-topped lesion >0.5 cm in diameter horizontally but lacking significant depth of height
Wheal: Edematous or fluid-filled area of dermal edema without epidermal changes; classic lesion of urticaria
Vesicle: Blister containing clear fluid
Bulla: Vesicle >0.5 cm
Pustule: Vesicle containing milky or purulent fluid
Papulosquamous: Sharply marginated scaly violaceous papules or plaques
Eczematous: Inflammatory lesions with oozing, crusting, or thickening (lichenification)

Table 11–2. Terminology: Secondary Skin Changes

Erosion: Disruption of the skin lacking part or all of the epidermis, which is usually moist and red; lesions are sometimes covered by a crust
Ulcer: Lesion deeper than an erosion in which part or all of the dermis (as well as the epidermis) is missing
Fissure: Linear, wedge-shaped erosion or ulcer
Scale: Visible flake of stratum corneum on the skin surface
Crust: Yellowish, firm covering on the skin surface consisting of dried plasma or exudate
Excoriation: Scratch mark, usually linear or oval depression in the skin
Lichenification: Thickening of the epidermis due to chronic rubbing
Atrophy: Area of depressed or thin skin
Sclerosis: Firm, smooth induration or thickening of the skin

skin is stroked lightly with an item such as the blunt end of a pen. The normal response is mild erythema at the stroked site. In patients with underlying urticaria, a linear wheal also develops at the stroked site; this is referred to as **red dermatographism.** In some patients with atopic dermatitis, a white wheal develops and is therefore referred to as **white dermatographism.** Although these signs are not pathognomonic, they can provide supportive evidence of the appropriate diagnosis.

The **Darier sign** refers to the elicitation of a hive or blister when one repeatedly strokes a lesion of mastocytosis. This results from the release of histamine from an excess number of mast cells present at the site. The **Auspitz sign** occurs when the adherent scale from a lesion of psoriasis is picked off, revealing multiple pinpoint areas of bleeding. It represents trauma induced to the increased numbers of dilated vessels found in the dermal papillae

of a psoriatic lesion. The **Nikolsky sign** refers to the ability to spread or enlarge a blister by applying pressure over the center of the lesion. This occurs in diseases such as staphylococcal scalded skin syndrome and pemphigus.

Potassium hydroxide preparation (KOH). This is probably the single most useful laboratory examination in dermatology. It can be used when searching for dermatophytes; yeasts, such as *Candida* and tinea versicolor; and parasites, such as scabies. A superficial cutaneous scraping is performed to obtain as much scale as is reasonably possible. In the case of scabies, one should always scrape the areas of highest yield (burrows, hands, feet, and, in teenagers, genitalia). It is often necessary to draw a bit of blood at the site, and it is always necessary to sample more than one lesion. The scrapings should be placed on a slide, a few drops of potassium hydroxide 10% solution applied, and a coverslip placed over the specimen. It is often advisable to do this immediately after obtaining the specimen because scales may blow off the slide. One should firmly press the coverslip against the sample and

Table 11–3. Terminology: Configuration (Pattern of Arrangement of Lesion)

Name	Characteristics	Example
Linear	In a straight line	Linear epidermal nevus
Grouped	Clustered	Herpes simplex virus
Annular	Ring-like, oval with central clearing	Tinea corporis
Discrete	Having well-defined distinct borders	Guttate psoriasis
Confluent	Individual lesions that are ill-defined and tend to merge	Urticaria, measles
Target	Having a bull's-eye appearance; concentric rings	Erythema multiforme
Zosteriform	Grouped in a dermatomal pattern	Zoster
Polycyclic	Oval lesions with multiple ringlike coalescent borders	Tinea cruris
Serpiginous	Twisted, spiral, or snake-like	Erythema marginatum

Table 11–4. Terminology: Distribution (Area of the Body Surface Involved)

Name	Characteristics	Example
Generalized	Involving the entire body	Varicella, measles
Localized	Dermatomal, segmental, or limited to a specific area	Zoster
Acral	Favoring face, distal extremities, hands, feet	Erythema multiforme minor, Rocky Mountain spotted fever
Photodistribution	Light-exposed areas	Lupus, photosensitivity eruption
Intertriginous	Where skin rubs against skin (i.e., groin, axillae, inframammary)	Seborrheic dermatitis, candidal dermatitis

Table 11–5. Pediatric Cutaneous Disorders: Neonates

Generalized vesicopustules
Erythema toxicum
Miliaria rubra, crystallina, profunda
Staphylococcal impetigo
Bacterial sepsis
Congenital cutaneous candidiasis
Congenital HSV
Scabies
Transient neonatal pustular melanosis
Incontinentia pigmenti
Congenital syphilis
Acne
Acropustulosis of infancy

Bullae
Sucking blister
Epidermolysis bullosa
Bullous impetigo
Mastocytosis
Burns
Acrodermatitis enteropathica

Papules
Red
Erythema toxicum
Acne
Candidiasis
Insect bites
Epidermal nevus
Furuncles
Brown
Congenital nevi
Epidermal nevi
Mastocytoma
Yellow
Nevus sebaceous
Juvenile xanthogranuloma
Epidermal nevi
Flesh-colored or white
Milia
Molluscum

Papulosquamous lesions
Tinea
Ichthyosis
Neonatal lupus
Candidiasis
Epidermal nevi
Psoriasis

Flat lesions
White
Ash-leaf macules
Hypomelanosis of Ito
Piebaldism
Nevoid (anemicus, depigmentosus)
Brown
Mongolian spots
Café-au-lait spots
Freckles
Lentigo
Transient neonatal pustular melanosis
Linear and whorled hypermelanosis
Incontinentia pigmenti

Eczematous disorders
Diaper dermatitis
Seborrheic dermatitis
Atopic dermatitis
Scabies
Leiner disease
Acrodermatitis enteropathica
Severe combined immunodeficiency syndrome
Histocytosis X

Vascular lesions
Purpuric
Congenital infections: STORCH (syphilis, toxoplasmosis, rubella, cytomegalovirus, HSV)
Autoimmune disorders
Coagulation defects, disseminated intravascular coagulation
Vasculitis
Blanching
Nevus simplex ("angel's kiss," "stork bite")
Hemangioma
Port-wine stain
Cutis marmorata

HSV = herpes simplex virus.

Table 11–6. Pediatric Cutaneous Disorders: Infants and Children

Papulosquamous
Psoriasis
Lichen planus
Pityriasis rosea
Tinea
Lupus
Parapsoriasis, mycosis fungoides
Secondary syphilis
Keratosis pilaris
Pityriasis rubra pilaris
Pityriasis lichenoides
  (Mucha–Habermann diagnosis)

Eczematous
Atopic
Contact
Nummular
Scabies
Polymorphous light eruption
HIV
Dermatitis herpetiformis
Histocytosis X
Seborrheic dermatitis

Pustular
Folliculitis
Bacteremia
Acne rosacea
Pustular psoriasis
Deep fungal infections
Impetigo
Acropustulosis of infancy
Scabies
Bug bites

Vesicular
Impetigo
Contact dermatitis
Herpes simplex virus
Varicella zoster virus
Other viral infection (e.g., Coxsackievirus)
Panniculitis (lupus, others)
Burns
Arthropod bites
Erythema multiforme
Toxic epidermal necrolysis
Staphylococcal scalded skin syndrome
Polymorphous light eruption
Bullous fixed drug eruption
Linear IgA disease
Dyshidrotic eczema
Epidermolysis bullosa

Bullous
Contact dermatitis
Impetigo
Erythema multiforme
Arthropod/bug bites
Burns
Pemphigus
Pemphigoid

Vascular reactions
Telangiectasias
Hemangiomas
Purpura
Venous lake

Papules
Red
  Acne
  Viral exantherns
  Arthropod/bug bites
  Drug reactions
  Urticaria
  Erythema multiforme
  Furuncles
  Secondary syphilis
  Cherry angiomas
  Pyogenic granuloma
White/flesh-colored
  Milia
  Keratosis pilaris
  Molluscum contagiosum
  Verrucae
  Angiofibroma
  Granuloma annulare
  Sarcoidosis
  Epidermal nevus
  Basal cell carcinoma
Yellow
  Juvenile xanthogranuloma
  Urticaria pigmentosa
  Nevus sebaceous
  Xanthomas
  Nevus lipomatosis
  Necrobiosis lipoidica diabeticorum
Brown
  Nevi
  Urticaria pigmentosa
  Dermatofibroma
  Melanoma

Nodules
Red
  Furuncles
  Abscesses
  Erythema nodosum
White/flesh-colored
  Keloid
  Epidermal inclusion cyst
  Lipoma
  Pilomatricoma
  Corn
Brown
  Burns
  Dermatofibroma

Flat lesions
White
  Pityriasis alba
  Vitiligo
  Tinea versicolor
  Ash-leaf macule
  Lichen sclerosus et
    atrophicus
  Postinflammatory
    hypopigmentation
  Scleroderma
Brown
  Freckle
  Lentigines
  Nevi (junctional, other)
  Café-au-lait spot
  Postinflammatory
    hyperpigmentation
  Tinea versicolor
  Becker nevus
  Incontinentia pigmenti

then gently heat the specimen. The slide is then examined under the microscope at low to medium power with the light source damped. Focusing up and down in the plane of the specimen is helpful because the walls of dermatophytes appear birefringent. Dermatophytes appear as septate hyphae, whereas yeasts appear as budding spores with short nonseptate hyphae. Scabies eggs and feces (scybala) are seen more often than the mite itself.

Skin biopsy. A skin biopsy specimen is particularly useful to identify inflammatory lesions and possible neoplasias. The involved area is carefully cleaned and anesthetized. An appropriate-sized incision or punch is made and the tissue gently removed, taking care never to squeeze the sample. The wound edges are then brought together and closed with suture material. In this manner, material can be obtained for routine histology (hematoxylin and eosin stain), immunofluorescence microscopy, or electron microscopy.

■ SKIN DISEASES OF THE NEONATE

Neonates possess distinct characteristics that must be considered when evaluating and treating dermatologic diseases. In addition, some disorders occur only or more commonly in the neonatal period. The newborn infant has less well-developed adnexal structures, no protective endogenous flora, and an increased susceptibility to external irritants. Of importance is the increased relative absorption of any topical agents. Neonates also differ in their ability to bind, metabolize, and excrete drugs.

Physiologic & Transient Changes

Newborns are subjected to a number of conditions that can lead to drying and damage. Skin irritation and subsequent breakdown can result from frequent manipulation, application of adhesive tapes and monitors, and exposure to phototherapy. Small breaks in the skin can then serve as portals of entry for bacteria or other organisms. Application of moisturizers can rehydrate the skin and may help decrease the incidence of skin-related infections in premature infants.

A number of "normal" changes occur in the first weeks of life. The most common are discussed briefly below. The following discussion reviews these disorders and other serious conditions with which they can be confused.

VASCULAR CHANGES

Acrocyanosis. A purplish-blue discoloration of the lips, hands, and feet is quite common in newborn infants. This is most noticeable during periods of chilling or crying and does not indicate any underlying pathology.

Cutis marmorata. A bluish-purple mottling of the trunk and extremities, which is reticulated, often occurs when newborns are chilled. It probably results from vasodilation of peripheral small vessels. This condition usually resolves after 2–3 weeks and usually is not serious. Persistence of this condition may occasionally be associated with an underlying condition, such as Cornelia de Lange, Down syndrome, or trisomy 18.

Cutis marmorata telangiectatica congenita. This consists of a persistent bluish mottling that extends during the first few weeks of life and is present on the trunk, extremities, and, occasionally, the face. Atrophy and ulcerations can occur; these tend to improve or resolve with time. This disorder has been associated with other vascular abnormalities, glaucoma, and a variety of other congenital abnormalities, such as cleft lip, syndactyly of the toes, and mental retardation.

Salmon patches. These vascular stains frequently are noted at birth and commonly occur on the nape of the neck, glabella, and eyelids. In contrast to port-wine stains, these lesions are usually centrally located and fade with time.

Port-wine stains. These stains are red, flat, and often unilateral (Figure 11–1). They may be more responsive to therapy early in life; if left untreated, they persist and deepen in color over time. If located on the face, the current therapy of choice is the pulsed dye laser, which is usually initiated in early infancy. The possibility of Sturge–Weber syndrome must be considered if such facial vascular stains involve the area of distribution of the trigeminal nerve. This disorder can include cerebral angiomatosis, seizures, and glaucoma, all of which should be considered when a port-wine stain occurs in the distribution of the first branch of the trigeminal nerve. Only a minority of children with port-wine stains in this area will actually have Sturge–Weber syndrome. All children with suspicious facial lesions must be evaluated for glaucoma because early treatment is crucial for this ophthalmologic complication (Table 11–7).

Hemangiomas. These vascular lesions develop within the first 2–4 weeks of life. They initially appear as flat red patches and subsequently darken and thicken over time. Occasionally they are surrounded by an area of pallor (see section on proliferative vascular lesions).

BENIGN PAPULAR LESIONS

Milia. These small (1–2 mm), discrete, smooth, white papules most frequently are located on the face. They represent small inclusion cysts and require no therapy. They usually resolve within the first few months of life. Persistent or extensive involvement raises the possibility of an underlying disorder, such as oral-facial-digital syndrome.

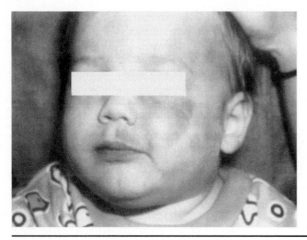

Figure 11–1. Port-wine stain.

Sebaceous gland hyperplasia. This condition presents as multiple, small, yellow papules on the nose, cheeks, and upper lip. It may be related to prenatal maternal hormonal stimulation and resolves spontaneously within the first months of life.

Infantile acne. Little is understood regarding the pathophysiology of "baby acne." It is thought to be the result of maternal hormonal stimulation of infantile sebaceous glands. Neonatal acne usually appears at 2–4 weeks of age and resolves by 6–8 months. Reassurance is the best therapy; in severe cases, however, a weak keratolytic agent, such as 2.5% benzoyl peroxide, may be used. Some believe that this eruption is caused by the commensal yeast *Pityrosporum,* and response to topical antifungals has been reported. Infantile acne is a more severe eruption that presents later (3–4 months of age) and may persist until

2–3 years of age. In this condition, other topical agents, such as topical or systemic antibiotics and topical retinoids, may be used if the severity warrants such therapy.

Subcutaneous fat necrosis. The etiology of these lesions is unknown but may relate to trauma in the neonatal period. Such lesions most often present as well-defined, firm, subcutaneous nodules on exposed surfaces and bony prominences. These lesions usually resolve spontaneously. Extensive calcification of the lesions can occur with liquification, spontaneous drainage, and, occasionally, scarring. Incision and drainage of persistent nodules are recommended. Hypercalcemia is a rare complication; therefore, evaluation of calcium levels is recommended, particularly in extensive cases.

Iatrogenic Lesions

Neonatal skin lesions can result from procedures performed ante- or postpartum.

Amniocentesis puncture marks. Approximately 1% of fetuses undergoing the procedure will have such lesions, which present as pits or depressions. They can occur anywhere, and multiple lesions may be apparent. Digital reductions or losses can occur after chorionic villus sampling undertaken before 10 weeks gestation.

Fetal scalp monitor trauma. Erythema, bleeding, abscesses, and hair loss can occur at the site of fetal scalp monitor placement. Application of a topical antibiotic may help prevent the development of some of these complications.

Noninvasive monitor lesions. Transcutaneous oxygen monitors and pulse oximeters can cause erythema and even blistering burns with necrosis at the site of placement. Careful observation and frequent rotation of the monitored site are important to avoid such complications.

Calcinosis cutis. These irregular, rock-hard subcutaneous nodules can present at any site of prior trauma but

Table 11–7. Differences in Port-wine Stains and Hemangiomas

Port-wine Stains	Hemangiomas
Present at birth	Usually first 2 months of life
Relatively rare (0.1–0.3%)	Common (10% of children)
Macular (flat)	Palpable
Growth proportionate with child	Rapid growth phase (1–6 mo)
	Plateau phase (6 to 12–18 mo)
No involution: hypertrophy, nodules in adulthood	Natural involution (30%, 3 y; 50%, 5 y; 80–90%, 9 y)
Pathology: dilated dermal capillaries; nonproliferative	Pathology: proliferating angioblastic endothelial cells
Treatment: laser ablation (pulsed-dye vascular laser)	Treatment: generally allow natural involution

are noted most frequently at the sites of prior heel sticks. The calcium in these lesions usually migrates to the skin surface and extrudes over time.

Vesicopustular or Bullous/Erosive Lesions

This category is extensive and best divided on the basis of benign, infectious, or mechanobullous disorders.

BENIGN VESICOPUSTULAR LESIONS

These lesions constitute the vast majority of vesicopustular neonatal skin lesions encountered (Table 11–8).

Erythema toxicum neonatorum. This condition presents within the first 2 weeks of life. During the first few days of life, a blotchy macular red eruption is noted; in time, papular or papulopustular centers appear in the eruption. The disorder requires no therapy. Palms and soles are usually spared. This condition occasionally is confused with more serious pustular disorders, such as congenital candidiasis or bacterial lesions; in such cases, evaluation of a pustule with Gram stain, KOH, or Wright or Giemsa stain will help differentiate among these disorders. A smear of erythema toxicum will show numerous eosinophils.

Transient neonatal pustular melanosis. This benign condition consists of very small and superficial vesicles present at birth or shortly thereafter. It is more common in African-Americans. Lesions rupture quite easily, leaving a collarette of scale. Hyperpigmented macules often develop at these sites. Occasionally only hyperpigmented macules will be noted at the time of birth. The lesions resolve spontaneously. The main difficulty with this disorder is in distinguishing it from more serious vesicopustular disorders. Evaluation of a smear will show a predominance of neutrophils without organisms.

Table 11–8. Differential Diagnosis: Vesicopustules in the Neonate

Type	Findings	Laboratory Tests
Infectious		
Herpes simplex virus	Blisters and erosions, often of the head	+ Tzanck stain + Wright stain } Multinucleate giant cells + Viral culture
Candidal (congenital = present at birth)	Morbilliform papulovesicles Pustules (often generalized, often involve palms and soles)	+ KOH + Gram stain } Pseudohyphae + Culture
Bacterial (e.g., staphylococcal, streptococcal, *Escherichia coli*)	Vesicles, pustules	+ Gram stain + Culture
Syphilis	Erosions, hemorrhagic bullae, mucous patches, petechiae, pustules, erosions	+ Serology + Darkfield examination: spirochetes
Scabies	Papules, nodules, acral and periumbilical predilection	+ Scabies preparation (mineral oil or KOH): mites, eggs, or scybala
Transient		
Erythema toxicum	Erythematous, blotchy macules ± central pustular component	+ Wright stain + Gram stain } Perifollicular eosinophils
Incontinentia pigmenti	Streaky, linear, clustered aggregates, ± verrucous or linear pigmentary changes	+ Wright and Gram stain for eosinophils + Eosinophilic pustules on biopsy specimen
Transient neonatal pustular melanosis	Pustules, vesicles, hyperpigmented macules with collarette of scale	+ Wright stain + Gram stain } PMNs
Miliaria	Nonfollicular papules and papulopustules	– Culture and Gram stain (usually no organisms, few cells)
Acropustulosis of infancy	Pruritic papules and vesicopustules favor acral sites	+ Gram stain for PMNs
Epidermolysis bullosa	Generalized blisters, bullae, erosions	+ Nikolsky sign – Gram stain

KOH = potassium hydroxide preparation; PMN = polymorphonuclear leukocytes.

Miliaria. "Prickly heat" is the result of destruction of the eccrine sweat ducts. The rash of this disorder can be vesicular, papular, or nodular, depending on the depth of involvement of the affected eccrine sweat ducts. The lesions are often small erythematous papules or vesicles present on the trunk. Treatment consists of decreasing sweating and relieving obstruction by airing out the skin and avoiding overheating in affected children. Cool baths are often useful therapeutic interventions.

Sucking blisters. These result from vigorous sucking of the affected site in utero. They are most common on the fingers, forearms, or wrists. The lesions may be vesicles, bullae, or erosions at the time of birth and usually resolve without need for treatment.

INFECTIOUS CAUSES OF NEONATAL VESICOPUSTULES

The list of possible infections in the newborn period is extensive and includes bacterial pathogens such as *Listeria, Staphylococcus aureus,* and *Streptococcus.* Viral infections, including herpes simplex and varicella, are possible pathogens, as are fungal etiologies, including *Candida.* As most of these conditions are addressed extensively elsewhere, we limit our discussion to candidiasis.

Congenital candidiasis. This infection is contracted in utero, and lesions may be present at birth. Small erythematous papules or papulopustules may be present on the trunk, extremities, palms, and soles. Microscopic examination of a skin scraping of a pustule will show budding yeast and pseudohyphae. In full-term healthy children, the infection usually poses no risk, and treatment involves local topical antifungal therapy or no intervention at all. In debilitated or premature infants, however, systemic antifungal therapy is usually recommended because severe systemic illness may result from congenital infection.

MECHANOBULLOUS DISORDERS

Epidermolysis bullosa. This disorder consists of a number of inherited disorders of the skin that result from defective structures in the epidermis or dermis. The skin's normal barrier function is compromised; therefore, friction or trauma to the skin leads to "lifting" of the epidermis from the underlying dermis. The level of separation depends on the type of epidermolysis bullosa present and the site of the defective structure (keratinocyte, hemidesmosome, or anchoring fibril). Blisters and erosions develop at the sites of trauma. Severely affected patients also may have nail, mucous membrane, and gastrointestinal complications. Newborns with erosions or blisters suspicious for epidermolysis bullosa should first be examined for the possibility of an infectious etiology for their blisters. A dermatology consultation should be procured so that biopsy specimens (which should include electron micrographic evaluation) can be obtained. In addition, these children require careful handling of the skin, sur-

veillance for infectious complications, and monitoring of fluid and electrolyte status.

OTHER BLISTERING DISORDERS IN THE NEONATAL PERIOD

Mastocytosis. This disorder of mast cells can present in the neonatal period with solitary lesions or a diffuse blistering eruption. Mast cells possess histamine and, when traumatized, release this cytokine with subsequent erythema, vasodilation, and edema. Severe reactions consist of blisters and erosions. When blistering and erosion are prominent, the disorder may be mistaken for an infectious process. Isolated lesions of mastocytosis may be flesh-colored, tan, pink, or hyperpigmented. They almost always possess the ability to swell or blister when stroked or rubbed vigorously (the Darier sign). Wheezing and gastrointestinal symptoms may result if enough histamine is released from such lesions. (For additional information, see section on raised [papular] pigmented lesions.)

Aplasia cutis congenita. This condition can appear as an oval or angular scar on the vertex of the scalp. It is a congenital defect in the epidermis and dermis and occasionally also involves the subcutis. It is commonly seen on or near the midline. The appearance of the lesions, which may be multiple, is variable. At times, the surface may look eroded and red; at other times, a thin blister or bulla will be present over the lesion. This condition usually will heal without complication, although alopecia commonly results at the involved site. Rarely, the defect may occur over the sagittal sinus and be complicated by bleeding and infection. A hydrocolloid dressing may be used when erosion is a major problem. These dressings expedite wound healing.

Papulosquamous Disorders in the Neonatal Period

Papulosquamous disorders (scaling red rashes) in the neonatal period are common and usually do not signify severe pathology. Occasionally, however, a scaling papular disorder in the neonatal period is a marker for severe systemic illness or a chronic cutaneous condition.

BENIGN PAPULOSQUAMOUS DISORDER

Seborrheic dermatitis. This greasy, red, scaly eruption is the most common scaling disorder of infancy. It presents shortly after birth and involves the scalp (cradle cap), postauricular areas, and groin. It can be confused with diaper dermatitis when it affects the groin area. Other sites of involvement include the intertriginous areas (neck, axillary, groin, and leg creases).

Well-circumscribed, discrete, and confluent erythematous patches with superimposed greasy or dry scale are the hallmark of seborrheic dermatitis. The rash can be bright red and, if severe enough, may ooze or become eroded. Adherent yellow scales may be present on the scalp, brows, and face. The condition usually resolves by 3–6 months of age.

Treatment consists of weak topical corticosteroids, if necessary. Hydrocortisone lotion 1% or 2.5% to the scalp twice a day for a short period is helpful, as is the use of a steroid cream, such as hydrocortisone, to the involved body surfaces twice a day. Secondary candidal infection is common. Simultaneous use of an antifungal agent, such as nystatin or clotrimazole cream, may help prevent this secondary fungal infection.

The scalp frequently responds to shampoos such as zinc pyrithione or selenium sulfide. The use of mineral oil to soften the scales before shampooing often will expedite removal of the scale and hasten response to therapy.

Children with severe findings should be evaluated for evidence of failure to thrive and gastrointestinal symptoms such as diarrhea. Hepatosplenomegaly and lymphadenopathy also should be ruled out. Such findings raise the possibility of more serious papulosquamous erythemas (caused by systemic diseases such as Leiner disease, Langerhans cell histiocytosis, and immunologic and nutritional deficiencies), which are discussed below.

Psoriasis. This disorder occasionally can present in the neonatal period and may lead to a diffuse erythrodermic condition. Family history, chronicity, and severity of the condition raise the suspicion of psoriasis. Treatment is similar to that for seborrheic dermatitis; however, stronger topical corticosteroids and other agents, such as tars and topical calcipotriene, may be required. The frequent use of emollients and avoidance of drying and irritation are crucial in patients with psoriasis. Patients may become secondarily infected with bacterial pathogens as a result of scratching, and antibiotic therapy will then be required.

Atopic dermatitis (eczema). Eczema does not usually present until 4–6 weeks of life. Discrimination between this disorder and seborrheic dermatitis in the first few months of life may be difficult; however, atopic dermatitis tends to be less well defined, with finer white scales. Atopic dermatitis more commonly involves the cheeks, trunk, and flexor surfaces, whereas seborrheic dermatitis favors the scalp and creases. Irritants and drying should be avoided. Moisturizers and weak topical corticosteroids are the mainstay of therapy. (This topic is covered in greater detail in the section on eczematous disorders.)

Ichthyotic disorders. Ichthyotic refers to fish-like scale and usually is used to describe four major categories of abnormal generalized scaling that can present at birth. Table 11–9 further describes these diseases.

More Serious Causes of Red, Scaly Eruptions in the Neonate

Red, scaling rashes in childhood occasionally signal a serious underlying illness.

Table 11–9. Ichthyoses

Type	Inheritance	Characteristics	Defect
Ichthyosis vulgaris	AD 1:250	Fine white scales on legs, face, back, extensor surfaces—flexural sparing, increased palmoplantar skin markings, keratosis pilaris, xerosis and atopy	Filaggrin or profilaggrin defect
X-Linked ichthyosis	X-Linked recessive 1:6000 male	Collodion membrane at birth; scales are dark and large, generalized; palms and soles spared; + corneal opacities	Steroid sulfatase deficiency
Lamellar ichthyosis	AR 1:300,000	Collodion membrane or erythema at birth, then thick, large, dark plate-like brown scales, then plaques. Nails absent; thick palms and soles; accentuated markings; severe ectropion and eclabion	Transglutaminase-I defect
NBCIE (nonbullous congenital ichthyosiform erythroderma)	AR < 1:100,000	Often collodion membrane at birth; persistent erythroderma, finer, whiter scales, also nail and palmar changes; less severe eye involvement	Probable increased n-alkanes; increased epidermal turnover
Epidermolytic hyperkeratosis (bullous congenital ichthyosiform erythroderma)	AD 1:300,000	Early childhood: Recurrent episodes of bullae formation; generalized erythroderma followed by large, thick, dark scales, often verrucous malodorous flexural involvement	Mutations of keratin 1 and 10 genes

AD = autosomal dominant; AR = autosomal recessive.

Immunologic disorders

Human immunodeficiency virus (HIV) infections (acquired immunodeficiency syndrome). Infants with HIV often have thrush and severe diaper rash. Severe generalized seborrheic dermatitis or recurrent bacterial skin infections also should raise a suspicion for HIV.

Any child with severe seborrheic, atopic, or diaper dermatitis should be evaluated for the presence of oral thrush, lymphadenopathy, and hepatosplenomegaly. Failure to thrive also should be ruled out. If indicated by history and clinical findings, appropriate laboratory evaluation should be performed to rule out HIV infection.

Severe combined immunodeficiency and Leiner disease. A number of immunodeficiency disorders can present with red scaling skin. Patients with severe combined immunodeficiency disorder often have recurrent infections and failure to thrive. Leiner disease was once thought to be a specific disorder of complement function that led to a severe generalized rash, infections, and diarrhea. It is no longer clear whether this is a specific disorder. Any infant with such symptoms should be examined for an underlying immunologic abnormality.

Graft-versus-host (GVH) disease. Maternal lymphocytes occasionally will engraft in neonates, leading to a GVH reaction. A scaling red rash, hepatosplenomegaly, and diarrhea can result. This can also occur if neonates receive transfusions of blood products that have not been irradiated.

Ommen disease. This is another neonatal immunodeficiency disorder that can present with a red, scaly rash and hepatosplenomegaly. The patient also may have alopecia and massive lymphadenopathy. In GVH and Ommen disease, skin biopsy specimens can help make the diagnosis as satellite cell necrosis within the epidermis will be present.

Metabolic deficiencies. These disorders often present with scaling red rashes and failure to thrive. Zinc deficiency causes a red and sometimes eroded rash that commonly occurs in the perioral, diaper, and acral areas. Diarrhea and failure to thrive also are common in this condition. Rarely, cystic fibrosis may have as its first obvious manifestation a red, scaly rash secondary to zinc malabsorption. Essential fatty acid, biotin, and multiple carboxylase deficiencies also can present in a similar fashion, although the erythema and scaling are usually more diffuse in these conditions.

Histiocytosis X (Langerhans cell histiocytosis). This histiocytic malignancy can present in infancy with a seborrheic dermatitis–like picture. The presence of infiltrated brown-yellow papules within the rash, purpuric lesions, and systemic findings of lymphadenopathy and hepatosplenomegaly point toward this diagnosis. A biopsy specimen must be obtained if this neoplastic disorder is suspected.

Diaper Dermatitis

The most common dermatologic condition occurring in infancy is diaper rash. This general category includes a number of distinct types of eruptions caused by a variety of agents.

Irritant contact dermatitis. If skin is directly irritated by an agent such as stool or urine, an irritant reaction will develop. This does not require an immunologic response. The occlusion offered by diapers and the humid environment provided by sweat and urine, combined with friction, lead to maceration and breakdown of the skin. This is the most common cause of diaper dermatitis.

Allergic contact dermatitis. This involves an allergic reaction to a contactant and can occur when a patient is exposed to cleansing wipes, perfumed talc, or an agent in the diapers. Occasionally, a medication being applied is the culprit.

Candidiasis. Yeast are found as normal residents in the oral cavity and stool and are not always pathogens. When skin is damaged, however, the yeast can become invasive and lead to the development of papular, erythematous, and, sometimes, erosive rashes.

It is usually fairly easy to distinguish between contact and candidal dermatitis. Contact rashes more commonly involve convex surfaces or areas rubbing against the diaper. The creases often will be spared. Candidiasis, in contrast, will involve the creases and scrotum and often manifests satellite papules and pustules; a beefy red appearance is not uncommon.

Initial therapy consists of frequent diaper changes, gentle cleansing with plain water or a mild soap, exposure to air of the affected area when possible, and application of zinc oxide or other protective agents after diaper changes. Cleansing wipes should be avoided because a contact dermatitis to their components may develop.

Severe cases may benefit from mild topical corticosteroids, such as hydrocortisone cream and topical antifungal agents. Potent steroid–antifungal combination agents are not recommended because they may lead to atrophy, striae, and telangiectases. The use of Mycostatin drops four times a day orally will help decrease the concentration of candidal infection in the gastrointestinal tract and may expedite improvement. Occasionally, the mother may need treatment of candidal infection of the nipples or genital tract, which may be contributing to the infant's disorder. Rarely, the infection may be severe enough to necessitate the use of a systemic fungal agent, such as fluconazole. This is reserved only for refractory cases.

Secondary infection with *Streptococcus* or *S. aureus* may occur in the affected areas. Group A β-hemolytic streptococcus can cause a severe red erosive condition, particularly in the intertriginous areas. Culture and systemic antibiotic therapy should be carried out in such cases.

Table 11–10. Differential Diagnosis of Diaper Dermatitis

Candidiasis
Irritant contact dermatitis
Seborrheic dermatitis
Atopic dermatitis
Allergic contact dermatitis
Bullous impetigo, streptococcal infection
Psoriasis
Histiocytosis X
Zinc deficiency
Scabies
Granuloma gluteale infantum
Tinea corporis
Essential fatty acid and biotin deficiency
Severe combined immunodeficiency
Graft-versus-host disease

The possibility of another diagnosis must be considered if a diaper rash does not improve despite appropriate therapy in a compliant family. Metabolic, infectious, and immunodeficiency disorders are major categories that must be ruled out in such cases (Table 11–10).

■ VASCULAR LESIONS

Vascular lesions are composed of blood vessels, including capillaries, veins, arteries, and/or lymphatics. Vascular lesions are usually red or blue; deeper lesions may be skin colored. These lesions are quite common, ranging from innocuous lesions, such as "stork bites," to those of significant medical consequence. A useful categorization is based on whether lesions are nonproliferative malformations or proliferative tumors.

Vascular Malformations (Nonproliferative)

Most nonproliferative vascular malformations are salmon patches (nevus simplex) or port-wine stains (nevus flammeus). These are described in the previous section, Skin Diseases of the Neonate.

Klippel–Trenaunay syndrome. This disorder is the association of a port-wine stain with hypertrophy of underlying soft tissue or bone. It usually occurs on an extremity or portion of the trunk and may have associated varicosities or phlebectasias. Lymphangiomatous components also may be present. Leg-length discrepancy may be functionally significant in lower-extremity lesions.

LYMPHANGIOMAS

Lymphangiomas are malformations of lymphatic origin; 70–90% are present at birth or develop within the first 2 years. Lesions may be flesh-colored dermal or subcutaneous tumors or thick-walled vesicles with a "frogspawn" appearance. Lesions may have a hemangiomatous component or deep cavernous component with large cystic areas of lymphatic tissue. There is no spontaneous regression. Surgical excision is difficult because multiple channels are often present, leading to difficulty with complete excision and a high recurrence rate.

Proliferative Vascular Lesions

HEMANGIOMAS

Hemangiomas, also known as "strawberry marks," are benign proliferative tumors of capillaries seen in 10% of infants (Figure 11–2). They may be present at birth but more commonly appear in the first few weeks. Classically, hemangiomas appear as raised, bright red, lobulated tumors with well-defined borders and prominent capillaries. Hemangiomas located superficially in the dermis have a "strawberry" appearance, whereas lesions deeper in the dermis may be skin-colored or bluish with indistinct borders. Lesions undergo a rapid growth phase in the first 6 months after birth, plateau usually from 6 to 12 months, and begin to involute between 12 and 18 months. Spontaneous regression usually occurs over several years. After year 3, approximately 10% of lesions

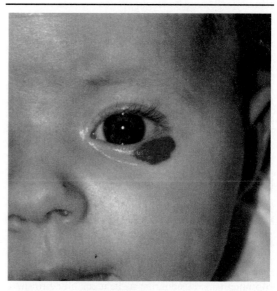

Figure 11–2. Hemangiomas.

clear per year (30% at 3 years, 50% at 5 years, 80% at 8 years).

Complications from hemangiomas are uncommon. They include ulceration and cutaneous infection, bleeding, functional organ compromise (e.g., periocular lesions), and high-output congestive heart failure from arteriovenous shunting. Platelet trapping and consumptive coagulopathy (Kasabach–Merritt syndrome), once thought to be complications of cavernous hemangiomas, are seen in hemangioma-like variants such as spindle cell hemangiomas and kaposiform hemangioendotheliomas. Owing to a low rate of complications and natural involution of most hemangiomas, conservative observation is the most reasonable plan of management. Therapy is appropriate for lesions that compromise function, such as vision, or cause airway obstruction or other complications. Oral or intralesional corticosteroids, α-interferon 2a or 2b, embolization, pulsed-dye laser therapy, or surgical excision may be used to treat these problematic hemangiomas.

PYOGENIC GRANULOMAS

Pyogenic granulomas are vascular, red, pedunculated papules and nodules that may appear anywhere on the skin or mucous membranes. Lesions most commonly occur on the head and neck. They usually occur in childhood rather than in infancy, with sudden onset and rapid growth over a period of several weeks. The surface of pyogenic granulomas is friable, causing bleeding with minimal trauma. Children often present with a "Band-Aid sign" from application of multiple adhesive bandages to stop hemorrhage. Despite the label "pyogenic," lesions are not thought to have an infectious origin and may be post-traumatic. Although benign, pyogenic granulomas usually persist, unlike capillary hemangiomas. Treatment consists of curettage, electrodesiccation, pulsed-dye laser, or full-thickness excision.

ADENOMA SEBACEUM (ANGIOFIBROMAS)

Adenoma sebaceum is a term used to describe multiple red-brown papules commonly seen on the central face or cheeks in patients with tuberous sclerosis. These lesions are angiofibromas and histologically show an increased number of fibroblasts and capillaries in the dermis. Lesions may begin in early childhood and are commonly misdiagnosed as "early acne." Isolated angiofibromas are benign growths of no medical significance.

■ FLAT PIGMENTED LESIONS & OTHER CUTANEOUS TUMORS

Most pigmented lesions that are light tan, blue-brown, or deep brown contain melanin. Increased concentrations of melanin may occur in the epidermis, as in freckles and lentigines; nests of melanocytes may be present in the epidermis or dermis, as in melanocytic nevi and melanoma; and melanin and/or melanocytes may be present deep in dermis, as in mongolian spots and nevus of Ota or Ito (Table 11–11).

CAFÉ-AU-LAIT SPOTS

Café-au-lait spots are even-colored, tan to brown, flat, pigmented lesions seen in 10–20% of children (Figure 11–3). Lesions may be present anywhere on the body and range in size from a few millimeters to larger than 20 cm. Lesions may be present at birth and may increase in size and number with age. Although most individuals with café-au-lait spots are healthy, multiple lesions may be seen with neurofibromatosis type 1 (NF-1) and other neurocutaneous disorders. The presence of six or more café-au-lait spots larger than 1.5 cm in adolescents or adults or 0.5 cm in prepubertal children raises a high degree of suspicion for NF-1. Multiple small (1–4 mm) café-au-lait spots in the axillary and inguinal area, termed "freckling," also may be a sign of NF-1 in children. Café-au-lait spots may also be seen with other syndromes including NF-2, polyostotic fibrous dysplasia (McCune–Albright syndrome), Watson's syndrome, and in patients with ring chromosome syndromes. Café-au-lait spots themselves are benign, and treatment is unneces-

Table 11–11. Differential Diagnosis of Flat Pigmented Lesions

Lesion	Clinical Appearance
Mongolian spots	Blue-gray macules; commonly lumbosacral area
Café-au-lait spots	Even-colored tan-brown macules with normal skin markings; multiple lesions seen in neurofibromatosis and other phakomatoses
Freckles/lentigines	Small light-tan to brown macules on sun-exposed skin
Nevus spilus	Circumscribed tan macule with darkly pigmented flat or raised spots; color is generally lighter than congenital nevi
Becker nevus	Gray-brown hyperpigmented area with hypertrichosis, commonly unilateral on shoulder, anterior chest, scapula; usually appears during early adolescence or adulthood
Nevus of Ota	Blue-gray macule of the face surrounding the eye, often involving sclerae and conjunctivae
Nevus of Ito	Blue-gray macule of the shoulder, clavicular area

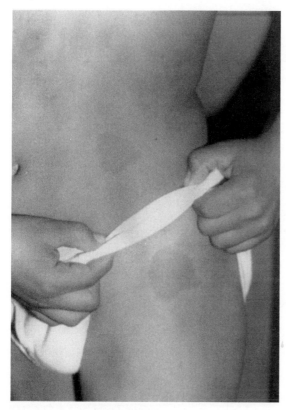

Figure 11–3. Café-au-lait spots.

sary. For lesions of cosmetic importance, laser therapy is effective.

MONGOLIAN SPOTS (DERMAL MELANOCYTOSIS OF INFANCY)

Mongolian spots are blue-gray, flat, macular lesions usually located on the lumbosacral area, buttocks, and, occasionally, limbs or trunk of normal infants. Lesions are present at birth and usually fade by late childhood. The lesions are composed of melanocytes in the dermis, and are presumed to be the result of embryonal failure of melanocytes to migrate from the neural crest to the epidermis. Occasionally, they may be mistaken for bruising associated with child abuse.

FRECKLES & LENTIGINES

"Freckles" **(ephelides)** are small (usually 2–4 mm), light tan to brown pigmented lesions that appear on sun-exposed skin. They are more common in early childhood, change seasonally with sun exposure, and usually fade during winter months. They are seen more commonly in children who have fair skin and red hair. Although lesions themselves are of cosmetic significance only, some stud-

ies have reported an increased number of freckles to be a risk factor for melanoma. The best treatment is prevention, with avoidance of the sun. **Lentigines** are usually darker tan, brown, or black, flat lesions seen in childhood and adult life. Lentigines acquired in early childhood may fade with time, whereas those acquired in later life tend to persist. Lentigines may be seen in several syndromes, including Peutz–Jeghers syndrome, Leopard (*l*entigenes, *e*lectrocardiographic conduction defects, *o*cular hypertelorism, *p*ulmonary stenosis, *a*bnormalities of genitalia, *r*etardation of growth, and *d*eafness) syndrome, and Lamb (*l*entigenes, *a*trial myxomas, *m*ucocutaneous myxomas, and *b*lue nevi) syndrome.

NEVUS OF OTA & ITO

Large blue-gray discoloration of the face surrounding the eye is seen with the nevus of Ota. Ipsilateral bluish coloration of the sclera is common. Nevus of Ito displays the same clinical features over the shoulder, neck, and clavicular area. Although both lesions have histology (dermal melanocytosis) and color similar to those of mongolian spots, nevi of Ota and Ito usually persist throughout life. Lesions are usually benign, with rare cases of malignant transformation recorded. Laser treatment may lighten or remove these lesions if desired.

■ RAISED (PAPULAR) PIGMENTED LESIONS

Pigmented nevi may appear light tan, brown, or brown-black. They are formed by collections of melanocytes, termed **nevus cells.** Although these lesions are usually benign in childhood, malignancy can occur. Nonmelanocytic cell collections may mimic pigmented lesions, such as urticaria pigmentosa, which is composed of mast cell skin infiltrates.

CONGENITAL MELANOCYTIC NEVI

Pigmented melanocytic nevi present at birth or in the first few months are termed **congenital nevi** (Figure 11–4). They appear in 1–2% of newborns as light tan, brown, or black plaques. Lesions are usually solitary but can appear in groups or clusters; they vary in size, ranging from 1 mm to larger than 20 cm ("giant nevi"). The vast majority are smaller than 3 cm. Nevi may be differentiated from other "dark spots" by shining a light from the side of the lesion; nevi have more prominent skin lines, a distorted surface, and speckling. These lesions may be classified on the basis of size: small congenital nevi, up to 1.5 cm; intermediate nevi, 1.5–20 cm; large (or giant) nevi, larger than 20 cm. However, because the lesions may grow over time, some define large congential nevi as greater than 5% of body surface area. Other names for large nevi include garment

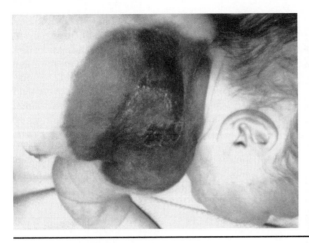

Figure 11–4. Large congenital nevus.

nevi, bathing trunk nevi, or giant hairy nevi. Classically, congenital nevi differ from acquired nevi histologically by involving deeper portions of the dermis, with nevus cells streaming around collagen bundles, nerves, vessels, and skin appendages.

The natural history of most congenital nevi is benign; they grow proportionately throughout the patient's life. Lesions may be flat, papular, nodular, with or without hair, firm, or warty. The risk of melanoma depends on the size of the congenital nevus. The lifetime risk of melanoma in giant congenital nevi is estimated at approximately 6% (with ranges of 2–42% documented in published studies). The risk of intermediate and small congenital nevi is uncertain. Lesions overlying the skull or spine may be associated with leptomeningeal melanosis or underlying spinal defects.

The management of congenital nevi is quite controversial. Giant nevi pose a significant health hazard but are difficult or, at times, impossible to excise prophylactically owing to involvement of vital structures and technical complexity. Many authorities recommend early excision, whereas others suggest serial observation for changes in morphology or color. The risk of complications from multiple surgical procedures should be balanced with the risk of development of melanoma. The risk of melanoma developing in intermediate and small congenital nevi is not known; malignant transformation in childhood is quite rare. Routine prophylactic excision, although recommended by some experts, is considered impractical and unnecessary by many. Clinical observation over time is reasonable, with consideration of elective excision when the child is old enough to cooperate with local anesthesia. Families should be taught how to recognize changes in nevi that are clinically important (Table 11–12).

Acquired Melanocytic Nevi

Acquired melanocytic nevi, or common moles, usually appear from early childhood to early adulthood. There is a large range in the number of lesions, with white adults having 10–40 nevi on average. Nevi are composed of melanocytic "nests" of cells and are classified by the predominant location of the cells. **Junctional nevi** are composed of nevus cells predominantly in the epidermis and clinically are smooth or minimally elevated, even-colored, tan to black macules. **Compound nevi** have melanocytic nests at the dermoepidermal junction and within the dermis. These lesions are similar in color to junctional nevi, with more prominent elevation. **Intradermal nevi** are formed by melanocytic nests fully within the dermis. These lesions are dome shaped, raised, or pedunculated; they may be pigmented or flesh-colored. It is believed that melanocytic nevi may progress from junctional nevi to compound nevi, and then to intradermal nevi as part of their normal biology. Nevi are seen predominantly on sun-exposed areas of the body, and evidence has linked sun exposure to subsequent development of an increased mole burden.

Table 11–12. ABCs of Worrisome Changes in Congenital Nevi

A = Asymmetry
B = Border irregularity
C = Color: Localized color variation to red, dark brown, blue, or black
D = Diameter: Changing size of atypical area
E = Elevation: Elevated, firm nodules

The clinical appearance of acquired moles is quite variable. Routine excision of acquired nevi is not necessary unless lesions have unusual characteristics. Lesions with pruritus, pain, rapid change in size or color, irregular borders, poor demarcation, or bleeding should be excised and evaluated histologically.

ATYPICAL (DYSPLASTIC) NEVI

Atypical nevi are clinically unusual moles that may connote an increased risk of malignant melanoma. Clinical characteristics are outlined in Table 11–13. Atypical nevi may be seen in families with a propensity for large numbers of atypical moles and malignant melanoma. This entity, the familial atypical mole syndrome (FAMS), is also known as **familial dysplastic nevus syndrome** or **BK mole syndrome.** Individuals with FAMS demonstrate multiple atypical nevi and have two first-degree relatives with malignant melanoma; lifetime risk of melanoma approaches 80–90%.

MELANOMA

Melanoma is quite uncommon in children, with only 2% of melanomas occurring in patients younger than 20 years. However, 10% of patients with FAMS develop melanoma before age 20 years. The possibility of melanoma must be considered in unusual congenital and acquired melanocytic nevi. Pediatricians also should be aware of the risk factors for melanoma (Table 11–14) and that childhood sun exposure, particularly a history of blistering sunburns, is a key risk factor for development of melanoma in adulthood.

SPITZ NEVI (SPINDLE & EPITHELIOID CELL NEVI)

Spitz nevi are dome-shaped, pink to reddish-brown nodules. Lesions are usually solitary but may be multiple or grouped. They usually appear in early childhood to adolescence, commonly on the face. Despite their original name, "juvenile melanoma," Spitz nevi are benign, with characteristic histopathologic features (spindle and epithelial cell nests). Lesions may be difficult to distinguish from true melanoma, and expert dermatopathologic review may be necessary. Recommended treatment is surgical excision.

Table 11–13. Clinical Characteristics of Atypical (Dysplastic) Nevi

Moles are large (6–15 mm)
Occur in usual sites as well as scalp, buttocks, other sun-protected sites
Irregular borders, mixed colors (tan, brown, dark brown, pink)
Indistinct margins
Macular component very common; may have "pebbly" or "fried-egg" appearance

Table 11–14. Risk Factors for Development of Melanoma

Fair skin
Blond/red hair
Freckling
Skin types I and II (easily burns, tans poorly)
History of sun exposure
Childhood
Cumulative
Intermittent
Blistering sunburns
Local environment (e.g., sunbelt states)
Increased number of benign-appearing moles
Atypical moles
Family history of melanoma or atypical moles
Large congenital nevi

URTICARIA PIGMENTOSA (MASTOCYTOSIS)

Mast cell infiltration of the skin and other organs is the hallmark of mastocytosis. Urticaria pigmentosa is the common form in childhood, presenting as solitary or multiple red-brown macules, papules, or nodules, usually 1–3 cm, and often found on the trunk. Lesions become hive-like when firmly stroked; this phenomenon is a positive Darier sign, a result of the release of histamines from the increased number of mast cells in these lesions. In the first few months after birth, lesions may become vesicular or bullous with vigorous contact. Repeated blistering at the same site or a nonhealing sore may be a clue to this diagnosis.

Lesions develop in more than 75% of patients by 2 years of age; most of these legions clear spontaneously by puberty. Systemic involvement is more common in older children and adults. Symptoms and signs include flushing, headaches, tachycardia, hypotension, cramps, and coagulation abnormalities. Fewer than 5% of children with onset of urticaria pigmentosa before age 10 years have systemic involvement, compared with 10–30% of older children. Mast cells may infiltrate bone marrow, liver, spleen, and gastrointestinal tract in the systemic form. Occasional familial forms of diffuse cutaneous, bullous mastocytosis have been reported.

An increased number of mast cells in the dermis and subcutaneous tissue on skin biopsy specimens can confirm the diagnosis. Toluidine blue or Giemsa stains will show metachromatic staining.

No effective therapy exists for mastocytosis. Patients should avoid mast cell degranulators such as aspirin, codeine, opiates, procaine, polymyxin B, and radiographic dyes. Scopolamine and pancuronium also may lead to exacerbation of symptoms. Hot baths and vigorous rubbing of the skin can lead to mast cell degranulation. H$_1$ and

H_2 antihistamines have been used with some success, as have oral cromolyn sodium and ketotifen. Psoralen and ultraviolet A therapy are reserved for severe cases. Topical fluorinated steroids may be beneficial for treatment of a small number of isolated cutaneous lesions.

■ RAISED NONPIGMENTED LESIONS

Nonpigmented raised papules and nodules may be skin-colored, tan, brown, or orange-yellow. Nonpigmented lesions in infants and children are associated with numerous different conditions, several of which are discussed below.

EPIDERMAL NEVI

Epidermal nevi are benign growths that can occur anywhere on the skin. Lesions usually are present at birth but may appear during childhood and adolescence. Lesions may be minimally elevated at birth but usually become more papular with a verrucous surface in later years. Color ranges from skin color to dark brown or black. Lesions grow proportionately with the child and often take on a linear appearance **(linear epidermal nevi).** Epidermal nevi may be mistaken for verrucae; persistence, proportionate growth, and linear configuration are useful differentiating features. Lesions may be large and expansive and arranged as spiral streaks, especially on the trunk. Extensive epidermal nevi may be associated with a congenitally acquired syndrome termed the **epidermal nevus syndrome.** Associated anomalies include central nervous system involvement (including seizures, mental retardation, and focal deficits), skeletal defects, hemihypertrophy, and renal and ocular anomalies.

NEVUS SEBACEOUS

Nevus sebaceous (nevus sebaceous of Jadassohn) is a benign epidermal tumor present at birth. Initially it appears as a flat or minimally raised, hairless plaque. The tumor has a characteristic waxy texture and yellow-orange or pink color and is most commonly present on the scalp or face. Nevus sebaceous lesions thicken with puberty, as the sebaceous glands that constitute much of the tumor are hormonally stimulated. Extensive nevus sebaceous may be associated with central nervous system disease and skeletal anomalies, as a variant of the epidermal nevus syndrome. Secondary neoplasia may occur in 15–20% of lesions, usually in adolescence or adulthood. Tricholemomas and syringocystadenoma papilliferum (a tumor of apocrine sweat glands) are the common tumors; rare basal cell carcinomas, squamous cell carcinomas and appendage tumors also have been reported. Because of the neoplastic risks, elective excision is recommended before or at puberty.

JUVENILE XANTHOGRANULOMAS

Juvenile xanthogranulomas are 2–10 mm, yellow, brown, or red-brown papules and nodules that typically occur in the first few months after birth. Lesions may be solitary or multiple; occasionally, hundreds of lesions are present. These histiocytic tumors usually are self-limited, and two thirds of lesions resolve spontaneously within 1 year. Associated iris xanthogranulomas may cause ocular hemorrhage or glaucoma. Xanthogranulomas also are associated with juvenile chronic myeloid leukemia; children with neurofibromatosis and juvenile xanthogranulomas seem to be at much greater risk. Xanthogranulomas do not require treatment, as lesions spontaneously regress.

PILOMATRICOMAS

Pilomatricomas (calcifying epitheliomas) are benign, firm, calcifying lesions that most often occur on the head and neck in the first two decades of life. Lesions may be skin-colored but often have a bluish color and stonelike consistency. Although these lesions are benign, surgical excision is recommended for prevention of discomfort and inflammation and for cosmetic reasons. Multiple pilomatricomas have been associated with myotonic dystrophy.

CONNECTIVE TISSUE NEVI

Connective tissue nevi are benign collections of dermal collagen or elastic tissue. These slightly elevated, firm or rubbery plaques are seen commonly on the trunk, buttocks, or extremities. Connective tissue nevus plaques may be seen in patients with tuberous sclerosis; these are termed **shagreen patches.** Connective tissue nevi are also associated with Buschke–Ollendorf syndrome, which consists of osteopoikilosis with bony dysplasia. Lesions may be hereditary without associated anomalies or sporadic. They are benign and require no treatment other than biopsy for diagnostic purposes.

DERMATOFIBROMAS

Dermatofibromas, which are firm, flesh-colored to tan, brown, or black papules or nodules often occurring on the extremities, are seen occasionally in children, although more often in adolescents and adults. They are fixed firmly to the skin but move freely above the subcutaneous fat.

NEUROFIBROMAS

Neurofibromas may be isolated growths or seen as a major finding of NF-1 (von Recklinghausen disease). Tumors vary greatly in size and consistency, ranging from smooth and soft to firm and polypoid. Although large, plaque-like, plexiform neurofibromas associated with neurofibromatosis may be present at birth, the vast majority of NF-1–associated fibromas present after age 10 years. Excision is recommended for lesions that enlarge rapidly, cause marked pain, are functionally significant, or are disfiguring.

■ HYPERSENSITIVITY REACTIONS

URTICARIA & ANGIOEDEMA

Urticaria is common in infancy and childhood. Often referred to as "hives," these lesions consist of erythematous, raised wheals, which may be present anywhere on the body. Lesions may range from a few millimeters to giant edematous plaques and typically have a pale or whitish center. These may be mistaken for lesions of erythema multiforme. Urticarial lesions occur suddenly, are quite pruritic, and persist for less than 24 hours. Although lesions shift or new lesions develop, individual lesions usually do not remain fixed. In contrast, lesions of erythema multiforme persist for a minimum of 1 week.

Extension of urticaria to deeper cutaneous tissue is termed **angioedema.** This may be associated with marked swelling of the face, hands, and feet. Laryngeal or bronchial edema can lead to life-threatening airway obstruction.

Urticaria is due to vasodilatation and increased permeability of capillaries and small blood vessels, with transudation of fluid into the upper dermis. This occurs when mast cells (often through antigenic stimulation) release a number of vasoactive substances, such as histamines, kinins, and prostaglandins. Urticaria results from a variety of causes, including foods, drugs, infections, bites and stings, physical agents, genetic diseases, and systemic diseases (Table 11–15).

Most urticarial reactions resolve spontaneously. Urticarial lesions that persist for more than 24 hours may rep-

resent urticarial vasculitis; skin biopsy is diagnostic. The term **chronic urticaria** is restricted to urticaria present for at least 6 weeks. Uncovering the instigating agent in these cases is often quite difficult. Physical urticarias should be considered (cholinergic, cold, and pressure urticaria). Unfortunately, an underlying cause can be found in only 20% of cases.

Treatment of urticaria depends on the severity of the condition and the presence or absence of airway involvement. Extensive skin or airway involvement should be treated with epinephrine and antihistamines. Oral antihistamines are usually effective in the treatment of urticaria. Systemic glucocorticoids are rarely necessary to manage urticaria or angioedema. It is appropriate to identify and eliminate any precipitating agent.

DRUG ERUPTIONS

Drug-induced rashes commonly occur in the pediatric age group. The morphologic diversity of these eruptions and their resemblance to other exanthems often lead to difficulty in diagnosis and management. Frequently, a patient with fever is treated with an antibiotic and subsequently has a rash; in such cases, it is difficult to discern whether the rash is infectious or drug induced. A variety of drug-related eruptions occur, ranging from benign macular or morbilliform eruptions to life-threatening entities, such as toxic epidermal necrolysis (Table 11–16). The time course for drug eruptions is typically 7–14 days into the course of initial exposure, with eruptions within a few days if there has been prior sensitization. However, there is great variability; some eruptions occur immediately on administration, whereas others develop weeks after discontinuation of the agent.

Morphologic features, although not diagnostic, may offer clues to both diagnosis and prognosis. Acneiform eruptions more commonly follow the ingestion of steroids, phenytoin (Dilantin), lithium, isoniazid (INH), or halogens and resolve after discontinuation of the offending agent. In contrast, toxic epidermal necrolysis (TEN) consists of severe sheet-like erosions of the skin and mucous membranes and has a more serious prognosis, with a significant mortality rate resulting from superinfection and sepsis. The most common agents associated with

Table 11–15. Causes of Urticaria

Infections
Bacterial: streptococcal
Viral: Epstein–Barr, hepatitis, adenovirus, enterovirus
Parasites
Other: Sinusitis
Foods
Eggs, nuts, milk, shellfish, berries, others
Drugs
Penicillins, cephalosporins, opiates, salicylates, nonsteroidal anti-inflammatory agents, blood products
Bites/stings
Hymenoptera (bees, wasps, hornets), spiders
Systemic diseases
Juvenile rheumatoid arthritis, systemic lupus erythematosus, dermatomyositis, Sjögren syndrome, Behçet syndrome, rheumatic fever

Adapted and reproduced, with permission, from Weston W, Lane A: *Color Textbook of Pediatric Dermatology.* Mosby–Year Book, 1991.

Table 11–16. Clinical Variation of Drug Eruptions

Urticaria	Exfoliative
Serum sickness–like	Erythema multiforme
Morbilliform	Erythema nodosum
Maculopapular	Toxic epidermal necrolysis
Macular	Fixed drug eruption
Scarlatiniform	Photosensitivity dermatitis vasculitis
Vesicobullous	Eczematous contact dermatitis

TEN are sulfonamides, anticonvulsants, and nonsteroidal anti-inflammatory drugs. The most frequently seen drug reaction is much less specific as to etiology and consists of a generalized erythematous morbilliform (macular and papular) eruption. Penicillins and cephalosporins are the most likely offenders, although a variety of other drugs and blood products also can induce these cutaneous findings. The eruption typically lasts 1–2 weeks and may be associated with moderate to severe pruritus.

Mild drug eruptions can progress to more severe processes, such as erythema multiforme, toxic epidermal necrolysis, or vasculitis. Drug hypersensitivity may involve multiple organs, including liver, kidneys, gastrointestinal tract, and central nervous system. Peculiar and life-threatening hypersensitivity reactions may be seen with phenytoin, phenobarbital, or carbamazepine. These reactions usually present 1–4 weeks after exposure to the drug and are characterized by fever, morbilliform eruptions, lymphadenopathy, and hepatitis. Drugs must be discontinued promptly. These medications appear to be cross-allergic; if anticonvulsants are needed, no agents of these three classes should be used. There is evidence of a possible enzymatic predisposition to this anticonvulsant hypersensitivity reaction.

Erythema Multiforme

Erythema multiforme (EM) is an acute hypersensitivity reaction characterized by distinctive skin lesions with or without mucosal involvement. There is a spectrum of disease, with EM minor and major as distinct syndromes; TEN may be a severe form of EM major. Erythema multiforme minor presents with symmetric erythematous macules or papules, often with superimposed vesicles, which evolve into annular target or iris lesions. Lesions occur primarily on the upper extremities and trunk. Erythema multiforme major, or Stevens–Johnson syndrome, is characterized by blistering of at least two mucosal surfaces accompanying typical cutaneous EM lesions. Toxic epidermal necrolysis presents with widespread erythema and necrosis of full-thickness epidermis that resembles deep scalding injury. Toxic epidermal necrolysis is complicated by fluid and electrolyte imbalance, severe mucosal injury, and sepsis and has an estimated mortality rate of 20–70%.

Lesions of EM may have central dusky areas from profound inflammation, termed "target" or "iris" lesions. Individual lesions persist for a minimum of 1 week, in sharp contrast to urticaria. Although urticarial wheals may appear "targetlike" because of central clearing or bluish color, they resolve within hours.

Erythema multiforme has been associated with a variety of infections and drugs. Erythema multiforme minor, especially when recurrent, is almost always associated with preceding herpes simplex virus (HSV) infection. Herpes virus antigens and DNA have been found in cutaneous lesions. Other precipitants of EM include *Mycoplasma pneumoniae* infections and drugs, especially sulfonamides, penicillins, anticonvulsants, and nonsteroidal anti-inflammatory agents.

The management of EM in children is controversial. Clearly, any instigating agent, such as a drug or infection, should be identified and eliminated if possible. Further treatment of EM is dictated by the type and extent of disease. EM minor is usually self-limited; it typically evolves over 1–2 weeks and completely heals by 3–4 weeks. Patients may be treated conservatively with cool compresses to lesions and oral antihistamines. Oral lesions may be painful, and patients may benefit from soothing mouthwashes (e.g., viscous lidocaine-diphenhydramine elixir-antacid combination). Acyclovir is not efficacious for treating established EM but may be effective prophylactically for those patients with HSV-associated EM minor. The use of steroids in EM is controversial. If they are to be used, they should be given early in the course of the disease, within the first 1–2 days of the rash. Mildly affected patients usually do well with supportive care only. For patients with extensive EM (>20% denudation) or TEN, the use of steroids remains controversial. The use of intravenous γ-globulin in this setting is also under investigation.

Erythema Nodosum

Erythema nodosum (erythema contusiformis) presents with distinctive tender erythematous nodules, classically on the pretibial surfaces. These nodules represent a hypersensitivity reaction to a variety of infections, drugs, and disease states (Table 11–17). These warm nodules are intensely painful and may be seen on any body surface, including the face and upper extremities. Lesions may evolve from pink-red to purple or yellow-brown and may appear bruise-like.

Lesions of erythema nodosum may be mistaken for cellulitis, bruises, bug bites, or other inflammatory diseases of subcutaneous tissue. Arthralgias and arthritis are commonly associated with erythema nodosum and do not necessarily suggest underlying rheumatic disease. A lesional

Table 11–17. Erythema Nodosum: Precipitating Factors

Infections	*Streptococcus*, tuberculosis, histoplasmosis, coccidioidomycosis, blastomycosis, cat-scratch disease, leptospirosis
Drugs	Oral contraceptives, sulfonamides, penicillin, tetracycline, halogens
Systemic diseases	Inflammatory bowel disease, sarcoidosis, connective tissue diseases, malignancies

biopsy specimen displays distinctive pathologic findings of inflammation of fatty tissue, primarily of the connective tissue surrounding fat lobules **(septal panniculitis).**

Erythema nodosum is usually self-limited, resolving in 2–3 weeks. Ibuprofen, salicylates, or other nonsteroidal anti-inflammatory agents may minimize the discomfort.

■ INFECTIOUS DISEASES

Many infectious diseases have cutaneous manifestations. This discussion is limited to important cutaneous diseases not discussed in Chapter 9. The infectious exanthems are summarized in Table 11–18.

Bacterial Infections

The skin serves as a common portal of entry for bacterial invaders. Excessive moisture or drying, friction, or trauma can damage the structural integrity of the epithelium or appendageal structures and predispose to infection.

Impetigo is the term for superficial bacterial infection of the epithelium (Figure 11–5). It occurs most commonly in young children, particularly in those exposed to conditions of crowding and poor hygiene. The lesions favor the periorificial areas and are initially erythematous macules that evolve into thin-roofed vesicles or pustules that quickly rupture. The erythematous erosion that results is often covered by a honey-colored crust. **Bullous impetigo,** another variant, is characterized by inflamed bullae that also eventually rupture, leaving a rim of epithelial roof and an eroded surface.

Ecthyma is the term for lesions with deeper bacterial penetration through the epidermis. Although these lesions initially consist of vesiculopustules, a firm, dark crust subsequently develops beneath which usually can be found a small amount of purulent exudate. **Cellulitis** is a bacterial infection that predominantly involves the dermis; it is characteristically a raised warm, erythematous plaque that can expand rapidly. **Necrotizing fasciitis** occurs if infection extends to the subcutaneous fat and fascia. This is a life-threatening process and is more common in patients with diabetes and immunocompromise.

Folliculitis occurs when bacteria superficially invade the hair follicle. Multiple erythematous follicular papules or papulopustules usually are noted. **Furuncles** are deeper infections of the follicles, with tender erythematous follicular nodules. **Carbuncles** are formed by multiple coalescent furuncles, which, if fluctuant, are referred to as **abscesses. Ecthyma gangrenosum** is a rare, deep cutaneous infection caused by *Pseudomonas aeruginosa.* It may look similar to streptococcal-induced ecthyma, although it is usually more necrotic and occurs in debilitated or immunocompromised patients.

ETIOLOGY & THERAPY

Staphylococcus aureus and group A β-hemolytic streptococci are the most commonly isolated organisms in skin infections. Ecthyma and cellulitis often harbor *Streptococcus,* whereas furunculosis is almost always secondary to *Staphylococcus* infection. Impetigo frequently harbors both organisms. *Haemophilus influenzae* cellulitis, which usually occurs in early childhood and may be accompanied by sinusitis or bacteremia, was a frequent cause of facial cellulitis prior to the introduction of *H. influenzae* type b conjugate vaccines in 1988. Invasive infections secondary to *H. influenzae* in this country now occur primarily in undervaccinated children or infants who have not completed the primary vaccination series. In neonates, colonization and infection with flora endogenous to the maternal perineum (e.g., group B streptococci and *Escherichia coli*) can occur. Therapy is directed toward the appropriate bacterial pathogens. Because impetigo commonly harbors *Streptococcus* and *Staphylococcus,* antibiotic therapy covering both organisms (e.g., a semisynthetic penicillin) is recommended. Although dicloxacillin would be a reasonable choice, most young children find its flavor offensive, and a cephalosporin is often substituted for improved treatment compliance. Topical mupirocin ointment may be used for treatment of localized lesions, eliminating the need for oral therapy. Children with recurrent *Staphylococcus* infections may be chronic nasal carriers and evaluation and treatment should be considered in such cases.

Viral Infections

MOLLUSCUM CONTAGIOSUM

Molluscum contagiosum is a relatively common cutaneous infection caused by the DNA pox virus. Lesions are single or multiple, white, opalescent, flesh-colored, or pink papules (Figure 11–6). They are often dome shaped with a central pinpoint core. Although usually 1–3 mm, they can occasionally be larger than 1 cm and are then referred to as **giant molluscum.** Lesions favor the face, neck, and trunk but can also involve the genitals. Genital lesions in children, especially those younger than 3 years, usually are not the result of abuse and may occur secondary to autoinnoculation from other affected sites. In addition, an eczematous eruption may occur around afflicted areas. Treatment is not necessarily required because the disease follows a natural course of spontaneous resolution. However, lesions often persist for months to years, and familial, school, and swimming pool transmission can occur. In addition, parents often become anxious concerning the cosmetic aspects of prolonged involvement. For these reasons, treatment is often prescribed. Because no uniformly efficacious treatment exists, multiple applications, and often multiple agents, are required. Needle extraction or curettage is often curative but is difficult to perform on multiple lesions. Cryotherapy and

(text continues on page 458)

Table 11–18. Exanthems

Disease (Etiology)	Usual Age	Season	Prodrome	Morphology
Measles (rubeola virus)	Infants to young adults	Winter/spring	High fever, URI Sx, conjunctivitis	Erythematous macules and papules, become confluent
Rubella (rubella virus)	Adolescents/ young adults	Spring	Absent or low-grade fever Malaise	Rose pink papules, not confluent
Erythema infectiosum (parvovirus B19)	70% 5–15 y	Winter/spring	Usually none	Slapped cheeks; reticulate erythema or maculopapular
Enteroviral exanthems (coxsackievirus, echovirus, other enteroviruses)	Young children	Summer/fall	Fever (occ.)	Variable maculopapular, petechial, purpuric, vesicular
Hand-foot-mouth syndrome (several coxsackieviruses)	Young children	Summer/fall	Fever (occ.), sore mouth	Gray-white vesicles 3–7 mm on normal or erythematous base
Adenovirus exanthems (adenoviruses)	5 mo–5 y	Winter/spring	Fever, URI Sx	Rubelliform, morbiform, roseolalike
Chickenpox (varicella zoster virus)	80% 1–14 y	Late fall/ winter/ spring	Usually none	Macules, papules rapidly become vesicles on erythematous base, then crusts
Roseola (human herpes virus 6 & 7)	99% 6 mo–3 y	Any season	High fever	Maculopapular rash appears after fever 3–6 d
Kawasaki disease	6 mo–6 y	Winter/spring	High fever, irritability	Polymorphous; papular, morbilliform, erythema with desquamation
Gianotti–Crosti syndrome (EBV, coxsackievirus, hepatitis B, others)	1–8 y	Any season	Usually absent	Papules or papulovesicles May become confluent
Scarlet fever (β-streptococcus)	School-aged children	Fall to spring	Acute onset with fever, sore throat	Diffuse erythema with sandpaper texture
Staphylococcal scalded-skin syndrome (Staphylococcus aureus/epidermolytic toxin)	Infants	Any season	None	Abrupt onset, tender erythroderma, scaling
Toxic-shock syndrome/ staphylococcal toxin	Adolescents/ young adults	Any season	None	Macular erythroderma
Meningococcemia/ meningococcus	<5 y	Winter/spring	Malaise, fever, URI Sx	Papules, petechiae, purpura
Unilateral laterothoracic exanthem	1–5 y (average 2 y)	Spring/winter	HX URI, fever, diarrhea	Morbilliform, eczematous erythema with late desquamation
Toxic shock syndrome/ streptococcal toxin	Young children	Any	None	Macular erythroderma

CMV = cytomegalovirus; Conv. = convalescent; EBV = Epstein–Barr virus; ER = emergency room; HAI = hemagglutinin; IM = intramuscularly; occ. = occasionally; Sx = symptoms; URI = upper respiratory tract infection.

Adapted and printed, with permission, from Frieden I, Williams ML. In: Dieckmann RA, Grossman M (editors): *Pediatric Emergency Medicine.* JB Lippincott, 1991.

Distribution	Associated Findings	Diagnosis
Begins on face and moves downward over whole body	Koplik spots, toxic appearance, photo-phobia, cough, adenopathy, high fever	Usually clinical: acute/conv. HAI serology
Begins on face and moves downward	Postauricular and occipital adenopathy Headache, malaise	Rubella IgM or acute/conv. HAI serology
Usually arms/legs; may be generalized	Rash waxes and wanes for weeks Occ. arthritis headache, malaise	Usually clinical; acute/conv. serology
Usually generalized, may be acral	Low-grade fever; (occ.) myocarditis, aseptic meningitis, pleurodynia	Usually clinical; viral culture from throat, rectal swabs in selected cases
Hands/feet most common; diaper area Occ. generalized	Oral ulcers (occ.), fever, adenopathy	Same as enteroviruses
Generalized	Fever, URI Sx occasionally pneumonia	Viral isolation or acute/conv. seroconversation
Often begin on scalp or face; More profuse on trunk than extremities	Pruritus, fever, oral lesions, occ. malaise	Usually clinical; Tzanck preparation, direct immunofluorescence, culture
Trunk, neck. May be generalized; fever declines	Cervical and postauricular adenopathy last hours to days	Clinical
Variable perineal accentuation common	Conjunctivitis, cheilitis, glossils, periph-eral edema, adenopathy	Clinical
Face, arms, legs, buttocks, spares the torso	Occasional lymphadenopathy, hepatomegaly, splenomegaly	Clinical; EBV, hepatitis B serologies
Facial flushing with circumoral pallor, linear erythema in skin folds	Exudative pharyngitis, palatal petechiae, abdominal pain	Throat cultures
Diffuse with perioral, perinasal systemic site (not skin)	Fever, conjunctivitis, rhinitis	Clinical; culture of *S. aureus* form
Generalized	Hypotension; fever, myalgias, diarrhea/vomiting	Clinical case definition criteria; isola-tions *S. aureus*, cervix, etc.
Trunk, extremities, palms, soles	2/3 temp >40°C meningismus circulatory collapse	Clinical, blood culture, spinal tap
Axillary/lateral thorax, periflexural, ini-tially unilateral, may generalized	Pruritus	Clinical
Generalized	Hypotension; necrotizing fasciitis	Clinical case definition criteria; isolation β *streptococcus*

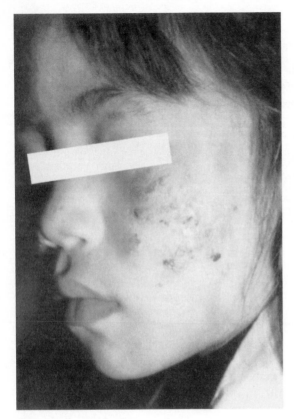

Figure 11–5. Impetigo.

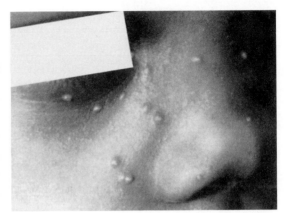

Figure 11–6. Molluscum contagiosum.

topical cantharidin can be effective treatments. Some investigators have reported a response to less invasive treatment, which involves nightly application of surgical or other thick tape to each lesion, with removal or stripping of the tape the following morning.

VERRUCAE (WARTS)

Verrucae are epidermal and mucocutaneous growths caused by human papillomavirus (HPV) (Figure 11–7). They are categorized predominantly on the basis of their most common locations.

Verrucae vulgaris lesions, also referred to as common warts, usually involve the hands and fingers. They are flesh-colored to brown, discrete, rough-surfaced papules and are particularly persistent when they involve the periungual or subungual area. **Digitate warts,** a variant seen more commonly on the face, tend to be filiform or fingerlike, with a narrow base. **Verrucae plantaris (plantar warts)** refer to lesions on the sole of the foot. These often are quite painful and difficult to eradicate. They can be single papules or may consist of multiple coalescent hyperkeratotic lesions. **Verrucae plana (flat warts)** are flatter,

often barely perceptible, 1–4 mm, flesh-colored to brown lesions that usually involve the face and legs. They often are spread by trauma, such as scratching or shaving. ***Condylomata acuminata*** **(genital warts)** most commonly involve the mucous membranes or perigenital area. They can be sexually transmitted or occur as a result of transmission via an infected birth canal.

Etiology & therapy. All warts are the result of infection with HPV. This viral agent is ubiquitous, and more than 80 types currently have been identified. Most types show a predilection for a particular body surface: HPV-1 affects the palmar and plantar surfaces, whereas HPV-6 and -11 commonly cause condylomata acuminata. Human papillomaviruses 16, 18, 31, 33, and 35 also have been isolated from genital warts and associated with cervical dysplasia and neoplasia. Human papillomavirus typing can be performed from tissue specimens, if necessary. Not all warts require treatment, and no completely effective therapy exists for any form of verrucae. Because 60–70% of common warts resolve spontaneously within 2 years, reassurance is often the best form of therapy. However, indications for treatment include discomfort, extensive spread on the digits or face, and genital involvement. Multiple therapies exist, but no ideal agent is available. Verrucae plana often respond to topical tretinoin, light electrodesiccation, or cryotherapy (freezing with liquid nitrogen). Genital warts may respond to topical therapies, such as podophyllin resin or trichloroacetic acid. Imiquimod, a topical immune response modifier that induces a variety of cytokines, is effective in some patients with genital warts. Treatment of common and plantar warts often initially consists of less invasive therapies, such as topical acetic or salicylic acid with or without occlusion. If required, paring of the lesion, cryotherapy, or curettage can be used subsequently. Multiple and repeated treatments are often required. In extensive or resistant cases, cimetidine may be

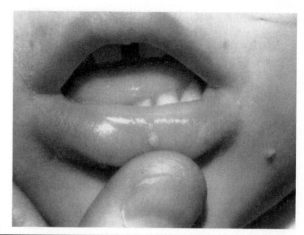

Figure 11–7. Warts, or verrucae vulgaris.

effective by virtue of its immunomodulating properties, especially if combined with topical therapy.

Fungal Infections

Superficial fungal infections may involve the scalp, nails, or skin. These dermatophyte infections use keratin as a metabolic substrate and can be quite difficult to eradicate. They are mildly infectious; many individuals can be exposed to the same inoculum (e.g., in locker room showers), yet only a few will be infected. Tinea infections are named by location (e.g., *capitis,* head; *corporis,* body; *manuum,* hand; and *pedis,* foot). Evaluation of possible tinea infections should include KOH preparations of scale and culture on appropriate media.

TINEA CAPITIS

Tinea capitis may take several forms: (1) a dry, scaling, dandrufflike involvement with mild or no hair loss;

(2) discrete areas of scarring alopecia with broken-off hairs and some element of scale; and (3) single or multiple erythematous, boggy masses, with overlying hair loss, known as **kerions** (Figure 11–8). The most common causative agent is *Trichophyton tonsurans,* which may be endemic and epidemic in some communities. Both *Microsporum* and *Trichophyton* species can be the causative agents in infections of the scalp. Family pets are sometimes the vehicle of transmission for *Microsporum* infections. Kerions reflect a more extensive inflammatory reaction. All forms of tinea capitis require systemic therapy. Griseofulvin is used most commonly, and concurrent topical selenium sulfide or ketoconazole shampoo therapy is recommended to decrease spore counts and expedite response to therapy. Itraconazole, fluconazole, and terbinafine, while not approved by the Food and Drug Administration (FDA) for this indication in children, may be useful as second-line therapy in tinea capitis.

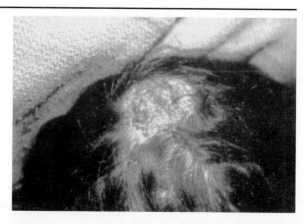

Figure 11–8. Tinea capitis.

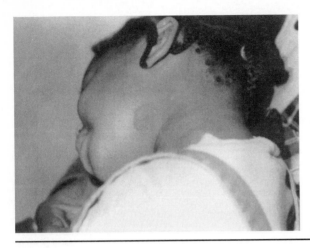

Figure 11–9. Tinea corporis.

TINEA CORPORIS, PEDIS, & MANUUM

Tinea corporis, pedis, and manuum represent infections of the skin, usually by a *Trichophyton* or *Microsporum* species. The lesions are annular, gyrate, and discrete or coalescent scaling papules or plaques (Figure 11–9). Lesions can be indolent or actively inflammatory, with erythema and erosions. Secondary bacterial infection is commonly seen in the interdigital web spaces of the feet. Treatment consists of topical antifungal therapy such as the imidazoles. Systemic griseofulvin or alternative antifungal therapy may be required for recalcitrant cases.

ONYCHOMYCOSIS

Onychomycosis is a fungal infection of the nails. Toenail involvement is most frequent and the most difficult to eradicate. Afflicted areas commonly exhibit distortion of the nail with whitening and subungual debris. The differential diagnosis for such findings includes trauma, psoriasis and lichen planus. The most common causative agent is *Trichophyton rubrum*. Whitening of the dorsal aspect of the toenail is seen in nail infections caused by *Trichophyton mentagrophytes*. Although superficial forms of onychomycosis may clear with topical antifungals, onychomycosis most often requires systemic therapy. Griseofulvin and ketoconazole have shown limited efficacy in this disease; fluconazole, itraconazole, and terbinafine appear more effective but currently are not approved by the FDA for onychomycosis in children.

■ INFESTATIONS

Pediculus humanus capitis and *corporis,* commonly known as lice, can infest the scalp and body, respectively. *Pthirus pubis,* the crab louse, usually infests areas with short hairs, such as the pubic area or eyelashes. Lice lay eggs (nits) on the hair shaft, with hatching occurring in 7–10 days. Head lice are becoming an important epidemiologic problem, with one-fourth of U.S. schoolchildren affected in 1999. Over-the-counter products such as 1% permethrin cream rinse (Nix) remain first-line treatment for head lice, although permethrin resistance has been documented recently in the United States. Meticulous removal of nits is helpful to prevent recurrences. Products with low ovicidal activity may require reapplication after 10 days. Alternative treatments include physical agents that suffocate the lice and nits, such as petrolatum and mayonnaise, or some aromatic hair oils that may be pediculotoxic. Overnight application of 5% permethrin cream (Elimite) can be used for resistant cases. Malathion lotion 0.5% (Ovide), now available in the United States, is very ovicidal and pediculocidal. However, it is flammable and not for use in neonates or infants. At this time, it may be wise to reserve its use for recalcitrant cases. Oral trimethoprim-sulfa may be used for resistant infestations. Oral and topical ivermectin are efficacious therapies and may become more important therapeutic options in the future.

Sarcoptes scabiei var hominis is the mite that causes human scabies. The mite burrows into the skin, producing an allergic reaction that is extremely pruritic in a sensitized host. Clinically, scabies can present as papules, nodules, vesicopustules, or classic burrows that are seen predominantly in the hands, feet, and body folds. Lesions tend to be more vesicular or nodular and generalized in young infants. Crusted scabies represents a massive scabies infestation that may be seen in immunocompromised or institutionalized individuals.

Scabies can be definitively diagnosed by microscopic examination of the mite itself or its eggs or feces (scybala). A burrow is the ideal site for a skin scraping, although the yield is higher when multiple areas are sampled.

Five percent permethrin cream (Elimite) currently is the treatment of choice. It is approved for use in infants as young as 2 months, and its use in neonates has been reported. It is applied from the neck to the toes overnight for 8–12 hours and washed off in the morning. Treatment of the head should be included in infants. It is important that all family members be treated simultaneously to prevent recurrences. A second application may be used 7–10 days later. Because the mite cannot live at high temperatures or away from its human host, all bed linens should be washed and machine dried the day after application or stored away for several days.

For crusted or persistent scabies, a single oral dose of 200 μg/kg of ivermectin has been shown to be effective; higher rates of efficacy can be achieved with a second dose 10 days later. However, it should not be used in infants under 15 kg or in pregnant females or nursing mothers. Further studies will influence whether ivermectin will assume a greater role in the treatment of scabies.

■ ACNE

Acne vulgaris is the most common skin disease of adolescence, with more than 90% of the population affected. Although not a life-threatening disease, acne may have substantial psychological effects on those afflicted. Acne lesions include closed comedones (whiteheads), open comedones (blackheads), papules, pustules, and nodules. Open comedones appear as pale, slightly raised skin-colored or white papules. Closed comedones are flat or slightly elevated lesions with a brown or black central opening. The dark color of "blackheads" is not due to dirt but to compact keratin and oxidized melanin pigment. Acne "cysts" are large suppurative nodular lesions that resemble inflamed epidermal cysts. Acne lesions may be followed by postinflammatory hyperpigmentation or a fibrous response causing pitted, hypertrophic, or papular scars. In severe cases, scarring can be substantial.

PATHOGENESIS

Acne pathogenesis is multifactorial. It is a disease primarily of the sebaceous follicle. Sebaceous follicles are cell-lined units with large sebaceous glands and a fine vellus hair. The follicles are most common in acne-prone areas (cheeks, nose, forehead, midline chest, and back). Sebaceous glands are responsive to androgenic hormones, which increase in early puberty. These hormones increase the mass and activity of sebaceous glands. Acne severity usually correlates with sebum production.

Cells lining the follicular canal are cornified keratinocytes. These cells normally slough into the canal and are carried out to the skin surface with sebum secretion. The normal epithelium is altered in active acne, and sloughed cells plug the follicle, forming a *microcomedone*. Subsequent dilation results in a thin-walled structure known as a *comedo*. In addition to sebum and shed follicular cells, the canal normally contains a population of organisms, including *Propionibacterium acnes,* an anaerobic diphtheroid. Follicular plugging facilitates a hospitable environment for bacterial proliferation. Chemotactic factors and cellular response to bacteria result in inflammatory lesions.

Genetic factors and the hormonal milieu may influence the tendency to form microcomedones. There is no evidence that chocolate, fatty foods, or other dietary indiscretions affect the development of acne.

TREATMENT

The ideal therapy would correct abnormal keratinization, decrease sebaceous gland activity (sebum secretion), inhibit the growth of *P. acnes,* possess an anti-inflammatory effect, and promote drainage of closed comedones and resolution of established inflamed lesions. It would be entirely topical to limit systemic effects and toxicities. It should have no adverse effects and cause no irritation or sensitization. Unfortunately, no such agent exists. On the basis of acne pathogenesis, treatment is directed at microcomedone formation, bacterial proliferation, inflammation, and hormonal or sebaceous gland activity. Therapy of acne begins with educating the patient about good skin care and attempting to dispel myths about acne being a disease of improper cleaning or poor diet. Vigorous scrubbing is to be avoided because it may aggravate acne and does not prevent further lesion formation.

Topical therapies are the mainstay of acne therapy for the vast majority of patients. Topical preparations include antibiotics, benzoyl peroxide, tretinoin, and tretinoinlike agents. Erythromycin, clindamycin, benzoyl peroxide, a benzoyl peroxide–erythromycin combination, and sulfacetamide are effective topical agents. Formulations include lotions, creams, and gels. Topical antibiotics effectively decrease inflammatory papules and pustules.

Tretinoin (Retin A, Avita). This topical vitamin A analog normalizes keratinization of the sebaceous follicle and decreases horny cell adhesion. It effectively promotes deplugging of comedones and prevents new microcomedone formation. Tretinoin requires appropriate patient education, counseling concerning the possibility of irritation and photosensitivity, and consistent use over several weeks for optimal tolerance and response to therapy. Nontretinoin retinoids and retinoidlike agents such as adapalene gel (Differin), tazarotene gel (Tazorac), and azelaic acid (Azelex) work similarly to diminish comedone production and prevent acne formation.

Antibiotics. Papulopustular, nodular, and nodulocystic acne may be treated with systemic antibiotics with activity against *P. acnes.* Tetracycline, minocycline, doxycycline, and erythromycin are effective agents, with anti-inflammatory effects as well. Treatment over many months is standard. There are increasing reports of *P. acnes* resistance to antibiotics. Because development of resistance may be hastened by the concommittant use of oral and topical antibiotics, this is usually avoided. To date, *P. acnes* resistance to benzoyl peroxide has not been observed.

Isotretinoin (Accutane). This systemic vitamin A analog is useful for severe papular, nodulocystic, scarring acne unresponsive to topical and systemic treatments described above. Isotretinoin is associated with serious side effects and potential toxicities and is a teratogen. It should be prescribed only by physicians skilled in its use. Use in women of childbearing age requires mandatory contraception and frequent screening for pregnancy during treatment.

An algorithm delineating the use of topical, systemic, or combination treatments, depending on type of acne, is presented in Figure 11–10.

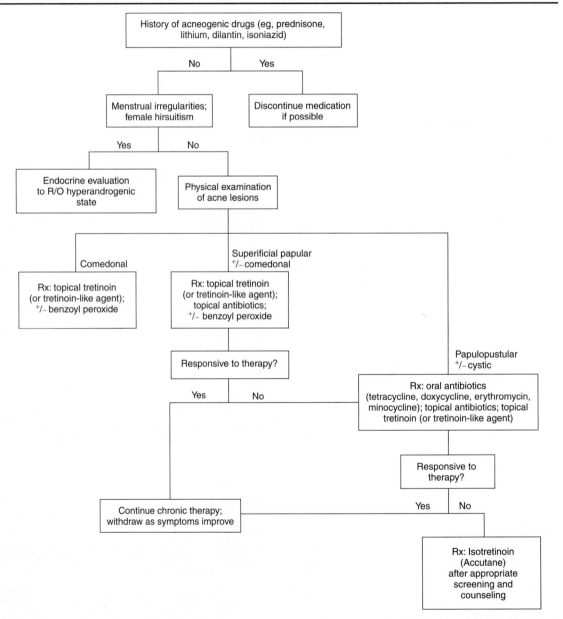

Figure 11–10. Approaches to the patient with acne.

■ ECZEMATOUS DISORDERS

Eczema is a term that is commonly misused and often confusing to the medical student. The term actually means "to boil over" and is used most correctly to describe a reaction pattern rather than a particular disease. This pattern consists of inflammation of the skin with the presence of intercellular edema (**spongiosis**), pruritus, erythematous papules, vesiculation, and oozing. The pattern can be seen in many disorders, including atopic dermatitis, contact dermatitis, seborrheic dermatitis, and dyshidrotic and nummular eczema. Although "eczema" is frequently used to denote atopic dermatitis, one must keep in mind that the reaction pattern it signifies can be noted in any of the diseases mentioned above. Table 11–19 lists the differential diagnoses for eczematous eruptions and their distinguishing characteristics.

ATOPIC DERMATITIS

Atopic dermatitis is an inherited skin disorder often found in association with asthma or hay fever. These three conditions or atopic states are characterized by an enhanced capacity to form immunoglobulin E in response to a variety of antigens. There is a strong genetic predisposition: a child with one atopic parent has a 60% chance of being affected; if both parents are afflicted, the odds increase to 80%. Atopic dermatitis affects approximately 10–20% of the childhood population and, because of its chronic nature, accounts for almost one third of pediatric dermatology visits.

The distribution of atopic dermatitis depends on age. It usually presents in children before the age of 5 years and frequently within 6–9 months after birth. In infancy, it favors the face and extensor surfaces of the extremities; in later childhood, it predominantly involves the antecubital and popliteal fossae. At all ages, the atopic skin tends to be dry and easily irritated. Acutely, the lesions are erythematous, papulovesicular, and oozing, with superimposed scale crust. With time, however, these lesions tend to become dry and thick from chronic rubbing (lichenification; Figure 11–11). It is customary to separate the disease into acute, subacute, and chronic states, depending on the degree of vesiculation and lichenification present. At all stages, pruritus is a cardinal finding; however, many have questioned whether pruritus is in fact the primary finding and whether the associated skin lesions are merely secondary changes caused by scratching ("an itch that rashes, rather than a rash that itches").

Associated findings include facial and especially perioral pallor, infraorbital folds (Dennie–Morgan lines), xerosis, increased linear markings of the palms, and keratosis pilaris. The differential diagnosis includes other eczematous disorders (see Table 11–19), scabies, Langerhans cell histiocytosis, and a variety of immunodeficiency disorders including Wiskott–Aldrich syndrome and ataxia-telangiectasia.

Table 11–19. Differential Diagnosis: Eczematous Disorders

Disorder	Clinical Appearance
Atopic dermatitis	Lesions ill defined distribution age dependent + xerosis/ lichenification (see text)
Contact dermatitis (diaper dermatitis)	Localized, usually with discrete margins
Tinea corporis	Usually annular, discrete borders, less pruritic, scale significant
Seborrheic dermatitis	Most common in infants and teens; greasy scale favors scalp, face, groin
Scabies	Severely pruritic, favors hands and feet; burrows, nodules, papules
Nummular eczema	Coin-shaped lesions, favor lower extremities, severely pruritic
Rare Ataxia-telangiectasia (see Chapter 7) Wiskott–Aldrich syndrome (see Chapter 7) Acrodermatitis enteropathica Leiner disease Cystic fibrosis (see Chapter 17)	

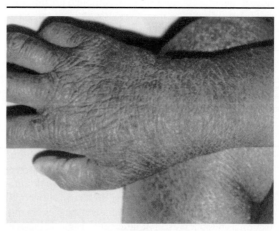

Figure 11–11. Chronic atopic dermatitis.

Although it has long been recognized that some immunologic abnormalities occur in patients with atopic dermatitis, the pathogenesis of the disease is still not clear. Current speculation rests on the presence of an immunologic maturational defect involving T-suppressor cells that allows for relatively unopposed immunoglobulin E synthesis. This is the basis for the experimental use of evening primrose oil (which contains high levels of γ-linoleic acid) and thymopoietin, which are thought to act as maturational factors for T cells. Although both modalities have shown some promise, neither has led to clear-cut, significant improvement in patients; thus, the pathogenesis and optimal treatment of the disease remain in question.

Fortunately, the course of the disease in most cases is one of progressive improvement and eventual resolution. Parents must be informed that, although there is no cure, it is possible to control disease manifestations and that the disease improves or resolves with time in most patients. Treatment rests on educating the patient and family regarding dry-skin care, as in many cases a change in bathing habits and increased use of emollients improve the patient's condition markedly. Other therapies include the use of low or moderate potency steroids and, occasionally, tar or oatmeal baths. New topical immunomodulating agents such as tacrolimus and pimecrolinias show promise in the treatment of atopic dermatitis.

One also must watch vigilantly for secondary bacterial infections because *S. aureus* colonization is common in patients with atopic dermatitis. If a patient does not respond to emollients and steroids, empiric treatment with a short course of antistaphylococcal therapy is sometimes appropriate. A semisynthetic penicillin or the more pleasant-tasting cephalosporins are the drugs of choice (Table 11–20). Elimination diets usually are not helpful, although the occasional patient responds to the elimination of egg, milk, or nut products. Although uncommon, secondary infection of atopic lesions with HSV can occur and lead to generalized, erosive lesions (**eczema herpeticum**). When appropriate, a Tzanck preparation should be performed and acyclovir administered.

■ PAPULOSQUAMOUS ERUPTIONS

Papulosquamous eruptions denote a group of diverse diseases unified by the physical characteristics of discrete papules or plaques with superimposed scale. Papulosquamous lesions, in contrast to eczema, are almost always well marginated and lack epidermal changes such as oozing, fissuring, and scale crust. The differential diagnosis includes pityriasis rosea, seborrheic dermatitis, psoriasis, parapso-

Table 11–20. Approach to Treatment of Atopic Eczema

Break the itch–scratch cycle: Wear long-sleeve clothes, cotton mittens at night, trim fingernails, use antihistamines liberally

Decrease inflammation: Avoid irritating substances (e.g., wool, coarse fibers) and fiction, apply topical steroids or non-steroidal immunomodulators and emollients

Moisturize the skin: Take short, infrequent baths with tepid water, use moisturizers (e.g., petroleum creams and lotions) frequently

Treat secondary bacterial or fungal infection: Consider empiric antistaphylococcal therapy when a patient's condition proves resistant to conventional therapy; use mupirocin ointment for localized, secondarily infected sites or treatment; culture for yeast and fungi in intertriginous areas when appropriate

Educate the family regarding the chronic (but gradually improving) nature of the disease and the need to avoid drying and irritation

riasis, and secondary syphilis. KOH preparation and the Venereal Disease Research Laboratory test for syphilis should be performed when doubt exists as to the diagnosis. Two disorders, psoriasis and pityriasis rosea, are briefly discussed.

Psoriasis

Psoriasis is a chronic inflammatory disease with a strong genetic predisposition that afflicts 1–3% of the population. The disease can present in four distinct forms: (1) discrete scaling papules and plaques that favor the scalp, sebum-producing areas, knees, and elbows; (2) small ovoid or guttate lesions, which tend to generalize and frequently occur after infection, particularly streptococcal pharyngitis; (3) groups of pustules that favor the palms and soles but can occur elsewhere; and (4) a diffuse erythematous or erythrodermic eruption, often with pustules. Nail findings are also common and include discrete pitting, onycholysis, yellow discoloration, and distortion with subungual debris. Psoriasis is thought to be a T-cell–mediated disorder; recent research has focused on the role of calcium in the control of cell proliferation and adhesion in this disease. It is evident that the disorder leads to hyperproliferation of keratinocytes, with impaired differentiation and a relative increase in certain forms of keratin. Genetics certainly plays a significant role in the development of the disorder, but stress, trauma, and infection clearly can exacerbate the course of the disease.

Treatment is less than optimal and consists of emollients, topical steroids, tars, vitamin D_3 (calcipotriene), and phototherapy. Fortunately, many patients respond to sunlight and a decrease in stressful conditions. If a patient does not respond to therapy, one must look for evidence of secondary bacterial or fungal infection and treat the infection appropriately.

PITYRIASIS ROSEA

Pityriasis rosea, a self-limited inflammatory disorder of probable infectious origin, most commonly occurs in winter. The first lesion often consists of a red scaling plaque known as the "herald patch." Although pityriasis rosea is usually asymptomatic, some patients report a preceding "flu-like" illness, and the skin lesions are sometimes pruritic. The lesions initially tend to involve the upper trunk and then gradually extend to the abdomen and legs. They are ovoid, erythematous, and scaly and follow the lines of cleavage in what is referred to as a "Christmas tree" pattern. The palms and soles are not involved, but oral lesions consisting of white or hemorrhagic patches may be seen. Resolution may take 6–12 weeks. Treatment is not required, but ultraviolet light sometimes shortens the course, and topical steroids and antipruritics may be used for pruritic cases.

REFERENCES

Cohen BA: *Atlas of Pediatric Dermatology.* Mosby-Yearbook, 1999.

Eichenfield LF, Frieden IJ, Esterzy NB: *Neonatal dermatology.* Saunders, 2001.

Friedlander SF, Suarez S: Pediatric antifungal therapy. Dermatol Clin 1998;16:527.

Harper J, Orange A, Pruse N: *Textbook of Pediatric Dermatology.* Blackwell Science, 2000.

Hurwitz S: *Clinical Pediatric Dermatology: A Textbook of Skin Disorders of Childhood and Adolescence.* Saunders, 1993.

Leyden JJ: Therapy for acne vulgaris. N Engl J Med 1997;336:1156.

Schachner LA, Hansen RC (editors): *Pediatric Dermatology.* Churchill Livingstone, 1995.

Singalavanija S, Frieden IJ: Diaper dermatitis. Pediatr Rev 1995; 16:142.

Thornton CM, Eichenfield LF: Treatment of common cutaneous vascular disorders of childhood. Dermatol Ther 1997;2:68.

Tucker MA et al: Clinically recognized dysplastic nevi: a central risk factor for cutaneous melanoma. JAMA 1997;277:1439.

Weston WL, Lane AT, Morelli JG: *Color Textbook of Pediatric Dermatology.* Mosby-Year Book, 1996.

Williams ML, Pennella R: Melanoma, melanocytic nevi, and other melanoma risk factors in children. J Pediatr 1994;124:833.

The Gastrointestinal Tract & Liver 12

Donald Wayne Laney, Jr, MD

Gastrointestinal symptoms account for a large portion of pediatric outpatient visits and hospital admissions. This chapter presents an approach to evaluating the most frequently encountered gastrointestinal (GI) complaints: vomiting, diarrhea, constipation, abdominal pain, GI bleeding, and jaundice. Each section includes a discussion of pathophysiology, clinical approach (history, physical examination, diagnostic studies), differential diagnosis, and management. Specific diseases are discussed within the context of their most common presenting sign or symptom.

■ VOMITING

Vomiting is a common occurrence among pediatric patients; yet, despite the frequency with which episodes of vomiting occur, they tend to provoke anxiety and apprehension on the part of the caregivers. This emphasis on the importance of vomiting is often justified because vomiting may be the cardinal manifestation of one of several serious and potentially life-threatening disorders.

Physiology

Vomiting is a highly complex event involving the coordinated responses of the abdominal and respiratory musculature to a variety of stimuli delivered through the nervous system. The first phase in an episode of vomiting is the sensation of nausea. This feeling of the need to vomit may be brought on by emotional stimuli, by labyrinthine stimuli (e.g., motion sickness), by unpleasant tastes or odors, or through stimulation of mechanoreceptors or chemoreceptors in the GI tract. If vomiting is due to a cause that does not involve any of these pathways (e.g., increased intracranial pressure), nausea may be absent. Nausea is not always followed by vomiting, but when it is, the second phase in the process is retching.

Retching consists of increasingly forceful movements of the chest and abdominal musculature. Inspiratory efforts are made by the respiratory muscles while the abdominal muscles contract, causing negative intrathoracic pressure. As these events are occurring, the gastric fundus dilates and the pylorus and distal stomach contract. Retching may or may not culminate in emesis.

Emesis occurs as a combined result of sustained contraction of the abdominal muscles and contraction (downward movement) of most of the diaphragm. The central portion of the diaphragm, which normally serves to aid the lower esophageal sphincter in preventing gastroesophageal reflux (GER), must relax for emesis to occur.

A much less violent retrograde passage of gastric contents into the esophagus occurs in regurgitation. Regurgitation occurs without the forceful muscular contractions that characterize emesis. The symptoms of nausea and retching also are usually absent. Typically, regurgitation appears to be relatively effortless and painless, causing only minimal distress. Because occasional regurgitation is almost universal among normal infants and decreases in frequency with maturation, it is more properly viewed as a physiologic rather than a pathologic process. It becomes pathologic when it occurs with excessive frequency, as with GER.

Clinical Approach

An algorithm presenting a logical method for evaluating a child with vomiting is shown in Figure 12–1 and incorporates elements of the patient's history and physical examination and pertinent diagnostic studies.

HISTORY

The clinical history of a patient with vomiting often provides information that is helpful in narrowing the otherwise extensive list of possible causes (Table 12–1). Initially, one should assess the relative severity of the problem, i.e., whether the patient is experiencing truly forceful emesis or whether the events are more accurately described as regurgitation or spitting. In an infant who appears to be otherwise healthy and is growing normally, regurgitation is far more likely than is frank emesis. Conversely, a description of emesis exiting the mouth with unusual force (projectile vomiting) is classically associated with hypertrophic pyloric stenosis.

The patient's age at onset of symptoms also can provide clues to the etiology. Vomiting in the first few days after birth may be caused by obstructive lesions in the GI tract. Vomiting in early infancy also may be caused by one of many metabolic diseases. In an older infant, acute gastroenteritis becomes more likely. The coexistence of fever and diarrhea is also consistent with the diagnosis of acute

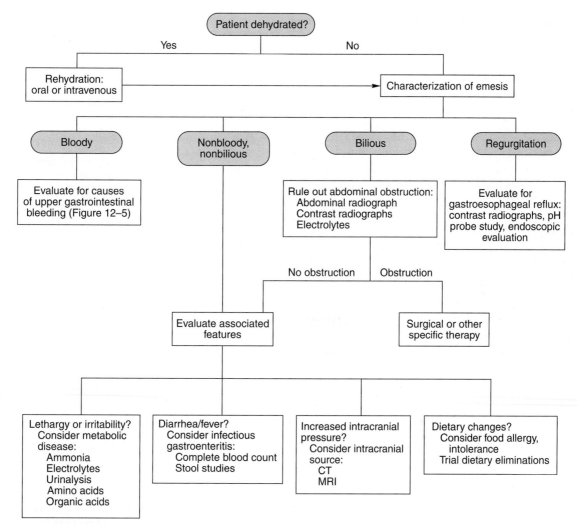

Figure 12–1. Algorithm presenting an approach to the evaluation of a patient with vomiting. CT = computed tomography; MRI = magnetic resonance imaging.

gastroenteritis. Food allergies or intolerances may present in children during the first year of life, as the composition of their diets becomes more varied. Children old enough to feed themselves may ingest inappropriate items, foods that have been contaminated or improperly prepared and/or stored, or nonfood items. In any of these situations, vomiting may occur.

Patients also should be asked about other symptoms associated with their vomiting. Abdominal pain associated with vomiting suggests the possibility of appendicitis or intestinal obstruction. Headache associated with vomiting may be due to migraine or to intracranial lesions.

Fever and diarrhea may be indicative of an infectious gastroenteritis.

A description of the vomitus itself also provides useful information. Bile staining of the emesis often indicates intestinal obstruction. The presence of blood in the vomitus (hematemesis) may be due to esophagitis, esophageal varices, gastritis, or peptic ulcers. Hematemesis also may occur secondary to swallowing blood from nasopharyngeal sources. A more thorough discussion of the clinical evaluation of patients with hematemesis is provided later in this chapter (see Upper Gastrointestinal Tract Hemorrhage, Clinical Approach).

Table 12–1. Differential Diagnosis: Vomiting

Anatomic causes	Infectious causes	Endocrinologic disorders
Malformations	Acute gastroenteritis[1]	Diabetes mellitus (especially with
Hypertrophic pyloric stenosis[1]	Meningitis	diabetic ketoacidosis)
Hiatal hernia	Sepsis	Diabetes insipidus
Intestinal duplications	Urinary tract infections	Congenital adrenal hyperplasia
Intestinal atresias	Hepatitis	**Dietary causes**
Malrotation	Appendicitis	Feeding problems[1]
Webs	Pneumonia	Overfeeding
Obstructions	Otitis media	Maternal anxiety or inexperience
Acquired gastric outlet obstruction	Oral candidiasis	Contaminated food or water
Chronic granulomatous disease	**Neurologic causes**	Food allergies and intolerances
Prostaglandin infusion	Intracranial neoplasms	Milk–soy protein intolerance[1]
Intussusception	Chronic subdural hematoma	Celiac disease
Volvulus	Hydrocephalus	**Toxin-induced**
Meconium ileus	Migraine	Poisons
Distal intestinal obstruction	Motion sickness	Pharmacologic and chemotherapeutic
syndrome	**Metabolic diseases**	agents
Bezoars	Urea cycle defects	Radiation
Hirschsprung disease	Aminoacidopathies	**Psychological**
Other	Organic acidurias	Cyclic (periodic) vomiting
Gastroesophageal reflux[1]	Galactosemia	Anorexia nervosa
Peptic ulcer disease	Hypercalcemia	Bulimia
Testicular torsion	Uremia	
Ménétrier disease		

[1] Frequently encountered causes of vomiting.

PHYSICAL EXAMINATION

Physical examination of a patient with vomiting should begin with an assessment of the patient's state of hydration (Figure 12–1). This is especially important in neonates and young infants because vomiting can rapidly lead to dehydration in those patients. Dehydration may be assessed by comparison of the patient's weight before the onset of illness, if available, with the weight obtained at the time of examination. If accurate weight comparison is not possible, the presence and degree of dehydration may be assessed using the clinical parameters listed in Table 12–9.

After assessing and addressing the patient's hydration status, other key features of the physical examination should be performed. Palpation of the abdomen may reveal abdominal distention or the presence of masses or organomegaly. The existence and site of tenderness or guarding should be noted. Jaundice may be observed in patients whose vomiting is due to hepatitis or to metabolic diseases involving the liver. Non-GI causes of vomiting often present with other characteristic physical findings (e.g., headaches and vision changes associated with vomiting due to disorders of the central nervous system).

DIAGNOSTIC STUDIES

Several laboratory investigations may be useful in the evaluation of a patient with vomiting. Evaluation of serum electrolytes is often beneficial. In hypertrophic pyloric stenosis, for example, a frequent characteristic finding is hypochloremic metabolic alkalosis. Metabolic acidosis may be due to dehydration or one of the many metabolic diseases associated with vomiting. Urine and serum evaluations for organic acids and amino acids may be indicated.

In patients in whom intestinal obstruction is suspected, abdominal radiographs can be useful. Contrast studies (barium swallow, upper GI series) and ultrasonography are two other potentially useful sources of information. Endoscopic visualization of the upper GI tract allows for direct mucosal visualization and the obtaining of biopsy specimens. Such studies may be helpful in the diagnosis of esophagitis, gastritis, or peptic ulcer disease. Esophageal pH monitoring can be used to document the reflux of acidic GI contents into the normally alkaline environment of the esophagus, as occurs in GER.

Differential Diagnosis

Vomiting may be the sole or major manifestation of a disease, as with GER, or may exist as one of a constellation of symptoms, as exemplified in several metabolic diseases. Table 12–1 lists many of the diseases known to cause vomiting. A thorough discussion of most of these entities may be found elsewhere in this text. In this chapter, we concentrate on those disorders in which vomiting is the predominant symptom and the GI tract is the site of the causative lesion.

HYPERTROPHIC PYLORIC STENOSIS

Hypertrophy of the circular muscle of the pylorus, which results in stenosis and gastric outlet obstruction, is a relatively common cause of vomiting, occurring in approximately 1 in 500 births. Male infants are affected more commonly than are female infants, and the incidence is far greater in full-term infants than in premature infants. The etiology of pyloric stenosis remains unknown, although several factors have been implicated. There is evidence suggesting that stenosis develops due to an intrinsic defect in enteric innervation. Nitric oxide serves as a vasodilator of vascular smooth muscle and has been shown to be deficient in the smooth muscle of the pylorus, thus facilitating contraction. Recent investigations have shown a localized increase in transforming growth factor α in the smooth muscle cells of the pylorus in patients with pyloric stenosis. This increase in transforming growth factor α may account for the hypertrophy of the pyloric muscle. In addition, edema due to the trauma of propelling the gastric contents against a narrowed pylorus probably adds to the degree of pyloric channel narrowing. Increased incidence of pyloric stenosis among infants whose siblings or mothers have pyloric stenosis suggests the existence of genetic factors in the etiology. It is likely that the disorder is a result of the combination of these and other factors.

Patients with hypertrophic pyloric stenosis typically experience the onset of nonbilious vomiting during the first few weeks after birth. The frequency of the episodes of vomiting increases, as does the force with which the vomitus is delivered, culminating in the projectile vomiting characteristic of this disorder. Affected infants are apparently hungry and initially take feedings eagerly. As the obstructed stomach is filled, reverse peristalsis begins; the rhythmic muscular contractions sometimes may be apparent on abdominal observation. As the disease progresses, emesis increases and dehydration develops.

In addition to those findings, the diagnosis of hypertrophic pyloric stenosis is supported by the palpation of the hypertrophied muscle itself, which has been described as an "olive" owing to similarities in size and shape. In a patient suspected of having pyloric stenosis, the finding of an olive is considered by some to be sufficient for diagnosis. The absence of a palpable olive, however, does not rule out the presence of stenosis. In cases where the diagnosis is not so clear-cut, radiologic studies may be helpful. Plain films of the abdomen may show absence of bowel gas distal to the pylorus, suggesting stenosis. Barium contrast studies are often more helpful and in patients with pyloric stenosis may show the passage of only a small amount of contrast material through the pylorus. This finding is referred to as a "string sign" and is illustrated by the radio-

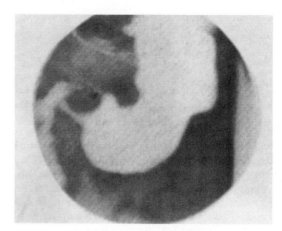

Figure 12–2. Characteristic radiographic findings in hypertrophic pyloric stenosis. The narrow, elongated pyloric channel causes the barium to appear as a thin "string," a finding often referred to as the "string sign." (Reproduced, with permission, from Rudolph AM [editor]: *Pediatrics*, 18th ed. Appleton & Lange, 1987.)

graph shown in Figure 12–2. Many clinicians rely on ultrasound for the diagnosis of pyloric stenosis. With ultrasound, the thickness of the pyloric muscle and its diameter may be measured. These measurements, or a ratio of the two, are then compared with established normal measurements. In experienced hands, ultrasound has proved to be sensitive and specific in the diagnosis of pyloric stenosis.

Management of patients with pyloric stenosis should begin with assessment of hydration and correction of fluid and electrolyte abnormalities. Hypochloremic hypokalemic metabolic alkalosis has been classically associated with pyloric stenosis, but with earlier diagnosis, this electrolyte disturbance is seen less often. Even without such severe fluid problems, however, patients often are found to have some degree of dehydration, and fluid deficits should be corrected before initiation of definitive therapy. Surgical correction of stenosis by pyloromyotomy, using an open or a laparoscopic approach, is the most commonly employed treatment method. Balloon dilatation also has been used. Although some investigators have reported resolution of stenosis and overall good outcome with gastric drainage and pharmacologic acid suppression, such noninterventional therapy currently is not widely accepted.

OTHER ANATOMIC MALFORMATIONS

Several other anatomic malformations of the GI tract can cause vomiting. **Hiatal hernias** occur when the abdominal esophagus and a portion of the gastric fundus protrude above the diaphragm into the thoracic cavity. This may lead to a decrease in the competence of the lower esophageal sphincter mechanism and be associated with vomiting or GER (see below, Gastroesophageal Reflux). In many patients, however, these hernias are asymptomatic.

Atresias are malformations in which the lumen normally present in an organ is not developed. **Stenoses** are similar disorders involving lumenal narrowing. Atresias occur in the esophagus and throughout the small and large intestine. Duodenal atresia is associated with Down syndrome and several other congenital malformations including intestinal malrotation, annular pancreas, and imperforate anus. Duodenal atresia is recognizable radiographically as the "double bubble" sign, consisting of air in the stomach and the distended first portion of the duodenum. There is absence of intraluminal gas distal to the duodenum (Figure 12–3). Atresia is more common in the jejunum and ileum than in the duodenum.

Patients with intestinal atresias present with bilious vomiting and abdominal distention, sometimes with palpable loops of bowel. In neonates, there may be failure to

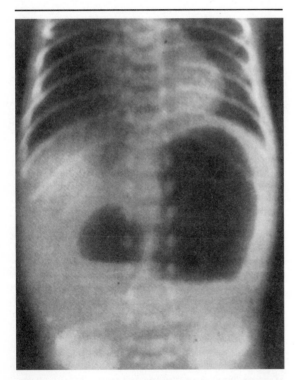

Figure 12–3. Abdominal radiograph demonstrating the "double bubble" characteristic of duodenal obstruction. (Reproduced, with permission, from Rudolph AM [editor]: *Pediatrics,* 18th ed. Appleton & Lange, 1987.)

pass meconium. Treatment begins with the restoration of fluid and electrolyte balance and relief of the obstructive symptoms through nasogastric suction. Definitive treatment is then accomplished surgically.

MALROTATION & VOLVULUS

During normal fetal development, the intestines undergo counterclockwise rotation and then are affixed to the posterior abdominal wall. When this process is not accomplished properly, malrotation results. The cecum lies in the right upper quadrant, and the duodenal–jejunal region is on the right side of the abdomen. Although malrotation itself may not cause symptoms, it allows for the occurrence of a volvulus, in which a segment of intestine twists on itself and causes obstruction. This may present in a manner similar to intestinal atresias, with bilious vomiting and abdominal distention. Radiographic studies may show the "double bubble" sign, as seen in duodenal atresia, or provide other information useful in determining the specific anatomic configuration. Volvulus is corrected surgically.

GASTROINTESTINAL OBSTRUCTIONS

In addition to anatomic obstructions, the GI tract may become obstructed by stasis of lumenal contents. In patients with **meconium ileus,** for example, the normally soft meconium is abnormally viscid and causes intestinal obstruction. This condition is seen almost exclusively in patients with cystic fibrosis (see Chapter 18, Respiratory Diseases). Patients demonstrate signs and symptoms typical of intestinal obstruction, including abdominal distention and vomiting. Rectal examination usually shows a narrow rectum empty of stool. When this diagnosis is suspected, a sweat test for cystic fibrosis is indicated. Barium enema studies may be useful in showing the presence of microcolon and simultaneously accomplishing removal of the meconium obstruction. If the obstruction is not relieved by barium enema, surgical removal is required. The **meconium ileus equivalent syndrome,** also known as **distal intestinal obstruction syndrome,** is a similar phenomenon that occurs in older patients with cystic fibrosis. In these patients, abdominal distention and pain are more common presenting symptoms than is vomiting.

Bezoars are collections of indigestible material found in the GI tract, usually the stomach. Bezoars may be composed of undigested milk solids (**lactobezoars**), hair (**trichobezoars**), or undigested vegetable matter (**phytobezoars**). Typically these masses cause gastric outlet obstruction and produce symptoms of vomiting with abdominal pain and distention, often accompanied by anorexia and weight loss. Examination may show an abdominal mass; halitosis is often noted. Lactobezoars are often digested if the stomach is kept otherwise empty for a few days and the patient nourished intravenously. Other bezoars may require surgical removal.

GASTROESOPHAGEAL REFLUX

Gastroesophageal reflux is probably the most common cause of vomiting among pediatric patients. It is distinguished from most other causes of vomiting in that episodes are typically effortless (without retching) and often unaccompanied by pain. It is probably more appropriate to refer to such symptoms as regurgitation rather than vomiting.

Gastroesophageal reflux occurs when gastric contents are propelled retrograde from the stomach into the esophagus. Reflux is a normal phenomenon in the postprandial period in adults and children and usually described as heartburn. It is also considered to be "physiologic" during the first few months of life because the lower esophageal sphincter mechanism is not yet functionally mature. This functional immaturity, coupled with the infant's liquid diet and recumbent posture, allows gastric contents to be regurgitated easily. In most patients, reflux episodes are little more than a nuisance necessitating frequent clothing changes, and their frequency gradually decreases during the first year of life.

For some babies, however, reflux is associated with other symptoms that are less benign than simple spitting up. If regurgitation is so severe that much of the feedings are lost, growth may be affected and failure to thrive may occur. Frequent or prolonged exposure of the esophagus to acid may produce esophagitis with pain (often manifested by fussiness), odynophagia, and even blood loss from the inflamed esophageal mucosa. If esophagitis is severe, the patient is at risk for the development of esophageal strictures. In addition to failure to thrive and esophagitis, reflux may be complicated by respiratory symptoms including cough, wheezing, recurrent upper respiratory disorders, apnea and cyanosis, and occasionally, aspiration pneumonia.

The diagnosis of GER often may be made solely on the basis of the patient's history and physical examination. A child who is growing normally, is otherwise healthy, and whose parents report spontaneous, effortless episodes of regurgitation almost certainly has GER. For patients with complicated reflux, as described above, a more rigorous diagnostic approach is often useful. A barium swallow or upper GI series is helpful in evaluating esophageal anatomy and ruling out anatomic defects. It is not uncommon for reflux of the contrast material into the esophagus to be observed during such studies. However, the absence of observed regurgitation episodes should not be interpreted as evidence that reflux is not occurring, but only that reflux was not occurring at the time of observation. For a more accurate assessment of the frequency and duration of reflux episodes, an intraesophageal pH probe study is appropriate. These studies may be continued for several hours and allow for correlation of clinical events (e.g., coughing, fussiness) with intraesophageal pH readings. Many consider the pH study to be the "gold standard" for the diagnosis of GER.

Several other diagnostic studies can be useful in the diagnosis of GER in children. Esophageal manometry allows for the measurement of esophageal sphincter pressures and may further aid in the diagnosis of reflux. Direct visualization of the esophageal mucosa is possible with endoscopy and allows one to obtain mucosal specimens for histologic evaluation. Mucosal biopsy is especially important if esophagitis has been chronic or severe and there is a possibility of metaplasia of the esophageal mucosa (Barrett's esophagus). If delayed gastric emptying is suspected as another factor in the patient's regurgitation, radionuclide (gastric emptying) scans may provide additional useful information.

The selection of treatment for GER should take into account the severity of the symptoms and their possible consequences. When reflux is so mild that normal growth and development are not impaired, minimal intervention is appropriate. Intervention may include changing the infant's sleeping position from supine (the position recommended by the American Academy of Pediatrics because of a decreased incidence of sudden infant death syndrome among infants sleeping in that position) to a side or prone position, with the head of the crib slightly elevated. In the prone position, aspiration is less likely; elevation of the head of the crib makes reflux mechanically more difficult and consequently less likely. Changes in feedings also may be beneficial; this includes the use of smaller volumes, offered at more frequent intervals, and the use of cereals and other foods to thicken the feedings.

In patients with more severe symptoms, pharmacotherapy is sometimes helpful. Antacids, histamine H_2-receptor antagonists, and proton-pump inhibitor drugs may be used to decrease the acidity of gastric contents, thus decreasing the risk of esophageal damage secondary to reflux. Metoclopramide has been commonly used in treating GER because it increases lower esophageal sphincter pressure and hastens gastric emptying. Cisapride, a promotility agent, had gained widespread use in the treatment of significant GER in children, although data documenting efficacy was largely lacking. Despite well-publicized warnings from the manufacturer regarding the possibility of potentially fatal cardiac arrhythmias occurring in a subgroup of patients (e.g., those with cardiac disease, those taking other medications metabolized through the hepatic cytochrome P-450 enzymes), several deaths were reported in relation to Cisapride and the drug has been withdrawn from the market.

In some patients who do not benefit from pharmacotherapy, surgical procedures aimed at improving the competence of the lower esophageal sphincter may be helpful. The Nissen fundoplication is the procedure most commonly used and may be done through a traditional open approach or laparascopically.

Management

Specific therapies have been mentioned in conjunction with the previously discussed disease entities. Regardless of the etiology of vomiting, several general management techniques are important.

Because of the possibility of dehydration resulting from vomiting, initial management should include restoration of adequate hydration. In patients with acute infectious gastroenteritis associated with vomiting, rehydration may be successfully achieved orally, as discussed later in this chapter (see Oral Rehydration). However, if the severity of the emesis precludes adequate fluid delivery orally, intravenous administration is necessary. Having addressed the patient's fluid status and simultaneously corrected any electrolyte abnormalities, further diagnostic studies may be performed.

With long-standing vomiting complicated by malnutrition and failure to thrive, nutritional replenishment is also important. In many instances, this requires parenteral delivery of nutrients.

Pharmacologic agents should be used with great caution to stop vomiting in children. This is especially true in children who cannot adequately communicate symptoms to their caregivers. In those children, antiemetic agents may mask the outward signs of disease even as the problem progresses. An exception to such limited use of antiemetics is in patients receiving chemotherapeutic agents and radiation therapy. In those and other situations in which the cause of vomiting is apparent, the use of antiemetics is indicated.

■ CONSTIPATION

Constipation is frequently encountered in children, especially in more developed countries where a diet composed largely of highly refined foods is the norm. Effective evaluation of constipation requires an understanding of normal defecation physiology and normal stooling patterns. This allows the clinician to determine whether a situation perceived to be a problem is truly abnormal or whether the patient's stooling pattern merely is not meeting the parents' expectations for normalcy.

Anatomy & Physiology

The colon terminates in the rectum, which in turn passes through the levator ani muscles and becomes the anal canal. The anal canal is circled by two groups of muscles, the internal and external anal sphincters. The internal sphincter, composed of smooth muscle, is under involuntary (reflex) control. The external sphincter provides a means of voluntary control over defecation. Also important in the control of defecation is the near 90-degree

angle formed at the junction of the rectum and the anal canal. This junction straightens with flexion of the hips, which explains the physiologic advantage of squatting for defecation.

The fecal mass is propelled distally through the intestine by peristalsis. In the colon, water is passively reabsorbed, making the feces more solid. Stools eventually reach the rectal ampulla, where they distend the rectum and activate a neuromuscular pathway resulting in relaxation of the internal anal sphincter and contraction of the external anal sphincter. Relaxation of the internal sphincter allows the rectal contents to come in contact with the sensory epithelium of the anal canal, where their nature (i.e., solid, liquid, or gas) is discernible. To defecate, the external sphincter and the puborectalis sling are voluntarily relaxed, allowing stool to pass the anus. A voluntary increase in intraabdominal pressure (Valsalva maneuver) assists the process.

A definition of "normal" stooling patterns involves several parameters, including stool size, consistency, and frequency. For more than 90% of adults, stooling occurs from three times per day to three times per week. For children, however, more frequent stooling may be normal. In infants, stooling is normally much more frequent, occurring from one to seven times per day in the first week. Stooling may continue at this frequency in breast-fed infants, but in formula-fed infants, stool frequency tends to decrease over subsequent weeks. In the toddler years, stooling typically decreases further in frequency, so that preschool children usually have bowel patterns more similar to those of adults.

Stool size and consistency are much more difficult to measure objectively than is stool frequency, yet even subjective information is useful in determining whether a patient has constipation. Stools that cause extreme discomfort in passing, because of excessive size or extreme firmness, are abnormal. Thus, constipation is present when stools are excessively large, uncomfortably large, or abnormally infrequent. It is important to keep in mind, however, that this definition allows for a broad range of "normal" and that which is perceived by a parent as abnormal in fact may be physiologic for a particular patient.

Clinical Approach

An algorithm outlining an approach to the evaluation of a patient with constipation is presented in Figure 12–4, and begins with a history and physical examination.

HISTORY

Several points are of special importance in the history of a patient with constipation. The child's age at the onset of symptoms may be significant. Patients with Hirschsprung's disease, for example, often have had symptoms since birth. Constipation due to other causes

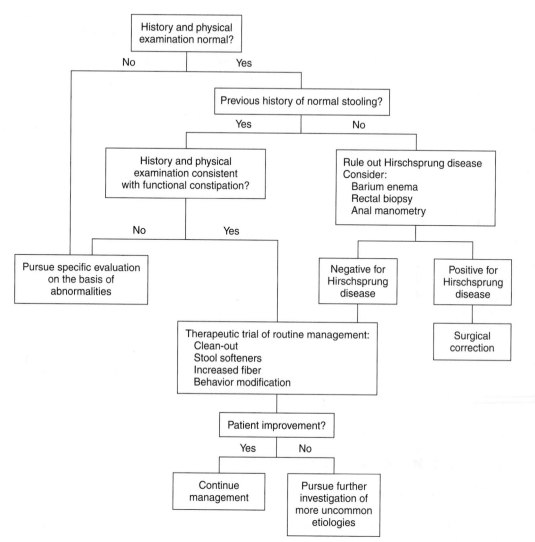

Figure 12–4. Algorithm presenting an approach to the diagnosis and management of the patient with constipation.

may present after a period of normal stooling. The history of the child's toilet training and subsequent fecal control is useful. Also important is the association of pain with defecation (**tenesmus**) or the passage of blood (**hematochezia).** The child's psychosocial situation also may be pertinent to the diagnosis.

The dietary history can provide helpful information. Breast-fed infants, at least in the first few weeks after birth, tend to have looser and more frequent stools than do formula-fed infants. Children who drink excessive amounts of cow's milk may be more prone to constipation. Diets low in fiber also can predispose the patient to constipation. Medications can be a factor because numerous pharma-

cologic agents, such as narcotics and anticholinergics, are known to cause constipation.

PHYSICAL EXAMINATION

The physical assessment should proceed with a thorough general examination. Inspection of the lower back, for example, may show a sacral dimple, possibly indicating the involvement of a spinal cord lesion. Examination of the abdomen should include palpation because large fecal masses often can be detected in the descending colon.

The rectal examination should begin with visual inspection of the anal skin, noting the presence of any skin tags, fissures, or other abnormalities. Evaluation of the neuromuscular integrity of the anus may be grossly gauged by attempting to elicit the reflex anal "wink" by lightly stroking the perianal skin with a cotton swab. Digital examination provides a means of evaluating the resting tone of the external sphincter and the relative capacity of the anal vault. Any stool present on the examining glove should be tested for the presence of occult blood.

DIAGNOSTIC STUDIES

The initial history and physical examination may show abnormalities or arouse suspicion of specific organic problems known to cause constipation. These possibilities should be evaluated with the appropriate diagnostic tests. In most patients with constipation, the initial history and physical examination will show no other problems.

Differential Diagnosis

A partial listing of the causes of constipation is given in Table 12–2. Despite this broad range of differential diagnosis, the vast majority of patients are found to have no discernible cause for their symptoms and thus are labeled

Table 12–2. Differential Diagnosis: Constipation

Anatomic defects
  Localized to the anus, rectum, or colon
    Aganglionosis
      Congenital (Hirschsprung disease)[1]
      Acquired (Chagas disease)
    Anal stenosis[1]
    Imperforate anus (postsurgical correction)
    Anterior ectopic anus
    Anteriorly located anus
    Anal fissures
    Dermatitis
    Colonic stricture
      Primary
      Secondary (e.g., secondary to inflammatory bowel
        disease or necrotizing enterocolitis)
  Localized to the gastrointestinal tract
    Malrotation
    Congenital intestinal bands
    Stenosis
    Gastric emptying defects (e.g., pyloric stenosis)
  Generalized
    Abnormal abdominal musculature
      Eagle–Barrett syndrome
      Gastroschisis, postrepair
      Postabdominal surgery
    Neurologic
      Spina bifida
      Meningomyelocele
      Spinal cord trauma
      Paraplegia
      Sacral teratoma

Endocrinologic or metabolic defects
  Hypothyroidism
  Hyperparathyroidism
  Pregnancy
  Diabetes insipidus
  Infantile renal acidosis
  Hypokalemia, hyponatremia
  Uremia

Neurologic defects
  Central nervous system defects (e.g., cerebral palsy)
  Spinal cord trauma
  Infectious polyneuritis
  Amyotonia congenita
  Neurofibromatosis
  Down syndrome
  Hypotonia

Neuromuscular/motility disorders
  Idiopathic slow transit constipation
  Pseudo-obstruction syndromes
  Infant botulism

Connective tissue disorders
  Lupus erythematosus
  Scleroderma

Psychological disorders
  Depression
  Anorexia nervosa
  Denial of bowel action
  Stool withholding[1]
  Sexual abuse

Dietary causes
  Inadequate dietary fiber
  Excessive cow's milk intake

Pharmacologic causes
  Antacids (especially those containing calcium and aluminum)
  Anticholinergics
  Bismuth
  Iron preparations
  Opiates

Idiopathic constipation[1]

[1] Frequently encountered causes of constipation.

as having chronic functional (or idiopathic) constipation. It is important to keep in mind, however, that the likelihood of diagnosing certain etiologies changes with the age of the patient. In children who are younger than 1 year of age, the possibility of Hirshsprung's disease (see below) and other secondary etiologies should be specifically considered. When constipation first presents in an older child, these diagnoses are far less likely and "functional" constipation is the most common diagnosis.

Several of the most common GI etiologies presenting with constipation are discussed below. Non-GI causes, such as hypothyroidism, infant botulism, and medication-induced constipation, always should be considered.

FUNCTIONAL CONSTIPATION & ENCOPRESIS

Patients with functional constipation may present with complaints of abdominal distention or recurrent abdominal pain in addition to a history of infrequent, often large stools. The results of the physical examination are usually entirely normal, with the exception of palpable fecal masses in the lower colon and an enlarged, stool-filled rectal vault.

Some patients with functional constipation also may have a lack of voluntary control over defecation (encopresis). Encopresis develops as a result of long-standing constipation with progressive enlargement of the rectal vault. Eventually, the sensation prompting an urge to defecate is lost. Large fecal masses accumulate in the rectum, allowing only liquid stool to pass. Soiling of the underclothing occurs commonly. When the large stool is finally passed, it is often associated with great discomfort. The association of pain with defecation discourages the patient from voluntarily passing stools, leading to continued stooling infrequency and perpetuation of the cycle. In addition to the physical unpleasantness of their condition, patients with encopresis are subject to social and behavioral problems. Understandably, other children often avoid them, making them social outcasts.

Although patients with encopresis are typically of early school age, the stool-withholding behavior that is often the initial cause of their problem may be seen in much younger children. This often occurs in 2- to 3-year-old children and may develop in response to attempts at toilet training or a previous episode of painful defecation (e.g., rectal fissures). Symptoms such as grimacing and grunting are often erroneously interpreted by the parents as signs of difficulty with defecation. In fact, these signs may accompany a child's voluntary withholding of stool. Appropriate treatment of stool withholding with agents such as fiber or simple laxatives (nonabsorbable carbohydrates or salts) may prevent the problems from progressing to chronic constipation.

Successful treatment of functional constipation and encopresis is almost always achieved by using a combination of therapies beginning with bowel evacuation and then followed by the use of stool softeners and the implementation of behavioral modification techniques. Treatment of the psychosocial aspects of the disease may require the involvement of experienced mental health personnel.

The first step in treatment is to remove fecal material from the colon. In many of these patients, the rectal vault has been stretched far beyond its normal capacity by the accumulation of stool. Removal of this material rarely may require manual disimpaction but is usually accomplished through the use of enemas. A variety of enema solutions have been used for this purpose. Plain water enemas have been associated with the development of water intoxication and are not recommended. Sodium biphosphate enemas are commercially available in adult and pediatric sizes; although these products are commonly used, caution is necessary because hyperphosphatemia and hypernatremia have occurred secondary to their administration. A preparation of equal parts of milk and molasses has long been used successfully in treating patients at Children's Hospital Medical Center in Cincinnati, Ohio, with no known side effects. Regardless of the preparation used, enemas should be continued on a twice-daily basis until the colon is evacuated (usually fewer than 3 days). Colonic clean-out also can be achieved through the use of oral laxatives or cathartics (magnesium citrate) or by the oral or nasogastric administration of polyethylene glycol–electrolyte solutions. The subsequent use of enemas or cathartics is usually not needed after the initial cleansing.

The second step in the management of constipation is aimed toward the production of smaller, softer stools so that frequent defecation is unavoidable. This more frequent stooling eventually leads to the return of the rectal vault to normal size and, consequently, to the return of sensation of the need to defecate. Multiple pharmacologic agents, including stool lubricants (mineral oil), osmotic agents (lactulose), and stimulants (senna, bisacodyl), have been shown to be effective in this stage of therapy. Mineral oil is an inexpensive and safe agent widely used for this purpose; however, because of the risks of aspiration, it should be used cautiously in the young child. The dose should be titrated so that the patient has bowel movements twice daily to every other day. Once stooling patterns have returned to normal, the medications should be tapered and eventually discontinued. Patients typically require these medications for several months. Increasing the dietary fiber content, with commercially available supplements or through dietary modification, is also beneficial in alleviating the symptoms of constipation.

Behavioral modification also plays an important role in the management of constipation. Patients should be encouraged to have established, routine periods of sitting on the toilet once or twice each day. Preferably, those times should be soon after meals to take advantage of the increased colonic motility induced by gastric activity (the gastrocolic reflex). For younger children, praise for the successful elimination of stool may be helpful. For all patients, the use of criticism or other negative approaches should be avoided. As part of behavior modification, the patient and family can be encouraged to improve their dietary habits by decreasing intake of highly refined foods and increasing intake of foods high in fiber.

Probably the most important facet of the treatment of constipation is education of the patient and family. Most are pleasantly surprised to learn that constipation is a common problem that can almost always be treated successfully. Involvement in support groups with other patients assists in the education process and may help to lessen those children's feelings of being abnormal. Patient education and encouragement should be an important part of the follow-up care of these patients.

HIRSCHSPRUNG'S DISEASE

In young children with constipation, especially those younger than 1 year of age, the diagnosis of Hirschsprung's disease must always be considered. This congenital disorder is characterized by an absence of ganglion cells from the myenteric (Auerbach) and submucosal (Meissner) plexuses of the rectum. The aganglionic segment includes the internal anal sphincter as its most caudal point and extends proximally for a variable distance. In most patients with Hirschsprung's disease, the aganglionic segment is limited to the sigmoid colon, but it may extend throughout the colon and has been known to extend as far as the duodenum. If the aganglionic segment involves only a few centimeters of the rectum, it is referred to as ultrashort segment disease.

The absence of ganglion cells causes the affected segment to be constantly contracted and without peristalsis. This creates a functional obstruction, which causes proximal intestinal dilatation and hypertrophy, manifested clinically as constipation, abdominal distention, and bilious vomiting. Hirschsprung's disease often is diagnosed soon after an infant is born because of the delayed passage of meconium (later than 48 hours after birth). When the disease is not diagnosed in the neonatal period, clinical features typically include failure to thrive in addition to the previously listed symptoms.

Fecal soiling is uncommon in patients with aganglionosis, except in those in whom only a very short segment of the colon is affected. Older patients with Hirschsprung's disease may report absence of sensation of the need to defecate because fecal contents do not come in contact with the sensory epithelium of the anal mucosa, where this sensation is triggered. Rectal examination usually is remarkable for increased sphincter tone, often described as a "sleeve effect." There may be little or no stool in the rectal vault, despite stool being palpable on abdominal examination. Frequently, withdrawal of the examining finger is followed by a sudden expulsion of stool.

The most severe complication of untreated Hirschsprung's disease is the development of enterocolitis. This condition, characterized by fever, heme-positive and watery stools, and abdominal distention, occurs in approximately one third of patients with Hirschsprung's disease. In some cases, the enterocolitis is mild and not detected until the time of surgical resection of the aganglionic segment. Typically, however, patients with enterocolitis are extremely ill, and about one third do not survive, making this the most likely cause of death in patients with Hirschsprung's disease. Enterocolitis associated with aganglionosis does not occur in patients older than 2 years.

The diagnosis of Hirschsprung's disease should begin with a very careful history, including a diligent attempt to determine the patient's age at onset of symptoms. Although Hirschsprung's disease may first be diagnosed in later childhood or even adulthood, careful history almost always shows the presence of symptoms from the neonatal period. Constipation symptoms that begin after the first few weeks of life are very unlikely to be secondary to aganglionosis.

The diagnosis of Hirschsprung's disease may be confirmed by information obtained from several studies. A plain radiograph of the abdomen, taken in the prone position, that shows the absence of intraintestinal air in the pelvis is suggestive of Hirschsprung's disease and necessitates further studies. A barium enema is often effective in delineating the location of the transition zone between the normal and aganglionic segments. It also may show a rectal diameter narrower than that of the sigmoid colon, which is typical of Hirschsprung's disease. To provide useful information in making this diagnosis, barium enemas should be done without prior evacuation of the colon by enemas or cathartics. Manometric studies of the anus are also useful in the diagnosis of aganglionosis. Distention of a balloon-tipped catheter in normal patients stimulates reflex relaxation of the internal anal sphincter. In patients with Hirschsprung's disease, however, the internal sphincter contracts. This study is especially useful in the diagnosis of patients whose aganglionic segment is 5 cm or shorter. Tissue obtained from rectal biopsy allows for a definitive diagnosis. Although this tissue may be obtained surgically, a more usual method is through the use of suction-assisted biopsy forceps. Histologic examination shows the absence of ganglion cells. Staining for acetylcholinesterase, an enzyme present in parasympathetic nerve fibers, shows abnormally prominent nerve fibers in the rectal mucosa of patients with Hirschsprung's disease.

Management should begin with stabilization of acutely ill patients, including restoration of fluid and electrolyte balance, administration of broad-spectrum antibiotics, and evacuation of the colon with enemas. Definitive treatment requires surgical intervention typically involving the creation of a colostomy to provide relief of the obstruction, followed by reanastomosis of the normal portion of the colon with the rectum at a later date. Recently, however, several pediatric surgeons have been successful in removing the aganglionic segment with a laparascopic and transanal approach. This procedure allows for a complete repair in one operation and alleviates the need for a colostomy. In patients with short-segment and ultrashort-segment disease, an anorectal myomectomy may provide effective relief of the obstruction.

OTHER GASTROINTESTINAL CAUSES OF CONSTIPATION

Several congenital anatomic defects of the anorectal region have been associated with constipation. **Anal stenosis** may cause stools to be of abnormally small caliber and thus lead to chronic stool retention. In mild cases, this may be corrected by progressive dilation of the anus with the examining finger. **Anterior ectopic anus** and **anteriorly located anus** are conditions that cause constipation, most often in females, beginning in early infancy. With an anterior ectopic anus, the anal canal and internal sphincter exit anterior to the normally located external sphincter. Rectal examination of patients with this disorder may show a "rectal shelf" posterior to the anal opening. With an anteriorly located anus, the anal canal and the external sphincter are located anterior to their normal position. In either disorder, the anal wink may be present in its normal location. Both conditions may require surgical repair for symptomatic relief.

Strictures of the colon also can cause obstruction and consequent constipation. These may be congenital anatomic defects or may occur later in life secondary to other disorders. In the neonate, strictures may arise secondary to necrotizing enterocolitis. In older children, inflammatory bowel disease (IBD) may be the cause. Correction usually entails surgical resection of the affected portion of the bowel.

Disorders of GI motility may also produce constipation. **Intestinal pseudo-obstruction** is a condition in which motility of all or portions of the intestine are abnormal. Patients experience symptoms of obstruction, including dysphagia and vomiting, in addition to constipation, without any anatomic obstruction. Management of patients with these disorders may require dietary modifications and the use of stool softeners and laxatives to prevent constipation. Prokinetic agents also are often used in the treatment of pseudo-obstruction.

Management

Management of constipation should be directed toward resolution of the specific underlying problem. In patients with idiopathic or functional constipation and in those with constipation secondary to causes that cannot be corrected (e.g., cerebral palsy), therapy must be directed toward lessening the symptoms. Treatment of functional constipation and encopresis have been described in detail above.

■ GASTROINTESTINAL TRACT HEMORRHAGE

Bleeding from the GI tract usually is classified as "upper" or "lower" on the basis of the location of the bleeding site proximal or distal, respectively, to the ligament of Treitz (near the duodenojejunal junction). Bleeding from upper tract lesions usually results in **hematemesis** (vomiting blood), whereas bleeding from lower tract lesions is more apt to present as loss of blood per rectum (**melena**: dark tarry stools containing digested blood; **hematochezia**: bright red blood in the stools). These two groups of disorders are sufficiently distinct that they are discussed as separate entities. We first consider the diagnosis and management of upper GI bleeding.

UPPER GASTROINTESTINAL TRACT HEMORRHAGE

Clinical Approach

An algorithm outlining a systematic approach for the evaluation of a patient with upper GI tract bleeding is presented in Figure 12–5. This pathway begins with assessment of the patient's hemodynamic status and relies mainly on data obtained from the physical examination and diagnostic studies. A thorough history, however, is also an essential part of the diagnostic process.

HISTORY

Hematemesis is a very frightening experience for the patient and the family. It is crucial to allay this anxiety and carefully obtain as much historical data as possible. History should include the time of the hematemesis and its relation, if any, to other events, including ingestion of food or other substances. One also should ask if the episode was preceded or accompanied by pain. An estimate of the amount of blood in the vomitus is another important fact, as is a description of its color (i.e., bright red vs. dark). One should ascertain whether the blood was truly vomited, or whether it was produced effortlessly, as can occur with bleeding from esophageal varices.

PHYSICAL EXAMINATION

The most important initial step in the physical examination of a patient with upper GI bleeding it to assess hemodynamic status: blood pressure decreases and pulse rate increases with acute blood loss. The hematocrit, in contrast, serves as a better measure of chronic blood loss and may not accurately reflect the patient's status during or soon after an acute bleed. Hemodynamic instability, if present, should be addressed immediately through administration of appropriate intravenous fluids and blood

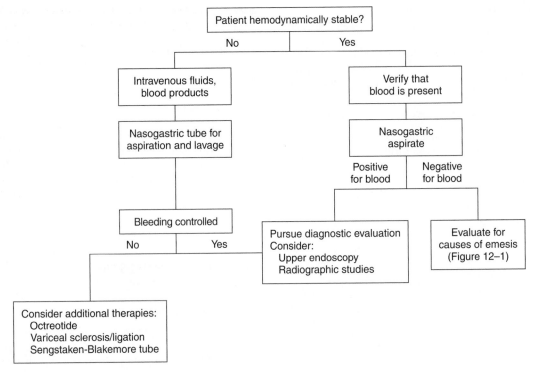

Figure 12–5. Algorithm presenting an approach to the evaluation of the patient with bleeding from the upper gastrointestinal tract.

products. Excessive administration of fluids and blood products, especially in patients whose bleeding is secondary to esophageal varices, actually may increase bleeding and forestall efforts at hemostasis.

After assessing and addressing the patient's fluid status, one may then proceed with a thorough examination. Any abnormal findings can provide clues as to the etiology of the bleeding. Hepatomegaly, for example, may indicate underlying liver disease and suggest a variceal source of the blood.

DIAGNOSTIC STUDIES

The next important step in the evaluation of a patient with hematemesis is to determine the site of bleeding. Placement of a nasogastric tube to aspirate gastric contents is useful in this step of the evaluation. Absence of blood in the gastric aspirate may indicate that the source of bleeding is in the nasopharynx; however, an aspirate that tests positive for hemoglobin does not rule out the nasopharynx as the source because blood may have been swallowed. Another potential explanation for a negative gastric aspirate is that the substance perceived to be blood is actually some other red substance. Food colorings found in beverages and gelatin products may impart a red color

to the vomitus and be mistaken for blood. The presence of apparently fresh, bright red blood in the gastric aspirate is evidence of an actively bleeding lesion. Blood that has been partly altered by the gastric contents may have the appearance of "coffee grounds."

In addition to evaluation of the gastric aspirate, radiographic studies may aid in the localization of bleeding. Contrast studies (barium swallow, upper GI series, small bowel follow-through) may provide evidence of ulcers and other gross mucosal lesions. The absence of visible lesions on radiographs should not be interpreted as ruling out mucosal lesions because lesions that are small or out of the plane of the image may not be detectable.

For most patients with hematemesis, upper endoscopy (esophagogastroduodenoscopy) is the diagnostic procedure of choice. Endoscopy allows not only for direct visualization of the mucosa but also for obtaining tissue for subsequent histologic evaluation. Information from biopsies is crucial in appropriately diagnosing gastritis and esophagitis. Endoscopy also may provide the best means of achieving hemostasis in a patient with ongoing upper GI tract bleeding. Techniques including injection of sclerosing agents and placing bands for ligation may be performed endoscopically under direct visualization.

Differential Diagnosis

Many diseases are known to cause bleeding localized to the upper GI tract (Table 12–3). Diseases that cause vascular lesions and coagulopathies may present with bleeding in the upper or lower GI tract and, with the exception of esophageal varices, are not specifically discussed in this chapter. The remaining causes of upper GI bleeding are attributable to mucosal damage in the duodenum, stomach, or esophagus.

ESOPHAGEAL MUCOSAL DISORDERS

Esophagitis describes a nonspecific inflammatory response of the esophageal mucosa to a variety of noxious stimuli. The diagnosis of esophagitis is suspected when endoscopic observation shows erythematous, eroded, or ulcerated mucosa. Biopsy specimens characteristically show increased numbers of intraepithelial eosinophils. Esophagitis varies in severity, and only the more severe cases present with upper GI bleeding.

Most cases of esophagitis in pediatric patients are secondary to the prolonged and recurrent exposure of the esophageal mucosa to acidic gastric contents that occurs with GER. In its most severe manifestation, this form of esophagitis not only results in upper GI bleeding but also potentiates the development of esophageal stricture.

Infectious microorganisms also can cause esophagitis. Most frequently, these infections occur in patients whose immune mechanisms are suppressed pathologically or pharmacologically. *Candida* is the most common agent identified in immunocompromised patients. In patients with intact immune response mechanisms, infectious esophagitis usually develops as a secondary phenomenon,

after esophageal mucosal damage due to another cause. Infectious esophagitis in and of itself is more likely to present as pain on swallowing than as upper GI bleeding. The presence of a foreign body in the esophagus and the ingestion of caustic substances are also possible causes of esophagitis.

Treatment of esophagitis relies on the diagnosis and management of the underlying condition responsible for the irritation. Antacids, histamine receptor antagonists, and proton-pump inhibitors decrease the acidity of gastric secretions and, consequently, decrease the amount of acid to which the esophageal mucosa is subjected. Sucralfate, a minimally absorbed disaccharide, serves as a cytoprotective agent and may provide symptomatic relief for esophageal discomfort secondary to esophagitis.

Mallory–Weiss syndrome involves the spontaneous laceration of the esophagus secondary to prolonged or forceful vomiting. The severity of bleeding associated with this lesion depends on the location and the depth of the mucosal tear. Diagnosis is made with upper GI endoscopy. The lacerations usually heal spontaneously, and only the most severe require surgical repair.

GASTRIC MUCOSAL DISORDERS

Gastritis describes nonspecific inflammatory changes in the gastric mucosa. These changes usually are manifested as abdominal pain and upper GI bleeding. When gastritis is attributable to one of the several known causes of gastric inflammation, it is referred to as **secondary gastritis.** When the cause is uncertain, it is considered **primary gastritis.** Primary gastritis may be associated with peptic ulcer disease (see subsequent discussion).

Table 12–3. Differential Diagnosis: Upper Gastrointestinal Tract Bleeding

Mucosal lesions	Vascular lesions
Esophagitis[1]	Esophageal varices[1]
Mallory–Weiss tear[1]	Hereditary hemorrhagic telangiectasia
Gastritis[1]	(Osler–Weber–Rendu syndrome)
Primary gastritis	
Secondary gastritis	**Coagulopathies**
Peptic ulcer disease	Hemophilia A or B
Duplications	Pharmacologically induced
Mucosal erosion	Vitamin K deficiency, including hemorrhagic disease
Foreign body	of the newborn
Caustic ingestion	Secondary to chronic liver disease
Stress-related ulceration	
Central nervous system lesion (Cushing ulcers)	**Miscellaneous**
Burn lesion (Curling ulcers)	Swallowed maternal blood[1]
Intramural hematoma (secondary to trauma,	Nasopharyngeal bleeding[1]
including physical abuse)	Rumination
Milk–soy protein intolerance	

[1] Frequently encountered causes of upper gastrointestinal bleeding.

Secondary gastritis has several causes. Stress-related gastritis may occur in patients with severe illnesses or injuries, including sepsis, severe burn injury, and head trauma, and in those who have undergone major surgical procedures. Many ingested agents are other known causes of gastritis. Alcohol is among the more common causes, but medications, including corticosteroids and nonsteroidal antiinflammatory agents, and corrosive substances, can produce gastric inflammation. Secondary gastritis can occur in patients with other inflammatory diseases, such as Crohn's disease, and in patients with allergic disease, as is seen in eosinophilic gastritis.

Primary gastritis has traditionally denoted cases in which no cause could be determined. In recent years, evidence has accumulated that many of these cases are actually due to infection with *Helicobacter pylori*. This organism also has been implicated in the pathogenesis of peptic ulcer disease.

Diagnosis of gastritis is based on histologic criteria and therefore necessitates obtaining mucosal biopsy specimens endoscopically. Cultures for *H. pylori* should be included in the evaluation. Pharmacologic treatment of gastritis with antacids, histamine H_2-receptor antagonists, or proton-pump inhibitors provides some benefit by reducing gastric acidity. Sucralfate and other agents designed to "coat" the gastric mucosa may be useful. When *H. pylori* is present, specific antimicrobial therapy should be added to the treatment regimen. For children, the combination of metronidazole, bismuth subsalicylate, and amoxicillin is often used, but many antibiotic combinations are apparently effective in eradicating the bacteria.

Peptic ulcer disease occurs when the normal balance between acidic gastric secretions and the mucosal protective elements is disrupted. The ulcers themselves are well-circumscribed regions of damaged tissue, with loss of mucosa, submucosa, and muscularis. The lesions are described as primary or secondary; the causes of secondary ulcers are similar to those of secondary gastritis. Important among those is the use of nonsteroidal antiinflammatory agents. The Zollinger–Ellison syndrome of excessive gastrin secretion from a gastrinoma and consequent peptic ulcer disease (another cause of secondary ulcers) is rare in children. There is increasing evidence that *H. pylori* also may cause peptic ulcer disease in the pediatric population.

Peptic ulcers may be found in the stomach or duodenum. In children younger than 6 years, most ulcers are located in the gastric antrum. These may present clinically with abdominal pain or GI bleeding. In older children, ulcers are located more commonly in the duodenum. Older boys are affected approximately four times as often as are older girls. Dramatic episodes of hematemesis are less likely to occur in these patients than in children younger than 6 years with peptic ulcer disease.

Diagnosis of peptic ulcer is best made through direct visualization of the lesions by upper GI endoscopy. Treatment involves the use of antacids, histamine H_2-receptor antagonists, proton-pump inhibitors, and mucosal coating agents. Surgical intervention is sometimes required in the management of severe hemorrhage or perforation occurring as a complication of peptic ulcer disease. Once healed, gastric ulcers are not likely to recur. Children with duodenal ulcers may experience recurrences throughout their lives, possibly as a result of persistent or recurrent infection with *H. pylori*.

VARICEAL BLEEDING

Varices are submucosal veins that become engorged as a result of obstructed outflow; they commonly develop in patients with portal hypertension, which in turn may be secondary to a variety of causes (Table 12–4). Veins in the esophagus and stomach are possible sites of varix formation, as are the internal hemorrhoidal veins and venous channels around the umbilicus (which, when engorged, are called the caput medusae).

Bleeding from esophageal varices is often massive and sudden in onset. Therefore, the restoration of hemodynamic stability through appropriate use of intravenous fluids and blood products is of utmost importance in managing these patients. The second priority is to stop the bleeding. Placement of a nasogastric tube allows aspiration of gastric contents and provides some gross measure of

Table 12–4. Etiology of Portal Hypertension

Prehepatic
  Portal vein obstruction (e.g., thrombosis)
    Congenital (cavernous transformation or portal vein thrombosis)
    Acquired
      Omphalitis
      Umbilical vein catheterization
      Coagulopathies
        Protein C deficiency
        Protein S deficiency
        Paroxysmal nocturnal hemoglobinuria

Intrahepatic
  Secondary to cirrhosis of any cause

Posthepatic
  Hepatic vein obstruction (Budd–Chiari syndrome)
  Inferior vena cava obstruction
    Congenital
    Acquired
  Trauma
  Tumor
  Clotting dysfunction
  Congestive heart failure
  Constrictive pericarditis

ongoing blood losses. The nasogastric tube is also useful therapeutically for gastric lavage. The administration of vasopressin is often used to decrease blood pressure and portal blood flow. Although usually effective, this medication should be used with great caution because of its many side effects, mainly related to ischemia. Mechanical tamponade of the bleeding varices may be accomplished through a special balloon catheter (Sengstaken–Blakemore tube). This tube should be placed only by those experienced in its use.

Patients with conditions associated with the development of portal hypertension and those who have previously experienced variceal bleeding often are monitored endoscopically for the development and progression of esophageal varices. Injection of the varices with sclerosing agents (sodium tetradecyl sulfate or sodium morrhuate) is often effective in preventing recurrent episodes of variceal bleeding. Ligation of varices using endoscopically placed constrictive bands also can be used to control variceal bleeding and is gaining wider acceptance among pediatric endoscopists. Surgical procedures aimed at shunting the blood flow away from the portal circulation are seldom required in the management of pediatric patients.

LOWER GASTROINTESTINAL TRACT HEMORRHAGE

The passage of blood from the rectum may be caused by a variety of disorders, some localized to specific sites along the GI tract and others more generalized in distribution. This section addresses those disorders that affect the lower (i.e., distal to the ligament of Treitz) GI tract.

Clinical Approach

An algorithm outlining a systematic approach that can be used in evaluating patients with blood loss per rectum is illustrated in Figure 12–6. As is the case with patients with upper GI tract blood loss, the initial evaluation should include an assessment of hemodynamic stability. If the patient is stable, the history can be obtained.

HISTORY

It is especially important to elucidate the duration of symptoms in patients with rectal bleeding. With IBD, the symptoms are sometimes acute in onset but more typically have a chronic course. Bleeding from anal lesions also may continue for an extended period.

The characteristics of the defecated blood may provide further etiologic clues. Bright red blood (hematochezia) is usually from a very distal source (anal fissure, hemorrhoid) or from a very active lesion at a more proximal site. Blood that has been partly degraded by the action of bacterial and digestive enzymes may cause the stool to appear black and tarry (melena). Blood that is present mainly on the outside of the feces is more likely to be of distal origin, whereas blood originating upstream likely will be mixed with the fecal material.

The history also should include an assessment of the feces with which the blood is passed. Loose, watery stools occurring in a previously healthy patient may be caused by infectious gastroenteritis. Several organisms that cause acute gastroenteritis also can cause bleeding, including *Salmonella, Shigella, Campylobacter,* and rotavirus. In contrast, the passage of extremely hard stools associated with bleeding suggests an external lesion (e.g., anal fissure) as a likely source. Mucus or white blood cells may be present in the stool as a result of intestinal inflammation. Mucus often is present in the stools of patients with IBD, but this finding is not specific for IBD and can be present in patients with bacterial or amebic infections.

Coexistence of other symptoms should be evaluated. Abdominal pain may be present when the bleeding is secondary to IBD. These patients may also report a feeling of urgency accompanying the need to defecate (tenesmus), especially when the disease affects the rectum. Acute abdominal pain may accompany rectal bleeding because of an obstructive intestinal lesion; episodic abdominal pain often is described with intussusception. Painless rectal bleeding may occur with rectal polyps. A history of recent use of medications is important because several drugs, notably aspirin, may be associated with bleeding disorders that present as blood in the stool.

PHYSICAL EXAMINATION

The physical examination should first assess the patient's hemodynamic status. A complete examination should then be done to detect any abnormalities or unusual features, such as dermatologic manifestations of Henoch–Schönlein purpura or the extraintestinal manifestations of Crohn's disease. The abdomen should be examined for signs of obstruction (e.g., rigidity, absence of bowel sounds), tenderness, or organomegaly. Rectal skin tags, fissures, or other abnormalities should be noted. If no gross blood is present on digital examination of the rectum, the fecal material should be tested for the presence of occult blood to verify that the apparent blood is not merely pigmentation caused by the ingestion of colored foods or beverages or medications (e.g., iron preparations, ampicillin, and bismuth preparations).

DIAGNOSTIC STUDIES

Testing of the stool to determine whether the observed pigmentation is actually blood is an important first step in the diagnostic evaluation. If blood is present, a decision must be made as to whether the source of the blood is in the lower or upper GI tract. If an upper tract source is suspected, nasogastric intubation for aspiration of gastric contents should follow. If the result is positive, evaluation may proceed as described in the previous section

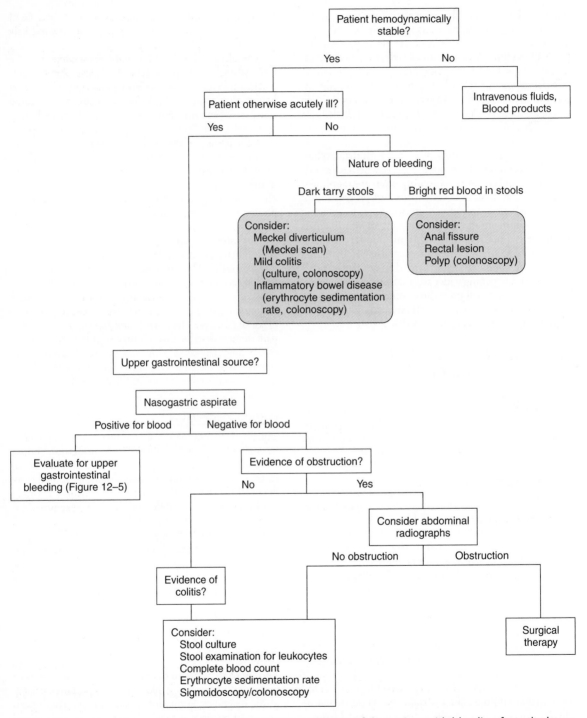

Figure 12–6. Algorithm presenting an approach to the evaluation of the patient with bleeding from the lower gastrointestinal tract.

(see Figure 12–5). If the aspirate is negative for blood, a lower tract source is likely responsible.

In patients with rectal bleeding who are ill, evidence of obstruction, including abdominal distention, tenderness to palpation, and vomiting, should be sought, and abdominal radiographs obtained. If obstruction is ruled out, investigation may continue with endoscopy and other studies such as stool cultures/smear and blood studies for evidence of inflammation (e.g., erythrocyte sedimentation rate, complete blood count). In those who are not acutely ill, the evaluation may progress with less urgency.

With passage of bright red blood per rectum, anal pathology, such as a fissure, is most likely. Rectal polyps also can cause painless passage of bright red blood. With a Meckel diverticulum, the blood may appear somewhat darker.

Conditions causing colonic inflammation, including the colitides and IBD, may present with mild bleeding associated with little or no pain. Evaluation of these disorders may require colonoscopy in addition to laboratory investigations.

Determination of the hematocrit is helpful in ascertaining the extent of blood loss in chronic disorders; patients who are anemic may benefit from iron supplementation. In those with acute loss of larger amounts of blood, blood products may be required.

Differential Diagnosis

The many etiologies of lower GI tract bleeding are listed in Table 12–5. Some of the more common causes are discussed below.

ANAL & RECTAL DISORDERS

Anal fissures are the most common cause of rectal bleeding in young children beyond the stage of infancy. Usually there is a history of constipation, with passage of excessively large or hard stools before development of the fissure. The amount of bleeding with a fissure is usually small, coating the outside of the stool or appearing as small amounts of bright red blood in the diaper or on the toilet tissue. The fissure often causes severe pain during defecation, which can lead to avoidance of defecation, worsening of constipation, and eventually the painful passage of yet another large, hard stool with further irritation of the fissure.

In patients with anal fissures not related to constipation, the possibility of perianal cellulitis, usually caused by *Candida albicans* or streptococci, should be considered. Patients with Crohn's disease (see Inflammatory Bowel Disease) also may have anal fissures, which may be accompanied by edema and purulent discharge. An anal fissure might be caused by sexual abuse.

The diagnosis of a fissure can be made by inspection. Digital examination causes great pain and usually is not

Table 12–5. Differential Diagnosis: Lower Gastrointestinal Tract Bleeding

Anorectal origin
  Anal fissure[1]
  Rectal prolapse
  Skin tags
  Hemorrhoids
  Foreign body
  Trauma/sexual abuse

Colonic origin
  Colitis[1]
    Infectious
    Antibiotic associated (pseudomembranous colitis)
    Allergic (e.g., cow's milk protein)
    Ulcerative colitis
    Necrotizing enterocolitis
    Secondary to Hirschsprung disease
  Polyposis[1]

Small intestinal origin
  Meckel diverticulum
  Intussusception
  Malrotation and volvulus

Generalized gastrointestinal origin
  Crohn disease[1]
  Transient ischemia related to vigorous exercise
  Upper gastrointestinal bleeding
    Varices
    Peptic ulcer disease
    Gastritis
    Foreign body and other ingestions
    Duplications
  Pharmacologically induced

Hematologic and vascular diseases
  Coagulopathies
  Hemangiomas and telangiectasias
  Henoch–Schönlein purpura
  Hemolytic–uremic syndrome

[1] Frequently encountered causes of lower gastrointestinal bleeding.

necessary. Treatment of uncomplicated anal fissures includes maintenance of good anal hygiene by washing or sitz baths and correction of constipation. Patients with perianal cellulitis should receive appropriate antimicrobial therapy. Persistence of painful defecation may indicate sphincter spasm, which is often alleviated by gentle digital dilation. Occasionally, surgical repair is necessary for treatment of chronic, extensive, or complicated fissures. The role of newer therapies for fissures such as Botulinum toxin and topical nitroglycerine ointment has not been well evaluated in pediatric patients.

In **rectal prolapse,** the rectal mucosa intermittently protrudes through the anus for brief or, less often, more protracted periods. It is associated most commonly with constipation, but prolapse also occurs in patients with cystic fibrosis or parasitic infestations. Rectal bleeding is not a prominent feature of prolapse and typically slight. Diagnosis must rely on the history because the physical findings are rarely persistent. Successful management is usually accomplished through treatment of the underlying disorder.

Hemorrhoids are a potential cause of rectal bleeding. They are usually exterior to the anus and associated with infection and edema related to an anal fissure. Minor rectal bleeding may occur; no treatment is required. Internal hemorrhoids are dilations of the rectal venous system; in children, they most often are secondary to portal hypertension. Although uncommon, bleeding from rectal varices may be substantial and ligation may be necessary.

COLONIC DISORDERS

Colitis is a general term used to describe inflammation in the colon; it may be associated with different degrees of rectal bleeding. In **infectious colitis,** the causative agents include *Salmonella, Shigella, Campylobacter, Yersinia,* enterohemorrhagic *Escherichia coli,* and rotavirus (see Chapter 9, Infectious Diseases). With colitis of bacterial etiology, the stool typically shows polymorphonuclear leukocytes in addition to gross or microscopic amounts of blood. Diagnosis usually is made from stool cultures. Rotavirus may be diagnosed with the use of a specific enzyme-linked immunoassay. For bacterial etiologies, treatment may include administration of appropriate antibiotics.

Pseudomembranous colitis is caused by the toxin produced by *Clostridium difficile.* It differs from the other infectious colitides in that its pathogenesis depends on colonization of the colon by *C. difficile* after eradication of the normal microflora by a course of antibiotics. Virtually all antibiotics have been implicated in this process.

Patients with pseudomembranous colitis present with symptoms ranging from mild, watery diarrhea to severe, bloody diarrhea, possibly associated with tenesmus and abdominal pain. In its most severe form, a fulminant colitis may develop, resulting in progressive loss of muscular tone in the colon. This condition, referred to as **toxic megacolon,** may progress to colonic perforation and peritonitis.

Diagnosis of pseudomembranous colitis may be made sigmoidoscopically by the identification of accumulations of inflammatory exudate (the pseudomembrane) on the colonic mucosa. Stool culture for the detection of *C. difficile* or assays for its toxin are useful in making a diagnosis in older children and adults because these markers may be positive in patients in whom pseudomembranes cannot be found. In infants, however, these studies are not useful because as many as 70% of patients in this age group have been shown to be asymptomatic carriers of *C. difficile.*

Allergic colitis may be associated with loss of blood in the stool; the most commonly implicated allergens are milk and soy proteins. Mucosal biopsy specimens in these patients may show increased numbers of eosinophils. Treatment is accomplished through elimination of the offending protein. Malabsorption, which may accompany allergic colitis, is discussed below.

Ulcerative colitis is a chronic IBD primarily affecting the colon. Because of its similarities to Crohn's disease, these two disorders are discussed together (see below, Inflammatory Bowel Disease).

Mucosal polyps commonly cause rectal bleeding. Polyps are defined as gross protrusions of intestinal mucosa into the lumen and, in children, occur most commonly in the colon. They occur less frequently in the small bowel and stomach. Polyps may cause abdominal pain by serving as the lead point for an intussusception or, less commonly, through luminal obstruction. More often, however, polyps are the source of painless rectal bleeding, which results from mucosal trauma from contact with passing stool or ischemic necrosis as the polyp outgrows its blood supply.

Although they may be neoplastic, more than 90% of polyps in children are inflammatory (**juvenile polyps)** and thought to carry little, if any, malignant potential. If left untreated, most polyps undergo self-amputation as they outgrow their blood supply. Diagnosis is best made through colonoscopy; this allows for definitive treatment by polypectomy. During examination, about half the patients with polyps are found to have more than one lesion.

Juvenile polyposis coli is a condition of multiple (more than 10) colonic polyps that occurs in familial and sporadic forms. In both conditions, the potential for malignant change is thought to be greater than that associated with isolated juvenile polyps. **Generalized juvenile polyposis** is a similar condition, with polyps not limited to the colon. **Familial polyposis coli** is an autosomal dominant disorder in which patients have hundreds to thousands of adenomatous polyps, usually not recognized until after puberty. In **Gardner's syndrome,** these polyps may occur throughout the small intestine and colon and are associated with tumors of bone and soft tissues as well as hypertrophy of the retinal pigment epithelium. In the **Peutz–Jeghers syndrome,** multiple hamartomatous polyps are associated with abnormal pigmentation of the lips and buccal mucosa.

DISORDERS OF THE SMALL INTESTINE

Meckel diverticulum is a vestigial remnant of the omphalomesenteric duct that, in the fetus, connects the gut to the yolk sac (Figure 12–7). It is the most common

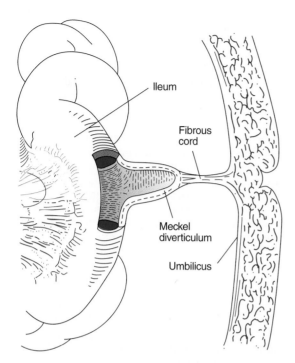

Figure 12–7. An illustration of a Meckel diverticulum, a persistent remnant of the omphalomesenteric duct, and its relationship to the normal gastrointestinal anatomy. (Reproduced, with permission, from Milov DE, Andres JM: Sorting out the causes of rectal bleeding. *Contemp Pediatr* 1988;5:80.)

Intussusception is the invagination of a segment of bowel into itself, sometimes described as "telescoping" (Figure 12–8). Although intussusception can occur in any segment of the small intestine or colon, most often it is near or includes the ileocecal junction. Most cases are idiopathic, but in some, an identifiable "lead point" causes the intussusception. Polyps, Meckel diverticula, parasites, and tumors are known to act as lead points.

Intussusception typically occurs in children older than 2 years of age, and presents with acute onset of episodic, crampy abdominal pain. In infants, pain is much less prominent. In time, the mucosa of the involved segments of bowel becomes edematous, and intestinal obstruction develops. Vomiting may occur, and an abdominal mass may be palpable. The classically described passage of maroon stools mixed with mucus ("currant-jelly" stool) occurs in only two thirds of patients.

An enema, using air or barium as the contrast agent, is the diagnostic modality of choice and when positive shows the so-called coiled spring appearance. Reduction of the intussusception can be accomplished in approximately 75% of cases through the use of hydrostatic or pneumatic pressure delivered through the enema catheter. These techniques carry a slight risk of intestinal perforation and a 10% risk of recurrence. When reduction is unsuccessful, surgical correction is indicated.

INFLAMMATORY BOWEL DISEASE

Idiopathic IBD is a term that encompasses ulcerative colitis and Crohn's disease. These disorders are similar in

congenital malformation of the GI tract, occurring in approximately 1.5% of the population, most of whom experience no symptoms.

The diverticulum is typically located on the antimesenteric side of the ileum, within 100 cm of the ileocecal valve, and is approximately 2 cm in length. Symptomatic diverticula occur in boys twice as often as in girls and usually present before 2 years of age. These features have been described as the "rule of 2's."

Ectopic mucosa, most often gastric, is found in approximately one third of Meckel diverticula. The acid secreted by this mucosa can cause ulceration and bleeding. In young children, bleeding is usually painless, but pain is a prominent feature in older children, especially when the diverticulum causes intestinal obstruction through intussusception or volvulus. Diagnosis of a Meckel diverticulum is made via radionuclide scanning in which radiolabeled technetium, concentrated by gastric mucosa, is visualized in an ectopic location. Treatment is by surgical resection.

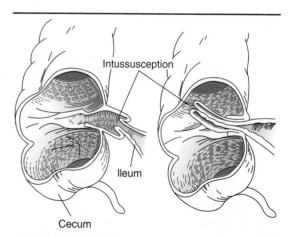

Figure 12–8. An illustration of the "telescoping" movement of one part of the bowel into another, which constitutes intussusception. (Reproduced, with permission, from Milov DE, Andres JM: Sorting out the causes of rectal bleeding. *Contemp Pediatr* 1988;5:80.)

that they tend to produce symptoms of diarrhea, often mixed with blood, and abdominal pain. Other features are sufficiently distinct to allow for the differentiation of the two diseases, as shown in Table 12–6.

Crohn's disease causes transmural inflammation of the GI mucosa at any point from the mouth to the anus, with the ileocecal region most commonly affected. Within a diseased segment of mucosa, areas of normal tissue ("skip lesions") may be interspersed. Noncaseating granulomas are often present, as are longitudinal ulcers, which create the characteristic cobblestone appearance. Progression of the inflammatory lesions may lead to bowel wall thickening, causing stenosis and obstruction, and the formation of fistulae.

The onset of Crohn's disease is often insidious. Patients may experience diarrhea, weight loss, or abdominal pain and tenderness. With ileal disease, rectal bleeding is often present. Signs of growth failure, delayed sexual maturation, arthritis, and unexplained fevers may also be among the initial manifestations.

The diagnosis may entail the use of multiple modalities. Contrast radiographic studies may show mucosal thickening, cobblestone features, ulcer formation, and areas of stenosis. Endoscopy provides direct mucosal visualization and the opportunity to obtain biopsy specimens for histologic diagnosis.

Medical therapy for Crohn's disease usually includes corticosteroids to reduce inflammation. When possible, steroid doses are tapered gradually to a dose sufficiently low to cause few side effects (hirsutism, fat deposition, cataract formation). In patients unresponsive to steroids or in those who are steroid dependent, 6-mercaptopurine and azathioprine are sometimes beneficial therapeutic alternatives. Despite effective medical therapy, many children with Crohn's disease eventually require surgical intervention to relieve an obstruction secondary to stenosis, remove an inflammatory mass, or repair a fistula. In addition to pharmacologic and surgical therapies, meticulous attention to the patient's nutritional status and dietary sup-

plementation, when needed, have been shown to have a significant impact on the patient's overall condition.

Ulcerative colitis causes inflammatory changes limited to the colon. The rectum is almost always involved, and different portions of the more proximal colon are often affected. In only about 15% of patients is disease confined to the rectum. The disease is recognized histologically by the presence of superficial ulcerations associated with increased numbers of polymorphonuclear leukocytes. Crypt abscesses also may be present.

Patients with ulcerative colitis often experience rectal bleeding and abdominal pain, which is relieved on defecation. Fever, anemia, and hypoalbuminemia are typical associated features. As in Crohn's disease, weight loss and growth failure may be noted. Occasionally, ulcerative colitis may present acutely as toxic megacolon.

Diagnosis of ulcerative colitis is sometimes made by barium enema, which may show the loss of normal haustral markings, but no abnormalities may be evident. Sigmoidoscopy or colonoscopy with biopsy is a preferable means of diagnosis. Endoscopically, the mucosa appears inflamed and friable. In contrast to Crohn's disease, the lesion is continuous, without intervening areas of normal mucosa. Barium enema and colonoscopy should be delayed in patients with severe disease because of the risk of precipitating toxic megacolon. Because the histologic changes of ulcerative colitis are similar to those seen in acute infectious colitis, appropriate bacterial cultures should be part of the diagnostic regimen.

Pharmacotherapy of ulcerative colitis usually includes sulfasalazine or 5-amino salicylic acid, which acts as an antiinflammatory agent affecting the colonic mucosa. Corticosteroids, administered orally or topically (as enemas), may be necessary in more severe disease. Nutritional supplementation frequently is required.

Despite optimal medical therapy, approximately 25% of children with ulcerative colitis do not respond adequately and require surgical intervention with colonic resection and construction of an ileostomy. Because of the

Table 12–6. Comparison of Characteristics of Crohn Disease and Ulcerative Colitis

	Crohn Disease	Ulcerative Colitis
Histology	Transmural involvement; noncaseating granulomas	Involvement of mucosa and submucosa only; crypt abscesses
Gross appearance	Longitudinal ulcerations; cobblestone features	Friable mucosa; pseudopolyps
Radiologic findings	Ulcers; "thumbprinting"; areas of stenosis	Loss of haustral markings
Location	Throughout the gastrointestinal tract; diseased areas interposed with areas of normal tissue	Rectum ± variable colonic involvement
Fistula formation	Possible	Not typical
Toxic megacolon	Not typical	Possible
Extraintestinal disease	Delayed maturation; arthralgias and arthritis; erythema nodosum; conjunctivitis and uveitis	Delayed maturation; erythema multiforme

increased risks of colon cancer in patients with ulcerative colitis, surveillance with colonic biopsies every 1–2 years is recommended beginning 8 years after the initial diagnosis. Colectomy is recommended when mucosal dysplasia is found. Patients with disease limited to the rectum or rectosigmoid are thought not to have an increased risk for colon cancer.

OTHER CAUSES OF LOWER GASTROINTESTINAL BLEEDING

Henoch–Schönlein purpura is a vasculitic syndrome of unknown cause characterized by arthritis, purpuric skin lesions, abdominal pain, and hematochezia (see also Chapter 8, Rheumatic Diseases). Skin lesions, which are typically the initial manifestation, often precede GI manifestations by several days. Gastrointestinal symptoms are provoked by edema and hemorrhage in the GI mucosa, which may be apparent endoscopically. Purpuric lesions also may be seen in the gastric, duodenal, and colonic mucosae. Treatment of the GI manifestations of Henoch–Schönlein purpura includes supportive measures beginning with nasogastric suction and the administration of intravenous fluids. The use of corticosteroids is thought by some to be beneficial in lessening abdominal pain and rectal bleeding and may decrease the risk of intussusception occurring as a complication.

The **hemolytic–uremic syndrome** is characterized by microangiopathic hemolytic anemia, uremia, and thrombocytopenia after enteric infection with one of several microorganisms including enterohemorrhagic *E. coli,* especially those of the serotype O157:H7. These *E. coli* may be carried in contaminated and insufficiently cooked hamburger and other food sources and have been implicated in multiple outbreaks of bloody diarrhea in which the hemolytic syndrome subsequently developed in some patients. Bloody diarrhea is often the presenting symptom and may be accompanied by abdominal pain and vomiting. Diagnosis is made by recognition of the characteristic combination of clinical symptoms. Treatment of the GI symptoms is largely supportive. The use of ampicillin, to which the often implicated *E. coli* strains are susceptible, is also frequently advocated even before a positive culture is obtained. There is no convincing evidence, however, that the use of antibiotics is effective in lessening the severity of the initial infection or decreasing the risk of developing the hemolytic–uremic syndrome or other sequelae (see Chapter 16, Kidneys & Electrolytes).

■ ABDOMINAL PAIN

Abdominal pain is frequently encountered in pediatric practice and often presents challenges in diagnosis and management. A wide variety of disorders may be associated with abdominal pain, ranging from acute, potentially life-threatening obstructions and infections to chronic functional disorders that, although difficult to tolerate, are not typically associated with dire consequences. An approach to the evaluation of patients with acute and chronic abdominal pain is presented in Figure 12–9.

ACUTE ABDOMINAL PAIN

Clinical Approach

HISTORY

In the patient suffering from an acute episode of abdominal pain, a description of the pain itself is most important. The time of onset and duration of the pain and its relation to any possible initiating event, especially trauma, should be determined. Also important is the character of the pain (e.g., burning or cramping) and any change in that character over time. In appendicitis, for example, pain is first vague and poorly localized and then gradually becomes more localized as the inflammation progresses to involve the visceral peritoneum. Pain also may be perceived to radiate to other sites.

The relation of the pain to other symptoms should be clarified. For example, vomiting that precedes pain may occur with acute gastroenteritis. With intestinal obstruction, pain typically precedes other symptoms. Bilious emesis should be considered to be due to intestinal obstruction until proved otherwise. Diarrhea, constipation, and fever commonly accompany abdominal pain. The medical history, especially in regard to surgical procedures, should be noted.

PHYSICAL EXAMINATION

Physical examination of patients with acute abdominal pain is often difficult because they are frequently in too much distress to cooperate. One should note whether the child prefers to lie motionless or writhes about. If children are not too ill, asking them to jump up and down may reproduce pain related to peritoneal inflammation.

Distention, gross asymmetry, or associated skin lesions should be noted on abdominal examination. Bowel sounds should be characterized on auscultation. Early in intestinal obstruction, sounds may be high pitched, but with long-standing obstruction, and as with ileus (i.e., nonmechanical obstruction), sounds are typically absent. Gentle palpation of the abdomen will localize areas of tenderness, reproduce the pain, and determine the presence of involuntary guarding. Deeper palpation may lead to the discovery of mass lesions. Digital rectal examination should be performed to localize possible areas of peritoneal irritation.

DIAGNOSTIC STUDIES

In evaluating the patient with abdominal pain, abdominal radiographs are frequently obtained and may be beneficial. Often, however, more specialized imaging including

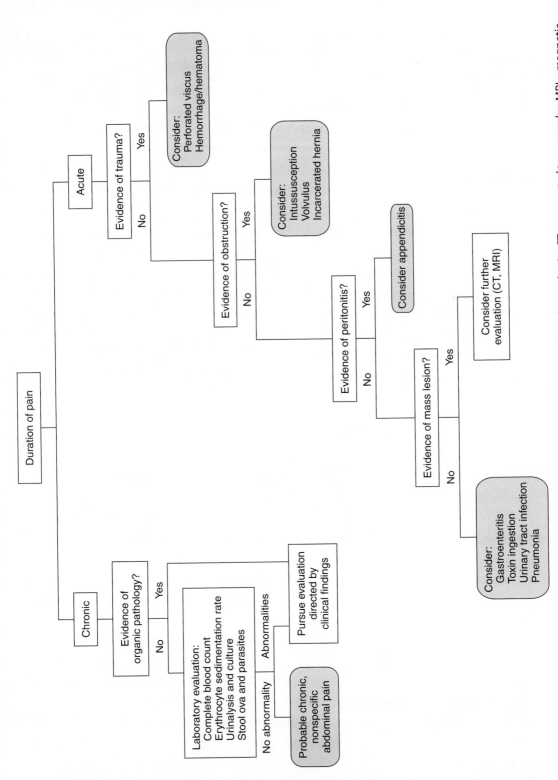

Figure 12–9. Algorithm presenting an approach to the evaluation of the patient with abdominal pain. CT = computed tomography; MRI = magnetic resonance imaging.

ultrasound and computed tomography are needed. These studies are discussed more specifically in regard to the various diagnoses in the differential.

As with imaging studies, laboratory tests should be chosen based on the specific etiologies under consideration. A complete blood count, including a white blood cell differential, helps to differentiate inflammatory from noninflammatory causes of acute abdominal pain and is usually indicated in most evaluations.

Differential Diagnosis

Diseases that may cause acute abdominal pain are listed in Table 12–7. Several of the more common GI etiologies are discussed below. Infectious gastroenteritis and colic are reviewed in Chapters 1, 3, and 9. Additional non-GI causes of acute abdominal pain are covered in their respective chapters.

APPENDICITIS

Inflammation of the appendix results from obstruction of the appendiceal lumen by factors such as fecaliths, foreign bodies, and lymphoid hyperplasia. Dilatation of the appendix follows, compromising the organ's blood supply and decreasing resistance to bacterial invasion. Untreated, this most often leads to appendiceal perfora-

tion and subsequent peritonitis. Appendicitis is approximately twice as frequent in males and more common in the adolescent–young adult group.

The initial symptom is usually vague abdominal pain, which is poorly localized, but with a periumbilical focus. With progression of appendiceal distention, the pain may become crampy and associated with nausea and vomiting. When the inflammatory process in the appendix becomes transmural, the parietal peritoneum becomes involved, and the pain becomes sharper in character and localized to the site of the appendix (usually in the right lower quadrant but potentially at any location in the abdomen or pelvis). With peritoneal inflammation, patients also may experience fever and chills.

The physical findings depend on the stage of the inflammation. Initially, when pain is poorly localized, findings may be equally nonspecific. When the parietal peritoneum is involved, the child usually prefers to lie fairly motionless in a supine position. There is localized tenderness over the site of the appendix, most commonly at McBurney's point (about 2 inches from the anterior superior iliac spine on a line to the umbilicus). Voluntary guarding is also common. Rectal examination often elicits tenderness.

With perforation of the appendix, peritoneal signs (involuntary guarding and rebound tenderness) are usually

Table 12–7. Differential Diagnosis: Acute Abdominal Pain

Infectious causes	**Intestinal obstruction**	**Vasculitic disease**
Gastrointestinal	Intussusception[1]	Henoch–Schönlein purpura
Appendicitis[1]	Volvulus[1]	Periarteritis nodosa
Mesenteric adenitis	Adhesions	Mucocutaneous lymph node
Infectious gastroenteritis[1]	Hernia with incarceration	syndrome (Kawasaki disease)
Food poisoning[1]		
Peritonitis	**Gallbladder**	**Renal disease**
Hepatitis	Cholecystitis	Nephrotic syndrome
Pancreatitis	Cholelithiasis	Renal colic
Nongastrointestinal	Hydrops	
Pharyngitis		**Miscellaneous**
(especially streptococcal)	**Abdominal trauma**	Ascites
Pneumonia	Abdominal wall muscle bruise/strain	Colic[1]
(especially right lower lobe)	Splenic rupture/hematoma	Toxin ingestion
Pyelonephritis/glomerulonephritis	Liver laceration or hematoma	Testicular torsion
Pelvic inflammatory disease	Pancreatic pseudocyst	Ovarian torsion
Abdominal abscess		Mesenteric artery occlusion
Pericarditis	**Hematologic disease**	Hypokalemia (causing paralytic ileus)
Serositis	Leukemia/lymphoma	Black widow spider bite
Epididymitis	Hemolytic crisis	
Generalized	Spinal cord tumors	
Herpes zoster		
Mononucleosis	**Endocrine disease**	
Acute rheumatic fever	Hypoglycemia	
	Diabetes mellitus (especially with	
	diabetic ketoacidosis)	

[1] Frequently encountered causes of acute abdominal pain.

present. If the inflammation is confined to the immediate area of the appendix, an abscess may develop. If uncontained, generalized peritonitis occurs.

Laboratory evaluation of patients suspected to have appendicitis includes a complete blood count with a differential count. Typically, there is a neutrophil leukocytosis, although the white cell count may be normal. Urinalysis is useful to exclude urinary tract infection. Evaluation of the serum electrolytes also may be useful, especially if vomiting has been a prominent feature.

Radiologic studies, although not usually helpful, may show a calcified fecalith, suggesting appendicitis, and may help to exclude intestinal obstruction. Abdominal ultrasound occasionally is useful in demonstrating dilatation of the appendix, a finding highly suggestive of appendicitis.

Treatment of appendicitis is by appendectomy. In patients who have experienced significant vomiting, rehydration and correction of associated electrolyte abnormalities should precede surgery. Many surgeons also advocate the use of preoperative antibiotics. If perforation and abscess formation have already occurred, operative incision and drainage may be instituted, or the infection may be treated with antibiotics, followed by elective appendectomy a few weeks later.

Pancreatitis

Although pancreatitis is not commonly encountered in children, it should be considered in the differential diagnosis of acute abdominal pain. Pancreatitis is a nonspecific inflammatory response of the pancreas to a variety of causes. In adults, biliary tract disease, especially gallstones, and ethanol toxicity are the most common precipitating factors. In children, the usual causes are systemic infections, notably mumps; abdominal trauma; pancreatic disease, including cystic fibrosis and diabetes mellitus; and pharmacologic agents.

Regardless of the etiology, the pathogenesis of pancreatitis involves the premature activation of trypsinogen to trypsin, which in turn catalyzes the activation of other proteolytic enzymes within the ductal lumen. The quantity of proteolytic enzymes generated is sufficient to overwhelm the protease inhibitors that are also normally present, and autodigestion of the pancreatic tissue ensues.

Patients with acute pancreatitis usually experience abdominal pain, which may be mild to severe. Classically the pain is sudden in onset, gradually increases in severity, and is localized to the right upper quadrant with radiation to the back. Many patients, however, describe their pain as periumbilical and may or may not experience radiation to other sites. Vomiting frequently accompanies the pain and sometimes may be bilious. Physical examination typically shows epigastric tenderness and absent or decreased bowel sounds. Fever, if present, is usually mild. Rarely, hypotension and shock may occur in severe cases of acute pancreatitis.

The laboratory evaluation of patients suspected of having pancreatitis usually includes measurement of serum amylase concentrations; in pancreatitis, values are three to four times normal or greater. Increased amylase concentrations are not specific for pancreatitis, and a normal value does not preclude the diagnosis. A more sophisticated test quantitates the various isoforms of amylase. In acute pancreatitis, the predominant pancreatic isoamylase is elevated. Measurement of the urinary amylase:creatinine clearance ratio is not helpful in differentiating elevated amylase levels due to pancreatitis from those due to other causes. Serum lipase levels also may be elevated in pancreatitis.

Radiologic studies of the abdomen may be helpful to exclude other causes of acute abdominal pain. They also may show areas of calcification within the pancreas, although this finding is more typical of chronic pancreatitis. Ultrasound studies are more helpful in detecting areas of abnormal density, cystic areas, or ductal dilatations. Computed tomography is sometimes useful to define pancreatic structure further. Endoscopic retrograde cholangiopancreatography allows precise visualization of the pancreatic ducts, but experience with this technique in children is limited.

Treatment of pancreatitis in children is directed primarily at eradicating the underlying disorder. Often the cause is not known or specific treatment is not available; consequently, only supportive measures can be provided. Withholding of enteral nutrition to "rest" the GI tract is presumably a beneficial means of decreasing pancreatic secretions and controlling the autodigestive process. Nasogastric suction to achieve gastric decompression is probably of no benefit unless persistent vomiting or ileus is also present. Analgesic agents may be necessary for severe pain. Morphine and codeine preparations should be avoided because they may cause spasm of the sphincter of Oddi, with consequent worsening of the pancreatitis. Surgery may be necessary in some patients, especially those whose pancreatitis is secondary to an obstruction.

The prognosis of patients with pancreatitis is variable, depending on the severity. Usually symptoms resolve with no long-term effects. With more severe disease, especially with accompanying hemodynamic instability and renal failure, pancreatitis may be fatal. In patients who survive the acute episode, inflammatory lesions, such as phlegmon (an area of pancreatic tissue with swelling, inflammation, and possible necrosis), abscess, or pseudocyst, may develop. Recurrent pancreatitis is rare in children but can lead to chronic pancreatitis and, ultimately, pancreatic insufficiency.

Gallbladder Disease

Diseases of the gallbladder are uncommon in children but, when present, tend to produce abdominal pain. **Cholecystitis,** an acute inflammation of the gallbladder, is usually accompanied by vague abdominal pain, which gradually localizes to the right upper quadrant. Obstruction of the cystic or common bile duct by stones, the most common inciting factor in adults with cholecystitis, is unusual in children. More commonly, cholecystitis is attributed to an intercurrent infectious illness. Ultrasound studies are useful in making the diagnosis of cholecystitis. Treatment is surgical.

Cholelithiasis, or gallstone disease, is far less common in children than in adults. Hemolytic diseases and conditions that lead to a low concentration of bile acids are the usual predisposing factors in children. Jaundice is often present, in addition to abdominal pain. Diagnosis is usually possible radiologically, and treatment of symptomatic patients is accomplished through cholecystectomy.

CHRONIC ABDOMINAL PAIN

Clinical Approach

Persistence or recurrence of abdominal pain over a period of 3 months or longer defines the condition as chronic abdominal pain. In contrast to acute abdominal pain, which demands rapid diagnosis and expeditious institution of therapy, evaluation of the patient with chronic pain requires patience, and treatment may consist largely of consolation and reassurance. A sequential plan for the evaluation of pediatric patients with chronic abdominal pain is outlined in Figure 12–9.

HISTORY

The history should be directed at differentiating between organic and functional pain. Inquiries should be made regarding changes in weight, appetite, energy level, or other symptoms such as vomiting or fever, which may accompany the episodes of abdominal pain. The character of the pain and its duration, severity, location, and quality should be determined, as should factors that alleviate or exacerbate it. Its relation to other events may be important; thus, pain that awakens the child from sleep is usually of organic origin, whereas pain that occurs only near school time is more likely to be functional. An important aspect of the history is to assess the patient's personality. Children who are especially tense, who are "worriers," or who are described as "overachievers" may experience abdominal pain as a manifestation of stress. Despite the relation of chronic abdominal pain to stress, the pain should be appreciated as real and not simply imagined.

PHYSICAL EXAMINATION

On physical examination, the general behavior of the child, such as facial expression, presence or absence of eye contact with the examiner, and other manifestations of "body language," should be observed. This could be helpful in determining whether psychological factors are contributing to the child's problems. On abdominal examination, the precise location of the pain should be noted. Apley and others have noted that functional pain is almost always localized to the umbilicus or central abdomen. Attention should be given to maneuvers that may elicit the symptoms. Abnormalities on physical examination increase the likelihood of an organic cause of the symptoms. With functional pain, the results of the physical examination are almost always entirely normal.

DIAGNOSTIC STUDIES

In the majority of children, chronic abdominal pain is functional in origin and the diagnosis is one of exclusion. If there is strong suspicion of functional pain, many clinicians choose to perform no diagnostic studies, believing that testing serves mainly to validate the patient's and family's suspicions that there is truly something anatomically or physiologically wrong. In general, diagnostic testing should be guided by pertinent positives in the history and physical examination.

Differential Diagnosis

Table 12–8 lists differential diagnoses of chronic abdominal pain. Many of these disorders are of non-GI origin and are discussed elsewhere in this text. Of the GI causes of chronic abdominal pain, most may also present with acute symptoms and are covered elsewhere in this chapter. Common GI conditions presenting primarily as chronic abdominal pain (and not covered elsewhere in this text) are discussed below.

LACTOSE INTOLERANCE

Lactose intolerance, a commonly recognized cause of chronic abdominal pain in adults, also can occur in pediatric patients. Lactose is a disaccharide found in the milk of cows and other mammals that is broken down in the intestine by the action of the brush-border enzyme lactase. In most of the world's population, lactase levels decline with maturation, corresponding to the natural process of weaning from mother's milk. As lactase levels decline, more and more lactose passes undigested to the colon. There it is digested by colonic bacteria, releasing hydrogen and carbon dioxide and giving rise to the abdominal discomfort, bloating, and "gassiness" often described in these patients. Diarrhea typically accompanies these symptoms.

Diagnosis of lactose intolerance may be made presumptively by eliminating lactose-containing foods from the diet and monitoring the patient for symptomatic improvement. A more definitive diagnosis may be made by using a lactose breath hydrogen test. After an overnight fast, patients are given a solution containing a known quantity of lactose. The amount of hydrogen expired in the patient's breath is measured. In patients who digest

Table 12–8. Differential Diagnosis: Chronic Abdominal Pain

Gastrointestinal causes	**Collagen vascular disease**	**Gynecologic disease**
Anatomic abnormalities	Juvenile rheumatoid arthritis	Dysmenorrhea[1]
Hiatus hernia	Systemic lupus erythematosus	Mittelschmerz
Linea alba hernia		Ovarian cyst
Duplications	**Endocrine disease**	Hematocolpos
Choledochal cyst	Hyperparathyroidism	Endometriosis
Mass lesions	Addison disease	
Hepatomegaly/splenomegaly		**Neurologic disease**
Bazoars	**Cardiovascular disease**	Migraine[1]
Constipation[1]	Superior mesenteric artery	Familial dysautonomia
Irritable bowel syndrome[1]	syndrome	Abdominal migraine
Peptic ulcer disease	Arrhythmias	Abdominal epilepsy
Inflammatory bowel disease	Coarctation of the aorta	
Parasitic infection		**Miscellaneous**
Lactose intolerance[1]	**Hematologic disease**	Chronic nonspecific abdominal
Heavy metal ingestion	Sickle cell anemia	pain of childhood[1]
Recurrent pancreatitis	Porphyrias	Aerophagia
Cystic fibrosis with meconium	Abdominal neoplasms	Familial Mediterranean fever
ileus equivalent	Wilms' tumor	Hereditary angioneurotic edema
	Neuroblastoma	Diskitis

[1] Frequently encountered causes of chronic abdominal pain.

lactose poorly, expired hydrogen concentrations increase within 2–3 hours. Hydrogen in the expired air is the product of colonic bacterial fermentation of lactose not digested in the small bowel.

In older children and adults, treatment of lactose intolerance is accomplished by eliminating lactose from the diet. In children for whom such elimination is undesirable or impractical, the addition of commercially available lactase enzymes to dairy products is often beneficial.

NONULCER DYSPEPSIA

Another subgroup of pediatric patients with chronic abdominal pain has symptoms that are predominantly peptic in nature. These symptoms include nausea, heartburn, and regurgitation. Excessive belching, bloating, and hiccups are also commonly described. When such symptoms are present and organic etiologies that may cause similar symptoms (e.g., esophagitis, gastritis, and peptic ulcer) have been excluded, the diagnosis of nonulcer dyspepsia may be made.

The pathogenesis of nonulcer dyspepsia remains elusive; consequently, treatment is symptomatic. Some patients note improvement with gastric acid reduction or neutralization agents, but this may be, at least in part, a placebo effect.

IRRITABLE BOWEL SYNDROME

The irritable bowel syndrome (IBS), also known as spastic colon, is a common cause of chronic abdominal pain in children and adults. Patients with IBS often complain of episodic pain, typically cramping in nature, that occurs with varying intensity and duration. The pain is frequently localized to the lower abdomen but may be perceived in any part of the abdomen, including the upper mid-abdomen. Some patients with IBS experience the onset of symptoms when eating and may feel the need to defecate soon after a meal. In many patients, diarrheal stools are passed on those occasions. After the passage of stool, patients frequently report alleviation or resolution of their pain.

The etiology of IBS is not thoroughly understood, but it is generally believed that the pain of IBS results from a disruption in peristalsis. Rather than normal, smooth, wavelike movements, peristalsis in patients with IBS is thought to be uncoordinated or spastic. This may account for the cramping nature of the pain that often occurs in IBS. Some speculate that IBS may be physiologically similar to infantile colic; a history of colic is not uncommon in patients with IBS.

The speed of intestinal transit is also apparently affected in IBS. Frequently, transit is rapid, giving rise to episodes of diarrhea with urgency. Transit time is not always rapid, however, and in some patients it may be slower than usual, giving rise to constipation.

Many patients with IBS note the clear relation between stressful situations and episodes of pain. Often the recognition of this connection by the physician, patient, and family relieves some anxiety associated with episodes of pain. Decreased anxiety in turn may be associated with a decrease in the severity and duration of painful episodes.

It is also reassuring to the patient and family to be informed of the lack of any known association between IBS and subsequent development of another, more serious medical problem.

In addition to reassurance, treatment of IBS should include counseling on the importance of a high-fiber diet. Dietary fiber, in fact, is the only intervention that has been proved consistently to be beneficial in the treatment of IBS. Fiber is equally efficacious whether provided through dietary sources or through commercially available supplements. Other dietary modifications, including the elimination of caffeine, may be associated with lessening of symptoms in some patients.

Pharmacotherapy for IBS is controversial. Multiple antispasmodic agents, including hycosamine, dicyclomine, and clidinium, are commonly used, and different degrees of efficacy in relieving symptoms have been reported. In limited amounts, these agents are probably safe and may have a role in the treatment of IBS.

CHRONIC NONSPECIFIC ABDOMINAL PAIN

Chronic, nonspecific abdominal pain (also referred to as recurrent abdominal pain) is thought to be caused by the interaction of physical or psychosocial stressors and the autonomically controlled motor activity of the intestinal tract. The child may complain of various types of abdominal pain but typically presents with gradual development of paroxysmal pain, often periumbilical in location, unrelated to meals or any other specific event but severe enough to interrupt normal activities. Some patients may describe their pain as upper abdominal in location, in association with features similar to those of nonulcer dyspepsia (see above). After excluding patients with IBS symptoms, those remaining may appropriately be said to have chronic nonspecific abdominal pain.

Some features of the history are characteristic of chronic nonspecific abdominal pain. Stressful events in the child's family or school environment often predate the onset of pain; the family is often unaware of the pain's relation to these events. Often the family is noted to be "enmeshed" and overly involved in minute details of the child's life. A family history of similar functional disturbances is also common.

The diagnosis of chronic nonspecific abdominal pain is difficult because the symptoms can change in severity and character, the physical findings are elusive or absent, and no specific tests can establish the diagnosis. However, the differential diagnosis of chronic abdominal pain is too extensive to attempt to exclude all possible causes before making the diagnosis of functional pain. A more reasonable approach is to conduct a thorough history and physical examination. If there are no indications for the presence of organic disease, and if the results of routine laboratory studies (including complete blood cell count, erythrocyte sedimentation rate, urinalysis and culture,

and stool specimen for ova and parasites) are normal, the diagnosis of functional pain may be considered. It is important to establish a definite diagnostic plan and adhere to it. Otherwise, the evaluation may be prolonged with multiple tests and procedures. In addition to possible discomfort and high costs, continuing diagnostic studies also may convey to the patient and family the message that the physician is concerned about the presence of occult organic disease.

Treatment of chronic nonspecific abdominal pain in a child should begin with a discussion of the problem with the patient and the parents, including affirmation that the pain is "real." The presumed relation of stressors and GI motility in the etiology of the pain should be explained. This information will make it easier for the diagnosis to be accepted as "legitimate."

If specific physical or psychosocial stressors have been identified, eliminating those factors may help to decrease the frequency and severity of the pain. When these stressors are psychosocial in nature, the assistance of mental health professionals may be beneficial to identify and then alleviated the stressors (see Chapter 3). Every attempt should be made to have the child reestablish a "normal" life. The child should go to school, despite the presence of pain. As little attention as possible should be given to the pain itself, and patients should be encouraged to deal with it on their own.

A high-fiber diet may be beneficial in treating functional abdominal pain. Excessive fiber, however, may cause colonic distention, increased gas, and increased pain. There is little evidence that antispasmodic agents are effective in the treatment of functional pain, but individual patients may report diminution or cessation of pain when these medications are used.

■ DIARRHEA

In less developed countries, diarrheal diseases contribute to problems of malnutrition and delayed growth and are responsible for several million deaths each year. In countries with better developed sanitation and more widely available health care, diarrheal diseases cause far fewer deaths but do cause significant morbidity. Among young children in the United States, approximately 20% of acute care medical visits and 10–15% of hospitalizations are prompted by diarrheal illnesses.

Diarrheal diseases, especially those of infectious etiology, are much more frequent in children than in adults. The reasons for this difference include a relatively immature immune system, greater likelihood for spread of organisms by the fecal–oral route, and clustering of children in group-care centers. In addition to the high incidence of diarrhea, children are more prone to have dehydration. Children have a greater fecal water loss due to incomplete reabsorption of water in the colon; this loss is increased during diarrhea. Fever, which often accompanies infectious diarrhea in children, also contributes to dehydration through an increase in evaporative fluid losses. An understanding of the physiology of fluid and electrolyte processing is important in the diagnosis and management of diarrheal diseases.

Physiology

The small intestine selectively absorbs required nutrients, electrolytes, and water and eliminates by secretion nonessential or indigestible substances. These complex processes are accomplished by the specialized functions of the various intestinal segments.

In the **duodenum,** partially digested foodstuffs are further mixed and their pH and osmotic pressure adjusted to achieve optimal conditions for nutrient and electrolyte absorption. The **jejunum** is the site of sodium-coupled active transport of amino acids and sugars accompanied by the passive absorption of water. Small peptides, which are the result of protein hydrolysis, are also absorbed in the jejunum, as are many vitamins and trace elements. In the **ileum,** additional sodium chloride is absorbed, as are bile acids and vitamin B_{12}. The colon is equipped to absorb additional sodium and chloride despite their relatively low concentrations in colonic fluid. Residual carbohydrates are metabolized by bacteria in the colon to absorbable short-chain fatty acids. The colon is also an important site of further absorption of water.

At each of these intestinal sites, the selective absorption of fluid and electrolytes depends on the intact functioning of cellular transport processes. Sodium–potassium adenosine triphosphatase, located on the basolateral membrane of enterocytes, "pumps" sodium out of the cells, creating a concentration gradient. Sodium enters the cells from lumenal fluid, causing passive intracellular movement of water. Other active transport processes important in normal intestinal functioning include sodium-coupled glucose transport, sodium-coupled amino acid transport, and the sodium–hydrogen exchange pump. Intestinal fluid secretion is achieved primarily by active transport of chloride ions.

On a macroscopic level, normal intestinal fluid and electrolyte processing rely on the existence of an adequate intestinal surface area. This is normally achieved through the microvillous and villous structure of the intestinal mucosa. If the villi are damaged or decreased in number, a decrease in effective absorptive surface area results. Normal intestinal motility is also necessary for optimal intestinal functioning. If intestinal motility is increased, fluid passage may be too rapid to allow for adequate absorption; if decreased, fluid stasis facilitates bacterial overgrowth and its consequent problems.

Normal intestinal function allows the body to process ingested fluid and foodstuffs and the significant volume of endogenously secreted fluids that accompany the digestive process. Diarrhea results when one or more components of the normal absorptive processes malfunction. Thus, from a physiologic basis, it is logical to define diarrhea as an excessive amount of water loss in the stool. This is easier to quantitate than is frequency, number, or liquidity of stools, and, indirectly, this definition encompasses each of those parameters. Under normal conditions, an infant produces approximately 5–10 g of stool/kg of body weight per day. Adults typically produce 100–200 g/d. Amounts in excess of these are usually abnormal and may have serious physiologic consequences.

Given the complex nature of normal intestinal fluid and electrolyte functioning, it is not surprising that disruption of any one of a number of parameters may upset fluid homeostasis, resulting in diarrhea. To simplify the study of these parameters, the abnormalities that cause diarrheal diseases traditionally have been classified as malabsorptive or secretory in nature on the basis of the predominant mechanism of action. In malabsorptive disorders, lumenal fluid osmotic concentration is greater than normal because of the presence of nonabsorbable substances. These substances may be unabsorbed owing to a variety of causes: decreased absorptive surface area, absence or impaired functioning of mucosal enzymes, or presence of normally nonabsorbable substances in increased amounts (e.g., sorbitol). Increased lumenal osmotic pressure causes more water to be retained in the lumen, which results in diarrhea.

In secretory disorders, the presence of certain substances within the intestinal lumen provokes an increase in chloride secretion by the intestinal crypt cells, resulting in increased luminal fluid. Certain bacterial enterotoxins (e.g., those of E. coli and Vibrio cholerae) and certain chemicals (laxatives, long-chain fatty acids) are known to be potent intestinal secretagogs. Secretory hormones, namely vasoactive intestinal peptide, have been demonstrated to provoke secretory diarrhea when excessively secreted, as occurs with some tumors.

From a clinical point of view, the physiologic mechanisms directly responsible for diarrhea may be less important—and certainly less readily accessible for investigation—than its physical manifestations. These physical and historical characteristics of diarrheal diseases are the major means through which etiologies can be determined and management strategies formulated.

Clinical Approach

History

As an initial step in the evaluation of a patient with diarrhea, the examiner must determine whether the problem is acute or chronic. Diarrheal illnesses are classified as acute if they have a duration of 2 weeks or less. Chronic cases are those that persist for longer than 2 weeks. Figures 10A and B provide an approach to the evaluation of patients with acute and chronic symptoms.

In addition to addressing the duration of symptoms, the patient history should include questions on several other pertinent topics. The coexistence of fever, for example, may indicate an infectious etiology. The presence of household contacts having similar symptoms also suggests infectious diarrheal illnesses, as does a history of day-care attendance. A history of recent travel or exposure to travelers may be relevant.

One should seek a description of the patient's stools and determine whether the complaint of diarrhea is based on increased numbers of stools or increased fluid content because either may be reported by the family as "diarrhea." The presence or absence of obvious blood and mucus should be investigated.

The patient's diet is another important component of the history. Not only might it show evidence of food-borne illnesses, but it also might aid in the diagnosis of other food-related illnesses. In celiac disease, for example, diarrhea begins after the introduction of gluten, usually from cereal, in the infant's diet. More general questions as to the patient's dietary preferences and overall nutritional health may be helpful.

PHYSICAL EXAMINATION

In examining a patient with diarrhea, assessment of the status of hydration is of primary importance. Among the most reliable measures of changes in a patient's state of hydration are changes in weight. Comparison of a child's normal weight and "dehydrated" weight shows the apparent "fluid deficit." Replacement of this fluid deficit can be accurately achieved through various techniques of rehydration (see below and Chapter 16, Kidneys & Electrolytes). If a comparison of weights is not possible, the fluid deficit may be estimated by the presence or absence of several clinical signs and symptoms (Table 12–9).

DIAGNOSTIC STUDIES

Stool examination often provides information that is useful in determining the etiology of diarrheal illnesses. If blood in the stool is suspected, evaluation for occult blood should be performed. This will exclude the possibility that the abnormal color is from ingested dyes or foods. If blood is present, an effort to determine the source of the bleeding in the upper or lower GI tract should be undertaken (see earlier in this chapter, Gastrointestinal Tract Hemorrhage). The stool should be examined for undigested vegetable matter, a finding characteristic of chronic, nonspecific diarrhea of childhood (see later in this chapter, Chronic Nonspecific Diarrhea of Infancy).

Microscopic examination of stool may provide additional useful information. The presence of leukocytes in the stool, which can be made visible more easily by the addition of a drop of methylene blue stain, is an indicator of colitis caused by bacterial infection or inflammation. Lymphocytes may be seen in the stool of patients with diarrhea due to chronic inflammatory causes, and eosinophils may be seen in patients with diarrhea due to food sensitivities. Fat in the stool, visualized with the assistance of a fat-specific stain such as Sudan red or black, suggests malabsorption or insufficiency of pancreatic enzymes. Microscopic examination may show parasites and cultures may be done to detect bacterial pathogens.

The presence of reducing substances in the stool is an indicator of carbohydrate malabsorption; this usually is assessed with the Clinitest reagent. This test underestimates the amount of carbohydrate present and does not recognize the presence of sucrose and other nonreducing sugars. Stool pH less than 5.5 also suggests carbohydrate malabsorption.

Evaluation of the electrolyte composition of stool has been used to differentiate malabsorptive from secretory causes of diarrhea. A stool sodium concentration greater than 70 mEq/L is usually indicative of a secretory etiology, whereas a concentration less than 50 mEq/L is more typical of malabsorptive diarrhea. The stool osmotic gap

$$\text{stool mOsm} - 2 \times ([\text{Na}] + [\text{K}])$$

provides another method for differentiating malabsorptive from secretory diarrheas; an osmotic gap of less than 100 mOsm/L indicates a secretory etiology, and an osmotic gap greater than 100 mOsm/L indicates a malabsorptive cause. All these measurements are merely estimates and must be interpreted with caution.

Differential Diagnosis

Causes of diarrhea in children are listed in Table 12–10. From a physiologic standpoint, it is logical to group these disorders, as they are in this table, on the basis of the organ or organ system that is primarily affected. Several of the more common causes of acute and chronic diarrhea are discussed below. A more indepth discussion of infectious gastroenteritis is found in Chapter 9.

ACUTE DIARRHEA

Infectious gastroenteritis. Acute diarrhea in children most frequently is caused by infection with viral, bacterial, or parasitic agents. Rotavirus is the single most common cause. Although several enteric viral pathogens can now be detected, no specific antiviral therapies are available. Treatment of diarrhea is limited to supportive (*text continues on page 498*)

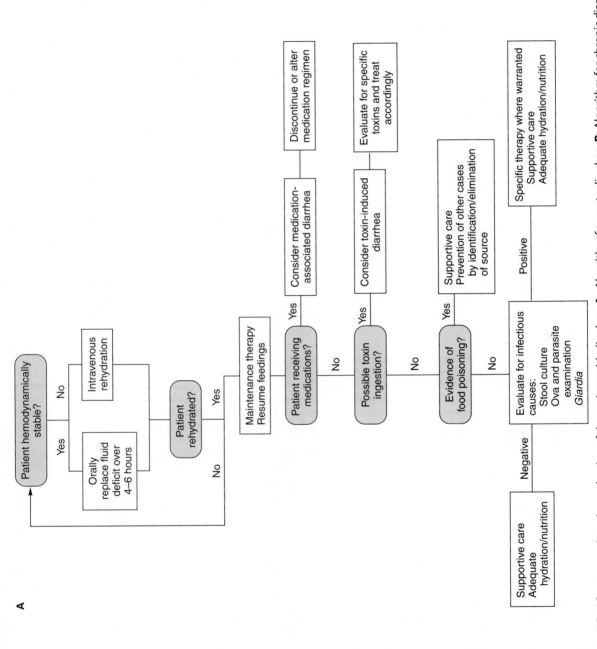

Figure 12–10. **Approach to the evaluation of the patient with diarrhea. A:** Algorithm for acute diarrhea. **B:** Algorithm for chronic diarrhea. RAST = radioallergosorbent test. (Adapted and reproduced, with permission, from Laney DW, Cohen MB: Approach to the pediatric patient with diarrhea. *Gastroenterol Clin North Am* 1993;22:499.)

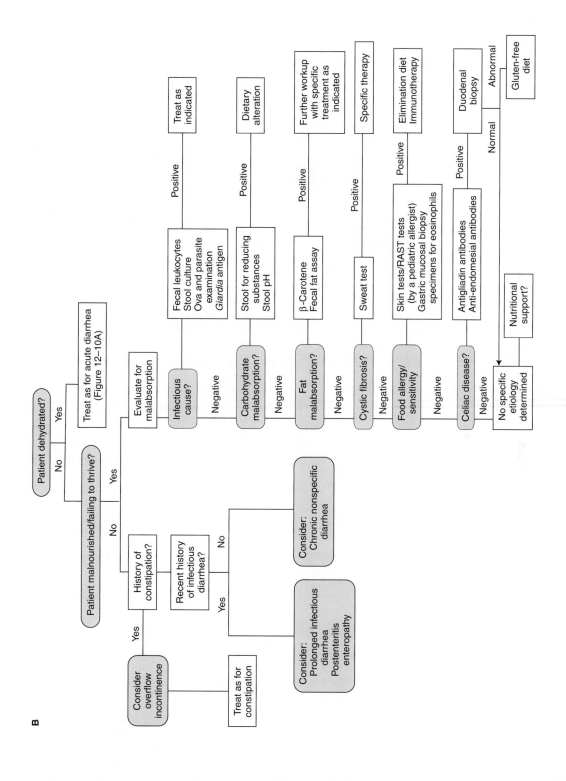

B

Patient dehydrated?

No → Patient malnourished/failing to thrive?

Yes → Treat as for acute diarrhea (Figure 12–10A)

Patient malnourished/failing to thrive?

No → History of constipation?

Yes → Evaluate for malabsorption

History of constipation?

Yes → Consider overflow incontinence

No → Recent history of infectious diarrhea?

Treat as for constipation

Recent history of infectious diarrhea?

Yes → Consider: Prolonged infectious diarrhea, Postenteritis enteropathy

No → Consider: Chronic nonspecific diarrhea

Evaluate for malabsorption

Infectious cause?
- Fecal leukocytes
- Stool culture
- Ova and parasite examination
- Giardia antigen

Positive → Treat as indicated

Negative → Carbohydrate malabsorption?
- Stool for reducing substances
- Stool pH

Positive → Dietary alteration

Negative → Fat malabsorption?
- β-Carotene
- Fecal fat assay

Positive → Further workup with specific treatment as indicated

Negative → Cystic fibrosis?
- Sweat test

Positive → Specific therapy

Negative → Food allergy/sensitivity
- Skin tests/RAST tests (by a pediatric allergist)
- Gastric mucosal biopsy specimens for eosinophils

Positive → Elimination diet Immunotherapy

Negative → Celiac disease?
- Antigliadin antibodies
- Anti-endomesial antibodies

Positive → Duodenal biopsy

Abnormal → Gluten-free diet

Normal → No specific etiology determined

Negative → No specific etiology determined

No specific etiology determined ← Nutritional support?

497

Table 12–9. Method of Estimating Degree of Dehydration on the Basis of Clinical Findings

5%	5–10%	>10%
Normal fontanelle	Sunken fontanelle	Deeply sunken fontanelle
Normal skin turgor	Normal or mildly reduced skin turgor	Reduced skin turgor
Moist mucous membranes	Tacky to dry mucous membranes	Very dry mucous membranes
Eyes with tears	Dry eyes; slightly sunken	Dry, sunken eyes
Normal urine output	Decreased urine output	No urine output
Normal peripheral circulation	Delayed capillary refill	Extremities cool and mottled
Normal mental status	Increased irritability or lethargy	Obtunded
Normal heart rate	Normal to increased heart rate	Rapid heart rate
Normal blood pressure	Orthostatic hypotension	Severe hypotension or shock

measures, including the effective use of rehydration techniques (see later in this chapter, Oral Rehydration). With bacterial infection, antibiotics may be beneficial in addition to rehydration. Viral and bacterial enteric pathogens and their treatment are discussed in Chapter 9.

Food poisoning syndromes. Acute diarrhea may result from food poisoning. Foods may be infected with bacteria or parasites or contain preformed bacterial toxins. *Staphylococcus aureus* is frequently implicated in the contamination of custards and cream-filled pastries that are insufficiently cooked or not properly refrigerated. Symptoms of staphylococcal poisoning, which include nausea, vomiting, and abdominal cramps in addition to diarrhea, develop within 4–6 hours of ingesting contaminated food. This short incubation period is characteristic enough that it is used to make a presumptive diagnosis. Symptoms usually resolve spontaneously within 24 hours.

Clostridium botulinum produces toxins that are among the most potent poisons known. Despite their potency, however, they are readily destroyed by boiling or thorough cooking of foods. Botulism may be acquired through home-canned foods and raw or commercially processed seafood. Nausea, vomiting, and diarrhea usually develop 12 hours to 3 days after ingestion of contaminated food. Symptoms associated with the central nervous system include dry mouth, dysphagia, blurred vision, and possibly paralysis of the respiratory muscles. Treatment includes administration of specific antitoxin and supportive measures, including ventilatory assistance when indicated. *Clostridium botulinum* infection in infants may be contracted through ingestion of contaminated foodstuffs. Of interest, in this age group, botulism tends to cause constipation rather than diarrhea (see Chapter 21, The Nervous System).

Clostridium perfringens, typically carried by contaminated meat and poultry products, causes a diarrheal illness within 8–15 hours of ingestion. *Vibrio parahaemolyticus* produces illness 8–22 hours after ingesting uncooked fish or shellfish. *Salmonellae, Shigellae, Yersinia,* and many other enteric pathogens can cause diarrhea.

Poisons & toxic ingestions. Ingestion of toxic substances is common in children. Because many of these agents provoke GI symptoms, toxins always should be considered in the differential diagnosis of acute diarrhea. The specific diagnosis and treatment of toxin ingestion is discussed in Chapter 10 (Injuries & Emergencies).

Pharmacologic agents. Pharmacologic agents are also frequently responsible for acute diarrhea. The temporal relation between administration of the medication and the onset of diarrhea suggests the drug's involvement. Discontinuation of the suspected medication may be sufficient treatment.

Medications may be given surreptitiously by a parent to provoke symptoms and make a child appear ill. This situation has been described as Münchausen syndrome by proxy. Laxatives and stool softeners may be given to the child to induce diarrhea. The possibility of Münchausen syndrome by proxy should be considered in a patient with diarrhea—acute or chronic—that cannot otherwise be explained.

CHRONIC DIARRHEA

Diarrhea lasting longer than 2 weeks may result from the same enteric infectious agents that cause acute diarrhea. If the child's resistance is decreased by other concurrent illnesses, the diarrhea may become chronic. There is also a risk for prolonged infectious diarrhea in patients with congenital or acquired immunodeficiencies. Coinfection with more than one enteric pathogen also can cause a more chronic diarrhea than would be expected with either organism alone.

Another related cause of chronic diarrhea is **postenteritis enteropathy**, in which transient mucosal damage is sustained secondary to an enteric infection. This mucosal damage often includes the loss of digestive enzymes, namely lactase. These patients experience transient carbohydrate intolerance and its accompanying

Table 12–10. Differential Diagnosis: Diarrhea

Gastrointestinal infections
  Viruses[1]
    Rotavirus
    Norwalk agent
    Enteric adenovirus
  Bacteria[1]
    Salmonella
    Shigella
    Campylobacter
    Yersinia
    Escherichia coli
    Clostridium difficile
    Vibrio cholerae
  Parasites[1]
    Giardia lamblia
    Amoeba
  Fungi
    Candida
    Cryptosporidium
  Disorders probably of infectious etiology[1]
    Necrotizing enterocolitis
    Inflammatory bowel disease

Dietary causes
  Contaminated food/water
  Malnutrition
  Overfeeding
  Inadequate dietary fat[1]
  Sorbitol, fructose, or other poorly
    absorbed carbohydrates[1]
  Nutrient deficiencies
    Niacin deficiency (pellagra)
    Zinc deficiency (acrodermatitis
      enteropathica)
    Folic acid deficiency
  Food allergies/intolerances[1]

Extraintestinal infections
  Urinary tract infections
  Otitis media
  Pneumonia
  Sepsis
  Pancreatitis

Toxins
  Boric acid
  Naphthalene (moth balls)
  Organophosphates
  Carbamates
  Iron overdosage
  Arsenic
  Lithium
  Mercury
  Poisonous mushrooms)

Pharmacologic agents
  Antibiotics[1]
  Decongestants
  Theophylline
  Chemotherapeutic agents
    (including irradiation)
  Liquid medications (containing
    poorly absorbed sugars)

Anatomic defects
  Malrotation
  Intestinal duplications
  Hirschsprung disease
  Intestinal lymphangiectasia
  Postoperative
    Short bowel syndrome
    Blind loop syndrome

Nutrient absorption disorders
  Pancreatic defects
    Cystic fibrosis[1]
    Schwachman syndrome
    Chronic pancreatitis
  Lipolytic defects
    Congenital lipase deficiency
    Congenital colipase deficiency
    Bile acid malabsorption
  Proteolytic defects
    Congenital trypsinogen deficiency
    Congenital enterokinase deficiency
  Hydrolytic defects
    Sucrase–isomaltase deficiency
    Lactase deficiency
  Transport defects
    Glucose–galactose malabsorption
    Familial chloride diarrhea
  Disorders causing villous atrophy
    Celiac disease[1]
    Protein intolerances[1]
      (milk, soya, rice, wheat)
    Autoimmune enteropathy
  Lymphatic obstruction
    Abetalipoproteinemia
    Intestinal lymphangiectasia
    Whipple disease

Metabolic defects
  Galactosemia
  Hartnup disease

Endocrine defects
  Thyrotoxicosis
  Addison disease
  Adrenogenital syndrome
    and hypoadrenalism
  Hypoparathyroidism
  Hyperparathyroidism
  Wolman disease

Neoplastic disease
  Neuroblastoma
  Ganglioneuroma
  Pheochromocytoma
  Carcinoid syndrome

Immunologic defects
  Immunoglobulin A deficiency
  Hypogammaglobulinemia/
    agammaglobulinemia
  Combined immunodeficiency
    syndrome
  Wiskott–Aldrich syndrome
  Ataxia–telangiectasia
  Defective cellular immunity
  Acquired immunodeficiency
    syndrome (AIDS)

Neurologic disorders
  Familial dysautonomia
  Neurofibromatosis

Miscellaneous etiologies
  Stress[1]
  Overflow diarrhea secondary
    to encopresis[1]
  Irritable bowel syndrome[1]

[1] Frequently encountered causes of diarrhea.

diarrhea. Treatment with lactose-free or elemental formulas is often adequate, and symptoms resolve in 4–8 weeks. Several additional causes of chronic diarrhea are discussed below.

Chronic nonspecific diarrhea of infancy. Chronic, nonspecific diarrhea of infancy describes an entity characterized by chronic diarrhea with no definitive cause in an otherwise healthy baby who is well nourished and who has grown normally. This condition, also called **"toddler's diarrhea"** and the "sloppy stool syndrome," typically affects children aged 6–24 months. The parents often note that stools contain particles of undigested food. Several factors have been implicated in the etiology of this disorder, including dietary fat restriction, excessive intake of fluids, excessive intake of poorly absorbed carbohydrates contained in fruit juice or sorbitol (a nonabsorbed sweetening agent), and abnormal small intestinal motility. Treatment may begin with the removal of any of these potential provocative agents. The mainstay of treatment, however, is reassurance to the parents that the problem usually resolves, spontaneously and without sequelae, when the child is 2–4 years old.

Protracted diarrhea of infancy. Protracted diarrhea of infancy is defined as diarrhea of greater than 2 weeks' duration in an infant younger than 3 months, in which three or more stools have had no ova or parasites and the cultures are negative. Unlike children with chronic, nonspecific diarrhea, these babies experience significant malabsorption and often fail to thrive. Protracted diarrhea may have its onset with an episode of acute infectious diarrhea; this emphasizes the importance of appropriate management and follow-up of infants with acute diarrhea. Bile acid malabsorption and the existence of antienterocyte antibodies have been proposed as possible mechanisms for protracted diarrhea. These infants are managed by administering elemental formulas enterally and providing parenteral nutrition when warranted.

Short bowel syndrome. The "short bowel syndrome" results from resection of significant portions of the intestine. The clinical features are attributable mainly to malabsorption and its consequences: diarrhea and growth failure. Conditions in which bowel resection is significant enough to cause symptoms of malabsorption are (1) congenital anomalies of the GI tract, including atresias, omphaloceles, gastroschisis, and vascular anomalies of the superior mesenteric artery; and (2) inflammatory or ischemic disorders, especially necrotizing enterocolitis (in neonates) and Crohn's disease.

After resection, the remaining intestine undergoes adaptation to maintain adequate absorption. Mucosal hyperplasia may be so great as to increase the effective surface area fourfold. This adaptive response appears not to occur without enteral nutrition. Therefore, it is important to initiate enteral nutrition as soon as possible after the fluid and electrolyte status has been stabilized in the initial postoperative period. As the patient's tolerance of enteral nutrition increases, the proportion of calories supplied parenterally may be decreased. The gradual change from parenteral to enteral nutrition may require months to years, depending on the amount and location of the initial bowel segment resection. Although many of these patients require extended hospitalizations, the increasing availability of nursing services that assist in the administration of home parenteral and enteral nutrition make earlier discharge possible. Intestinal transplantation is being explored as a means of therapy for patients with the short bowel syndrome.

Bacterial overgrowth is a common complication of the short bowel syndrome. Disruption of the normal anatomy and changes in normal motility allow for intestinal fluid stasis and increased colonization by bacteria normally present in the intestine. The bacteria cause deconjugation of bile acids and mucosal inflammation, both of which cause malabsorption. This problem may also lead to elevation of serum D-lactate levels. Diagnosis of bacterial overgrowth is possible by aspiration and culture of the intestinal fluid or by use of breath hydrogen testing. Treatment with broad-spectrum antibiotics is recommended.

Diarrhea due to malabsorption. Chronic diarrhea may be caused by one or more defects in processing of nutrients. These disorders are characterized by the symptoms of chronic diarrhea, abdominal distention, and failure to thrive.

The normal digestion and absorption of nutrients is a complex process involving separate mechanisms for carbohydrate, protein, and fat. It would be logical to classify problems of malabsorption on the basis of the affected nutrient. Unfortunately, isolated defects affecting the absorption of only one class of nutrients are the exception rather than the rule. An alternative method of classification, which considers the site of the defect itself, has been devised: intralumenal, at the intestinal mucosal surface, or at a site encountered after absorption into the enterocyte. Both models are presented schematically in Figure 12–11.

Intraluminal defects (Figure 12–11A). Disorders of intraluminal digestion with malabsorption are most commonly caused by pancreatic insufficiency and may affect all three classes of nutrients. **Cystic fibrosis,** an autosomal recessive inherited defect of chloride secretion, causes exocrine pancreatic insufficiency. This process apparently begins in utero with decreased rate of fluid flow through the pancreatic ducts with consequent plugging, which leads to a loss of exocrine function with inadequate production of amylases, proteases, lipases, and colipases. In addition to severe malabsorption, GI manifestations include meconium ileus and meconium ileus equivalent, focal biliary cirrhosis, and hypofunctioning of the gallbladder with the possible development of gallstones. Once recognized, these symptoms may be remedied through the

scaled to 94%

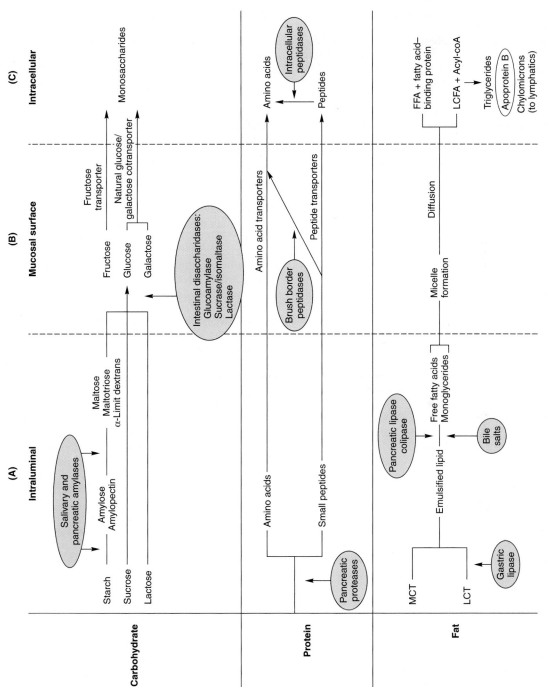

Figure 12–11. Chart representing the major components involved in the digestion of carbohydrates, proteins, and fats. FFA = free fatty acids; LCFA = long-chain fatty acids; LCT = long-chain triglycerides; MCT = medium-chain triglycerides.

use of pharmacologic pancreatic enzyme supplements. Rectal prolapse also occurs at increased frequency in patients with cystic fibrosis and may be the presenting symptom.

The diagnosis of cystic fibrosis usually is confirmed by use of the sweat chloride test. Pancreatic function tests and measurements of pancreatic enzymes in the stool are much more difficult to perform and are also of more limited utility. The pulmonary manifestations and other aspects of this disease are discussed in Chapter 18.

Schwachman's syndrome is another disorder of exocrine pancreatic function. Pancreatic function is not as severely affected as in cystic fibrosis, and significant fat malabsorption may not be present. The results of sweat chloride tests in these patients are normal. In addition to GI manifestations, patients with Shwachman's syndrome typically have short stature, skeletal abnormalities, bone marrow dysfunction, neutropenia, and, consequently, recurrent infections. Those with significant fat malabsorption benefit from pancreatic enzyme replacement. Of interest, the need for these supplements may decrease with age.

Isolated pancreatic enzyme deficiencies, which result in the malabsorption of only one class of nutrient, are rare. Intraluminal fat malabsorption may result from congenital lipase or colipase deficiency, disorders of bile acid synthesis and absorption, and disorders of bile acid excretion (e.g., biliary atresia). Selective protein malabsorption is rare but occurs with congenital enterokinase deficiency.

Mucosal surface defects (Figure 12–11B). Malabsorption may be caused by defects in the intestinal mucosae. The most common group of these disorders is associated with intestinal villous atrophy and includes celiac disease, milk and soy protein intolerance, *Giardia lamblia* infection, and postenteritis enteropathy.

Patients with **celiac disease** are intolerant of gluten, a protein found in wheat and rye but not in corn and rice. Exposure to gluten-containing foods leads to small intestinal mucosal damage and eventually to villous atrophy. The mechanism by which this protein intolerance develops is not yet known. With loss of normal intestinal villous structure, production of brush-border enzymes (disaccharidases, peptidases) is impaired and nutrients cannot be properly absorbed.

Preliminary evaluation in patients suspected to have this disorder may include testing for antiendomesial antibodies. Presence of these antibodies suggests celiac disease and usually warrants further diagnostic testing. A presumptive diagnosis of celiac disease may be made on the basis of a small intestinal mucosal biopsy specimen demonstrating characteristic villous atrophy. Patients are then treated with a gluten-free diet. Resolution of symptoms of malabsorption and the return of normal villous morphology on a subsequent biopsy specimen add more evidence to the diagnosis.

Cow's milk protein allergy, the most common food allergy in children, can induce villous atrophy and malabsorption. Patients may exhibit other allergic symptoms such as rhinorrhea, cough, and eczema. Infants also frequently present with symptoms of colitis such as blood in their stools (see above, Lower Gastrointestinal Tract Hemorrhage). Treatment necessitates removal of the offending allergen; soy-based formulas are often tried first. However, as many as 25% of infants with cow's milk allergy are also allergic to soy-based products. These patients may be fed formulas containing hydrolyzed proteins. Milk protein allergy should be differentiated from milk intolerance, which may be due to lactase deficiency (see below), fat intolerance, and other causes.

Intracellular defects (Figure 12–11C). The third group of malabsorptive disorders is associated with defects at the cellular level. These disorders typically do not cause alteration of the intestinal mucosa or other morphologic changes but are due to absent or abnormal digestive enzymes. Patients with **sucrase–isomaltase deficiency** have complete or almost complete absence of sucrase activity accompanied by a variable decrease in maltase and isomaltase activities. The disease, inherited in an autosomal recessive manner, leads to the onset of watery diarrhea when affected individuals are exposed to sucrose or starch-containing foods. Diagnosis is made presumptively with a sucrose hydrogen breath test and definitively by assay for the specific enzymes in intestinal mucosal biopsy specimens. Treatment involves elimination of sucrose and starch from the diet. Dietary restriction is usually necessary only during the first few years of life. **Congenital lactase deficiency,** a similar but even rarer disorder, causes malabsorption of lactose, the major sugar in milk. **Hypolactasia,** which refers to the normal decline in lactase activity occurring with maturation, is much more common.

Malabsorption may be due to defective nutrient transport in the mucosa (Figure 12–11B and C). **Glucose–galactose malabsorption** occurs when the sodium-coupled transport protein for those sugars is absent. Typically, these patients present with profuse, watery diarrhea in the first few days after birth; if untreated, severe dehydration and acidosis develop. Treatment is based on the elimination of the malabsorbed sugars from the diet by use of commercially available formulas designed especially for patients with this defect.

Another mechanism for malabsorption involves abnormal nutrient passage away from the absorptive cells. In **intestinal lymphangiectasia,** the lymphatics that drain the intestinal villi are dilated because of a congenital structural defect or an obstructed lymphatic drainage. These dilated lymphatics are evident in intestinal biopsy specimens of affected individuals. As dilatation progresses, lymphatic rupture occurs, with ensuing loss of serum proteins and possible development of edema and ascites. This condition may be mitigated by the use of diets enriched in medium-chain triglycerides.

Abetalipoproteinemia, another defect of nutrient transport, may lead to malabsorption. Congenital inability to synthesize apoprotein B leads to defective chylomicron synthesis and subsequent transport from the absorptive cells into the lymphatics. Intestinal biopsy specimens show accumulated lipid droplets. Non-GI manifestations of this disease include ataxia and progressive neuromuscular degeneration, ocular disease including retinitis pigmentosa, and acanthocytosis, all of which are related to vitamin E deficiency. Relief of the symptoms of malabsorption may be accomplished through dietary restriction of long-chain fatty acids. Supplementation with medium-chain triglycerides and fat-soluble vitamins may be beneficial.

Management

ORAL REHYDRATION

In almost all cases of diarrheal illness, the most crucial facet of management is the timely determination of the patient's degree of dehydration (see Diarrhea, Clinical Evaluation) and the restoration of normal hydration. Rehydration may be accomplished orally or intravenously; for a variety of reasons, however, the oral route is usually preferable. Oral rehydration solutions are widely available and may be safely administered at home. Oral therapy is less invasive than intravenous therapy and, consequently, less painful to the patient. The simplicity and safety of oral rehydration make it far more advantageous.

The selection of appropriate fluids is of crucial importance in oral rehydration. Home remedies, including carbonated beverages and liquid gelatin, do not provide the appropriate concentrations of glucose and electrolytes necessary for the most efficient and safe restoration of fluid balance. It is recommended that commercially available oral rehydration solutions be used. Much attention has been given to the development of optimal oral rehydration solutions. Acceptable products are formulated to provide an isotonic combination of sodium and glucose to which potassium and bicarbonate are added. Glucose, in concentrations of 110–140 mmol/L (yielding 2–2.5% glucose), takes advantage of glucose-coupled sodium transport mechanisms by maximize sodium absorption. The concentration of sodium in currently available oral rehydration solutions ranges from 30 to 90 mEq/L. These products, regardless of their sodium concentration, have been shown to be effective and safe in the reestablishment of hydration. Because of concern regarding the possibility of iatrogenic hypernatremia, however, the American Academy of Pediatrics recommends that solutions with sodium concentrations in the range of 70–90 mEq/L be used only for initial replacement of the water and sodium deficit. Solutions with lower sodium concentra-

tions (40–60 mEq/L) are then recommended as maintenance fluids until the patient resumes a normal diet. For most patients in developed countries, however, solutions that have a sodium concentration in the 40–60 mEq/L range may be used safely for rehydration and maintenance. Contraindications to oral rehydration therapy are (1) severe dehydration (>10%) and hemodynamic instability, (2) stool output greater than 10 mL/kg/h, and (3) the coexistence of ileus. Vomiting is not a contraindication to the use of oral rehydration therapy. Complications in the use of oral rehydration solution are uncommon.

Once it has been determined that a patient is an appropriate candidate for oral rehydration, an estimate of the fluid deficit is needed. This may be determined from documented weight loss since onset of illness or from the estimated degree of dehydration (Table 12–9). For example, in a patient weighing 7.0 kg with 5% dehydration, the deficit is $(0.05 \times 7.0) = 0.35$ L, or 350 mL. The deficit amount, in addition to the normal maintenance requirement, should be replaced over 4–6 hours by offering the patient frequent small amounts from a spoon, bottle, or cup. After the initial deficit is replaced, the patient's hydration status should be reevaluated. If the patient is appropriately hydrated, maintenance therapy only should be continued. If significant dehydration persists, the deficit amount should again be determined and replaced. Only if the patient's clinical status deteriorates should the oral route be abandoned and intravenous therapy substituted. Intravenous therapy for dehydration is discussed in Chapter 15 (Kidneys & Electrolytes).

REFEEDING

After restoration of a normal state of hydration, it is necessary to restore normal diet. Common practice has been to withhold feedings in the early phases of treatment of acute diarrhea. This offers some benefit by shortening the severity and duration of diarrhea. The benefits of more rapid reintroduction of foods, however, seem to outweigh those of withholding. These include stimulation of intestinal digestive enzymes and increased mucosal cell growth. In the breast-fed infant, it is also advantageous to resume nursing as soon as possible. In light of these advantages, many recommend resumption of feedings as soon as rehydration has been achieved. In the formula-fed infant, use of lactose-free formula in the first 48 hours of feeding may be of some advantage. In the nursing infant, breast milk is normally well tolerated. In older children, reintroduction of solid foods may begin with complex carbohydrates and the addition of other foods as the patient returns to normalcy. Feedings initially should be in small amounts offered at frequent intervals.

OTHER THERAPIES

The techniques of oral rehydration and reintroduction of a normal diet are applicable to all patients with diarrhea and dehydration, regardless of the cause. In patients with chronic diarrhea, management may be more difficult. This may involve dietary modifications and the use of specific or general nutritional supplementation. Efforts should focus on achieving as nearly normal growth and development as is possible.

■ JAUNDICE IN THE NEONATE

Jaundice may be associated with benign, self-limiting conditions or progressive disorders that lead to cirrhosis and end-stage liver disease. Many of these disorders become apparent in the neonatal period and are discussed in this section. Causes of jaundice more often presenting in childhood or adolescence are discussed in the next section.

Physiology

Bilirubin is the major product of the breakdown of heme. Heme is first converted to biliverdin, which is then reduced to bilirubin. This "free," or unconjugated, bilirubin is released into the plasma, where it combines with albumin, making it water soluble and facilitating transport to the liver. Unconjugated bilirubin is taken up by the hepatocytes, where it is conjugated with glucuronic acid by the action of enzymes in the microsomal and canalicular membranes. Most of this conjugated, lipid-soluble bilirubin is then excreted as a component of bile into the intestine. A small portion of the conjugated bilirubin reenters the blood.

In the intestine, bilirubin is catabolized to urobilinogen by the action of the indigenous bacterial flora. A portion of this water-soluble urobilinogen is reabsorbed from the intestine and returns to the liver (the enterohepatic circulation). A small percentage of the reabsorbed urobilinogen is excreted by the kidneys as urobilin. The urobilinogen remaining in the intestine is converted to stercobilin and excreted in the feces. Urobilin and stercobilin, respectively, are largely responsible for the pigmentation of the urine and stool, thus explaining the association of acholic (unpigmented) stool and dark urine with disorders that impair bilirubin metabolism or excretion.

Several aspects of bilirubin metabolism are not fully developed in the newborn infant. The shorter life span of erythrocytes and the higher red cell mass are responsible for an increased bilirubin load in the neonate. Binding of albumin to unconjugated bilirubin is less efficient in the neonate, as are the mechanisms of conjugation. Bile flow is decreased owing to a combination of factors, including inefficient bile acid uptake and conjugation and decreased hepatocellular excretion. The physical structure of the neonatal liver may add to the decreased efficiency of bile excretion. The enterohepatic recirculation of unconju-

gated bilirubin may be increased in the neonate, in part because of the relative sparseness of bacterial colonization of the neonatal intestine and consequent decreased conversion of bilirubin to urobilinogen.

Clinical Approach

HISTORY

The history may provide important clues regarding the cause of jaundice in the neonate. Prenatal course, gestational age, and delivery history should be noted. The infant's behavior should be evaluated because irritability, vomiting, or poor feeding often accompany metabolic disturbances. The appearance of the stools is important; acholic stools often indicate extrahepatic biliary obstruction. The family history should be explored for possible genetic or inherited defects.

PHYSICAL EXAMINATION

In addition to a detailed physical examination, certain specific features should be noted, such as the degree of jaundice in the skin and sclera, the presence of distinctive or unusual facial appearance, and presence of organomegaly or abdominal masses. The chest should be examined for murmurs; peripheral pulmonic stenosis may be associated with arteriohepatic dysplasia.

DIAGNOSTIC STUDIES

Figure 12–12 presents an algorithm outlining an approach to the diagnosis of neonatal jaundice. In this evaluation, a crucial first step is the differentiation of **unconjugated bilirubin** (indirect hyperbilirubinemia) from that due to increased **conjugated bilirubin** (direct hyperbilirubinemia). This is important not only for diagnostic purposes but also because there is some urgency in recognizing direct hyperbilirubinemia and cholestasis (reduction of bile flow). When the conjugated bilirubin concentration is 2 mg/dL, or 20% or more of total bilirubin, the child should be evaluated for disorders of conjugated hyperbilirubinemia.

Examination of the peripheral blood smear and Coombs testing is useful in determining whether hemolysis is a causative factor. In the absence of hemolysis or infection, unconjugated hyperbilirubinemia is most likely physiologic or related to intake of breast milk. For patients whose jaundice does not fit the typical pattern of physiologic or breast milk jaundice (see below), enzyme defects that lead to alterations in bilirubin uptake and storage should be considered.

A far more complex evaluation usually is necessary to determine the etiology of conjugated hyperbilirubinemia. Because of the importance of early intervention in some of these disorders, this evaluation should be accomplished as expeditiously as possible. Initially, a group of studies should be undertaken to look for evidence of one of the

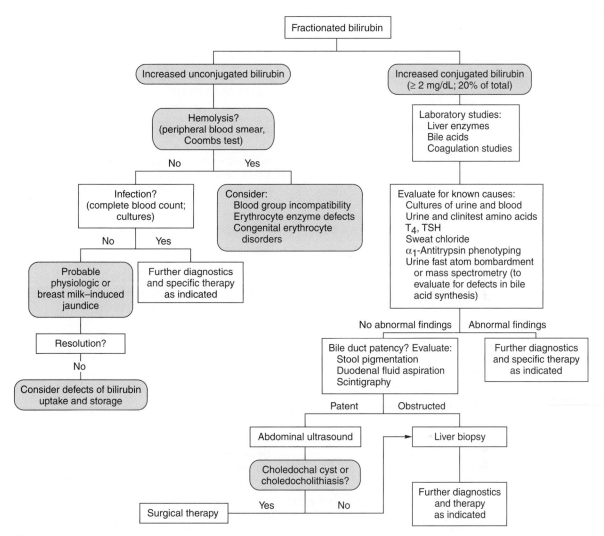

Figure 12–12. Algorithm presenting an approach to the evaluation of the neonate with jaundice. TSH = thyroid-stimulating hormone.

several known causes of neonatal cholestasis. These studies may include cultures of blood and urine, viral titers, thyroid hormone levels, sweat chloride concentrations, and α_1-antitrypsin phenotype. A urine Clinitest should be done to check for reducing substances; a positive test suggests galactosemia, the diagnosis of which can be confirmed by finding reduced levels of galactose-1-phosphate uridyl transferase activity in erythrocytes. Positive findings may then be confirmed with additional studies, as indicated. Specific therapy can then be initiated.

In most patients, the initial screening studies do not show the etiology. Evaluation should then proceed to de-termine the patency of the bile ducts. This includes observation of the presence or absence of stool pigmentation, examination of duodenal fluid pigmentation, and investigation of biliary uptake and excretion with scintigraphy. In patients with evidence of decreased or absent excretory function, biliary atresia is likely and evaluation should proceed accordingly. Ultrasound is useful to investigate the possibility of choledochal cyst or cholelithiasis as a cause of extrahepatic biliary obstruction.

In patients in whom extrahepatic causes of cholestasis have been ruled out, liver biopsy should be performed. Histologic findings in many of these patients will be consistent with the diagnosis of idiopathic neonatal hepatitis. Alternatively, biopsy findings may be consistent with another cause of cholestasis.

Differential Diagnosis

The differential diagnosis of neonatal jaundice is presented in Table 12–11. Several of the more common and important disorders are discussed below.

Unconjugated Hyperbilirubinemia

Physiologic jaundice. Inefficient bilirubin metabolism and increased bilirubin production combine to make unconjugated hyperbilirubinemia a physiologic phenomenon of the newborn. Bilirubin concentrations are somewhat elevated in newborn infants and continue to increase to maximal levels of 8–9 mg/dL by 3–5 days postnatally. The concentrations then gradually decrease, reaching normal values (approximately 2 mg/dL) by the end of the second week. In premature infants, the peak value may be somewhat higher, and hyperbilirubinemia may persist somewhat longer than 2 weeks.

Without evidence of an underlying disorder, normal term infants with unconjugated bilirubin concentrations of 10–12 mg/dL or less do not usually require further evaluation or treatment. If the bilirubin concentration is

Table 12–11. Differential Diagnosis: Neonatal Jaundice

Unconjugated hyperbilirubinemia	
Increased bilirubin production	Decreased bilirubin uptake or storage
Hemolytic disease[1]	Crigler–Najjar syndrome, type I
Isoimmune hemolysis (Rh, ABO, or other incompatibility)	Crigler–Najjar syndrome, type II (Arias syndrome)
Erythrocyte defects[1]	Gilbert's syndrome
Congenital spherocytosis	Lucey–Driscoll syndrome
Hereditary elliptocytosis	Drug inhibition
Infantile pyknocytosis	Hypothyroidism/hypopituitarism
Erythrocyte enzyme defects[1]	Congestive heart failure
Glucose-6-phosphatase dehydrogenase	Portacaval shunt
Pyruvate kinase	Hypoxia
Hexokinase	Acidosis
Infection[1]	Sepsis[1]
Enclosed hematoma[1]	Altered enterohepatic circulation
Polycythemia[1]	Breast milk jaundice[1]
Drugs (e.g., vitamin K)	Intestinal obstruction
	Antibiotic administration
Conjugated hyperbilirubinemia	
Intrahepatic disorders	Hepatitis
Idiopathic neonatal hepatitis[1]	Infectious (including cytomegalovirus, ECHO virus, rubella)
Intrahepatic persistent cholestasis	Toxic (secondary to total parenteral nutrition or sepsis)
Arteriohepatic dysplasia (Alagille syndrome)	Genetic/chromosomal (trisomy E, Down syndrome, Donahue
Byler's disease (persistent familial intrahepatic cholestasis)	syndrome)
Zellweger's syndrome	Miscellaneous disorders
Anatomic disorders	Histiocytosis X
Congenital hepatic fibrosis/infantile polycystic disease	Shock/hypoperfusion
Caroli disease	Intestinal obstruction
Metabolic disorders	Polysplenia syndrome
Disorders of amino acid metabolism (e.g., tyrosinemia)	Extrahepatic disorders
Disorders of lipid metabolism (e.g., Wolman disease,	Biliary atresia[1]
Niemann–Pick disease, Gaucher disease)	Bile duct stenosis
Disorders of carbohydrate metabolism (e.g., galactosemia,	Anomalies of the choledochopancreaticoductal junction
fructosemia, glycogen storage disease type IV)	Mass (neoplasia, stone)
Disorders in which the defect is uncharacterized	Bile/mucous plug
α_1-Antitrypsin deficiency	
Cystic fibrosis[1]	
Neonatal iron storage disease	

[1] Frequently encountered causes of neonatal jaundice. ECHO = enteric cytopathogenic human orphan (virus).

higher or remains elevated for more than 2 weeks, the possibility of hemolytic disease, impaired bilirubin conjugation, or other causes of indirect hyperbilirubinemia, including breast feeding, must be investigated.

With physiologic jaundice and indirect hyperbilirubinemia due to other causes, the major concern is the development of kernicterus. **Kernicterus** is the staining of the basal ganglia, pons, or cerebellum caused by the accumulation of unconjugated bilirubin. This condition may manifest clinically with a variety of neurologic symptoms, ranging from lethargy and hypotonia to severe encephalopathy. Kernicterus is often fatal; in survivors, some degree of neurologic insult is usually present. Kernicterus apparently does not develop unless the serum concentration of unconjugated bilirubin exceeds 20 mg/dL. Therapy should be instituted when levels are in this range. Unconjugated bilirubin is subjected to photochemical reduction by light with a wavelength of 450 nm. Phototherapy is useful in decreasing the levels of unconjugated bilirubin, regardless of the cause.

Breast milk jaundice. Breast-fed infants commonly have higher plasma concentrations of unconjugated bilirubin than do bottle-fed infants. Typically, these infants show a slow progression of jaundice, with peak bilirubin values of 10–20 mg/dL occurring 2–3 weeks after birth. In some breast-fed infants, especially those with poor caloric intake or inadequate hydration, jaundice may be noted somewhat earlier.

The mechanism of breast milk–associated jaundice is not well understood but may involve increased intestinal bilirubin reabsorption. Treatment of breast milk jaundice usually is not necessary. If levels of unconjugated bilirubin are increasing rapidly and nearing 20 mg/dL, therapy is often instituted, even though kernicterus has not been documented to occur in association with breast milk jaundice. Brief interruption of breast feeding is often sufficient to allow for reduction in serum bilirubin levels. When nursing is resumed, bilirubin levels typically increase, but with a peak value lower than previously.

Other causes of unconjugated hyperbilirubinemia. Several enzymatic defects cause hyperbilirubinemia as a result of alterations in uptake, storage, or conjugation of bilirubin. **Crigler–Najjar syndrome** is characterized by absent (type I) or deficient (type II) hepatic glucuronyl transferase activity and consequent hyperbilirubinemia with levels of unconjugated bilirubin in the range of 20–40 mg/dL. Kernicterus develops unless the disorder is treated aggressively, usually with bilirubin binding agents, phenobarbital, or phototherapy. Orthotopic liver transplantation may be necessary in patients with type I Crigler–Najjar syndrome.

Patients with **Gilbert's syndrome** have mildly elevated levels of unconjugated bilirubin secondary to decreased hepatic bilirubin uptake, the exact mechanism of which remains poorly understood. These patients will be found to have bilirubin diglucuronide in their bile, which helps to differentiate them from those with Crigler–Najjar syndrome. Typically, patients with Gilbert's syndrome experience fluctuating levels of bilirubin, with increases secondary to stressors including illness and fasting. Often the disorder is so mild that it is not diagnosed until puberty or later; the sole physical finding may be scleral icterus. No treatment is necessary.

Lucey–Driscoll syndrome (transient familial neonatal hyperbilirubinemia) is a rare disorder characterized by the presence of marked (>60 mg/dL) hyperbilirubinemia, usually beginning on the first day after birth. This condition is thought to be caused by the transient presence of a glucuronyl transferase inhibitory factor. Kernicterus commonly develops if the disorder is not treated. With the use of exchange transfusions, however, most infants recover and have no permanent sequelae.

CONJUGATED HYPERBILIRUBINEMIA

Unlike conditions associated with elevations of unconjugated bilirubin, which are often transient, elevations of conjugated bilirubin concentrations tend to be prolonged. These conditions are referred to collectively as **neonatal cholestasis.** The extent of possible differential diagnoses of neonatal cholestasis and the similarity of the clinical presentations of many of the disorders make diagnosis a challenge. Further, arriving at the correct diagnosis should be undertaken with urgency to identify diseases for which there are effective therapies and institute treatment in a timely manner.

Idiopathic infantile cholangiopathies. After the known causes of cholestasis have been ruled out, most patients are found to have one of the idiopathic infantile cholangiopathies: biliary atresia or neonatal hepatitis. Neither of these terms denotes a specific etiology. Rather, they describe recognizable groups of signs and symptoms.

Neonatal hepatitis, the most common cause of neonatal cholestasis, tends to be more frequent in low-birth-weight infants. Jaundice usually develops within the first week and is always present before 2 months of age. Acholic stools are uncommon, but hepatomegaly may be present. Vitamin K malabsorption and deficiency may lead to a bleeding diathesis.

The diagnosis of neonatal hepatitis can be made only after excluding metabolic and infectious causes of cholestasis. Once this has been done, a liver biopsy may be performed. The histologic features necessary for diagnosis include disturbance of the normal hepatic architecture, increased presence of inflammatory cells in the portal areas, and evidence of increased extramedullary hematopoiesis. Multinucleated giant cells are also often present. However, these features are not pathognomonic.

There is no specific therapy for neonatal hepatitis; general measures used in treatment of cholestasis are applied (see Management, below). The condition is heterogeneous, making it difficult to define the prognosis. However, the prognosis is worse in the familial than in the sporadic form.

Approximately one third of cases of neonatal cholestasis are due to **extrahepatic biliary atresia.** The defect involves obliteration of all or part of the extrahepatic biliary ductular system. In the early stages of disease, hepatic architecture may be relatively normal; with progression, however, there is bile stasis and proliferation of the intrahepatic bile ducts. These findings and the presence of bile plugs in the portal ducts are characteristically noted in biopsy specimens. The progression of hepatic lesions associated with this disorder has suggested that an inflammatory process may be involved, which leads to fibrosis and eventual ductal obliteration.

Biliary atresia, unlike neonatal hepatitis, occurs almost exclusively in full-term infants. Jaundice may be present from birth or develop in the first few weeks. Stools are often acholic. Hepatomegaly is common and may be associated with splenomegaly as a result of portal hypertension. Progression of disease is associated with the development of cirrhosis and the consequent problems of failure to thrive and nutritional deficiencies.

When extrahepatic biliary atresia is suspected, radioisotope scanning may be performed. With biliary atresia, uptake of isotope by the liver is usually normal, but no excretion into the intestine is visualized, thereby confirming the presence of an obstructive lesion. This is in contrast to neonatal hepatitis, in which isotope uptake is delayed because of parenchymal disease, but excretion is normal. Characteristic findings on radionuclide scanning and liver biopsy specimens necessitate confirmation of the diagnosis by exploratory laparotomy with intraoperative cholangiography. With cholangiography, the gallbladder is filled with contrast material; if no reflux into the proximal ductular system is apparent, the diagnosis is confirmed. This procedure is performed intraoperatively so that, if the diagnosis is confirmed, the appropriate surgical procedure can be performed. In approximately one fifth of patients, the proximal extrahepatic duct is patent to the level of the porta hepatis and the obstruction is distal. In these patients, surgical correction allows resumption of adequate bile drainage. In most patients, however, the obstruction is proximal and not correctable. For these patients, the Kasai procedure (hepatoportoenterostomy with Roux-en-Y enteroanastomosis) is performed to allow some biliary drainage. The success of this procedure is directly related to the patient's age at the time of surgery, with patients younger than 2 months experiencing the best results. After this procedure, ascending cholangitis is the most common complication.

Even in those patients in whom the Kasai procedure is successful in relieving extrahepatic obstruction, progression of intrahepatic disease may lead to cirrhosis and portal hypertension. The availability of orthotopic liver transplantation for patients with end-stage liver disease has improved their prognosis remarkably.

α_1**-Antitrypsin deficiency.** α_1-Antitrypsin is a protease inhibitor, synthesized in the liver, that acts as the major inhibitor of potentially destructive enzymes such as trypsin. When deficient, hepatic disease (neonatal cholestasis or cirrhosis) or pulmonary disease (emphysema) may result. Clinically, patients with hepatic disease secondary to α_1-antitrypsin deficiency may be indistinguishable from those with idiopathic neonatal hepatitis; they present with jaundice, acholic stools, and hepatomegaly. The histologic findings of the two disorders are also similar, with giant cell transformation, bile stasis, inflammation, and portal fibrosis often present.

Phenotyping should be performed to confirm the diagnosis. The protease inhibitor (*Pi*) phenotype *PiMM* is present in most individuals and therefore is considered "normal." Patients with the phenotype *PiZZ* are much more likely to have low serum concentrations of the enzyme and clinically apparent symptoms. Individuals with the heterozygous phenotype (*PiMZ*) may or may not have a clinically significant enzyme deficiency. The presence of the *ZZ* or *MZ* phenotype in an infant with cholestasis is diagnostic of this disorder. Another test that may be helpful is periodic acid Schiff staining of liver biopsy tissue that, with α_1-antitrypsin deficiency, may show intrahepatic globules that are resistant to the effects of diastase. α_1-Antitrypsin concentrations can be measured, but these must be interpreted with caution because α_1-antitrypsin is an acute phase reactant, and concentrations may be increased by various stressors, including inflammation.

Treatment of patients with α_1-antitrypsin deficiency is supportive and consists of measures aimed at minimizing cholestasis and its complications (see Management). Gene therapy for the disease is an area of active investigation. If the condition progresses to end-stage liver disease, orthotopic liver transplantation is a therapeutic option and converts the recipient to the *Pi* phenotype of the donor liver.

Alagille's syndrome. Alagille's syndrome, or arteriohepatic dysplasia, describes a constellation of symptoms associated with paucity of intralobular bile ducts and, consequently, neonatal cholestasis. In addition to having liver abnormality, these patients may have some or all of the following characteristic manifestations: (1) unusual facies (prominent forehead, flat, wide nasal bridge, antimongoloid ocular slant, and relatively small forward-jutting chin); (2) ocular abnormalities, such as posterior embryotoxon; (3) cardiovascular abnormalities, including peripheral pulmonic stenosis; and (4) vertebral arch defects, including anterior vertebral arch fusion and the presence of butterfly vertebrae.

Because the paucity of bile ducts is progressive and other findings may be subtle or not present, the diagnosis of Alagille's syndrome in early infancy may be difficult. It is crucial, however, that this disorder be differentiated from extrahepatic causes of cholestasis, such as biliary atresia, so that unnecessary portoenterostomy is avoided. Treatment of these patients is limited to efforts to minimize the effects of cholestasis.

Byler's disease. This progressive familial disorder causing intrahepatic cholestasis is differentiated from Alagille's syndrome by the absence of extrahepatic manifestations and the less frequent occurrence of bile duct paucity. These patients experience progressive cholestasis, which eventually reaches end-stage liver disease.

Management

For most neonates with **unconjugated hyperbilirubinemia**, no specific therapy is necessary because the bilirubin level will gradually return to normal without intervention. In patients with hemolytic disease, exchange transfusions may be required. For those with erythrocyte enzyme defects, transfusion may be necessary to correct anemia.

Because of the association of kernicterus with plasma concentrations of unconjugated bilirubin in excess of 20 mg/dL, infants with unconjugated hyperbilirubinemia in this range of any etiology are often treated with phototherapy. This process involves the photoisomerization of bilirubin to forms that are less lipophilic and thus more readily excreted, even without conjugation. During phototherapy, dehydration due to the accompanying increase in insensible water losses must be avoided. The eyes also must be protected to avoid retinal injury. The use of phototherapy in infants with conjugated or mixed hyperbilirubinemia may result in the "bronze baby syndrome," in which the skin assumes a bronze discoloration because of the retention of photo-oxidation products of bilirubin; this may last for several months.

In patients with **conjugated hyperbilirubinemia**, treatment is tailored to the specific etiology, if known. Symptomatic treatment also should be provided. Malnutrition may occur in patients with cholestasis because of poor caloric intake and malabsorption of fat. Nutritional deficiencies should be treated appropriately. Fat-soluble vitamin deficiencies may result from malabsorption due to diminished intestinal bile acid concentration. Vitamin D deficiency may present as rickets, and progressive neuromuscular disease, including areflexia and peripheral neuropathy, may occur with vitamin E deficiency. Deficiencies of vitamin K, leading to hypoprothrombinemia, and vitamin A, resulting in visual impairment, may also be present. Thus, supplementation of the fat-soluble vitamins should be routine in the management of patients with cholestasis.

Pruritus is another common complication of cholestasis. Medications intended to increase choleresis (e.g., phenobarbital) and those designed to bind bile acids (e.g., cholestyramine) may be useful in treating pruritus. More recently, ursodeoxycholic acid has been found to be useful in diminishing pruritus.

Hepatic cirrhosis and portal hypertension often develop in patients with cholestatic disorders. Ascites, which may accompany portal hypertension, may be diminished by sodium restriction and diuretic administration. The development of esophageal varices may necessitate the use of sclerotherapy or band ligation. Despite these temporizing measures, patients typically progress to end-stage liver disease. In these patients, the possibility of orthotopic liver transplantation should be strongly considered.

■ THE CHILD WITH JAUNDICE

Clinical Approach

An approach to the evaluation of the child presenting with jaundice outside of the neonatal period is presented in Figure 12–13.

HISTORY

The history of a patient with jaundice should include the duration of symptoms and any coexistent symptoms that preceeded or began with the clinical jaundice. In the rare event that the child's symptoms have been present since infancy, the possibility of previously unrecognized congenital defects should be entertained.

If the patient reports having symptoms of fever or malaise, infectious causes of jaundice should be considered. The viruses that cause hepatitis may present in this way. If hepatitis is suspected, a history of blood transfusion should be investigated. Sexual contact, voluntarily or through sexual abuse, should also be identified because some of the viral hepatidides may be spread through sexual contact.

The history also should address any medications the patient may be taking acutely or chronically. In addition, one should investigate the possibility of illicit drug use or of overdosage of prescription medications. A history of alcohol intake is important for patients old enough to consume alcoholic beverages. In many instances of jaundice in pediatric patients, there is no accompanying abdominal pain. If pain is present, one should consider the possibility of gallbladder disease (including choledocholithiasis) in the differential diagnosis.

PHYSICAL EXAMINATION

In addition to a complete physical examination, the evaluation should include an assessment of the distribution and degree of skin discoloration. In patients with Gilbert's syndrome, for example, icterus may be limited to the sclerae. Children with carotenemia have yellow-orange skin pigmentation resulting from absorption of pigments from carrots and other yellow vegetables. This may be

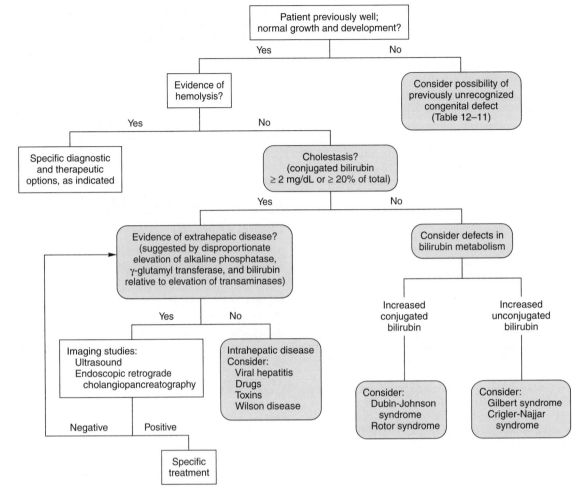

Figure 12–13. Algorithm presenting an approach to the evaluation of the child in whom jaundice develops after the neonatal period.

differentiated from bilirubin pigmentation by its absence from the sclerae. Abdominal examination should include an assessment of the size and texture of the liver and determination of the presence of abdominal masses.

DIAGNOSTIC STUDIES

As is true in evaluating neonatal jaundice, the fractionated bilirubin is an important first step in determining underlying etiology. If the bilirubin is predominantly unconjugated, hemolysis should be considered and a complete blood count and peripheral smear done. If there is no hemolysis, unconjugated hyperbilirubinemia in a child is most likely due to Gilbert's syndrome (see above).

Conjugated hyperbilirubinemia is present when the conjugated fraction is greater than or equal to 2 mg/dL or

is greater than or equal to 20% of the total bilirubin. Investigation of conjugated hyperbilirubinemia usually warrants obtaining liver enzymes including alkaline phosphatase, γ-glutamyl transferase (GGT), aspartate aminotransferase(AST), and alanine aminotransferase (ALT). Extrahepatic diseases typically are associated with disproportionate increases in alkaline phosphate and GGT in relation to AST and ALT. When extrahepatic disease is suspected hepatic, ultrasound and other imaging studies may provide helpful information. Alternatively, if the AST and ALT are more elevated than the other hepatic enzymes, intrahepatic causes are more likely.

When studies suggest intrahepatic disease, the possibility of viral hepatitis should be considered and appropriate serologic tests ordered. Drugs, prescription and illicit, may cause intrahepatic damage as can drug overdoses and toxic ingestions.

Heavy metals, especially copper, as with Wilson's disease, may cause intrahepatic disease and jaundice. When this diagnosis is suspected, laboratory studies should include serum ceruloplasmin and copper levels and urinary copper levels.

In all patients in whom chronic or severe liver disease is suspected, as assessment of the synthetic function of the liver is important. Clotting studies (protime, partial thromboplastin time) are often abnormal with severe liver dysfunction because those factors are produced in the liver. Serum albumin often is also decreased with impaired hepatic protein synthesis.

Differential Diagnosis

Table 12–12 provides a partial list of disorders that can cause jaundice in childhood. Many are similar to those that cause jaundice in the neonate (see Table 12–11). In older children with a previously unremarkable medical history and evidence of normal growth and development, the likelihood of diagnosing a previously undetected congenital disorder as the cause of jaundice is low. Congenital disorders that are undetected and asymptomatic during the neonatal period are included in the differen-

tial diagnosis outlined in Table 12–12. Most disorders that cause jaundice in children and adolescents are discussed elsewhere in this chapter. Additional coverage of the infectious hepatitities is found in Chapter 9 (Infectious Diseases).

INFECTIOUS HEPATITIS

Infection with the hepatotropic viruses (hepatitis A, B, C, etc.) causes a variety of clinical presentations, depending on the specific virus and the age of the patient. Serum transaminase concentrations are often increased, and jaundice and hepatomegaly may be associated. Viral hepatitis is discussed in Chapter 9.

HEPATOLENTICULAR DEGENERATION

Hepatolenticular degeneration, or **Wilson's disease,** is an autosomal recessive disorder associated with inadequate biliary excretion of copper. The metabolic defect remains unknown but may involve impaired synthesis of the copper-binding protein ceruloplasmin. Regardless of the defect, the result is the accumulation of copper in the liver, leading to hepatocyte necrosis. Copper is then released into the circulation and may be deposited in the eyes, central nervous system, and kidneys.

Patients with Wilson's disease rarely manifest symptoms in early childhood. More commonly, they are well

Table 12–12. Differential Diagnosis: The Child Presenting With Jaundice After the Neonatal Period

Disorders causing increased bilirubin production	
Hemolytic diseases	Reabsorption of hematoma
Erythrocyte enzyme defects[1]	Transfusion
Hemaglobinopathies	

Disorders causing decreased bilirubin clearance	
Hereditary defects of bilirubin metabolism	Hepatocellular disease
Gilbert's syndrome[1]	Infectious hepatitis[1]
Crigler–Najjar syndrome	Toxin-induced liver disease[1]
Dubin–Johnson syndrome	Total parenteral nutrition
Rotor syndrome	Pharmacologic agents (acetaminophen, phenytoin)
Disorders causing cholestasis	Intrahepatic persistent cholestasis
Metabolic diseases	Alagille syndrome
Tyrosinemia	Byler disease (persistent familial intrahepatic cholestasis)
Wilson disease[1]	Sepsis
Disorders of carbohydrate metabolism	Biliary tract obstruction
Galactosemia	Congenital hepatic fibrosis/infantile polycystic disease
Hereditary fructose intolerance	Caroli disease
Glycogen storage disease (types I, III, and IV)	Bile duct stenosis
Disorders of lipid metabolism	Anomalies of the choledochopancreaticoductal junction
Wolman's disease	Choledocholithiasis
Niemann–Pick disease	Tumors
Disorders in which the defect is uncharacterized	Sclerosing cholangitis
α_1-Antitrypsin deficiency	Pancreatitis
Cystic fibrosis[1]	

[1] Frequently encountered causes of jaundice.

throughout childhood and begin to experience hepatomegaly, jaundice, and other symptoms commonly associated with acute infectious hepatitis in early adolescence. If these are untreated, cirrhosis and portal hypertension gradually develop. Occasionally patients may present with acute hepatic failure associated with hemolytic anemia.

Diagnosis of Wilson's disease requires evidence of abnormal copper metabolism. Slit-lamp examination may show copper deposition in the eye (Kayser–Fleischer rings). A neurologic evaluation should be done to determine the presence of subtle neurologic findings, including changes in school performance. More severe neurologic disease is typically seen in older patients. Serum transaminase levels may be low, especially with the fulminant form of the disease. Decreased plasma ceruloplasmin levels are present in most patients homozygous for Wilson's disease. Ceruloplasmin levels also may be low in heterozygotes and patients with other liver diseases or with malnutrition. Measurement of urinary copper excretion from a 24-hour collection should be performed if Wilson's disease is suspected. Although urinary copper excretion typically is low in patients with Wilson's disease, this may not be a consistent finding. A more reliable test in those in whom the diagnosis is uncertain involves measurement of urinary copper before and after treatment with chelating agents. An increase in copper excretion after treatment is typical of Wilson's disease. The finding of elevated copper content in liver tissue obtained by biopsy is diagnostic.

Treatment of Wilson's disease relies on the use of D-penicillamine, or other copper-chelating agents, to increase urinary copper excretion. Dietary restriction of copper to less than 1 mg/d should be instituted. These therapies usually lead to resolution of symptoms as the extrahepatic sites of copper deposition are gradually cleared. In patients with fulminant disease, plasmapheresis and possibly liver transplantation are indicated. If untreated, Wilson's disease is always fatal.

REFERENCES

Vomiting

Fonkalsrud EW, Ament ME: Gastroesophageal reflux in childhood. Curr Probl Surg 1996;33:1.

Garcia VF, Randolph JG: Pyloric stenosis: diagnosis and management. Pediatr Rev 1990;11:292.

Hillemeier AC: Gastroesophageal reflux. Diagnostic and therapeutic approaches. Pediatr Clin North Am 1996;43:197.

Orenstein SR, Izadnia F, Khan S: Gastroesophageal reflux disease in children. Gastroenterol Clin North Am 1999; 28:947.

Constipation

Baker SS et al: Constipation in infants and children: evaluation and treatment. J Pediatr Gastroenterol Nutr 1999;29:612.

Loening-Bauke V: Encopresis and soiling. Pediatr Clin North Am 1996;43:279.

Rudolph C, Benaroch L: Hirschsprung disease. Pedatr Rev 1995;16:5.

Tietelbaum DH, Coran AG: Enterocolitis. Semin Pediatr Surg 1998;7:162.

Gastrointestinal Tract Hemorrhage

Arain Z, Rossi TM: Gastrointestinal bleeding in children: an overview of conditions requiring nonoperative management. Semin Pediatr Surg 1999;8:172.

Hyams JS: Crohn's disease in children. Pediatr Clin North Am 1996;43:255.

Kirschner BS: Ulcerative colitis in children. Pediatr Clin North Am 1996;4:235.

Lehmann CU, Elitsur Y: Juvenile polyps and their distribution in pediatric patients with gastrointestinal bleeding. W V Med J 1996;92:133.

Mezoff AM, Balistreri WF: Peptic ulcer disease in children. Pediatr Rev 1995;16:257.

Abdominal Pain

Apley J: *The Child with Abdominal Pains,* 2nd ed. Oxford: Blackwell, 1975.

Blecker U, Gold BD: Gastritis and peptic ulcer disease in childhood. Eur J Pediatr 1999;158:541.

Gauderer MW: Acute abdomen. When to operate immediately and when to observe. Semin Pediatr Surg 1997;6:74.

Jones NL, Sherman PM: *Helicobacter pylori* infection in children. Curr Opin Pediatr 1998;10:19.

Diarrhea

Burkhardt DM: Management of acute gastroenteritis in children. Am Fam Phys 1999;60:2555.

Laney DW, Cohen MB: An approach to the pediatric patient with diarrhea. Gastroenterol Clin North Am 1993;22:499.

Sherman PM et al: Infectious gastroenterocolitides in children: an update on emerging pathogens. Pediatr Clin North Am 1996;43:391.

Troncone R et al: Gluten-sensitive enteropathy. Pediatr Clin North Am 1996;43:355.

Vanderhoof JA: Chronic diarrhea. Pediatr Rev 1998;19:418.

Vanderhoof JA et al: Short bowel syndrome in children and small intestinal transplantation. Pediatr Clin North Am 1996;43:533.

Jaundice

Balistreri WF: Liver disease in infancy and childhood. In: Schiff ER et al (editors): *Schiff's Diseases of the Liver,* 8th ed. Lippincott-Raven, 1999.

Bates MD et al: Biliary atresia: Pathogenesis and treatment. Semin Liver Dis 1998;18:281.

Burton BK: Inborn errors of metabolism in infancy: a guide to diagnosis. Pediatrics 1998;102:E69.

Cuthbert JA: Wilson's disease: Update of a systemic disorder with protean manifestations. Gastroenterol Clin North Am 1998;27:655.

Lasker MR, Holzman IR: Neonatal jaundice: When to treat, when to watch and wait. Postgrad Med 1996;99:187.

Schwarzenberg SJ, Sharp HL: Pediatric gastroenterology: update on metabolic liver disease. Pediatr Clin North Am 1996;43:27.

Blood

Caroline A. Hastings, MD, & Bertram H. Lubin, MD

The diagnosis of hematologic problems in the pediatric age group poses several challenges to health care practitioners. One must not only take into account variation in normal hematologic values for different age groups, but must be able to decide which of the many paths of testing to follow from basic examination results. To facilitate this process, careful attention must be given to the family history, history of the current illness, and physical examination. Similarly, the blood smear should be evaluated before ordering more specific laboratory tests or obtaining a consultation with a pediatric hematologist. This chapter discusses diagnosis and care of the more common hematologic problems in the pediatric age group.

RED CELLS: ANEMIA

Mature red cells are derived from the stem cells, which exist within bone marrow. Erythrocytosis is regulated by erythropoietin, cytokines, and growth factors. During the maturation of red cell progenitors, hemoglobin (Hb) synthesis increases, the nucleus is extruded from the cell, membrane remodeling occurs, and cell volume decreases.

Anemia, the most common hematologic problem diagnosed in children, is a condition in which tissue hypoxia occurs because of inadequate oxygen-carrying capacity of the blood. Failure to produce red cells or an imbalance between red cell production and red cell destruction causes anemia. The diagnosis is most often made by comparing the patient's Hb or hematocrit value with age-matched normal values. Although practical and effective in most cases, this approach does not take into consideration the physiologic, and more accurate, definition of anemia. This point is exemplified by studies of patients with cyanotic heart disease or of patients with Hb variants characterized by a high oxygen affinity, in which the Hb level may be elevated or within the normal range, although tissue hypoxia exists.

History and Physical Examination

Important clues about the underlying cause of anemia can be obtained by obtaining a careful medical history, including age, sex, race, ethnicity, neonatal history, diet, drug exposure, infections, inheritance, and history of gastrointestinal dysfunction. The obstetric, perinatal, and birth history should be reviewed carefully, and questions should be asked regarding perinatal blood loss, maternal illness

or risk factors, and maternal history of transfusion. Information regarding a family history of splenectomy, red cell transfusions, jaundice, and cholecystectomy are useful in evaluating patients suspected of having a hemolytic anemia (Table 13–1).

The symptoms of anemia depend on the degree of reduction in the oxygen-carrying capacity of the blood, the change in blood volume, the rate at which these changes occur, and the ability of the cardiovascular and hematopoietic systems to compensate. General signs of anemia in childhood can include poor feeding or dyspnea, irritability, inactivity, faintness, change in behavior, and poor school performance. Pallor and jaundice, in association with dark urine, suggest hemolytic anemia (Table 13–2).

Cardiac enlargement and signs of congestive heart failure may be present with either acute blood loss or chronic anemia. Tachycardia, prominent arterial pulses, bruits, tachypnea, dyspnea, and postural hypotension can be detected in patients with modest to severe anemia. Hemic murmurs reflect an increase in cardiac output, stroke volume, and heart rate associated with decreased peripheral resistance and decreased blood viscosity. Gallop rhythm may also be present in a hemodynamically compromised state. These abnormalities disappear after blood transfusion or treatment of the anemia.

Patients in whom marrow hyperplasia develops to compensate for their hemolytic anemia may have frontal bossing and prominent malar eminences. Specific dysmorphic features can be seen with certain inherited anemias, such as radial limb abnormalities in Diamond-Blackfan anemia and Fanconi anemia.

Splenomegaly may be a prominent finding in infants and children with hemolytic anemia, storage diseases, infections, and malignancies. The spleen is occasionally enlarged in patients with iron deficiency anemia or megaloblastic anemia of infancy. In pathologic states, the edge of the spleen is hard and occasionally tender. In contrast, if the spleen is palpable in normal children, it has a soft edge and is nontender. If lymphadenopathy is detected, infection or leukemia should be excluded.

The liver may be enlarged in patients with anemia because of acute or chronic congestive heart failure. Hepatomegaly is also noted in patients who have received frequent blood transfusions for diseases such as aplastic anemia, sickle cell anemia, and β-thalassemia as a consequence of iron overload.

Table 13–1. Important Historical Points in Evaluation of Anemia

History	Consider
Prematurity	Anemia of prematurity (erythropoietin-responsive) Iatrogenic blood loss
Perinatal risk factors	
Maternal illness (autoimmune)	Hemolytic anemia
Drug ingestion	
Infections (TORCHES, hepatitis)	
Mechanical problems at delivery	Acute blood loss Fetal-maternal hemorrhage
Ethnicity	
African American	HbS, C; G6PD deficiency
Mediterannean	α, β-Thalassemia; G6PD deficiency
Southeast Asian	α, β-Thalassemia; HbE
Family history	
Gallstones, cholecystectomy	Inherited hemolytic anemia
Splenectomy, jaundice	Spherocytosis, elliptocytosis
Isoimmunization (Rh or ABO)	Hemolytic disease of newborn Predisposed to iron deficiency
Male sex	X-linked enzymopathies (G6PD)
Early jaundice (<24 h)	Isoimmune, infectious
Persistent jaundice	Hemolytic anemia
Diet (usually >6 mo)	
Pica (ice, dirt)	Lead toxicity, iron deficiency
Excessive milk intake	Iron deficiency
Macrobiotic diets	Vitamin B_{12} deficiency
Goat's milk	Folic acid deficiency
Drugs	
Sulfa, anticonvulsants	Hemolytic anemia (G6PD deficiency)
Chloramphenicol	Aplastic anemia
Low socioeconomic status	Pica (lead, iron deficiency) Iron deficiency
Malnutrition	
Malabsorption	Anemia of chronic disease
Environmental	Iron, vitamin B_{12} deficiency Vitamin E, K deficiency
Liver disease	Shortened red cell survival
Renal disease	Shortened red cell survival Decreased red cell production (decreased erythropoietin)
Infectious diseases	
Inflammation, acute gastroenteritis, otitis media, pharyngitis	Transient mild decreased Hb
Bacterial, viral, mycoplasma	Hemolytic anemia

G6PD = glucose-6-phosphate dehydrogenase; Hb = hemogloblin; TORCHES = toxoplasmosis, other (congenital syphilis and viruses), rubella, cytomegalovirus, and herpes simplex.

Table 13–2. Physical Examination of Anemic Children

General signs		
Skin	Pallor	Severe anemia
	Jaundice	Hemolytic anemia, acute and chronic
		Hepatitis, aplastic anemia
	Petechiae, purpura	Autoimmune hemolytic anemia with thrombocytopenia
		Hemolytic uremic syndrome
		Bone marrow aplasia or infiltration
	Cavernous hemangioma	Microangiopathic hemolytic anemia
Head and neck	Frontal bossing, prominent malar and maxillary bones	Extramedullary hematopoiesis (thalassemia major, sickle cell anemia, other congenital hemolytic anemias)
	Icteric sclerae	Congenital hemolytic anemia and hyperhemolytic crisis associated with infection (red cell enzyme deficiencies, red cell membrane defects, thalassemias, hemoglobinopathies)
	Angular stomatitis	Iron deficiency
	Glossitis	Vitamin B_{12} or iron deficiency
Chest	Rales, gallop rhythm, tachycardia, murmur	Congestive heart failure, acute or severe anemia
Extremities	Radial limb dysplasia	Fanconi anemia
	Spoon nails	Iron deficiency
	Triphalangeal thumbs	Red cell aplasia
Spleen	Splenomegaly	Congenital hemolytic anemia, infection, hematologic malignancies, portal hypertension

Laboratory Procedures

Normal hematologic values reported from birth to adolescence are shown in Table 13–3. Changes occur dramatically during the first few weeks after birth and then more gradually over the next 5 to 7 years. Use of automated electronic cell counters provides information on Hb, hematocrit, red cell count, red cell indices [mean corpuscular volume (MCV), mean corpuscular Hb (MCH), and mean corpuscular Hb concentration (MCHC)], and red cell distribution width (RDW).

An examination of the peripheral blood smear is perhaps the simplest, most often overlooked, laboratory procedure in the evaluation of anemic patients. The morphology of the red cells can serve to identify children with nutritional anemias, red cell membrane defects, and hemoglobinopathies. Figure 13–1 demonstrates several of these characteristic morphologic changes in the more common forms of anemia in childhood.

The reticulocyte count is useful in determining the rate of red cell destruction and in monitoring response to treatment. The normal value in the newborn is $3.2 \pm 1.4\%$ and in children $1.2 \pm 0.7\%$. Anemia is classified as hemolytic if red cell survival is less than 120 days. In these cases, the reticulocyte count is elevated and the Hb concentration is normal, in the case of compensated hemolytic anemia, or low. Additional laboratory tests that can be used to document hemolysis include serum haptoglobin and hemopexin concentrations. These proteins bind Hb and heme released from red cells after their destruction. The complexed proteins that are formed after intravascular hemolysis are removed from the circulation. As a consequence, haptoglobin and hemopexin levels are low in patients who have hemolytic anemia. When haptoglobin is saturated, free plasma Hb can be detected. The indirect bilirubin level frequently is determined to provide evidence for a hemolytic process; however, it is an insensitive measurement of hemolysis and is elevated only when liver function is impaired or when hemolysis is extensive. Another means of detecting hemolysis is by measuring endogenous carbon monoxide production. When Hb is degraded, the α-methyl group of heme becomes carbon monoxide. Determination of endogenous production of carbon monoxide may be useful to detect hemolysis in the neonatal period but is of limited value in older children owing to the background levels of carbon monoxide in the environment.

When nutritional anemias are suspected, measurements of iron status, vitamin B_{12}, and folic acid may be indicated. The red cell indices, free erythrocyte protoporphyrin (FEP), and red cell distribution width (RDW) can be used efficiently to diagnose iron deficiency with minimal cost to patients.

The osmotic fragility test is used to measure the osmotic resistance of red cells. Red cells are incubated under hypotonic conditions, and their ability to swell before

(*text continues on page 518*)

Table 13–3. Red Blood Cell Values at Various Ages: Mean and Lower Limit or Normal

Age	Hemoglobin (g/dL)		Hematocrit (%)		RBC (10¹²/L)		MCV (fL)		MCH (pg)		MCHC (g/dL)	
	Mean	–2 SD	Mean	–2 SD	Mean	–2 SD	Mean	–2 SD	Mean	–2 SD	Mean	–2 SD
Birth (cord blood)	16.5	13.5	51	42	4.7	3.9	108	98	34	31	33	30
1–3 d (capillary)	18.5	14.5	56	45	5.3	4.0	108	95	34	31	33	29
1 wk	17.5	13.5	54	42	5.1	3.9	107	88	34	28	33	28
2 wk	16.5	12.5	51	39	4.9	3.6	105	86	34	28	33	28
1 mo	14.0	10.0	43	31	4.2	3.0	104	85	30	28	33	29
2 mo	11.5	9.0	35	28	3.8	2.7	96	77	30	26	33	29
3–6 mo	11.5	9.5	35	29	3.8	3.1	91	74	30	25	33	30
0.5–2 y	12.0	10.5	36	33	4.5	3.7	78	70	27	23	33	30
2–6 y	12.5	11.5	37	34	4.6	3.9	81	75	27	24	34	31
6–12 y	13.5	11.5	40	35	4.6	4.0	86	77	29	25	34	31
12–18 y: female	14.0	12.0	41	36	4.6	4.1	90	78	30	25	34	31
male	14.5	13.0	43	37	4.9	4.5	88	78	30	25	34	31
18–49 y: female	14.0	12.0	41	36	4.6	4.0	90	80	30	26	34	31
male	15.5	13.5	47	41	5.2	4.5	90	80	30	26	34	31

MCH = mean corpuscular hemoglobin; MCHC = mean corpuscular hemoglobin concentration; MCV = mean corpuscular volume; RBC = red cell count.

Compiled from the following sources: Dutcher: Lab Med 1971;2:32; Koerper et al: J Pediatr 1976;89:580; Marner: Acta Paediatr Scand 1969;58:363; Matoth et al: Acta Paediatr Scand 1971;60:317; Moe: Acta Paediatr Scand 1965;54:69; Okuno: J Clin Pathol 1972;25:599; Oski, Naiman: *Hematological Problems in the Newborn*. Saunders, 1972, p 11; Penttilä et al: Suomen Lääkärilehti 1973;26:2173; and Viteri et al: Br J Haematol 1972;23:189. Emphasis is given to studies using electronic counters and to the selection of populations that are likely to exclude individuals with iron deficiency. The mean ± 2 SD can be expected to include 95% of the observations in a normal population. Cited in: Rudolph AM (ed): *Rudolph's Pediatrics*, 16th ed. Appleton & Lange, 1977.

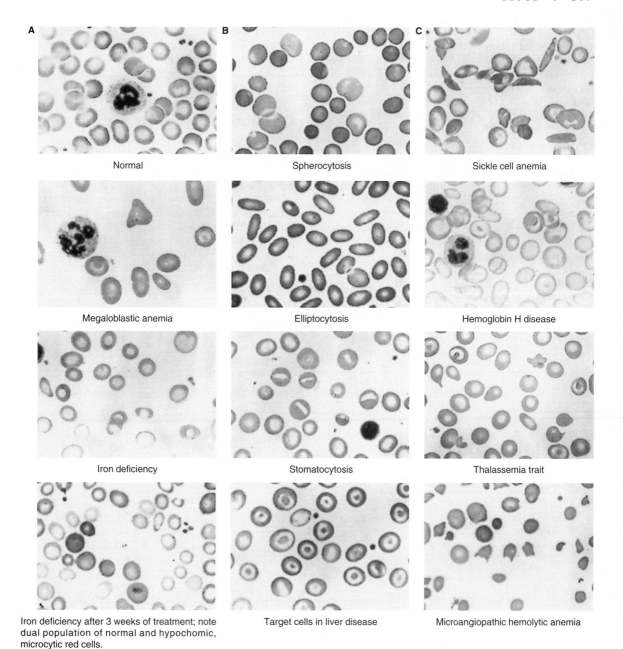

A

Normal

Megaloblastic anemia

Iron deficiency

Iron deficiency after 3 weeks of treatment; note dual population of normal and hypochomic, microcytic red cells.

B

Spherocytosis

Elliptocytosis

Stomatocytosis

Target cells in liver disease

C

Sickle cell anemia

Hemoglobin H disease

Thalassemia trait

Microangiopathic hemolytic anemia

Figure 13–1. Red cell appearance in various diseases. **A:** Peripheral blood morphology, various anemias. **B:** Membrane abnormalities. **C:** Hemoglobinopathies and other conditions.

lysis is determined. The osmotic fragility of red cells is increased when the surface area:volume ratio of the cell is decreased, as in hereditary spherocytosis, in which membrane instability results in membrane loss and decreased surface area. Conversely, it is decreased in liver disease and in iron deficiency, in which the surface area:volume ratio of the red cell is increased. A test performed on an Ektacytometer measures the deformability of red cells subjected simultaneously to shear stress and osmotic stress.

In patients in whom hemolytic anemia is suspected, immunologic tests, such as the direct and indirect Coombs tests, are required to exclude antibody-mediated red cell destruction. Intrinsic defects in the red cell can be assessed by analysis of red cell membrane proteins, Hb electrophoretic tests, and specific enzyme or cations and water determinations. Details of these disorders are presented in the later section, "Extracorpuscular Defects."

Examination of bone marrow is useful in the assessment of anemia associated with reticulocytopenia, neutropenia, or thrombocytopenia. Histologic examination of the stained bone marrow aspirate allows one to identify red cell precursors as well as myeloid and megakaryocytic

precursors, and to detect malignant or infiltrating cells. The bone marrow sample also can be used to determine iron stores by using a Prussian blue stain. In certain cases of familial anemias, cytogenetic analysis of bone marrow samples can be useful.

Age-Related Causes of Anemia

The causes of anemia in children vary with age. Understanding the age-related causes can simplify diagnosis by quickly excluding factors not generally associated with each age group.

Figure 13–2 demonstrates a useful diagnostic approach to the diagnosis of anemia in newborns. An Hb concentration less than 13.5 g/dL during the first week after birth is 2 SD below the norm for that age and requires investigation. If the reticulocyte count is elevated, a hemolytic anemia or blood loss should be suspected. Performance of a Coombs test is necessary to exclude immune hemolytic anemia. With a negative Coombs test result, blood loss, an intrinsic red cell disorder, or an infection must be excluded. If the reticulocyte count is low, either a

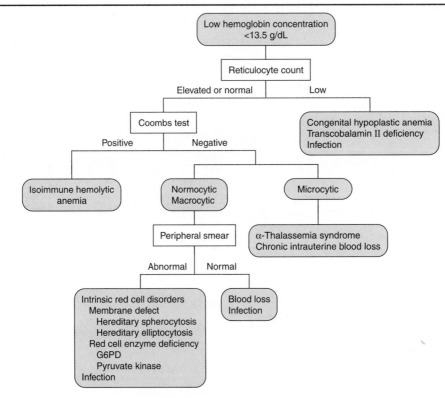

Figure 13–2. Algorithm diagramming an approach to the assessment of the newborn with anemia. G6PD = glucose-6-phosphate dehydrogenase.

defect in erythropoiesis or a congenital infection must be considered. The MCV is also useful to categorize the cause of anemia. Low values are seen with iron deficiency owing to intrauterine hemorrhage or to α-thalassemia. Infection can produce hemolysis (elevated reticulocyte count) or inhibit erythropoiesis (decreased reticulocyte count). When associated with hemolysis, the peripheral smear is abnormal, showing microangiopathic changes. Laboratory diagnosis in patients with congenital hemolytic anemias should include procedures to identify defects in membrane structure or function, abnormal cell metabolism, or defects in Hb structure and function. The specific laboratory tests are described in the sections dealing with these disorders.

Blood loss can occur before delivery in association with abruptio placentae or twin-to-twin transfusion, or can occur through the gastrointestinal tract. Internal bleeding can occur within the cranium or within organs, such as the liver or lung. If extensive blood loss has occurred in utero, as might be the case with fetal-maternal transfusion or partial placental abruption, infants may be in congestive heart failure at birth. When fetal-to-maternal hemorrhage is suspected, a prompt search for fetal cells in the maternal circulation is indicated, using the Kliehauer-Betke staining technique.

When the Coombs test produces a positive result, the various causes of immune hemolysis should be pursued. Although the Coombs test result is positive in cases of Rh incompatibility, some cases of ABO incompatibility may not give a positive test result. If the reticulocyte count is elevated and the Coombs test result is negative, hereditary red cell membrane defects (e.g., spherocytosis, pyropoikilocytosis, or elliptocytosis) or enzyme deficiencies [e.g., glucose-6-phosphate dehydrogenase (G6PD) deficiency or pyruvate kinase (PK) deficiency] should be considered. Intrauterine or acquired infections may produce either hemolytic anemia or hypoplastic anemia. Infants with either of these conditions often have splenomegaly, may have petechiae, and are jaundiced.

A physiologic decrease in the Hb concentration is reached by approximately 2 months after birth. The decrease in Hb concentration is most dramatic in premature infants, in whom this condition has been called anemia of prematurity. Although the relative reticulocyte count may be elevated, if corrected for anemia, the absolute reticulocyte count is often low. Most infants tolerate this anemia and recover without intervention. With cardiorespiratory distress, however, red cell transfusion may be required. Recovery is heralded by an increase in the reticulocyte count and a subsequent increase in the Hb value. Red cell transfusion may delay this process. It is not unusual to confuse the recovery period, associated with reticulocytosis, with a hemolytic anemia. When one observes patients over the following 6 to 8 weeks, the Hb will increase and the reticulocyte count will decrease. In contrast, children with congenital hemolytic anemia have persistent reticulocytosis and anemia. Anemic infants, particularly those with anemia of prematurity, benefit from the administration of erythropoetin. Infants with extreme prematurity need high doses of erythropoetin to overcome the relative resistance to erythropoetin.

Nutritional anemias, particularly due to iron deficiency, peak between ages 6 months and 2 years. Because premature infants have limited iron stores at birth, iron deficiency likely will occur unless the diet contains sufficient iron. A similar situation is noted in full-term infants who are neither breast-fed nor fed iron-fortified formulas. Although most often related to nutritional inadequacy, iron deficiency anemia in childhood can also occur as a result of gastrointestinal blood loss, as with Meckel diverticulum or gastroenteritis due to milk protein intolerance.

Pure red cell aplasia (Diamond-Blackfan syndrome) is usually detected by 3 months of age. Although initially it may be confused with physiologic anemia, in Diamond-Blackfan syndrome, the reticulocyte count does not increase over time, nor does the anemia resolve without therapeutic interventions. Examination of the bone marrow in children with pure red cell aplasia reveals few, if any, erythroid progenitors. Megaloblastic anemia of infancy occurs chiefly between 2 and 18 months of age. Macrocytic red cells are seen in the peripheral blood, and megaloblastic red cell precursors are found in the bone marrow. Fanconi anemia, an inherited form of progressive pancytopenia, can present with anemia early in life, but usually not until 3 to 4 years of age. Transient erythroblastopenia of childhood usually occurs in the first few years after birth. Clinical and hematologic features of the hemoglobinopathies, such as β-thalassemia and sickle cell anemia, are usually evident by 6 months, when the switch from fetal Hb to adult Hb synthesis is complete.

By early adolescence, the causes of anemia are similar to those in adulthood, with the exception of the high incidence of iron deficiency. This is usually related to the pubertal growth spurt or to a diet lacking in essential nutrients. Pregnant adolescents are at particular risk for nutritional deficiencies because of greater nutritional requirements during pregnancy.

Classification of Anemia

Anemias are classified on either a physiologic or a morphologic basis. The physiologic classification includes anemias due to increased red cell loss, increased red cell destruction, and impaired red cell production. Table 13–4 illustrates the types of anemias grouped according to these approaches. The morphologic classification schema, based on red cell size, red cell indices, and red cell morphology, is presented later in this chapter.

BLOOD LOSS

The symptoms associated with blood loss are related to its acute or chronic pattern. Acute blood loss may follow

Table 13–4. Physiologic Classification of Anemia

Increased Red Cell Loss	Increased Red Cell Destruction	Inadequate Red Cell Production
Blood loss	Inherited intracorpuscular defects	Abnormalities of cytoplasmic maturation
Acute	Defective red cell membrane	Iron deficiency
Chronic	Hereditary spherocytosis	Lead poisoning
Milk protein	Hereditary pyropoikilocytosis	Sideroblastic anemias
intolerance	Hereditary stomatocytosis	Abnormalities of nuclear maturation
Ulcers	Hereditary xerocytosis	Vitamin B_{12} deficiency
Iatrogenic	Abnormal glycolysis	Folic acid deficiency
(blood sampling)	Red cell enzyme deficiencies	Orotic aciduria
	Hexose monophosphate shunt	Dyserythropoietic anemias
	Embden-Myerhof pathway	Hereditary erythrocytic multinuclearity with a
	Glucose-6-phosphate dehydrogenase	positive acidified serum test, types I, II, III
	Pyruvate kinase	Impaired erythropoietin production
	Others	Renal disease
	Hemoglobinopathies	Chronic infection
	Sickle cell disease and other structural	Hypothyroidism, hypopituitarism
	variants	Protein malnutrition
	Unstable hemoglobins	Liver disease
	Thalassemias	Defective marrow response
	Thalassemia syndromes	Aplastic anemia
	Thalassemia	Congenital (Fanconi anemia)
	Extracorpuscular defects	Acquired
	Isoimmune hemolytic anemia	Pure red cell aplasia
	Autoimmune hemolytic anemia	Congenital (Diamond-Blackfan, Aase syndromes)
	Mechanical hemolysis and microangiopathic	Acquired (transient erythroblastopenia
	hemolytic anemia	of childhood)
		Marrow replacement
		Malignancies
		Myelofibrosis

trauma or surgery. Chronic blood loss may be due to gastrointestinal tract bleeding, as is seen with inflammation, ulcers, or recurrent nose bleeds. Chronic blood loss can also occur into the lungs or through the kidney in diseases such as idiopathic pulmonary hemosiderosis and nephritis.

The medical history often provides important clues to the site of blood loss. Examination of the stool and urine for occult blood is essential. Specialized radiographic tests and endoscopy may be required. An underlying bleeding disorder, such as von Willebrand disease (VWD) or a defect in platelet function, should be considered, especially in patients with recurrent, severe epistaxis.

The degree of anemia after blood loss depends on the amount and rate of loss and the ability of the bone marrow erythroid pool to respond. The Hb concentration may not fall until 24 h *after* acute blood loss, when fluid equilibrium is established. Changes in vital signs, such as increased pulse rate, tachypnea, and decreased blood pressure, occur when blood loss is significant. In cases of anemia secondary to acute blood loss, the red cell indices are normal. Within

3 to 5 days after the bleed, erythrocyte production can be detected, as evidenced by an elevated reticulocyte count. Leukocytosis and thrombocytosis may also occur. With chronic blood loss, iron deficiency may develop, and red cells may become microcytic and hypochromic.

INCREASED RED CELL DESTRUCTION

The normal life span of the erythrocyte is 120 days. In newborns, normal survival rates for red cells are reduced to 80 to 100 days, and survival rates as low as 45 to 60 days have been reported in the literature. Any anemia in which the life span of the red cell is shortened is classified as a hemolytic anemia. A useful approach in considering these types of anemia is shown in Figure 13–3. Each of these disorders is reviewed briefly.

Inherited intracorpuscular defects
Red cell membrane disorders
Hereditary spherocytosis. Hereditary spherocytosis (HS) is the most common congenital red blood cell membrane disorder. Patients with HS are often of northern European descent. The usual patient with HS has

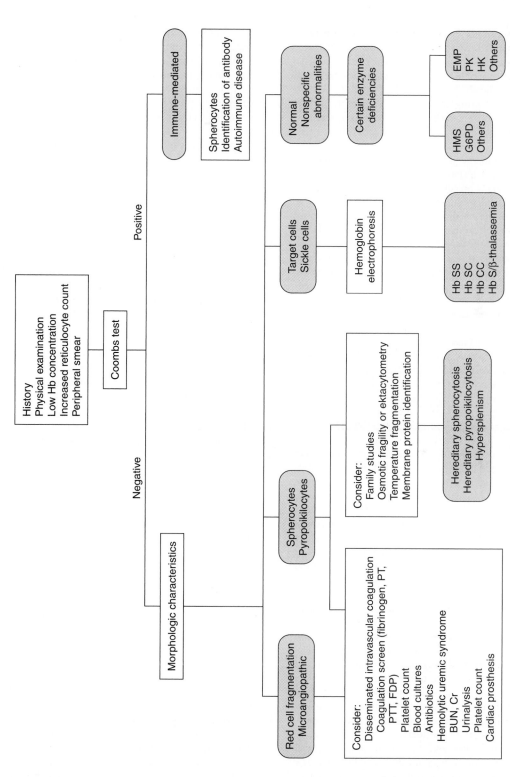

Figure 13–3. Algorithm diagramming an approach to the assessment of children with hemolytic anemia. BUN = blood urea nitrogen; Cr = creatinine; EMP = Embden-Meyerhof pathway; FDP = fibrin degradation products; G6PD = glucose-6-phosphate dehydrogenase; Hb = hemoglobin; HK = hexokinase; HMS = hexose monophosphate shunt; PK = pyruvate kinase; PT = prothrombin time; PTT = partial prothrombin time.

intermittent jaundice, as well as hemolytic and/or red cell aplastic episodes associated with viral infection, splenomegaly, and cholelithiasis. However, the clinical presentation is quite variable, with the most severe cases presenting in the newborn period or early childhood and milder cases presenting in adulthood. The family history is positive in only 20% of cases, and autosomal dominant and autosomal recessive inheritance patterns have been reported.

Several membrane protein defects are responsible for HS. Most result in instability of spectrin, one of the major skeletal membrane proteins. This skeletal defect is classified as a vertical defect in membrane stability because the attachment of the extrinsic (cytosolic skeleton) to the intrinsic membrane proteins is altered. There is a good correlation between the extent of spectrin deficiency and the degree of hemolysis. Structural changes that result as a consequence of protein deficiency lead to membrane instability, loss of surface area, abnormal membrane permeability, and decreased red cell deformability. Metabolic depletion accentuates the defect in HS cells, which accounts for an increase in osmotic fragility after a 24-h incubation of whole blood at 37°C (98.6°F). The splenic sinusoids prevent passage of nondeformable spherocytic red cells. This explains the occurrence of splenomegaly in HS and the therapeutic effect of splenectomy.

Patients with HS have a mild to moderate chronic hemolytic anemia. Red cell indices reveal a decreased MCV. Cellular dehydration increases the MCHC (characteristically >36%). The RDW is elevated because of the variable presence of microspherocytes, and the reticulocyte count is increased in proportion to the degree of hemolysis. Osmotic fragility tests and Ektacytometry studies are characteristic for HS, with increased fragility in hypotonic environments. In unusual cases, in which patients have bile stones related to obstructive liver disease, the red cell surface area may increase because of the accumulation of unesterified cholesterol in the membrane. This clinical point must be considered, as such patients have normal osmotic fragility curves. When the obstructive jaundice clears, the osmotic fragility again becomes abnormal.

As with other hemolytic anemias, affected individuals are susceptible to hypoplastic crises during viral infections. Human parvovirus B19, a frequent pathogen and the organism responsible for erythema infectiosum, selectively invades erythroid progenitor cells and may result in a transient arrest in red cell proliferation. Recovery begins within 7 to 10 days after infection and is usually complete within 4 to 6 weeks. If the initial presentation of patients with HS is during an aplastic crisis, a diagnosis of HS might not be considered because the reticulocyte count will be low and the peripheral blood smear may be undiagnostic. The family history of HS should be explored; if it is positive, patients should be evaluated for HS after recovery from the aplastic episode.

Splenectomy is often considered for patients who have had severe hemolysis requiring transfusions or repeated hospitalization. In patients with mild hemolysis, the decision to perform splenectomy should be delayed; in many cases, it is not required. For pediatric patients who have excessive splenic size, an additional consideration for splenectomy is to diminish the risk of traumatic splenic rupture. The risk of splenectomy must be considered before any clinical decision is made regarding this procedure.

Red cell survival returns to normal values after splenectomy unless an accessory spleen develops. Although an increased number of spherocytes can be seen in the peripheral blood smear after splenectomy and the osmotic fragility is worse, the Hb value is normal. Platelet counts frequently increase to more than 1,000,000/mL immediately after splenectomy but return to normal levels over several weeks. No therapeutic interventions are required for postsplenectomy thrombocytosis in patients with HS.

To minimize the risk of sepsis due to *Haemophilus influenzae* and *Streptococcus pneumoniae,* the splenectomy procedure (when necessary) is often postponed until after the child's fifth or sixth birthday. Patients should be immunized against streptococcal pneumonia and *H. influenzae* with pneumococcal and *H. influenzae* type B vaccines, and prophylaxis with penicillin is often recommended after splenectomy. The duration of penicillin prophylaxis depends on evaluation of the patients' and families' ability to recognize and promptly seek medical attention for febrile episodes. In some cases, penicillin prophylaxis is continued for several years. The increase in penicillin-resistant strains of *Strep. pneumoniae* has raised questions regarding the use of prophylactic penicillin. No studies have determined the frequency of this problem in children receiving prophylactic penicillin after splenectomy.

Hereditary elliptocytosis. Hereditary elliptocytosis (HE) is a congenital red cell disorder in which the red cells appear elliptical on peripheral blood smears (see Figure 13–1). The membrane protein abnormalities that cause these disorders result in lateral defects in membrane stability. These refer to side-to-side protein interactions that stabilize the membrane cytoskeleton; the abnormalities involve primarily the α and β chains of spectrin. Considerable clinical heterogeneity exists depending on the effect of the structural spectrin defect on membrane stability.

In autosomal dominant HE, elliptocytes can be detected in the peripheral blood smear, but patients are not anemic, the reticulocyte count is normal, and red cell indices are normal. Although the osmotic fragility may be normal, the membrane abnormality in HE can be detected by the fragmentation patterns of red cell membrane preparations using an Ektacytometer. Elliptocytes also can be seen in the blood smear of patients with thalassemia, iron deficiency anemia, and megaloblastic anemia. In these cases, the abnormal red cell morphology is secondary to an acquired membrane defect. Protein electrophoresis patterns of spectrin show abnormalities, and functional studies reveal defects in tetramer formation.

In cases in which HE is coinherited with another skeletal protein defect, the red cell morphology may show elliptocytes and poikilocytes. These patients have a moderate to severe hemolytic anemia, and their red cells fragment in vitro as the incubation temperature is increased above 37°C (98.6°F). As a consequence, this disorder is called *hereditary pyropoikilocytosis (HPP)*.

Depending on the precise molecular defect, newborns with HE may have a transient, moderate to severe hemolytic anemia similar to that seen in patients with HPP. This anemia corrects in 4 to 6 months, at which time elliptocytes are seen on the peripheral blood smear and the Hb and reticulocyte counts are normal. An interesting mechanism has been proposed to explain this transition. Because fetal Hb does not bind 2,3-diphosphoglycerate (2,3-DPG), the concentration of unbound 2,3-DPG inside the neonatal red cell is increased. Because 2,3-DPG can weaken skeletal protein interactions, it is possible that the combination of a hereditary protein defect with a weakened skeletal network results in the poikilocytes noted in the peripheral blood smear. As adult Hb increases, the unbound 2,3-DPG associates with the Hb and no longer weakens the membrane. This hypothesis might also explain why some patients with hereditary spherocytosis have problems in the newborn period, whereas most do not.

Other inherited membrane defects. Several other less common forms of inherited membrane defects include *hereditary stomatocytosis* and *hereditary xerocytosis*. These rare congenital hemolytic anemias are associated with permeability defects in the membrane leading to abnormalities in red cell water and cation content. The stomatocyte is characterized by a "stoma" fish mouth-like appearance, excess water, and a marked cation permeability defect that lowers intracellular K^+ and increases intracellular Na^+. The MCV is greater than 110 fL. Patients with hereditary xerocytosis have dense, dehydrated red cells and mild to moderate hemolytic anemia. The MCHC is greater than 36%, the MCV is low, and the cells are depleted of intracellular cations. Both of these disorders result in severe hemolytic anemia that is only partially corrected by splenectomy.

Abnormalities in red cell glycolysis. Glucose is the primary metabolic substrate for the red cell. Because the mature red cell does not contain mitochondria, it can metabolize glucose only by anaerobic mechanisms. The two major metabolic pathways within the red cell are the Embden-Meyerhof pathway (EMP) and the hexose monophosphate shunt (HMS). Other minor metabolic pathways involve the reduction of oxidized Hb, the methemo-

globin reductive pathway, and the reutilization of purines, the purine salvage pathway. A flow diagram of red cell metabolism is shown in Figure 13–4.

In the EMP, which accounts for 90% of the glucose used by the red cell, two molecules of adenosine triphosphate (ATP) are generated for each molecule of glucose consumed. Adenosine triphosphate is the high-energy phosphate required for phosphorylation reactions in cellular functions such as deformability, membrane permeability, membrane lipid turnover, and protein phosphorylation. The inability to maintain ATP results in shortened red cell survival. In the HMS, where the remaining 10% of the red cell glucose is metabolized, substrates required to protect against red cell oxidation are generated. Defects in this pathway render the cell susceptible to oxidative injury. As a consequence, oxidized Hb (Heinz bodies), lipids, and membrane proteins accumulate in the red cell, resulting in hemolysis.

Genotypic and phenotypic variations have been reported for almost every red cell enzyme. The clinical manifestations associated with these disorders are determined by the net effect of the enzyme abnormality on ATP production, 2,3-DPG content, or red cell antioxidant capacity. Several of the enzyme deficiencies affect tissues in addition to the erythrocyte and have associated symptoms (Table 13–5).

In cases in which the enzyme abnormality is distal to the synthesis of 2,3-DPG, 2,3-DPG accumulates in the red cell and its interaction with Hb facilitates oxygen delivery. This explains why patients with pyruvate kinase deficiency, who have elevated red cell 2,3-DPG, can tolerate anemia much better than do patients with hexokinase deficiency, who, although they exhibit a similar inability to maintain normal levels of red cell ATP, have lower levels of 2,3-DPG.

Red cell morphologic changes are minimal in patients with red cell enzyme deficiency involving the EMP. Red cell indices are usually normochromic and normocytic. The reticulocyte count is elevated in proportion to the extent of hemolysis. The diagnosis may require measurement of multiple red cell enzyme activities, as well as determination of the concentration of glycolytic intermediates. The latter is important, as certain enzyme deficiencies are more likely to be detected by the accumulation of a particular intermediate than by a dramatic change in enzyme activity. Because many enzyme activities are normally increased in young red cells, a mild deficiency in one of these may be obscured by the reticulocytosis. Under these circumstances, techniques to eliminate the effects of red cell age must be used, and a relative deficiency in the enzyme of interest signifies that this enzyme is responsible. Family studies can facilitate diagnosis. As many of the enzyme deficiencies have been characterized at the molecular level, molecular techniques can be used to establish a diagnosis and provide the option of intrauterine

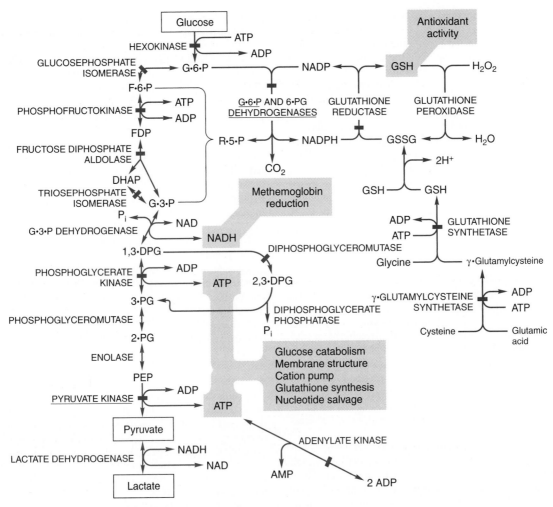

Figure 13–4. Glucose metabolism in mature erythrocytes. The hexose monophosphate shunt and glutathione metabolism are shown within the shaded area. Reactions involved in the synthesis of glutathione are indicated at the lower right. Solid bars indicate enzymatic deficiencies the association of which with hereditary hemolytic disorders is well established. ADP = adenosine diphosphate; AMP = adenosine monophosphate; ATP = adenosine triphosphate; DHAP = dihydroxyacetone phosphate; DPG = diphosphoglycerate; FDP = fructose diphosphate; F-6-P = fructose-6-phosphatase; G-3-P = glucose-3-phosphate; G-6-P = glucose-6-phosphate; GSH = glutathione (reduced); GSSG = glutathione (oxidized); NAD = nicotinamide-adenine dinucleotide; NADH = reduced NAD; NADP = nicotinamide adenine nucleotide (oxidized); NADPH = nicotinamide adenine nucleotide (reduced); PEP = phosphoenolpyruvate; PG = phosphoglycerate; Pi = inorganic phosphate; R-5-P = ribose-5-phosphatase.

diagnosis. Except in the case of pyruvate kinase or G6PD deficiency, the two most common enzyme deficiencies responsible for hemolytic anemia, reference laboratories should be used to measure the panel of red cell enzymes and glycolytic intermediates.

Pyruvate kinase deficiency. This is the most common enzyme deficiency in the EMP. The inheritance pattern of this disorder is autosomal recessive. Homozygotes usually have hemolytic anemia with splenomegaly, whereas heterozygotes are usually asymptomatic. The disorder is found worldwide, although it is most common in whites of northern European descent. The range of clinical expression is variable, from severe neonatal jaundice to a fully compensated hemolytic anemia. Anemia is

Table 13–5. Enzyme Deficiencies of the Embden-Meyerhof Pathway

Enzyme		Tissues Involved	Clinical Features	Red Cell Metabolites		Other Remarks
				ATP	2,3-DPG	
Hexokinase	AR	RBC	CNSHA	↓	↓	Increased hemoglobin O₂ affinity, decreased exercise tolerance for degree of anemia
Glucose phosphate isomerase	AR	RBC, WBC, skin fibro-blasts	CNSHA	↓, N	N	Spiculated microsphe-rocytes sometimes observed
Phosphofructokinase	AR	RBC, muscle	CNSHA, myopathy (muscle glycogen storage disease)	↓	↓	
Aldolase	AR	RBC	CNSHA	N	↑	Fructose-1,6-diphosphate accu-mulates in RBC
Triosephosphate isomerase	AR	RBC, WBC, muscle, serum, CSF	CNSHA, severe pro-gressive neuro-logic disorder	↓	—	Dihydroxyacetone phosphate accu-mulates in RBC, in-creased susceptibil-ity to infection
Phosphoglycerate kinase	Sex-linked	RBC, WBC	CNSHA, mental retardation, myopathy	N	N, ↑	
2,3-DPG mutase	AR, AD	RBC	?CNSHA or polycythemia	N, ↑	↓	Increased hemoglobin O₂ affinity
Pyruvate kinase	AR	RBC, liver	CNSHA	N, ↓	↑	Decreased hemoglobin O₂ affinity, increased exercise tolerance for degree of anemia

AR, autosomal recessive; AD = autosomal dominant; ATP = adenosine triphosphate; CNSHA = congenital nonspherocytic hemolytic anemia; CSF = cerebrospinal fluid; 2,3-DPG = 2,3-diphosphoglycerate; N = normal; RBC =red blood cell; WBC =white blood cell.

Reproduced with permission from Mentzer WC: Abnormalities of erythrocyte metabolism. In Rudolph AM (editor): *Rudolph's Pediatrics,* 19th ed. Appleton & Lange, 1991.

usually normochromic and normocytic, but macrocytes may be present shortly after a hemolytic crisis, reflecting erythroid hyperplasia and early release of red cells from the marrow. In severe cases, the morphologic examination of the peripheral smear shows polychromasia, aniso-cytosis, poikilocytosis, and nucleated red cells. The os-motic fragility of red cells is normal or slightly reduced. Diagnosis is confirmed by a quantitative assay for pyru-vate kinase, by the measurement of enzyme kinetics and glycolytic intermediates, and by family studies. It may be necessary to measure enzyme kinetics using several sub-strates, because in some PK-deficient patients with un-usual forms of the disease, the enzyme defect cannot be identified using one substrate.

Splenectomy is a therapeutic option for PK-deficient patients. As with HS, the decision should be made on the basis of patients' clinical courses. Unlike HS patients, PK-deficient patients, although they improve after splenec-tomy, do not have complete correction of their hemolytic anemia. Because reticulocytes contain mitochondria, they are capable of oxidative metabolism and have a selective survival in patients with PK deficiency. The spleen, with its hypoxic and acidotic environment, results in destruc-tion of reticulocytes as well as mature red cells in PK deficiency. When the spleen is removed, the Hb count increases slightly, but the reticulocyte count increases dramatically. Thus, it is not uncommon to have a reticu-locyte count greater than 50% in a PK-deficient patient after splenectomy. In contrast to HS, Kupffer cells in the liver are also capable of destroying PK-deficient cells, par-tially explaining why splenectomy is not as effective in PK deficiency as in HS. As with all hemolytic anemias, these patients should have dietary supplementation with folic acid (5 mg/d) to prevent megaloblastic complications associated with relative folate deficiency and immunization against *Strep. pneumoniae* and *H. influenzae*, as well as consideration for lifelong prophylactic penicillin for splenectomized patients.

Glucose-6-phosphate dehydrogenase deficiency. Glucose-6-phosphate dehydrogenase, the most common red cell enzyme deficiency, is sex-linked, with partial expression in the female population and full expression in the affected male population. The distribution of G6PD deficiency is worldwide, with the highest incidence in Africans and African Americans. Mediterraneans, American Indians, Southeast Asians, and Sephardic Jews are also affected. In African Americans, 12% of the male population have the deficiency, 18% of the female population are heterozygous, and 2% of female population are homozygous. In Southeast Asians, G6PD deficiency is found in approximately 6% of the male population. One hypothesis for the prevalence of this enzyme abnormality is that it confers resistance to malaria. Once the malaria parasite invades a red cell, it generates oxidants during metabolism. The inability of G6PD-deficient cells to detoxify these oxidants may result in red cell death and, along with it, death of the parasite.

Many variants of G6PD deficiency are known and have been characterized at the biochemical and molecular levels. Depending on the molecular defect and the ability of the mutant enzyme to stabilize cellular enzymes required for antioxidant defense, some of the enzyme deficiencies result in extreme depletion of enzyme and auto-oxidant reserve (reduced glutathione, in particular) and are associated with chronic hemolytic anemia. These are often found in Mediterraneans. Other variants are associated with an unstable enzyme that has normal levels in young red cells. These result in hemolysis only in association with an oxidant challenge; this is the type found in African Americans. In some cases of G6PD deficiency, the defect can be identified in both granulocytes and erythrocytes. In addition to having chronic hemolytic anemia, such patients may be susceptible to bacterial infections.

In the African American type of G6PD deficiency, hemolysis may be triggered by the oxidant intermediates generated during viral or bacterial infections or after ingestion of oxidant compounds (Table 13–6). Shortly after exposure to the oxidant, Hb is oxidized to methemoglobin and eventually denatured, forming intracellular inclusions called Heinz bodies. Heinz bodies attach to the red cell membrane and aggregate certain intrinsic membrane proteins, in particular band 3. The reticuloendothelial cells recognize this perturbation in the membrane as a new antigenic site and ingest this portion of the cell. The resulting cell, often called a *bite* cell as a consequence of this unusual phagocytic process, has a shortened survival owing to its loss of membrane components. To compensate for hemolysis, red cell production is increased and the reticulocyte count is elevated.

In normal red cells, G6PD is an age-dependent enzyme. Because the molecular basis of G6PD deficiency in African Americans is due to enzyme instability and not enzyme deficiency, as is the case of Mediterranean variants of the enzyme, levels of G6PD are normal in the reticulocyte but decreased in older red cells. Therefore,

Table 13–6. Some Agents Reported to Produce Hemolysis in Patients with Glucose-6-Phosphate Dehydrogenase (G6PD) Deficiency

Drugs and chemicals clearly shown to cause clinically significant hemolytic anemia in G6PD deficiency:	
Acetanilid	Pentaquine
Methylene blue	Sulfanilamide
Nalidixic acid (NegGram)	Sulfacetamide
Naphthalene	Sulfapyridine
Niridazole (Ambilhar)	Sulfamethoxazole
Nitrofurantoin (Furadantin)	(Gantanol)
Phenylhydrazine	Thiazolesulfone
Primaquine	Toluidine blue
Pamaquine	Trinitrotoluene

Drugs probably safe in normal therapeutic doses for G6PD-deficient individuals (without nonspherocytic hemolytic anemia):	
Acetaminophen (Paracetamol Tylenol, Tralgon Hydroxyacetanilid)	para-Aminobenzoic acid
	Phenylbutazone
	Phenytoin
Acetophenetidine (Phenacetin)	Probenecid (Benemid)
Acetylsalicylic acid (aspirin)	Procaine amide hydrochloride (Pronestyl)
Aminopyrine (Pyramidone, Amidopyrine)	Pyrimethamine (Daraprim)
Antazoline (Antistine)	Quinidine
Antipyrine	Quinine
Ascorbic acid (vitamin C)	Streptomycin
Benzhexol (Artane)	Sulfacytine
Chloramphenicol	Sulfadiazine
Chlorguanidine (Proguanil, Paludrine)	Sulfaguanidine
	Sulfamerazine
Chloroquine	Sulfamethoxypyriazine (Kynex)
Colchicine	Sulfisoxazole (Gantrisin)
Diphenhydramine (Benadryl)	Trimethoprim
L-Dopa	Tripelennamine (Pyribenzamine)
Menadione sodium bisulfite (Hykinone)	Vitamin K
Menaphtone	

Reproduced with permission from Beutler: *Hemolytic Anemia in Disorders of Red Cell Metabolism.* Plenum, 1978. Cited by Mentzer WC: Abnormalities of erythrocyte metabolism. In Rudolph AM (editor): *Rudolph's Pediatrics,* 19th ed. Appleton & Lange, 1991, p 1138.

after an oxidant exposure, only the older cell is destroyed and hemolysis is limited. This can cause a diagnostic problem, as cells not destroyed by the oxidant are reticulocytes in G6PD-deficient African Americans and have normal or elevated enzyme levels. Methods are available to sort out the older red cells, however, so that they can be analyzed for enzyme activity. Once patients have been removed from the oxidant challenge, the hemolytic anemia will resolve, at which time the enzyme assay can readily be performed.

Individuals with the Mediterranean or Asian forms of G6PD deficiency, in addition to being sensitive to infections and certain drugs, often have a chronic, moderately severe anemia, with nonspherocytic red cells and jaundice. Hemolysis usually starts in early childhood. Reticulocytosis is present and can increase the MCV. This severe variant is most common in the Greek population. Molecular studies of these variants may show complete absence of the enzyme in all red cells.

In Asian newborns with G6PD deficiency, stress related to delivery, infection, or antibiotics can precipitate hemolysis. Indeed, G6PD deficiency can be a cause of hemolytic jaundice and kernicterus in the newborn period, and many hospitals where susceptible populations are born (e.g., in Hawaii) have instituted newborn screening programs for this enzyme deficiency. Jaundice is particularly common in premature infants who are G6PD deficient.

Favism, a severe form of G6PD deficiency, occurs after ingestion or inhalation of materials released from the fava bean. It has been reported in Asians and Mediterraneans but not in African Americans. After exposure to the bean, acute, life-threatening hemolysis can appear within 24 h. The pathophysiology of favism appears to involve both G6PD deficiency and an undefined susceptibility of the red cell membrane to damage secondary to a toxin released by the fava bean. Although hemolysis may be sufficient to cause severe anemia, requiring transfusion to prevent cardiorespiratory distress, most cases resolve spontaneously and will not recur if patients are not exposed to the fava bean.

When a hemolytic crisis occurs in G6PD deficiency or favism, pallor, scleral icterus, hemoglobinemia, hemoglobinuria, and splenomegaly may be noted. Plasma haptoglobin and hemopexin concentrations are low. The peripheral smear shows the fragmented bite cells and polychromatophilic cells. Red cell indices may be normal. Special stains can detect Heinz bodies in the cells during the first few days of hemolysis.

A diagnosis of G6PD deficiency should be based on family history, ethnicity, laboratory features, physical findings, recent exposure to oxidants, and acute hemolytic event. It can be confirmed by a quantitative enzyme assay or by molecular analysis of the gene. Treatment is directed toward supportive care for the acute event and counseling

regarding prevention of future hemolytic crises. In patients with chronic hemolysis, dietary supplements with folic acid, 1 to 5 mg/d, are recommended. Use of vitamin E, 500 mg/d, may improve red cell survival in patients with chronic hemolysis.

Hemoglobinopathies. Disorders in Hb structure and synthesis, collectively called the hemoglobinopathies, are due to molecular defects that result in changes in the structure or synthesis of a particular globin chain. The clinical manifestations of the structurally abnormal Hb depend on the charge and location of the amino acid substitution. Alterations in oxygen transport or HHb stability or physical changes in the Hb molecule can occur. Hemoglobinopathies due to defective synthesis of either α- or β-globin chains are called *thalassemia.* Partial or complete absence of globin synthesis results in an imbalance of globin chain synthesis. The excess globin chains, either α or β, that accumulate within the developing red cell interact with the red cell membrane, alter cellular properties, and ultimately shorten red cell survival. Depending on the degree of imbalance, red cell destruction can occur within the bone marrow.

The structure of the predominant Hbs is shown in Table 13–7. Adult Hb (HbA) is composed of two α-globin chains and two β-globin chains. Fetal Hb (HbF), the predominant Hb in the newborn, contains two α-globin chains and two γ-globin chains. HbA_2, which represents no more than 3.6% of the total Hb in adults, consists of two α-globin chains and two δ-globin chains. HbH (β4) and Bart Hb (γ4) are found in α-thalassemia.

The chromosomal location and organization of the genes responsible for globin-chain synthesis are shown in Figure 13–5. The two genes responsible for β-globin production are located on chromosome 11, whereas the genes responsible for α-globin production are located on chromosome 16. Because there are four genes for α-globin–chain production, the clinical manifestations and laboratory diagnosis of disorders involving the α-globin genes are quite variable. If one gene is structurally abnormal, approximately 25% of the Hb will be altered. Because there are only two β-globin genes, a defect in one will affect approximately 50% of the Hb.

The molecular mechanisms responsible for the switch from HbF to HbA begin during the second to third trimester of pregnancy; at birth, the predominant Hb is HbF. Rare, structural defects in γ-globin have been reported, although most of these are benign. They can result in hemolysis, however, if the γ-chain variant is unstable. Therefore, a Hb disorder should be considered in the workup of newborns with a hemolytic anemia. When the switch from fetal to adult Hb is complete, the clinical manifestations associated with these γ-chain variants disappear.

In newborns, defects in α-globin are much more common than are defects in γ-globin. These can result in a structurally abnormal Hb or in an α-thalassemia–like

Table 13–7. Hemoglobin Composition

Hemoglobin	Structure	Percentage of Total Hemoglobin	Increased	Decreased
A	$\alpha_2\beta_2$	Adult 98 Newborn 10–40		
A$_2$	$\alpha_2\delta_2$	Adult 1.6–3.5 Newborn < 1	β-Thalassemia	α-Thalassemia Iron deficiency
F	$\alpha_2\gamma_2$	Adult < 1 Newborn 60–90	β-Thalassemia Hereditary persistence of fetal hemoglobin Stress erythropoiesis	
H	β^4	20	Hemoglobin H disease Hydrops fetalis due to homozygous thalassemia	
Bart	γ^4	10 5–30	Hydrops fetalis α-Thalassemia syndromes	

pattern. The structural defects are usually benign, as they are caused by mutations affecting only one of the four α-globin genes. In contrast, the consequences of synthetic defects in α-globin chains (α-thalassemia) can be quite significant.

Sickle cell disease. Structural defects involving the β-globin genes are the most frequent types of hemoglobinopathies affecting children in the United States. Sickle cell disease is the most common of these. Sickle cell anemia (homozygous inheritance of the sickle gene), sickle cell–HbC disease [doubly heterozygous for sickle cell Hb (HbS) and HbC], and sickle cell–β-thalassemia (either β⁺ or β⁰) are classified as the sickle cell diseases. In the United States, the sickle cell diseases primarily affect African Americans. However, as distribution of the sickle gene is worldwide because of the selective advantage that individuals with sickle cell trait have when infected by malaria, sickle cell disease quite possibly will be detected in a number of white or Hispanic newborns as experience is gained with newborn screening.

The sickle cell diseases are inherited in an autosomal, codominant manner. The molecular defect in HbS is due to the substitution of valine for glutamic acid in the sixth position of the β-globin chain. The charge and location of this substitution cause HbS to be converted from a soluble state into a polymer when it undergoes the structural changes that accompany release of oxygen. Hypoxia, acidosis, and hypertonicity facilitate polymer formation. The polymerization of Hb causes the red cell to transform from a deformable, biconcave disk into a rigid, sickle-shaped cell. The process of sickling and loss of cell deformability is reversible to a point, at which time the cell is permanently damaged. At this point, it is called an *irreversibly sickled cell (ISC)*. Even under completely oxygenated conditions, ISCs remain sickled. The sickled red cells seen on examination of the peripheral blood smear are examples of ISCs.

Clinical manifestations. The clinical manifestations of sickle cell disease are due to anemia and vascular occlusion. Sickled cells are rigid and fragile, and these properties contribute to the moderate to severe hemolytic anemia characteristic of this disease. The life span of the erythrocyte may be as short as 20 days. For unexplained reasons, these cells are very sticky. This abnormal adhesive

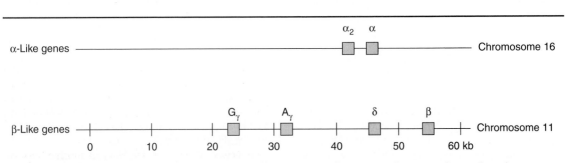

Figure 13–5. Chromosomal organizations of the globin genes. The β-like gene clusters are located on chromosome 11, and the α-like gene clusters on chromosome 16.

property causes them to stick to endothelial surfaces, as well as to other cells, and contributes to the vascular occlusive events, pain, and organ damage characteristic of this disease. Vascular obstruction within the spleen results in loss of splenic function and increases the susceptibility of patients to bacterial sepsis. Vascular obstruction in cerebral vessels can lead to stroke, and all organs can be damaged by vascular obstruction.

In African Americans, the frequency of the sickle cell gene is 8%; the HbC gene, 4%; and β-thalassemia gene, approximately 1%. Approximately 1:600 African American infants has sickle cell anemia.

The clinical severity of sickle cell diseases is quite variable. Although several factors have been recognized that contribute to variations in clinical severity (Table 13–8), many additional factors likely remain to be identified. The most important of these is the type of the sickle cell disease. The frequency and severity of both anemic and vasoocclusive complications is highest in patients with homozygous sickle cell anemia (HbSS), whereas patients with sickle cell-β$^+$ and sickle cell–HbC disease have the least severe forms of disease. These variations have been explained on the basis of the ease with which Hb polymerization and sickling occur in these disorders.

In sickle cell anemia, the level of HbF within each red cell affects the polymerization of HbS: Pain crises, as well as life span, have an inverse correlation with the level of HbF. A genetic polymorphism, determined by analysis of the DNA in proximity to the sickle globin gene, has identified four categories of patients whose genetic origins are Bantu, Benin, Indian, and Senegalese. HbF levels are highest in the India and Senegal haplotypes.

The polymerization of HbS is logarithmically proportional to the MCHC. Thus, if the MCHC is reduced, the chance that polymers will form as the red cell releases oxygen in the capillary bed is reduced. When α-thalassemia is coinherited with sickle cell trait or disease, the MCHC and MCV of the red cell are decreased. The frequency of α-thalassemia trait is 1 to 3% in African Americans. Patients who have both α-thalassemia and sickle cell anemia are less anemic than are those who have sickle cell anemia alone. However, α-thalassemia trait does not appear to prevent the frequency or severity of vasoocclusive complications or organ damage.

The coinheritance of both HbC and HbS results in a mild form of sickle cell disease. Nevertheless, patients with sickle cell–HbC disease can have all of the complications found in patients with sickle cell anemia. This includes vascular as well as infectious complications.

When the sickle cell gene is coinherited with a β-thalassemia–trait gene, patients have sickle cell–β-thalassemia. Clinical severity depends on the type of β-thalassemic gene, either β^0-thalassemia, in which no HbA is synthesized, or β$^+$-thalassemia, in which a variable amount of HbA is made. In sickle cell–β$^+$-thalassemia, due to the thalassemic gene, the Hb electrophoresis shows more HbS than HbA. This contrasts with sickle cell trait, in which the amount of HbA is greater than that of HbS. This distinction is extremely important as individuals with sickle cell trait do not have a disease, whereas those with sickle cell–β$^+$-thalassemia have sickle cell disease. Patients with sickle cell–β^0-thalassemia have only HbS on electrophoresis and can have symptoms identical to those in patients with sickle cell anemia. Analysis of Hb in the parents of these patients should show sickle cell trait in one parent and normal Hb in the other. Rather than consider nonpaternity, it is important to exclude β-thalassemia trait in the parent who has HbA only. This can be done by determining the MCV and by measuring the level of HbA$_2$.

As a result of early diagnosis, comprehensive medical care, and education of families and health care providers, the mortality in the first decade of life from sickle cell disease has decreased dramatically over the past several years, from approximately 25% to less than 3%. Most states have instituted newborn screening for hemoglobinopathies. Because HbF is the predominant Hb in newborns, the electrophoretic pattern in newborns with sickle cell disease is FS. A similar FS pattern is seen in newborns with sickle cell–β^0-thalassemia, sickle cell–hereditary persistence of fetal Hb (HPFH), or sickle cell–HbD or HbG. Family studies or repeated testing at 4 to 6 months of age may be necessary to confirm the diagnosis. Molecular biology techniques can also be used to distinguish these disorders at birth.

Hematologic values for each of the sickle cell diseases are shown in Table 13–9. In sickle cell anemia, the hematocrits can vary from 18 to 28%. The reticulocyte count is elevated (12 to 25%), reflecting the rate of hemolysis. The MCV is elevated as the result of the young red cell population. If the MCV is low, coinheritance of α- or β-thalassemia trait or iron deficiency should be suspected. The coinheritance of α-thalassemia trait with sickle cell disease increases the hematocrit, lowers the reticulocyte

Table 13–8. Factors that Affect Clinical Severity of Sickle Cell Disease

Type of sickle cell disease:
  SS > S β^0-thalassemia > SC > S β$^+$-thalassemia
Fetal hemoglobin concentration
β-Globin gene cluster haplotype
α-Thalassemia
Nonerythroid factors
  Adhesive molecules and their interaction
    with plasma proteins
  Regulators of microcapillary tone
  Psychosocial

Table 13–9. Hematologic Values in Sickle Cell Disease

Syndrome	Hematocrit (%)	Reticulocyte (%)	MCV (mm³)	Electrophoresis (%)
SS	18–28	12–25	86	80–100 S 0–20 F
SC	30–36	5–10	77	50 S 50 C
S β⁰-thalassemia	20–30	10–15	66	75–100 S 0–20 F 3–6 A₂
S β⁺-thalassemia	30–36	3–6	70	50–80 S 0–20 F 10–30 A 3–6 A₂
SS α-thalassemia	25–30	5–10	70	80–100 S 0–20 F

MCV = mean corpuscular volume.

Reproduced with permission from Platt OS, Nathan DG: Disorders of hemoglobin: Sickle cell disease. In Nathan DG, Oski FA (editor): *Hematology of Infancy and Childhood*, 3d ed. Saunders, 1987.

count, and lowers the MCV. The amount of HbS, A, or C is shown for each of the sickle cell diseases. Note the similar levels of HbS in sickle cell anemia and sickle cell–β⁰-thalassemia.

The white cell count is elevated (12,000 to 18,000/mL), but the differential count remains normal. Platelet counts are also elevated. Leukocytosis and thrombocytosis represent the products of a hyperplastic marrow in asplenic persons who have a persistent chronic hemolytic process. HbF levels vary among the different disorders and between patients.

The clinical manifestations of sickle cell disease are related to the degree of hemolytic anemia and to the frequency and location of vasoocclusive events. Almost every organ of the body can be affected. Susceptibility to infection is increased primarily because of splenic infarction, but also because of other acquired immunologic abnormalities. This can result in life-threatening episodes of sepsis. Recognition of this susceptibility and aggressive medical management have resulted in an increased life span for most patients.

Complications in sickle cell disease are characterized by sudden, unexpected onset, including vascular occlusion (pain), splenic sequestration, hyperhemolysis, and infections. Associated chronic medical complications due to organ damage increase with age. The kidney is frequently affected, and many adult patients require dialysis or renal transplantation. Cerebrovascular occlusion is a devastating complication and can present as clinically manifest strokes or silent cerebral infarctions in children and as cerebral hemorrhage in adults. Acute medical complications in young children can occur because of splenic sequestration.

A major cause of morbidity and mortality in sickle cell disease is the acute chest syndrome, a complication in which pulmonary function is rapidly compromised owing to vascular obstruction, changes in ventilation-perfusion ratios, atelectasis, infection, and pulmonary fat embolism secondary to sickling-related bone marrow infections.

Management. Although details of appropriate treatment for complications of sickle cell disease are beyond the scope of this chapter, general guidelines are described briefly. A National Institutes of Health monograph, available from the Sickle Cell Disease Branch of the National Heart, Lung & Blood Institute, records an excellent description of treatment in sickle cell disease. First, it is important to deliver comprehensive care. Prophylactic penicillin, immunizations, attention to growth and development, and concern regarding psychosocial issues are necessary. One must always consider patients with sickle cell infection as compromised hosts, and, if patients are febrile, the infection should be aggressively diagnosed and treated with antibiotics. The possibility of penicillin-resistant *Strep. pneumoniae* should be considered. Underlying causes must be sought for vasoocclusive complications. Prompt attention should be given to changes in hematologic status, such as a decrease in Hb (aplastic crisis), as seen with parvovirus infections. In addition, parents and family members should be taught to palpate the spleen and recognize early signs of splenic sequestration. Any pulmonary complication requires careful monitoring and aggressive intervention if progressive pulmonary dysfunction is detected.

Adequate hydration is an important component of therapy for many complications of sickle cell disease.

Dehydration occurs frequently in these patients because of inadequate fluid intake and sickle cell hyposthenia. Because renal function is altered, urine specific gravity measurements cannot be used to assess hydration. Comparison of patients' weights with baseline values is the best method to assess fluid requirements. Except for pulmonary complications, in which excess hydration should be avoided as it can lead to pulmonary edema, 1.5 times maintenance fluid therapy is generally used. Red cell transfusions should be given for conditions recognized to benefit from this treatment. Abuse of transfusion therapy can lead to iron overload and alloimmunization. Pain management should be aggressive; combinations of narcotic with nonnarcotic drugs may be beneficial. Concerns regarding potential for drug addiction can result in inadequate therapy for painful complications and lead to secondary "chronic pain" behavior patterns while having no impact on the incidence of drug addiction. Current trials with agents to stimulate Hb production, such as hydroxyurea, are encouraging. This drug should be used only in a setting that provides appropriate monitoring for drug toxicity. Bone marrow transplantation may have a role for selected patients when appropriate donors can be identified. The future holds the promise of gene therapy as methods have become available to target genes to erythroid progenitors.

Sickle cell trait. Individuals who have sickle cell trait do not have a disease. They are not anemic, their red cell indices and reticulocyte counts are normal, and they do not have painful vasoocclusive complications. However, hyposthenuria and hematuria may occur in individuals with sickle cell trait because of the harsh metabolic conditions within the kidney, which induce polymer formation even in conditions in which the intracellular concentration of HbS is less than 50%. Other rare complications have been reported in individuals with sickle cell trait, primarily as a consequence of these persons exposing themselves to conditions in which oxygen tension is low (e.g., at high altitudes, skiing, mountain climbing, or high pressures, diving) and during extreme exertion associated with dehydration during basic training in the military.

Homozygous HbC disease. HbC is due to a different mutation at the same site as seen in HbS, with lysine, rather than valine, substituted for glutamic acid. The inheritance of two genes for HbC is associated with a mild hemolytic anemia and splenomegaly. Oxyhemoglobin C can crystallize within red cells when they are dehydrated. Typical red cell morphology includes a few fragmented red cells, a few microspherocytes, and target cells. Patients with homozygous HbC disease usually do not require therapy for their hemolytic anemia, nor do they have evidence of vascular obstruction as do patients with sickle cell disease. Individuals with HbC trait have normal hematologic laboratory parameters except for high numbers of target cells, which can be seen in the peripheral blood smear.

HbE disease. HbE, the second most common Hb variant worldwide, is the result of an amino acid substitution of glutamic acid for lysine at the twenty-sixth position of the β-globin chain. Besides the charge difference in HbE, the synthesis of HbE is decreased when compared with HbA. This results in a β-thalassemia-minor-like phenotype with mild anemia and microcytosis in individuals with HbE trait. Because of its charge, the electrophoretic pattern of HbE is similar to that of HbC is rarely seen in Asians; therefore, a laboratory report of HbC in a person of Asian background should be repeated, and a specific request made to identify HbE. In homozygous HbE, patients have mild hemolytic anemia (Hb concentrations, 11 to 14 g/dL) with moderate to severe microcytosis (MCV, 50 to 65 fL). The reticulocyte count is not particularly abnormal (approximately 2%), and target cells, microcytes, and hypochromic cells are seen on the peripheral blood smear. The RDW is normal.

In contrast to these mild disorders, the coinheritance of HbE (which has a mild defect in β-globin synthesis) with β-thalassemia trait (a more severe defect in β-globin synthesis) results in significant hematologic problems. These patients with HbE–β-thalassemia are phenotypically similar to those with β-thalassemia intermedia and have ineffective erythropoiesis and anemia. They often become transfusion dependent and require chelation therapy. The degree of anemia depends on the type of β-thalassemia globin gene (β⁰ or β⁺). The distinction between homozygous HbE and HbE–β⁰-thalassemia is important, as the former requires no specific medical attention, whereas the latter is a disease associated with complications. This distinction can be made on the basis of hematologic changes in patients by 1 year of age. Moderate to severe anemia (Hb levels >3 g/dL below normal) is noted in HbE–β-thalassemia, and mild anemia is noted in homozygous HbE. Family studies, as well as molecular techniques, can help to establish a diagnosis. Molecular techniques are of particular value if both parents are not available for study. Furthermore, molecular techniques can be used to distinguish readily homozygous HbE from HbE–β-thalassemia in the newborn and to facilitate subsequent counseling and medical care.

Other structural Hb variants. In addition to the common Hb variants described above, several rare, structural heterozygote Hb defects are associated with clinical findings. In one group, the oxygen affinity (P_{50}) of whole blood is increased. The electrophoretic mobility of the Hb may be affected on the basis of the charge conferred by the amino acid substitution. In cases in which the oxygen affinity is increased, the Hb concentration is above normal because of erythrocytosis. The differential diagnosis of erythrocytosis should include hypoxia (pulmonary or cardiac-related) or hereditary erythrocytosis. Patients with low-oxygen-affinity Hb variants have Hb levels below normal. They are not anemic from a physiologic standpoint, however, because the Hb can deliver more oxygen to the tissue at a given partial pressure of oxygen (PO_2) than does normal Hb. Measurements of arterial blood gas, serum erythropoietin levels, and Hb oxygen affinity are required to establish a diagnosis in patients with high- or low-oxygen-affinity variants. Familial erythrocytosis due to an abnormality in the erythropoietin receptor on erythroid progenitors has been reported.

Another structural group of Hb variants that can give rise to hemolysis is the unstable Hb variants. In these disorders, the amino acid substitution in the globin chain weakens the Hb tetramer and causes it to dissociate and oxidize, resulting in intracellular methemoglobin and Heinz bodies. This process is accelerated by exposure of the red cell to oxidant stress. Unstable Hb variants can be detected by their charge, instability in the presence of isopropanol, and the presence of intracellular Heinz bodies after oxidant stress. The interaction between Heinz bodies and the cell membrane is believed to result in perturbations in membrane structure and function and to lead to both intravascular and extravascular cell destruction.

Patients with unstable Hb variants display a wide range of clinical severity, ranging from no symptoms to severe hemolytic anemia. This is determined by the site of the mutation, its charge, and its location on an α- or β-globin gene. The inheritance pattern is autosomal dominant, and symptoms occur in the heterozygote state. β-Globin variants are associated with more symptoms than are α-globin variants, as a greater proportion of Hb is affected when one of the two β-globin genes, rather than one of the four α-globin genes, is involved. When the disease is severe, it usually presents with hemolytic anemia in childhood. Severe intravascular hemolysis, jaundice, extensive reticulocytosis, and hemoglobinuria can occur. In some patients, the oxygen affinity of the Hb is also affected.

Normal Hb transports oxygen without becoming oxidized by maintaining its iron in the reduced state. However, 3% of Hb is oxidized to methemoglobin each day. Methemoglobin reductase, an intracellular enzyme, reduces this methemoglobin to oxyhemoglobin. Methemoglobin can be formed when there is a deficiency in methemoglobin reductase or when the red cell's antioxidant capacity is overwhelmed, as noted in G6PD deficiency, favism, and unstable Hb disorders. Hb can also undergo oxidation to methemoglobin if there is an amino acid substitution in α- or β-globin chains in the vicinity of the heme pocket.

Methemoglobinemia. Methemoglobinemia can be hereditary or acquired. The hereditary disorders are associated with a deficiency of the cytoplasmic enzyme, NADPH-methemoglobin reductase, or a structural defect in Hb that facilitates oxidation of the iron molecule. These Hb variants are called HbM, and several types have been identified. Methemoglobin reductase deficiency is rare

and is inherited in an autosomal recessive mode. There are few associated physical findings other than cyanosis and erythrocytosis. Methemoglobin levels are usually 15–30%; methemoglobin cannot transport oxygen, and when the level exceeds 15%, erythrocytosis and cyanosis result. In HbM disorders, mild hemolysis may be present because of the unstable nature of the Hb. Specific electrophoretic techniques can be used to identify HbM, and structural characterization will establish a diagnosis.

In acquired cases of methemoglobinemia, exposure to certain chemicals, such as nitrates (found in well water, certain foods, hemodialysis), aniline dyes, and sulfonamides, causes the rate of Hb oxidation to exceed the reductive capability of methemoglobin reductase. The clinical features are usually mild and include cyanosis, fatigue, and tachycardia. Newborns in whom methemoglobinemia develops often are considered to have pulmonary or cardiac disease and are extensively examined for these conditions. A diagnosis can be made by quantitation of methemoglobin using spectrophotometric methods. Treatment involves identification and avoidance of the toxic agent. Reducing compounds, such as ascorbic acid or methylene blue, can be used if clinically indicated.

Disorders of hemoglobin synthesis. The thalassemias are a heterogeneous group of inherited disorders characterized by a defect in synthesis of normal globin chains that leads to an intracellular imbalance in the α:β chain ratio. The excess globin chains bind to the cell membrane and cause significant damage, resulting in ineffective erythropoiesis and shortened red cell survival. The geographic distribution of the thalassemia gene includes areas near the Mediterranean, Southeast Asia, Middle East, and Orient. This distribution suggests a selective advantage, and resistance to malaria has been the underlying factor.

α-Thalassemia. In α-thalassemia, there may be a deletion or defect in the regulation of 1 to 4 α-globin genes. The spectrum of clinical manifestations depends on the nature and number of affected genes. The genetic basis for the spectrum of α-thalassemias is shown in Figure 13–6.

The most severe form of α-thalassemia, in which there is complete suppression of α-globin synthesis, causes hydrops fetalis. Although intrauterine transfusion has been successful in a few cases and could provide benefit if the fetus survives and is placed on chronic transfusion or has bone marrow transplantation, this condition is usually incompatible with extrauterine life and results in stillbirth.

The clinical picture is that of a pale, premature, edematous (hydropic) baby with massive splenomegaly and severe anemia. Hb electrophoresis reveals no HbF, no HbA, and approximately 90–100% Hbγ^4, which is called Hb Bart. Hbγ^4 has a high oxygen affinity and lacks the Bohr effect; although it readily picks up oxygen, it cannot release it to the tissues under physiologic conditions.

The Asian parents of infants born with homozygous α-thalassemia have the type of α-thalassemia trait with

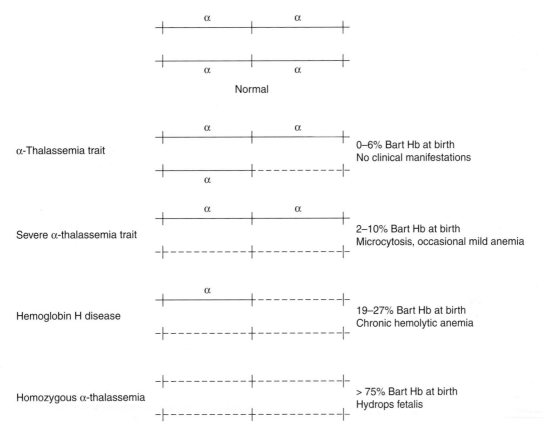

Figure 13–6. Genetic origins of the "classic" α-thalassemia syndromes due to gene deletion, with associated Bart hemoglobin (Hb) expression and clinical manifestations. (Reproduced and modified with permission from Schwartz E, Benze EJ: The thalassemia syndromes. Page 385 in: Hoffman B (editor): *Hematology: Basic Principles and Practice.* Churchill Livingstone, 1991.)

two α-globin gene deletions on the same chromosome. Because Hb electrophoresis is normal in α-thalassemia trait, the microcytic anemia associated with α-thalassemia trait can be confirmed only by gene mapping techniques. Because of the high frequency of α-thalassemia among Southeast Asians, prenatal programs have been encouraged to screen pregnant women for α-thalassemia trait. If the trait is detected, the male partner should be tested, and, if the test result is positive, the option for intrauterine diagnosis should be reviewed with the family. In contrast to Asians, African Americans who have α-thalassemia trait (6%) have the two gene deletions on separate chromosomes. This might explain why homozygous α-thalassemia does not occur in African Americans.

HbH disease. HbH disease is due to deletion of three α-globin genes. Family studies reveal that one parent has α-thalassemia trait, whereas the other has completely normal hematologic findings (silent carrier). Using molecular techniques, a variety of defects in the α-globin genes can be detected. The most common is a two-gene deletion in one parent and a one-gene deletion in the other. Occasionally, an Hb called *constant spring* can be detected in association with HbH disease, as this structural abnormality is associated with a decrease in α-globin synthesis similar to that seen in individuals who are silent carriers.

The pathophysiology of HbH disease is due to the accumulation of excess β chains within the red cell. These β⁴ tetramers are very unstable and readily oxidized. When this occurs, the red cell membrane is damaged, and the survival of the red cell is shortened. The clinical picture is quite similar to that of patients with mild to moderate HS. Significant variation exists among patients. Reports suggest that patients with HbH disease who have constant spring have more severe hemolysis than do those with HbH caused by the three α-globin gene deletion alone. The identification of constant spring requires molecular techniques in most patients, as the amount of the variant may be too small to detect by electrophoretic methods. In some cases, splenectomy is useful to diminish hemolysis.

Infants who have HbH disease are anemic at birth. The Hb electrophoresis shows Hb γ^4 (Hb Bart) and some HbH (β^4). Over the first few months after birth, Hb γ^4 disappears, and HbH (approximately 20%) and HbA are seen. Hb concentration ranges from 9 to 12 g/dL, and the red cell morphology is abnormal. Evident on the smear are hypochromia, microcytosis, target cells, and polychromasia. The reticulocyte count is slightly elevated except during a hemolytic crisis, during which it increases in response to the worsening anemia.

α-Thalassemia minor is characterized by deletions of two of the four α-globin genes and is fairly benign, with little or no anemia. Red cell morphology shows microcytosis, and, as with β-thalassemia trait, the RDW is normal. The reticulocyte count is normal to slightly increased. HbA_2 levels are low (1 to 2%). α-Thalassemia minor can be diagnosed in infancy (Hb γ^4, 3 to 10%). After the first few months of life, the diagnosis can be established by the use of gene mapping or α : β globin chain ratios. Fig. 13–7 illustrates the use of laboratory tests to distinguish the most common forms of microcytosis, including α- and β-thalassemia trait.

The silent carrier state (heterozygous α-thalassemia-2) is a variant that does not produce any clinical or hematologic abnormalities. Suspected carriers are the parents or siblings of children affected with HbH disease, and confirmation is made by gene mapping. In the newborn, Hb γ^4 levels may be as high as 3%. By 3 months of age, Hb γ^4 can no longer be detected.

β-*thalassemia*. The clinical manifestations of the β-thalassemia disorders vary, and classification into thalassemia major, intermedia, and minor has been made. Laboratory measurements, age of onset of anemia, course of the disease, and severity of the clinical manifestations make it possible to distinguish between these forms.

Many of the molecular defects are well characterized and include more than 100 recognized abnormalities of the globin genes or their regulatory sequences. There are two genes for β-globin production, and the location of the mutations within the β-globin gene or in regulatory sequences on chromosome 11 determines the clinical pictures. In the β^0-thalassemias, β-chain synthesis is lacking, often despite the presence of intact β genes. In the β^+-thalassemias, β-chain synthesis is present but reduced. In thalassemia trait, one β-globin gene has normal function and the other is affected.

The β-thalassemias, like the α-thalassemias, produce a wide range of clinical and hematologic findings. These disorders are characterized by decreased rates of β-chain synthesis and, consequently, reduced amounts of HbA in the red cells. Individuals with homozygous β-thalassemia

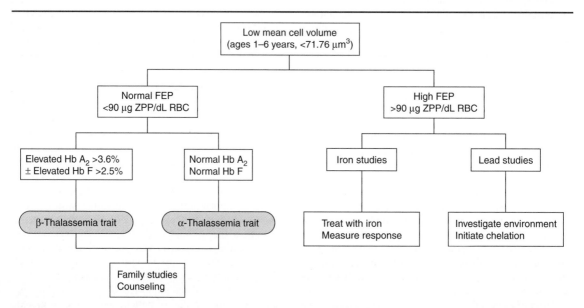

Figure 13–7. Algorithm diagramming the evaluation of microcytosis. FEP = free erythrocyte protophyrin; RBC = red blood cell; ZPP = zinc protoporphyrin.

require lifelong transfusion therapy and iron chelation to prevent iron overload. If iron accumulation from chronic transfusion exceeds iron loss because of chelation, parenchymal damage can be detected, most notably in cardiac, liver, and endocrine organs. Skeletal deformities occur as a consequence of massive ineffective erythroid hyperplasia in patients who do not receive adequate transfusions. Splenomegaly occurs because of extramedullary hematopoiesis and entrapment of abnormal cells not destroyed in the marrow.

β-Thalassemia major, or homozygous β-thalassemia, is not clinically expressed in the first few months after birth because of the protective effects of γ-globin synthesis, which is able to balance α-globin synthesis. Within 2 to 3 months, however, progressive pallor associated with anemia develops, and, in patients who have not received transfusion therapy, growth retardation may become a prominent feature. Hepatosplenomegaly occurs as a consequence of extramedullary hematopoiesis and transfusion-related organ damage. Infections are frequent owing to iron overload (*Yersinia enterocolitica*) and acquired splenic dysfunction.

The laboratory features of β-thalassemia major include severe, microcytic anemia with marked anisocytosis, poikilocytosis, and hypochromia and numerous target cells. There is a paucity of reticulocytes, although nucleated red cells are common. A slight leukocytosis and thrombocytosis can be seen, related to bone marrow stimulation. Serum iron and the free plasma Hb concentrations are elevated. Serum transferrin is often fully saturated. Ferritin levels are elevated as a consequence of transfusion therapy and must be monitored to adjust chelation therapy. Haptoglobin concentrations and red cell survival are decreased. The bone marrow aspirate shows a normoblastic, erythroid hyperplasia and increased iron stores, especially in patients who have received transfusion therapy. Ringed sideroblasts occasionally can be seen as a consequence of disordered globin synthesis. Iron kinetics reflect ineffective erythropoiesis with rapid uptake into the marrow and minimal return to the peripheral blood. HbF is the predominant Hb, and HbA_2 concentrations are elevated (typically 3.5–8.0%).

In the heterozygous form of β-thalassemia, or thalassemia minor, mild anemia with slight reticulocytosis is present. The peripheral blood smear shows microcytosis, hypochromia, poikilocytosis, basophilic stippling, and target cells. The degree of microcytosis is disproportionate to the degree of anemia. The marrow is normal or may show mild erythroid hyperplasia from a slight degree of ineffective erythropoiesis. The Hb electrophoresis shows elevations of HbA_2 (>3.6%) and HbF. Figure 13–7, which shows the diagnostic approach to microcytosis, demonstrates the laboratory procedures that can distinguish β-thalassemia trait from iron deficiency or α-thalassemia trait.

Thalassemia intermedia is characterized by an intermediate depression in β-globin chain synthesis when compared with thalassemia major and thalassemia trait; as a consequence, hematologic and clinical parameters are relatively mild compared with β-thalassemia major. Transfusion therapy usually is not required. The genetic defect does not result in elevated HbA_2 in heterozygotes. The degree of anemia and the hematologic characteristics are determined by the molecular defects causing the disorder. Treatment of thalassemia includes transfusions at 3- to 4-week intervals with leukocyte-depleted packed red cells and aggressive iron chelation. Comprehensive treatment guidelines are followed in established thalassemia treatment centers. Hydroxyurea and other agents to increase fetal hemoglobin are currently being evaluated. In addition, studies are being conducted with oral iron-depleting agents. These agents will be especially important in view of the difficulty related to compliance with subcutaneous deferoxamine chelation.

Hereditary persistence of fetal Hb. This disorder, found principally in the African American and Mediterranean populations, is characterized by persistence of HbF throughout adult life in the absence of any clinical stigmata. HPFH is classified by the type of HbF present (γA, fetal, or γG, adult) and frequently is a result of large deletions of the β-globin gene on chromosome 11. It does not result in unbalanced globin chain synthesis, a fact that sets it apart from α and β-thalassemia. The association of HPFH trait with other β-globin chain structural variants, such as HbS, results in a benign disorder, with no anemia or vascular obstruction. The benign nature of this disorder is most likely because HbF is homogeneously distributed in the red cells, inhibiting the polymerization and sickling of the cells. Proper identification of newborns with sickle cell trait–HPFH is important, as these infants do not have a disease. Family studies, longitudinal evaluation, and molecular biology studies can be used to confirm the diagnosis.

Extracorpuscular defects. Plasma and vascular factors can cause premature destruction of red cells. Immune hemolytic anemias result in early red cell destruction by the interaction of antibodies with the red cell. Mechanical trauma, such as that induced by prosthetic heart valves, and vasculitis secondary to inflammation can also cause premature red cell destruction. The clinical severity of these disorders is determined by the type and amount of antibody that binds to the red cell.

Isoimmune hemolytic anemia. Although transfusion reactions are rare because of ease of detection of the ABO blood group system, cross-matching, and scrutiny of the labels on the bags of blood before transfusion, isoimmune anemias can result from the sensitization to specific blood-group antigens after a blood transfusion. Depending on the extent of sensitization, the clinical features result from massive intravascular hemolysis and include chills, rigors, fever, jaundice, hypotension, and oliguria.

Immediate or delayed reactions can occur. Laboratory findings include an elevated plasma Hb concentration, hemoglobinuria, reduced serum haptoglobin, and hyperbilirubinemia. Renal function may be reduced owing to haptoglobinemia. The timing of these studies is important to detect this, and they may need to be done serially. Elevated plasma Hb and hemoglobinuria are seen shortly after a transfusion reaction (within 1 to 2 h) and, in severe cases, may not peak for 24 h. Blood urea nitrogen and creatinine concentrations can also be abnormal within 24 h but may take a week to become mildly elevated if hemolysis is mild and prolonged. A positive result with the direct antiglobulin (Coombs) test is common. In this test, the antibody is detected on the surface of the patients' red cells using heterologous antisera prepared against human immunoglobulin.

The usual form of transfusion-induced hemolytic reactions involves IgG antibodies produced during an anamnestic response. Antibodies frequently are directed against the Rhesus (Rh), Kell, Kidd, and Duffy antigens. The antibodies coat the red cells, which are then sequestered by splenic macrophages or lysed in the intravascular space because of complement activation. The clinical and laboratory features of hemolysis are similar to those seen with IgM antibodies although they are less severe in nature. Fever and chills are common and can be delayed for several hours after completion of the transfusion. Laboratory results reflecting Hb catabolism can also be delayed, and hemolysis may be milder than that described in intravascular hemolysis associated with ABO incompatibility. Transfusion reactions due to alloimmunization represent a particular problem in patients with sickle cell anemia, as the donor pool of African Americans is often limited for patients requiring red cell transfusion. By increasing the pool of African American blood donors, transfusing with phenotypically marked blood, and carefully monitoring patients who received chronic transfusion therapy for alloantibodies or autoantibodies, this problem can be minimized.

Reactions due to IgM red cell abnormalities are less frequent, although they are dramatic and can be life-threatening; they usually begin after receipt of only small amounts of transfused blood. These antibodies cause rapid activation of complement on the cell membrane. This type of transfusion reaction is mainly associated with incompatibilities of the ABO blood group, and the degree of red cell destruction is proportionate to the amount of antibodies in the recipient's plasma, the quantity of A or B antigen on the transfused cells, and the volume of incompatible blood transfused. Red cells containing complement-activated antibodies on their surface are destroyed intravascularly or by the liver macrophages.

Hemolytic anemia of newborns. Isoimmune hemolytic anemia in newborns results from contamination of the maternal circulation with fetal red cells, and subsequent maternal sensitization and transplacental passage of maternal anti-fetal red cell antibody. This is most often the result of ABO or Rh incompatibility between the mother and the fetus but can also occur with minor blood group incompatibility because of Kell, Kidd, Duffy, and other rarer blood groups.

In hemolytic disease of newborns (HDN), fetal red cells cross the placenta to the maternal circulation. If the mother lacks the antigen, IgG antibodies are produced and passively transfer back across the placenta to the fetal circulation. The fetal red cells become coated and hemolyze. In theory, any blood group that can produce IgG molecules and possesses sufficient antibody avidity potentially can cause the anemia.

ABO incompatibility. In the case of anti-A and anti-B HDN, a mother with type O blood is specifically at risk for HDN. In most institutions, determining blood type and performing a Coombs test on umbilical cord blood are standard practice. Clinically, most cases go undetected. Frequently, the indirect Coombs test (which measures antibodies in plasma by incubating patients' plasma with a panel of red cells and subsequently with rabbit antihuman γ globulin) yields a positive result, and the direct Coombs test result is negative or weakly positive. The findings within 24 h after birth are hyperbilirubinemia and hemolysis. The peripheral smear shows moderate anisocytosis, microspherocytes, and a mild reticulocytosis. Except for the positive findings on the direct antibody test, these infants cannot be distinguished from children with hereditary spherocytosis. Disease caused by ABO antibodies differs from that caused by Rh incompatibility in that infants from the first pregnancy can be affected in ABO incompatibility.

Rh disease. The antibody that binds to newborns' red cells in this type of hemolytic anemia is produced by the mother's immune response to fetal red cells. It causes a more severe clinical hemolytic anemia than that seen in ABO disease. Rh disease does not usually affect first-born children unless the mother has been sensitized previously from transfusion or abortion and already possesses alloantibodies. Screening for these antibodies is performed on all Rh-negative pregnant women during their first trimester to identify pregnancies that require careful monitoring. Methods have been reported to identify the Rh type of the fetus using molecular analysis of fetal amniocytes.

Hemolytic disease due to maternal–fetal Rh incompatibility is most commonly associated with anti-D, alone or in combination with anti-C or anti-E. Laboratory diagnosis depends on a strong positive result on Coombs testing of infants' cord blood cells. The C, D, E phenotype can influence the variability of expression of the disease by affecting the potency of the D antigen. Therefore, knowledge of the maternal genotype may be predictive of disease severity. Serial titers of maternal antibody can be predictive of severe HDN. Rh sensitization and subsequent hemolytic disease of newborns can be prevented or decreased in severity by careful monitoring of the Rh-negative mother. Rh immune globulin, when given in the second trimester, inhibits production of maternal Rh antibody. Detailed protocols for fetal monitoring during pregnancies affected by Rh sensitization are available and should be followed. Treatment of affected newborns may require intrauterine transfusion or exchange transfusion at birth. Immune hemolysis can continue for several months after birth, requiring careful monitoring and occasional red cell transfusion.

Autoimmune hemolytic anemia. The term *autoimmune hemolytic anemia (AIHA)* is used to refer to a variety of warm antibody-mediated hemolytic anemias associated with various disorders, including postviral infection, systemic lupus erythematosus, lymphomas, and autoimmune disease. Autoimmune hemolytic anemia is associated with a wide variety of antibodies, the most common belonging to the Rh blood group. Red cell destruction is primarily due to macrophages in the spleen, which recognize the antibody and remove it, along with parts of the cell membrane, resulting in spherocytes. Extent of hemolysis is determined by the amount of IgG bound to the cell. When large amounts are found, complement (C3b) is also bound to the membrane, and red cells are thus sequestered in both the spleen and the liver.

Autoimmune hemolytic anemia can occur abruptly, usually after an acute viral infection. It often represents a pediatric emergency, as the decrease in Hb may be rapid and severe and immunocompatible blood is frequently impossible to obtain. When a milder, chronic picture is observed, it is important to rule out a defect in immune surveillance, which may be a consequence of primary immunodeficiency diseases, a malignancy, or a collagen vascular disease.

The clinical features of AIHA include pallor, jaundice, and splenomegaly. The peripheral blood picture often shows a normal MCH and a variable MCV (depending on the reticulocyte count). Anisocytosis, polychromasia, and reticulocytosis are common, and spherocytes, schistocytes, and nucleated red cells can be present. In the acute form, children younger than 2–4 years are affected. Onset of hemolysis usually occurs after a viral infection. Children may have severe anemia, jaundice, hemoglobinemia, and cardiorespiratory distress. The Hb concentration may be extremely low (<2 g/dL). When red cells are needed to correct the severe anemia, blood is found to be incompatible, as evidenced by the strong positive Coombs test result. High and prolonged doses of corticosteroids are often required to treat this disease.

Products of Hb catabolism are present and include an elevated bilirubin, increased urinary urobilinogen, and increased serum lactic dehydrogenase. The direct Coombs test result is positive, and, in most cases, red cell coating with IgG molecules or complement binding can be demonstrated by using specific antisera. The component of complement most frequently involved is C3b.

Some antibodies react most efficiently with red cells at temperatures less than 37°C (98.6°F) and may optimally agglutinate at temperatures ranging from 4°C (39.2°F) to 25°C (77°F). These antibodies are often IgM; they cause aggregation of red cells when blood is placed in the cold and, therefore, are called *cold agglutinins.* The antibodies are usually formed after viral infection (e.g., *Mycoplasma pneumoniae*) or infection with the Epstein-Barr virus; formation has been reported in cases of lymphomas and systemic lupus erythematosus. An association between the virus and the red cell agglutinin has been implicated in responsibility for the creation of a new antigenic site.

Clinical hemolysis can occur in patients with cold antibodies when the thermal range of the antibody is broad, and antibody binding can be demonstrated at temperatures up to 30°C (86°F). The serologic findings show extremely high titers of a cold agglutinin often having anti-I (a red-cell-associated antigen) specificity. The result of the direct Coombs test is positive, especially when an antiserum containing anticomplement components is used.

Another form of autoimmune hemolytic anemia in childhood is called *paroxysmal cold hemoglobinuria.* The IgG antibody responsible for this disease is the Donath-Landsteiner antibody. When this antibody is exposed to the cold, antigen-antibody complexes are formed; as the cells return to a normal temperature, these complexes bind complement, resulting in hemolysis. This uncommon disorder has been associated with syphilis and viral and bacterial infections. The specificity of this antibody is against the P antigen. The laboratory features include a smear showing spherocytes, elevated reticulocyte count, and erythrophagocytosis. Hemoglobinuria is common. The direct result of the Coombs test is positive under cold conditions, 4°C (39.2°F) to 12°C (53.6°F), and negative in warm conditions if antisera against IgG are used. However, complement can be detected on the red cell surface. This type of antibody is not uncommon in children.

Drug-related mechanisms must be considered in the differential diagnosis of immune hemolytic anemia. Certain drugs can induce an immune hemolytic anemia by causing the formation of antibodies, either against the drug itself, which subsequently cross-reacts with the red cells, or against drug–red cell membrane complexes by possibly altering membrane antigenic structures (penicillin, cephalosporins, and methadone). Other drugs (antihistamines, insulin, rifampin, quinidine, quinine, chlorinated hydrocarbons, insecticides, sulfonamides) cause immunocomplex adsorption to red cells and activate complement. The result of the Coombs test may be positive for antibody or complement in these situations. If patients found to have an immune hemolytic anemia are taking medication that could cause an immune response, the medication should be discontinued. When a causal relation exists, hemolysis will subside.

Mechanical hemolysis and microangiopathic hemolytic anemia. A hemolytic anemia can occur when red cells are fragmented by mechanical trauma, vascular inflammation, or thermal injury. A hemolytic anemia may develop in patients who have required heart-valve prostheses as a result of mechanical blood flow problems that cause red cell damage, a condition called the *Waring blender syndrome.* In certain inflammatory states associated with infection or collagen vascular disease, fibrin deposition can occur across the microvascular bed; as a consequence, red cells are sheared as they pass through the fibrin meshwork. Notable findings on the peripheral smear include fragmented and distorted red cells (schistocytes), microspherocytes, and moderate thrombocytopenia due to platelet trapping in the fibrin strands. This type of hemolysis has been called *microangiopathic hemolytic anemia.* It can be found in the hemolytic uremic syndrome, thrombotic thrombocytopenic purpura, disseminated intravascular coagulation (DIC), systemic lupus erythematosus, acute glomerulonephritis, giant hemangiomas, and malignancies.

Acute hemolysis can also occur after thermal injury. The degree of hemolysis is often related to the severity of the burns and is believed to be caused by the irreversible denaturation of the red cell-membrane protein spectrin. Schistocytes and spherocytes are seen in the peripheral blood in these conditions, and spontaneous resolutions occur.

INADEQUATE RED CELL PRODUCTION

Processes that cause anemias as a result of inadequate cell production include nutritional deficiencies, dyserythropoiesis, chronic inflammatory diseases, and bone marrow atrophy or infiltration.

Nutritional deficiencies

Iron deficiency anemia. Iron deficiency is the most common form of anemia and exceeds all other causes in childhood by a factor of at least three. As the amount of iron in newborns is approximately 75 mg/kg, a 3-kg infant will have approximately 225 mg total body iron at birth. If there is no iron in the diet, or if iron loss is greater than iron intake, by 6 months in full-term infants and as early as 3 to 4 months in premature infants, the iron stores present at birth will be depleted. The most common cause of iron deficiency is inadequate intake of iron during the rapidly growing childhood years. Excessive consumption of cow's milk associated with gastroenteritis and chronic blood loss and blood loss due to underlying diseases through the gastrointestinal tract, lungs, or kidney should be considered.

Iron reserves begin to decrease during the early stages of iron deficiency, resulting in a low serum ferritin concentration. Values less than 12 mg/mL have been considered diagnostic of iron deficiency. Normal ferritin levels can exist in iron-deficient states, however, when coexisting with a bacterial or parasitic infection, malignancy, or chronic inflammatory condition, as ferritin is an acute-phase reactant. As serum iron concentrations decrease, transferrin [total iron binding capacity (TIBC)] synthesis is stimulated, and the iron-transferrin ratio, called the *transferrin saturation,* decreases. A transferrin saturation less than 10% is consistent with iron deficiency.

The FEP concentration increases when the iron supply is low enough to impede Hb synthesis. The FEP is a simple, sensitive test for iron deficiency and can provide a guide to the adequacy of iron replacement therapy. Although the FEP was originally designed to detect lead poisoning, FEP levels in lead poisoning are usually very high. A careful environmental history should be taken to exclude lead poisoning as it can coexist with iron deficiency. Blood lead determination should be performed if there is any concern regarding lead poisoning.

With pronounced iron deficiency, the peripheral blood smear is remarkable for a microcytic, hypochromic anemia with severe anisocytosis and poikilocytosis. Basophilic stippling can occur, making such cases quite similar to thalassemia trait. Iron deficiency occurs over time; therefore, the red cell size is varied and the RDW is very high (>14). This is in contrast to the thalassemia traits, in which the RDW is normal.

Physical findings associated with iron deficiency include pallor, lethargy, tachycardia, and tachypnea. Because iron deficiency develops over time, cardiorespiratory compensation is often quite remarkable, and some patients can tolerate Hb concentrations as low as 4 g/dL. In some cases of iron deficiency, growth retardation and neurodevelopmental delay can occur. In addition, protein-losing enteropathy can result as a consequence of iron depletion in the cells lining the gastrointestinal tract. Iron stores will be depleted before development of anemia, placing infants at risk for the nonhematologic effects of iron deficiency.

Treatment of iron deficiency requires identification and correction of nutritional inadequacies, search for blood loss, and therapy with iron (2 mg elemental iron per kilogram twice daily). Iron therapy should be continued for several months after the red cell indices return to normal. Failure to respond to iron often reflects poor compliance. However, it may mean that the response is blunted by infection or that the diagnosis is incorrect. An adequate response to iron therapy is reflected by an increase of Hb concentration greater than 1 g/dL in 10 days. If measured, a reticulocytosis is usually evident within 3 to 5 days after starting oral iron supplementation. The FEP returns to normal when iron deficiency is corrected.

Megaloblastic anemia. Vitamin B_{12} and folic acid deficiency are the most common causes of megaloblastic anemia. Rarely, megaloblastic anemia is due to inborn defects of pyridine (hereditary orotic aciduria) or purine metabolism (Lesch-Nyhan syndrome). Chemotherapeutic drugs such as methotrexate, cytosine arabinoside, and 5-fluorouracil commonly result in megaloblastic anemia.

The common biochemical abnormality in both folate and B_{12} deficiency is a defect in DNA synthesis, with lesser alterations in RNA and protein synthesis, leading to a state of unbalanced cell growth and impaired cell division. These cells, called *megaloblastic,* have greater quantities of DNA than do normal cells and are morphologically larger than normal. Nuclear maturation is dissociated from cytoplasmic maturation.

Megaloblastic anemia reflects only one component of the global cellular defect in DNA synthesis. Careful identification of the cause of megaloblastosis is required before initiation of therapy; these anemias can be confused with aplastic anemia or leukemia because they may lead to pancytopenia. Vitamin B_{12} deficiency causes severe neurologic disturbances in addition to its hematologic effects. Misdiagnosis and treatment of vitamin B_{12} deficiency as folate deficiency will result in hematologic improvement but will not correct the neurologic abnormality and can lead to permanent neurologic impairment.

Folic acid deficiency. Folic acid (pteroylmonoglutamate) is the commercially available parent compound for more than 100 compounds collectively referred to as *folates.* These are synthesized by microorganisms and by plants and are very thermolabile; thus, they are generally destroyed when food is boiled. A balanced Western diet can sustain folate balance because the daily requirement in children is approximately 0.3 mg/d. In the absence of dietary intake, folate stores can be depleted in weeks.

Food folates are hydrolyzed to an absorbable form by enzymes in the brush-border membranes of the small intestine; brush-border membrane folate-binding proteins facilitate active transport of folate into epithelial cells. Passive transport across the intestinal epithelium occurs with pharmacologic ingestion of folates. Ingested milk, which contains folate-binding proteins, can inhibit this process and decrease folate transport. Folate balance is maintained by both intestinal absorption and by an active enterohepatic circulation. Folate coenzymes are essential for the thymidylate cycle and for the methylation cycle, and defects in either of these cycles affect formation of methionine and inhibit DNA synthesis.

Folate receptors are present on all cells and are required for folate incorporation. These receptors can be upregulated or downregulated in various disease states. Congenital abnormalities in folate structure and function also exist. In newborns, the concentrations of folate are maintained despite deficiencies in maternal folate. Once inside the red cell, folate is polyglutamated; this form associates with Hb. The level of intracellular folate is a more accurate predictor of folate status than is serum folate concentration, and normal red cell folate levels can occur in conditions in which plasma levels are low.

Deficiencies of folate can occur in the following conditions: dietary intake is inadequate, demand is increased relative to intake (e.g., during periods of active growth or in hemolytic anemias, there are increased requirements for hematopoiesis), drugs impair folate metabolism and inhibit absorption or use, gastrointestinal absorption of the vitamin is limited, and genetic abnormalities exist in the structure or activity of folate receptors or binding proteins.

Infant formulas and breast milk provide adequate folate for term and probably for low-birth-weight infants. Goat's milk is an extremely poor source of folate. In low-birth-weight infants who are given proprietary multivitamin supplements, folate must be administered separately because it is relatively unstable on storage. Infants require at least 10 times more folate for body weight than do adults. The recommended daily intake for infants is 20 to 50 µg/kg/d. Intestinal bacteria may augment folate supply, but prolonged use of antibiotics inhibits this source.

Folate deficiency occurs in chronic diarrheal states because of a secondary deficiency in intestinal conjugase, the enzyme required to convert dietary folate into an intestinally absorbable form, or interference with the enterohepatic circulation of folate. An extremely rare cause of congenital malabsorption of folate, manifested by 2 to 3 months of age, is the absence of cellular folate receptors. Folate analogues, such as methotrexate, and certain antibiotics, such as trimethoprim (Septra and Bactrim), can cause folate deficiency by reacting with dihydrofolate reductase and interfering with the conversion of normal dihydrofolate substrates to the active tetrahydro forms. Oral contraceptives, phenytoin, and other anticonvulsants can interact with polyglutamates in the intestinal lumen and interfere with their digestion to the absorbable monoglutamate form. Understanding these mechanisms is important so that an appropriate form of folic acid is used to treat folate deficiency.

Folate deficiency should be considered in the evaluation of macrocytic anemia (see Fig. 13–8). The reticulocyte count is normal or low, and neutropenia and thrombocytopenia may be found. The RDW is elevated, and red cell morphology is macrocytic and ovalocytic. The number of lobes within the granulocytes, called the *Arneth count,* is increased above the average of 3.4 nuclear lobes per cell if 100 cells are counted. Megaloblastic changes can be seen in all cell lines within the bone marrow, most notably in erythroid progenitors, in which nuclear maturation is markedly delayed compared with cytoplasmic maturation. A definitive diagnosis can be made by measuring the red cell folate content. Values less than 140 ng/mL are diagnostic. Although a serum folate content less than 3 ng/mL is also consistent with the diagnosis, serum levels are too sensitive to dietary fluctuations to be useful in many cases. If it is clear that megaloblastic

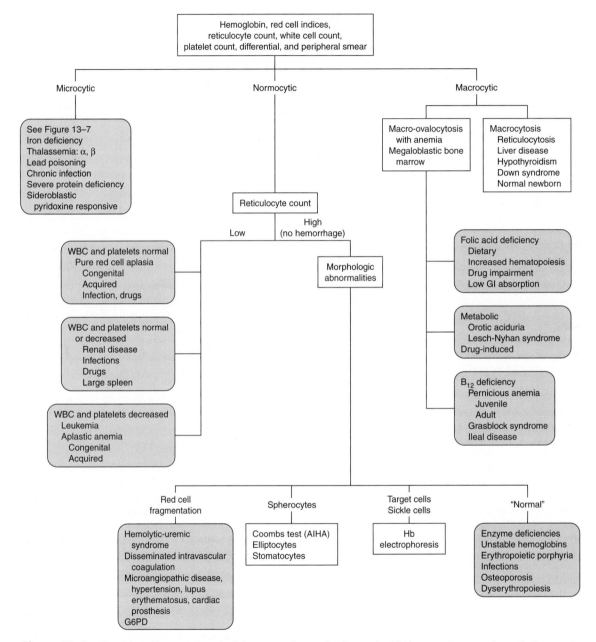

Figure 13–8. Algorithm diagramming the laboratory diagnosis of anemia. AIHA = autoimmune hemolytic anemia; GI = gastrointestinal; G6PD = glucose-6-phosphate dehydrogenase; Hb = hemoglobin; WBC = white blood cell count.

anemia is secondary to folate deficiency and not vitamin B_{12} deficiency, folate can be given (0.5 to 1.0 mg/d). A response can be seen within several days. In cases in which it is not clear whether vitamin B_{12} deficiency has been excluded, the dose of folate should be reduced to 0.05 to 0.10 mg/d parenterally or 0.1 mg/d orally; this is adequate to produce a prompt reticulocyte response. A larger dose will cause a hematologic response in patients with B_{12} deficiency, although it will not affect the neurologic consequences of B_{12} deficiency.

Vitamin B_{12} deficiency. Vitamin B_{12} deficiency is uncommon in children; however, identifying and treating it is important because it can produce irreversible neurologic complications in addition to its hematologic effects. Humans receive their vitamin B_{12} exclusively from the diet, primarily from animal protein. Unlike folate, vitamin B_{12} is stable at high temperatures. The liver is the primary organ for B_{12} storage, and stores in children are capable of sustaining B_{12} needs for months. An efficient enterohepatic circulation preserves endogenous vitamin B_{12} and helps to prevent deficiencies when dietary inadequacy exists.

Once released by proteolysis from dietary protein, B_{12} is bound to a protein called *R protein* [so-called because it migrates more rapidly in an electrophoretic field than does the intrinsic factor (IF)] in the stomach. Pancreatic proteases digest R protein; as a consequence, B_{12} is released and rapidly combines with IF, which is resistant to digestion by pancreatic enzymes. The intrinsic factor is secreted in response to food in the stomach in a manner analogous to secretion of acid. In patients with pancreatic insufficiency, this process does not occur, and the B_{12} bound to protein is not absorbed. Specific receptors for IF exist in the ileum and account for the absorption of B_{12} by endocytosis. Within the enterocyte B_{12} is released from IF and is rapidly bound by transcobalamin II, which then transports B_{12} throughout the body. Vitamin B_{12} is incorporated into cells by a process of endocytosis.

The function of vitamin B_{12} within cells is to coordinate, with folate, the transfer of methyl groups required for DNA, RNA, and protein synthesis. Intracellular vitamin B_{12} is bound to methylmalonyl-CoA mutase and methionine synthetase and is required for their functions. This explains why patients with B_{12} deficiency have methylmalonic aciduria and why measurement of the concentration of this organic acid in the urine can be useful for the diagnosis of this vitamin deficiency. The polyglutamal form of tetrahydrofolate plays a central role in one-carbon metabolism required for these synthetic steps, and production of this important intermediate depends on both folate and vitamin B_{12}. Deficiencies of either vitamin result in similar defects in cell maturation and megaloblastic anemia; however, only vitamin B_{12} deficiency causes posterior lateral column disease and progressive neurologic impairment.

Vitamin B_{12} deficiency may be caused by nutritional inadequacy or by abnormal intragastric events. These include poor dissociation of food, deficient or defective IF, disordered mucus, or IF receptors, transenterocytic transport, and abnormal events in the small bowel (e.g., inadequate pancreatic protease or usurping of luminal B_{12} by bacteria or intestinal worms).

If children are fed a diet that completely lacks B_{12}, neonatal stores will be depleted by 6 months of age. Dietary inadequacy can be related to maternal deficiency, as seen in a breast-feeding mother who is a strict vegan and does not take B_{12} containing supplements and whose child has megaloblastic anemia and neuropathy by 4 months of age.

The term *pernicious anemia* is applied to the anemia that results from a deficiency of IF. Juvenile pernicious anemia occurs in older children and is similar to pernicious anemia of adults. Gastric atrophy and decreased secretion of acid and pepsin are commonly associated with antibodies to intrinsic factor or to parietal cells. Selective immunodeficiencies appear to contribute to the endocrinopathies associated with pernicious anemia and may be responsible for the entire clinical picture. Congenital pernicious anemia is usually manifest by 3 years of age. Although secretion of normally active IF is absent, other gastric functions and gastric morphology are normal. Furthermore, this disease has no immunologic component.

Because vitamin B_{12} is selectively absorbed by the distal half of the ileum, surgical removal of this portion of the small bowel for treatment of necrotizing enterocolitis, intussusception, regional enteritis, or congenital malformation results in a severe lifelong deficiency. Chronic regional enteritis can also cause B_{12} deficiency. Other rare causes of B_{12} deficiency are congenital absence or abnormal function of transcobalamin II and hereditary defects in enterocyte uptake of the B_{12}-IF complex.

The diagnosis of vitamin B_{12} deficiency is based on a high index of suspicion after a careful history and physical examination. Neurologic signs due to posterior and lateral column demyelinization in the spinal cord include parathesias, sensory deficits, loss of deep tendon reflexes, slowing of mental processes, confusion, and memory defects. Neurologic defects may precede anemia. Inappropriate administration of folate can result in a hematologic response in B_{12} deficiency but will have no effect on, or may aggravate, the neurologic effects.

Laboratory studies show macrocytic anemia and often pancytopenia. As with folate deficiency, the neutrophil lobe count is elevated. The serum B_{12} concentration is depressed to less than 100 pg/mL. The serum folate level is usually normal, but the red cell folate concentration may be decreased. Consequently, all three measurements—serum B_{12}, serum folate, and red cell folate—should be performed. When pernicious anemia is considered, a Schilling test should be performed, in which radiolabeled

B_{12} is given with or without IF. Intrinsic factor can also be measured in gastric juice. Absence of gastric acid after histamine stimulation, and gastric mucosal morphology can distinguish forms of pernicious anemia.

The long-term treatment of vitamin B_{12} deficiency depends on its cause. In all cases, 25 to 100 μg/day vitamin B_{12} for several days may be used to initiate therapy followed by monthly injections of 50 to 100 μg. Hematologic improvement is prompt, and the extent of neurologic improvement depends on the extent of damage before onset of therapy.

Congenital dyserythropoietic anemias. The congenital dyserythropoietic anemias are a rare group of hematologic disorders inherited in either an autosomal recessive or an autosomal dominant mode. They are characterized by anemia (usually hemolytic) and abnormal morphology in peripheral red cells and bone marrow erythroid progenitors. They affect all ethnic groups. Among the three major subtypes, there is marked clinical variability, ranging from mild to severe, life-threatening anemia. The central characteristic of the dyserythropoietic anemias is the failure to produce mature red cells in an orderly manner. Anemia with an inadequate reticulocyte response is often seen. Red cell destruction often occurs in the marrow. Type II, the most common form, is known by the acronym HEMPAS (*h*ereditary *e*rythroblastic *m*ultinuclearity with a *p*ositive *a*cidified *s*erum test), because multinucleated red cell precursors are seen in the marrow. The peripheral smear shows tear-drop cells and may demonstrate nucleated red cells. After incubation in an acid media, red cells are destroyed owing to their inability to prevent complement-mediated lysis. This laboratory picture is similar to that in patients with paroxysmal nocturnal hemoglobinemia.

Anemia secondary to inflammation. The anemia of chronic inflammation is due to impaired iron use, impaired production of erythropoietin, and hemolysis. Serum erythropoietin concentrations are often low, and serum iron is elevated because of a block in iron metabolism. Bone marrow iron stores are increased. The anemia is usually normochromic and normocytic with mild anisocytosis. The bone marrow shows mild normoblastic erythroid hyperplasia and elevated iron stores. In some cases, the diagnosis of anemia in chronic inflammatory conditions may be complex, as both iron deficiency and chronic inflammation may occur. For example, in cystic fibrosis, a combination of blood loss resulting in iron deficiency and chronic inflammation may be present.

Anemia that occurs during chronic inflammatory states develops within a few months of the primary disease. Red cell morphology is normochromic and normocytic, although hypochromia can develop over time. Anisocytosis is present, and FEP may be elevated. In contrast, the Hb concentration may be reduced by 1.0 to 1.5 g/dL during acute inflammation. This anemia is normochromic and normocytic, and its cause is unknown. During acute inflammatory conditions, it is prudent to delay investigation of anemia, as the Hb concentration will increase to normal levels when the infection subsides. The anemia due to chronic inflammation will respond to treatment with erythropoietin. It will also resolve as the inflammatory condition resolves.

Anemia associated with defective bone marrow response

Pancytopenia. The term *pancytopenia* refers to a reduction of erythrocytes, leukocytes, and thrombocytes. Pancytopenia may be due to bone marrow failure associated with the loss of stem cells; to inflammatory states that decrease stem cell production; to conditions that "crowd out" stem cells, such as malignancy, leukemia, or storage diseases; or to hypersplenism, which increases the number of peripheral blood cells residing in the spleen.

Acquired aplastic anemia refers to a situation of inadequate or complete cessation of hematopoietic activity within the marrow. It is often associated with bone marrow fibrosis. The cause is uncertain, but theories include acquired deficiencies of stem cells, deficiencies of environmental factors required for stem cell survival and function in the marrow, and immune-related disorders. Chemical and physical agents that have been associated with temporary or prolonged marrow suppression include cytotoxic drugs used for chemotherapy, benzene, sulfonamides, and chloramphenicol. Ionizing radiation also can cause injury to the bone marrow. Infections (e.g., viral hepatitis and tuberculosis) can lead to marrow hypoplasia and aplastic anemia, and these must be excluded in a differential diagnosis. Most often, the cause of acquired aplastic anemia is idiopathic.

Quantitative abnormalities of all cell lines exist, as do qualitative abnormalities of maturation. The red cells exhibit anisocytosis, poikilocytosis, and macrocytosis, with an associated reticulocytopenia. The platelets appear small on a peripheral smear, if they are present at all. There is a concomitant increase in the bleeding time, and clot retraction is poor. Leukopenia is present; however, leukocyte morphologic abnormalities are not. Erythropoietin levels are markedly elevated, and the percentage of HbF may be increased. Serum iron concentrations are often high, as are the TIBC and transferrin saturation. The diagnosis is established on the appearance of the bone marrow aspiration and biopsy specimens.

Treatment depends on the cause. In idiopathic cases, bone marrow transplantation is performed when compatible donors are available. Immunosuppressive agents are used if transplantation is not possible. Supportive care includes appropriate transfusions and aggressive treatment of infectious illness. Prognosis is poor if bone-marrow transplantation is not available.

Congenital aplastic anemia (Fanconi anemia) is a rare, autosomal recessive hereditary disorder characterized by chromosome fragility and bone marrow hypoplasia. It is associated with a variety of congenital anomalies, including short stature, bony abnormalities associated with displacement of the thumb, abnormal skin pigmentation, and congenital abnormalities, such as single or horseshoe kidney. Affected individuals also have an increased predisposition to the development of leukemia. The bone marrow may be normocellular early in the disease, with a mild plasmacytosis, but ultimately becomes hypocellular. A normochromic and normocytic anemia is present at the outset, but macrocytosis can develop. There is an absolute reticulocytopenia. HbF concentrations usually are elevated, and nucleated red cells and immature leukocytes can be seen in the peripheral blood. The diagnosis of congenital aplastic anemia is usually not apparent until the end of the first decade, when thrombocytopenia is evident. If physical or radiographic findings are suggestive, however, specific cytogenetic abnormalities, such as chromosome breaks and abnormal cytogenetic changes after exposure to specific chemical agents, can be determined.

It is important to distinguish Fanconi anemia from idiopathic aplastic anemia, as Fanconi anemia has a better response to therapy with androgens and prednisone. In addition, the increased susceptibility to malignant transformation and associated clonal chromosomal abnormalities in Fanconi anemia must be recognized. Several reports of transplantation using cord blood, which is enriched in hematopoietic stem cells, obtained from siblings of patients with Fanconi anemia are encouraging. In all cases in which marrow transplantation might be indicated, this source of donor tissue should be considered.

Pure red cell aplasia. Red cell aplasia is characterized by a selective decrease in red cell precursors in the presence of normal production of leukocytes and platelets. The two major groups of red cell aplasia in children are Diamond-Blackfan anemia and transient erythroblastopenia of childhood (TEC).

Diamond-Blackfan anemia. This congenital form of red cell aplasia is characterized by a slowly progressive anemia usually beginning in infancy, like Fanconi anemia. Physical anomalies involving the skeletal and urogenital systems can be present in up to 25% of affected individuals. Children with this condition are often identified by 3 to 6 months of age, when anemia is detected and the reticulocyte count is very low. The presence of the low reticulocyte count is an important clue for suspecting the diagnosis. The anemia is eventually severe and is normochromic and normocytic. Macrocytosis may be seen, consistent with dyserythropoiesis. Other findings consistent with disordered erythropoiesis are elevated HbF levels, elevated fetal "i" antigen, and a fetal pattern of red cell glycolytic and hexose-monophosphate shunt enzymes. Bone marrow examination reveals diminished or absent erythroid precursors and normal myeloid or erythroid precursors. The course is severe and prolonged, and patients are usually dependent on red cell transfusion, iron chela-

tion, and steroids. Acute myelocytic leukemia has been reported in some patients. As immunologic mechanisms may be responsible for Diamond-Blackfan anemia, cyclosporin has been used with some success in patients not responsive to prednisone. Bone marrow transplantation is also an option if a suitable donor is available.

Transient erythroblastopenia of childhood. Transient erythroblastopenia of childhood, a relatively common, acquired form of pure red cell aplasia, usually presents in the 6-month to 4-year age group and is often preceded by a viral infection. Parvovirus B19 has been implicated in both normal children and in those affected by a hereditary hemolytic anemia. Patients with sickle cell anemia and HS may have aplastic episodes secondary to parvovirus infection. No physical stigmata are present, and spontaneous recovery occurs usually within weeks. Anemia is normochromic and normocytic. Neither macrocytosis nor elevated concentrations of HbF are noted, and fetal red cell antigens and enzymes are absent. Bone marrow aspirates show depressed or absent erythropoiesis but are otherwise normal. In patients with parvoviral infection, platelet counts may be elevated. Except for red cell transfusion, no therapy is required, and patients usually have complete remission within 4 to 6 weeks.

Morphologic Classification of Anemia

An approach to the diagnosis of anemia on the basis of red cell volume and Hb concentration is shown in Fig. 13–8. As all patients have red cell indices performed during the evaluation for anemia, use of this information may facilitate the diagnostic evaluation.

MICROCYTIC ANEMIA

Microcytic hypochromic anemias encompass a subgroup of disorders involved with decreased Hb production, including iron deficiency, thalassemia, lead poisoning, sideroblastic anemia, and chronic blood loss. These anemias are characterized by an MCV less than 80 fL and MCHC less than 31%. The association of low cell volume with decreased Hb concentration suggests a relation between these two parameters.

The first step in the evaluation of a microcytic, hypochromic anemia is to take a careful history. A history of adequate dietary iron intake and a family history of refractory iron deficiency suggest thalassemia trait. Red cell indices and RDW will help to determine the subsequent workup. If the MCV is proportionately depressed for the degree of anemia and the RDW is elevated, iron deficiency should be considered. If the MCV is disproportionately depressed for the degree of anemia (i.e., Hb concentration, 8.5; MCV, 60) and the RDW is normal, consider α- or β-thalassemia trait. An elevated FEP level suggests iron deficiency or lead poisoning and is not consistent with α- or β-thalassemia trait. Blood lead levels will exclude lead poisoning. Elevated FEP levels can also

Table 13–10. Laboratory Assessment of Common Forms of Microcytic Anemia in Children[1]

	Iron Deficiency	α-Thalassemia Trait	β-Thalassemia Trait	Hemoglobin E Trait
Hemoglobin	Low/very low	Low	Low	Low
Mean cell volume	Low/very low	Very low	Very low	Very low
Red blood count	Low	High	High	Low
Relative distribution width	High	Normal	Normal	Normal
Free erythrocyte protoporphyrin	High	Normal	Normal	Normal
Hemoglobin electrophoresis	Normal	Normal	More A$_2$	Normal
Cord blood	Normal	Bart	Normal	F, A, E
Iron studies: ferritin	Low	Normal	Normal	Normal

[1] Relative scale: very low→low→normal→high.

be seen in children with heterozygote or mild forms of erythropoietic porphyria (Table 13–10).

NORMOCHROMIC NORMOCYTIC ANEMIA

Anemia associated with normal red cell indices can occur in diseases in which red cell production is decreased, or by increased red cell loss through hemorrhage or hemolysis. Included in this category are a wide range of primary or secondary bone marrow disorders, including hypoplastic anemias due to the bone marrow suppression from drugs, alcohol intoxication, infection, and bone marrow replacement (fibrosis, storage diseases, and malignancies). Anemias associated with a normal bone marrow response include acute blood loss, acute hemolysis, and hemoglobinopathies. Depression of erythropoietin production is usually secondary to renal disease or liver disease (impaired source of production), anemia of endocrine disorders (reduced stimulus), or anemia of chronic disease.

The reticulocyte count is the first decisive point in the investigation of normochromic, normocytic anemias. A corrected reticulocyte count should be calculated, as it is a prime indicator of bone marrow activity and, more specifically, of red cell production. Normal or reduced reticulocyte counts are present in situations with bone marrow suppression or replacement; consequently a bone marrow aspirate may help clarify the situation. Decreased reticulocyte counts with a normal marrow examination indicate a lack of marrow response in the presence of anemia.

MACROCYTIC ANEMIA

This subgroup includes the megaloblastic anemias that result from an asynchronous nuclear cytoplasmic maturation, such as vitamin B$_{12}$ deficiency, folate deficiency, pernicious anemia, drug-induced states, and the congenital dyserythropoietic anemias. Macrocytic red cells develop in sickle cell patients treated with hydroxyurea. Bleeding disorders associated with reticulocytosis and liver disease may also show macrocytic characteristics. Newborns or individuals with elevated HbF values have

macrocytic cells. Red cell macrocytosis is a common finding in individuals with Down syndrome, but it is usually not associated with anemia.

WHITE CELLS

Leukocytes include granulocytes, macrophages, and lymphocytes. Lymphocyte biology, function, and pathology are reviewed in Chapter 7. Leukocytes originate from premature stem cells in the bone marrow, and their production and function are regulated by growth factors and cytokines. Leukocytes can be classified as *granulocytes*, the primary function of which is to ingest and kill bacteria, or as *mononuclear phagocytes*, which function as an important component in the reticuloendothelial system to remove abnormal cells or particles and participate in the immune response. Two pools of granulocytes exist in the circulation: One (which adheres to blood vessel walls) is called the *marginating pool*, and the other is the *circulating pool*. Fifty percent of white cells are usually found in each pool.

The phagocytes originate in the bone marrow from stem cells, circulate briefly in the blood stream, and exit to peripheral tissues. The neutrophils mature from myeloblast to mature polymorphonuclear neutrophils in 7 days and have an average half-life of 6 to 7 days in the peripheral circulation. Mononuclear phagocytes mature in 13 h and have a circulating half-life of 8 h. Survival in the tissues as macrophages may be as long as several months.

The macrophages reside principally in the spleen, liver, lymph nodes, lungs, and bone marrow; to a lesser extent, they are in the alimentary tract, central nervous system, mammary glands, and skin. In the spleen, the macrophages reside in close association with the lymphocytes in the germinal centers that make up the red pulp. The sluggish blood flow through the pulp allows sufficient time for the macrophages to perform a clearance function. Although the hepatic circulation is less sluggish than the splenic circulation, the contact time between the blood and the liver macrophages, the Kupffer cells, is still considerable. In the lymph nodes, macrophages are present throughout but are most abundant in the medullary zones, close to blood capillaries and efferent lymphatics. Here, macrophages play an important role in antigen presentation to T lymphocytes and, possibly, in the generation of specific immune response. Pulmonary macrophages reside in the alveolar sacs and within air spaces and clear inhaled microorganisms and inhaled matter. Macrophages reside abundantly in the bone marrow and may serve a clearance function in normal states or in pathologic states of ineffective erythropoiesis.

Granulocyte functions include phagocytosis and destruction of foreign particles. The process begins with stimulus recognition, then chemotaxis, adhesion, extravasation from the vascular space, activation of metabolic pathways to create microbicidal oxidative products, and phagocytosis of the smaller particles, with discharge of the lysosomal contents into the media. Defects in any of these processes can result in an impaired ability to fight infection.

Quantitative Disorders of Granulocyte Function

Little is known at the molecular level about the clinical conditions associated with abnormalities in the numbers of circulating granulocytes. Much, however, is known about the molecular basis of the pathophysiologic processes involved in ingestion and killing of bacteria.

NEUTROPENIA

Neutropenia is a condition in which inadequate numbers of granulocytes are produced. Normal neutrophil counts vary for age and race (Table 13–11). The absolute neutrophil count (ANC) is found by multiplying the white blood cell count by the total percentage of bands plus segmented (mature) neutrophils. *Mild neutropenia* is defined as an ANC of 1000 to 1500 cells per microliter, *moderate neutropenia* as an ANC of 500 to 1000 cells per microliter, and *severe neutropenia* as an ANC less than 500 cells per microliter. This division into three categories is useful for determining the individual's risk for infection and the urgency of medical intervention. In severely neutropenic patients, endogenous bacteria are the most frequent pathogens, but neutropenic hosts often become colonized with a variety of nosocomial organisms.

Susceptibility to bacterial infection in neutropenic patients is quite variable and depends on the cause of the neutropenia and other associated problems. Many patients with chronic neutropenia have an elevated circulating monocyte count, which provides limited protection against pyogenic organisms. Patients who are neutropenic as a result of cytotoxic therapy (e.g., chemotherapy or radiation) may be at an increased risk of infection because of the rate of decline of the neutrophil count, even before the ANC is reduced to less than 500 cells per microliter. In addition, these patients can have altered phagocytic function related to their therapy and defects in cell-mediated, humoral, and macrophage-monocyte immunity.

Table 13–11. Normal Leukocyte Counts[1]

Age	Total Leukocytes		Neutrophils[2]			Lymphocytes			Monocytes		Eosinophils	
	Mean	*Range*	*Mean*	*Range*	%	*Mean*	*Range*	%	*Mean*	%	*Mean*	%
Birth	—[3]	—	4.0	2.0–6.0	—	4.2	2.0–7.3	—	0.6	—	0.1	—
12 h	—	—	11.0	7.8–14.5	—	4.2	2.0–7.3	—	0.6	—	0.1	—
24 h	—	—	9.0	7.0–12.0	—	4.2	2.0–7.3	—	0.6	—	0.1	—
1–4 wk	—	—	3.6	1.8–5.4	—	5.6	2.9–9.1	—	0.7	—	0.2	—
6 mo	11.9	6.0–17.5	3.8	1.0–8.5	32	7.3	4.0–13.5	61	0.6	5	0.3	3
1 y	11.4	6.0–17.5	3.5	1.5–8.5	31	7.0	4.0–10.5	61	0.6	5	0.3	3
2 y	10.6	6.0–17.0	3.5	1.5–8.5	33	6.3	3.0–9.5	59	0.5	5	0.3	3
4 y	9.1	5.5–15.5	3.8	1.5–8.5	42	4.5	2.0–8.0	50	0.5	5	0.3	3
6 y	8.5	5.0–14.5	4.3	1.5–8.0	51	3.5	1.5–7.0	42	0.4	5	0.2	3
8 y	8.3	4.5–13.5	4.4	1.5–8.0	53	3.3	1.5–6.8	39	0.4	4	0.2	2
10 y	8.1	4.5–13.5	4.4	1.8–8.0	54	3.1	1.5–6.5	38	0.4	4	0.2	2
16 y	7.8	4.5–13.0	4.4	1.8–8.0	57	2.8	1.2–5.2	35	0.4	5	0.2	3
21 y	7.4	4.5–11.0	4.4	1.8–7.7	59	2.5	1.0–4.8	34	0.3	4	0.2	3

[1] Numbers of leukocytes are in × 10⁹/L or thousands per μL; ranges are estimates of 95% confidence limits, and percentages refer to differential counts.
[2] Neutrophils include band cells at all ages and a small number of metamyelocytes and myelocytes in the first few days of life.
[3] Insufficient data for a reliable estimate.

Reproduced with permission from Dallman PR: Page 1222 in: Rudolph AM et al (editor): *Rudolph's Pediatrics,* 20th ed. Appleton & Lange, 1996.

Malnutrition, splenectomy, and increased exposure to pathogens further weaken the host. All these factors must be considered when assessing patients with neutropenia.

Neutropenia may be caused by defects in myelopoiesis, congenital or acquired, or may be secondary to factors extrinsic to the bone marrow. Intrinsic defects of myelopoiesis are rare but should still be included in the differential diagnosis of newly identified patients with neutropenia, especially infants.

Intrinsic disorders of myelopoiesis. *Reticular dysgenesis* is a rare disorder in which the early stem cells committed to myeloid and lymphoid lineages fail to differentiate. Infants with this disorder are vulnerable to fatal bacterial and viral infections and survive a few months at most. Although they lack neutrophils, T lymphocytes, B lymphocytes, and immunoglobulin formation, their erythroid and megakaryocytic lines are spared. Bone marrow transplantation has been successful in treating this inherited disorder.

Disorders of immunoglobulin formation, such as *X-linked agammaglobulinemia* and *dysgammaglobulinemia type I,* have been associated with neutropenia. Examination of the bone marrow reveals a maturation defect at the myelocyte stage. Clinical manifestations are variable and commonly include failure to thrive, frequent bacterial infections, and early death.

Severe congenital neutropenia, also known as *Kostmann syndrome,* is characterized by a lack of maturation of myeloid progenitors to the promyelocyte or myelocyte stage in the bone marrow. This is an autosomal recessive disorder in which chronic neutropenia exists with an ANC usually less than 200 cells per microliter. Patients with this disorder tend to have a monocytosis and moderate eosinophilia, yet frequent life-threatening infections develop starting from the first month of life. They have frequent febrile episodes, skin infections, stomatitis, and perineal abscesses and are susceptible to infection with the host's flora and opportunistic organisms. Since the introduction of granulocyte-colony-stimulating factor (G-CSF) into the treatment of this disorder, quality and length of survival have dramatically improved. Studies have shown that these patients have normal levels of G-CSF, but the defect seems to reside at the level of the G-CSF receptor that can be overridden by pharmacologic doses of G-CSF. The therapy is well tolerated, and most patients maintain an ANC greater than 1000 cells per microliter and do not have bacterial infections.

Cyclic neutropenia is a rare disorder characterized by regular periodic oscillations of the absolute neutrophil count every 19 to 21 days. Other blood cells, such as the platelets and reticulocytes, can also follow this oscillatory path. During the periods of neutropenia, patients may have oral ulcers, lymphadenopathy, and, at times, serious infections including perineal ulcerations. The severity of the neutropenia determines the severity of the infection. During these episodes, bone marrow aspirates show maturation arrest at the myelocyte stage or myeloid hypoplasia. Between these episodes, patients usually are infection free and have normal neutrophil counts. The symptomatic periods tend to become fewer with age. There has been some evidence for a familial occurrence of this disorder, but most cases are sporadic. Animal studies support the hypothesis that cyclic neutropenia involves a regulatory defect in hematopoietic stem cells, although the exact nature of this defect has yet to be elucidated. Evaluation and management of these patients should start with determination of the individual's neutrophil cycle. A range of 14 to 36 days has been reported, with a median of 21 days. Infections during the neutropenic times should be treated aggressively, and appropriate precautions, especially good dental hygiene, should be taken to avoid infection. Preliminary studies using G-CSF to treat cyclic neutropenia appear promising.

Chronic benign neutropenia of childhood. A particular group of children with chronic idiopathic neutropenia likely represents several poorly understood disorders. Many of these children have a benign course, hence the name *chronic benign neutropenia of childhood.* They often have mild to moderate neutropenia; the susceptibility to infection is roughly proportionate to the degree of neutropenia. The blood neutrophil count remains stable over years; however, in a subset of children the count becomes elevated in response to an infection. Spontaneous remissions at 2 to 4 years of age have been reported. Some cases appear to be familial. Affected individuals have normal life expectancies. Evaluation of the marrow shows decreased myelopoiesis (often with monocytosis), and there is considerable variability in the stage at which maturation is arrested. These patients are at low risk for development of serious infections, and no treatment is required except during infectious episodes. Some of these children resemble those with the lazy leukocyte syndrome, in which profound neutropenia is present with an apparently normal bone marrow and a characteristically poor response of the peripheral blood leukocytes to chemical or inflammatory stimuli. Some of the more symptomatic children may benefit from treatment with corticosteroids. Treatment with G-CSF is also being investigated.

Absolute neutrophil counts are significantly lower in African Americans than in whites. The explanation for these differences is unclear. Absolute neutrophil counts may be as low as 800/μL, yet they are not associated with infection, as an increase in ANC occurs in response to infection. Furthermore, bone marrow aspirate is normal with respect to myelopoiesis. Red cell and platelet counts are also normal. If the history for infections is unremarkable, neutropenia with counts greater than 500/μL in African Americans require no further investigation. If bacterial infections are present, these patients should have complete evaluation for neutropenia.

Extrinsic causes of neutropenia. Replacement of the bone marrow (as occurs with hematologic malignancies, glycogen storage diseases, granulomas associated with infection, and fibrosis related to chemical or radiation injury or osteoporosis) results in neutropenia. Frequently, the erythroid and megakaryocytic lines are also affected. Ineffective granulopoiesis can be seen in states of vitamin deficiency (vitamin B_{12} or folate), malnutrition (anorexia nervosa and marasmus), copper deficiency, and the Chédiak-Higashi syndrome (CHS).

The most common cause of transient neutropenia in childhood is viral infection. Viruses known to cause neutropenia include hepatitis A and B, influenza A and B, measles, rubella, varicella, and respiratory syncytial virus. Neutropenia corresponds to the period of acute viremia—the first 24 to 48 h of the illness—lasting up to 1 week. Neutropenia occurring 1 to 2 weeks after viremia suggests an immune-mediated mechanism of neutrophil destruction or sequestration, and it should be determined whether titers of antineutrophil antibodies are elevated.

Bacterial sepsis is one of the more serious causes of neutropenia. Phagocytosis of microbes leads to release of toxic metabolites, which then activate the complement system, inducing neutrophil aggregation and adherence of leukocytes to the pulmonary capillary bed. Tumor necrosis factor and interleukin-1 (IL-1), released by the macrophages, likely accelerate this process. Activated granulocytes sequestered in the lungs may cause acute cardiopulmonary complications. Neonates have a limited granulocyte pool in their bone marrow, which can be exhausted rapidly during overwhelming bacterial sepsis. These infants may benefit from granulocyte transfusions or treatment with G-CSF.

Drug-induced neutropenia is a common and expected side effect of anticancer therapy. Many chemotherapeutic agents have a direct toxic effect on the early marrow stem cells. The severity and duration of the neutropenia depend on the particular medication, dosage, method of delivery, underlying disease, and state of nutrition and general health. These children should follow general supportive care guidelines for chronic neutropenia by taking prophylactic trimethoprim-sulfamethoxazole to prevent *Pneumocystis carinii* and antifungal medication; adhering to vigorous mouth care; avoiding exposure to crowds and sick individuals; and receiving prophylactic immunoglobulin for varicella exposures. Therapy with G-CSF or other granulocyte-mobilizing cytokines may shorten the period of severe neutropenia after chemotherapy.

Many other medications can induce neutropenia, including antibiotics (chloramphenicol, cephalosporins, penicillins, and sulfonamides), anticonvulsants (phenytoin and valproic acid), anti-inflammatory agents, cardiovascular agents, tranquilizers, and hypoglycemic agents. The severity and duration of drug-induced neutropenia are variable. The underlying mechanism is not known, although studies with certain drugs have led to various hypotheses: immune-mediated, toxic effect of the drug or metabolites on the marrow stem cells, and toxic effects on the marrow microenvironment. After withdrawal of the drug, the marrow can repopulate with early myeloid forms in 3 to 4 days and appear morphologically normal by 1 to 2 weeks. The duration of neutropenia is likely related to the underlying mechanism; some chronic idiosyncratic drug reactions can last from months to years. Immune-mediated neutropenia usually resolves within 6 to 8 days of withdrawal of the offending agent.

Some cases of acquired neutropenia may represent an autoimmune disease with neutrophil specificity. Unlike in adults, immune neutropenia in children usually occurs in the absence of other diseases. These children have elevated titers of antineutrophil antibodies. The neutropenia is variable, ranging from mild to severe, and is often accompanied by monocytosis. Examination of the bone marrow usually shows myeloid hyperplasia, a response expected with increased peripheral destruction of the neutrophils. Treatment consists of aggressive management of infections with antimicrobials; in addition, steroid therapy is used for patients with severe neutropenia associated with recurrent infections. Splenectomy may be of only transient benefit and is not recommended. Use of high-dose intravenous immunoglobulin has been tried, but its efficacy remains unproved. Autoimmune neutropenia can also be a part of other autoimmune diseases such as Felty syndrome, a triad of rheumatoid arthritis, splenomegaly, and leukopenia. Immune neutropenia can also be associated with immune hemolytic anemia and thrombocytopenia (Evans syndrome).

Isoimmune neonatal neutropenia, analogous to Rh hemolytic anemia, can occur as a result of maternal sensitization to fetal neutrophil antigens during gestation. This results in the formation of IgG antibodies that cross the placenta and destroy the infant's neutrophils. The infants usually recover within 6 to 7 weeks, but fever and life-threatening infections can develop within the first few days after birth. Treatment of these infections may include use of antibiotics, plasma exchange, and infusion of maternal neutrophils known to lack the antigen to which the antibody is directed.

Organomegaly, in particular splenic enlargement from any cause, can cause sequestration of circulating neutrophils, resulting in neutropenia. Anemia and thrombocytopenia may also occur. Treatment of the underlying disease process often ameliorates the neutropenia.

Diagnostic approach to children with neutropenia. Evaluation of children with neutropenia begins with a thorough history and physical examination. Included should be the children's family history, medication list, recent illnesses, age, and ethnicity. On examination, attention should be paid to any phenotypic abnormalities, adenopathy, splenomegaly, evidence of a chronic or underlying disease, and meticulous evaluation of the skin and mucous membranes (oral and perirectal). The laboratory evaluation helps establish the severity and duration (using periodic blood cell counts) of the neutropenia. Patients with chronic neutropenia should have blood cell counts checked twice a week for 6 weeks to evaluate for cyclic neutropenia. Additional studies include antineutrophil antibodies, assessment of cellular and serum immune status, and careful review of the peripheral smear for morphologic abnormalities of the white cells. Hematologic values, red cell indices, and platelet studies should also be done. A bone marrow aspirate and biopsy specimen may be necessary to identify granulocyte precursors and to search for defects in myeloid maturation. In addition, the bone marrow aspirate and biopsy specimen can be used to exclude hematologic malignancies, marrow infiltration, or fibrosis (Fig. 13–9).

Management of children with neutropenia. The management of neutropenia depends on many factors, including the nature of the neutropenia (acute or chronic), its severity, and the association with immune defects, underlying illnesses, or malignancies. Patients with acquired neutropenia arising from malignancy or chemotherapeutic drugs have a diminished inflammatory capability and are unusually susceptible to sepsis. Fever may be the earliest and only warning sign. Sepsis related to induced neutropenia remains a leading cause of mortality in these patients. Aggressive management of febrile, neutropenic patients in the hospital has markedly reduced morbidity and mortality associated with infection.

In neutropenic patients, the definition of fever is one episode of a temperature of 38.5°C (101.3°F) or higher or two temperatures of 38°C (100.4°F) or higher in a 24-h period. The initial evaluation of children with fever and neutropenia includes meticulous physical examination with particular attention to sites of occult infection (the oral cavity and perineum); peripheral and indwelling catheter blood cultures; urinalysis and urine culture; chest roentgenogram, if pulmonary symptoms are present; and cultures from sites of suspected infection, such as skin, throat, and stool. Blood cultures should be obtained every 24 h in persistently febrile patients. Broad-spectrum antibiotics must be started immediately and provide coverage for gram-negative and gram-positive organisms. A combination of an aminoglycoside and a β-lactam antibiotic provides initial broad coverage and is synergistic for *Pseudomonas* species. If the fever subsides, the cultures remain negative, and the clinical course improves, the antibiotics can be discontinued after 72 h. Documented bacteremia should be treated with a full course of antibiotics. In the patient in whom infection of an indwelling catheter is a recurrent problem or the bacteremia persists beyond 48 to 72 h, the catheter should be removed. In persistently febrile, neutropenic patients, antifungal therapy with amphotericin should be begun by the fifth to seventh day and continued until the patients are no longer neutropenic and febrile. Many oncologists continue antibiotic therapy until the neutropenia resolves or there is some evidence of marrow recovery.

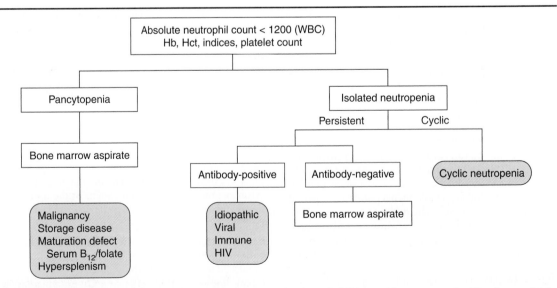

Figure 13–9. Algorithm diagramming the laboratory evaluation of children with neutropenia. Hb = hemoglobin; Hct = hematocrit; WBC = white blood cell count.

EVALUATION OF PATIENTS WITH RECURRENT INFECTIONS

The differential diagnosis for patients with recurrent infections is extensive. Although most of these patients will not have identifiable phagocytic disorders, defects of the host immune system should be considered. The algorithm in Figure 13–10 is presented to help organize this complicated workup.

NEUTROPHILIA

Neutrophilia refers to a circulating neutrophil count greater than 7500/μL in children and 13,000/μL in infants. Neutrophilia may result from increased marrow production or changes between the circulating and marginating pools of neutrophils. Acute neutrophilia occurs after administration of epinephrine or corticosteroids, as

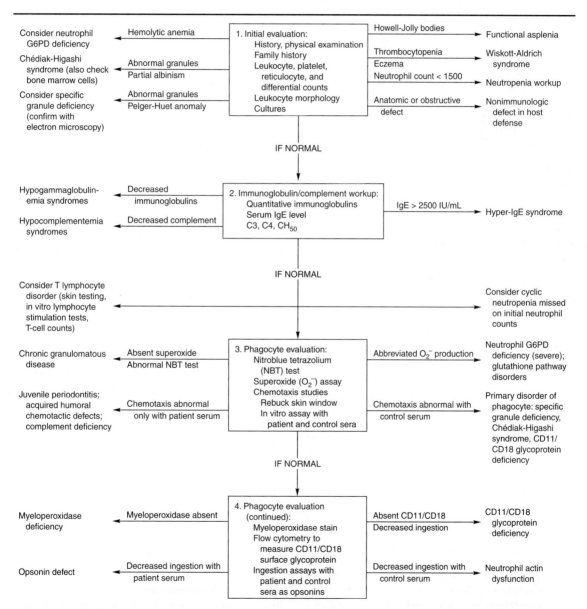

Figure 13–10. Algorithm diagramming laboratory evaluation of patients with recurrent infections. G6PD = glucose-6-phosphate dehydrogenase. (Reproduced with permission from Lehrer RI: Neutrophils and host defense. *Ann Intern Med* 1988;109:127.)

well as after splenectomy. Chronic neutrophilia may be related to defective feedback mechanisms between circulating neutrophils and the marrow and may follow periods of prolonged administration of corticosteroids, infection, chronic inflammation, and chronic blood loss. A transient neutrophilia is seen after blood transfusions. Infections such as tuberculosis, herpes simplex, and varicella may cause prolonged elevated neutrophil counts. Leukemoid reactions and leukocytosis resembling leukemia have been observed in neonates with Down syndrome and in association with sepsis. The benign neutrophilia of infancy resolves by the end of the first few weeks after birth.

Qualitative Disorders of Granulocyte Function

Numerous rare inherited and acquired disorders have been described that are caused by abnormalities in one or more steps of phagocytic function, such as chemotaxis, adhesion, ingestion, degranulation, and oxidative metabolism. Affected individuals may have recurrent bacterial and fungal infections.

DISORDERS OF ADHESION

Leukocyte adhesion deficiency. *Leukocyte adhesion deficiency (LAD)* is a rare, autosomal recessive disorder of impaired phagocyte adhesion, chemotaxis, and ingestion of complement (C3bi)-opsonized microbes. The molecular basis for this disease has been investigated, and mutations of the genes coding for specific neutrophil glycoprotein subunits have been found. Carriers can be identified, and prenatal diagnosis can be made if the genetic locations of the parental mutations are known.

To date, approximately 60 cases of LAD have been reported in the literature. Clinically, the disorder is characterized by repeated bacterial or opportunistic infections, severe gingivitis and periodontitis, frequent superficial bacterial infections with an invasive predisposition, and slow wound healing that is often first manifested as delayed umbilical cord separation. *Staphylococcus aureus* and gram-negative enteric bacteria are the most common pathogens. Laboratory features include a persistent granulocytosis and failure of the neutrophils to accumulate at sites of infection.

The diagnosis of LAD should be suspected in any infants or newborns who have an unusually severe bacterial infection in the face of a striking granulocytosis (up to 100,000/μL). A leukemoid reaction may be mistakenly deemed the cause of the elevated white cell count. Treatment depends on the clinical severity of the disorder, with phenotypes ranging from moderate to severe. In all patients, granulocytosis is the hallmark. Cutaneous and oral infections should be treated promptly. Prophylaxis with trimethoprim-sulfamethoxazole has been beneficial. Aggressive dental hygiene is advisable, with antimicrobial

rinses such as chlorhexidine gluconate. Patients with LAD can have unusually severe infections, and the mortality rate is high, especially in patients younger than 2 years. Bone marrow transplantation has been used successfully to treat several cases and, at this time, may provide the only chance for survival.

Acquired disorders of adhesion. Exposure to a wide array of drugs can cause *decreased adhesiveness* of the neutrophils. Epinephrine and corticosteroids, the most common offenders, cause a dramatic increase in the total neutrophil count as the blood cells from the marginating pool within the vascular tree are released into the circulation. Epinephrine causes endothelial cells to release cyclic adenosine monophosphate (AMP), which impairs the neutrophil's ability to adhere. The mechanism by which corticosteroids alter adherence is unknown.

A variety of clinical situations can result in *increased neutrophil adherence* by complement activation. Such situations include thermal injuries, gram-negative bacterial sepsis, trauma, pancreatitis, and exposure to artificial membranes during hemodialysis and cardiopulmonary bypass. Neutrophils experience increased aggregation, and neutrophil clumps become trapped within small capillary beds, such as in the lung. These aggregated neutrophils generate toxic oxygen radicals and release proteases that damage structural proteins, such as collagen and elastin. These events can contribute to acute respiratory distress syndrome.

DISORDERS OF CHEMOTAXIS

Many mechanisms regulate the directed migration of phagocytes from the circulation to sites of infection and inflammation. Chemotactic factors must be generated in sufficient quantities to establish chemotactic gradients that promote granulocyte mobility. The phagocytes must have receptors for these agents as well as mechanisms for discerning the direction of the gradient. When these receptors are engaged, a series of intracellular metabolic events occurs that regulates the increased surface expression of adhesion-promoting molecules. Inflammatory mediators, such as IL-1, further direct the migration of phagocytes. Phagocyte-endothelial cell interactions play a central role in directing the tissue localization of neutrophils and monocytes during inflammation.

Many conditions may impair chemotaxis; this may be due to complement deficiency (C1, C2, C3, C4, and C5), immunodeficiency syndromes (e.g., Wiscott-Aldrich), or disorders of phagocyte function (LAD, CHS, and specific leukocyte granule deficiencies).

Chemotaxis in the neonate. In the first few weeks after birth, infants are at an increased risk for the development of severe bacterial infections. The risk is even greater in preterm infants. Neonates may have defects in specific immunity and phagocyte-mediated immunity including splenic function. Defects in neutrophil adherence, chemotaxis, phagocytosis, and bacteriocidal activity have all been reported. The directed migration of neonatal neutrophils toward a variety of chemotactic agents (C5a and bacterial extracts) is reduced by 50% compared with adult neutrophils because of a defect in upregulation of cell-adhesion molecules. Neonatal neutrophils also display a diminished fusion of the specific granules within the plasma membrane after stimulation. Compounding these defects is a deficiency of antibodies directed against organisms that typically infect infants. Furthermore, with severe pyogenic infections, neonates can quickly exhaust their bone marrow granulocyte reserves. In addition to these granulocyte defects, the susceptibility of newborns to infections is further accentuated by defects in cellular and antibody-mediated immunity as well as in functional asplenia. Finally, as mentioned previously, the bone marrow reserve of granulocyte precursors is elevated in newborns, and neutropenia can occur with stress. All these abnormalities appear to correct within the first few months of life.

DISORDERS OF DEGRANULATION

Chédiak-Higashi syndrome. *Chédiak-Higashi syndrome* is a rare, autosomal recessive disease characterized by recurrent bacterial infections, partial oculocutaneous albinism, giant cytoplasmic inclusions in the granulocytes, and, in some patients, a mild bleeding diathesis. Peripheral and cranial neuropathies have also been described. A variety of tissues are affected. In melanocytes, the giant inclusions *(melanosomes)* prevent the even distribution of melanin, resulting in hypopigmentation of the hair, skin, iris, and ocular fundus. There are approximately 200 known cases of CHS; its rarity has made elucidation of the underlying molecular defect difficult. The lysosomal defect involves all blood cells. The neutrophils are most characteristic and contain giant coalesced azurophil-specific granules. The absolute neutrophil count ranges from 500 to 2000 cells per microliter, reflecting intramedullary granulocyte destruction. Monocytes and lymphocytes are also affected, and the combined effects may contribute to abnormalities in specific immunity. Although the platelet count is normal, the platelets have a decreased number of dense granules and a storage pool deficiency of adenosine diphosphate (ADP) and serotonin. Platelet aggregation is often defective, and patients bruise easily and may have epistaxis and intestinal bleeding.

Individuals with CHS have recurrent infections involving the skin, respiratory tract, and mucous membranes, usually caused by both gram-positive (*Staph. aureus*) and gram-negative bacteria, as well as fungi. Impaired bactericidal activity is a result of neutropenia and defective neutrophil function. Chemotaxis is markedly depressed. The large granules may impede the neutrophil's ability to travel through tight passages, such as between endothelial cells.

Degranulation is delayed and incomplete, and there is a deficiency of antimicrobial protein production in the CHS neutrophils.

Affected individuals who survive beyond the first decade have a high risk of progressing to an accelerated phase of the disease, perhaps because of infection by Epstein-Barr virus. This phase is heralded by the onset of hepatosplenomegaly, lymphadenopathy, bone marrow infiltration by lymphohistiocytic cells, hemophagocytosis, and high fevers not attributable to infections. Thrombocytopenia develops and can worsen the bleeding disorder already present. The risk of overwhelming sepsis during this period is high, and many patients succumb.

The diagnosis of CHS is usually made by the history and physical examination and the finding of giant granules in the peripheral blood or bone marrow myeloid cells. In severely neutropenic patients, a bone marrow aspirate may be needed to confirm the diagnosis.

Management involves treatment of infections and supportive care measures as described for immunocompromised patients. The accelerated phase may respond to chemotherapeutic intervention but is frequently fatal. Bone marrow transplantation has been successfully performed on several patients during the chronic phase of the disease.

DISORDERS OF OXIDATIVE METABOLISM

Neutrophils contain a group of antimicrobial polypeptides that act as endogenous antibiotics. These are called *defensins*. Another class of microbicidal agents called *free radicals* is generated within the cell by the phagocyte respiratory burst pathway. In a series of reactions, molecular oxygen is converted initially to superoxide, and then to hydrogen peroxide (H_2O_2), hypochlorous acid (HOCl), and hydroxyl radical. The enzyme responsible for this burst of respiration is NADPH oxidase. Before this series of reactions, the neutrophil consumes little oxygen and relies primarily on anaerobic glycolysis for energy. Several clinically significant defects in the respiratory burst pathway have been identified and involve deficiencies of the regulatory enzymes: NADPH, G6PD, myeloperoxidase, glutathione reductase, and glutathione synthetase.

Chronic granulomatous disease. Chronic granulomatous disease (CGD) is a rare, genetically heterogeneous disorder, caused by a failure of respiratory burst activation in the phagocytes. At the molecular level, the defect has been localized to a defect in one of the NADPH subunits in the membrane or cytoplasm of the granulocyte. The symptoms of CGD appear during the first year and are characterized by recurrent purulent bacterial and fungal infections. The most common pathogens are *Staph. aureus,* *Aspergillus* species, and gram-negative bacilli, including *Serratia marcescens,* various *Salmonella* species, and *Pseudomonas cepaci.* Typical infections include pneumonia, complicated by empyema or lung abscess; suppurative lymphadenitis, usually involving the cervical nodes; cutaneous abscesses, paronychia, and perinasal impetigo; hepatic abscesses; osteomyelitis; and perirectal infections. In addition to pyogenic infections, a chronic inflammatory state is present with resultant formation of granulomas, one of the hallmarks of CGD. Hyperglobulinemia, short stature due to chronic illness, and anemia of chronic disease are evident in many affected individuals.

The unique susceptibility of CGD patients to specific infections is based on the inability of CGD phagocytes to produce hydrogen peroxide. Many bacteria, such as *Strep. pneumoniae,* produce hydrogen peroxide and lack catalase, an enzyme that breaks down hydrogen peroxide. As a consequence, these organisms can be killed by CGD granulocytes.

The diagnosis of CGD is suspected from the history of infections, particular pathogens and sites of infection, and a family history of disease. A useful diagnostic test is the nitroblue tetrazolium (NBT) test. In dormant cells, NBT remains oxidized and is soluble and yellow. When normal neutrophils are stimulated to undergo a respiratory burst in the presence of NBT, which creates superoxide, this reduces the NBT and converts it to a deep purple color. Stimulated CGD neutrophils cannot reduce NBT dye, as they do not generate superoxide. Carrier states can also be identified using this method, with intermediate levels of NBT reduction seen in the phagocytes of autosomal recessive carriers. However, NBT reduction may vary with the degree of X inactivation of the affected chromosome, and some carriers may be missed because of the selective advantage of the normal X chromosome. Molecular techniques can definitely establish a diagnosis and can be used for prenatal diagnosis as well.

The prognosis for patients with CGD is improving steadily. Many patients survive into their adult years with aggressive management of infectious episodes with antibiotics, antifungal agents, surgical drainage of abscesses, and prophylactic trimethoprim-sulfamethoxazole. The use of human recombinant interferon-g has been shown to be useful in some patients and is a well-tolerated treatment that reduces the frequency of serious infections. Allogenic bone marrow transplantation has been used successfully in several cases of CGD.

Glucose-6-phosphate dehydrogenase deficiency. Leukocyte and erythrocyte G6PD are encoded by the same gene; however, clinically significant neutrophil G6PD deficiency is rare. This is explained in part by the neutrophil's high tolerance: Respiratory burst function is not adversely affected until the G6PD level is less than 5%. In addition, low levels of respiratory burst activity can be sufficient for host protection. In most types of G6PD deficiency, the neutrophil level is 20 to 75% of normal. Because of the neutrophil's short half-life, the effect of enzyme decay is not as significant as it is in the erythro-

cytes. This explains why leukocyte G6PD deficiency is not associated with clinical problems in African Americans. The diagnosis of G6PD deficiency should be suspected in any patients with known erythrocyte G6PD deficiency, or in patients with congenital nonspherocytic hemolytic anemia in association with recurrent infections. Treatment is aimed at prevention of infections with prophylaxis and with antimicrobials as indicated.

Myeloperoxidase deficiency. Myeloperoxidase deficiency, a rare disorder, is inherited in an autosomal recessive mode. The deficiency of myeloperoxidase from the azurophilic granules of the neutrophils results in a pronounced delay in the killing of both catalase-positive and catalase-negative intracellular bacteria. Myeloperoxidase deficiency is the most common inherited disorder of phagocyte function, with a complete deficiency in 1 : 4000 individuals. Expression is variable and very mild. Neutrophils and monocytes are affected, but eosinophils show normal activity. The neutrophils have large residual stores of myeloperoxidase, and the respiratory burst seems to be augmented in these patients. In addition, the other oxidants produced by the respiratory burst, the various lysosomal antimicrobial proteins, and the activity of the normal eosinophils all contribute to provide sufficient host defense against most microorganisms. Usually, no treatment is required. Infections should be treated as in normal individuals, although these patients do have an increased susceptibility to candidal infections.

Basophils and Eosinophils

Eosinophils are leukocytes that are identified by their characteristic intracellular, refractile, eosinophilic staining granules. Eosinophils can be found in the bloodstream, as well as in many body tissues. The epithelial lining of the intestine, especially the colon, is one of the most heavily populated areas. Eosinophils are capable of ingesting and killing bacteria and can enhance or suppress acute inflammatory reactions.

In normal children, the absolute circulating eosinophil count is 150 to 700/μL. Eosinopenia may occur as a result of adrenocortical hyperfunction or after the administration of pharmacologic doses of corticosteroids. Eosinophilia may be hereditary, but is most often due to allergy; asthma, hay fever, skin rashes, and allergic drug reactions are among the causes. Invasive parasitic infections, such as toxocariasis, trichinosis, echinococcal disease, ascaris, and, less commonly, intestinal parasites, can cause eosinophilia. Visceral larval migrans results in a large increase in the number of circulating eosinophils. Eosinophilia can be seen in premature infants and often occurs in infants who have chlamydial pneumonia. Gastrointestinal disorders, such as ulcerative colitis, Crohn disease, chronic hepatitis, and milk precipitin disease, may have an associated eosinophilia. Immunodeficiency syndromes, such as Wiscott-Aldrich syndrome, have associated eosinophilia. Cases of Hodgkin disease in which an eosinophilic factor is produced have moderate to severe eosinophilia. Acute lymphocytic leukemia may present with eosinophilia and should be considered when common causes have been eliminated. A rare group of hypereosinophilic syndromes of unknown etiology involves the cardiopulmonary system and includes disseminated eosinophilic collagen disease, Loeffler disease, endocarditis with endomyocardial fibrosis, and pulmonary infiltration with eosinophils.

Basophils are leukocytes that contain a few densely staining, basophilic granules. They account for less than 1% of the circulating leukocytes. Basophil granules are rich in histamine and heparin. Like eosinophils, basophils participate in allergic reactions. If basophilia is associated with leukocytosis and thrombocytosis, chronic myelogenous leukemia should be suspected. Basophilia can also occur with ulcerative colitis and myxedema.

PLATELETS

Megakaryocytes derive from the early stem cells, which are called colony-forming unit stem cells (CFU-S); a molecule called *thrombopoietin (TPO)* has been identified. TPO regulates the number of circulating platelets. Once the CFU-megakaryocyte becomes committed, the transitional megakaryocytes go through four stages of maturation. The megakaryoblasts are large and have globulated nuclei and basophilic cytoplasm-containing granules and dense bodies. These cells then develop indented, horseshoe-shaped nuclei with more abundant and less basophilic cytoplasm with increased numbers of organelles. In the third stage of maturation, the megakaryocytes appear large with abundant granular eosinophilic cytoplasm. Finally, the megakaryocytes mature into cells with compact, dense nuclei and homogenous, intensely stained eosinophilic cytoplasm. The state of cytoplasmic maturation and its ploidy level determine the number of platelets contained by the megakaryocyte. Where and under what circumstances the platelets are released from the megakaryocytes have not yet been determined.

Mature platelets are small cells, approximately 1 to 4 μm in diameter. They are crucial in the initiation of hemostasis, forming the platelet plug. Excessive bleeding can occur if the platelets are dysfunctional or deficient in number. Bleeding secondary to platelet insufficiency typically involves the skin or mucous membranes and includes petechiae, ecchymoses, epistaxis, menorrhagia, hematuria, and gastrointestinal bleeding. Intracranial hemorrhages can occur but are rare. In response to marrow stress or thrombocytopenia, large platelets can be seen in the peripheral blood.

There are normally 150,000 to 400,000 platelets per μm in the peripheral circulation. Platelet mass is maintained at a constant rate under the control of TPO. Approximately one third of the platelets are sequestered in the spleen and serve as a reserve pool, released in times of hemostatic stress. The proportion of platelets sequestered is related directly to spleen size. Splenomegaly or asplenia must be considered when interpreting the circulating platelet concentration. Platelets survive 7 to 10 days once released from the marrow. Transfused platelets survive for a considerably shorter period, even if patients' thrombocytopenia is due to decreased platelet production.

When the endothelial cell lining of the vessel wall is interrupted, platelets bind to the exposed adhesive proteins in the subendothelium. Primary hemostasis, or platelet plug formation, is initiated. During platelet adhesion, von Willebrand factor acts as a bridge between the platelet glycoprotein (GP) Ib/IX complex and the subendothelial matrix proteins. Platelets contract, extend pseudopods, and, during this activation process, release the contents of their granules (ADP, calcium, and serotonin), thereby drawing other platelets to form a platelet aggregate. A network of platelet–platelet linkages via GP Ib/IIIa receptors results in formation of a platelet plug. Fibrinogen and von Willebrand factor are also important participants in this interaction. Arachidonic acid is released from the platelet membrane during the activation process, and its metabolic products initiate release of platelet granules. More platelets are recruited to the site of adherence, and the platelet framework facilitates the clotting cascade with the formation of a fibrin clot.

As with erythrocytes and leukocytes, disorders of platelet numbers can be secondary to increased destruction or storage in the spleen or decreased production. Qualitative platelet defects can also occur. Conversely, elevated platelet counts can be seen when the rate of production exceeds the rate of destruction or storage, as noted in acute inflammation, in postsplenectomy st ates (when the storage site for platelets is removed), or in acute hemorrhagic states.

Quantitative Abnormalities of the Platelets

The initial evaluation of thrombocytopenia requires the confirmation of the platelet count on review of the peripheral smear, especially in nonsymptomatic children. False values for platelet counts can result from aggregation of platelets in the syringe or collection tube; counting of small, nonplatelet particles (fragmented red or white cells) by automated cell counters; and pseudothrombocytopenia due to in vitro platelet agglutination by anticoagulant-dependent ethylenediamine tetra-acetic acid (EDTA) antibodies. In the latter case, review of the blood film may show clumps of agglutinated platelets at the periphery of the slide. The diagnoses of thrombocytopenia in children are shown in Table 13–12, and the approach to managing children with thrombocytopenia is presented in Figure 13–11.

Table 13–12. Diagnoses of Thrombocytopenia in Pediatrics

Destructive thrombocytopenias		Impaired production	
Immunologic	Idiopathic thrombocytopenic purpura	Congenital and hereditary disorders	Thrombocytopenia-absent radius syndrome
	Drug-induced		Fanconi anemia
	Infection-induced		Bernard-Soulier syndrome
	Posttransfusion purpura		Wiscott-Aldrich syndrome
	Autoimmune disease		Glanzmann thrombasthenia
	Neonatal alloimmune		May-Hegglin anomaly
	Posttransplant		Amegakaryocytosis
Nonimmunologic	Microangiopathic disease	Associated with chromosomal defects	Trisomy 13 or 18
	Hemolytic anemia and thrombocytopenia		
	Hemolytic uremic syndrome	Metabolic disorders and acquired processes	Marrow infiltration
	Thrombotic thrombocytopenia purpura		Malignancies
	Cyanotic heart disease		Storage disease
			Myelofibrosis
Platelet consumption	Disseminated intravascular coagulation		Aplastic anemia
	Giant hemangiomas		Drug-induced
	Meconium aspiration	**Sequestration**	
		Hypersplenism	
Neonatal problems	Pulmonary hypertension		Hemolytic anemia, chronic
	Polycythemia		Portal hypertension
	Respiratory distress syndrome		Glycogen storage disease
	Sepsis		
	Prematurity		

DESTRUCTIVE THROMBOCYTOPENIA

Immune-mediated thrombocytopenia. The most common cause of destructive thrombocytopenia is immune-mediated platelet destruction. Shortened platelet survival can result from an IgG antibody directed against a platelet membrane antigen—either an autoantigen or, possibly, neoantigen resulting from infection with a microorganism or drug exposure. IgM antibodies and complement activation are less frequently found but can also be seen in childhood immune idiopathic thrombocytopenia purpura (ITP).

Idiopathic thrombocytopenia purpura. Idiopathic thrombocytopenia purpura is an acute, self-limited disease of isolated thrombolytic thrombocytopenia that usually occurs in children aged 2 to 4 years; it usually resolves within 6 months. When ITP occurs in children younger than 1 year or older than 10 years, the course is often chronic and associated with a generalized immune disorder. Otherwise healthy children have sudden onset of severe thrombocytopenia, manifest by petechiae, purpura, epistaxis, and, less frequently, hematuria and gastrointestinal hemorrhage. There may be a history of an antecedent viral illness within the preceding 1 to 3 weeks. Death from ITP is rare (<1%) and usually due to intracranial hemorrhage.

Initial evaluation of children with suspected ITP begins with a complete history and physical examination. Other than a possible antecedent illness and the acute onset of minor bleeding and bruising, children are otherwise well. There is no hepatosplenomegaly or significant adenopathy (other than that seen with a mild viral illness). There should be no evidence of chronic disease, weight loss, fevers, or bone pain.

Review of the peripheral blood smear confirms a low platelet count, and the few remaining platelets are large. If platelet size is determined by an automated cell counter, it is elevated, consistent with young platelet age and rapid platelet destruction. The erythrocyte and leukocyte counts are normal, and there is no evidence of hemolysis or microangiopathic disease. Lymphocyte morphology may reflect the recent viral infection.

If any findings suggest another diagnosis, consideration should be given to performing bone marrow aspiration. The presence of immature megakaryocytes in normal or increased numbers in the marrow with normal erythroid and myeloid lineages confirms that the thrombocytopenia is due to increased peripheral destruction

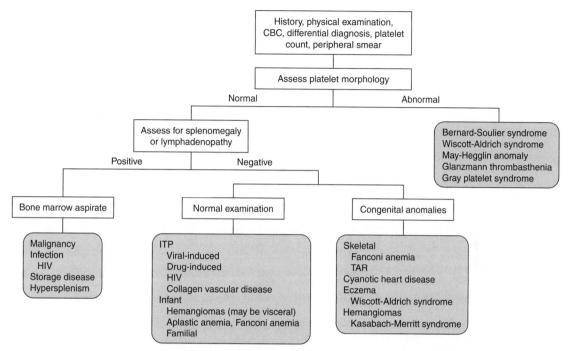

Figure 13–11. Algorithm diagramming the approach to the management of children with isolated thrombocytopenia. CBC = complete blood count; ITP = idiopathic thrombocytopenic purpura; TAR = thrombocytopenia-absent radius syndrome.

and supports the diagnosis of ITP. By convention, bone marrow aspiration is done on individuals with suspected ITP if steroids are to be part of the treatment plan, because of the small possibility that steroids may interfere with the diagnosis of leukemia.

A careful drug history should be obtained to identify agents that can cause thrombocytopenia, with particular attention to heparin, aspirin, aspirin-containing cold medications, and seizure medications. Agents that alter platelet function must be avoided. Clinicians should consider HIV infection when evaluating patients with isolated thrombocytopenia, as this may be a first manifestation. One should screen for risk factors and test for HIV, if appropriate.

The physical examination should include particular attention to the presence of skeletal anomalies, as can be seen in thrombocytopenia-absent radius syndrome (TAR) and Fanconi anemia (short stature, radial limb dysplasia), diseases that can present with thrombocytopenia. Evidence of microangiopathic disease on the smear, fever, and central nervous system symptoms can be seen in thrombotic thrombocytopenia purpura and hemolytic uremic syndrome. Small platelets are seen in Wiscott-Aldrich syndrome, an X-linked disorder characterized by immuno-

logic abnormalities, eczema, and recurrent infections. Patients with aplastic anemia may present initially with thrombocytopenia before progressing to pancytopenia.

A search for platelet antibodies should be conducted on all patients with acute thrombocytopenia. Assays for direct antibody measurement involve determining the antibodies coating the platelets, whereas indirect assays measure antiplatelet immunoglobulin in the plasma.

As the natural history of acute ITP is to resolve gradually and completely, the decision whether to treat the disorder becomes controversial. Many patients who have been observed carefully without pharmacologic intervention have done well. All patients and families should be counseled regarding rough play, contact sports, and the use of protective gear (helmets) and seat belts; intramuscular injections should be withheld until platelet counts increase.

For children with platelet counts below 20,000/μL, extensive oral or nasal mucosal hemorrhage, or retinal petechiae, the risk of central nervous system hemorrhage may be increased, and therapy with intravenous γ globulin (IVIG) or corticosteroids is usually given. Treatment with IVIG, 1 g/kg over 4 to 6 h, is often therapeutic. This treatment may need to be repeated 2 to 3 times for a total dose of 2 to 3 g/kg; doses should be given 24 hours apart.

An increase in the platelet count is usually seen within 24 to 72 h and peaks at approximately 9 days. γ Globulin is thought to saturate the Fc receptors on the reticuloendothelial cells and therefore decrease the clearance of opsonized platelets. Side effects of IVIG are usually immediate and related to the rate of infusion and include nausea, light-headedness, and headache. These symptoms can be alleviated with further doses by slowing the rate of infusion. Fever may also occur, and premedication with acetaminophen before the infusion is advisable.

Corticosteroids, rather than IVIG, have also been used in the medical management of ITP. Response is slightly slower than with IVIG. The usual steroid prescribed is prednisone, 1 to 2 mg/kg/d for 10 to 20 days, tapering the dosage over 2 weeks. Many patients respond to this treatment, but side effects may occur with repeated treatment or chronic use. An alternative to oral steroids has been pulse high-dose infusion of intravenous methylprednisolone. Some patients become thrombocytopenic after therapy and require retreatment. A relapse may be managed safely by observation and restriction of activity and medications, or with intermittent IVIG or pulse steroids.

If patients have evidence of central nervous system hemorrhage and remain severely thrombocytopenic and unresponsive to IVIG and steroids, an emergency splenectomy should be considered. Continuous infusion of platelets is advised to control bleeding, and plasmapheresis should be considered, although the response is very limited.

Anti-Rh(D) immunoglobulin has been used in the treatment of acute ITP but caution should be exercised because hemoglobinemia and hemoglobinuria, which may be severe, have been reported with its use.

Chronic idiopathic thrombocytopenia purpura. In approximately 10 to 20% of children with acute ITP, chronic, persistent thrombocytopenia develops beyond 6 months. Children with chronic ITP may have an associated autoimmune disease or immunodeficiency state. Many patients with chronic ITP may not need treatment as the platelet count is often greater than 20,000/μL. Spontaneous remission can occur in these patients, and some remissions have been reported 2 years after the original diagnosis. Platelet count alone does not correlate with the risk of hemorrhage, as platelets are large and, consequently, have greater than normal procoagulant activity. In rare patients with chronic, refractory ITP who have clinical hemorrhage or cannot tolerate the living restrictions imposed by the thrombocytopenia, splenectomy should be considered. Up to 85% of patients respond to splenectomy. Vinca alkaloids (vincristine and vinblastine); danazol, a nonvirilizing androgen; immunosuppressive agents (e.g., azathioprine and cyclophosphamide); and infusion of RhoGAM, or anti-Rh (D) immunoglobulin, to individuals who are Rh-positive have been used with some success in selected patients requiring therapy. Ascor-

bic acid, cyclosporin, and interferon α-2b are other agents currently being investigated for use in chronic ITP.

Neonatal alloimmune thrombocytopenia. Neonatal alloimmune thrombocytopenia is a rare syndrome that occurs in approximately 1:5000 newborns. Immunization against platelet alloantigens can occur through either pregnancy or transfusion and can lead to severe thrombocytopenia in the fetal–newborn period, with a high risk of fatal hemorrhage. Several platelet antigens have been implicated, but the greatest number of cases can be related to PL^{A1} incompatibility. PL^{A1} is a platelet antigen that resides on the GP IIb/IIIa complex (the complex responsible for the fibrinogen receptor activity of platelets and important in aggregation and platelet-plug formation). Development of anti-PL^{A1} antibodies, therefore, not only can decrease platelet number, but can also interfere with normal platelet aggregation, resulting in a qualitative defect in the platelets in addition to thrombocytopenia. This likely explains the high incidence of serious bleeding in these infants after birth or in utero as compared with infants born to mothers with ITP who have antibodies that are not directed against PL^{A1}.

The typical presentation of the affected infant is an otherwise healthy newborn, without perinatal complications and with a normal maternal hematologic history, in whom petechiae, purpura, and extreme thrombocytopenia develop. For a mother with a previous low platelet count, the differential diagnosis includes maternal autoimmune or drug-dependent thrombocytopenia, infection, and preeclampsia. Infants who have birth asphyxia, infection, or congenital bone marrow hypoplasia, or who are premature, can also be thrombocytopenic. The presence of hepatosplenomegaly, intrauterine growth retardation, or intracranial calcifications with thrombocytopenia suggests a congenital viral infection. However, it is also important to exclude alloimmune thrombocytopenia by appropriate immunologic testing in these infants, as there is a potential recurrence of this complication in future pregnancies.

Most affected infants are first-born offspring, suggesting that antigenic exposure occurs early in pregnancy. The incidence of death and serious central nervous system disease is 10 to 15%, and many of these infants have had prenatal or perinatal intracranial hemorrhage. Evidence of intrauterine intracranial hemorrhage can be made by ultrasound. Even a platelet count less than 50,000/μL warrants concern, especially if infants were delivered vaginally. Complications of early central nervous system hemorrhage include hydrocephalus, porencephaly, seizures, and fetal loss. Hyperbilirubinemia may occur owing to resolution of intracranial or intraorgan hemorrhage.

The thrombocytopenia is transient, lasting up to 4 to 6 weeks after delivery. An early platelet alloantigen evaluation of newborns and parents is important, both to offer affected infants treatment and to prevent such devastating complications with future pregnancies. Platelet typing should be done on the mother and father, looking for antigens responsible for alloimmunization in particular, as well as other platelet antigens frequently involved in alloimmune thrombocytopenia. The serum from the mother and infant should also be screened for antiplatelet antibodies. Studies should be done with maternal plasma and paternal or neonatal platelets to screen for antibodies.

Several treatment options are available for infants with neonatal alloimmunization. Transfusion with antigen-negative platelets has been the mainstay of treatment. Because PL^{A1} antigen-negative platelets are present in only 2% of the population, the most available source of platelets is from the mother. Random platelets may provide a transient increase, lasting 1 to 2 days, and should be used in cases of serious hemorrhage while antigen-negative platelets are obtained and prepared. An alternative treatment is the administration of IVIG. The recommended dose is 1 g/kg/d for 1 to 3 days until the platelet count is 50,000 to 100,000/µL. Platelet transfusion may still be necessary with IVIG if immediate correction of the thrombocytopenia is needed.

Mothers who have had one infant with neonatal alloimmune thrombocytopenia are at high risk for having subsequent infants with the same disease. The severity of antenatal and perinatal hemorrhage is also increased. Maternal antiplatelet antibody titers cannot be used to predict affected fetuses accurately. Fetal cord blood samples should be obtained periodically for determination of the platelet count starting at about 20 weeks of gestation, with ultrasound monitoring for hemorrhage. Studies done on mothers treated with IVIG 1 g/kg/w from midgestation until near term have shown increases in fetal platelet count in most cases; this approach should be considered. Delivery should be planned near term with an elective cesarean section or by planned, induced vaginal delivery after documented increase in the fetal platelet count after administration of maternal IVIG. Antigen-negative platelets should be obtained and prepared before delivery in the event of extreme thrombocytopenia or hemorrhage. Mothers can undergo platelet phoresis before delivery to obtain PL^{A1}-negative platelets. Infants' platelet counts should be checked at birth and every 6 to 12 h for 1 to 2 days, then daily, and be kept at or greater than 20,000/µL.

Drug-induced thrombocytopenia.
In addition to immune-mediated mechanisms for thrombocytopenia induced by drugs, many bone marrow–suppressive agents used in chemotherapy cause thrombocytopenia, usually in the face of pancytopenia. Management is usually with platelet transfusion to prevent or treat bleeding. The bone marrow effects of these agents define their dose-limiting toxicities, and thrombocytopenia is a common and anticipated problem. These patients usually respond well to platelet transfusion, but their condition can become refractory because of the underlying illness, organomegaly and sequestration, sepsis, and other medications.

Nonimmune-mediated platelet consumption.
Several nonimmune-mediated processes involve increased platelet consumption. Generalized platelet activation with trapping of microaggregates in the small vasculature contributes to the microangiopathic hemolytic anemia occurring in the hemolytic uremic syndrome and thrombotic thrombocytopenia purpura. Increased use of platelets may occur in active bleeding or infection. In DIC, there is an imbalance between intravascular thrombosis and fibrinolysis, with increased platelet consumption, depletion of plasma-clotting factors, and formation of fibrin. Disseminated intravascular coagulation can be activated by many etiologic events, including sepsis due to bacteria, viruses, or fungi; malignancy, particularly acute promyelocytic leukemia and neuroblastoma; hemolytic transfusion reactions; and trauma. Therapy is aimed at the underlying etiologic process; supportive care consists of platelet transfusion and plasma protein replenishment (cryoprecipitate, fresh-frozen plasma).

Thrombocytopenia can occur in sick newborns for many reasons, most commonly infection, prematurity, asphyxia, respiratory distress syndrome, pulmonary hypertension, or meconium aspiration. These infants appear to have normal to increased platelet production but a decreased platelet life span for reasons that are unclear. Thrombocytopenia is a frequent occurrence in congenital cyanotic heart disease associated with compensatory polycythemia. Therapeutic phlebotomy may lessen the thrombocytopenia.

The association between thrombocytopenia and giant hemangiomas occurs in infants with Kasabach-Merritt syndrome. The hemangiomas may be multiple and may involve only viscera. Therefore, in infants with unexplained thrombocytopenia, imaging studies should be done to look for a vascular anomaly. Hemangiomas are proliferative lesions that grow rapidly for several months and then regress spontaneously. Platelet thrombi may develop in these lesions, and platelet life span may be decreased. These infants may also have a consumptive coagulopathy with low fibrinogen levels and elevated concentrations of fibrin degradation products. The lesions are prone to necrosis and infection. The size or location of a particular hemangioma cannot predict whether it will lead to platelet trapping and thrombocytopenia. These infants should be managed by close observation and hematologic monitoring, waiting for regression to occur. The lesions may become large enough, however, to compromise infants (impinge on the airway or vital organs and lead to compartment syndrome) resulting in serious illness or death. Corticosteroid treatment may be beneficial in a dose of 1 to 2 mg/kg/d until regression of the lesion and normalization of the platelet count occur, with subsequent tapering. Interferon-α_2 has been reported to be beneficial in correcting the platelet count and shrinking the lesion; it has been given in doses of 1 to 3 million U/m²/d. This treatment, used alone or in combination with steroids, is under further investigation. Supportive transfusion therapy may be necessary when infants are at risk of hemorrhage; platelet transfusions are given 1 to 2 times daily, as are plasma and cryoprecipitate if there is fibrinogen consumption. Antiplatelet medications (aspirin and dipyridamole) have been used to interfere with platelet trapping within the hemangioma, but they carry the risk of causing platelet destruction in addition to the thrombocytopenia.

THROMBOCYTOPENIA FROM DECREASED PLATELET PRODUCTION

Congenital amegakaryocytic thrombocytopenia, a rare cause of neonatal thrombocytopenia, may be caused by a congenital viral infection or an inherited disorder or may be idiopathic. Cytomegalovirus, rubella, and HIV all have been associated with hypoproductive thrombocytopenia. Neutropenia and anemia are often associated findings. The TAR syndrome is an autosomal recessive disorder with variable thrombocytopenia despite normal erythroid and myeloid lineages. Many patients are transfusion dependent but may experience a spontaneous increase in megakaryocytopoiesis after 1 year of age. Fanconi anemia is another inherited disorder with both skeletal anomalies and hypoproductive thrombocytopenia, although other cell lines are affected. The cytopenia begins in early to late childhood and is associated with chromosomal instability. Infants with hypoproductive states without evidence of skeletal abnormalities may have other reasons for isolated thrombocytopenia, including Wiscott-Aldrich syndrome, viral infection, or an inherited giant platelet syndrome, such as the May-Hegglin anomaly or Bernard-Soulier syndrome. Evaluation of the peripheral smear and possibly a bone marrow aspirate may help confirm the diagnosis. Bone marrow transplantation, when a suitable HLA donor is available, should be considered for these disorders.

Qualitative Abnormalities of the Platelets

A number of molecular defects in platelet GP, receptors, and granules have been described and have furthered our understanding of platelet function. Some drugs and certain acquired metabolic conditions, such as renal failure, can affect platelet function.

The most useful screening test for qualitative platelet disorders in patients with normal platelet counts is the bleeding time, which measures the length of time required for a platelet plug to form and cease bleeding from a small cut. This process requires normal platelet adhesion, activation, and aggregation in addition to normal vascular endothelium. In syndromes with defective blood vessels, such as Ehlers-Danlos and Marfan, the bleeding time may be prolonged despite normal platelet function. Also important is review of a peripheral blood smear with regard to platelet size and morphology. A number of con-

genital qualitative disorders are associated with either small or large platelets. Specific platelet aggregation studies can be done to measure the formation of platelet clumps in response to a variety of stimuli, which usually include ADP, epinephrine, collagen, arachidonic acid, and ristocetin. Normal agglutination requires that the platelet secretory granules (dense, a, lysosomes) respond appropriately to the stimulus. An intact platelet membrane and presence of normal GP and receptors are also necessary. These platelet reactions also initiate the coagulation cascade.

CONGENITAL DISORDERS OF PLATELET FUNCTION

Glanzmann thrombasthenia. Glanzmann thrombasthenia is an autosomal recessive disorder, with a normal platelet count and morphology, in which platelet deficient-type bleeding occurs (i.e., epistaxis, petechiae, ecchymoses, menorrhagia, and gastrointestinal and mucous membrane bleeding). The surface-membrane GP IIb and IIIa are decreased (partially or completely), leading to inadequate platelet-plug formation. On platelet aggregation studies, platelet aggregation is completely absent with all agonists. The diagnosis can be confirmed by documenting the absence of GP IIb/IIIa by sodium dodecyl sulfate polyacrylamide gel electrophoresis. The treatment of severe hemorrhage is platelet transfusion. Isoantibodies against the GP IIb/IIIa protein complex can develop in these patients after platelet transfusion, which limits the benefit of platelet transfusion.

Bernard-Soulier syndrome. Bernard-Soulier syndrome is an autosomal recessive disorder characterized by mild thrombocytopenia, very large platelets (5 to 6 μ), and a clinical syndrome of easy bruising and severe hemorrhage after trauma or surgery. These patients have deficiencies in the platelet GP Ib/IX and GP V. Challenge with ristocetin in platelet aggregation studies is abnormal, because the presence of von Willebrand factor and GP Ib is necessary for this stimulant. Treatment is the use of platelet transfusion at times of bleeding, but isoantibodies may develop against the glycoproteins missing from their own platelets and present on the transfused platelets.

Wiscott-Aldrich syndrome. The Wiscott-Aldrich syndrome is a rare X-linked recessive disorder characterized by thrombocytopenia, very small platelets, severe eczema, and immunodeficiency. The clinical features, in particular the eczema and immunodeficiency, may be mild at birth but become florid by 6 to 12 months of age. Management of these patients includes aggressive local therapy for the eczema, treatment of infections, and ultimately bone marrow transplantation.

PLATELET GRANULE DEFECTS

Platelets may be dysfunctional because of deficient granule content or lack of release of their contents on activation. Several families have been reported with severe forms of platelet-dense granule deficiency, also known as storage pool deficiency, reflecting an absence of ADP and ATP in the granules. Another rare defect involves absence of the contents of the a granules, resulting in a gray appearance of the platelet on Wright-stained smears. The gray platelet syndrome appears to be a result of a lack of packaging of the contents rather than a lack of synthesis of the platelet-specific proteins. These patients can also have myelofibrosis caused by local effects of platelet-derived growth factor.

DRUG-INDUCED PLATELET DYSFUNCTION

A number of drugs impair platelet function, in particular aspirin and other nonsteroidal anti-inflammatory agents. Acetylsalicylic acid is a potent, irreversible inhibitor of the cyclooxygenase enzyme. When normal platelets are stimulated with an agonist (e.g., ADP, epinephrine) arachidonic acid is released from the platelet membrane and then converted by cyclooxygenase to thromboxane A_2, a potent stimulant of platelet aggregation. Prostacyclin (PGI_2), an inhibitor of platelet aggregation, is released from the endothelial cells by the same mechanism. A balance exists between the platelet stimulatory effects of thromboxane production by platelets and the inhibitory effects of prostacyclin formation by the vascular endothelium. Aspirin interferes at both sites, and its effects on the platelets are permanent, for the duration of their life span (7 to 10 days). Aspirin in doses of 5 to 10 mg/kg causes a slightly prolonged bleeding time, without clinical sequelae. Individuals with mild intrinsic platelet defects may be particularly sensitive to an aspirin challenge, as measured by bleeding time before and after ingestion. Several nonsteroidal anti-inflammatory agents may also affect platelet function, although their inhibitory effects on platelet cyclooxygenase are reversed approximately 6 hours after removal of the drug. Anti-inflammatory agents that do not inhibit platelet function include choline salicylate and sodium salicylate.

SYSTEMIC DISEASES ASSOCIATED WITH PLATELET ABNORMALITIES

Uremia and chronic liver disease have been associated with severe hemorrhage and platelet dysfunction. Uremic patients have prolonged bleeding times and abnormal platelet aggregation, although the precise mechanism is unknown. The platelet receptor Ib may be defective, or there may be an inhibition of the platelet von Willebrand factor and GP Ib receptor interaction in uremic patients. These patients usually have normal or increased von Willebrand factor with normal activity. Nevertheless, administration of DDAVP (1-deamino-18-D-arginine vasopressin) increases levels of von Willebrand factor and transiently corrects the bleeding time. The bleeding time may also be corrected with cryoprecipitate infusion. Dial-

ysis is a necessary part of the treatment of uremic patients; should they require surgery, they should undergo dialysis and receive DDAVP or cryoprecipitate to reduce the risk of hemorrhage.

Patients with liver disease have a multifactorial bleeding diathesis. Synthesis of all the plasma coagulation factors is markedly decreased. These patients may have associated portal hypertension with splenomegaly and shortened platelet survival. In addition, they may have an abnormality of platelet function, which may be transiently corrected with DDAVP or platelet transfusion.

HEMOSTASIS

Hemostasis requires the coordinate interaction between platelets, vascular endothelial cells, and plasma-clotting factors. Hemostatic mechanisms can be classified into primary and secondary. In primary hemostasis, the platelets serve an important function in conjunction with the vascular endothelial cells. The clinical disorders that are associated with abnormalities of primary hemostasis are vascular abnormalities, qualitative abnormalities of the platelets, and VWD. An aberration in primary hemostasis is characterized by bleeding of the mucous membranes, epistaxis, and superficial ecchymoses. Typical manifestations are prolonged oozing from minor wounds or abrasions, or abnormal intraoperative bleeding. Abnormalities of secondary hemostasis are most frequently the result of coagulation factor deficiencies. Bleeding characteristically occurs from large vessels with subcutaneous, palpable hematomas, hemarthroses, or intramuscular hematomas. Patients with severe factor VIII or IX deficiency may bleed after trauma or surgery but may also have spontaneous bleeding.

History

Assessment of children with suspected or known bleeding diathesis begins with a complete history. A summary of important points in the history of children with a bleeding disorder is presented in Table 13–13. The nature of the bleeding should be explored, with particular attention to location, duration, and frequency and the measures necessary to stop it. A previous history of bleeding associated with events such as trauma or surgery, dental extraction, circumcision, appendectomy, and tonsillectomy is also important. Inquiry should be made into a history of rash (petechial) or arthritis, with hemarthrosis, and of blood transfusion. The first episode of bleeding should be documented, and a careful history of bruising during the toddler age is important. In girls, the duration and severity of menstrual bleeding should be documented.

A family history and pedigree are crucial, as many bleeding disorders are hereditary (see Chap. 5). The history should also address the use of over-the-counter and

Table 13–13. Obtaining a Bleeding History

Medical history
  Spontaneous bleeding
    Age of onset
    Bruising, petechiae (location)
    Joint bleeding, muscle bleeding
    Mucous membrane bleeding (epistaxis)
  Induced bleeding
    Injuries
      Duration of bleeding, nature of injuries
      Wound healing
      History of transfusions
    Surgical procedures
      Circumcision
      Tonsillectomy and adenoidectomy
      Dental work
      Appendectomy
  Menstrual history (duration and amount)
  Medications (over-the-counter, prescription, aspirin)

Family history
  Known bleeding diathesis
  Excessive hemorrhage after childbirth
  Gender of affected members
  Prepare family tree

prescription drugs that can induce bleeding. The most common offender is aspirin; it is important to ask patients specifically about the use of medications for colds, sinus trouble, muscle aches, or headaches, as these drugs may contain aspirin. Some antibiotics, penicillin in particular, can affect platelet function or be associated with specific inhibitors of clotting. Anticonvulsants can cause thrombocytopenia, and procainamide has been associated with an acquired lupus anticoagulant.

Physical Examination

In addition to the routine examination, the skin should be scrutinized carefully for petechiae, purpura, and venous telangiectasias. The joints should be examined for swelling or chronic changes, such as contractures or distorted appearance with asymmetry related to repeated bleeding episodes. Mucosal surfaces, such as the gingiva and nares, should be examined for bleeding.

Laboratory Evaluation

An attempt should be made to classify the bleeding abnormality as related to primary or secondary hemostasis. The following tests provide most of the information needed to make a laboratory diagnosis of a bleeding diathesis: examination of the peripheral smear, platelet count, bleeding time, prothrombin time (PT), partial thrombo-

plastin time (PTT), and thrombin time (TT). Confirmatory tests include specific coagulation factor assays, fibrin degradation products, fragment F1.2, fibrinogen, inhibitor assays, and multimeric analysis of the factor VIII complex. The laboratory evaluation of children with bleeding is presented in Figure 13–12.

The peripheral smear should be examined for morphology and number of platelets. It can also provide evidence of microangiopathic hemolytic anemia. The bleeding time is the single best test for evaluating primary hemostasis, as it requires a normal platelet count and normal platelet function in addition to normal vascular integrity. Patients with abnormal bleeding times may be thrombocytopenic, have qualitative platelet abnormalities (inherited or acquired), or have VWD. If bleeding time is abnormal, further studies include platelet aggregation studies and quantification of the components of the factor VIII complex (factor VIII:Ag, factor VIII:C, and factor VIII:RCoF). The bleeding time is not determined in patients with platelet counts less than 50,000/μL, as it is expected to be abnormal.

Measurement of PT evaluates the extrinsic system of secondary hemostasis (factors VII, X, V, II, and fibrinogen). Factor VII is unique to the extrinsic system, and PT is prolonged with a normal PTT in isolated factor VII deficiency. Factor VII is the first coagulation factor to be affected by oral anticoagulants, so PT is an excellent test for monitoring oral anticoagulant therapy. Deficiencies in factors VII, X, V, II (prothrombin), or fibrinogen cause a prolongation of PT.

The PTT assesses the integrity of the intrinsic system of coagulation. For PTT to be normal, the coagulation factors involved need to be present with at least 30% activity. Patients with a normal PT but an abnormally elevated PTT typically have deficiencies of the factors unique to the intrinsic system (factors XII, XI, VIII, and IX, Fletcher factor, and Fitzgerald factor). Patients with the lupus anticoagulant can also have a normal PT but a prolonged PTT. Partial thromboplastin time is widely used for monitoring heparin therapy, and a time 1.5 to 2.5 times longer than the upper limit of the normal range is desired for heparinization.

Thrombin time is abnormal when the plasma level of fibrinogen is decreased, when the fibrinogen is dysfunctional (hereditary or acquired), or when there are circulating anticoagulants (heparin) or fibrin degradation products. A modified thrombin test, because of its extreme sensitivity to heparin, is frequently used as a control for heparin contamination in assessing the coagulation status of patients.

In the approach to patients with prolonged PTTs, a circulating anticoagulant should be considered as the cause. To evaluate for an inhibitor, a 1 : 1 mixture of the patient's plasma and normal pooled plasma is prepared, and the PTT repeated. If the PTT is not corrected, the

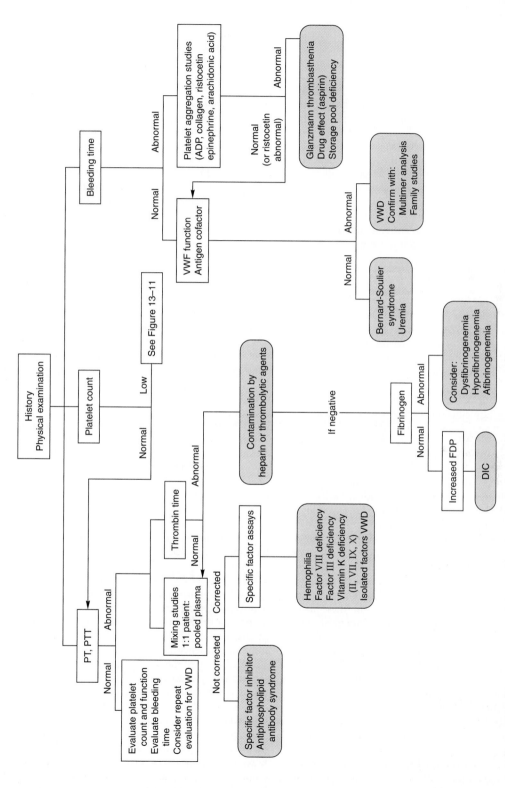

Figure 13–12. Algorithm diagramming the laboratory evaluation of children with bleeding. ADP = adenosine diphosphate; DIC = disseminated intravascular coagulation; FDP = fibrin degradation products; PT = prothrombin time; PTT = partial prothrombin time; VWD = von Willebrand disease; VWF = von Willebrand factor.

presence of an inhibitor can be assumed. If the PTT corrects, a deficiency of one or more coagulation factors probably exists, and specific factor assays should be performed. Some inhibitors are time dependent, such as factor VIII, and an incubation period before the PTT can assist in the diagnosis. The most frequent inhibitor encountered is heparin, and the second most frequent is the lupus anticoagulant. This inhibitor is present in 10% of patients with systemic lupus erythematosus, but lupus anticoagulant is common in patients with no evidence of underlying collagen vascular disease. Paradoxically, this anticoagulant is associated with clinical thrombosis rather than hemorrhage in up to 30% of patients. Therefore, an attempt to identify the nature of the anticoagulant is important. The anticardiolipin antibody test and lupus anticoagulant test can help with this distinction.

Inherited Bleeding Diatheses

VON WILLEBRAND DISEASE

Von Willebrand disease is a common, heterogeneous disorder of a thoroughly characterized GP called von Willebrand factor. This GP is responsible for the adherence of platelets to damaged endothelium and for the transport of factor VIII in the circulation. Von Willebrand disease is usually inherited in an autosomal codominant manner, but at least two variants of this disorder have been recognized: a rare autosomal recessive form and an X-linked recessive type. The heterogeneity results from a variety of genetic defects, ranging from congenital absence of the von Willebrand protein to major dysproteinemias in which the molecular structure is abnormal. Von Willebrand factor is a large multimeric GP that is synthesized in megakaryocytes and endothelial cells. The activation of either endothelial cells or platelets at local sites results in a greatly increased local concentration of von Willebrand factor, thereby facilitating normal hemostasis. Desmopressin (DDAVP) can induce the release of von Willebrand factor from storage sites in the platelets and increase plasma levels in those whose levels were previously decreased. Once the von Willebrand factor causes the platelets to adhere via its GP Ib receptor, these platelets are activated, with subsequent recruitment of more platelets and platelet plug formation. Absence of von Willebrand factor leads to insufficient formation of both the platelet plug and fibrin clot. Von Willebrand factor also serves as a carrier protein for the plasma factor VIII molecule, and deficiency of this factor also results in a secondary deficiency of factor VIII. Infusion of plasma from patients deficient in factor VIII causes an increase in the factor VIII level in patients with VWD because hemophiliac plasma contains von Willebrand factor.

The clinical picture is variable, depending on whether the defect is a quantitative or qualitative deficiency of the von Willebrand factor. Males and females are similarly affected, and symptoms can be mild or as severe as hemophilia. There are several subtypes, categorized on the basis of factor VIII levels (antigen, ristocetin cofactor, and von Willebrand factor) and multimer structure. Those affected with VWD have mucocutaneous bleeding and post-traumatic and postsurgical bleeding. VWD should be suspected in the patient with platelet-type bleeding and a family history of a bleeding diathesis. The laboratory evaluation is summarized in Figure 13–12.

Treatment of VWD requires knowledge of the clinical subtype. Desmopressin is the treatment of choice in mild type I disease (the most common form) and may be of benefit with some of the other variants. Desmopressin is contraindicated in certain variants (type IIB), however, as it may cause thrombocytopenia due to platelet activation and may fail to generate a therapeutic response. A therapeutic trial of desmopressin is usually given with measurement of the bleeding time, PTT, and factor VIII levels before and after administration. A standard dose of 0.3 µg/kg is administered intravenously over 15 to 30 min, and follow-up studies are done 30 to 60 min after the infusion is completed. Patients who have severe VWD or the type IIB variant, or who are unresponsive to the desmopressin challenge, require replacement of von Willebrand factor from plasma-derived sources for bleeding episodes. Currently, no genetically engineered products are available. Humate P, a commonly used concentrate, has normal multimeric structure of von Willebrand factor and nearly normal levels of the protein. Treatment with factor concentrate is based on attaining a factor VIII level of 30 to 50%, with 1 IU/kg body weight of von Willebrand factor required to increase the plasma level by 2 IU/dL. If treatment is required for a prolonged period (e.g., after trauma or surgery), treatment with desmopressin can result in tachyphylaxis and is therefore alternated with factor concentrate. Antifibrinolytics, such as epsilon amino caproic acid, are often used for oral bleeding and as an adjunct to therapy with dental surgery.

HEMOPHILIA A, FACTOR VIII DEFICIENCY

Classic hemophilia, or hemophilia A, is the most common hereditary clotting factor deficiency. The recessive gene is located on the X chromosome and linked closely to the genes for color blindness and G6PD. The disorder results from the deficiency of factor VIII antigen (factor VIII:Ag), a small subunit of the factor VIII molecule. Female carriers are usually unaffected, and the disease is seen almost exclusively in the male population.

Clinically, the first indication that a bleeding disorder is present may be from hemorrhage after circumcision or separation of the umbilical cord. A number of affected male infants have no difficulty during the neonatal period, however, and a negative history of bleeding after circumcision does not rule out the diagnosis of hemophilia. Mild hemophilia may go unsuspected for years until patients experience trauma or have surgical procedures. Hemorrhage can occur spontaneously and be internal or external. Large hematomas can result in secondary conditions, such as hemarthrosis, disability, and joint degeneration. Significant blood loss can occur with muscular bleeds, and the leading cause of death is intracranial hemorrhage.

The diagnosis of factor VIII deficiency should be suspected in males with bleeding characteristic of factor deficiency, a family history of males with bleeding diatheses, and abnormal clotting studies (prolonged PTT). It can be confirmed by specific factor assays. The clinical severity range depends on the level of factor VIII present. Patients with mild hemophilia (factor VIII level, 10 to 30%) may experience bleeding only with surgery or trauma. Moderate hemophilia (factor VIII level, 2 to 10%) can be associated with severe hemorrhage after trauma, or occasionally with spontaneous hemorrhage. Spontaneous joint and soft tissue bleeding is characteristic of severe hemophilia (factor VIII level, 0 to 1%).

Treatment of patients with hemophilia and bleeding is by replacement of factor in a concentrated form. Many preparations are available, including recombinant products. Duration, frequency, and dosages of the treatments depend on the severity of the hemophilia and bleeding episode. Studies are being conducted on gene replacement therapy for Factor VIII.

In all children with hemophilia, in addition to replacement of appropriate factor levels when bleeding has occurred and use of physical therapy programs to prevent or minimize chronic joint disease, comprehensive medical care must be given. Immunizations to prevent hepatitis B should be given as soon as possible after birth; appropriate consideration and screening procedures for HIV, prophylactic dental care, and aggressive management of hemarthrosis are required. Emotional support is essential to assist patients and families in coping with the emotional and social burden imposed by the disease. Prevention of chronic joint complications is crucial for the health and well-being of patients with hemophilia, and home care treatment should be used when possible.

Unfortunately, in approximately 10% of patients with severe hemophilia, antibody develops to administered concentrate containing the specific factor required for treatment. This prevents response to therapy and requires specific steps, such as consideration of immunosuppressive therapy, exchange transfusion, administration of prothrombin complex, and, in most cases, administration of sufficient factor product to block circulating antibody and still provide procoagulant activity.

HEMOPHILIA B, FACTOR IX DEFICIENCY

Factor IX deficiency is inherited as an X-linked recessive trait and is much less common than is factor VIII deficiency, accounting for 12% of all patients with hemophilia. The clinical findings and initial evaluation are similar to factor VIII deficiency, although factor IX deficiency can be milder. Treatment of acute bleeding episodes is with specific factor concentrate. During the initial evaluation of bleeding patients, if the identity of the specific coagulation factor deficiency has not been made, fresh-frozen plasma can be used to stop hemorrhage, as it contains all of the clotting factors. Attempts at gene replacement have yielded some promising preliminary results.

HEMOPHILIA C, FACTOR XI DEFICIENCY

Factor XI deficiency, a coagulation defect, is transmitted as an autosomal recessive trait and occurs in both sexes, primarily in patients of Jewish ancestry. The homozygotes can have severe factor XI deficiency although the clinical manifestations are milder than those in patients with factor VIII or IX deficiency. Bleeding episodes can be managed by infusion of 10 mL/kg of fresh-frozen plasma.

FACTOR XIII DEFICIENCY (FIBRIN-STABILIZING FACTOR)

Factor XIII deficiency, a coagulation abnormality, is unique in that patients bleed soon after birth similar to the types seen with classical hemophilia. Standard laboratory assays such as PT, PTT, and TT, however, are normal. A high index of suspicion is essential to establish the diagnosis, which can be accomplished by determining the solubility of the patients' clots in 5-M urea. Normal clots are insoluble because of the action of fibrin-stabilizing factor. Clots from patients with this deficiency are readily dissolved. The disorder can be treated with plasma infusions.

OTHER RARE COAGULATION ABNORMALITIES

a_2-Antiplasmin deficiency, factor XII deficiency, prekallikrein deficiency (Fletcher factor), high-molecular-weight kininogen (Fitzgerald factor) deficiency, hereditary afibrinogenemia or dysfibrinogenemia, and deficiencies of isolated prothrombin as well as factors V, VII, and X have all been identified using appropriate clotting measurements. Prekallikrein deficiency, high-molecular-weight kininogen deficiency, and factor XII deficiency all cause laboratory abnormalities but are not associated with clinical hemorrhage.

Evaluation and Management of Children with Thrombophilia

Venous thromboembolism has been recognized as a rapidly increasing secondary complication in children treated for serious, life-threatening, primary diseases. There is still limited information on the relative importance of congenital and acquired risk factors, appropriate diagnostic tests and optimal use of antithrombotic agents for the prevention and treatment of venous thromboembolism. Most recommendations are extrapolated from adult trials, but optimal prevention and treatment in pediatric patients may differ for several reasons. These include physiologic age-dependent differences in the hemostatic system that influence the risk for venous thromboembolism, differing underlying etiologies and location of clots, and differing responses to antithrombotic agents.

Patients with a tendency to thrombosis are defined as having thrombophilia. Thrombophilia is usually suspected in patients with one or more of the following clinical features: idiopathic thrombosis, thrombosis at a young age, family history, recurrent thrombosis, or thrombosis at an unusual site. The incidence of venous thromboembolism is estimated at 53/100,000 hospitalized children and 240/100,000 hospitalized neonates. The greatest risk for thrombosis is in infancy and the teen years, usually in association with acquired prothrombotic conditions.

The single most common acquired risk factor for venous thromboembolism is the presence of a central venous catheter. Other acquired risk factors include trauma, surgery, nephrotic syndrome, diabetes, inflammatory bowel disease, collagen vascular disease and malignancy (acute leukemia in association with the use of L-Asparaginase).

Children may develop thrombosis in any vein. The most common sites are the large proximal veins of the upper and lower extremities. Unusual sites for thrombosis include renal vein, portal vein and pulmonary vessels. Many clots are related to the presence of central venous catheters, which are primarily located in the upper venous system. Symptoms of thrombosis include failure to aspirate blood or flush the line, swelling, pain, superior vena cava syndrome, chylothorax, recurrent bacteremia, and pulmonary embolus. Chronic thrombosis can result in development of collateral circulation in the neck, chest, arm, and abdomen.

Several variables affect the incidence of central venous catheter related deep venous thrombosis, such as the presence of an underlying disease, damage to the vessel wall with insertion, use of large catheters in small veins, duration of use, and injection of potentially thrombogenic substances (such as blood products or hyperalimentation). Many clots are asymptomatic. The frequency of reported thrombosis may relate to the sensitivity of the radiographic method for screening or evaluation.

There are several congenital and acquired prothrombotic disorders that are linked to thromboembolism during childhood. The most well characterized are the deficiencies in the naturally occurring anticoagulants anti-thrombin III (AT III), protein C and protein S. These deficiencies may be genetic or acquired, such as in consumptive processes DIC, clots, hemorrhage, inflammatory states, and use of oral anticoagulants. Two surprisingly common, genetic prothrombotic conditions are the Factor V Leiden gene mutation and the prothrombin gene mutation. The factor V Leiden mutation is a result of a single point mutation resulting in the activated pro-

coagulant Factors V and VIII becoming more resistant to inactivation by protein C. This mutation is now believed to be the most common inherited risk factor for development of venous thromboembolism. Another cause of activated protein C resistance is inheritance of a prothrombin gene mutation. This is recognized as the second most common inherited defect linked to venous thromboembolism in adults. This abnormality in children has also been reported but requires further study. Other hereditary deficiencies causing thrombosis are hypofibrinogenemia, dysfibrinogenemia, homocystinuria (often seen with methylene tetrahydrofolate reductase deficiency), and heparin cofactor II deficiency. Hypofibrinogenemia may be acquired secondary to consumptive states or decreased production, such as seen with the used of L-asparaginase in the treatment of acute lymphocytic leukemia (Table 13–14).

EVALUATION OF CHILDREN WITH THROMBOSIS

An algorithm for evaluation of children with venous thromboembolism is shown in Figure 13–13.

The evaluation begins by obtaining a complete medical history. The assessment should consider the presence of prothrombotic stimuli such as trauma, surgery, immobilization, presence of a catheter, and any underlying medical or inflammatory condition. The medication history should be reviewed, including an inquiry about the use of estrogens or oral contraceptives. An extensive family history should include an assessment of family members with venous thromboembolism or known congenital thrombophilia.

The physical examination should include a careful assessment of the skin and any catheter sites. Patients may have subtle signs or symptoms, even with such conditions as pulmonary emboli, renal vein thrombosis, and portal vein thrombosis. Clinically, there may be pain, swelling, warmth, or erythema in the area of the clot. A clot in the "upper" venous syndrome may lead to signs of superior vena cava syndrome.

Table 13–14. Alterations of Coagulation Proteins Associated with a Prothrombotic State

Factor V Leiden mutation (activated protein C resistance)
Prothrombin gene 20210 gene mutation
Antithrombin III deficiency
Protein C deficiency
Protein S deficiency
Homocystinuria (methylene tetrahydrofolate reductase mutation)
Plasminogen deficiency
Dysfibrinogenemia/hypofibrinogenemia
Lupus anticoagulant

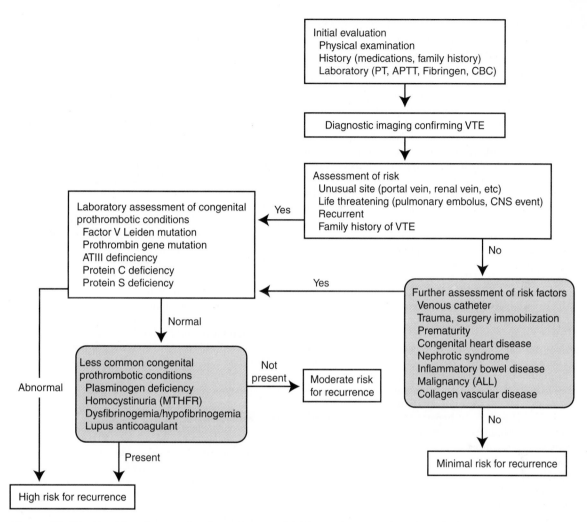

Figure 13–13. Algorithm diagramming the evaluation of children with venous thromboembolism. MTHFR = methylene tetrahydrofolate reductase mutation; VTE = venous thromboembolism.

The presence of a thrombus should be confirmed radiographically. Diagnostic methods include Doppler ultrasound, computed tomography, impedance plethysmography, venography, and magnetic resonance imaging.

GUIDELINES FOR ANTICOAGULATION THERAPY FOR VENOUS THROMBOEMBOLISM IN CHILDREN

The general principles of the treatment of thromboembolism incorporate heparin for treatment and prophylaxis. Additionally, acute events should be treated with a thrombolytic agent. *Acute events* are defined as events likely to have occurred within hours to 3 to 5 days. When thrombolytic therapy is initiated early, there is a good chance the clot will be completely lysed. The most commonly used thrombolytic agents are tissue plasminogen activator (t-PA) and urokinase. Tissue plasminogen activator should be given at a rate of 0.5 mg/kg/h IV for 6 h. Plasminogen levels should be monitored and replacement with FFP may be necessary. If urokinase is used, the standard dose is a loading dose of 4000 U/kg IV over 10 min followed by 4000 U/kg/h for 6h. Heparin (20 U/kg/h) should be given concomitantly with the thrombolytic agent. Careful monitoring of patients should be done. This includes laboratory assessment with PT, APTT, fibrinogen, and d-dimers prior to therapy and every 6 h. Fibrinogen, AT III, and plasminogen levels, in addition to the platelet count, should be checked prior to therapy and at least daily during the infusions as replacement may be necessary. Minor bleeding may occur (i.e., oozing from venipuncture sites) but major bleeding will necessitate termination of thrombolytic and heparin therapies. If needed, the fibrinolytic process can be reversed with aminocaproic acid (Amicar) given as a bolus in a dose of 100 mg/kg (maximum 5 g), then 30 mg/kg/h (maximum 1.25 g/h) until the bleeding stops. Protamine sulfate may be required to reverse the effect of heparin.

Standard heparin is part of the classic regimen for the treatment of acute venous thromboembolism. Heparin complexes to the physiologic inhibitor anti-thrombin III and accelerates the inhibition of thrombin and other coagulant proteins. It is therefore important to ensure adequate levels of AT III when administering heparin. There are several problems with the use of standard heparin in children. These include its rapid clearance, low ATIII levels in the first few months of life, greater variability in dosing compared to adults, and lack of clinical trials assessing the optimal target APTT range for the prevention and treatment of venous thromboembolism.

Heparin is given as a loading dose of 75 U/kg IV over 10 min, followed by a maintenance dose of 20 U/kg/h in children over 1 year of age and 25 U/kg/h in children under 1 year of age. It is given for a minimum of 5 days, up to 10 to 14 days for extensive deep venous thrombosis or pulmonary embolus. Laboratory monitoring may be done by determining anti-factor Xa levels (0.30 to 0.70 units/mL) or APTT levels (150% of normal). Complications of heparin therapy include bleeding, heparin-induced thrombocytopenia, and in long-term use, osteoporosis. Oral anticoagulation (Coumadin) should overlap 4 to 5 days with therapeutic INRs (2 to 3) on 2 successive days.

Low-molecular-weight heparin (LMWH) is a therapeutic option rapidly gaining popularity due to its ease of use and fewer complications, especially in children. The starting dose is 1 mg/kg every 12 h subcutaneously; infants may require higher doses. Anti-factor Xa levels are monitored and should be drawn 4 h after the injection, with a target range of 0.5 to 1.0 U/mL. Low-molecular-weight heparin can be used both in the acute therapeutic

regimen and as prophylaxis. It is considered to be a safe alternative to Coumadin for prophylaxis. Furthermore, LMWH does not require as frequent laboratory monitoring as does Coumadin.

The decision regarding who should received prophylactic anticoagulation, when, and for how long should be made after considering risk factors, family history, age at presentation, site of the clot (life-threatening), and documentation of a congenital defect predisposing to thrombophilia. Patients at the highest risk for thrombosis are those with recurrent clots and the presence of an on-going risk factor (see Fig. 13–13). These patients should receive anticoagulation indefinitely. Those at moderate risk are children with two or more idiopathic clots, young age, unusual site, familial carriers of known thrombophilic conditions, and a family history of clotting, or thromboembolism following a trivial provocation such as trauma, surgery, immobilization, or estrogen therapy. Prophylaxis in these patients should be limited to a defined risk period, usually 3 to 6 months, though if the event was life-threatening, there should be consideration for indefinite anticoagulation. The lowest risk patients are those with thromboembolism following no known provocation, with no family history, and no known thrombophilic condition. These patients should receive short-term prophylaxis (less than 3 months) following treatment for a venous thromboembolism.

REFERENCES

Andrew M, Monagle PT, Brooker L (editors): *Thromboembolic Complications during Infancy and Childhood.* B.C. Decker Inc., 2000.

Bain B (editor): *Blood Cells: A Practical Guide.* Lippincott, 1989.

Hoffman B, et al (editors): *Hematology: Basic Principles and Practice,* 3rd ed. Churchill Livingstone, 2000.

Mentzer WC, Wagner GM (editors): *The Hereditary Hemolytic Anemias.* Churchill Livingstone, 1989.

Nathan DG, Oski FA (editors): *Hematology of Infancy and Childhood,* 5th ed. Saunders, 1998.

Reid CD, et al (editors): *Management and Therapy of Sickle Cell Disease,* 3rd ed. National Institutes of Health, Bethesda, MD, 1995.

Cancer in Children

Daniel C. West, MD

Fortunately the occurrence of cancer in children is relatively uncommon and, when it does occur, it is usually treatable and potentially curable. Nevertheless, a practicing general pediatrician is likely to encounter children with cancer on many occasions and will often have the opportunity to assist in the management of these patients. This chapter is designed to provide a general overview of childhood cancer focusing on the basic principles of diagnosis and therapy of the most common childhood cancers. The chapter is organized according to the major problems in which one might consider cancer highly in the differential diagnosis. In addition, a discussion of the general principles of chemotherapy and the approach to the families of children with cancer is included.

ABNORMAL BLOOD CELL PRODUCTION

The most common childhood cancer in the developed world is acute leukemia, which accounts for 30% of cancer in children less than 15 years of age. It usually presents with manifestations of the abnormal proliferation of immature white blood cell precursors in the bone marrow leading to impaired hematopoiesis. The most common presenting sign of acute leukemia is pallor, secondary to decreased red blood cell production. Impaired production of normal white blood cells, especially phagocytic cells such as neutrophils and monocytes, can lead to fever and/or infection. A reduced number of megakaryocytes can result in thrombocytopenia and associated hemorrhage, such as petechiae or purpura in the skin. Bone pain, arthritis, and arthralgias, presumably secondary to bone marrow infiltration and expansion, are quite common and can present as irritability and refusal to bear weight or walk. Hepatosplenomegaly and lymphadenopathy from leukemic cell infiltration are commonly found on physical examination.

Typical laboratory findings in acute leukemia include thrombocytopenia, anemia, and an elevated white blood cell count (WBC) with a significant percentage of circulating leukoblasts (lymphoblasts or myeloblasts) in the peripheral blood. Serum markers of rapid cell turnover, such as lactic dehydrogenase (LDH) and uric acid, are frequently elevated as well. Often the laboratory findings are subtle, such as when children have an isolated cytopenia (one cell line decreased). In this situation, the differential diagnosis can include immune thrombocytopenic purpura (ITP), viral bone marrow suppression, or autoimmune disorders, such as autoimmune hemolytic anemia.

If acute leukemia is suspected, a bone marrow aspirate and biopsy is the critical diagnostic test. The diagnosis of acute leukemia requires the presence of immature myeloid or lymphoid blast cells in numbers equaling at least 25% of the total bone marrow cells. In most cases of childhood acute leukemia, the bone marrow findings are not subtle, with the normal bone marrow often almost completely replaced by leukemia cells. Acute lymphoblastic leukemia (ALL) accounts for 70 to 80% of acute leukemia, and acute myelogenous leukemia (AML) comprises the remaining 20 to 30%. Distinguishing between these two major classes of acute leukemia is not always easy, but it is critical because therapy and prognosis are very different. Children occasionally develop chronic leukemias, but this is rare and almost always in the form of chronic myelogenous leukemia (CML). Chronic leukemias will not be discussed in this chapter.

Acute Lymphoblastic Leukemia

Thirty-five years ago, children diagnosed with ALL almost always died of the disease. Today, about 70% of children with ALL are cured and are expected to live relatively normal and productive lives. This tremendous progress is due to large, successive clinical trials involving multiple centers that have systematically compared therapies. These studies serve as a testimony to what can be achieved through well-organized clinical research.

EPIDEMIOLOGY AND ETIOLOGY

The annual incidence of ALL in the United States is between 3 to 4 cases per 100,000 children less than 15 years of age, and, overall ALL accounts for 25% of all childhood cancer. The incidence peaks between 3 to 4 years of age, and evidence points to a 1.6% annual increase (20% cumulative) in incidence from 1974 to 1991. The reason for this rising incidence is unknown, but some speculate that unknown environmental exposures are to blame. Acute lymphoblastic leukemia occurs more often in boys (1.2:1) and in Caucasians as compared with African-Americans (1.8:1).

With rare exception, the specific cause of ALL in any particular individual is unknown. However, there are several well-known constitutional genetic syndromes linked to an increased risk of developing ALL, such as Down syndrome, neurofibromatosis, and ataxia-telangectasia. Numerous potential environmental factors have also been implicated but not confirmed, such as exposure to tobacco smoke, marijuana, pesticides, ionizing radiation, and electromagnetic fields. Other implicated risk factors include advanced maternal age, high socioeconomic status, parental occupational exposures, high birth weight, and first-born status. Infections, especially viral infections, have been suspected to cause acute leukemia; however, the only known infectious causative agent is the adult T-cell leukemia virus, which primarily occurs in Japan. Cancer family syndromes have been described in which family members carry a germline gene mutation that makes them more likely to develop leukemia. An example of this is the Li-Fraumani syndrome in which affected individuals carry a mutation in the p53 gene (the protein product of which is important in regulating the cell cycle).

PATHOLOGY AND BIOLOGY

In general, ALL arises from a monoclonal proliferation of immature lymphocytes, either B-cell or T-cell precursors. The typical microscopic appearance of ALL is sheets of monotonous small round cells with a large nucleus with fine (not clumped) nuclear chromatin and a thin rim of cytoplasm. These "blast" cells replace most, if not all, of the normal bone marrow hematopoietic cells. While the lymphoblast of ALL usually has a very characteristic microscopic appearance, distinguishing it from AML on the basis of morphology alone is unreliable. Therefore, additional histochemical stains are performed that are relatively specific for certain types of leukemia. For example, ALL usually stains positively for periodic acid-Schiff (PAS), while AML is often positive for myeloperoxidase or nonspecific esterase (NSE). The classic diagnostic criteria for ALL relies on cell morphology coupled with histochemical staining patterns. This information is often, but not always, adequate to make the diagnosis.

Because most leukemia cells share some features with the normal hematopoietic precursor cells from which they originate, it is usually possible and, in fact, useful to classify them according to their cell of origin. This is accomplished by establishing the leukemia cell's surface antigen expression pattern using a panel of antibodies and comparing that with expression patterns normally seen during B- or T-lymphocyte development. Although this can be done using immunohistochemical stains of bone marrow biopsy sections, it is best accomplished using flow cytometry on a bone marrow aspirate cell suspension sample. At least two different lineage specific antigens should be detected in order to classify confidently a leukemia cell in a given lineage. For example, B-precursor ALL usually expresses immature B-cell markers, such as CD10 (CALLA) and CD19 (B4), while T-cell ALL would express some combination of CD5, CD3, CD4, or CD8.

Surface marker expression can also differentiate between ALL and AML, because AML expresses myeloid markers, such as CD13 (My7) and CD33 (My9). In situations where the diagnosis is not clear from morphology and histochemical stains alone, establishing the cell surface expression pattern can be invaluable.

Acute lymphoblastic leukemia often demonstrates relatively specific chromosomal abnormalities that can be detected by cytogenetic analysis of bone marrow aspirate material. Numerous cytogenetic abnormalities in ALL have been described and many of the genes involved in these rearrangements identified, but a detailed discussion of these is beyond the scope of this chapter. However, the t(9;22)(q34;q11) and the t(4;11)(q21;q23) are particularly noteworthy since they are associated with forms of ALL that are particularly difficult to successfully treat. In addition to providing some prognostic information, chromosomal abnormalities can sometimes provide important diagnostic information, especially in particularly difficult and ambiguous cases. Thus, the diagnosis of ALL usually involves the assimilation of data from morphologic appearance, histochemical staining pattern, surface antigen expression, and cytogenetic abnormalities.

CLINICAL PRESENTATION

While there are many clinical features previously described that are common to both ALL and AML, adenopathy, organomegaly, bone pain, arthralgias, and arthritis are more typically characteristic of ALL. In addition, the T-cell form of ALL often presents with a very high WBC, hyperuricemia, and massive lymphadenopathy, including an anterior mediastinal mass (enlarged thymus). All patients with a suspected diagnosis of ALL should have a chest radiograph to rule out an anterior mediastinal mass, since its presence places them at risk for airway obstruction.

TREATMENT

Modern treatment for ALL usually consists of four basic elements: remission induction, intensification and consolidation, maintenance or continuation therapy, and central nervous system (CNS) therapy. With the notable exception of mature B-cell ALL, the treatment of B-precursor and T-cell ALL requires a prolonged course of therapy ranging from 2 to 3 years. The basic principle of therapy is to use combinations of chemotherapy designed to prevent the emergence of drug-resistant leukemia cells.

Several factors related to patients' clinical presentations carry prognostic significance, and the therapeutic plans are usually adjusted to take these into account. The two most important factors are a patient's age and initial WBC. Patients with a high WBC (>50,000 cells/mm³) and children younger than 1 year or older than 10 years of age at the time of diagnosis have the worst prognosis. Children with T-cell ALL and those with certain chromosomal abnormalities, such as t(9;22)(q34;q11) or t(4;11)(q21;q23), are also at higher risk for relapse. Therefore, a typical standard risk patient would be a child between 1 to 10 years of age with B-precursor ALL presenting with a WBC <50,000 cells/mm³. Specific therapeutic alterations are used for high-risk patients such as infants, children with T-cell ALL, and those with ALL carrying a cytogenetic abnormality known to be associated with a poor prognosis.

The goal of induction therapy is to achieve a remission, which is defined as the absence of overt disease based on a normal physical exam (e.g., resolution of adenopathy or organomegaly), the presence of normal peripheral blood cell counts, and no evidence of leukemia on examination of the bone marrow (<5% blasts) and cerebrospinal fluid. With appropriate therapy, one can expect about 98% of patients to achieve a complete remission within 4 weeks of starting therapy. Typical induction chemotherapy includes systemic treatment with vincristine, glucocorticoids (prednisone or dexamethasone), and L-asparaginase, as well as CNS treatment with methotrexate, cytarabine, and hydrocortisone delivered directly into the cerebrospinal fluid. Additional induction drugs, such as the anthracyclines (doxorubicin or daunomycin), are often added to the regimen of high-risk patients, since there is evidence that early intensive therapy can improve the outcome of these patients.

Remission induction is usually followed by a period of consolidation and/or intensification therapy. The intent of this phase is to "consolidate" the gains of remission by further eliminating remaining leukemia cells with different drugs or higher doses of previously delivered drugs. A typical approach in this phase of treatment is to prescribe several cycles of high dose methotrexate or intermittent pulses of L-asparaginase and doxorubicin. Such intensification and consolidation regimens have been credited with improving the outcome of high-risk patients, especially those with T-cell disease.

Once the consolidation and intensification phase is completed, all patients must move on to some form of maintenance or continuation therapy. Typical maintenance therapy includes combinations of weekly methotrexate and daily 6-mercaptopurine with intermittent pulses of vincristine and prednisone to complete a total of 2–3 years of therapy.

Effective treatment of the CNS is necessary for long-term survival. The CNS is a well-known sanctuary site for leukemia cells and without specific treatment directed to this area almost all patients would eventually suffer a relapse there. Leukemia in the CNS can be treated with irradiation, intrathecal chemotherapy, and high-dose systemic therapy, alone or in various combinations. As one might guess, cranial irradiation, especially in the growing and developing brain of young children, is associated with significant morbidity, such as short stature, developmental delay, and learning disabilities. In addition, there is an increased risk of developing a secondary malignancy, such as brain tumors. For these reasons, recent clinical trials have focused on replacing radiation with intrathecal chemotherapy consisting of methotrexate/cytosine arabinoside/hydrocortisone and high doses of systemic chemotherapy (such as high-dose methotrexate). Most treatment protocols now limit CNS irradiation to the highest risk patients, such as those with overt CNS leukemia, T-cell ALL, high initial WBC, or adverse chromosomal markers.

While there is no doubt that the treatment of ALL is a long and difficult road to travel, the trip is worth it. Results from clinical trials indicate that approximately 70% of children diagnosed with ALL today can expect to be cured of their disease. Children in the lowest risk groups (e.g., age 1 to 10 years, WBC <50,000 cells/mm³, and B-precursor disease) have an even better prognosis. Clinical trials are focusing on improving methods of identifying patients at the highest risk for relapse and developing more effective therapy for those patients, as well as minimizing treatment toxicity for patients with the best prognosis.

RELAPSE

Unfortunately, the initial therapy in some children will be unsuccessful and they will suffer a relapse of ALL. The most common site of relapse is the bone marrow, usually manifested by the reappearance of leukemia blast cells on the peripheral blood smear. Relapse can also occur in extramedullary sites such as the CNS (as indicated by the presence of leukemia blast cells on examination of the cerebrospinal fluid) or in the testes (presenting as a diffuse enlargement or an isolated palpable testicular mass). An ALL relapse can present in any one or all of these sites and an isolated extramedullary relapse usually indicates an impending bone marrow relapse. The prognosis after relapse depends on the timing of relapse. Children relapsing after 2 years of complete remission (late relapse) have an intermediate prognosis when treated with additional conventional chemotherapy, while those relapsing before 2 years (early relapse) have a poor prognosis despite therapy. Numerous investigators have explored the role of bone marrow transplantation (either autologous or allogeneic) in the treatment of relapsed ALL. Current data indicate that there is probably no advantage to using bone marrow transplantation instead of conventional chemotherapy in late-relapsing patients. However, for those children who relapse early, most oncologists would suggest some form of bone marrow transplantation. In any case, the prognosis for early-relapsing patients is poor, presumably because the leukemia cells are drug resistant.

Acute Myelogenous Leukemia

Acute myelogenous leukemia (AML), also referred to as acute nonlymphocytic leukemia (ANLL), is a heterogeneous group of disorders in which there is a clonal proliferation of hematopoeitic (other than lymphocytic) precursor cells. This proliferation appears to result from a maturation arrest in the normal differentiation pathway of the affected cell type and can occur at any point in hematopoeisis from the pluripotent stem cell to a committed stem cell or precursor cell. The molecular mechanisms that lead to the development of AML is an area of active investigation in many research laboratories but will not be further discussed in this chapter.

EPIDEMIOLOGY AND ETIOLOGY

Acute myelogenous leukemia accounts for approximately 20 to 25% of childhood leukemia and about 5% of childhood cancer. In contrast to ALL, the incidence of AML is constant through the first 10 years of life, with a slight peak in adolescence. The incidence then remains steady until around 55 years of age when it progressively increases.

While the cause of AML is unknown, there are several known acquired and congenital risk factors. For example, the occurrence of AML is more frequent in children with underlying disorders of DNA repair such as Fanconi anemia syndrome and Bloom syndrome. In addition, children with congenital disorders of hematopoiesis such as Kostmann syndrome (congenital neutropenia), Diamond-Blackfan anemia, and dyskarytosis congenitae have an increased risk of developing AML. Children with acquired disorders of hematopoiesis, such as myelodysplastic syndromes, myeloproliferative disorders, or aplastic anemia, are also at great risk of progressing to overt AML. There can be a significant risk of developing a second malignant neoplasm with AML many years after treatment with chemotherapy or radiation for other forms of cancer. This risk is greatest in patients who received high doses of alkylating agents (e.g., cyclophosphamide and nitrogen mustard) or drugs that inhibit DNA repair such as topoisomerase inhibitors (e.g., etoposide).

There are certain genetic syndromes that also are associated with the development of AML. Down syndrome, or trisomy 21, is associated with a greatly (>15 times) increased risk of developing acute leukemia. In the first few years of life this leukemia is more likely to be AML, but later the ratio of ALL to AML mirrors that seen in normal children. A fascinating association of AML with neurofibromatosis type I has been described, particularly arising after myelodysplastic syndromes and myeloproliferative disorders. There is evidence that the *NF-1* gene functions as a tumor suppressor in this situation.

Despite the numerous known disorders and predisposing factors associated with the development of AML, much remains to be learned about the true cause. The majority of children who develop AML have no known predisposing condition.

PATHOLOGY AND CLASSIFICATION

The diagnosis of AML is made by finding at least 25% of leukemia blasts cells in the bone marrow on light microscopy. The differential diagnosis is usually quite limited although there can be situations that can represent diagnostic challenges. For example, newborns with Down syndrome can develop a transient myeloproliferative disorder, or leukamoid reaction, that is virtually indistinguishable from AML. Myeloproliferative disorders, such as juvenile chronic myelogenous leukemia or myelodysplastic syndromes, can sometimes also cause diagnostic confusion; however, the skilled morphologist usually can tell the difference.

Cell morphology, histochemical stains, cell surface antigens, cytogenetic abnormalities, and gene rearrangements are all used in the classification of AML. Several years ago the French-American-British (FAB) cooperative group classified AML into subtypes based on morphology and histochemical staining patterns. The subtypes along with key distinguishing features are shown in Table 14–1. M0 is the most undifferentiated leukemia and is usually negative for the typical histochemical markers of AML. Increasing degrees of myeloid maturation are seen in M1, M2, and M3 subtypes. M4 represents a leukemia cell that demonstrates both myeloid and monocytic differentiation, while M5 is a pure monocytic leukemia. M6 represents a malignant clone of the erythroblast (red blood cell precursor), and M7 is a megakaryoblastic leukemia (platelet precursor). Myeloperoxidase is a useful histo-

Table 14–1. The French-American-British (FAB) Classification System for Acute Myelogenous Leukemia

FAB Type	Definition	Key Features
M1	Myeloblastic without differentiation	Undifferentiated blasts, MPO+/−
M2	Myeloblastic with differentiation	Blasts with granules, MPO+
M3	Promyelocytic	Abundant granules and auer rods, MPO+
M4	Myelomonocytic	Mix of myelocytic and monocytic, MPO+, NSE+
M5	Monocytic	Monoblast morphology, NSE+
M6	Erythroblastic	Large erythroid appearing blasts, PAS+
M7	Megakaryoblastic	Large blasts with cytoplasmic blebs, gpIIB/IIIA+

gp = glycoprotein; MPO = myeloperoxidase; NSE = nonspecific esterase; PAS = periodic acid-Schiff stain.

chemical stain for identifying myeloid leukemias, whereas nonspecific esterase (NSE) is positive in monocytic leukemia. There is no specific histochemical stain for erythroid leukemia, although these tumors stain strongly with PAS. (ALL and many other childhood cancers stain positively for PAS as well.) The definitive diagnosis of M7 leukemia requires the detection of platelet peroxidase by electron microscopy or reactivity with specific monoclonal antibodies directed against platelet surface antigens, such as glycoprotein IIB/IIIA.

As in ALL, determination of cell surface antigen expression patterns can sometimes be diagnostically useful in AML. Depending on the subtype, AML usually expresses cell surface markers typical of early myeloid precursors such as CD13 or CD33. There are many other surface antigens that are expressed in other forms of AML. The AML leukemia cells can also demonstrate coexpression of both myeloid and lymphoid antigens with these leukemias, sometimes referred to as mixed lineage AML (found in as many as 10 to 15% of cases).

Most cases of AML demonstrate chromosomal aberrations, which can provide useful clinical and biological information. Examples of the most common chromosomal abnormalities include t(8;21), t(15;17), inv 16, trisomy 8, and rearrangements of the chromosomal locus 11q23. Most of the genes involved in these and other chromosomal rearrangements have been cloned, and this information has enhanced the understanding of the biology of AML. One of these chromosomal abnormalities deserves special mention. The t(15;17)(q22;p11) rearrangement, which is seen in almost all cases of M3 AML, results in the fusion of the retinoic acid receptor (*RAR*) gene to the *PML* gene. The result is a specific genetic marker that can be used to detect submicroscopic levels of leukemia cells using polymerase chain reaction techniques. It is important to note that treatment of M3 AML cells with retinoic acid (the all trans form) induces leukemia cells to differentiate and is now an important treatment modality in such patients.

CLINICAL PRESENTATION

As noted earlier, the common presenting features of all acute leukemias include pallor, fatigue, fever, bleeding, bruising, petechiae, and purpura. Bone pain and arthralgias can occur, but are more characteristic of ALL than AML. Skin involvement (leukemia cutis) also can be seen, especially in infants with AML. Primary CNS AML is possible, but much less likely than it is in ALL. Some patients with very high WBC and most patients with M3 AML (acute promyelocytic leukemia) have disseminated intravascular coagulation (DIC). In the case of M3 AML, the DIC is due to the procoagulant activity in intracellular granules of the leukemia cells. Unlike those with ALL, children with AML who have WBCs greater than 100,000 cells/mm^3 are at risk for leukostasis when the white blood cells impair blood flow to vital organs. In the worse case, leukostasis results in stroke or multiorgan failure (especially pulmonary and renal), although such complications usually occur only when the WBC is greater than 200,000 cells/mm^3. Leukocytopheresis (removing white blood cells using an apheresis machine) plus the institution of chemotherapy is the treatment of choice in this situation.

TREATMENT

Therapy for AML usually begins by addressing any immediate life-threatening complications such as fever and infection, leukostasis, or bleeding from thrombocytopenia or DIC. The backbone of treatment is intensive systemic chemotherapy, with the goal of attaining a complete remission and reestablishing normal hematopoiesis within the first 30 days. Induction therapy consists of some combination of an anthracycline (usually daunorubicin) plus cytosine arabinoside (ara-C). Other drugs, such as 6-thioguanine (6-TG) or etoposide, are sometimes added, but clinical trials have shown that they offer no increase in remission rates as compared to the daunorubicin/ara-C combination alone. While CNS leukemia is much less common in AML than it is in ALL, it does occur, especially in the M4 and M5 subtypes; therefore, some specific CNS treatment is required. Patients usually receive intrathecal ara-C once or twice during induction and periodically throughout the remainder of therapy.

The chemotherapy necessary to induce remission for AML is more intensive than that used for ALL, and, accordingly, patients are at very high risk of developing life-threatening complications. Severe bone marrow suppression with prolonged neutropenia and thrombocytopenia is expected, and breakdown of mucosal surfaces (mucositis) is very common. Patients are supported through this phase with frequent red blood cell and platelet transfusions, and many require parenteral nutrition and pain management. Undoubtedly the most life-threatening risk is developing an infection with gram-negative bacteria or fungal organisms secondary to the prolonged period of neutropenia. Over 90% of patients will require prolonged administration of antibiotics, and many will need antifungal therapy as well. Current intensive induction regimens have achieved a remission rate of 80 to 85%. Some children will fail to achieve remission because their leukemia is resistant to chemotherapy, while a substantial percentage will die from complications of their therapy.

After remission is achieved, postremission therapy is necessary to maintain the remission, but long-term maintenance or continuation therapy, a fundamental principle in the treatment of ALL, is unnecessary. There are two possible choices for postremission therapy: several more courses of intensive chemotherapy similar to that given during induction or an allogeneic bone marrow transplant.

If patients have a complete HLA sibling match, then bone marrow transplant is the treatment of choice, since survival in children with AML is better with transplantation (the same is not true for adults with AML). If patients lack a complete match, then intensive chemotherapy, usually 6 courses given over 6 months, is appropriate. Typical drugs might include high doses of ara-C alone or in combination with etoposide or additional courses of daunomycin with etoposide.

Unfortunately, the prospects for long-term survival of children with AML are not as promising as are those with ALL. The overall survival for children with AML is about 40%, but if children achieve remission, the probability of survival increases to about 50% with intensive chemotherapy and close to 70% with bone marrow transplantation. As in ALL, there are certain clinical and biological characteristics of AML that are associated with good or bad outcomes. Those presenting with a high WBC (>100,000 cells/mm³), extramedullary disease (other than CNS disease), or who require more than one course of therapy to achieve complete remission tend not to do as well. In addition, AML arising from myelodysplastic syndrome or as a second malignant neoplasm is particularly difficult to treat successfully. The presence of monosomy 7 on cytogenetic analysis, which is often associated with myelodysplastic syndromes, is a poor prognostic sign. Favorable predictors include the presence of certain cytogenetic abnormalities, such as the t(15;17) in M3 AML, the t(8;21), and the inversion 16 chromosome usually seen in M4 AML. The FAB M1 AML subtype is also associated with a good outcome. For unknown reasons, children with Down syndrome who have AML have a favorable prognosis. All children with AML require intensive chemotherapy if they are to have any hope of survival, so information regarding prognosis is usually used to help decide whether to use intensive conventional chemotherapy or to choose more experimental and riskier forms of bone marrow transplantation.

When children with AML relapse, they usually do so within 2 years of diagnosis. It is possible to achieve a second remission after relapse, but it is usually short-lived. The treatment of choice once a second remission has been obtained is bone marrow transplantation using the best available donor. This may involve using matched unrelated donors through the bone marrow registry or even partially mismatched donors.

LYMPHADENOPATHY

The presence of persistent adenopathy in children can be a source of worry for both parents and primary care physicians alike. The differential diagnosis of lymphadenopathy in children is quite large; however, the overwhelming majority is due to infectious processes rather than cancer (see Chapter 9, "Infectious Diseases"). *Lymphadenopathy* is defined as a nontender lymph node greater than 10 mm in diameter. Exceptions include the epitrochlear area, where lymph nodes larger than 5 mm are considered abnormal, and the inguinal area, where a lymph node must be larger than 15 mm in diameter.

Lymphadenopathy, especially when it persists longer than 6 weeks, often raises the concern of cancer. It is sometimes difficult for the clinician to differentiate infectious from malignant lymphadenopathy, but several clues should raise one's suspicion of a malignancy. Although many of the systemic symptoms of infection are similar to those of a malignancy, in general, weight loss (greater than 10% of body weight), recurrent fever, malaise, bone pain, and bleeding (e.g., petechia, purpura, or epistaxis) should suggest a malignancy rather than a simple infectious process. On physical examination, matted nodes, particularly in the low cervical or supraclavicular regions, are more consistent with cancer. The lymphadenopathy associated with Hodgkin lymphoma (HL) and metastatic neuroblastoma or sarcoma, is characteristically hard, immobile, and localized; however, in the case of non-Hodgkin lymphoma (NHL) or leukemia, the lymph nodes can be rubbery, mobile, and more generalized. A key distinguishing feature is that cancer lymphadenopathy is not usually associated with tenderness, erythema, or warmth unless a secondary infection is present. Most lymphadenopathy associated with a viral process resolves without treatment within 2 to 6 weeks, while a bacterial adenitis requires antibiotic therapy.

An oncologist's approach to patients with persistent lymphadenopathy is diagrammed in Figure 14–1. Certain laboratory studies can often be helpful in either providing reassurance that all is well or in increasing the level of concern for cancer. Initial studies should include a complete blood cell count with differential looking for evidence of likely infection versus leukemia or bone marrow infiltration. Other important screening tests include markers of cell turnover, such as lactic dehydrogenase (LDH) and uric acid. If these are significantly elevated, cancer becomes a much more likely possibility. Although an erythrocyte sedimentation rate (ESR) is an indicator of inflammation, it is not particularly helpful in distinguishing cancer from an infectious process. A chest radiograph is potentially quite helpful, since the presence of significant mediastinal adenopathy, especially an anterior mediastinal mass, is very suggestive of a lymphoma or leukemia. A posterior mediastinal mass coupled with low cervical adenopathy suggests a diagnosis of neuroblastoma.

If the preceding screening tests suggest a low likelihood of malignancy, then simple observation or perhaps a trial of oral antibiotics is indicated. If the lymphadenopathy persists for greater than 6 weeks or the clinical signs and symptoms change (i.e., lymph nodes continue to enlarge) in a way that increases the likelihood of cancer, a fine-needle aspirate with cultures should be considered. How-

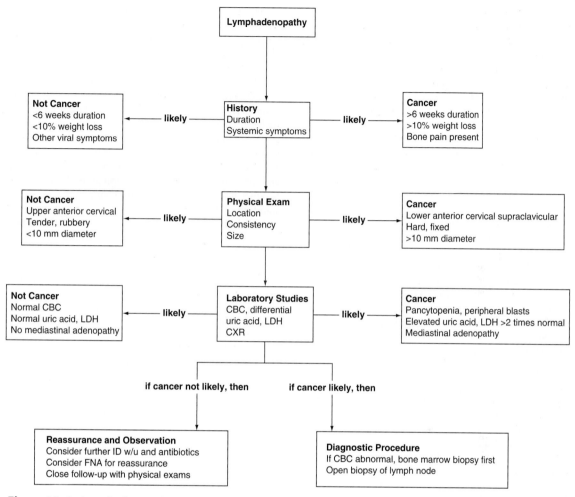

Figure 14–1. Lymphadenopathy in children. This diagram outlines the key features on history, physical examination, and laboratory studies that can be used to help differentiate cancer-associated lymphadenopathy from that of other causes. CBC = complete blood cell count; CXR = chest radiograph; FNA = fine-needle aspirate; ID = infectious disease; LDH = lactate dehydrogenase.

ever, if cancer seems likely, an open lymph node biopsy should be performed so that the lymph node architecture can be assessed and adequate tissue will be available for other diagnostic studies. Probably the most important rule to avoid missing adenopathy associated with malignancy is to take a very careful history and to follow the patient's status closely with repeated physical examinations.

Non-Hodgkin Lymphoma

Lymphomas are the third most common malignancy in children and adolescents after acute leukemias and brain tumors. As in adults there are two major types, HL and

NHL, and they collectively account for about 12 to 15% of childhood cancer.

EPIDEMIOLOGY AND ETIOLOGY

The NHLs account for approximately 60% of childhood lymphomas, with an annual incidence of 7.1 cases per million children. Males are affected more often than are females (3:1) with a peak age of incidence between 7 to 11 years. In the United States and Europe about 50% of NHLs are of the small noncleaved cell type (Burkitt lymphoma), 30% are lymphoblastic, and 20% are large cell, but this distribution can vary substantially in other regions of the world. For example, in equatorial

Africa, Burkitt lymphoma accounts for 50% of all child-hood cancer.

Children with congenital or acquired dysfunction of the immune system have a greater-than-expected risk of NHL. In particular, congenital disorders, such as ataxia-telangiectasia, Wiskott-Aldrich, Chédiak-Higashi, and Bloom syndromes, are associated with the development of NHL. Children receiving chronic immunosuppressive therapy after organ transplantation and those with AIDS also have an increased risk of NHL. The Epstein-Barr virus (EBV) is implicated in the development of ende-mic forms of Burkitt lymphoma in African children, but appears to be uninvolved in the sporadic forms seen in the United States.

PATHOLOGY AND BIOLOGY

Unlike NHL in adults, which has been classified into an overwhelming array of subtypes, NHL in children can essentially be classified in three histologic types, all of which are high-grade lymphomas. The three categories include lymphoblastic, small noncleaved cell (Burkitt and non-Burkitt), and large cell lymphomas. The dis-tinction between types is based on a combination of his-tologic features, surface antigen expression, and chro-mosomal abnormalities.

Lymphoblastic lymphomas. Lymphoblastic lympho-mas are microscopically indistinguishable from ALL. The cells have a uniform appearance with a high nuclear to cytoplasmic ratio, weakly basophilic cytoplasm, and occa-sional nucleoli. The distinction between lymphoma and ALL is based on the degree of bone marrow involvement; thus, if malignant cells involve 25% or more of the bone marrow, it is considered leukemia regardless of the degree of lymph node involvement. Typically, lymphoblastic lymphomas arise from T-lymphocyte precursors, which express early thymocyte surface antigens such as CD5, CD7, and other T-cell antigens (e.g., CD3, CD4, and/or CD8) depending on the degree of differentiation. Much less commonly, lymphoblastic lymphomas will arise from a B-precursor cell and express related surface antigens (e.g., CD10, CD19, or HLA-DR). Chromosomal abnormali-ties are common in lymphoblastic lymphoma and usually mirror those found in acute lymphoblastic leukemia.

Small noncleaved cell lymphoma. Small noncleaved cell lymphomas are all of mature B-cell origin character-ized by the expression of immunoglobulins on the cell surface (usually IgM). Morphologic features include a high nuclear and cytoplasmic ratio with a deep, intensely basophilic cytoplasm with numerous vacuoles and several well-circumscribed nucleoli in the nucleus. The intersper-sion of occasional macrophages between these cells gives rise to the classic "starry sky" appearance of a Burkitt lymphomas. Small noncleaved cell lymphomas can be further divided into classic Burkitt lymphoma, charac-terized by small uniformed cells and Burkitt-like lym-phomas in which the cells are larger and more pleo-morphic. Clinically, the distinction is irrelevant, since all small noncleaved cell lymphomas behave and respond to therapy in a similar manner.

The characteristic chromosomal abnormality of small noncleaved cell lymphoma is the (8;14) translocation, which results in the rearrangement of the immunoglobu-lin heavy chain gene on chromosome 14 with the *MYC-C* gene on chromosome 8. The result is a loss of normal reg-ulatory control resulting in constitutive expression of *MYC-C,* a DNA transcription factor. This observation and subsequent study of the function of the *MYC-C* gene product has led to tremendous advances in the under-standing of the pathogenesis, not only of Burkitt lym-phoma, but of carcinogenesis in general. A full discussion of the molecular genetics of Burkitt lymphoma is beyond the scope of this chapter; suffice it to say that while the t(8;14) and subsequent dysregulation of *MYC-C* is a vital event in the oncogenesis of Burkitt lymphoma, it is insufficient by itself. Additional genetic events are neces-sary to result in full transformation into the Burkitt lymphoma phenotype.

Large cell lymphoma. Large cell lymphomas share many morphologic features with small noncleaved cell lympho-mas. As one might guess from the name, when compared with a macrophage nuclei, the nuclei of large cell lym-phomas is larger, while small noncleaved cell nuclei are smaller. For the most part, large cell lymphomas are of B-cell origin, although some arise from T cells or, more rarely, histiocytic lineage. Approximately 25% of large cell lymphomas demonstrate unusual morphologic or anaplas-tic features. These anaplastic large cell lymphomas usually express T-cell surface markers and/or CD30 (Ki-1 anti-gen) and are usually more difficult to treat successfully.

Chromosomal rearrangements and other abnormali-ties are common in large cell lymphomas, but none are specific for a given tumor type. Interestingly, a small per-centage of large cell lymphomas will also have *MYC-C* rearrangements.

CLINICAL PRESENTATION

Fever, weight loss, malaise, and night sweats are systemic symptoms common to children with all three types of NHL. Beyond these symptoms, the clinical presentation can be quite varied depending on the location of the tumor mass (Table 14–2). Patients usually have a local-ized mass, most commonly in the form of lympha-denopathy. A common feature of all three types of NHLs in children is that they are, almost without exception, fast-growing tumors, in which signs and symptoms can change quickly as the tumor mass grows.

While the clinical presentation can be quite varied, it often follows patterns that correlate well with the type

Table 14–2. Site Distribution of Primary Non-Hodgkin Lymphoma

Site	Percentage
Mediastinum	26
Abdomen	35
Head and neck	3
Peripheral nodes	14
Other	22

of NHL. For example, children and adolescents with T-cell lymphoblastic lymphoma usually have adenopathy above the diaphragm involving the tonsils, nasopharynx, Waldeyer ring, cervical lymph nodes, and, especially, the anterior mediastinum. Symptoms usually result as the massive adenopathy begins to compress vital structures. Lymphoblastic lymphoma can also infiltrate organs below the diaphragm resulting in hepatosplenomegaly, retroperitoneal adenopathy, or enlarged kidneys. The superior vena cava (SVC) syndrome is a dangerous situation in which the SVC is extrinsically compressed by the tumor mass. These patients typically have plethora and edema of the face, neck, and upper chest, as well as visible, dilated collateral veins over the chest, abdomen, and neck (such as jugular venous distention). Respiratory distress can occur from compression of the tracheobronchial tree and/or from either sympathetic or malignant pleural effusions. In a manner similar to ALL, lymphoblastic lymphoma can involve the CNS and present with signs such as cranial nerve palsies, cerebrospinal fluid pleocytosis, or, rarely, as an epidural mass with spinal cord compression. Bone marrow involvement is common, although involvement of more than 25% of the bone marrow would be classified as ALL.

In the typical African or endemic form of Burkitt lymphoma, children have a massive and rapidly enlarging mass arising from the jaw (maxilla or mandible) with or without orbital involvement. In sporadic cases in the United States or Europe, children often have a rapidly enlarging abdominal mass that causes pain, constipation, nausea, and vomiting. Intestinal involvement leading to intussusception or a right iliac fossa mass, which can be mistaken for acute appendicitis, can also occur. About 20% of the time Burkitt's lymphoma arises outside of the abdomen in places such as cervical or tonsilar lymph nodes, bone, testes, breasts, and salivary and thyroid glands. Again, bone marrow involvement is possible, but greater than 25% would be classified as a Burkitt leukemia. Since Burkitt lymphoma grows so rapidly, symptoms and signs may be present for only a very short time (days to weeks), therefore appearing to represent an infectious process rather than a malignancy.

Large cell lymphomas have the most unusual and unpredictable behavior among the childhood NHLs. These tumors can present with the mediastinal masses typically seen in T-cell lymphoblastic lymphomas or with abdominal masses seen in Burkitt lymphoma. Large cell lymphomas are more likely to involve the skin than are the other two types, and CNS and bone marrow involvement is less common.

Despite the association of the preceding clinical patterns with particular types of NHL, the diagnosis can only be made by biopsy of involved areas. Such a biopsy can be accomplished in a variety of ways, but usually involves an open biopsy. Undertaking heroic measures to excise a large mass (especially an abdominal mass) is not only unnecessary, but also unwise, since it provides no therapeutic advantage and may lead to substantial complications. The role of surgery is essentially limited to obtaining adequate tissue for diagnostic studies. That having been said, a significant amount of tissue must be collected since the classification (and therefore the correct treatment) depends on not only histopathology, but immunophenotypic and cytogenetic/molecular studies as well.

Staging of NHL is related to whether there is tumor involvement that extends to regional lymph nodes, whether there is disease present both above and below the diaphragm, and whether there is distant metastatic tumor in the bone marrow or CNS. In addition to radiographic imaging studies of the involved area, additional staging studies such as chest radiograph, computed tomography (CT) scan of the chest, abdomen, and pelvis, and gallium scan or technetium bone scan (if indicated) should be obtained for accurate staging. Additional laboratory studies include a complete blood cell count and differential, serum chemistries including lactate dehydrogenase and uric acid, bone marrow biopsy and aspirate, and lumbar puncture to examine the cerebrospinal fluid.

TREATMENT

Treatment is based on the principle that NHL is a systemic disease with widespread, although usually not clinically apparent, disease at the time of presentation. Therefore, the primary therapeutic modality is systemic chemotherapy and intrathecal chemotherapy to treat the CNS. Radiation therapy is reserved for urgent situations where rapid tumor shrinkage is required to eliminate symptoms of mass compression, such as SVC syndrome or cord compression.

Tremendous advances have been made in the overall survival of children with NHL over the past 25 years through the development of multiagent chemotherapy regimens. The actual drug combinations and length of therapy is relatively specific for the type of NHL. For example, therapy of lymphoblastic lymphomas is essentially identical to that of ALL, which includes combinations of prednisone, L-asparaginase, vincristine, anthracyclines, antimetabolites (such as 6-MP), and methotrexate. Long-term event-free survival in the 50 to 70% range and better has been reported. In B-cell NHL, such as Burkitt lymphoma, therapy is much more intensive, shorter in duration, and relies on high doses of alkylating agents and drugs such as methotrexate and/or cytosine arabinoside (ara-C). Outstanding long-term event-free survival in the range of 90% or better can be expected. The optimal treatment of large cell lymphomas is not clear, primarily because of the heterogeneity of this group of lymphomas. Large cell lymphomas with B-cell phenotype are best treated in a manner similar to Burkitt lymphoma. The anaplastic large cell lymphoma and T-cell large cell lymphoma are more difficult to treat, although there are reports of good long-term outcomes using ALL-like protocols. Patients with NHL who relapse after treatment have a poor prognosis, although a few patients have been successfully treated with autologous or allogeneic bone marrow transplantation.

It is important to be aware that patients with NHL can have problems that can represent true emergencies. Most complications are related to tumor compression of vital organs such as in SVC syndrome or spinal cord compression. The development of tumor lysis syndrome is common, especially in patients with Burkitt lymphoma, and can evolve rapidly into a life-threatening situation. Please refer to the section on oncologic emergencies for more details on the management of these problems.

Hodgkin Lymphoma

EPIDEMIOLOGY AND ETIOLOGY

In the United States and other industrialized countries, HL, also referred to as Hodgkin disease, has a bimodal age-specific incidence with a peak in young adulthood and again after 50 years of age. The appearance of HL prior to age 5 years is rare. Compared with the general population, HL is more common in close relatives of affected patients. This familial risk is associated with certain human leukocyte antigens (HLA). In the United States, HL occurs less commonly in nonwhites and more often in high socioeconomic groups. There is also an increased incidence in children with congenital and acquired immunodeficiencies, such as ataxia-telangiectasia, inherited hypogammaglobulinemia, and AIDS.

The preceding observations, coupled with epidemiological studies, suggest that HL may have an infectious etiology. Interest has centered primarily on EBV, the same virus responsible for endemic Burkitt lymphoma in Africa. Patients with HL have been shown to have high EBV titers, and experimental evidence has demonstrated the presence of the EBV genome in Reed-Sternberg cells. While this information is interesting and suggestive, the true etiology of HL remains an enigma. It appears likely that genetics, environmental factors, and the relative immunocompetence of the individual plays a role in the susceptibility to this disease.

PATHOLOGY

The light microscopic appearance of HL consists of stromal elements with reactive infiltrates of normal lymphocytes, plasma cells, and eosinophils, and the Reed-Sternberg cell. The Reed-Sternberg cell, which accounts for less than 1% of the cellular elements, is usually a large cell with abundant cytoplasm and characteristic multinucleated or multilobed nuclei. Reed-Sternberg cells can occur in isolation or in clusters and are surrounded by stromal cells, which together destroy the normal architecture of the lymph node. The Reed-Sternberg cell appears to be the malignant cell in HL, but the origin of this cell is controversial. For the most part, Reed-Sternberg cells express antigens consistent with B or T lymphocytes, but in the nodular sclerosing type, Reed-Sternberg cells often express markers characteristic of monocytic lineage.

Depending on the degree of fibrosis and the predominant type of stromal cells present, four histologic types have been described: lymphocyte-predominant (LP), mixed cellularity (MC), lymphocyte-depleted (LD), and nodular sclerosing (NS). The prognosis for patients with one of the first three types has historically correlated with the relative proportion of lymphocytes to abnormal cells—the more lymphocytes the better the prognosis. However, advances in therapy have improved the outlook for patients with LD types and reduced the prognostic significance of histologic features.

The LP types occur in approximately 10 to 15% of childhood cases and are characterized by destruction of the lymph node architecture and significant infiltrates of normal lymphocytes surrounding relatively rare Reed-Sternberg cells. Fibrosis is usually not seen. In the MC type, Reed-Sternberg cells are plentiful, there is some fibrosis, and the lymph node architecture is often completely effaced. This type occurs in about 30% of cases, especially those occurring in children younger than 10 years of age and those with immunodeficiencies such as AIDS. The distinguishing histologic feature of the LD type is a relative paucity of lymphocytes and significant fibrosis and necrosis. It is uncommon in children and can sometimes be confused with anaplastic large cell lymphomas, but when it does occur it is often widespread and found infiltrating distant metastatic sites, such as bone marrow. The NS type is by far the most common in the pediatric population affecting 40% of children and 70% of adolescents. It is characterized by thick capsules with proliferating bands of collagen that divide the lymph node into distinct nodules.

CLINICAL PRESENTATION

The vast majority of children with HL have a history of asymptomatic, nontender enlargement of cervical or supraclavicular lymph nodes. The degree of nodal enlargement can wax and wane over time, and patients with mediastinal or perihilar nodal involvement can have symptoms of tracheal or bronchial compression. However, airway compression with HL does not usually present as an acute airway emergency in the same way that airway compression from NHL can. Constitutional symptoms of fever, drenching night sweats, and weight loss of greater than 10% of body weight (referred to as "B" symptoms) occur in 25 to 30% of children, and their presence is associated with a less favorable prognosis.

One of the most characteristic and unique features of HL is its tendency to arise in a single group of lymph nodes and subsequently spread in an orderly and sequential fashion to adjacent nodal groups. Therefore, if it arises in an inferior anterior cervical lymph node, one can expect the orderly spread of disease inferiorly to involve first the mediastinal and perihilar lymph nodes followed by the spleen and periaortic lymph nodes. The more widespread the nodal involvement, the more likely there is distant metastatic disease involving bone marrow and other extranodal organs, such as the liver, lungs, and bone. Early involvement of extranodal structures is usually associated with contiguous spread from adjacent lymph nodes.

Cellular immunodeficiency is present in greater than 50% of patients with HL based on delayed hypersensitivity reactions with skin testing and the increased tendency of these patients to develop certain bacterial, viral, and fungal infections. There is limited evidence to suggest that these cellular immunodeficiencies precede the development of HL and can persist after successful treatment.

DIAGNOSIS AND STAGING

The diagnostic workup of HL begins with a careful history and physical examination. The presence of persistent (over a period of several months), relatively slow-growing unilateral cervical and/or supraclavicular adenopathy in older children or adolescents makes the diagnosis of HL more likely than other typically faster growing malignancies, such as NHL. Because the histologic assessment of nodal architecture is essential to making a definitive diagnosis, open biopsy of the affected lymph node is required. Needle biopsy or fine-needle aspiration is insufficient because it does not adequately preserve nodal architecture.

Other useful laboratory tests include a complete blood cell count, which may demonstrate signs of anemia (usually due to chronic disease) or thrombocytopenia (there may be an associated immune-mediated thrombocytopenia purpura), and an erythrocyte sedimentation rate (ESR), which is usually elevated. Assessment of liver transaminase levels and function is sometimes helpful and, if abnormal, can suggest liver metastatic disease. A chest radiograph is especially important in order to look for evidence of mediastinal or perihilar lymphadenopathy and tumor involvement.

Once the diagnosis of HL has been confirmed, clinical staging is necessary to choose appropriate therapy and counsel patients regarding potential treatment outcomes. The staging criteria are outlined in Table 14–3. The important determinants of the staging system are whether the disease involves more than one lymph node group and, if so, if it involves nodal groups on both sides of the diaphragm. In addition, noting the presence of B symptoms (defined as fever, night sweats, and weight loss >10% of body weight) is critical. As in almost all forms of cancer, the more disease that is present, the higher the stage and the poorer the prognosis.

To determine the stage, CT of the chest, abdomen, and pelvis; bone marrow aspiration and biopsy; and gallium scan should be performed. Lymphangiography can be helpful in the staging workup because of its ability to detect retroperitoneal lymphadenopathy; however, many institutions lack the necessary expertise to use it reliably, especially in children. Several years ago a staging laparotomy, which includes a sampling of all node groups, biopsy of the liver, and splenectomy was routinely used to assess the extent of intraabdominal disease. Currently, a staging laparotomy is only performed if the information gained will affect treatment. For example, patients who could receive radiation therapy alone, such as those with stage I or II disease, probably should at least undergo lymphangiography, if not laparotomy, to rule out occult splenic or intraabdominal nodal involvement. However, if chemotherapy is planned regardless of what is found, a laparotomy is not needed.

TREATMENT

The method of treating children and adolescents with HL is influenced by several factors related not only to

Table 14–3. Staging of Hodgkin Lymphoma[1]

Stage I	Involvement of a single lymph node region or a single extralymphatic site
Stage II	Involvement of two or more lymph node regions on the same side of the diaphragm or localized involvement of extralymphatic organ or site, and of one or more lymph node regions on the same side of the diaphragm
Stage III	Involvement of lymph node regions on both sides of the diaphragm, which may also be accompanied by localized involvement of extralymphatic organ or site or by involvement of the spleen or both
Stage IV	Disseminated involvement of one or more extralymphatic organs or tissues with or without lymph node enlargement

[1] Patients with B symptoms (weight loss, fever, and night sweats) have a worse prognosis.

which therapy choices are most effective, but also how it might impact patients years after the cure is obtained. Historically, HL has been curable using high-dose radiation therapy for more localized disease and chemotherapy with or without radiotherapy in high-stage disease. While these therapies are effective, they can result in unacceptable side effects many years later, such as inhibition of musculoskeletal development in growing children or adolescents and second cancers arising within the radiation field. Chemotherapy (usually with alkylating agents) can result in infertility (especially in postpubertal males) or acute leukemias as second cancers. For these reasons, choices of therapy often involve combinations of lower doses of chemotherapy and radiotherapy designed to achieve cure, but maintain the lowest risk of late toxicity possible.

Hodgkin lymphoma responds to a variety of chemotherapy agents, but there is a long track record of success using two particular combination chemotherapy regimens: MOPP (nitrogen mustard, vincristine, prednisone, and procarbazine) and ABVD (doxorubicin, bleomycin, vinblastine, and dacarbazine). The typical duration of therapy with these drugs is 6 to 8 months. The advantages of chemotherapy in early stages of the disease are that it obviates the need for a splenectomy and avoids the late effects of radiation therapy. The major disadvantages of using chemotherapy alone are the higher risk of late relapses at the primary site and long-term side effects of infertility, cardiomyopathy, and other types of second malignancies. Combined modality therapy with chemotherapy and radiotherapy provides many potential benefits including improved local control and the ability to use less and lower doses of chemotherapy and radiation.

With these issues in mind, one might chose chemotherapy alone for growing children and adolescents, and additional low-dose involved-field radiation to enhance local control if bulky mediastinal disease is present. High-dose "extended-field" radiotherapy without chemotherapy should be reserved for fully grown adolescents (growth plates fused) and adults with low-stage disease without B symptoms. Current clinical investigations are exploring whether fewer cycles of chemotherapy with low-dose radiotherapy will be an equally effective treatment.

After completing the treatment plan, patients should be observed closely for signs of relapse both at the primary site and distantly. If relapse is to occur, it will usually happen within 2 years of diagnosis, but can occur more than 4 years after diagnosis. If patients have a relapse, different chemotherapy plus radiation or bone marrow transplantation might still be effective in achieving a cure.

The acute side effects of treatment for HL are similar to those for other cancers. However, because most patients with HL can expect to live full lives, the long-term side effects of radiation and chemotherapy take on greater meaning. Impaired growth and reproductive function is common, and the risk of second malignant neoplasms

(either sarcomas in the radiation field or acute leukemias) is significant. Of particular concern is increased risk of breast cancer in women who received mediastinal radiation during adolescence. These women should have frequent breast exams and start mammograms earlier than normal. In addition, depending on the chemotherapy drugs used and which organs were included in the radiation field, long-term organ damage can occur, especially in the heart and lungs. Survivors should be monitored for these effects so that appropriate and timely interventions can be made.

ABDOMINAL MASSES

An abdominal mass in children or adolescents is usually a cause for great alarm because of the fear that it may represent cancer. These masses are often discovered inadvertently by a parent or during a routine physical examination. On other occasions, children will have pain and obstruction of vital organs. The differential diagnosis depends on the age of the child and the location of the mass. A good first step in the workup of such children is an abdominal ultrasound or CT scan to characterize better the extent of the mass and the organ from which it appears to arise. (See Table 14–4 for a review of the differential diagnosis of abdominal masses in children.) Extensive discussion of all the possible abdominal cancers of childhood is beyond the scope of this chapter. Instead this chapter will focus on the two most common abdominal malignancies: neuroblastoma and Wilms tumor (WT). Both tumors may appear to arise from the kidney, although a neuroblastoma actually arises from the adrenal gland or paravertebral sympathetic ganglia. Other abdominal tumors include hepatoblastoma, which arises from the liver, and germ cell tumors, which usually originate in the ovaries.

Neuroblastoma

Neuroblastoma is one of the most fascinating of all childhood cancers. The tumor derives from the primordial neural crest cells that populate the adrenal medulla and sympathetic ganglia. Perhaps the most intriguing aspect of neuroblastoma is that some tumors can undergo spontaneous maturation or regression with little or no therapy. Over the past 2 decades great progress has been made in the understanding of the biology of this neoplasm and in developing effective treatment for localized or regional disease.

EPIDEMIOLOGY AND ETIOLOGY

Neuroblastoma is the most common solid tumor in children occurring outside the CNS. The annual incidence of neuroblastoma in the United States is approximately 8 cases per 1 million children accounting for 8 to 10% of all childhood cancer and 50% of cancer in infants. The median age at diagnosis is approximately 2 years with more than 95% of cases diagnosed before 10 years of age.

Table 14–4. Differential Diagnosis of Abdominal Masses

Location	Differential Diagnosis	Common Age
Upper abdomen	Multicystic kidney	Infants/young children
	Hydronephrosis	Young children
	Neuroblastoma	Young children
	Wilms tumor	Young children
	Adrenal hemorrhage	Neonates
	Normal kidneys	Young children
	Choledochal cyst	Neonates through older children
	Hepatoblastoma	Young children
	Hepatocellular carcinoma	Older children
Middle abdomen	Cysts (duplication, urachal, mesenteric)	Neonates through older children
	Non-Hodgkin lymphoma	Young children through adolescents
	Ovarian/testicular mass	Older children/adolescents
	Ectopic kidney	Any age
Lower abdomen/pelvis	Fecal impaction	Young children
	Ovarian/testicular mass	Older children/adolescents
	Ovarian cyst	Adolescents
	Sacrococcygeal teratoma (germ cell tumor)	Young children
	Rhabdomyosarcoma	Young/older children
	Neuroblastoma (organ of Zuckerkandl)	Young children
	Ewing sarcoma (from pelvic bones)	Older children/adolescents
	Abscess (tuboovarian)	Adolescents
	Abscess (appendix)	Young children through adolescents

Neonates = <2 months of age; infants = 2 to 12 months; young children = 1 to 5 years; older children = 6 to 12 years; adolescents = >12 years.

Rare occurrences in twins and siblings imply that a small number of patients have a hereditary predisposition for neuroblastoma. In this situation the tumor is more likely to present at an earlier age and with multiple primaries.

The cause of neuroblastoma is unknown, although there are studies that suggest that exposure to a variety of environmental factors, such as prenatal drug exposures, may play a role. Since neuroblastoma arises from neural crest cells, laboratory investigators have focused on trying to understand whether problems in the cellular regulation of neuronal differentiation may play a role in the development of this tumor.

PATHOLOGY AND BIOLOGY

The classic light microscopic appearance of neuroblastoma is that of dense nests of immature, small round cells separated by fibrillar bundles often forming pseudorosettes of cells surrounding a pink fibrillar center. Often tumors demonstrate variable degrees of maturation toward ganglion cells. A neuroblastoma is a very undifferentiated tumor, while a ganglioneuroblastoma demonstrates a mixture of mature and immature elements. A fully mature tumor is referred to as ganglioneuroma. The issue is important because the spectrum of differentiation correlates with clinical behavior. Less mature tumors (i.e., neu-

roblastoma) behave in a more malignant fashion, while more mature tumors (i.e., ganglioneuroma) are progressively benign.

Neuroblastoma is one of the small round cell tumors (SRCT) of childhood and distinguishing it from other SRCT can sometimes be difficult. The usual approach is to look for evidence of neuronal maturation with special stains such as S100 or neuron specific enolase. Immunohistochemistry using antibodies to various neuron-specific cellular components, such as synaptophysin and neurofilaments, can be helpful. In addition, electron microscopy can demonstrate specific cellular structures such as neurosecretory granules, microfilaments, and microtubules specific for neuroblastoma.

Neuroblastoma is unique among the SRCT in that 90 to 95% of tumors secrete the catecholamine metabolites, homovanillic acid (HVA) and vanillylmandelic acid (VMA). Neuroblastoma cells produce these metabolites because, unlike adrenal chromaffin cells and pheochromocytomas, neuroblastoma tumor cells lack the enzyme to produce epinephrine from norepinephrine and dopamine. Instead these catechols are converted to HVA and VMA and excreted in the urine where they can be measured.

The great majority of neuroblastomas have cytogenetic abnormalities, with a deletion in the short arm of chromosome 1 (1p deletion) being most common. Presumably this region of chromosome 1 contains a tumor suppressor gene. Amplification of the oncogene MYC-N is also common, especially in more advanced stages, and its presence has been associated with a poor prognosis.

CLINICAL PRESENTATION

Neuroblastoma can develop anywhere along the sympathetic chain. The most common primary site in children older than 1 year of age is the adrenal gland or paraspinal sympathetic ganglion in the abdomen. The remainder arise from the sympathetic ganglion in the thorax or, more rarely, the cervical region or pelvic region. Infants are more likely to have primary tumors arising in the thorax. About 50% of infants and 70% of older children have tumor spread beyond the primary site (either regional or distant). The most common metastatic sites are regional lymph nodes, bone marrow, bone, liver, and, less frequently, subcutaneous tissue.

The clinical presentation depends on the primary site and the degree of spread. Often the presence of a hard, irregular abdominal mass discovered on routine physical exam can be the first sign of disease. Thoracic primaries in the posterior mediastinum can go undetected for extended periods of time until a chest radiograph is obtained for other reasons. Metastatic disease can present as inferior cervical adenopathy, often associated with Horner syndrome. The presence of bowel or urinary tract obstruction can result directly from tumor compression of the affected organ or indirectly from spinal cord compression. Liver metastatic disease can result in massive hepatomegaly leading to respiratory compromise, especially in infants. Large retroperitoneal masses arising from the adrenal medulla often cause vascular compression resulting in edema of the lower extremities and compression of the renal artery with associated hypertension. Paraspinal tumors at any site may extend through the vertebral foramina resulting in spinal cord compression. Skin and subcutaneous involvement can also occur, primarily in infants, and usually in the form of nontender, bluish, and mobile nodules. Bone and bone marrow disease is often manifest by bone pain and limping with subsequent infiltration of the bone marrow resulting in pallor, bleeding, and susceptibility to infection because of pancytopenia. Sphenoid and retroorbital bone involvement is common, resulting in orbital ecchymosis, referred to as "raccoon eyes."

In older children, presenting symptoms can be less specific including intermittent fever, weight loss, and lethargy. One unusual presentation of neuroblastoma is the syndrome of opsoclonus/myoclonus in which children demonstrate acute cerebellar and truncal ataxia and rapid eye movements. The pathophysiology of this syndrome is not understood, and it is usually associated with a localized, not metastatic, tumor. Even though such a localized tumor is usually cured with surgery alone, 75% of patients are left with some permanent neurologic disability, such as ataxia and mental retardation.

DIAGNOSIS AND STAGING

Usually the diagnosis of neuroblastoma is suspected based on clinical features, such as age, location of tumor, metastatic spread, and appearance on imaging studies. Laboratory abnormalities, other than elevated urine catecholamine concentrations, are nonspecific, but may include a normocytic anemia from chronic disease, thrombocytosis for unknown reasons, or pancytopenia due to bone marrow infiltration. Liver and renal functions are usually normal at the time of diagnosis, although they can be compromised from the local effects of a large abdominal primary or massive liver metastatic disease.

The definitive diagnosis usually requires tissue biopsy of the primary tumor or a conveniently accessible metastatic site. The exception to this approach is the patient who has bone marrow involvement, in which the presence of clumps of tumor cells in the bone marrow biopsy coupled with elevated urine HVA or VMA levels is adequate to establish a diagnosis. For this reason, if a diagnosis of neuroblastoma is suspected, bilateral bone marrow aspirates and biopsies along with urine VMA and HVA should be obtained prior to any surgery, since it may obviate the need for a risky open biopsy.

In addition to CT or magnetic resonance imaging (MRI) of the primary tumor and bone marrow studies, an appropriate staging workup includes imaging of likely areas of regional and distant metastatic disease. At a minimum, this should including CT or MRI of the entire cavity in which the tumor arises, such as thorax or abdomen and pelvis. Regardless of the tumor's primary location, an abdominal CT scan is required to rule out liver metastatic disease. Bone metastatic disease is common and often involves long bones, orbit, and skull. A technetium bone scan is usually adequate to detect most lesions, but any areas that are suspicious based on history of pain or physical exam findings should be imaged with CT or MRI. Imaging with radiolabeled metaiodobenzylguanidine (MIBG), which is incorporated into catecholamine-producing cells, provides a specific and sensitive method of detecting neuroblastoma. This imaging technology is becoming more widely available and can substitute for a bone scan.

Historically, the staging system for neuroblastoma has varied among different clinical research groups. In last few years an international group has developed a uniform staging system, referred to as the International Neuroblastoma Staging System (INSS), that is now widely employed and is useful in predicting treatment outcome. In general, the system is based on three principles: the local and regional extent of the primary tumor, the completeness of surgical resection, and the presence or absence of distant metastatic disease. Details of the INSS are outlined in Table 14–5.

Table 14–5. International Staging for Neuroblastoma

Stage I	Localized tumor confined to area of origin; complete gross excision, with or without residual disease; identifiable ipsilateral and contralateral lymph nodes negative microscopically
Stage 2A	Unilateral tumor with incomplete gross excision; identifiable ipsilateral and contralateral lymph nodes negative microscopically
Stage 2B	Unilateral tumor with complete or incomplete gross excision; positive ipsilateral regional lymph nodes; identifiable contralateral lymph nodes negative microscopically
Stage 3	Tumor infiltrating across the midline with or without regional lymph node involvement, or unilateral tumor with contralateral regional lymph node involvement, or midline tumor with bilateral regional lymph node involvement
Stage 4	Disseminated tumor to distant lymph nodes, bone, bone marrow, liver, or other organs (except as defined in stage 4S)
Stage 4S	Localized primary tumor as defined for stage 1 or 2 with dissemination limited to liver, skin, or bone marrow (limited to infants <12 months of age)

One clinical situation deserves special mention. Infants with distant metastatic disease limited to skin, liver, and/or bone marrow and a primary tumor that would otherwise be considered stage 2 or 3, are grouped into a unique subset of patients defined as *stage 4S*. These infants, despite the presence of widely metastatic disease, usually do well with minimal or sometimes no therapy at all.

TREATMENT

The fundamental principle of treating neuroblastoma is the coordination of multimodality therapy, including surgery, chemotherapy, and radiotherapy. Whether to use any or all of these modalities depends on many factors related to the patient's age, site of primary tumor, stage, and risk of recurrence.

Surgery is required in almost all cases, not only to gather tissue for diagnostic purposes, but also to adequately stage the patient, to obtain tumor tissue for biology studies, and to resect the primary tumor. Many children with localized disease who have their tumor completely removed, or those with only microscopic residual disease have a high likelihood of cure without the need for other therapy. For this reason, if it is possible to resect the tumor at diagnosis, it should be done, provided it can be done without undue risk. If the tumor cannot be safely or completely removed, a second-look operation after several courses of chemotherapy can be done to assess response to therapy and to potentially remove any residual tumor.

Radiotherapy is limited to treating gross residual tumor that cannot be safely resected. It also can play an important role in treating metastatic sites with palliative intent. In infants with stage 4S disease, radiation in low doses can be useful to help induce earlier regression of the tumor than would otherwise occur.

Multiagent chemotherapy is the mainstay of treatment for neuroblastoma. The most commonly used drugs are alkylating agents (cyclophophamide and ifosfamide), anthracyclines (doxorubicin), epipodophyllotoxins (etoposide and teniposide), and platinum-based agents (carboplatinum and cisplatinum). Although improved survival has been seen with combinations of these chemotherapy agents in infants with disseminated and older children with lower stage disease, the same is not true for older children with stage 4 disease. For these high-risk patients, high-dose chemotherapy and total body irradiation followed by bone marrow or hematopoietic stem cell rescue has been used with promising early success. However, since neuroblastoma can recur many years after therapy, it is not yet known whether these treatments will result in sustained improvement in long-term survival.

Experimental therapies designed to deliver specific therapy targeted to neuroblastoma cells have been attempted. Examples include monoclonal antibodies that recognize specific antigens on the surface of neuroblastoma cells and radioactively labeled drugs (^{131}I and metaiodobenzylguanidine) that are taken up preferentially by cells producing adrenergic neurotransmitters. In addition, drugs such as retinoic acid, which cause differentiation of neuroblastoma cells into mature cells, show some promise. Treatment with retinoic acid after bone marrow transplantation has been shown to improve the outcome for high-risk patients.

Over the past two decades, the coupling of clinical and biological research in neuroblastoma has led to therapeutic approaches that are related to an individual patient's predicted risk of developing recurrent disease. The most important variables for predicting outcome are the stage of disease and age at diagnosis. For example, the survival rate for all children with stage 1, 2, or 4S disease is 75 to 90%. In stages 3 and 4 disease, children have an expected cure rate of 50 and 15%, respectively, while infants (less than 1 year of age) have cure rates of approximately 80 and 70%, respectively. Other variables have also been shown to be associated with outcome, such as genetic aberrations (e.g., *MYC-N* amplification, chromosome 1p deletions, and abnormal DNA index) and histopathology. While most of these variables appear to have predictive value independent of stage and age, no study has yet been done to test all of these factors together. However, future studies are being designed to do just that.

Wilms Tumor

EPIDEMIOLOGY AND ETIOLOGY

Wilms tumor (WT), tumor of the developing kidney, is the second most common malignant solid tumor in children outside the CNS and the most common malignant renal tumor. It accounts for 6 to 7% of all childhood cancer with an annual incidence of approximately 8 cases per 1 million white children younger than 15 years of age. This translates into approximately 400 new cases per year in the United States. The peak age of diagnosis is between 2 to 4 years and 80% of cases will be diagnosed in children less than 5 years of age.

Most cases of WT are sporadic, that is, they are not associated with a particular genetic disorder or positive family history. Familial forms of WT, however, do occur in about 1 to 2.5% of cases and are especially likely in cases of bilateral WT. The familial forms of WT include those associated with genitourinary abnormalities such as hypospadias, cryptorchidism, ureteral duplication, and horseshoe, fused, and polycystic kidney. Wilms tumor also occurs as part of genetic syndromes such as Beckwith-Wiedemann syndrome, unilateral hemihypertrophy, WAGR (*W*T, *a*niridia, *g*enitorurinary anomalies, and mental *r*etardation), isolated aniridia, and Denys-Drash syndrome.

The cause of WT is unknown. Numerous studies have been performed searching for environmental causes, but results have been mixed and inconsistent. Based on the known associations of WT with a variety of genetic syndromes, DNA abnormalities appear to play a major role in its development. A two-hit mutational model of a classic tumor suppressor gene has been proposed. According to this model, all at-risk individuals have a mutation in one of two WT suppressor genes. Those individuals who go on to develop WT develop a "second-hit" mutation in the other WT suppressor gene. For those with the familial forms of WT, the first hit is present in the germline inherited from parents and the second hit occurs postzygotically in somatic tissues. For those with sporadic forms, both mutations are somatic (postzygotic). Children with WT and associated aniridia or WAGR have been noted to have constitutional deletions in the region of chromosome 11p13. Based on this information, a WT suppressor gene (WT-1) has been cloned, and the gene product is a transcription factor that plays a critical role in normal kidney and gonadal development. There is evidence that there are other WT genes located in other areas of the genome, such as the short arm of chromosome 11.

PATHOLOGY AND BIOLOGY

Classically, the histopathologic appearance of WT is composed of three elements: primitive metanephric blastema, dysplastic tubules, and supporting mesenchyma or stroma. The simultaneous occurrence of all three of these elements is referred to as triphasic, but each individual tumor may have varying amounts of each element. Each of these elements can demonstrate varying degrees of cellular atypia, differentiation, and maturation. Given such histopathological diversity, WT can be categorized as demonstrating favorable or unfavorable histology based on the degree of nuclear atypia and differentiation—the more atypical and less differentiated, the more unfavorable the histology. Obviously, children with tumors that demonstrate favorable histology have a better prognosis than do those with unfavorable histology.

CLINICAL PRESENTATION

The most common clinical presentation is the discovery of an asymptomatic abdominal mass, often discovered by a parent. Other potential signs and symptoms include abdominal pain, malaise, gross hematuria, and hypertension. Hematuria can be significant enough to cause anemia with associated pallor and fatigue. Occasionally a tumor thrombus can form in the inferior vena cava resulting in occlusion of the inferior vena cava and distention of superficial abdominal veins. As mentioned earlier, WT can occur in association with specific genetic syndromes; therefore, it is important to specifically look for signs of aniridia, hemihypertrophy, and macroglossia.

DIAGNOSIS AND STAGING

Wilms tumors can arise anywhere within the kidney and usually spread beyond a tumor pseudocapsule into the renal sinus, intrarenal lymphatics, and blood vessels. With this in mind, the radiographic evaluation of a suspected WT should begin with an ultrasound examination to establish the organ from which the tumor mass arose, the extent of renal involvement, and whether blood vessels, such as the inferior vena cava, are free of tumor thrombus. A CT scan of the abdomen also helps to define the extent of the tumor and any associated regional adenopathy. Approximately 10 to 15% of children with WT have distant metastatic spread, most commonly to lung, liver, or lung and liver. The abdominal CT scan can usually reveal liver metastases and a posteroanterior and lateral chest radiograph can demonstrate most pulmonary metastatic disease. While a chest CT scan is even more sensitive in detecting the presence of pulmonary metastatic lesions, it is not clear whether this information offers any advantage over a simple chest radiograph. This is based on results from clinical trials that found excellent outcomes for children with pulmonary metastasis seen by CT only (and with negative chest radiographs) when these children are treated as if they do not have pulmonary metastatic disease. Evaluation of bone, bone marrow, and brain is unnecessary, unless there are signs and symptoms at presentation to suggest involvement of these organ systems.

With the great success of current therapy for WT, accurate staging is more important for choosing the appropriate therapy rather than predicting the outcome. In general, the staging system for WT incorporates clinical, surgical, and pathological criteria. The system includes five stages that are outlined in Table 14–6. It is important to note that the presence of diffuse anaplastic histology features (which occurs in about 5% of cases) imparts a poor prognosis regardless of stage.

Treatment

Modern therapy is based on results from 4 successive clinical trials from the National Wilms Tumor Study Group (NWTS). A central feature of therapy is the need for initial radical nephrectomy in most patients, which allows for appropriate surgical staging. The exceptions to this approach are children with extensive bilateral renal disease or advanced-stage unilateral disease in whom performing a nephrectomy would pose excessive risk. In these situations, preoperative chemotherapy and/or radiotherapy are used to decrease tumor size and, subsequently, the risk of intraoperative tumor hemorrhage or rupture, or, in the case of bilateral disease, increase the likelihood of preserving some normal renal parenchyma.

Definitive therapy for WT is based on stage. Patients with lower stage disease (I or II) and favorable histology can be treated with surgery and combination chemotherapy with vincristine and actinomycin D. Patients with stage III disease should be treated with surgery, radiotherapy to the tumor bed, and the addition of doxorubicin to the preceding chemotherapy regimen. Children presenting with pulmonary metastatic disease and favorable histology require the addition of whole lung irradiation. Children with stage II-IV disease and unfavorable histology do better with the addition of cyclophosphamide to the vincristine, actinomycin D, and doxorubicin regimen.

Table 14–6. Clinicopathologic Staging of Wilms Tumor

Stage I	Tumor limited to kidney and completely excised; no invasion through renal capsule, no kidney rupture, no distant spread
Stage II	Tumor extends through capsule and into perirenal soft tissue and may infiltrate vessels outside the kidney, but is completely excised; there may be local spill of tumor into flank
Stage III	Residual nonhematogenous dissemination of tumor confined to abdomen; tumor may extend beyond surgical margin at resection and may involve lymph node tumor spill or peritoneal implants
Stage IV	Hematogenous dissemination of tumor to lungs, liver, bone, brain, or distant lymph node dissemination
Stage V	Bilateral renal involvement at diagnosis

Relapse-free survival rates for children with favorable histology of any stage is 80% or greater. Most relapses will occur within 2 years of diagnosis, usually in the lung, but also at the site of the original tumor. A significant percentage of these children can still be cured, especially those who have not received prior radiation therapy or only vincristine and actinomycin D chemotherapy. Overall survival is greater than 90% for patients (including those who have relapsed and been treated again) with a favorable histology and stage I-III WT and about 80% for those with stage IV disease.

Ongoing clinical trials now focus on improving cure rates for children with unfavorable histology and trying to minimize acute and long-term toxicity for the great majority of children with a more favorable outlook. Many of the late side effects are related to radiotherapy, such as scoliosis and trunk underdevelopment secondary to irradiation of vertebral bodies, and secondary malignant neoplasms arising from organs in the radiation field (e.g., thyroid cancer, breast cancer, and sarcomas).

SOFT TISSUE TUMORS

Most soft tissue neoplasms in children are sarcomas, which arise from primitive mesenchymal cells that normally differentiate into muscle, cartilage, ligaments, and bone. Soft tissue sarcomas are divided into two broad groups—rhabdomyosarcomas (RMSs) and non-RMSs. Non-RMS soft tissue sarcomas do occur in children and adolescents, but they are rare and heterogeneous (e.g., fibrosarcoma, neurofibrosarcoma, and synovial cell sarcoma). Treatment usually consists of surgical excision with or without radiotherapy, and successful therapy depends on the ability to completely resect the tumor. Chemotherapy, in general, has little role in therapy. These tumors will not be discussed further here, but rather, the focus will be on RMSs, which are more common and constitute one of the small round cell tumors of childhood.

Rhabdomyosarcoma

Rhabdomyosarcoma is the most common soft tissue sarcoma in children under 15 years of age. Like many other childhood cancers, great progress has been made over the last three decades in treating RMS—so much so that with current multimodality therapy, the 5-year survival of all patients is about 70%.

Epidemiology and Etiology

Rhabdomyosarcoma is one of the four main classes of small round cell tumors of childhood and accounts for 5 to 8% of cases of childhood cancer. It is the third most common extracranial tumor, after WT and neuroblastoma, occurring at a rate of 8 cases per 1 million white children in the United States. Interestingly the incidence in African American children is about 50% that of white children. More than one half of all cases occurs in children younger than 5 years of age.

Rhabdomyosarcoma is a heterogeneous group of tumors but they all appear to arise from common precursor cells that normally give rise to striated muscle. Accordingly, the tumor often occurs in areas of the body where striated muscle is found; however, it can arise almost anywhere in the body. Common sites include the bladder and vagina (primarily in infants and young children), the head and neck region, and skeletal muscle of extremities.

The etiology of RMS is unknown, but clearly genetics plays a major role. There is an association between the development of RMS and neurofibromatosis, Beckwith-Wiedemann syndrome, and a few other rare genetic syndromes. Some studies have suggested a causative role for certain environmental factors in the oncogenesis of RMS, but none have been proved conclusively. Rhabdomyosarcoma does occur as a second malignant neoplasm years after radiation therapy, therefore implicating ionizing radiation as an etiologic factor.

PATHOLOGY AND BIOLOGY

Rhabdomyosarcomas consist of four types: embryonal, botryoid (a variant of embryonal), alveolar, and undifferentiated. About 60% are embryonal, 5% botryoid, 20% alveolar, and the remainder undifferentiated. Establishing a diagnosis of RMS can sometimes be difficult. The key histologic feature is the presence of small round blue cells that show evidence of skeletal muscle differentiation, such as cross-striations similar to striated muscle. More specific studies include immunohistochemical stains with antibodies directed against specific components of skeletal muscle, such as myosin, desmin, and actin. Electron microscopy can be particularly helpful, especially with undifferentiated sarcomas, since it can often demonstrate sarcomeres with Z bands, actin, and myosin filaments and other ultrastructural features reminiscent of skeletal muscle.

The embryonal type demonstrates variable amounts of spindle and primitive round cells that appear to "float" in a myxoid matrix. The botryoid variant is characterized by subepithelial aggregates of tumor cells that invariably arise from mucosal surfaces such as the nasopharynx, external auditory canal, or the genitourinary tract (classically the vagina). The alveolar type demonstrates small round cells with abundant eosinophilic cytoplasm on background fibrovascular septa that resemble the alveoli of the lung. The undifferentiated type lacks light microscopic evidence of skeletal muscle differentiation.

CLINICAL PRESENTATION

Rhabdomyosarcomas usually present with an enlarging mass. Other signs and symptoms, such as pain or organ obstruction, depend on the site of the primary tumor. For example, orbital tumors can present with proptosis and,

sometimes, ophthalmoplegia. Nonorbital head and neck tumors tend to arise from parameningeal sites, such as the nasopharynx, middle ear, mastoid region, pterygoid infratemporal fossa, and paranasal sinuses. These tumors often present with nasal, aural, or sinus obstruction, and a mucopurulent or sanguineous discharge. The presence of cranial nerve palsy may suggest involvement of the adjacent meninges, while headache, vomiting, and systemic hypertension may result from intracranial tumor extension. The head and neck tumors are most commonly of embryonal type.

Bladder, prostate, or paratesticular sites are the most common sites in the genitourinary tract. These tumors also tend to be of embryonal-type histology. Bladder tumors arise intraluminally, usually in or near the trigone. Hematuria, urinary obstruction, and occasionally extrusion of mucosanguineous tissue can occur. Bladder primaries tend to occur most commonly in children less than 4 years of age. A prostate primary usually presents as a large pelvic mass with or without accompanying urethral obstruction, constipation, or spinal cord compression. Paratesticular tumors are often discovered as painless unilateral masses in the inguinal or scrotal region in prepubertal and postpubertal males. Up to 40% of these patients have regional lymph node involvement at the time of diagnosis.

Rhabdomyosarcomas of the trunk and extremities most commonly present with a painless mass. About 50% have the alveolar histology, and regional lymph node involvement is relatively common in that situation. Intrathoracic and retroperitoneal tumors can become quite large, with local invasion of adjacent tissues and lymph nodes often occurring before they are diagnosed.

DIAGNOSIS AND STAGING

The initial evaluation of patients with a suspicious mass should start with an MRI or CT scan of the primary tumor site to determine the extent of the tumor. A staging workup to assess metastatic disease includes a CT scan of the chest, a technetium bone scan, and bilateral bone marrow biopsy. When parameningeal sites are involved, cerebrospinal fluid should be obtained for cytology, looking for tumor cells. Baseline laboratory work includes a complete blood cell count; liver and renal function studies; and measurements of serum electrolyte, calcium, phosphorus, and uric acid concentrations in anticipation of chemotherapy. Establishing the diagnosis usually requires an open biopsy.

The staging of RMSs can be very confusing because it relies on both surgical grouping and clinical staging systems. Thus, each patient is given a group and stage classification, and the distinction is important since therapy and prognosis are based on this information. Table 14–7 outlines the staging and grouping system for RMSs as defined by the Intergroup Rhabdomyosarcoma Study Committee (IRS).

Table 14–7. Surgical-Pathologic Grouping System for Rhabdomyosarcoma

Group I	Localized disease, completely resected A. Confined to organ or muscle of origin B. Infiltration outside organ or muscle of origin; regional nodes not involved
Group II	Total gross resection with evidence of regional spread A. Grossly resected tumors with microscopic residual disease B. Regional disease with involved nodes, completely resected with no microscopic residual disease C. Regional disease with involved nodes, grossly resected, but with evidence of microscopic residual disease and/or histologic involvement of the most distal regional node (from the primary site) in the dissection
Group III	Incomplete resection or biopsy specimen with presence of gross residual disease
Group IV	Distant metastasis present at onset

TREATMENT

The initial step in treating RMS is surgical resection provided it can be accomplished without undue morbidity. If microscopic or gross residual tumor remains, or if the histology is unfavorable (e.g., alveolar histology), then radiation therapy should be used at the primary tumor site. Active chemotherapy drugs include vincristine, actinomycin D, cyclophosphamide, doxorubicin, ifosfamide, and cisplatinum. A typical approach would be to use the combination vincristine and actinomycin D for the low stage and tumors with favorable histology and add cyclophosphamide and perhaps doxorubicin or other agents for more advanced disease or unfavorable histology. Chemotherapy is typically given over the course of 1 year. Decisions about specific therapy are complex and depend greatly on group, stage, histology, and tumor location. A more detailed discussion of treatment options is beyond the scope of this chapter, and interested readers are referred to the references listed at the end of this chapter.

Several prognostic variables have been defined for RMS. Patients who have localized disease fare much better than do those with metastatic disease at the time of diagnosis. The histologic type also carries prognostic significance, for example, those with alveolar histology do worse than do those with embryonal type. The primary tumor site is also important prognostically. For example, patients with extremity or retroperitoneal tumors have a worse prognosis than those with orbital or genitourinary primaries.

BONE TUMORS

Benign and malignant tumors of bone usually present with pain localized to a particular site. Soft tissue swelling may or may not be present and sometimes patients develop pathologic fractures through the involved site. Plain radiographs of the affected bone can have a variety of appearances depending on the type of tumor, but lytic bone lesions, especially with cortical destruction and soft tissue extension make malignancy more likely. The differential diagnosis of lytic bone lesions includes osteosarcoma, Ewing sarcoma, Langerhans cell histiocytosis (LCH), metastatic cancer, and, potentially, osteomyelitis. There are also a variety of benign neoplastic tumors to consider such as giant cell tumor, aneurysmal bone cyst, unicameral bone cyst, osteoblastoma, osteochondroma, and chondroblastoma. This rather broad differential diagnosis can be narrowed substantially based on the radiographic appearance of the bone abnormality. In this section, the focus will be on the two most common cancers of bone, osteosarcoma and Ewing sarcoma, and the fascinating group of disorders known as histiocytosis.

Osteosarcoma

EPIDEMIOLOGY AND ETIOLOGY

Osteosarcoma occurs most frequently in the second and third decades of life, so it is primarily a disease of adolescents and young adults. While it can occur in younger children, it is extremely rare in children less than 5 years of age. Each year there are about 600 new cases of osteosarcoma diagnosed in the United States.

The fact that the peak age of onset occurs during the adolescent growth spurt leads many to hypothesize that the development of osteosarcoma is related to rapid bone growth, although there is no direct evidence to support such a notion. However, one mechanism for the oncogenesis of osteosarcoma is clearly related to radiation exposure, since a significant percentage of cases occur in the treatment field of long-term cancer survivors who were treated with radiotherapy. The incidence of osteosarcoma is also greatly increased among survivors of retinoblastoma and in certain cancer family syndromes, such as Li-Fraumeni syndrome. This risk is related to the presence of germline gene mutations in the retinoblastoma (Rb) and p53 tumor suppressor genes, respectively. Both genes are important regulators of the cellular mechanisms that determine whether a cell continues through the cell cycle to cell division or proceeds to programmed cell death (apoptosis).

PATHOLOGY AND BIOLOGY

The diagnosis of osteosarcoma is usually suspected based on clinical history and the radiographic appearance of the bone lesion. Establishing the correct diagnosis, however, requires biopsy of the involved area. The light microscopic appearance of osteosarcoma is that of pleomorphic spindle tumor cells that are trying to form an osteoid matrix or, in other words, malignant cells that attempt to make bone. Several histologic variants have been described, such as osteoblastic, chondroblastic, fibroblastic, and telangiectatic, but these have no real therapeutic or prognostic significance.

The understanding of the biology of osteosarcoma has grown significantly in the past two decades. The most common genetic alterations occur in the tumor suppressor genes p53 and Rb, which appear to play an important role in the tumorogenesis of osteosarcoma. Other abnormalities of oncogenes have also been described. Thus, while acquired abnormalities in tumor suppressor genes are clearly important in the development of osteosarcoma, it is not clear which of these represents the seminal event in its development.

CLINICAL PRESENTATION

The most common presentation of osteosarcoma is a painful hard mass that appears to be arising from the bone. The pain often leads to other associated signs or symptoms, such as a limp or decreased use of an affected extremity. A history of trauma at the affected site is common and often leads to a delay in diagnosis. Osteosarcoma can occur in any bone in the body, but usually develops in the metaphysis of long bones. The most common sites are on either side of the knee (distal femur or proximal tibia), which account for more that 50% of tumors. The proximal humerus is the third most common site. Systemic symptoms, such as fever, night sweats, and weight loss, are rare, and the presence of such should lead one to consider other diagnoses, such as osteomyelitis or Ewing sarcoma. About 20% of osteosarcoma patients will have overt metastatic disease at diagnosis. Pulmonary metastatic disease is by far the most common, although metastatic disease in other bones or soft tissues occur.

DIAGNOSIS AND STAGING

A plain radiograph of the suspected site is the first step in the diagnostic workup. The usual radiographic appearance is that of a lytic and/or sclerotic bone abnormality. A "sunburst" appearance is the classic finding for this tumor. A soft tissue mass along with evidence of cortical destruction and periosteal reaction is a key feature distinguishing malignancy from other benign bone tumors. The extent of bone and soft tissue involvement is best assessed with a MRI scan, which should be done, if possible, prior to biopsy. While radiographic and clinical information can be suggestive, a biopsy of the tumor mass is mandatory in order to establish the correct diagnosis.

Even though needle biopsies can be adequate to establish the diagnosis, an open biopsy should be done whenever possible to obtain adequate tissue for diagnostic and biologic studies. It is also important that an expert do the biopsy in order to ensure that the incision is placed in such a way as not to limit future limb salvage possibilities. The remainder of the staging workup, which can be done before or after the biopsy, includes a CT of the chest to look for pulmonary disease and a technetium bone scan to look for other sites of bone involvement.

TREATMENT

Successful therapy for osteosarcoma requires not only local control of the primary tumor, but also systemic therapy to eradicate microscopic metastatic disease at distant sites. After biopsy confirms the diagnosis, the typical approach would be to use preoperative (neoadjuvant) chemotherapy for 10 to 12 weeks followed by surgery to resect the primary tumor. The use of preoperative chemotherapy allows one to assess tumor response to chemotherapy (which has important prognostic implications) and often reduces tumor bulk, making surgical resection easier. The surgical approach varies depending on the tumor location, extent of tumor involvement, and patient preferences, but undoubtedly will involve either amputation or some form of limb salvage surgery. Osteosarcoma is usually resistant to conventional doses of radiotherapy, thus limiting its role in local control. After surgical resection of the primary tumor, patients usually receive additional postoperative chemotherapy for a total of approximately 12 months. Standard chemotherapy includes high-dose methotrexate, alternating with the combination of doxorubicin and cisplatinum. Ifosfamide is also active against osteosarcoma, but it is unclear whether it provides any additional survival advantage. As one might guess, therapy for patients with metastatic disease is more complex and, usually, less successful. The usual approach is still preoperative chemotherapy followed by resection of the primary tumor mass. Resection of any metastatic disease is also important and usually performed after resection of the primary tumor.

With the therapeutic approach described earlier, approximately 65 to 70% of patients with nonmetastatic disease can expect to be cured. If such patients are going to relapse, it usually occurs within 2 years of the diagnosis. Determining which patients will do well and which will not is difficult to do; however, there are several variables that are predictive. The presence of metastatic disease at diagnosis indicates a poor prognosis, and the outlook for these patients depends on the extent of metastatic disease and how easily it can be surgically resected. For example, patients with only limited pulmonary metastatic disease have an intermediate prognosis (40% disease-free survival), but those with multiple bone metastatic disease have a uniformly poor prognosis (less than 5% disease-free survival). Within the nonmetastatic group, individuals with tumor primaries located in the axial skeleton appear to do better (compared with pelvic tumors), while those with elevated lactate dehydrogenase or alkaline phosphatase levels, and younger children (<10 years of age) generally do worse. Histologic response to preoperative chemotherapy (based on light microscopy assessment of percentage of tumor cell kill) is an excellent predictor of outcome. Patients with good responses, or high percentage of tumor cell kill, do much better.

Research in the treatment of osteosarcoma is now focusing on finding more effective therapies to help the 30 to 35% of patients who still die from this disease. Much of this effort is directed at understanding the biology of this neoplasm in hopes of identifying novel therapeutic targets.

Ewing Sarcoma

Ewing sarcoma is one of a group of tumors referred to as the Ewing sarcoma family tumors (ESFT). This tumor family consists of classic Ewing sarcoma of bone, soft tissue Ewing sarcoma, and peripheral primitive neuroectodermal tumors (PNET) of bone and soft tissue. They are grouped together because they arise from primitive neuroectodermal precursor cells and share the same chromosomal abnormalities. The key distinguishing feature of the different subtypes is the degree of neural differentiation: PNET demonstrates substantial neural differentiation compared with the undifferentiated Ewing sarcoma.

EPIDEMIOLOGY AND ETIOLOGY

Ewing sarcoma family tumors are the second most common malignant bone tumors in children and adolescents in the United States and Europe. While ESFT can occur at any age, greater than 80% of patients are less than 20 years of age at diagnosis, with approximately 50% between 10 and 20 years of age. The annual incidence in the United States is about 2.7 cases per million children less than 15 years of age. Interestingly, there is a marked ethnic disparity with ESFT occurring predominately in white children and those of Hispanic origin, but only rarely in African and Asian American children.

The cause of ESFT is unknown. However, in contrast to osteosarcomas, ESFT appear unrelated to radiation exposure, since they only rarely occur as a second malignant neoplasm after cancer therapy. Likewise, ESFT appear not to be inherited or associated with any cancer family syndromes.

PATHOLOGY AND BIOLOGY

The light microscopic appearance of ESFT is characterized by sheets of small to moderate round cells with scant cytoplasm, a round to oval nucleus, and little evidence of differentiation. Atypical variants are common and can present a significant diagnostic dilemma, especially in tumors that arise in the soft tissue. Neuroectodermal differentiation, based on positive staining for neural markers such as S100 and the presence of rosettes by light-microscopy or dense granules by electronmicroscopy, is the hallmark of the PNET variant. The distinction

between Ewing sarcoma and PNET variants, however, are not clinically important, since they do not appear to behave clinically or respond to therapy differently. Since greater than 90% of ESFT express the cell surface marker CD99 (MIC2 protein), immunohistochemical staining with antibodies (such as 013, HBA71, and 12E7) to CD99 can be helpful in distinguishing Ewing tumors from other small round cell tumors.

In the last decade, tremendous progress has been made in our understanding of the tumor genetics and biology of ESFT. Essentially all ESFT have in common a rearrangement of the *EWS* gene on chromosome 22. The most common is the *EWS/FLI1* rearrangement that is expressed cytogenetically as t(11;22)(q24;q13). This rearrangement creates an aberrant DNA transcription factor that plays a major role in the oncogenesis of ESFT.

CLINICAL PRESENTATION

Similar to osteosarcoma, pain and swelling at the site of the primary tumor are the most common presenting symptoms in patients with ESFT. Unlike osteosarcoma, systemic symptoms, such as fever and weight loss, are relatively common at presentation making it easy to confuse ESFT with osteomyelitis or histiocytosis. In general, systemic symptoms are more likely to occur in patients with metastatic disease. The time from onset of symptoms to diagnosis varies, but periods of 4 to 6 months are common, especially in those children with primaries arising in the pelvis.

Ewing sarcoma family tumors can develop in any bone in the body. The femur is the most common site, but ESFT arise in almost equal frequency from long bones of the extremities and bones of the axial skeleton. In contrast to osteosarcoma, which usually arise in the diaphysis or end of long bones, ESFT often occur in the metaphysis, or midshaft of long bones. The classic radiographic appearance is that of a lytic bone lesion with cortical destruction and laminating elevation of the periosteum (referred to as "onion skinning"). Soft tissue masses are common and can become quite massive, especially with pelvic tumors. The ESFT arising from the chest wall represent a special case and are historically referred to as Askin tumors. About 25% of patients with ESFT will present with overt metastatic disease. Lung parenchyma (most commonly), distant bone, and bone marrow are the most common sites.

DIAGNOSIS AND STAGING

The workup of patients with suspected ESFT begins with radiographic imaging of the presumed primary site followed by a detailed search for metastatic disease. Plain radiographs can be helpful in localizing and identifying the tumor, especially if they reveal the classic appearance. An MRI scan of the primary site is necessary to determine the extent of bone and soft tissue involvement. An open surgical biopsy is the preferred method of obtaining tissue for the diagnosis and, like osteosarcoma, should be done in a way as to not compromise later limb salvage surgery options. A chest radiograph and CT scan is important to rule out pulmonary metastatic disease, and a bone scan helps rule out distant bone metastatic disease. All patients should have a bone marrow aspirate and biopsy to search for bone marrow metastatic disease.

<u>TREATMENT</u>

The cornerstone of therapy for ESFT is local control of the primary tumor with surgery and/or radiotherapy and systemic chemotherapy to eradicate micrometastatic disease at distant sites. A standard approach is to start with chemotherapy for 10 to 12 weeks followed by local control with surgery or radiation therapy. The decision to use surgery or radiation depends on the location of the tumor and the likelihood of obtaining a complete resection. While ESFT are very radiosensitive neoplasms, surgery is usually the preferred option because it avoids the late effects of radiotherapy on bone growth and reduces the risk of radiotherapy-related second malignant neoplasms. After local control is complete, patients undergo more chemotherapy for a total of 12 months. The best treatment results have been obtained using combination chemotherapy with vincristine, doxorubicin, and cyclophosphamide, alternating with ifosfamide and etoposide.

Using the preceding approach, the 5-year event-free survival for patients with nonmetastatic disease is approximately 60 to 70%. For the most part, patients who are disease-free at 5 years are likely to be cured, but some very late relapses (as late as 17 years) have been reported. The presence or absence of metastatic disease at diagnosis is the best predictor of outcome. Patients with pulmonary-only metastatic disease have an intermediate prognosis between 30 to 40%, while those with widely metastatic disease involving bone and/or bone marrow do poorly. Very high dose chemotherapy with autologous bone marrow or stem cell rescue has been used with mixed results for patients with metastatic disease. Similar to osteosarcoma, patients with tumors that respond well to initial chemotherapy have a better outcome.

Histiocytosis

The histiocytoses are a fascinating constellation of disorders characterized by abnormal infiltrations and accumulations of cells from the monocyte-macrophage lineage. In the past decade a new classification system has been adopted based on the relation of these disorders to normal histiocytes and reticulocytes. This system consists of three classes of histiocytoses, which provide a conceptual framework for diagnosis and treatment.

<u>CLASS I HISTIOCYTOSIS</u>

This group of disorders, formerly known as histiocytosis X, includes those syndromes whose cell of origin has the features of Langerhans cell histiocytes. Langerhans cells are normal tissue histiocytes in skin and serve an important antigen processing and presentation function (dendritic cells). The class I histiocytoses, best referred to as Langerhans cell histiocytosis (LCH), are not true malignancies, but rather represent a clonal proliferation of Langerhans cells probably due to abnormal immune regulation. Eosinophilic granuloma, Hand-Schüller-Christian disease, and Letterer-Siwe disease, known from the previous nomenclature, fit into this category.

The light microscopic appearance of the LCH is that of granulomatous lesions with histiocytic infiltration usually with eosinophils. Langerhans cells stain positively for S100, and electronmicroscopy demonstrates the characteristic finding of Birbeck granules (granules shaped like "tennis rackets") in the cytoplasm. The pathophysiologic significance of Birbeck granules is not known.

Clinical presentation. As Langerhans cell histiocytosis can involve almost any organ system, it therefore can present in a variety of ways. Typical signs and symptoms include skin rash, chronic ear drainage from external canal or middle ear involvement, fever, adenopathy, bone pain, diabetes insipidus from pituitary gland involvement, hepatosplenomegaly, and cytopenias from bone marrow involvement. The clinical hallmark is the presence of lytic bone lesions on plain radiograph. When LCH presents in infants, it tends to be severe and involve multiple organs systems, while in older children it is usually more limited. It is important to note that children with skull involvement are especially likely to also have pituitary involvement manifested as diabetes insipidus.

The initial evaluation of children with suspected histiocytosis includes taking careful history, especially regarding the presence of polyuria and polydypsia. All such patients should have a urinalysis to check the urine-specific gravity. The diagnosis of LCH is made by tissue biopsy of the most accessible involved site.

Treatment. The treatment of LCH should take into account that the disease will usually resolve on its own. Unfortunately, resolution of the disease can take many years and during this time children can develop substantial and potentially life-threatening morbidities. Therefore, treatment is designed to use the least therapy possible in order to limit or eliminate symptoms and morbidity. Children with local disease, such as an isolate bone lesion, are best treated with surgery or low dose radiotherapy. Those with more extensive disease require systemic chemotherapy. A typical treatment plan might include an induction phase with prednisone and vinblastine followed by continuation therapy with weekly vinblastine. After the symptoms resolve, it is usually possible to gradually taper the dose frequency of vinblastine. Children with multiorgan system disease may require additional chemotherapy agents such as etoposide.

The likely treatment outcome depends on the age at diagnosis and the degree of organ system involvement.

Children younger than 2 years of age tend to have a more severe form of disease with higher mortality rates compared with older children. The presence of multiple organ system dysfunctions is also a poor prognostic sign.

CLASS II HISTIOCYTOSIS

The class II histiocytoses are a fascinating and, fortunately, very rare group of disorders characterized by an abnormal proliferation of normal monocyte-macrophage cells. The class II disorders differ from the class I disorders in that they involve the true phagocytic macrophages. They are nonmalignant because there is no cytological atypia; in other words, the macrophages appear normal under the microscope. The two most significant disorders in this group are infection-associated hemophagocytic syndrome (IAHS)(also referred to as viral-associated hemophagocytic syndrome) and familial erythrophagocytic lymphohistiocytosis (FEL).

Clinical presentation. The class II histiocytoses appear to be due to abnormal macrophage regulation secondary to an underlying immunodeficiency. Typical presenting features include fever, adenopathy, organomegaly with organ dysfunction or potentially failure, and pancytopenia. Often these patients are very ill appearing with multiorgan system failure. The diagnosis is made by biopsy of involved organs, usually a lymph node, or by the demonstration of erythrophagocytosis on bone marrow aspirate (morphologically normal macrophages with red blood cells inside them).

Familial erythrophagocytic lymphohistiocytosis is very rare and, as indicated by its name, patients usually have a positive family history. More common, IAHS is associated with a variety of infectious organisms and immunodeficiencies. The most common situation is an EBV infection in patients with an underlying T-cell immunodeficiency (either acquired or congenital). It also can sometimes occur in association with T-cell malignancies.

Treatment. Treatment of these disorders is difficult and usually successful only if the underlying immunodeficiency can be corrected. In the case of FEL, bone marrow transplant is essentially the only way to achieve a cure. With IAHS it is sometimes possible to change the course of the disease if the underlying immunodeficiency can be corrected with drug therapy (either withdrawing immunosuppression or treating the T-cell malignancy).

CLASS III HISTIOCYTOSIS

Class III histiocytosis comprises the true malignant disorders of the monocyte and macrophage lineage, such as acute monoblastic leukemia (M5 AML), malignant histiocytosis, and histiocytic lymphoma. Acute monoblastic leukemia is derived from bone marrow monoblasts and is the most common histiocytic cancer in childhood. True malignant histiocytosis is almost exclusively a disease of adults and represents a malignant clone that is partially differentiated from a monocyte toward a tissue histiocyte. Histiocytic lymphoma is malignant at the stage of the tissue histiocyte and, at least in childhood, can be considered a type of large cell lymphoma.

The typical presentation includes fever, weight loss, hepatosplenomegaly, and lymphadenopathy. The diagnosis is usually made by lymph node biopsy. Histiocytic malignancies are usually treated with chemotherapy and potentially bone marrow transplantation, as described in the earlier sections on AML and NHL.

CHEMOTHERAPY BASICS

Most chemotherapeutic agents produce cytotoxic effects by interfering with the synthesis or function of DNA (Table 14–8). Only actively proliferating cells are susceptible to the effects of these agents; therefore, cancer chemotherapy drugs are most effective in cancers with a high growth fraction. Because growth fraction decreases as tumor size increases, most chemotherapy is more effective against microscopic disease than bulk disease.

Developing a rational approach to the use of chemotherapy drugs in children has been difficult since pharmacokinetic studies in children are limited and the mechanism of action of many anticancer drugs are not well understood. Combination chemotherapy using drugs with different mechanisms of action and nonoverlapping toxicities however, is almost always superior to single drug therapy. Such an approach appears to provide the greatest range of coverage against naturally occurring chemotherapy resistance and decreases the chance of acquired resistance. Most drug dosages and combination schedules have been determined empirically, usually through a series of clinical trials. Phase I trials involve determining the dose-limiting toxicity of a new anticancer drug, while phase II trials focus on empirically determining which types of cancer the drug is active against. Phase III trials involve the comparison of a particular treatment regimen to another control regimen, usually in the form of a randomized trial.

Acute toxicities of chemotherapy include myelosuppression, nausea and vomiting, alopecia, mucositis, allergic or cutaneous reactions, and local tissue burn from subcutaneous extravasation of the drug. Some drugs have unique toxicities, such as cardiotoxicity with anthracyclines and neuropathy with vincristine. Fever is particularly dangerous during periods of myelosuppression since the absence of neutrophils puts patients at increased risk of developing a life-threatening bacterial or fungal infection. Transfusions with platelets and packed red blood cells are necessary for many patients during treatment. Nausea and vomiting secondary to the chemotherapy can usually be controlled with antiemetic drugs.

The late effects of chemotherapy on children who survive cancer are a growing concern. The major adverse side effects include impaired musculoskeletal growth, developmental and learning disabilities, impaired reproductive

Table 14–8. Summary of Commonly Used Chemotherapy Agents

Class	Mode of Action	Examples
Alkylating agent	Covalently binds alkyl group, leads to DNA-protein and DNA-DNA cross-links, leads to DNA damage	Cyclophosphamide, ifosfamide, nitrogen mustard, nitrosureas, cisplatinum
Antimetabolites	Structural analogues of enzyme substrates in a variety of biosynthetic pathways that inhibit the synthesis of nucleic acids and proteins	Methotrexate (folate analogue) 6-mercaptopurine and 6-thioguanine (purine analogue), cytosine arabinoside, and 5-fluorouracil (pyrimidine analogue)
Antitumor antibiotics	Binds to DNA by intercalation, interferes with DNA synthesis and transcription, inhibits topo-isomerases (DNA repair mechanism)	Doxorubicin, daunorubicin, bleomycin
Microtubule inhibitors	Disrupts intracellular microtubular system, inhibits mitotic spindle	Vincristine, vinblastine, taxol
Topoisomerase II inhibitors	Interacts with DNA to inhibit topoisomerase II, which leads to impaired DNA repair	Etoposide (VP-16), teniposide (VM-26)
Topoisomerase I inhibitors	Inhibits topoisomerase I blocking DNA repair	Topotecan
Corticosteroids	Lympholytic agents used in ALL and lymphomas	Prednisone, dexamethasone
Enzymes	Selectively depletes pool of the amino acid L-asparagine that ALL and NHL cannot readily synthesize	L-Asparaginase

ALL = acute lymphoblastic leukemia; DNA = deoxyribonucleic acid; NHL = non-Hodgkin lymphoma.

function, and the possibility of permanent cardiac, pulmonary, or renal damage. In addition, patients treated with chemotherapy for a malignancy are at a greater risk than the general population for developing a second malignancy. The long-term toxicities of radiation are of particular concern for children, not only because of the increased risks of second malignancies, but also because of impaired growth of the musculoskeletal system.

Over the past decade, there have been significant advances in the understanding of how anticancer drugs kill cancer cells and how cancer cells develop drug resistance. The cytotoxic action of most cancer chemotherapy appears to be related to the apoptosis (programmed cell death) regulatory systems in cells. Drug resistance most likely develops from alterations in these pathways that result in a cancer cell circumventing chemotherapy-induced apoptosis. A great deal of research is currently directed at finding ways to bypass this drug resistance.

ONCOLOGIC EMERGENCIES

While there are many problems encountered in the care of children with cancer that require urgent attention, there are four clinical situations that constitute true medical emergencies: tumor lysis syndrome, SVC syndrome, spinal cord compression, and leukostasis. Table 14–9 summarizes the oncological emergencies, situations in which they are likely to occur, and appropriate interventions. Timely and appropriate intervention can mean the difference between life and death.

Tumor lysis syndrome is a metabolic derangement caused by rapid lysis of leukemic cells with release of intracellular phosphate, uric acid, and potassium at a rate that exceeds renal clearance. It is most commonly encountered during the initial 48 h of treating children with rapidly growing tumors, such Burkitt lymphoma or T-cell ALL (with high WBC). Usually the first signs are hyperkalemia, hyperphosphatemia, hypocalcemia, and hyperuricemia in serum laboratory studies. The electrolyte abnormalities can rapidly worsen if uric acid, phosphate, and calcium precipitate in the renal tubules, which can lead to acute renal failure. The best treatment for tumor lysis syndrome is to prevent problems by maintaining a high urine output with aggressive hydration and allopurinol to limit the production of uric acid and by creating an alkaline urine pH to increase the solubility of uric acid. Frequent monitoring of serum electrolytes, uric acid levels, and urine pH are mandatory. The basic management plan is summarized in Table 14–9.

Another important emergency is SVC syndrome, which is described in the section on NHL. The SVC syndrome is most often caused by an anterior mediastinal

Table 14–9. Summary of Most Common Oncology Emergencies

Emergency	Situation	Management
Tumor lysis syndrome	Fast growing cancer (Burkitt lymphoma, leukemias/NHL), related to tumor burden	IV hydration at 3000 mL/m^2, monitor intake and output; alkalinization of urine with Na bicarbonate NaHCO$_3$ 150–200 mEq/m^2 d; allopurinol 300 mg/m^2 divided q8h; cardiac monitor; monitor electrolytes/uric acid/calcium/phosphorous q4–8 h; oral aluminum phosphate binders as necessary; standard potassium reduction measures as necessary; mannitol, if urine output decreases; renal dialysis as required
Superior vena cava syndrome	Mediastinal mass	ICU monitoring airway and venous return; corticosteroids and/or radiotherapy; prompt institution of chemotherapy
Spinal cord compression	Tumor extension into intervertebral foramina (Ewing's sarcoma or neuroblastoma); primary CNS tumor; CNS tumor drop metastasis	Meticulous neurologic exam; dexamethasone 8–40 mg divided q6h depending on patient size; emergent radiotherapy; emergent surgical decompression
Leukostasis	Hyperleukocytosis (>100,000–200,000 WBC/mm^3); occurs in AML primarily	IV hydration at 3000 mL/m^2; leukocytopheresis (apheresis of WBCs); prompt institution of chemotherapy (watch for and prevent tumor lysis syndrome)

AML = acute myelogenous leukemia; CNS = central nervous system; ICU = intensive care unit; NHL = non-Hodgkin lymphoma; WBC = white blood cell count.

mass that compresses not only the SVC, but vital airway structures as well. Children with SVC syndrome should be monitored in the hospital (usually the intensive care unit), with a diagnosis made and treatment begun as soon as possible. Great care should be taken in sedating these patients since it can be very difficult for them to maintain an open airway once they fall asleep. Sometimes patients will need immediate treatment to reduce tumor compression prior to establishing a diagnosis. In this situation, steroids or a few doses of radiotherapy are usually enough to decrease tumor bulk until a biopsy can be performed.

Spinal cord compression can occur from a variety of different cancer types. The most common situation in children results from extension of a tumor, such as Ewing's sarcoma or neuroblastoma, into the intervertebral foramina. It is also possible for a metastatic tumor in the vertebral body or subarachnoid metastases from a primary CNS tumor to cause cord compression. One must always consider the possibility of cord compression in any cancer patient that complains of back pain, paresthesias, bladder or bowel problems, or muscle weakness. A meticulous physical exam including neurological exam must be done and an emergent MRI performed if cord compression is possible. If spinal cord compression is confirmed, immediate treatment with high-dose dexamethasone, followed by decompression with surgery or radiotherapy, must be instituted. Failure to recognize spinal cord compression might result in permanently paralyzed patients.

Leukostasis can occur in children with AML or CML who have WBCs over 100,000 cells/mm^3, although the risk is highest above 200,000 cells/mm^3. The elevated WBC results in increased blood viscosity, leukemia blast cell aggregates, and microthrombi formation that can compromise blood perfusion and lead to organ failure or stroke. Signs and symptoms include dyspnea, mental status changes, blurred vision, hypoxia, and acidosis. Often hydration alone will be adequate to drop the WBC to a safe level. If the WBC continues to climb or patients develop symptoms, however, leukocytopheresis (removal of WBCs by an apheresis procedure), followed by treatment of the underlying malignancy, is the next step.

THE FAMILY AND CHILD WITH CANCER

The diagnosis of cancer in children is an incomprehensible tragedy for families. Reactions of fear, anger, denial, and disbelief are common and expected. Approaching the family with sensitivity and care is crucial to establishing a long-term working relationship. Once the possibility of a cancer diagnosis is raised, the greatest source of anxiety is usually that of uncertainty and lack of control. When the diagnosis is confirmed, even if the long-term prognosis is poor, there is some relief from at least knowing what one is dealing with. Thus, one of the most compassionate things a physician can do for a family is proceed with the diagnostic workup in a timely and efficient manner. During this phase, a thorough and thoughtful explanation of the upcoming diagnostic evaluation and procedures are crucial for preparing the child and family and play an instrumental role in building trust.

Once the workup is complete and the diagnosis is confirmed, a family conference should be held to discuss the findings and the possibilities for treatment. This conference should include members of the family, key caretakers, and the health care team, comprising the oncology nurse specialist, social worker, pediatric oncologist, and primary care physician. Encouraging the family to bring a tape recorder or take notes at the session provides the opportunity for them to review the discussion at a later time. It is also wise to provide the family with educational materials before the conference so that they may prepare questions in advance. The family conference should cover the cause of the disease, the outcome without treatment, treatment options, possible clinical trials, and the team's specific recommendations for treatment. Information should be given on how chemotherapy works, acute and chronic effects of chemotherapy, and the side effects of the specific chemotherapy to be used. In addition, the psychological impact of the experience on the patient and the family should be discussed. This is also the time when consent is obtained to proceed with treatment. Perhaps the most important function of the meeting, besides conveying information about the disease and treatment, is to emphasize that treating a child with cancer is a team effort in which the family plays a crucial role. The family should be told that, besides curing cancer, the goal of treatment is to promote and maintain as normal a childhood as possible for patients and their siblings. Emphasizing the importance of the family's role as educated advocates for the child not only ensures knowledge of the treatment and expected side effects, but also allows the family to experience some sense of control and usefulness. An educated and reliable family is invaluable for everyone involved.

The family and child will usually manifest a myriad of behaviors and emotions in response to the diagnosis of cancer and helping guide the family to find productive coping strategies can greatly improve the child's overall well-being. Particular attention to the special needs and responses of the patient's siblings are important. It is not uncommon to see school problems, acting out, and depression in the siblings of children in whom cancer is diagnosed. The combined insights of the medical team members should be shared in regular discussions with the family to ward off predictable and anticipated problems throughout the course of treatment. Involving the family in a support group may be helpful and should be recommended to all families.

In summary, responding to both the child and the family with respect, patience, and honesty is crucial to succeed in the complicated, often lengthy and stressful process of treating cancer in a child.

REFERENCES

Bleyer WA: The U.S. pediatric cancer clinical trials programmes: International implications and the way forward. Europ J Cancer 1997;33:1439.

Rubnitz JE, Crist WM: Molecular genetics of childhood cancer: implications for pathogenesis, diagnosis, and treatment. Pediatrics 1997;100:101.

Acute Leukemia

Ebb DH, Weinstein HJ: Diagnosis and treatment of childhood acute myelogenous leukemia. Pediatr Clin North Am 1997;44:847.

Pui CH: Acute lymphoblastic leukemia. Pediatr Clin North Am 1997;44:831.

Shu XO: Epidemiology of childhood leukemia. Curr Opin Hematol 1997;4:227.

Smith M, et al: Uniform approach to risk classification and treatment assignment for children with acute lymphoblastic leukemia. J Clin Oncol 1996;14:18.

Lymphadenopathy

Perkins SL, Segal GH, Kjeldsberg CR: Work-up of lymphadenopathy in children. Semin Diagnos Pathol 1995;12:284.

Non-Hodgkin Lymphoma

Sandlund JT, Downing JR, Crist WM: Non-Hodgkin's lymphoma in childhood. New Engl J Med 1996;334:1238.

Hodgkin Lymphoma

Hudson MM, Donaldson SS: Hodgkin's disease. Pediatr Clin North Am 1997;44:891.

Neuroblastoma

Maris JM, Matthay KK: Molecular biology of neuroblastoma. J Clin Oncol 1999; 17:2264.

Matthay KK, et al: Treatment of high risk neuroblastoma with intensive chemotherapy, radiotherapy, autologous bone marrow transplantation, and 13-*cis*-retinoic acid. New Engl J Med 1999;341:1165.

Wilms Tumor

Petruzzi MJ, Green DM: Wilms tumor. Pediatr Clin North Am 1997;44:939.

Rhabdomyosarcoma

Arndt CA, Crist WM: Common musculoskeletal tumors of childhood and adolescence. New Engl J Med 1999;341:342.

Bone Tumors

Link MP, et al: The effect of adjuvant chemotherapy on relapse-free survival in patients with osteosarcoma of the extremity. N Engl J Med 1986;314:1600.

Granowetter L, West DC: The Ewing's sarcoma family of tumors: Ewing's sarcoma and peripheral primitive neuroectodermal tumor of bone and soft tissue, in *Diagnostic and Therapeutic Advances in Pediatric Oncology.* Boston, Kluwer Academic Publishers, 1997.

Kidneys & Electrolytes

15

Anthony A. Portale, MD, Robert S. Mathias, MD, Donald E. Potter, MD, & David R. Rozansky, MD, PhD

EVALUATION OF RENAL FUNCTION

In healthy individuals, the kidneys excrete water, solutes, and metabolic wastes in amounts that permit the maintenance of a relatively constant internal milieu despite the consumption of a widely varied diet. Cellular integrity depends on the maintenance of a tightly regulated extracellular fluid (ECF) osmolality. In response to information from osmoreceptors and volume receptors, the brain and kidneys produce hormones and vasoactive substances that allow rapid and precise regulation of salt and water excretion by the kidney.

The kidneys produce urine via glomerular ultrafiltration of plasma and selective tubular reabsorption of water and solutes; tubular secretion of solutes also plays an important but lesser role. The kidneys receive approximately 20% of the cardiac output via the renal arteries. In individuals with a cardiac output of 5 L/min, renal blood flow is 1 L/min and renal plasma flow is 550 mL/min, assuming a hematocrit of 45%. As a consequence of the Starling forces, which favor filtration, and a highly permeable glomerular capillary membrane of large surface area, approximately one fifth of the plasma flowing through the glomerular capillaries is filtered into Bowman's space. The rate of formation of ultrafiltrate is termed the *glomerular filtration rate (GFR)*. In a 70-kg adult man, the GFR is approximately 125 mL/min, or 180 L/d. Because the GFR is determined in part by cardiac output and renal plasma flow, both of which are a function of body size and gender, the GFR in children is lower than that in adults. Rather than establishing normative values for children of various ages and sizes, it is customary for the measured GFR to be normalized to a body surface area of 1.73 m^2 using the following formula:

$$GFR(mL/min/1.73m^2) = \frac{GFR(mL/min) \times 1.73m^2}{SA(m^2)}$$

where SA equals the surface area of the patient.

Within each nephron, the ultrafiltrate of plasma passes from Bowman's space into the renal tubule, where its composition is changed by reabsorptive and secretory transport processes. More than 99% of the filtered water, sodium, chloride, and bicarbonate is reabsorbed by the renal tubule and returned to the blood. The daily filtered

load of sodium is approximately 25,000 mEq; the tubules reabsorb this amount minus an amount equal to the daily dietary intake of sodium, 100–250 mEq/d, which is excreted. Failure to reabsorb nearly all the sodium filtered would quickly result in life-threatening sodium and volume depletion. The kidneys also excrete the daily load of endogenous acid produced from diet and metabolism and remove metabolic wastes, such as urea nitrogen, creatinine, phosphorus, and uric acid.

GLOMERULAR FILTRATION RATE

The need to assess renal function in children arises when they have symptoms or signs suggestive of renal disease, such as abnormal urinary findings, peripheral edema, or hypertension. The GFR is an important measure of renal function, as it reflects the overall excretory function of the kidney and, therefore, the number of functioning nephrons. Glomerular filtration rate is not measured directly, but can be estimated by measuring the clearance from plasma of a marker substance such as inulin. Inulin, a low-molecular-weight sugar, is an ideal substance for estimating GFR because it is not bound to plasma proteins, is freely filtered by the glomerulus, and is not reabsorbed, secreted, or metabolized by the renal tubules. *Renal clearance* of any substance is defined as the volume of plasma completely cleared of that substance per unit time. When inulin is infused intravenously at a constant rate to achieve a steady-state plasma inulin concentration, all the inulin filtered by the glomerulus is excreted in the urine, thus completely clearing the volume of plasma filtered.

The clearance of inulin (C_{inulin}) is calculated according to the following equation:

$$GFR \cong C_{inulin}(mL/min) \frac{U_{inulin} \times V(mL/min)}{P_{inulin}}$$

where U_{inulin} equals urinary inulin concentration, V equals the volume of urine passed during a given time, and P_{inulin} equals the plasma inulin concentration. Normative values for GFR (corrected to 1.73 m^2), measured by inulin clearance in children, are listed in Table 15–1.

The clearance of creatinine (C_{creat}), the metabolic end-product of normal muscle metabolism, is commonly used to estimate GFR in the clinical setting. At steady state,

593

Table 15–1. Glomerular Filtration Rate (GFR) Measured by Inulin Clearance at Different Ages

Age	GFR (Inulin Clearance) Mean and Range (± 2 SD) (mL/min/1.73 m²)
Premature	47 (29–65)
2–8 d	38 (26–60)
4–28 d	48 (26–68)
35–95 d	58 (30–88)
1–6 mo	77 (41–103)
6–12 mo	103 (49–157)
12–19 mo	127 (63–191)
2–12 y	127 (89–185)
Adult men	131 (88–174)
Adult women	117 (87–147)

the rate of creatinine produced from muscle metabolism remains relatively constant from day to day and is equal to the rate of creatinine excretion. In normally proportioned individuals, the rate of creatinine excretion ranges from approximately 15 mg/kg/d in young children to 20 to 24 mg/kg/d in adults; this difference reflects the proportionate increase in muscle mass that occurs with growth. The C_{Creat} is usually measured from a urine specimen collected over a 24-h period; the plasma creatinine value is determined at the end of the urine collection period. The C_{Creat} is calculated according to the following equation:

$$C_{Creat}(mL/min) = \frac{U_{Creat}(mg/dL) \times V(mL/min)}{P_{Creat}(mg/dL)}$$

The C_{Creat} tends to overestimate the GFR because, in addition to being filtered across the glomerulus, creatinine also is secreted into the renal tubular lumen. When renal function is normal, C_{Creat} overestimates the GFR by approximately 10 to 20%; the degree of overestimation increases substantially, however, as renal function worsens, because a greater percentage of the creatinine excreted derives from tubular secretion. Despite these limitations, C_{Creat} determination remains a useful and readily obtainable estimate of the GFR. Repeated measurements made over time provide useful information about the rate of disease progression or regression.

Radionuclide imaging studies also can be used to estimate the GFR. The low-molecular-weight filtration markers, diethylenetriaminepenta-acetic acid (DTPA) and iothalamate, can be conjugated to radioisotopes and then injected intravenously into the patient. Their rate of appearance in and disappearance from the kidneys is monitored by external radiation counters. Estimates of GFR obtained with this technique are comparable to those obtained by inulin clearance measurements. Performance of a radionuclide study requires less time than does a C_{Creat} deter-mination and does not necessitate blood or urine collection; its disadvantages are a relatively high cost, the need for intravenous access, and the radiation exposure, albeit low.

In clinical practice, the plasma creatinine concentration is the most commonly used index of kidney function. It can be seen from the following equation that the C_{Creat}, which estimates the GFR, varies inversely with the plasma creatinine (P_{Cr}) concentration:

$$C_{creat} = \frac{Constant}{P_{Creat}}$$

where Constant equals the daily amount of creatinine excreted in urine. To see how C_{Creat} and P_{Creat} are inversely related, consider a patient with a GFR of 120 mL/min and serum creatinine concentration of 1.0 mg/dL. A decrease in GFR to 60 mL/min (a 50% decrease) will be accompanied by an increase in serum creatinine concentration to 2.0 mg/dL. An important hazard of using P_{Creat} to monitor renal function is that the largest actual reduction in GFR is accompanied by the smallest numerical increase in the serum creatinine concentration. For example, in a healthy 4-year-old child in whom the serum creatinine concentration normally is 0.4 mg/dL, a 50% decrease in GFR (from 120 mL/min/1.73 m² to 60 mL/min/1.73 m²) will result in a doubling of the serum creatinine concentration to 0.8 mg/dL, an increase of only 0.4 mg/dL. A further limitation of use of the serum creatinine concentration to monitor GFR is that a mild to moderate decrease in GFR is accompanied by an increase in the rate of tubular secretion of creatinine. The increased tubular secretion of creatinine limits the increase in serum creatinine concentration that would be expected from the decrease in GFR. When creatinine secretory activity is maximally increased, further decreases in the GFR are more directly associated with increases in serum creatinine concentration.

An easily obtainable estimate of GFR often is needed when evaluating patients with renal disease or determining the correct drug dosage for medications that undergo renal metabolism or excretion. Various formulas have been developed that allow for an estimation of the C_{Creat} from the serum creatinine concentration and some parameter of body size. The following formula (Schwartz formula), which was derived from measurements of height, serum creatinine concentration, and C_{Creat} values, can be used in children:

$$C_{Creat}(mL/min/1.73m^2) = \frac{K \times Height\,(cm)}{P_{Creat}(mg/dL)}$$

where K is a coefficient that accounts for differences in body size and thus in muscle mass in children of different ages and sexes. The appropriate values of K to be used in this equation are listed in Table 15–2.

Table 15–2. K Values for Children of Various Ages for Use in Schwartz Formula

Age	K Value
Low-birth-weight infants <1 y	0.33
Full-term infants <1 y	0.45
Children 2–12 y	0.55
Girls 13–21 y	0.55
Boys 13–21 y	0.70

URINALYSIS

A complete urinalysis includes both chemical and microscopic examination of a urine specimen; the specific determinations of which are listed in Table 15–3. The general appearance of urine can provide useful information, as frothy or foamy urine may indicate proteinuria; pink, red, or tea-colored urine usually indicates hematuria.

The urine *specific gravity* is a measurement of the density of urine compared with that of water. Under most circumstances, the urine specific gravity reflects the osmolality of the urine, which in turn reflects the action of antidiuretic hormone (ADH; arginine vasopressin) on the renal tubule. The normal range of urine specific gravity is 1.001 to 1.030, corresponding to a urine osmolality of approximately 40 to 1200 mOsm/kg. In patients with diabetes insipidus, the urine specific gravity is very low, usually 1.000 to 1.005, whereas in those with the syndrome of inappropriate antidiuretic hormone (SIADH) secretion, urine specific gravity is high, 1.015 to 1.030. Osmolality is the preferred measurement of renal con-

centrating capacity, as the presence of glucose, protein, or contrast media in urine can give rise to an increase in the measured specific gravity without a change in osmolality.

Chemical tests can be performed on urine specimens using reagent-impregnated dipsticks that yield semiquantitative results. Urinary *pH,* measured with the dipstick, or less commonly with a pH electrode, ranges from approximately 4.5 to 8.0 throughout the course of the day; first morning specimens typically are acidic (i.e., <6.0). Measurement of urinary pH during acid or bicarbonate loading of patients with suspected renal tubular acidosis can help to delineate the precise location of the renal tubular defect.

The dipstick detects urinary *protein concentration.* A positive result by dipstick can reflect either an increased quantity of urinary protein or a normal quantity of protein in a concentrated specimen. Collection of a timed urine specimen is necessary to quantitate urinary protein excretion precisely (see section "Proteinuria").

The presence of *glucose* in the urine, in the absence of hyperglycemia, suggests an impairment in the tubular handling of glucose, as occurs in the Fanconi syndrome, a disorder in which proximal tubular reabsorption of phosphate, amino acids, and bicarbonate also is impaired.

Urine dipsticks yield a positive test for blood when either hemoglobin or myoglobin is present in the urine. Hemoglobin is detected when either erythrocytes or free hemoglobin are present; the latter can occur in patients with intravascular hemolysis. Myoglobinuria occurs during rhabdomyolysis. On microscopic examination of urine, the finding of erythrocytes confirms the presence of hematuria, and the finding of red blood cell (RBC) casts confirms that the kidney is the source of the hematuria. The presence of white blood cells (WBCs) suggests an infection of the urinary tract; WBC casts accompanied by a positive urine culture are diagnostic of urinary tract infection. Other types of casts, such as hyaline or granular casts, can be found in normal individuals and are therefore nondiagnostic.

Crystals can form in the urine in a pH- and temperature-dependent manner. In acid urine, calcium oxalate and uric acid crystals are most commonly seen; both may be present in the urine of normal individuals. Cystine crystals are always abnormal and indicate that patients have either cystinosis or cystinuria. In alkaline urine from healthy individuals, calcium carbonate, calcium phosphate, and triple phosphate crystals can be seen. Triple phosphate crystals are also seen in patients with urinary tract infections (UTIs) caused by urease-producing bacteria.

Table 15–3. Components of a Urinalysis

General Appearance	
Color	Odor
Turbidity	Foam
Specific Gravity Chemical Tests (Dipstick)	
pH	Bilirubin
Protein	Urobilinogen
Glucose	Nitrite
Ketones	Leukocyte esterase
Blood	
Microscopic Examination	
WBC, WBC casts	Hyaline, granular casts
RBC, RBC casts	Bacteria
Epithelial cells	Crystals

RBC = red blood cell; WBC = white blood cell.

FLUIDS AND ELECTROLYTES

Disorders of Plasma Sodium

The kidneys are responsible for maintaining plasma osmolality within a narrow range and for regulating the body's overall fluid balance. Parallel regulatory systems have evolved to achieve these goals. Plasma osmolality is monitored by osmoregulatory sensors in the hypothalamus and regulated by the actions of ADH on the kidney. Extracellular fluid volume is monitored by low pressure (cardiac atria) and high pressure (aortic arch, carotid sinus, and renal juxtaglomerular apparatus) baroreceptors, and is sensitively regulated via complex interactions of the renin-angiotensin-aldosterone system, atrial natriuretic factor (ANF), sympathetic nervous system, and, to a lesser extent, intrarenal hemodynamics and ADH. Although sodium and its associated anions account for 97% of plasma osmolality, abnormalities of plasma sodium concentration—whether increased or decreased—represent disorders of water balance. Since both hyponatremia and hypernatremia can result in serious and permanent neurologic sequelae, an approach to diagnosis and appropriate treatment is essential.

HYPONATREMIA

Hyponatremia is defined as a plasma sodium concentration of <135 mEq/L. Life-threatening neurologic symptoms can develop when the plasma sodium decreases to <120 mEq/L, but symptoms can be present at higher sodium concentrations, if the rate of decrease of the sodium concentration is rapid or other intracerebral hemodynamic factors are deranged.

Hyponatremia represents a decrease in the ratio of total body sodium relative to total body water. Hyponatremia can occur if (1) total body sodium content is reduced with a lesser reduction in total body water; (2) total body sodium content is normal with excess total body water; or (3) total body sodium content is increased with a greater excess of total body water. Hyponatremia can occur with either suppression or stimulation of ADH release. The most common causes of hyponatremia are listed in Table 15–4.

Hyponatremia occurs when water intake exceeds the kidney's capacity for water excretion; under these circumstances, plasma ADH is usually appropriately suppressed. The capacity of normal kidneys to excrete water is substantial, approximately 8 L per day in a healthy 40-kg child with normal solute excretion, thus hyponatremia due to excessive water intake is uncommon. The capacity for water excretion, however, can be significantly impaired in patients with low GFR, such as in premature infants or patients with acquired renal disease, or in individuals with a greatly reduced solute load for excretion, such as in malnutrition. Diuretics, especially thiazide diuretics, also can impair maximum renal diluting capacity. Thus, excessive water intake is more likely to induce hyponatremia when these conditions are present.

More commonly, hyponatremia occurs in settings in which plasma ADH concentrations are increased. Antidiuretic hormone release is stimulated by baroreceptor-mediated mechanisms when the effective circulating

Table 15–4. Causes of Hyponatremia

Decreased ADH
  Reduced GFR
  Greatly increased water intake/polydipsia
  Very low solute intake (malnutrition)
  Thiazide diuretics

Increased ADH
  Hypovolemia
    Renal: Mineralocorticoid deficiency or resistance, diuretic excess
    Extrarenal: hemorrhage, dehydration, capillary leak syndrome
  Normovolemia
    Glucocorticoid deficiency, hypothyroidism
  Hypervolemia
    Nephrotic syndrome, congestive heart failure, hepatic cirrhosis
  SIADH

ADH = antidiuretic hormone; GFR = glomerular filtration rate; SIADH = syndrome of inappropriate ADH secretion.

volume is decreased. As depicted in Table 15–4, decreased effective circulating volume can be associated with hypovolemia, as with dehydration or hemorrhage, normovolemia, as with adrenal or thyroid insufficiency, or hypervolemia, as with congestive heart failure, hepatic cirrhosis, or nephrotic syndrome. Plasma ADH concentrations also can be increased in the absence of changes in effective circulating volume by the so-called syndrome of inappropriate ADH secretion (SIADH), which has multiple etiologies (a partial list is shown in Table 15–5). For an additional discussion of ADH, see Chapter 19, "Endocrinology."

Table 15–5. Causes of SIADH

Increased secretion of ADH from posterior pituitary gland
  Disorders of CNS
    Tumors, meningitis, vasculitis, subarachnoid hemorrhage, postcranial surgery, psychosis
  Pulmonary disease
    Asthma, tuberculosis, pneumonia
  Drugs stimulating ADH release
    Morphine, nicotine, tricyclic antidepressants, cyclophosphamide

Ectopic ADH secretion
  Carcinoma of lung
  Carcinoid tumor
  Lymphoma
  Thymoma
  Hepatoma

ADH = antidiuretic hormone; CNS = central nervous system; SIADH = syndrome of inappropriate ADH secretion.

The diagnosis of hyponatremia requires a careful assessment of water intake (both oral and parenteral) and water loss (including skin, gastrointestinal, and renal), a physical examination, and review of relevant laboratory data. Figure 15–1 depicts one strategy toward narrowing the diagnosis. Initially, it is important to rule out pseudohyponatremia as the cause of hyponatremia by determining whether severe hyperproteinemia or hyperlipidemia is present. Hyperglycemia can reduce plasma sodium concentration; the magnitude of the effect can be estimated by noting that for each 100 mg/dL increase in glucose, the measured sodium level is decreased by approximately 1.6 mEq/L. In most cases of hyponatremia, determining whether osmoregulation is normal or abnormal can help narrow the diagnosis. This is accomplished by measuring the urine osmolality. If the urine osmolality is low (<100 mOsm/kg H_2O), then osmoregulation is appropriate and hyponatremia reflects the kidney's failure to excrete the excess free water, due to excessive intake, reduced GFR, or diuretic usage. If the urine osmolality is high (>100 mOsm/kg H_2O), then osmoregulation is not appropriate. A patient's effective circulating volume should then be evaluated to delineate the diagnosis. If the effective circulating volume is normal, then SIADH is the likely etiology; if it is decreased, then hyponatremia is due to one of the causes of reduced ECF volume status (see Table 15–4).

Treatment of hyponatremia is directed toward the severity of the condition. Asymptomatic mild hyponatremia usually can be corrected by water restriction in patients with normal or increased ECF volume. In patients with hypovolemia, adrenal insufficiency, or excessive use of diuretics, sodium replacement may be necessary. In such cases, the sodium deficit can be corrected slowly at a rate not to exceed 0.5 mEq/L/h. Symptomatic hyponatremia, regardless of volume status, should be corrected more rapidly at a maximal rate of 1.5 mEq/L/h to achieve a serum sodium concentration of 125 mEq/L or cessation

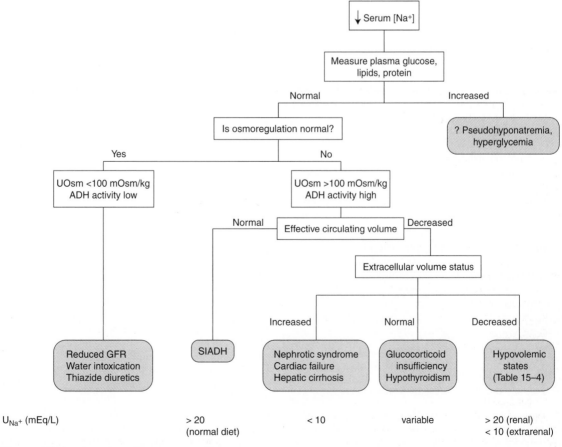

Figure 15–1. Algorithm of assessment of hyponatremia.

of symptoms, whichever comes first. This latter strategy seeks to prevent long-term neurologic damage associated with very low serum sodium levels, while also reducing the risk of osmotic demyelination, which can arise if the correction is too rapidly performed.

HYPERNATREMIA

Hypernatremia is defined as a plasma sodium concentration greater than 145 mEq/L. Common initial presenting symptoms of hypernatremia are lethargy and fatigue, with the potential for progression to seizures or even death in severe cases. Much of the morbidity associated with hypernatremia is attributed to rapid shifts in osmolality, which can damage neurons and blood vessels. In children, severe symptoms can occur when plasma sodium concentrations are greater than 158 mEq/L.

Hypernatremia represents an imbalance of total body sodium and water such that the ratio of total body sodium to total body water is increased. When plasma sodium levels increase due to either an increase in sodium intake or a loss of free water, the body's normal physiologic response is to activate thirst behavior and to stimulate ADH secretion. When both of these mechanisms acting in concert are unable to maintain the normal balance of sodium and water, hypernatremia results.

Common causes of hypernatremia are listed in Table 15–6. Excessive or inadvertent administration of large amounts of sodium chloride, though uncommon, can cause hypernatremia. Infants are particularly susceptible because their GFR is low and access to free water limited. More often, hypernatremia is due to loss of free water in excess of intake, such as with increased insensible water loss through the skin or respiratory tract, hypoosmolar diarrheal losses, or reduced capacity to concentrate urine. Rarely, a resetting upward of the hypothalamic osmotic sensor can occur, usually due to an intracranial abnormality. All of these conditions are associated with high plasma ADH and a concentrated urine

(>300 mOsm/kg H_2O). If plasma ADH and urine osmolality are not appropriately increased, then one must consider that patients have diabetes insipidus (DI), either central or nephrogenic.

An approach to the diagnosis of hypernatremia is outlined in Figure 15–2 according to the ability of patients to mount a physiologic osmoregulatory response. If urine osmolality is less than 300 mOsm/kg H_2O, then patients may have DI. The more common causes of DI in children are listed in Table 15–7. Administration of exogenous ADH (Pitressin) after a period of water deprivation can differentiate between central and nephrogenic DI.

If patients with hypernatremia have a urine osmolality greater than approximately 300 mOsm/kg H_2O, then at least a partial renal response to ADH is present. Evaluation of patient's ECF volume status can then narrow the diagnosis further. For children with clinical signs of reduced ECF volume, a determination can be made of the cause of the free-water loss by the history and physical examination and by evaluating urine output, urine sodium concentration (UNa), and fractional excretion of sodium (FENa). Oliguria with a low Una (<20 mEq/L) and low FENa (<1%) indicates appropriate renal conservation of sodium and water, and a nonrenal origin of water loss should be sought. Polyuria with UNa >20 mEq/L or a FENA >1% indicates an osmotic diuresis. It should be noted that the threshold values for FENa and UNa are often higher in young infants, whose renal tubules are less mature.

To correct hypernatremia, one should estimate a patient's water deficit. The rate and method of correction depends on the etiology. The risk of occurrence of cerebral edema during treatment is minimized if plasma sodium is lowered at a rate less than 12 mEq/L/d; Dehydrated patients should have their ECF volume status restored with isotonic saline prior to replacement of free water. Patients with central DI may require treatment with DDAVP or chlorpropamide, and patients with nephrogenic DI may require treatment with thiazide diuretics.

Table 15–6. Causes of Hypernatremia

Low ADH activity
Central diabetes insipidus
Nephrogenic diabetes insipidus
High ADH activity
Excessive sodium intake
Excessive water loss via sweat glands, lungs
Gastrointestinal loss (viral enteritis, lactulose)
Adipsia (absence of thirst)
Reset osmostat (hyperaldosteronism, hypothalamic damage)
Osmotic diuresis (hyperglycemia, radiocontrast dye)

ADH = antidiuretic hormone.

Disorders of Plasma Potassium

Maintenance of potassium balance is essential for basic cellular functions, including contraction of heart and skeletal muscle. Potassium homeostasis depends upon a complex interplay between dietary intake, renal and gastrointestinal excretion, and dynamic fluxes between intracellular and extracellular compartments. Approximately 98% of total body potassium is located in the intracellular compartment. Potassium is the most abundant intracellular cation whose concentration ranges from 100 to 150 mEq/L. In contrast, extracellular potassium concentrations are much lower, normally 3.5 to 5.5 mEq/L, and are exquisitely controlled. The potassium concentration differences between these compartments is maintained

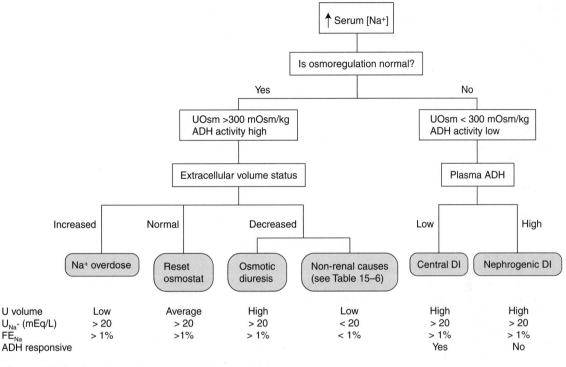

Figure 15–2. Algorithm of assessment of hypernatremia.

by the Na^+K^+ ATPase, which, in addition to yielding high extracellular and low intracellular sodium concentrations, sets up an important electrochemical gradient necessary for proper cellular function.

The regulation of plasma potassium concentration is an extremely efficient process. A rapid influx of potassium into the extracellular compartment (e.g., from dietary sources, cellular breakdown, or metabolic acidosis) invokes a rapid shunting of potassium into cells, so that untoward sequelae are avoided. Potassium balance is regulated by two sets of processes: (1) mechanisms that respond within minutes to changes in plasma potassium concentration and that promote the import to or export from intracellular compartments, or (2) mechanisms that respond within hours and that regulate potassium excretion from the body. The factors that rapidly alter potassium distribution between intracellular and extracellular compartments are insulin, β_2 adrenergic agonists, acidosis or alkalosis, aldosterone, and hyperosmolality. These factors act (Table 15–8) by inducing secondary messenger systems that alter the activity of Na^+K^+ATPase, as well as other ion transporters and channels.

The kidney plays a critical role in maintaining total body potassium balance, accounting for 90% of potassium excretion. Stool and skin losses account for approximately 10% of potassium excretion. Non-renal potassium loss can increase significantly under certain circumstances, such as heat, dehydration, and diarrhea, and thus children are particularly susceptible to such nonrenal potassium losses. Renal potassium excretion occurs by secretion from the distal renal tubule. Since more than 90% of filtered potassium is reabsorbed prior to the distal nephron, net potassium excretion is governed by the actions of several factors on the distal nephron. The most important factors promoting renal K^+ secretion are increased plasma aldosterone and potassium concentrations, increased luminal sodium concentration and its delivery to the distal nephron, and high tubular flow rates.

HYPOKALEMIA

Hypokalemia is defined as a plasma potassium concentration less than 3.5 mEq/L, although severe symptoms usually do not occur until the plasma concentration is less than 2.5 mEq/L. Hypokalemia may be associated with a deficit in total body potassium or may be due to a redistribution of potassium from the extracellular to the intracellular compartment. Symptoms of hypokalemia (Tables 15–9 and 15–12) include paresthesias, muscle cramps, cardiac

Table 15–7. Major Causes of DI in Children

Central DI (ADH deficiency)
Head trauma
Brain tumor
Infarction
Tuberculosis
Nephrogenic DI (ADH resistance)
Chronic renal failure
Obstructive uropathy
Chronic pyelonephritis
Sickle cell nephropathy
Lithium intoxication
Familial
Vasopressin type 2 receptor defect (X-linked)
Aquaporin 2 defect (autosomal recessive)

ADH = antidiuretic hormone; DI = diabetes insipidus.

arrhythmias with characteristic changes in the electrocardiogram, glucose intolerance, and impaired renal tubule function, such as a diminished capacity to concentrate or dilute urine and to reabsorb sodium. Rarely, prolonged hypokalemia may compromise renal excretion of ammonia, leading to an accumulation of total body ammonia and to the potential development of encephalopathy.

A partial list of the causes of hypokalemia is shown in Table 15–10. The four general categories are insufficient intake, excessive nonrenal losses, excessive renal losses, and redistribution of potassium intracellularly. A careful history usually can help determine whether the cause of hypokalemia is due to inadequate intake or gastrointestinal or skin losses, and this can be confirmed, if necessary, by a low (<5%) fractional excretion of potassium. In children, the common causes of hypokalemia include excessive gastrointestinal losses due to diarrhea or excessive renal losses due to hyperaldosteronism and metabolic alkalosis during episodes of severe emesis. In newborn in-

Table 15–8. Major Factors Influencing Potassium Distribution between Intracellular and Extracellular Compartments

Increases extracellular potassium
Acidosis
Hyperosmolality
Exercise
Decreases extracellular potassium
Alkalosis
Insulin
β_2-adrenergic agonists
Aldosterone

Table 15–9. Signs and Symptoms of Hypokalemia

Muscle weakness
Paresthesias, ileus
Renal dysfunction
Metabolic alkalosis; impaired urinary concentration, sodium reabsorption and ammonia excretion
Cardiac arrhythmias
Sinus bradycardia, paroxysmal atrial and junctional tachycardia, atrioventricular block

fants, hypokalemia is commonly caused by diuretics or impaired renal handling of potassium due to immaturity of the renal tubules.

Treatment of hypokalemia usually requires administration of potassium either orally or intravenously, with the notable exception being those etiologies due exclusively to intracellular redistribution. Potassium chloride is the most commonly used potassium salt, but the route, dosage, and duration of administration depend on the underlying etiology and the severity of the hypokalemia.

HYPERKALEMIA

Hyperkalemia is defined as plasma potassium levels greater than 5.5 mEq/L. Hyperkalemia dampens neuromuscular and cardiac conduction, resulting in symptoms of muscle weakness and cardiac arrhythmias (Table 15–11). As the plasma potassium level approaches or exceeds 7.0 mEq/L, life-threatening arryhthmias including ventricular fibril-

Table 15–10. Causes of Hypokalemia

Insufficient intake
Low dietary intake
Starvation
Nonrenal losses
Sweat
Diarrhea
Renal losses
Loop and thiazide-type diuretics
Osmotic diuretics
Mineralocorticoid excess, primary or secondary
Renal tubular acidosis (proximal or distal)
Metabolic alkalosis
Drugs (amphotericin, diamox)
Redistribution of potassium intracellularly
Increased β_2-adrenergic activity (asthma treatment or stress)
Alkalosis (metabolic or respiratory)
Hyperinsulinemia

Table 15–11. Causes of Hyperkalemia

Pseudohyperkalemia
  Inadvertent hemolysis following phlebotomy

Increased load, exogenous sources
  Intravenous infusion

Increased load, endogenous sources
  Cell lysis (trauma, tissue catabolism, hemolysis,
    rhabdomyolysis, tumor lysis syndrome)
  Redistribution (metabolic acidosis, severe exercise,
    hyperosmolality, hyperglycemia, insulin resistance)

Decreased renal excretion
  Severe renal insufficiency, especially acute renal failure
  Primary and secondary hypoaldosteronism

lation may ensue; therefore, elevated plasma potassium levels require prompt evaluation and treatment.

The causes of hyperkalemia can be divided into four general categories: pseudohyperkalemia; increased potassium load from exogenous sources; increased potassium load from endogenous sources, due to either cell lysis syndromes or redistribution of potassium from intracellular to extracellular pools; and decreased renal excretion. A partial list of etiologies is found in Table 15–11. In children, pseudohyperkalemia is the most common cause of elevated potassium levels; this can often occur due to venous stasis or hemolysis during blood drawing. Thus, while any diagnostic workup is underway, the concentration of potassium should be remeasured with these causes in mind. A chronic increase in plasma potassium concentration indicates impairment in renal potassium excretion, while an increased potassium load, due to exogenous sources or cell lysis, usually is associated with appropriate urinary potassium excretion.

Hyperkalemia should be treated immediately with the level of severity guiding the choice of intervention. In severe

Table 15–12. Electrocardiographic Changes in Hypokalemia and Hyperkalemia

Hypokalemia
  ST depression
  Flattened T wave with prominent U wave
  Increased P-wave amplitude[1]
  Increased duration of QRS[1]

Hyperkalemia
  T-wave narrowing and peaking
  QT-wave shortening
  Decreased P-wave amplitude[1]
  Widened QRS[1]

[1] Seen with more severe changes in potassium.

cases, particularly with cardiac arrhythmias, treatments that induce a rapid redistribution of potassium into intracellular compartments (insulin/glucose, sodium bicarbonate, and β_2 adrenergic agonists) and that stabilize myocardial conduction (calcium) should be initially employed. Electrocardiographic monitoring for arrhythmias is essential (Table 15–12). Such treatments should be followed by strategies that reduce the overall potassium load of the body. These include diuretics, kayexalate, or hemodialysis. Recommendations regarding dosage and route of administration for these treatments are listed in Table 15–13.

Calcium and Phosphorus Metabolism

Calcium and phosphorus are essential for normal growth and mineralization of bone and for other important metabolic processes. The plasma concentrations of calcium and phosphorus are maintained by the interaction between three major organ systems—bone, intestine, and kidney—and are regulated within a narrow physiologic range by the actions of three hormones—1,25-dihydroxyvitamin D $(1,25(OH)_2D)$, parathyroid hormone (PTH), and calcitonin (CT). Abnormalities of calcium and phosphorus metabolism are often seen in the context of reduced renal function and, therefore, are discussed in this chapter.

Calcium in plasma exists in three fractions: protein-bound calcium (40%), which is not filtered by the renal glomerulus, and ionized calcium (48%) and complexed calcium (12%), which are filtered. Albumin accounts for 90% of the protein-bound calcium in plasma, and conditions that affect the serum albumin concentration, such as nephrotic syndrome or hepatic cirrhosis, will affect the measurement of total calcium concentration. Ionized calcium is the fraction of plasma calcium that is important for a variety of physiologic processes. Phosphorus exists in plasma in two forms, an organic form (57%) and an inorganic form (43%); in clinical settings, only the inorganic form is routinely measured. Most inorganic phosphorus (85%) is freely filterable by the kidneys.

VITAMIN D

The major source of vitamin D in humans is the cutaneous conversion of 7-dehydrocholesterol to vitamin D_3 *(cholecalciferol)*, which occurs on exposure of the skin to ultraviolet light. Little vitamin D is present naturally in foods, and fortification of certain foods, such as milk, with vitamin D_2 *(ergocalciferol)*, or administration of supplemental vitamin D_2 often is necessary to prevent the occurrence of vitamin D deficiency in infants and adolescents and in those with limited exposure to sunlight. Vitamin D is subsequently hydroxylated in the liver to 25-hydroxyvitamin (25OHD), the major circulating form of vitamin D. Both vitamin D and 25OHD represent storage, not active forms, of this hormone. Conversion of 25OHD to its physiologically active form, $1,25(OH)_2D$, occurs in the kidney. The principal factors that stimulate renal syn-

Table 15–13. Treatment of Hyperkalemia

Drug	Effect	Onset of Action	Duration of Action	Dose	Comments, Complications
Calcium	Stabilizes myocardium	Immediate	Minutes	10% calcium gluconate, 0.5 mL/kg intravenously over 2–4 min	Bradycardia, hypercalcemia; requires ECG monitoring
NaHCO$_3$	Shifts K$^+$ into cells with increased blood pH	30–60 min	Hours	2–3 mEq/kg over 30–60 min	Hypernatremia, hypervolemia, alkalosis, hypocalcemia
Glucose and insulin	Shifts K$^+$ into cells	30 min	Hours	Glucose 0.5 g/kg with insulin 0.3 U/g glucose over 30 min	Hyperglycemia or hypoglycemia
Sodium polystyrene sulfonate	Exchanges Na$^+$ for K$^+$ in gut and thus removes K$^+$ from patient	1 h	Hours	1 g/kg orally or 1.5 g/kg rectally, with 3 mL 70% sorbitol per gram resin; repeat at 4 to 6-h intervals	Fecal impaction; hypernatremia with repeated doses

ECG = electrocardiogram.

thesis of 1,25(OH)$_2$D are hypocalcemia, increased serum concentrations of PTH, and hypophosphatemia. The active hormone 1,25(OH)$_2$D acts primarily on the intestine to increase its absorption of calcium and phosphorus on the skeleton to increase calcification of osteoid and mobilization of skeletal mineral and on the parathyroid gland to decrease synthesis and secretion of PTH.

PARATHYROID HORMONE

Parathyroid hormone is an 84–amino acid polypeptide that is synthesized and secreted by the four parathyroid glands, which are derived from the third and fourth pairs of branchial pouches, usually located just posterior to the thyroid gland. In healthy adults, the total weight of the four glands is less than 200 mg. The plasma ionized calcium concentration is the principal regulator of PTH secretion. A decrease in ionized calcium induces a rapid increase in synthesis and secretion of PTH, whereas an increase in ionized calcium induces a decrease in PTH secretion. Severe hypomagnesemia can impair PTH secretion in response to hypocalcemia. Parathyroid hormone secretion also is inhibited by increased concentrations of 1,25(OH)$_2$D. Hyperphosphatemia, often seen in patients with severe renal insufficiency, can directly stimulate PTH secretion; conversely, hypophosphatemia can suppress PTH secretion.

Parathyroid hormone testing. Whereas the intact PTH molecule has a plasma half-life of only minutes, metabolites of PTH can remain in the circulation for hours. Such fragments of PTH are biologically inactive, are excreted by the kidneys, and thus are retained in the circulation in patients with renal insufficiency. With the

development of PTH assays that measure the "intact," biologically active hormone, clinical determination of serum PTH concentrations is readily performed. Because PTH release is regulated by plasma calcium concentration, rational interpretation of serum PTH concentrations requires knowledge of the simultaneously measured calcium concentration (Figure 15–3).

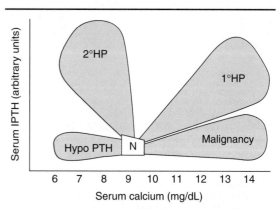

Figure 15–3. Interpretation of measured parathyroid hormone (PTH) concentrations and simultaneous calcium concentration. 1°HP = primary hyperparathyroidism; 2°HP = secondary hyperparathyroidism; IPTH = inactive parathyroid hormone; N = normal; Hypo PTH = hypoparathyroidism. (Reproduced with permission from Andreoli TE, et al: Page 521 in: *Cecil Essentials of Medicine*, 2nd ed. Saunders, 1990.)

CALCITONIN

Calcitonin is a 32–amino acid peptide synthesized and secreted by the parafollicular or C cells of the thyroid gland. Secretion of CT is stimulated by hypercalcemia and inhibited by hypocalcemia. Calcitonin acts primarily on bone to decrease bone resorption, and the principal physiologic effect of the hormone is to decrease the serum calcium concentration.

EXTRACELLULAR CALCIUM HOMEOSTASIS

A decrease in the plasma calcium concentration induces a rapid increase in secretion of PTH from the parathyroid gland. Parathyroid hormone acts on the kidney to decrease excretion of calcium, increase excretion of phosphorus, and stimulate production of $1,25(OH)_2D$. Together with $1,25(OH)_2D$, PTH acts on bone to stimulate release of calcium and phosphorus. Alone, $1,25(OH)_2D$ acts on the intestine to promote absorption of calcium and phosphorus. These actions of PTH and $1,25(OH)_2D$ on their target issues result in an increase in plasma calcium concentration to normal values. Because of the phosphaturic effect of PTH, phosphorus released from bone is excreted in the urine; thus, there is little change in serum phosphorus concentration. Conversely, with an increase in plasma calcium concentration, release of PTH and production of $1,25(OH)_2D$ are decreased, and release of CT is stimulated. The combined effects of these hormonal changes on bone, kidney, and intestine are opposite to those occurring with hypocalcemia; the result is a decrease in calcium concentration to normal values.

DISORDERS OF CALCIUM HOMEOSTASIS

Rickets. In growing children, rickets can occur when the availability of calcium and phosphorus are not sufficient to permit normal mineralization of newly formed bone osteoid. In the most common form of rickets, calcium and phosphorus deficiency are secondary to deficiency of vitamin D, which results from inadequate dietary intake of vitamin D combined with limited exposure to sunlight. Congenital or acquired disorders of vitamin D metabolism (Table 15–14) also can give rise to deficiency of the hormone. Vitamin D deficiency results in impaired intestinal absorption of calcium and phosphorus, hypocalcemia, secondary hyperparathyroidism, increased bone resorption, hyperphosphaturia, hypophosphatemia, and impaired bone mineralization. In industrialized countries, the incidence of vitamin-D-deficient rickets has been greatly reduced because of the routine fortification of foods, such as milk and supplementation of breast-fed infants, with vitamin D. Nevertheless, vitamin-D-deficient rickets remains a major public health problem in many countries.

The clinical and radiographic signs of rickets vary greatly with age of onset, duration, and severity of vitamin D deficiency. The signs predominate in those areas in which bone growth is rapid, namely, the epiphyses of long bones and the costochondral junctions. Palpable enlargement at the wrists and ankles and at the costochondral junctions ("rachitic rosary") are characteristic clinical signs of florid rickets. With weight-bearing in older infants and children, bowing of the femur and tibia can be seen. Radiographs reveal characteristic abnormalities of the epiphyseal regions of the long bones. There is widening of the radiolucent space between the metaphyseal lines and the epiphysis that reflects the accumulation of uncalcified cartilage. The metaphyseal lines often are irregular, frayed, and hollowed ("cupping"). The shafts of the long bones usually reveal thinning of the cortices. The biochemical findings in patients with rickets, noted earlier, vary greatly depending on the etiology, duration, and severity of the disease.

Hyperparathyroidism. Disorders of increased PTH production are uncommon in children. The clinical manifestations of these disorders are varied and are summarized in Table 15–15. There are many causes of hypercalcemia (Table 15–16). Primary hyperparathyroidism may result from an adenoma, hyperplasia, or carcinoma; can occur in either familial or nonfamilial patterns; and may be isolated or occur in association with multiple endocrine adenomatoses syndromes I and II. Treatment of primary hyperparathyroidism usually involves surgical removal of adenomatous, hyperplastic, or carcinomatous parathyroid glands. Secondary hyperparathyroidism typically occurs in

Table 15–14. Differential Diagnosis of Rickets

Abnormalities of vitamin D metabolism
    Deficient dietary vitamin D and lack of sunlight exposure
    Fat malabsorption with reduced vitamin D absorption
    Increased metabolic clearance secondary to anticonvulsant therapy
    Liver disease (impaired 25-hydroxylation of vitamin D)
    Renal insufficiency
      (impaired 1-hydroxylation of 25-hydroxy-vitamin D)
    1α-hydroxylase deficiency
      (vitamin D-dependent rickets type 1)
    Vitamin D receptor/postreceptor defect
      (vitamin D-dependent rickets type 2)
Dietary calcium deficiency (rare)
Dietary phosphorus deficiency (rare after infancy)
Impaired renal reabsorption of phosphorus
    X-linked hypophosphatemic rickets
    Hereditary hypophosphatemic rickets with hypercalciuria
    Fanconi syndrome (renal proximal tubular dysfunction)
    Renal tubular acidosis
    Postrenal transplantation hypophosphatemia
    Tumor-induced hyperphosphaturia
      (oncogenic osteomalacia)

Table 15–15. Signs and Symptoms of Hyperparathyroidism

General	Renal
Weakness	Polyuria/polydipsia
Fatigue	Stones
Weight loss	**Bones**
Gastrointestinal	Pain
Peptic ulcer	Osteopenia
Chronic pancreatitis	
Nausea/vomiting	
Pain	
Central nervous system	
Headache	
Depression	
Delusion/confusion	
Lethargy/coma	

Table 15–17. Clinical Signs of Hypocalcemia

Tetany
Convulsions
Muscle cramps
Carpopedal spasm, Trousseau sign
Facial twitching, Chvostek sign
Laryngeal stridor
Paresthesias

patients with chronic renal insufficiency or nutritional deficiency of vitamin D, and treatment involves administration of vitamin D or its active metabolites.

Hypoparathyroidism. Most patients with inadequate secretion of PTH present with symptoms associated with hypocalcemia and hyperphosphatemia (Table 15–17). These include tetany, convulsions, muscle cramps, laryngeal stridor, and paresthesias. Because the ability to secrete PTH can be limited even in normal infants, feeding of a high-phosphorus-containing formula, such as cow's milk, can give rise to hypocalcemia. A number of disorders are associated with decreased secretion of PTH (Table 15–18). Di George's syndrome results from the abnormal embryologic development of the third and fourth pharyngeal pouches. Most infants (60%) with Di George's syndrome present within 48 h after birth with cardiovascular defects, most often an interrupted aortic arch or truncus arteriosus, and have hypocalcemia secondary to PTH deficiency at a median of 8 days after birth. Other associated findings include hypertelorism, antimongoloid slant of the eyes, cleft palate, carp-shaped mouth, and micrognathia. Some affected infants have

thymic dysplasia with a variable degree of cellular immunodeficiency. The prognosis of such infants depends on the severity of and ability to correct their immunodeficiency and cardiac anomalies.

Pseudohypoparathyroidism. Pseudohypoparathyroidism (PHP) results from a failure of end-organ responsiveness to PTH. In patients with PHP, serum concentrations of PTH are increased, but hypocalcemia and hyperphosphatemia occur, similar to that seen in patients with hypoparathyroidism. Three types of PHP have been described. Pseudohypoparathyroidism type Ia is associated with variable dysmorphic features, including short stature, round face, and short metacarpal bones; many patients are mentally retarded. This type of PHP, which is often familial, is associated with deficient activity of the G_S protein, which couples the PTH receptor to adenylate cyclase, resulting in defective stimulation of cyclic adenosine monophosphate (cAMP) in response to PTH. Patients with PHP Ib have normal G_S activity and are often normal in appearance. Patients with PHP type II appear to have a defect in PTH signaling distal to the formation of cAMP.

Parenteral Fluid Therapy

BODY COMPOSITION

Water is the major constituent of the body; total body water (TBW) accounts for approximately 70 to 75% of body weight in the term newborn infant, approximately 65% of body weight in infants and children, and approx-

Table 15–16. Causes of Hypercalcemia

Hyperparathyroidism	Adrenal insufficiency
Excessive vitamin D intake	Sarcoidosis
Hypervitaminosis A	Milk-alkali syndrome
Hypercalcemia of malignancy	Thiazide diuretics
Immobilization	Williams syndrome
Familial hypocalciuric	(idiopathic hypercalcemia of infancy)
hypercalcemia	
Hyperthyroidism	Subcutaneous fat necrosis

Table 15–18. Conditions Associated with Hypoparathyroidism

Parathyroid destruction
  Surgery
  Autoimmune
    Polyglandular autoimmune syndromes, type 1
Magnesium deficiency
Di George syndrome
Transient
Familial

imately 60% of body weight in adult men. Because the water content of fat is low, TBW represents a smaller fraction of body weight both in obese individuals and in women (55%), in whom body content of fat is higher than in men. Body water has two components: intracellular fluid (ICF), which constitutes 35 to 40% of body weight, and ECF, which constitutes 25% of body weight in children and about 20% in adults. The ECF is composed of intravascular (plasma) fluid (5%), interstitial fluid (15%), and transcellular fluid (1 to 3%), the last of which consists of gastrointestinal secretions and pleural, peritoneal, and synovial fluids.

The amount of water in the body is precisely regulated to maintain the plasma osmolality constant at 285–295 mOsm/kg water, despite daily fluctuations in water and solute intake. This regulation occurs via a close feedback interaction between the hypothalamic osmoreceptors and volume receptors in the aortic arch and cardiac atrium, the posterior pituitary, and the collecting ducts of the kidney. When a decrease in water intake or an increase in solute intake induces an increase in plasma osmolality of 1 to 2%, thirst is stimulated, which leads to an increase in water intake and release of ADH, and thereby to increased water retention by the renal collecting ducts. Both thirst and release of ADH also are stimulated by a decrease in ECF volume of approximately 8% or more, as can occur with hemorrhage or dehydration. Conversely, a decrease in plasma osmolality of approximately 1 to 2% results in suppression of ADH release. These homeostatic responses result in a return of plasma osmolality to normal values. In certain circumstances, the stimulatory effect of reduced intravascular volume on ADH release can override the suppressive effect of a reduction in plasma osmolality.

MAINTENANCE PARENTERAL FLUID THERAPY

The goal of *maintenance parenteral fluid therapy* is to provide water and electrolytes in amounts that equal their daily physiologic losses from the body. The daily requirements for water and electrolytes depend on the body's metabolic rate and thus the caloric expenditure of the individual. For example, an increase in the rate of metabolism results in an increase both in heat production, which increases evaporative water loss from the skin, and in endogenous generation of solutes requiring renal excretion, which increases urine water loss at any given urine osmolality.

The energy expenditure of the average hospitalized patient can be estimated from the body weight (Table 15–19). These estimates, which include basal metabolic expenditure plus an average increment for activity in bed, are higher per kilogram body weight in younger patients than they are in those who are older. The initial estimate must be modified in patients whose metabolic rate is affected by a specific circumstance; for

Table 15–19. Calculation of Energy Expenditure in Children

Body Weight (kg)	Energy Expenditure (kcal/kg/d)
3–10	100
10–20	1000 + 50 kcal/kg for weight >10 kg
>20	1500 + 20 kcal/kg for weight >20 kg

example, with fever, the caloric expenditure is increased by 12% per °Celsius increase in body temperature above normal and, with hypermetabolic states (hyperthyroidism, salicylate intoxication), the caloric expenditure is increased by 25 to 75%. Conversely, caloric expenditure is reduced in patients with hypothermia or hypometabolic states.

Water. Water is lost from the skin owing to evaporation and from the lungs owing to normal respiration; these losses are referred to as *insensible water loss (IWL).* Daily insensible water loss is approximately 45 to 50 mL for each 100 kcal of energy expended; of this, approximately one third is lost through the lungs and approximately two thirds through the skin. *Daily urine water loss* can vary widely and depends on the amount of solute requiring excretion and on renal concentrating ability. When the urinary solute load is relatively low and the urine osmolality is approximately equal to that of plasma (i.e., there is neither significant concentration nor dilution of urine), the average urine water loss is approximately 65 mL/100 kcal/d. These insensible and urinary water losses are offset in part by water that is generated endogenously during metabolism, an amount estimated at 12 to 15 mL/100 kcal/d. Losses of water in formed stools usually are negligible. Thus, the daily provision of approximately 100 mL water per 100 kcal energy expended meets physiologic water losses in most patients (Table 15–20). In the presence of significant sweating, an additional 10 to 25 mL/100 kcal/d should be added.

Electrolytes. Electrolytes (sodium, potassium, and chloride) are provided in amounts that approximate their

Table 15–20. Maintenance Water Requirements

	mL/100 kcal/d
Insensible water loss	45–50
Lungs	30
Skin	15
Urine water loss[1]	60–80
Hidden intake (water of oxidation)	12–15
Usual requirements	100

[1] Urine water loss depends on renal solute load and renal concentrating ability.

average daily urinary losses in healthy infants and children, thus avoiding the need for either maximal renal conservation or maximal excretion of these substances. It is customary to provide 3 mEq of sodium and 2 mEq of potassium per 100 kcal/d as the chloride salts (i.e., as sodium and potassium chloride).

Energy. In patients with only brief illness and without preexisting malnutrition, full replacement of caloric needs is not necessary. Rather, provision of approximately 20% of the estimated caloric expenditure as glucose will prevent ketosis and minimize endogenous catabolism of protein. This is accomplished by administering 5% dextrose in water.

For example, the daily maintenance fluid requirements in a healthy 9-year-old girl who weighs 30 kg are as follows: energy expenditure, 1700 kcal; water, 1700 mL; sodium, 54 mEq; potassium, 34 mEq; chloride, 88 mEq; and glucose, 85 g. These would be provided by administering 5% dextrose in water containing 30 mEq/L of sodium chloride and 20 mEq/L of potassium chloride, at a rate of 70 mL/h for 24 h. It is customary and convenient to use a solution of 5% dextrose in 0.25% NaCl, which contains 38 mEq/L NaCl, plus 20 mEq/L potassium chloride, as the maintenance solution in pediatrics. These guidelines are appropriate for use in infants, children, and adolescents; the exception is newborn infants, in whom insensible and renal losses vary depending on gestational and postnatal age.

Abnormal losses. In certain circumstances or disease states, ongoing insensible and renal losses of water and electrolytes differ from those estimated, and their replacement during maintenance therapy must be adjusted accordingly. Examples of states of abnormal loss and the appropriate modifications to maintenance therapy are given in Table 15–21.

Approach to Patients with Dehydration

CLINICAL FEATURES

The normal rate of turnover of water, electrolytes, and foodstuffs in infants and children is about three times that in adults; as a consequence, infants and children are more susceptible to the adverse effects of abnormalities of fluid balance. Deficits of water, sodium, and potassium can occur in a wide variety of clinical disorders that affect children; the most common of these is acute gastroenteritis, in which diarrhea and vomiting lead to dehydration. In children with acute gastroenteritis, water and electrolytes are lost from the gastrointestinal tract in considerable excess of their intake, which leads to contraction of the ECF volume and the appearance of clinical signs of dehydration.

The patient's state of hydration is evaluated by the physical examination, although historical information, such as

Table 15–21. States of Abnormal Loss and Modifications in Maintenance Therapy

Fever	Increase caloric estimate by 12% per 1°C (1.8°F) increase in body temperature
Hypermetabolism Salicylism Hyperthyroidism	Increase caloric estimate by 25–75%
Sweating	Increase water allowance by 10–25 mL/100 kcal; increase Na and Cl allowance by 0.5–1 mEq/100 kcal
Obligatory oliguria Renal insufficiency Congestive heart failure Edematous states Syndrome of inappropriate ADH secretion	Decrease water allowance by 20–50%
Obligatory polyuria Diabetes insipidus Renal tubular disease High solute load	Increase water allowance
Gastrointestinal loss Nasogastric suction Small bowel drainage Diarrhea	Replace with equal volume of solution with equivalent electrolyte composition
Third space loss Postoperative, burns, trauma	Replace with isotonic solution

ADH = antidiuretic hormone.

the frequency of urination or the patient's prior body weight, can be helpful. Based on the physical findings (Table 15–22), the magnitude of dehydration is judged to be mild, moderate, or severe, which corresponds to a loss of body weight in the infant of approximately 5%, 10%, or 15%, respectively, or in older children, of 3%, 6%, or 9%, respectively. The physical findings described and the corresponding estimates of the degree of dehydration apply to patients in whom dehydration develops over 3 to 5 days and in whom the serum sodium concentration is relatively normal (130 to 150 mEq/L), so-called isotonic dehydration. In such patients, approximately 60% of body fluid is lost from the extracellular space and approximately 40% from the intracellular space. With hypertonic dehydration (serum sodium concentration >150 mEq/L), the ECF volume is better maintained owing to greater movement of water from the intracellular to the extracellular space. As a

Table 15–22. Clinical Assessment of Hydration

	Magnitude of Dehydration		
	Mild	**Moderate**	**Severe**
Body weight loss (<2 y of age)	5%	10%	15%
(>2 y of age)	3%	6%	6%
Skin turgor	nl, sl ↓	↓↓	↓↓↓
Mucous membranes	nl, sl dry	very dry	parched
Skin color	pale	gray	mottled
Urine output	sl ↓	oliguria	marked oliguria and azotemia
Blood pressure	normal	± normal	reduced
Pulse rate	↑	↑↑	↑↑↑, weak

nl = normal; sl = slight.

consequence, the clinical signs of dehydration are less severe for a given loss of body weight. Conversely, with hypotonic dehydration (serum sodium <130 mEq/L), the ECF volume is less well maintained; thus, the clinical signs of dehydration are more severe for a given loss of body weight.

LABORATORY FINDINGS

Patients with severe dehydration who are hospitalized should have the following laboratory tests performed: complete blood cell count; serum electrolyte, total carbon dioxide content, urea nitrogen, and creatinine concentrations; venous blood gas determination; and complete urinalysis. Based on the serum sodium concentration, dehydration is judged to be isotonic, hypertonic, or hypotonic; this information assists in the clinical assessment of patients, as noted earlier, and in therapy. Patients with diarrheal dehydration frequently have metabolic acidosis, which can have several causes, including loss of bicarbonate ion via the gastrointestinal tract, reduced urinary excretion of acid due to oliguria, and poor peripheral perfusion with accumulation of lactic acid. The urinalysis should be consistent with the diagnosis of dehydration (i.e., the urine osmolality should be >500 mOsm/kg or the specific gravity >1.020). Dilute urine (specific gravity <1.010, osmolality <300 mOsm/kg) in dehydrated patients with frequent urination suggests that a defect in the urine-concentrating mechanism is present.

TREATMENT

The objectives of treatment are to provide water, electrolytes, calories, and other nutrients in amounts that will rapidly replace the existing deficits of these substances and meet their ongoing losses, both normal and abnormal. These objectives should be accomplished safely and over a relatively brief period. Rehydration therapy can be administered either orally or intravenously.

Oral rehydration therapy is safe and effective for treatment of children with dehydration caused by diarrhea, and is appropriate and recommended for patients with mild to moderate dehydration. The oral solution used should contain 75 to 90 mmol/L sodium, 20 mmol/L potassium, approximately 30 mmol/L as base (acetate, citrate, lactate, or bicarbonate), 65–85 mmol/L chloride, and 2% to 2.5% (110–140 mmol/L) glucose. For prevention of dehydration and maintenance of hydration after dehydration treatment, it is recommended that a solution similar in composition be used except for a lower sodium content (40 to 60 mmol/L). Alternatively, the solution used to treat acute dehydration can be used during maintenance by alternating this solution with one much lower in sodium, such as water, low-carbohydrate juices, or human milk. Infants with mild or moderate dehydration should be rehydrated with 50 ml/kg or 100 ml/kg, respectively, of oral rehydration solution over approximately 4 h, plus replacement of stool losses. If clinical signs of dehydration are still present, rehydration therapy should be repeated until dehydration is corrected. As soon as dehydration is corrected, feeding of age-appropriate diets should be begun.

For patients with severe dehydration (≥10%) or with shock, isotonic fluid (saline, Ringer lactate) should be rapidly administered intravenously until intravascular volume is restored and clinical signs of dehydration are substantially improved or reserved. Treatment of such patients is traditionally viewed as occurring in three phases:

1. Phase 1: The goal of this phase is the rapid expansion of the intravascular volume to treat or prevent shock, to improve peripheral perfusion, and to restore normal renal function. This helps to improve acidosis and electrolyte imbalance if present. This phase lasts 1 hour or less.

2. Phase 2: The goal of this phase is the replacement of the remaining deficits of water and sodium, ongoing abnormal stool losses, and normal physiologic losses of water and electrolytes. The deficits of potassium are partially replaced, and acid-base status is normalized.

This phase lasts several (4 to 8) hours. Oral rehydration therapy can be considered when the child is more stable and mental status is satisfactory.

3. Phase 3: Refeeding of age-appropriate diets should be initiated when rehydration is complete. This helps to replace the remaining body deficits of potassium and nutritional deficits. This phase lasts several days to weeks.

Patients should be monitored closely during the first two phases of therapy. Parenteral therapy of severe dehydration is outlined in Table 15–23.

HEMATURIA

Evaluation of Hematuria

Hematuria is defined as the excretion of an excessive number of erythrocytes in the urine. Normal individuals may excrete as many as 1 million RBCs per day, which gives rise to 1 to 2 RBCs per high-power field (HPF) on microscopic examination of centrifuged urine. Hematuria in children is the finding of more than 3 to 5 RBCs/HPF. In large study populations of healthy, school-aged children, the incidence of hematuria, when only a single urinalysis is performed, is 4 to 5%. When hematuria is detected on at least 2 of 3 consecutive urinalyses, the incidence is significantly lower, 0.5 to 1%, indicating that hematuria is frequently transient. Most children with hematuria have benign conditions that require no intervention and have an excellent prognosis. Thus, time-consuming and expensive diagnostic studies should be reserved for patients who,

Table 15–23. Intravenous Treatment of Dehydration

I. Restore circulating blood volume:
A. Administer *isotonic* fluid, 20–40 mL/kg over 20–40 min: lactated Ringer 0.9% saline, plasma
B. Monitor perfusion, blood pressure, urine output; give additional isotonic fluid until these normalize
II. Calculate and replace deficits of water and electrolytes:
A. With isotonic or hypotonic dehydration, replace deficits over 4–8 h. For severe hyponatremia, serum Na <115 mEq/L, or seizures, infuse 3% NaCl to increase serum Na to 120 mEq/L (3% NaCl contains 0.5 mEq/mL Na). With hypernatremic dehydration, replace deficits over 48–72 h (rate of serum sodium correction is <5 mEq/L per 12 h)
B. Replace ongoing abnormal losses with appropriate fluid
C. Provide normal maintenance requirements
III. Restore K+ deficit over 2–4 d and nutritional deficit over days to weeks

by history, physical examination, and initial laboratory screening tests, are deemed to be at high risk for serious renal or extrarenal disease. Fortunately, a determination of risk can be readily made during the initial evaluation.

Hematuria may be readily apparent as a bright red or brownish discoloration of the urine, in which case it is termed *macroscopic* or *gross hematuria*. Visible hematuria is usually alarming to patients and families and often prompts medical evaluation. In contrast, microscopic hematuria usually is detected in asymptomatic children undergoing routine dipstick screening of urine. Commercially available dipsticks are impregnated with reagents that change color in the presence of hemoglobin, yielding a positive result for blood. Using this methodology, the presence of as few as 5 RBCs/HPF will yield a positive test for blood. A positive dipstick test for blood indicates the presence of RBCs, hemoglobin, or myoglobin but cannot distinguish among them. For this reason, a positive dipstick must be followed by microscopic examination of a properly centrifuged, freshly obtained urine specimen (15 mL of urine spun at 2000 RPM for 5 min) to confirm the presence of RBCs before the diagnosis of hematuria is made.

Once the diagnosis of hematuria is confirmed, an attempt should be made to determine the site of blood loss. Macroscopic hematuria of renal origin is classically brownish, tea-colored, or Coca-Cola–colored and usually is not associated with pain or blood clots. The findings of proteinuria, hypertension, edema, or azotemia suggest IgA nephropathy or acute postinfectious glomerulonephritis. Additional disorders include thin basement membrane disease, lupus nephritis, Alport's syndrome, or idiopathic hypercalciuria. Conversely, macroscopic hematuria of extrarenal origin is bright red and frequently associated with pain and blood clots. Such disorders include trauma, hemorrhagic cystitis, hemoglobinopathies, or tumor.

On microscopic examination, the morphologic appearance of urinary RBCs has been shown to reflect their site of origin (i.e., glomerular versus nonglomerular). Presumably because of their deforming journey through small disruptions in the glomerular capillary wall, RBCs of glomerular origin become dysmorphic. They are smaller than their isomorphic counterparts and have distorted, irregular contours. Phase contrast microscopy is the traditional method for examining RBC morphology in urine specimens. Red blood cells of nonglomerular origin display a normal morphologic appearance. The finding of urinary RBC casts is diagnostic of glomerular or tubular origin for the hematuria and is not seen with extrarenal bleeding. A mild degree of proteinuria due to the release of hemoglobin from RBCs may be found in patients with macroscopic hematuria. The most common causes of hematuria in children are listed in Table 15–24.

Table 15–24. Causes of Hematuria

Renal diseases, glomerular
  Benign familial hematuria (thin basement membrane
    disease)
  Postinfectious glomerulonephritis (poststreptococcal)
  IgA nephropathy
  Chronic glomerulonephritis (focal segmental glomerulo-
    sclerosis, membranoproliferative glomerulonephritis,
    membranous nephropathy)
  Systemic vasculitis (Henöch-Schonlein purpura, systemic
    lupus erythematosus)
  Alport syndrome
  Hemolytic uremic syndrome

Renal diseases, extraglomerular
  Interstitial nephritis
  Pyelonephritis
  Acute tubular necrosis
  Polycystic kidney disease
  Thrombosis, renal artery or vein
  Sickle cell nephropathy
  Wilms tumor
  Hydronephrosis
  Papillary necrosis

Nonrenal disease
  Cystitis, urethritis
  Hypercalciuria
  Vigorous exercise
  Nephrolithiasis
  Vesicoureteral reflux
  Trauma
  Foreign body (urethra)
  Hemorrhagic cystitis (cyclophosphamide)
  Tumors (sarcoma botryoides, rhabdomyosarcoma)
  Coagulopathy
  Vascular malformations

Patient Evaluation

HISTORY

Evaluation of children with confirmed hematuria begins with a thorough history. Important historical features and physical findings and the most likely corresponding diseases are listed in Table 15–25.

PHYSICAL EXAMINATION

The physical examination begins with the accurate recording of blood pressure in all children regardless of age, using an appropriately sized cuff. Height and weight measurements should be plotted on standardized growth charts. The patient's skin should be assessed for rash, petechiae, purpura, pallor, and edema. The abdominal examination

Table 15–25. Evaluation of Children with Hematuria

Historical Features	Associated Disease
Recurrent gross hematuria	IgA nephropathy Henöch-Schonlein purpura Alport syndrome Benign familial hematuria Idiopathic hypercalciuria
Dysuria, urinary frequency, suprapubic or flank pain	Urinary tract infection Pyelonephritis Urolithiasis
Recent upper respiratory tract infection or sore throat, impetigo	Postinfectious glomerulonephritis IgA nephropathy
Recent therapy with penicillin, nonsteroidal anti-inflammatory drugs	Interstitial nephritis
Trauma	Kidney contusion, hydronephrosis
Family History	
Hearing loss	Alport syndrome
Microscopic hematuria	IgA nephropathy Benign familial hematuria Idiopathic hypercalciuria Alport syndrome
Renal insufficiency or failure	Alport syndrome Polycystic kidney disease
Nephrolithiasis	Idiopathic hypercalciuria
Sickle cell disease or trait	Sickle cell nephropathy
Physical Findings	
Edema	Proteinuria/nephrotic syndrome Fluid retention/acute renal failure
Petechiae, purpura, malar rash	Henöch-Schonlein purpura Systemic lupus erythematosus
Abdominal mass	Polycystic kidney disease Hydronephrosis Tumor (Wilms)
Costovertebral or suprapubic pain	Urinary tract infection Pyelonephritis Idiopathic hypercalciuria with renal stone

should evaluate for palpable masses (hydronephrosis, polycystic kidney disease, and Wilms tumor) and areas of pain or tenderness (UTI). The external genitalia should be inspected for signs of inflammation or trauma or the presence of a foreign body.

LABORATORY EVALUATION

A complete urinalysis should be obtained for each patient with hematuria. Of particular importance are the findings of leukocytes (infection, interstitial nephritis), WBC casts (pyelonephritis), RBC casts (acute glomerulonephritis, other glomerular diseases), proteinuria (quantity, nephrotic versus nonnephrotic amount), and dysmorphic RBCs (renal versus nonrenal origin). Renal biopsy is not recommended for patients with microscopic hematuria and no other clinical or laboratory abnormalities. A similar conservative approach can be recommended for asymptomatic patients with gross hematuria. In contrast, a renal biopsy is indicated for patients with microscopic or gross hematuria with moderate proteinuria, elevated serum creatinine concentration, or hypertension.

Etiology of Hematuria

The more commonly encountered diseases causing hematuria in children are discussed later in detail. With the information obtained from the history, physical examination, and urinalysis, a differential diagnosis can be made for individual patients based on the knowledge of the likely etiologies and their characteristic features. Figure 15–4 provides an algorithm for the evaluation of children with persistent hematuria.

THIN BASEMENT MEMBRANE DISEASE (BENIGN FAMILIAL/NON-FAMILIAL HEMATURIA)

Thin basement membrane disease manifests in children and young adults as persistent microscopic hematuria with or without proteinuria. If proteinuria occurs, it is usually mild and rarely results in the nephrotic syndrome. Although this disease is known to cluster in families, no particular mode of inheritance has been elucidated. Hematuria found in thin basement membrane disease differs from Alport's syndrome in several important ways: (1) deafness and ocular abnormalities are not seen, (2) deterioration of renal function is rare, and (3) thickening and splitting of the glomerular basement membrane are not seen in renal biopsy specimens examined by electron microscopy (EM).

The diagnosis of benign familial hematuria should be strongly considered in patients with persistent microscopic hematuria in whom dipstick screening of family members reveals microscopic hematuria or in whom the family history reveals the presence of hematuria without deafness or progressive renal insufficiency. Although rarely performed in the setting of isolated microscopic hematuria, a defini-

tive diagnosis requires EM examination of renal tissue obtained by biopsy. The distinctive finding is decreased thickness (265 nm or less) of the peripheral glomerular capillary basement membranes. The light microscopic appearance of the glomerulus is normal. Despite the persistence of microscopic hematuria for many years, this condition is benign and nonprogressive in virtually all patients and thus requires no therapy.

IDIOPATHIC HYPERCALCIURIA

Ionized and complexed calcium is freely filtered by the renal glomerulus, and 98 to 99% of the filtered calcium load is reabsorbed by the renal tubules. In healthy children, urinary calcium excretion is less than 4 mg/kg/day. *Hypercalciuria,* defined as urinary calcium excretion in excess of this amount, is present in approximately 3% of healthy children. Increased dietary intake of calcium-containing foods does not cause hypercalciuria because the normal gastrointestinal tract limits absorption of calcium. Idiopathic hypercalciuria is the result of either excessive gastrointestinal absorption of dietary calcium or decreased renal tubular reabsorption of calcium. With increased gastrointestinal absorption of calcium, the resultant increase in filtered load of calcium results in hypercalciuria, which appropriately returns the serum calcium level to normal.

In one report, 25% of children with isolated hematuria were found to have idiopathic hypercalciuria as a cause. The hematuria is painless and can be either microscopic or rarely macroscopic; the bleeding is thought to result from mechanical trauma to tubular and uroepithelial cells caused by calcium crystals. Invariably, RBC casts and proteinuria are absent. Although hematuria does not occur in all children with hypercalciuria, such children are at increased risk for the development of calcium-containing stones and frequently have a positive family history of nephrolithiasis. The inheritance pattern of hypercalciuria resembles that of an autosomal dominant trait.

An easily performed screening test for hypercalciuria is the calculation of the ratio of urine calcium to creatinine concentration, determined in a randomly obtained urine sample. A ratio greater than 0.22 in a fasting morning specimen suggests excessive urinary calcium excretion, although infants may have ratios as high as 0.80. If the result of the screening test is positive, a confirmatory 24-h urine collection should be obtained to determine the calcium excretion rate quantitatively. All children with isolated hematuria of unknown etiology should be screened for hypercalciuria.

For children with hypercalciuria without a history of renal stones, conservative therapy is appropriate. This includes dietary salt restriction, which decreases urinary calcium excretion. In children whose dietary intake of calcium greatly exceeds the Recommended Dietary Allowance (RDA), limitation of calcium intake to the RDA level may decrease calcium excretion. Restriction of calcium intake

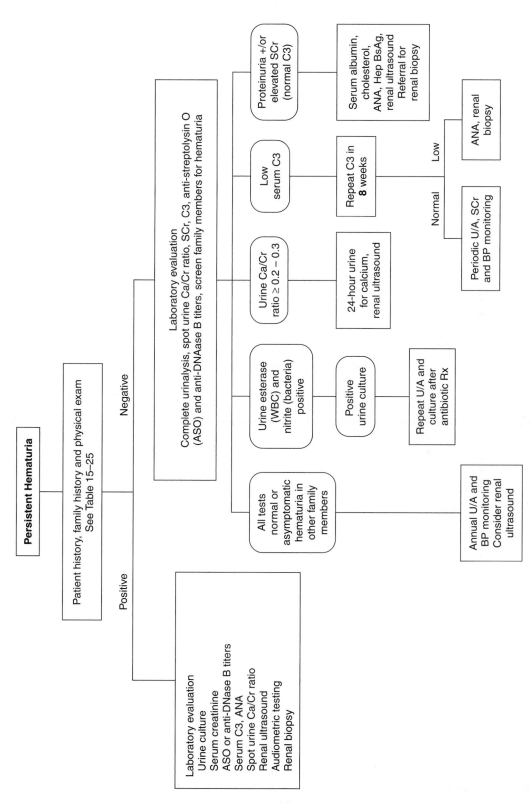

Figure 15–4. Algorithm for the diagnostic evaluation of children with persistent hematuria. ANA = antinuclear antibody; Ca/Cr = calcium, creatinine; HBs Ag = hepatitis B surface antigen; SCr, serum creatinine; Serum C3 = serum complaint 3; U/A = urinalysis.

611

below the RDA is inadvisable in growing children. In all patients with hematuria and hypercalciuria, a renal ultrasound should be performed to look for the presence of nephrocalcinosis or renal stones. In hypercalciuric children with a history of renal stones, high fluid intake is advisable, as this will dilute urinary calcium and avoid supersaturation, a condition necessary for stone formation. Such patients may also require a thiazide diuretic, if limitation of the intake of salt and calcium (to the RDA) do not result in resolution of the hypercalciuria. Thiazide diuretics reduce calcium excretion by increasing calcium reabsorption in the distal tubule.

URINARY TRACT INFECTION

Both cystitis and pyelonephritis are common causes of hematuria, either microscopic or macroscopic. Symptoms of cystitis include dysuria, frequency, urgency, and suprapubic abdominal pain. Pyelonephritis in infants is distinguished by fever, vomiting, and irritability and in older children by the additional findings of costovertebral angle tenderness, flank pain, and dysuria. The presence of urinary RBCs, if due to infection, should be accompanied by leukocytes. Urine dipsticks that test positive for nitrite and leukocyte esterase suggest the presence of infection. A urine culture should be performed in all patients with hematuria to rule out bacterial infection, even in the absence of dysuria.

Diagnosis of UTI depends on the isolation of more than 100,000 bacterial colonies per milliliter from the culture of a clean-catch urine specimen. Colony counts of less than 100,000 organisms per milliliter are considered to be positive if the urine has been obtained by either suprapubic aspiration or urethral catheterization. Cultures obtained from U-bag specimens are unreliable unless meticulous skin preparation is insured and the specimen is delivered promptly to the laboratory for processing. With antibiotic therapy and resolution of the infection, urinary tract discomfort and hematuria resolve. Viral cystitis also may cause gross hematuria, dysuria, and suprapubic pain. In this case, the urine culture is negative for bacteriologic pathogens, and the hematuria usually resolves within 1 week without specific therapy.

GLOMERULONEPHRITIS

Glomerulonephritis is defined histologically as inflammation of the glomeruli. There is proliferation of one or more of the glomerular cell types—mesangial cells, endothelial cells, and epithelial cells—and exudation of leukocytes. Other glomerular diseases, which are not characterized by inflammation, are often included under the term *glomerulonephritis* but are more properly known as glomerulopathies (e.g., minimal change disease and membranous glomerulopathy). Hematuria and proteinuria are nonspecific clinical expressions of all glomerular diseases and cannot reliably distinguish between proliferative and non-proliferative types. In this section, *glomerulonephritis* is used as a generic term for both types of disease. Only those glomerulonephritides that occur with some frequency in children are considered.

Glomerulonephritis can be acute, subacute, or chronic. Clinical features of acute glomerulonephritis are both gross and microscopic hematuria, including the presence of RBC casts, proteinuria, pyuria, edema, oliguria, hypertension, flank pain, and increased serum concentrations of both urea nitrogen and creatinine (azotemia) (Table 15–26). Although the classic form of glomerulonephritis, acute poststreptococcal glomerulonephritis (APSGN), often presents as a serious illness with many of these features, glomerulonephritis also may be detected incidentally by the findings of microscopic hematuria or proteinuria on a routine urinalysis.

Glomerulonephritis occurs in many forms, which have been classified according to characteristic patterns observed by light, immunofluorescence, and electron microscopy. These types can exist as primary renal diseases or as renal manifestations of systemic diseases. For example, diffuse proliferative glomerulonephritis can be a primary renal disease, such as APSGN, or it can be the renal manifestation of a systemic disease, such as systemic lupus erythematosus. In addition, systemic diseases such as systemic lupus erythematosus can be associated with glomerulonephritis of different histology types (e.g., focal glomerulonephritis, membranous glomerulopathy, or diffuse proliferative glomerulonephritis), either in different patients or in the same patient at different times. Because of this variability, hybrid classifications of the glomerulonephritides, on the basis of both clinical and histological descriptions, are commonly used (Table 15–27).

The causes of most forms of glomerulonephritis, whether intrinsic to the kidney or part of a systemic disease, are unknown, but their pathogenesis often involves immune mechanisms, such as the deposition of antigen-

Table 15–26. Clinical and Laboratory Features of Acute Glomerulonephritis

Clinical Features	Laboratory Findings
Gross hematuria	Microscopic hematuria
Edema	Red blood cell casts
Hypertension	Proteinuria
Flank pain	Pyuria
Oliguria	Increased antistreptolysin O, anti-hyaluronidase, and anti-DNAse-B titers
Fever (uncommon)	Decreased CH_{50} and C3 levels
	Increased erythrocyte sedimentation rate
	Leukocytosis
	Azotemia

Table 15–27. Classification of Glomerulonephritis

Intrinsic Renal Diseases
Diffuse proliferative glomerulonephritis
Postinfectious, poststreptococcal glomerulonephritis
Mesangial proliferative glomerulonephritis
IgA nephropathy
Focal segmental glomerulosclerosis
Membranoproliferative glomerulonephritis
Membranous glomerulopathy
Rapidly progressive glomerulonephritis
Systemic Diseases
Systemic lupus erythematosus
Henöch-Schonlein purpura
Hepatitis B virus infection
Chronic infection; infective endocarditis, ventriculoatrial shunts
HIV type 1 infection
Polyarteritis nodosa
Goodpasture syndrome
Wegener granulomatosis
Diabetes mellitus
Sickle cell disease

antibody complexes in the glomeruli. Anti-inflammatory and immunosuppressive drugs, such as corticosteroids and cytotoxic agents, are frequently used to treat these diseases. However, for many glomerular diseases, controlled studies have not been performed to test the efficacy of these drugs. The prognosis of most of the glomerulonephritides is better in children than it is in adults; nevertheless, chronic glomerulonephritis is one of the most common causes of end-stage renal disease in older children and adolescents. The three most common forms of glomerulonephritis in children, acute poststreptococcal glomerulonephritis, IgA nephropathy, and systemic lupus erythematosus (SLE) nephritis are discussed later in this chapter.

ACUTE POSTSTREPTOCOCCAL GLOMERULONEPHRITIS

The occurrence of glomerulonephritis after streptococcal infection has been recognized for more than 150 years. After pharyngeal or skin infections with certain strains of group A streptococci, glomerulonephritis may develop after a latent period of 1 to 3 weeks. A number of nephritogenic strains of streptococci have been identified, but the occurrence rate of nephritis after infection with any one of these strains is variable. Primarily a disease of children, with a peak incidence at age 7 years; acute poststreptococcal glomerulonephritis (APSGN) is rare in infants. Boys are affected twice as often as girls are. The incidence of the disease in North America decreased after 1940 due to a decreased incidence and severity of strep-

tococcal infections in general, but there has been an apparent resurgence in recent years. The disease can occur in either sporadic or epidemic forms.

Clinical features. There is marked variability in the clinical presentation and course of the disease. Patients usually seek medical attention because of the onset of periorbital edema or gross hematuria, which is often described as tea-colored or brown urine. Hypertension, oliguria, urinary RBC casts, and proteinuria are also common, and children may complain of headache, malaise, flank pain, and fever. Renal failure severe enough to necessitate the use of dialysis occurs in a small percentage of patients, as does the nephrotic syndrome. In contrast, many cases are so mild as to go unnoticed, as evidenced by the fact that urinalyses performed on apparently healthy siblings of index cases often show microscopic hematuria and proteinuria. Therefore, in patients with microscopic hematuria who report a recent pharyngeal or skin infection, serologic evidence of streptococcal infection should be sought.

Laboratory findings include leukocytosis, mild anemia, elevated erythrocyte sedimentation rate, increased serum levels of creatinine and urea nitrogen, decreased serum levels of complement 3 (C3), and increased serum levels of antibodies against streptococcal antigens. The most sensitive tests of the latter are the antihyaluronidase and anti-DNAse B titers for skin infections and the antistreptolysin O (ASO) titer for pharyngitis.

The overt signs and symptoms of nephritis usually subside within 1 to 2 weeks, although microscopic hematuria and, especially, low-grade proteinuria may persist for months or even years. Complete recovery occurs in more than 95% of children but in only 70 to 85% of adults.

Pathogenesis and pathology. The pathogenesis is incompletely understood but appears to involve the deposition of a streptococcal antigen, streptokinase, in the glomeruli with subsequent activation of plasminogen and complement leading to an inflammatory reaction. A diffuse proliferative glomerulonephritis, APSGN, is the classic example of this pathologic form, although the same pathology also can be observed in glomerulonephritis that follows pneumococcal, staphylococcal, and viral infections, including mumps and varicella. There is proliferation of all three types of glomerular cells—mesangial, endothelial, and epithelial—as well as accumulation and exudation of polymorphonuclear leukocytes in the glomerulus. In severe cases, proliferating cells can obliterate glomerular capillary lumens, or the glomerular tuft can be compressed by epithelial cell crescents. Electron microscopy demonstrates the presence of electron-dense humps, which are thought to be immune complexes, on the epithelial side of the glomerular basement membrane. Immunofluorescence microscopy reveals a granular pattern of staining of immune globulins, primarily IgG and complement, outlining the capillary loops.

Diagnosis. The diagnosis of APSGN depends on the demonstration of elevated serum titers of antibodies against streptococcal antigens and decreased serum complement levels in children with glomerulonephritis. Antibody titers to streptococcal antigens remain elevated for 4 to 6 months, whereas serum complement levels return to normal within 10 days to 8 weeks after the onset of nephritis. The finding of persistently decreased complement levels for longer than 8 weeks suggests the diagnosis of membranoproliferative glomerulonephritis.

Treatment. Most patients can be managed at home. Indications for admission to the hospital are hypertension, which usually is caused by oliguria with fluid retention, and acute renal failure. The treatment is symptomatic and includes salt and fluid restriction and the use of diuretics, such as furosemide, and antihypertensive drugs, such as hydralazine and nifedipine. Antibiotics are indicated if a streptococcal infection is still present, but they do not alter the course of the nephritis. Corticosteroids may be beneficial in severe cases.

IgA Nephropathy

IgA nephropathy, or Berger disease, was first described in 1968 and has subsequently been recognized as the most common form of glomerulonephritis in both children and adults. Because the diagnosis of IgA nephropathy is dependent on a renal biopsy specimen, its incidence is unknown, but it has been found in approximately 20% of children undergoing biopsy for evaluation of hematuria. IgA nephropathy is primarily a disease of children and young adults and is rare in infants. Males are involved twice as frequently as females. The etiology and pathogenesis are unknown. The finding of identical patterns of deposition of IgA both in glomeruli and in subdermal capillaries in patients with IgA nephropathy or Henoch-Schönlein purpura suggests that these two entities may be different expressions of the same disease.

Pathology. Immunofluorescence microscopy reveals the characteristic feature, which is the predominant deposition of IgA throughout the mesangial areas of the glomerulus. IgG, IgM, C3, and properdin may also be present, but in lesser amounts. By light microscopy, the glomeruli may appear normal but, more frequently, exhibit focal or diffuse mesangial cell proliferation and increased mesangial matrix, sometimes accompanied by focal necrotizing lesions, segmental glomerulosclerosis, capsular adhesions, or epithelial crescents. Patchy areas of tubular atrophy and interstitial mononuclear cell infiltration often accompany glomerular disease.

Clinical features. The most common presenting feature is the occurrence of intermittent and recurrent episodes of gross hematuria, or the finding of microscopic hematuria with or without proteinuria on urinalysis. Gross hematuria characteristically occurs during or a few days after an upper respiratory tract infection and resolves spontaneously after several days. This is in contrast to the hematuria of poststreptococcal glomerulonephritis, in which pharyngitis precedes the onset of hematuria by 1 to 2 weeks. Loin pain may be present. Between episodes, the urine may be clear or contain small numbers of red blood cells and, occasionally, protein. In most children with IgA nephropathy, blood pressure and renal function are normal at the time of diagnosis.

The natural history is incompletely characterized. In the largest pediatric experience, 15 years after the onset of disease 11% of the children had chronic renal failure, whereas 71% were in complete remission. Features of the disease predicting a poor prognosis include heavy proteinuria and pathologic findings of diffuse mesangial proliferation and a high percentage of glomeruli with sclerosis or crescents. Although there is a high recurrence rate of IgA nephropathy in patients who receive renal transplants, the disease in the transplanted kidney is invariably mild and nonprogressive.

Diagnosis. Although definitive diagnosis depends on histologic findings, the pattern of gross hematuria occurring in association with upper respiratory infection is so characteristic of IgA nephropathy that a presumptive diagnosis can be made without a renal biopsy. This pattern also occurs in children with hereditary nephritis (Alport syndrome) and benign familial hematuria, but these entities usually can be excluded on the basis of a negative family history and the fact that many children with Alport syndrome have sensorineural hearing loss. The renal histologic findings in IgA nephropathy are indistinguishable from those in patients with nephritis due to Henoch-Schönlein purpura, a systemic vasculitis characterized by a purpuric rash, abdominal pain, joint swelling or pain, and glomerulonephritis.

Treatment. Since IgA nephropathy is a benign disease in most children, treatment usually is reserved for patients with poor prognostic features. Treatments with demonstrated effectiveness have been fish oils (omega-3 fatty acids) in adults and corticosteroids, with or without cyclophosphamide, in children.

Systemic Lupus Nephritis

Systemic lupus erythematosus (SLE) is a systemic disease characterized by weight loss, fever, rash, hematological abnormalities, arthritis and involvement of the lungs, heart, central nervous system, and kidney. The general features of this disease are discussed in more detail in Chapter 8. The renal manifestations of SLE will be described in this section.

Clinical manifestations. Over 50% of patients with SLE have evidence of renal disease. The most common presentation includes microscopic hematuria, however, patients may also present with hematuria and proteinuria, and, less commonly, overt nephritis with or without nephrotic syndrome. Most patients show evidence of multiorgan disease, but a few patients may only have renal involvement. The various clinical presentations correlate generally with the various histologic patterns that are seen with this condition (see later). In rare instances, however, patients with type IV proliferative glomerulonephritis have been found to have a normal urinalysis.

Pathogenesis and pathology. The clinical manifestations of lupus nephritis may be mediated by immune complexes, which are formed in the systemic circulation and deposited in various target organs. The most commonly used classification system describing the renal histology in SLE nephritis was devised by the World Health Organization, based on light immunofluorescence and EM findings. The five major categories are "normal" with or without immunofluorescence findings (type I), mesangial glomerulonephritis (type II), focal proliferative glomerulonephritis (type III), diffuse proliferative glomerulonephritis (type IV), and membranous glomerulonephritis (type V). More often, patients with milder histologic abnormalities (types I, II, and some type III) typically have hematuria, mild proteinuria, and normal renal function. In contrast, patients with types III and IV histologic changes typically have hematuria, heavy proteinuria and abnormal renal function. Type IV is the most common and serious lesion of lupus nephritis. Type V lupus nephritis is predominantly associated with the nephrotic syndrome. It has been observed that the renal histology can change from one class to another, either from mild to more severe lesions, from severe to milder lesions.

Diagnosis. The diagnosis of lupus nephritis is based on both clinical findings and laboratory measurements. If patients are found to have renal involvement and evidence of systemic SLE disease, the presence of increased levels of serum antinuclear antibodies (ANA) and antibodies to double-stranded DNA (anti-dsDNA) and depressed levels of both C3 and C4 confirm the diagnosis. All patients with SLE and renal involvement should have a renal biopsy to determine the severity of the renal histology and, in most cases, to provide guidance to the physician in selecting an appropriate therapy.

Treatment. Therapy for lupus nephritis includes the administration of corticosteroids, cyclophosphamide, and azathioprine in various combinations. The goal of treatment is to reverse the clinical manifestations of disease and to correct the serologic abnormalities (depressed C3 and elevated anti-dsDNA). Most patients with mild renal disease and less severe renal histology are treated with daily oral prednisone. In patients with more severe nephritis (type III), intravenous methylprednisolone may be given in high doses for a brief period (usually 1 to 3 days) followed by the administration of high-dose oral prednisone. If clinical and serologic remission is achieved, the dosage of prednisone is reduced. In patients with type III nephritis who do not respond initially to steroids or in those with type IV disease, a combination of intravenous methylprednisolone and cyclophosphamide has been used.

Cyclophosphamide typically is administered monthly for 6 months followed by every 3 months for varying lengths of time. Azathioprine has been used as a steroid-sparing medication to maintain remission in patients who exhibit signs of steroid toxicity, which include hypertension, diabetes mellitus, or growth retardation. There is limited experience with the use of cyclosporine, tacrolimus, or mycophenolate mofetil in the treatment of lupus nephritis. For patients with type V lesions, there is controversy as to the appropriate therapy. Patients with lupus nephritis should be managed in conjunction with specialists who have expertise in the management of renal and extrarenal lupus (i.e., nephrologists and rheumatologists).

Prognosis. Over the past 20 years, aggressive immunosuppressive therapy has dramatically improved the long-term outcome of lupus nephritis in children. Patients with types I, II, and III lupus nephritis generally have a better outcome than those with type IV nephritis. A number of patients with type IV nephritis can progress to renal failure and require either hemodialysis or transplantation. The long-term outcome of type V lesions is more variable, but renal failure develops slowly in such patients.

ALPORT SYNDROME

Alport syndrome, also known as *progressive hereditary nephritis,* is characterized by glomerulonephritis, sensorineural deafness, and ocular abnormalities, including anterior lenticonus and perimacular pigmentary changes. Symptoms of the disease include hematuria, proteinuria, and progressive renal insufficiency. The hearing deficit, which is usually in the high-frequency range, may not appear until the teenage years and may require formal audiologic testing for detection.

Since the first description of Alport syndrome in the early 1900s, many kindreds have been identified. Pedigree analysis most commonly indicates the presence of X-linked dominant patterns of inheritance and less often, autosomal dominant or autosomal recessive inheritance in families. Males are more severely affected than are females, even within the same family. In most females with Alport syndrome, persistent microscopic hematuria is the only manifestation of the disease, and progression to end-stage renal failure is rare. In affected males, in contrast, persistent microscopic or recurrent macroscopic hematuria typically is observed in early childhood, and progression to end-stage renal failure occurs by 20 to 30 years of age.

No specific laboratory findings aid in the diagnosis. Alport syndrome should be strongly considered in children with microscopic hematuria in whom a positive family history is obtained for either Alport's syndrome, sensorineural deafness, or progressive renal insufficiency. Such children should undergo audiologic evaluation. The definitive diagnosis requires a renal biopsy. The diagnostic findings of Alport syndrome are seen by EM rather than by light microscopy. On EM, the lamina densa of the glomerular basement membrane appears thickened and split and is sometimes referred to as having a "basket weave" appearance.

The management of patients with Alport syndrome includes close attention to fluid, electrolyte, and acid-base status and treatment of hypertension, as with other forms of progressive glomerulonephritis (see later section, "Chronic Renal Failure"). To date, there is no specific therapy to alter the progressive course of Alport nephritis. Dialysis and renal transplantation are appropriate for patients whose disease progresses to end-stage renal failure. Alport nephritis does not recur in the transplanted kidney; however, a small percentage of patients with Alport syndrome who undergo transplantation have developed antiglomerular basement membrane nephritis, which can result in loss of the transplanted kidney.

MISCELLANEOUS

Isolated hematuria also may be due to strenuous exercise, blunt trauma, a bleeding disorder, or sickle-cell trait or disease. The first three of these should be apparent from a careful history. Although blunt trauma to an otherwise normal kidney can cause hematuria, the occurrence of macroscopic hematuria after minimal trauma should raise the possibility of a hydronephrotic or cystic kidney. Any patients at risk for carriage of the sickle-cell trait, particularly African Americans, should be tested for the presence of hemoglobin S. Heterozygotes, as well as homozygotes for hemoglobin S, can have hematuria secondary to medullary ischemia, which is caused by the sickling of RBCs within the renal medulla.

Hematuria also is seen in allergic interstitial nephritis, a condition usually caused by exposure to certain medications and characterized by hematuria, proteinuria, sterile pyuria, and a decreased GFR. The medications most often responsible for this condition are nonsteroidal anti-inflammatory agents, penicillin, methicillin, cephalosporins, phenytoin, cimetidine, furosemide, and thiazide diuretics. A history of recent or current use of one of these medications in patients with hematuria should raise the possibility of this diagnosis. A positive Wright stain demonstrating urinary eosinophils lends further support for this diagnosis. Therapy for allergic interstitial nephritis is withdrawal of the offending medication. In most patients, urinary abnormalities resolve and the GFR returns to normal after the medication has been discontinued.

PROTEINURIA

Evaluation of Proteinuria

In healthy individuals, protein is excreted in the urine in very small amounts; the amount varies with age (Table 15–28). The composition of urinary proteins is complex and consists of albumin (40%), immunoproteins

Table 15–28. Urinary Protein Excretion in Healthy Infants, Children, and Adolescents

Age	Mean (Range) (mg/m^2/d)
5–30 d	182 (88–377)
7–30 d	145 (68–309)
2 mo–4 y	100 (37–244)
5–10 y	85 (21–234)
11–16 y	63 (22–181)

(15%), Tamm-Horsfall proteins (40%), and various peptides (5%). Important immunoproteins that appear in the urine are IgA, IgG, and β_2-microglobulin. Tamm-Horsfall proteins are mucoproteins derived from tubular epithelium of the distal nephron. Peptides or hormones that are present in the urine include parathyroid hormone, vasopressin, insulin, vitamins, and various binding proteins.

Mechanisms of Renal Handling of Protein

The composition and quantity of urinary protein are determined by a number of renal and extrarenal factors. The GFR influences the filtration of protein macromolecules by affecting both the glomerular capillary plasma flow rate and the transcapillary hydraulic pressure gradient. The glomerular capillary wall permits free passage of water and small solutes but restricts the passage of plasma proteins depending on their size, charge, and overall configuration. The clearance of proteins is inversely related to their molecular size. Moreover, negatively charged proteins, such as albumin, are repulsed by the negatively charged glomerular capillary wall, thus preventing their filtration and excretion. The proximal tubule not only reabsorbs most filtered amino acids, but also reabsorbs and degrades albumin and low-molecular-weight proteins that have traversed the glomerular barrier. Most of these proteins are absorbed from the tubular lumen by either endocytic or pinocytic processes and then transferred to lysosomal compartments where they are catabolized by proteolytic enzymes.

Detection and Quantification of Proteinuria

The dipstick method is the most commonly used screening test for detection of proteinuria. With this method, protein in the urine induces a color change of the indicator dye tetrabromphenol; the change is proportionate to the concentration of the protein. The results are graded from negative (yellow) to 2+ (100 mg/dL green) to 4+ (>2000 mg/dL, dark green). The lower limit of detection for urinary protein by the dipstick method is 10 to 20 mg/dL. A false-negative result can occur when the urine is very dilute (specific gravity <1.005) or contains a non-albumin-like protein, and a false-positive result can occur when the urine is strongly alkaline (pH >7.0) because the indicator dye is buffered to maintain a pH of 3.0. Because of the variability of daily urine flow rates and the limit of detection of urinary protein, the dipstick method is not useful as a quantitative test for urinary protein.

Urinary protein can also be detected by the turbidimetric method in which reagents such as sulfosalicylic acid, trichloroacetic acid, or heat cause a denaturation of urinary proteins, resulting in their precipitation. The degree of turbidity of the urine sample is compared against a set of standards, thus permitting semiquantification of the urinary protein concentration. For precise measurements, a third method using spectrophotometry can be used (biuret, Coomassie blue, or Lowry methods).

Etiology of Proteinuria

In healthy children aged 3 weeks to 18 years, the prevalence of asymptomatic proteinuria varies from 1.8 to 11.6% on a single random urine test and is 0.6% when two or more consecutive urine specimens are analyzed. The prevalence is highest in adolescence and appears to be greater in girls than it is in boys. The causes of proteinuria in children are listed in Table 15–29.

Diagnostic Approach to Isolated Proteinuria

The finding of isolated proteinuria (Figure 15–5) in children should be confirmed on at least two subsequent urinalyses. Urine for analysis is preferably obtained in the morning when it is concentrated (specific gravity >1.018) and acidic (pH <6.0). If neither of the repeated urinalyses is positive for protein, transient proteinuria is likely and further evaluation is not warranted. If proteinuria is confirmed, however, a detailed medical history and physical examination are required. A history of recent infections, signs and symptoms of other renal or systemic disease, previous abnormal urinalysis results, exposure to potential renal-toxic medications (e.g., aminoglycosides and ifosfamide), and a family history of renal disease or deafness are important pieces of information that assist in differentiating among the various glomerular diseases. The physical examination should focus on the detection of growth retardation and hypertension, as these can be the first signs of renal dysfunction. Generalized edema and signs of respiratory difficulty may occur when proteinuria is severe.

If the urine dipstick reveals proteinuria of 1+ or less and the findings on the physical examination and the remainder of the urinalysis are normal, children should be observed, with a physical examination and complete urinalysis performed annually. If the urine dipstick reveals proteinuria of 2+ or greater, however, one should evalu-

Table 15–29. Causes of Proteinuria in Children

Transient	
Fever	Extreme cold
Orthostatic	Epinephrine
Exercise	Seizures
Stress	Congestive heart failure

Persistent
Orthostatic
Benign (sporadic or familial)
Increased plasma concentration of protein
Lymphoma, chronic lymphocytic leukemia
Decreased tubular reabsorption of protein
Hereditary: Fanconi syndrome, Wilson disease, cystinosis, Lowe syndrome
Acquired: drugs (aminoglycosides, phenacetin, lithium), acute tubular necrosis, interstitial nephritis, radiation nephritis
Glomerular
Primary: Minimal change disease, focal segmental glomerulosclerosis, mesangial proliferative glomerulonephritis, membranous nephropathy, membrano-proliferative glomerulonephritis, IgA nephropathy
Secondary
Infectious: Poststreptococcal glomerulonephritis, endocarditis, hepatitis B
Immune/multisystem: Systemic lupus erythematosus, Henöch-Schonlein purpura, Wegener granulomatosis, polyarteritis nodosa, Goodpasture syndrome
Metabolic: diabetes mellitus
Hereditary: Alport syndrome
Drugs: nonsteroidal anti-inflammatory agents
Structural abnormalities of the urinary tract, congenital or acquired
Polycystic kidney disease: autosomal recessive or dominant
Hydronephrosis: posterior urethral valves, ureterovesical or ureteropelvic obstruction
Hypoplastic-dysplastic disease
Reflux nephropathy

ate patients (children and adolescents) for orthostatic proteinuria. This is performed by collecting the first urine specimen (specimen 1) when the patients have arisen in the morning and the second specimen after the patients have ambulated for 4 h (specimen 2). Both specimens are checked for protein by the dipstick method. If specimen 1 is free of protein and specimen 2 contains protein, the test result is positive for orthostatic proteinuria. A confirmatory test should be performed in all patients. If orthostatic proteinuria is confirmed and renal function is normal, the patients can be observed with an annual physical examination and urinalysis. If both specimens are positive

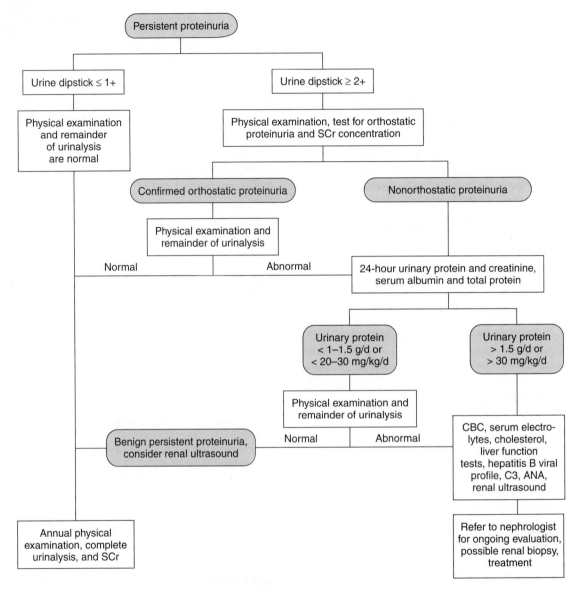

Figure 15–5. Algorithm for the diagnostic evaluation of children with persistent proteinuria. ANA = antinuclear antibody; C3 = serum complement 3; CBC = complete blood cell count; SCr = serum creatinine.

for protein, however, orthostatic proteinuria is probably not the cause. A serum creatinine level should be determined in all patients.

If proteinuria is persistent and not orthostatic, further evaluation is warranted. The proteinuria should be quantitated, and the 24-h urine collection permits the most precise determination of total protein excretion. Proteinuria is considered abnormal when it exceeds the upper limit of normal for age (see Table 15–28). In the same

collection, a creatinine clearance (C_{Creat}) should be determined not only to estimate the GFR but also to verify the adequacy of the collection. In addition to obtaining a serum creatinine specimen for C_{Creat} measurement, a serum albumin and total protein concentration should be determined. One can estimate the magnitude of proteinuria on a random, untimed urine sample by computing the ratio of the urinary total protein concentration to the urinary creatinine concentration. As a guide, values <0.1

are considered normal, 0.1 to 1 mild, >1.0 to 3.0 moderate, and >3.0 severe proteinuria; the last category correlates with nephrotic range proteinuria.

If urinary protein is <1.0 to 1.5 g per day or <20 to 30 mg/kg/d, and if the findings from serum chemistries, remainder of urinalysis, and physical examination are normal, patients can be observed with an annual physical examination, urinalysis, and serum creatinine determination. Patients with more severe proteinuria, with or without edema, require further diagnostic tests and should be referred to a nephrologist. Such tests should include a complete blood cell count; serum electrolyte and cholesterol levels; liver function tests, hepatitis B virus profile, C3 level, and ANA test (see below). A renal ultrasound study should be performed to determine whether cystic disease or structural abnormalities are present (e.g., polycystic, dysplastic, or reflux nephropathy), although nephrotic range proteinuria is rare in these patients. The decision whether to intervene with therapy or to perform a renal biopsy is determined by the clinical presentation and the initial evaluation.

TRANSIENT PROTEINURIA

Transient proteinuria can be associated with many conditions, such as stress, heavy exercise, extreme cold, heart failure, fever, seizures, and epinephrine administration. Under these conditions, the proteinuria is postulated to result from hemodynamic changes that produce a decrease in renal plasma flow out of proportion to GFR. These hemodynamic changes result in an increase in the protein concentration in glomerular capillaries, which enhances its concentration gradient and thus its movement into the urinary space. With resolution of these conditions, the proteinuria disappears.

ORTHOSTATIC PROTEINURIA

Orthostatic proteinuria is a condition in which protein excretion is considerably greater in the standing than in the recumbent position. Although this phenomenon occurs in most healthy individuals, the amount of protein excreted in the standing position is below the detection limit of the dipstick method. In patients with orthostatic proteinuria, the amount of proteinuria ranges from 0.5 to 1.5 g per 24 h. Orthostatic proteinuria is found most commonly in the adolescent population. Renal biopsy specimens of affected individuals have revealed either normal glomeruli or mild glomerular changes; the long-term clinical course is benign. Although the mechanism is not completely understood, orthostatic proteinuria is believed to result from increased transglomerular passage of albumin. This condition may be transient or long-standing.

PERSISTENT PROTEINURIA

Persistent proteinuria typically is a sign of glomerular disease, although it can also be caused by conditions associated with renal tubular disease or an increased filtered load of protein. Both the site and degree of injury are important determinants of the magnitude of proteinuria. With tubular injury, the amount of proteinuria is usually less than 2 g per 24 h. Proteinuria can occur in patients with proximal tubular dysfunction, such as with the Fanconi syndrome, or in patients receiving aminoglycoside antibiotics, which are known to be toxic to the proximal tubule. Removal of the toxin usually restores tubular function to normal, and the proteinuria resolves. In adult patients with multiple myeloma, in which the proteinuria is due to an increased filtered load of low-molecular-weight proteins (immunoglobulin light chains), measurement of serum proteins and the urinary immunoelectrophoresis pattern are useful for diagnosis.

Persistent proteinuria can be due to primary glomerular disease (disorders in which the glomeruli are the sole or predominant tissue involved) or secondary to a systemic disease (see Table 15–29). Depending on the severity of the glomerular injury, urinary protein excretion can range from less than 1 g to more than 20 g per day. The clinical course, response to therapy, and prognosis of patients with proteinuria vary greatly depending on the underlying cause. In patients with benign persistent proteinuria, the outcome is excellent and no therapy is warranted; in postinfectious glomerulonephritis, the outcome usually is favorable, and only supportive therapy is necessary for the acute complications. By contrast, in certain primary glomerular diseases, moderate proteinuria or severe proteinuria associated with the nephrotic syndrome (protein excretion >50 mg/kg/d, hypoalbuminemia, edema, and hyperlipidemia) can be persistent and unresponsive to therapy, and progression to renal insufficiency can occur, requiring dialysis and subsequent transplantation. Congenital disease with or without associated structural anomalies of the urinary tract can also cause persistent proteinuria. Diagnosis of these conditions usually is made on the basis of their clinical, radiological, or, rarely, histologic features.

Nephrotic Syndrome

The *nephrotic syndrome* is defined by a constellation of clinical and laboratory findings that includes severe proteinuria, hypoalbuminemia, edema, and hyperlipidemia. The severe proteinuria usually is a result of glomerular injury that leads to increased glomerular capillary wall permeability to serum proteins. In contrast, the hypoalbuminemia, edema, and hyperlipidemia are a consequence of the heavy urinary protein loss. Over the years, it has become clear that nephrotic syndrome has diverse etiologies with distinct glomerular histopathology and clinical courses. Tables 15–30 lists the causes of primary nephrotic syndrome in children. The following discussion focuses on primary or idiopathic nephrotic syndrome in children.

Table 15–30. Causes of Primary Nephrotic Syndrome in Children

Acquired
  Minimal change disease
  Focal segmental or global glomerulosclerosis
  Mesangial proliferative glomerulonephritis
  Membranous nephropathy (idiopathic)
  Membranoproliferative glomerulonephritis
  IgA nephropathy
Hereditary
  Congenital nephrotic syndrome
    Finnish type
    Diffuse mesangial sclerosis
  Alport syndrome

Secondary causes of nephrotic syndrome are shown in Table 15–31; some of these conditions are discussed in the section on glomerulonephritis.

EPIDEMIOLOGY

In patients younger than 16 years, the nephrotic syndrome is the most frequent presentation of persistent glomerular disease; the incidence is 2 to 7 new cases per 100,000 persons per year. The prevalence is approximately 16 cases per 100,000 children. In early childhood, cases in boys predominate with a ratio of 2 : 1; however, in adolescence and adulthood, the distribution between genders is equal.

CLINICAL AND LABORATORY FEATURES

Most children with nephrotic syndrome come to medical attention because of the onset of edema, expressed

Table 15–31. Secondary Causes of Nephrotic Syndrome in Children

Multisystemic disease: systemic lupus erythematosus, Goodpasture syndrome, Henoch-Schönlein purpura, Wegener granulomatosis, amyloidosis
Malignancy: Hodgkin disease, leukemia, multiple myeloma
Drugs: mercurial compounds, gold, penicillamine, captopril, nonsteroidal anti-inflammatory agents
Toxins: bee sting, diphtheria, pertussis, tetanus toxoid
Infectious:
  Bacterial: poststreptococcal glomerulonephritis, infective endocarditis, tuberculosis
  Viral: hepatitis B, cytomegalovirus, HIV type 1, Epstein-Barr virus
Metabolic disease: diabetes mellitus
Miscellaneous: massive obesity, reflux nephropathy, chronic renal graft rejection, sickle cell anemia

as swelling of the eyes in the morning and of dependent areas, such as the genitals, legs, and feet, later in the day. In most cases, the swelling is preceded by a nonspecific prodromal illness. A few children have a history of allergies and previous treatment with antihistamines; on rare occasions, there is a history of edematous periods followed by spontaneous remissions. On physical examination, the peripheral edema is characteristically soft and pitting. With an increase in the severity of the edema, ascites and pleural effusions can occur.

The "gold standard" laboratory test for determining the degree of proteinuria is the timed 24-h urine collection, although less precise estimates can be made from a single untimed urine specimen (see earlier, "Proteinuria"). *Nephrotic-range proteinuria* is defined as a urinary protein excretion rate of >40 mg/m^2/h or >50 mg/kg/d in children, or >3.5 g per 24 h in adults. When the rate of urinary protein loss exceeds the capacity of the liver to synthesize new protein, hypoalbuminemia occurs.

One important function of albumin is to generate oncotic pressure within the intravascular compartment. When the plasma albumin concentration decreases significantly, a decrease in plasma oncotic pressure promotes the movement of fluid from the intravascular to the interstitial space, which results in the development of edema. The intravascular depletion leads to activation of the renin-angiotensin system, retention of sodium and water, and worsening of the edema. Clinically apparent edema usually does not occur until the plasma albumin concentration decreases to less than approximately 2 g/dL. In some patients with nephrotic syndrome, there is primary renal retention of sodium and water, which results in expansion of the plasma volume and suppression of the renin-angiotensin system. The expanded plasma volume increases capillary hydrostatic pressure, which further promotes loss of fluid into the interstitial space and the development of edema (Figure 15–6).

EXTRARENAL COMPLICATIONS

In most patients with nephrotic syndrome, serum concentrations of total cholesterol and triglycerides are increased. Data suggest that either the hypoalbuminemia and consequent reduction in plasma oncotic pressure or the enhanced urinary loss of an unknown regulatory factor, or both, result in enhanced hepatic production of very-low-density lipoproteins (VLDL) and reduced peripheral use and catabolism of lipoproteins. In nephrotic syndrome, plasma protein, in addition to albumin, are lost in the urine. Decreased concentrations of IgG and factor B, important components of the alternate pathway of complement activation, may play a role in the unusual susceptibility to infection by encapsulated bacteria observed in patients with massive proteinuria.

In patients with nephrotic syndrome, there is an increased risk of thrombosis of the renal vein, pulmonary ar-

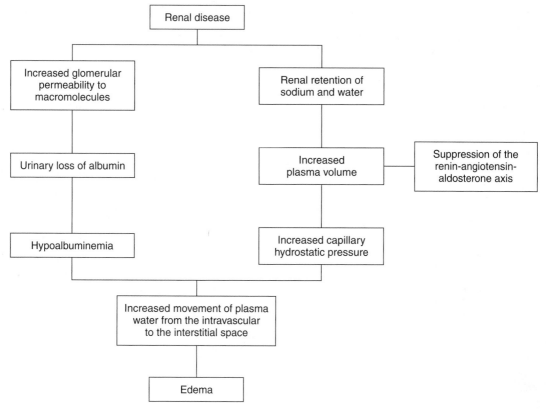

Figure 15–6. Proposed mechanisms of edema formation in nephrotic syndrome.

tery or vein, or peripheral arteries or veins, and of pulmonary emboli. The mechanisms responsible for the hypercoagulable state of these patients are not well understood. Antithrombin III levels may be severely depressed because of urinary losses and may play an important role. Plasma protein C and protein S levels may be normal or elevated, but their functional activity may be reduced. Factors IX and XII concentrations are reduced in nephrotic syndrome, whereas factors V, VII, VIII (von Willebrand factor), and X are elevated. In addition to these disturbances in the coagulation system, increased platelet aggregation or enhanced erythrocyte aggregation may play a role. Another contributing factor is volume depletion with its associated stasis, hyperviscosity, and hyperlipidemia.

The most common site of thrombosis is the renal vein, and affected patients may have flank pain, hematuria, and an acute decline in GFR. Acute pain or other symptoms at other sites, such as the leg or chest, may suggest the development of thrombosis. Useful diagnostic studies include renal ultrasound, peripheral venous Doppler, arteriogram, pulmonary ventilation-perfusion (V/Q) scan, or magnetic resonance imaging.

Another group of proteins that may be lost in the urine is the important metal and hormone-binding proteins. For example, zinc deficiency may contribute to poor wound healing and impaired cell-mediated immunity. Deficiency of thyroxine-binding globulin may lead to a hypothyroid state. Urinary losses of vitamin-D–binding globulin may cause a vitamin D deficiency state.

PRIMARY IDIOPATHIC NEPHROTIC SYNDROME

In the next section, the clinical spectrum, histopathology, natural history, and response to therapy of the more common diseases classified as primary idiopathic nephrotic syndrome are discussed (see Table 15–30). The frequency of the different diseases varies according to the age at the time of presentation. For example, minimal change disease (MCD) is found in 80 to 85% of young children with nephrotic syndrome, whereas membranous glomerulonephritis is the most common cause in patients older than 60 years. The classification of renal diseases is based on the histologic appearance of renal tissue obtained by biopsy.

Minimal change disease. Minimal change disease, also known as *lipoid nephrosis,* is the most common cause of primary idiopathic nephrotic syndrome in children, with a peak occurrence between the ages of 2 and 6 years. In many cases, a viral upper respiratory illness precedes the onset of the proteinuria, and, occasionally, there is a history of allergies or previous immunizations. Although the pathogenesis of MCD is unknown, considerable evidence suggests that a disorder of the immune system is involved (Table 15–32).

The initial clinical manifestation of nephrotic syndrome typically is the appearance of edema. Edema usually is dependent and demonstrated by swollen eyes in the morning and swelling of the feet at the end of the day. With progression of the disease, more severe edema, marked weight gain, abdominal distention with ascites, and respiratory distress with pleural effusion are commonly seen. Both blood pressure and renal function are normal in most patients; however, a subset of patients may have mild hypertension and azotemia. In addition to heavy proteinuria, approximately 10% of patients have microscopic hematuria, whereas gross hematuria or the presence of RBC casts is not consistent with the diagnosis of MCD. The serum C3 level is normal. Thus, the diagnosis of MCD should be strongly considered in children younger than 6 years with nephrotic syndrome in whom hematuria, hypertension, azotemia, and hypocomplementemia are absent.

On pathologic examination of the kidney, the characteristic feature on light microscopy is the absence of glomerular alterations. Immunofluorescence studies fail to demonstrate IgG or complement; however, occasional mesangial deposits of IgM are seen. Patients with increased mesangial cellularity and mesangial deposits have been distinguished from pure MCD and are now classified as *mesangial proliferative glomerulonephritis*. In both diseases, EM reveals effacement of the foot-processes of the glomerular capillary epithelial cells. As the proteinuria resolves, the epithelial cells resume their normal ultrastructural appearance.

Therapy. Most children with a diagnosis of MCD can receive treatment on an outpatient basis. Indica-

tions for hospitalization include severe anasarca requiring aggressive diuretic therapy, inability to take oral medications, infections such as peritonitis, or the need for a renal biopsy. The management of edema includes dietary salt restriction and the judicious use of diuretics. Salt restriction is accomplished by eliminating foods with a high salt content and by not adding salt during preparation or serving of food. A high protein intake offers no advantage in compensating for the severe urinary protein loss. The most commonly used diuretics are loop diuretics, such as furosemide. One should be familiar with the known side effects of prolonged use of loop diuretics, such as hypokalemia, hypochloremic metabolic alkalosis, hypercalciuria, and, rarely, interstitial nephritis; their occurrence necessitates frequent monitoring of these patients.

The striking feature of MCD is its characteristic response to steroid therapy; specifically, an accelerated diuresis and the elimination of proteinuria. The International Study of Kidney Diseases in Children revealed that 93% of 363 patients with MCD responded to 8 weeks of therapy, defined as 3 or more days of "protein-free" urine (<1+ by Albustix). A suggested protocol for the treatment of MCD with prednisone is shown in Table 15–33; other similar protocols have been used. In patients with minimal change nephrotic syndrome who receive an initial 8 to 12-week course of prednisone therapy, approximately 93% respond with resolution of the proteinuria (Figure 15–7). Several patterns of responsiveness to subsequent courses of prednisone in such children have been observed, including (1) nonrelapsers—complete remission without relapses; (2) relapsers—complete remission, with relapses of proteinuria occurring when prednisone has been discontinued for at least 2 weeks; (3) steroid dependence—complete remission with relapse of proteinuria occurring when prednisone is tapered; and (4) steroid resistance—failure to induce complete remission of proteinuria. In patients with frequent

Table 15–32. Evidence for a Disorder of Immune Function in the Pathogenesis of Minimal Change Nephrotic Syndrome

Remission associated with measles infection
Remission induced by corticosteroids and cytotoxic drugs
Occurrence in Hodgkin disease
Sera from nephrotic patients inhibits lymphocyte proliferation in response to mitogens; no inhibition during remission
Increased incidence of allergic disease
Decreased immunoglobulin levels

Table 15–33. Treatment of Nephrotic Syndrome with Corticosteroids

Initial treatment	Month 1: Prednisone, 2 mg/kg (~60 mg/m^2) orally daily
	Month 2: Prednisone 2 mg/kg orally every other day
	Month 3: Taper over 2–4 weeks
	Total duration is ~10–12 weeks
Treatment of first relapse	Same as above
Treatment of frequent relapses	Same as above
	Tapering schedule should be extended over 8–16 weeks, depending on clinical response

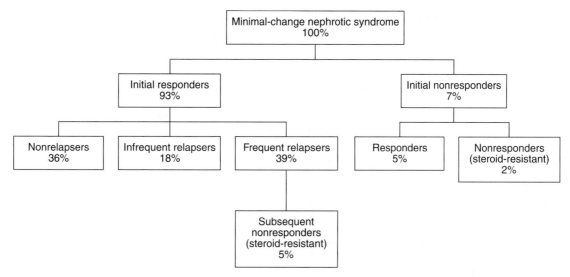

Figure 15–7. Response to prednisone therapy in children with minimal change nephrotic syndrome.

relapses (>3 per year), a prolonged course of alternate-day low-dose steroids may be beneficial in preventing further relapses.

In patients with frequent relapses or steroid dependency, untoward effects of long-term steroid therapy can occur, such as growth suppression, obesity, striae, gastritis, or bleeding, and, less commonly, hypertension, diabetes mellitus, osteoporosis, or cataracts. When these occur, most pediatric nephrologists recommend that a renal biopsy should be performed (Table 15–34) and that therapy with either cyclophosphamide or chlorambucil be initiated. In addition to determining the renal histology, the biopsy specimen provides information regarding the response to therapy and long-term prognosis. Cyclophosphamide is the most frequently used cytotoxic agent. Studies have shown that treatment with 2 to 3 mg/kg/day for 8 to 12 weeks is effective in inducing a sustained remission of proteinuria. Cyclophosphamide toxicity includes both acute effects, such as bone marrow sup-

pression, gastritis, alopecia, and hemorrhagic cystitis, and the potential long-term effects of cancer and gonadal dysfunction. The latter complications appear to be minimal when the total cumulative dose administered is less than 168 mg/kg. The long-term follow-up of children with biopsy-proved minimal change nephrotic syndrome is highly favorable. The estimated 10-year survival rate of steroid-responsive patients with MCD is greater than 95%. Progression to renal failure and hypertension do not occur, and any increased morbidity or mortality is attributed to the side-effects associated with corticosteroid therapy, such as infection and diabetes mellitus. Similar to patients with MCD, patients with mesangial proliferative glomerulonephritis typically respond to corticosteroids. There is some suggestion, however, that this latter lesion has a worse prognosis than MCD.

Focal segmental glomerular sclerosis. Most patients with focal segmental glomerular sclerosis (FSGS) present in a fashion similar to those with minimal change nephrotic syndrome. However, a subset of patients may have asymptomatic proteinuria noted on routine urinalysis. Focal segmental glomerular sclerosis is found in about 7 to 15% of children with primary nephrotic syndrome and is the second most common lesion seen in such children. Typically, the diagnosis is made when a renal biopsy is performed in children with presumed minimal change nephrotic syndrome who do not respond to corticosteroids or who have a history of frequent relapses or steroid dependency.

The pathogenesis of FSGS is unknown. It may be idiopathic or associated with other glomerular or systemic diseases. On light microscopy, the lesion is characterized

Table 15–34. Relative Indications for Renal Biopsy in Nephrotic Syndrome

Secondary causes of nephrotic syndrome
Age > 10–12 y
Significant hematuria, hypertension, or azotemia
Low C3 for more than 8 weeks
Initial nonresponse to corticosteroids
Before using cytotoxic agents
Steroid toxicity

by focal and segmental sclerosis of the glomerular tuft associated with increased mesangial matrix. Lesions preferentially affect the juxtaglomerular glomeruli. IgM and C3 can often be seen in the affected glomerular segments, but IgG and IgA are less common. Electron microscopy reveals effacement and diffuse or segmental alterations of the foot processes of the epithelial cells.

Most patients with FSGS (50 to 70%) demonstrate persistent proteinuria, progressive decline in GFR, and hypertension that are unresponsive to therapy. However, spontaneous remission without progressive renal failure can occur in approximately 10 to 15%, and exacerbation of proteinuria and nephrotic syndrome with a late onset of renal failure can occur in 10 to 15%. Treatment with cytotoxic agents, cyclosporine, or nonsteroidal anti-inflammatory agents has been ineffective in altering the course of this disease. However, two uncontrolled studies—one in which prolonged high-dose intravenous corticosteroids combined with cytotoxic therapy was administered and another in which high-dose oral cyclosporine A was used—have demonstrated some effectiveness in inducing and maintaining remission in patients previously resistant to conventional corticosteroid therapy. For patients who progress to renal failure, dialysis and transplantation are therapeutic options. Unfortunately, the risk of recurrence of FSGS in the transplanted kidney is reported to be as high as 40%.

Membranoproliferative glomerulonephritis. Although membranoproliferative glomerulonephritis (MPGN) is an uncommon cause (7%) of primary nephrotic syndrome in childhood, more than 50% of patients with this disease will have nephrotic syndrome. Other patients with MPGN can present with hematuria, hypertension, and mild azotemia. A persistently reduced serum C3 level is a characteristic finding in MPGN, in contrast to the transient reduction observed in patients with acute poststreptococcal glomerulonephritis.

The clinical course of MPGN in children is variable. In patients with serum creatinine concentrations of 2 mg/dL or greater at the time of diagnosis, most progress to endstage renal failure within 3 years. Some patients may have prolonged periods of hematuria and proteinuria followed by the development of edema, subsequent azotemia, and end-stage renal failure. Only a small percentage of patients go into complete remission.

Pathologically, two major variants of MPGN have been described (although some groups have reported a third variant). Both variants demonstrate increased mesangial cellularity and matrix and C3 deposition in both the mesangium and glomerular capillary wall. In type I MPGN, the glomerular capillary wall is thickened, with a "tram-track" appearance, and EM reveals electron-dense deposits in subendothelial and mesangial areas. In type II MPGN, EM reveals widened glomerular basement membranes associated with the presence of dense deposits. The pathogenesis of type I MPGN is thought to involve chronic glomerular deposition of immune complexes; the pathogenesis of type II is unknown.

Poor prognostic indicators in MPGN are hypertension, reduced GFR, and the nephrotic syndrome. Various therapeutic regimens have been used in an attempt to slow the progression of disease. There is some evidence that low-dose, long-term, alternate-day corticosteroid therapy with close observation may be beneficial.

Membranous glomerulopathy. The histologic lesion of membranous glomerulopathy (MGN) is rare in the pediatric age group; when present, it is more common in older children and adolescents, although it can occur at any age. Most patients are asymptomatic and are often referred to the pediatric nephrologist because of significant proteinuria detected on routine urinalysis or nephrotic syndrome unresponsive to corticosteroid steroid therapy. Other patients may have edema and hematuria, either microscopic or macroscopic. The pathogenesis of MGN is unknown; however, there is evidence that immune complex–mediated mechanisms are involved. Membranous glomerulopathy has been associated with various infections, the most frequent being the hepatitis B virus.

The clinical course of patients with MGN is highly variable. Most patients have persistent proteinuria; however, isolated hematuria has been reported. Edema and the nephrotic syndrome can occur. In most patients, serum complement concentrations are normal.

The histologic lesion is characterized by diffuse and uniform thickening of the glomerular capillary wall without significant mesangial proliferation. Immunofluorescence microscopy reveals diffuse granular staining along the capillary loops with IgG and C3. Electrton microscopy reveals immune complexes as dense deposits in the subepithelial space.

Even though the clinical course of MGN is variable in children, the overall prognosis is excellent, with spontaneous remission of proteinuria occurring in 50 to 60%. Renal failure has been reported to occur in 13 to 30% of patients. Children with nephrotic syndrome are at greatest risk of long-term complications; alternate-day steroid therapy may improve their prognosis.

In summary, the underlying histologic lesion is the principal determinant of the clinical course, and the ultimate outcome of primary idiopathic nephrotic syndrome in children. As discussed, one often cannot determine the underlying histologic lesion on the basis of the presenting symptoms alone. After consultation with a pediatric nephrologist, a reasonable therapeutic approach to children with nephrotic syndrome who have no risk factors for serious underlying diseases (see Table 15–34) would be a short course of treatment with oral prednisone. In patients in whom the nephrotic syndrome resolves with prednisone therapy, the most likely lesion is MCD. Unfortunately, such patients can later become unresponsive to corticosteroids and, when a renal biopsy is performed, can be shown to have FSGS.

HYPERTENSION

Hypertension is uncommon in children. Mild hypertension may be secondary to obesity or have no demonstrable cause, but severe hypertension, especially in prepubertal children, is almost always secondary to some medical condition. When defining and evaluating hypertension in children, special attention must be paid to techniques of blood pressure measurement and to recognizing that blood pressure levels normally increase with age throughout childhood. The goal of the evaluation of children with hypertension is primarily to discover the cause of the hypertension and, secondarily, to determine whether the hypertension has resulted in damage to other organs.

Measurement of Blood Pressure

The size of the blood pressure cuff must be appropriate to the size of the child. The bladder of the cuff should encircle, or nearly encircle, the upper arm, and the width of the cuff should be at least two-thirds the length of the upper arm. A smaller cuff results in spuriously high blood pressure measurements.

Children must be quiet when blood pressure is measured. The measurement of blood pressure in infants and toddlers is often difficult. In this age group, as well as in older children, it may be easier to obtain accurate measurements of blood pressure by machines that use oscillometric or Doppler techniques than by traditional auscultatory techniques. The blood pressure should be taken three times, and the last measurement, or the mean of the last two measurements, should be recorded.

Definition of Hypertension

Hypertension is defined as a systolic or diastolic blood pressure, or both, determined on three separate occasions, equal to or greater than the 95th percentile of the blood pressure of normal children of the same age and sex (Table 15–35). In adolescents, a blood pressure of 140/90 mmHg or greater is also considered to represent hypertension, although it may be less than the 95th percentile for normal children.

Etiology of Hypertension

Hypertension in children can be primary (essential) or secondary. Studies of blood pressure in large school populations have identified small numbers of mildly to mod-

Table 15–35. Classification of Significant Hypertension by Age Group

Age Group	Blood Pressure (mm Hg)	
	Systolic	Diastolic
Newborn		
7 d	≥96	—
8–30 d	≥104	—
Infant <2 y	≥112	≥74
Children		
3–5 y	≥116	≥76
6–9 y	≥122	≥78
10–12 y	≥126	≥82
Adolescents		
13–15 y	≥136	≥86
16–18 y	≥142	≥92

erately hypertensive children; in many of these children, no cause for the hypertension could be found. In contrast, in studies of children admitted to tertiary care hospitals because of severe hypertension, a cause has almost always been discovered. Primary hypertension is rare in young children but becomes more common in adolescents, especially in black males and in children with a strong family history of hypertension.

Secondary hypertension can be associated with a variety of acute illnesses but is more often a consequence of obesity or of chronic diseases, congenital malformations, or tumors of organs known to affect the regulation of blood pressure (Table 15–36). Hypertension can also result from the ingestion of drugs and toxins and can occur in children with Turner syndrome and Williams syndrome; in the latter conditions, the hypertension usually is related to renal or vascular anomalies. The most common causes of severe persistent hypertension are chronic pyelonephritis and glomerulonephritis, renal anomalies, coarctation of the aorta, and renal artery stenosis. Endocrine causes of hypertension are much less common.

Evaluation of Hypertensive Children

A careful history and physical examination and a few laboratory tests usually are sufficient to diagnose the common causes of hypertension or to indicate the need for further evaluation of a suspected cause. Many of the causes of acute hypertension listed in Table 15–36 are identified by the clinical setting. If the cause is not apparent after this basic evaluation, further tests for less common causes can be performed. The need for extensive or invasive testing is determined by the age of children and the severity of the

Table 15–36. Causes of Hypertension in Children

Persistent Causes by Organ System	Acute and Miscellaneous Causes
Obesity	Ingestions
Renal	Contraceptives, steroids, cocaine, amphetamines, phencyclidine
Chronic glomerulonephritis, pyelonephritis, renal failure	Lead intoxication
Malformations (cystic, etc.)	Turner syndrome
Obstructive uropathy	William syndrome
Renal artery stenosis or thrombosis	Bronchopulmonary dysplasia
	Acute renal disease
Endocrine	Burns
Cushing's syndrome	Orthopedic traction
Congenital adrenal hyperplasia	Poliomyelitis
Primary hyperaldosteronism	Guillian-Barré syndrome
Dexamethasone-suppressible hyperaldosteronism	Cyclic vomiting
	Hypercalcemia
Apparent mineralocorticoid excess	Genitourinary surgery
Hyperthyroidism (systolic)	
Cardiovascular	
Coarctation of the aorta	
Takayasu arteritis	
Central nervous system	
Increased intracranial pressure	
Dysautonomia	
Tumors	
Pheochromocytoma	
Neuroblastoma	
Wilms tumor	

Table 15–37. History and Physical Examination of Hypertensive Children

Historical Features	Relevance
Family history of hypertension	Essential hypertension Dexamethasone-suppressible hypertension
Ingestion of contraceptive pills, steroids, amphetamines, cocaine, phencyclidine, lead	Drug or toxin-induced hypertension
Heat intolerance, restlessness	Hyperthyroidism
Headaches, sweating, pallor, palpitations	Pheochromocytoma
Previous urinary tract infections	Chronic pyelonephritis

Physical Findings	Relevance
Obesity	Obesity-related hypertension
Signs of increased intracranial pressure	
Moonface, buffalo hump, striae	Cushing syndrome
Webbed neck, low hairline, widely spaced nipples	Turner syndrome
Elfin facies, mental retardation	Williams syndrome
Café-au-lait spots	Renal artery stenosis Pheochromocytoma
Warm skin, hyperactive reflexes, large thyroid	Hyperthyroidism
Decreased blood pressure and pulses in legs	Coarctation of the aorta
Abdominal masses	Wilms tumor, neuroblastoma, cystic or obstructed kidney
Abdominal bruits	Renal artery stenosis
Virilization, hypogonadism, pseudohermaphroditism	Congenital adrenal hyperplasia
Retinal arteriolar changes	Severity, chronicity of hypertension

hypertension. Items in the history and physical examination that are important in establishing the cause of hypertension are listed in Table 15–37, and useful laboratory and imaging tests are listed in Table 15–38. A schema for evaluation is given in Figure 15–8.

HISTORY

It is important to elicit a family history of hypertension. The presence of a strong family history of essential hypertension in an adolescent with mild to moderate hypertension suggests that the adolescent's hypertension is primary and decreases the need for evaluation of secondary causes. A rare form of hypertension, dexamethasone-suppressible hypertension, is an autosomal dominant condition that is suggested by the early onset of hypertension in family members. In adolescent girls, the use of contraceptive pills should be ascertained, because this is the most common cause of hypertension in this population.

PHYSICAL EXAMINATION

Determination of blood pressures and pulses in the arms and legs is important to exclude coarctation of the aorta. Hyperthyroidism, Cushing syndrome, and adrenogenital syndrome should be suggested by the characteristic physical signs of these disorders, and the presence of an

Table 15–38. Laboratory and Imaging Evaluation of Hypertensive Children

Test	Relevance
Initial Evaluation	
Urinalysis	Chronic pyelonephritis, glomerulonephritis, renal anomalies
Urine culture (girls)	Chronic pyelonephritis
Serum blood urea nitrogen, creatinine	Renal insufficiency
Serum electrolytes	Hypokalemia and alkalosis (hyperaldosteronism)
Renal ultrasound	Renal anomalies, hydronephrosis, renal scars, Wilms tumor, neuroblastoma
Extended Evaluation	
Plasma renin concentrations	Increased: renal artery stenosis Decreased: primary hyperaldosteronism, dexamethasone-suppressible hypertension
Plasma aldosterone concentrations	Increased: renal artery stenosis, primary hyperaldosteronism, dexamethasone-suppressible hypertension
Plasma deoxycorticosterone	Increased: congenital adrenal hyperplasia
Urinary steroids	Apparent mineralocorticoid excess Congenital adrenal hyperplasia
Urinary catecholamines, metanephrines, VMA	Pheochromocytoma, neuroblastoma
DMSA scan	Chronic pyelonephritis
Renal Doppler ultrasound	Renal artery stenosis
Captopril renal scan	Renal artery stenosis
Renal arteriography	Renal artery stenosis

DMSA = dimercaptosuccinic acid; VMA = vanillylmandelic acid.

abdominal mass suggests Wilms tumor, neuroblastoma, or a hydronephrotic or cystic kidney. Café-au-lait spots suggest neurofibromatosis, which is associated with an increased incidence of renal artery stenosis and, less commonly, of pheochromocytoma.

BASIC LABORATORY EVALUATION

Laboratory tests used to diagnose the causes of hypertension are divided into two categories in Table 15–38: basic and extended evaluations. The basic tests are those used to detect structural abnormalities or chronic diseases of the kidneys, which are the most common causes of severe hypertension in children and which are often occult. A decreased serum potassium level and an increased serum carbon dioxide level suggest hyperaldosteronism, which may be primary or may be secondary to increased renin-angiotensin levels associated with renal artery stenosis. In the absence of other evidence of renal disease, it is not necessary to perform a renal ultrasound study when evaluating adolescent patients with mild or moderate hypertension and a family history of essential hypertension.

EXTENDED EVALUATION

If the history, physical examination, and basic laboratory evaluation have not revealed the cause of the hypertension and the hypertension is mild, no further testing is indicated, but the child's blood pressure should be checked periodically. If the hypertension is severe or if there is evidence of damage to the heart, as determined by echocardiography, or to the eyes, as determined by examination of the ocular fundi, extended testing should be performed to detect occult renal disease, renal artery stenosis, disorders of adrenal steroidogenesis, or catecholamine-secreting tumors. Chronic pyelonephritis without a history of UTIs is diagnosed by dimercaptosuccinic acid (DMSA) renal scan. The definitive test for renal artery stenosis, which is much more common than either hyperaldosteronism or pheochromocytoma, is renal arteriography. Less invasive screening tests for renal artery stenosis are available, such as plasma renin activity, Doppler imaging of the renal arteries, and the captopril renal scan, but their sensitivity is less than 90% and they cannot reliably exclude the diagnosis of this condition. Primary hyperaldosteronism, which is rare in childhood and may be associated with familial dexamethasone-suppressible hypertension, is diagnosed by elevated plasma aldosterone levels and decreased plasma renin activity. Pheochromocytoma, which is also rare, is diagnosed by elevated levels of catecholamines in a 24-h urine specimen. The interpretation of tests in the extended evaluation can be difficult and often requires consultation with an endocrinologist or a nephrologist.

TREATMENT

In children with mild hypertension, nonpharmacologic intervention is indicated; this includes restriction of dietary salt intake, weight reduction, and an increase in physical exercise. In adult patients with essential hypertension, approximately 50% appear to respond to salt restriction with a lowering of blood pressure. Data also suggest that weight loss is effective in lowering blood pressure in obese patients. In the adolescent population, however, both motivation and compliance with dietary restrictions are poor. Therefore, patient education, along with a dietary regimen of moderate sodium allowance, in contrast to strict salt restriction, increases the likelihood of compliance.

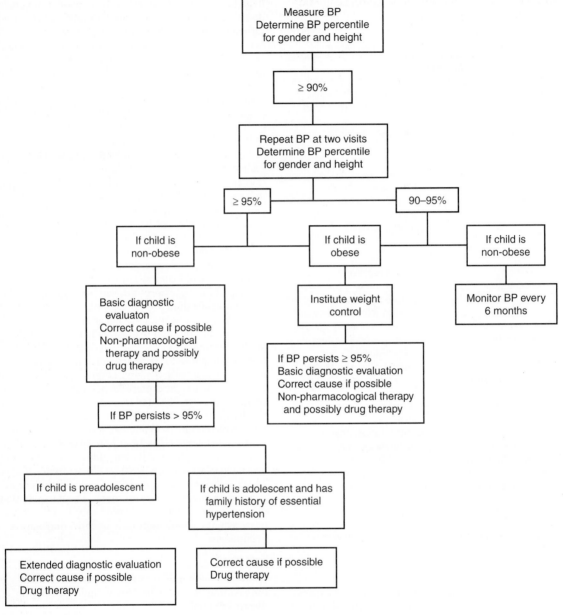

Figure 15–8. Algorithm for the evaluation of children with hypertension.

In children with moderate or severe hypertension, pharmacologic therapy is indicated, especially in patients with evidence of damage to other organs (left ventricular hypertrophy, change in optic fundi, proteinuria). For acute and long-term treatment of hypertension, agents used in children are shown in Tables 15–39 and 15–40, respectively.

Once optimal lowering of blood pressure has been achieved (diastolic blood pressure <90th percentile) with a minimum of side effects, it is recommended that antihypertensive medication be continued for 6 to 12 months. At that time, a trial reduction in the amount of medication can be attempted with close monitoring of the blood pressure.

Table 15–39. Pharmacologic Treatment of Acute Hypertension

Agent	Mechanism of Action	Dose/Route	Onset of Action	Comments/Side Effects
Nifedipine	Calcium channel blocker	0.25–0.5 mg/kg po or sl; may repeat q 10–20 min × 1	10 min	Flushing, headache, nausea, tachycardia, edema
Labetalol	α- and β-adrenergic blocker	0.25–2 mg/kg/h IV	3–5 min	Dizziness, tiredness, nausea
Diazoxide	Direct arteriolar vasodilator	2 mg/kg IV push, may repeat q 5–10 min × 2	3–5 min	Nausea, vomiting, flushing, hyperglycemia
Hydralazine	Direct arteriolar vasodilator	0.2–0.4 mg/kg IV; repeat q 4 h	5–10 min	Tachycardia, palpitations, flushing, headache
Sodium nitroprusside	Arteriolar and venous vasodilator	0.5–6 μg/kg/min by continuous IV infusion	Instantaneous	Monitor serum thiocyanate concentrations in ICU setting

ICU = intensive care unit; IV = intravenous; po = oral; sl = sublingual.

Table 15–40. Pharmacologic Treatment of Chronic Hypertension in Children

Class of Drug	Examples	Dosage, mg/kg/day		Comments/ Doses (h)	Side Effects
		Initial	Interval Between Maximum		
Calcium channel blockers	Amlodipine	0.1	0.3	24	Flushing, nausea, headache, tachycardia, edema
	Nifedipine extended release	30[1]	120[1]	12–24	
β-adrenergic blockers	Propranolol			8–12	Dizziness, tiredness, avoid in asthma
	Atenolol	1	8	24	
		0.5	4		
α- and β-adrenergic blocker	Labetalol			8–12	
		3	20		
Central α-adrenergic agonists	Clonidine			12	Dry mouth, tiredness, rebound hypertension on withdrawal
	Clonidine skin patch	0.003	0.02	One every 7 d	
		No. 1[2]	No. 3[3]		
Vasodilators	Hydralazine			6–8	Tachycardia, palpitations, flushing, headache
	Minoxidil			24	
		0.75			
		0.1	7.5		
			1		
Angiotensin-converting enzyme inhibitors or receptor blockers	Captopril				Cough, hyperkalemia, can lower GFR
	Children			8–12	
	Neonates	1		6–12	
	Enalapril	0.03	6	12	
	Lisinopril	0.1	2	24	
	Losartan	0.1	1	12–24	
		1	1		
Diuretics	Chlorothiazide			12–24	Hypokalemia, hyperuricemia, hyperglycemia (thiazides), hypokalemia, hypercalciuria, ototoxicity (furosemide)
	Hydrochlorothiazide	10	2	12–24	
	Furosemide	0.5	20	12–24	
		1	2		
			4		

GFR = glomerular filtration rate.
[1] Total daily dose in mg.
[2] Delivers 0.1 mg per day.
[3] Delivers 0.3 mg per day.

ACID-BASE DISORDERS

Normal Renal Acidification

In healthy individuals, the kidneys participate in regulating the acid-base composition of extracellular fluid by regulating the plasma concentration of bicarbonate at normal levels. To do this, the kidneys must reabsorb nearly all the bicarbonate filtered at the glomerulus and must excrete acid as titratable acid ($H_2PO_4^-$) and ammonium (NH_4^+). In the proximal tubule, secretion of hydrogen ion (H^+) results in reabsorption of approximately 80 to 90% of the filtered load of bicarbonate at normal plasma bicarbonate concentrations. In the distal nephron, principally the cortical and medullary collecting tubules, secretion of H^+ results in reabsorption of the remaining 10 to 15% of filtered bicarbonate, thereby decreasing the pH of tubular fluid to less than approximately 6.4. As the pH of tubular fluid decreases further to 4.5–5.5, the secreted H^+ titrates further the major urine buffers, HPO_4^{2-} and ammonia (NH_3), to form $H_2PO_4^-$ and NH_4^+. The amount of H^+ excreted as titratable acid and ammonium is referred to as *net acid excretion*. Excretion of net acid results in the generation of new bicarbonate in an amount equal to that lost in buffering the endogenous load of noncarbonic acid generated from diet and metabolism; this amount averages approximately 1 mEq/kg/day in normal adults ingesting typical North American diets and approximately 1 to 3 mEq/kg/day in healthy infants and young children.

Renal Tubular Acidosis

Renal tubular acidosis (RTA) is a clinical syndrome in which the kidneys fail to maintain a normal plasma concentration of bicarbonate in the setting of a normal rate of acid production from diet and metabolism. The syndrome is characterized by metabolic acidosis with hyperchloremia and often an inappropriately high urine pH. When the acidification disorder results in reduced reclamation of filtered bicarbonate by the proximal nephron, the disorder is called *proximal RTA,* or *type 2 RTA.* When the disorder results in reduced excretion of $H_2PO_4^-$ and NH_4^+ (net acid) by the distal nephron, it is called *distal RTA,* or *type 1 RTA;* when the reduction in net acid excretion is accompanied by hyperkalemia, the disorder is called *hyperkalemic RTA,* or *type 4 RTA.* The disordered renal acidification can occur with little or no reduction of renal mass, which distinguishes RTA from the acidosis that accompanies chronic renal insufficiency.

PROXIMAL (TYPE 2) RENAL TUBULAR ACIDOSIS

In patients with proximal RTA, the capacity of the proximal tubule to reabsorb bicarbonate is reduced. Thus, at normal plasma bicarbonate concentrations, substantial bicarbonaturia occurs, net acid excretion ceases, and metabolic acidosis ensues. As the plasma bicarbonate concentration decreases, the amount of bicarbonate that escapes reabsorption by the impaired proximal tubule becomes sufficiently small that it can be completely reabsorbed by the otherwise normal distal nephron. Bicarbonaturia then ceases, urine pH decreases to less than 5.5, and net acid excretion becomes equivalent to acid production. The excessive urinary loss of bicarbonate stimulates secretion of potassium by the distal nephron and results in hypokalemia; the hypokalemia often worsens when sodium bicarbonate is given.

Proximal RTA occurs in a variety of diseases, usually as part of the Fanconi syndrome, a generalized dysfunction of the proximal tubule characterized by impaired reabsorption of bicarbonate, amino acids, phosphate, glucose, low-molecular-weight proteins, and, sometimes, uric acid. The causes of proximal RTA are listed in Table 15–41.

Children with proximal RTA associated with the Fanconi syndrome typically have hypophosphatemia and sometimes mild hypocalcemia and hypomagnesemia; bone age may be retarded, rickets or osteomalacia often occur, and nephrocalcinosis and nephrolithiasis typically are not observed.

CLASSIC DISTAL (TYPE 1) RENAL TUBULAR ACIDOSIS

In patients with classic distal (type 1) RTA, the collecting tubule is unable to lower urine pH appropriately to less than approximately 6.0, which results in incomplete reabsorption of bicarbonate and a reduction in urinary excretion of $H_2PO_4^-$ and NH_4^+; metabolic acidosis thus ensues. The value of the urine anion gap, which reflects the urine NH_4^+ concentration (see later), is zero or positive during acidosis, whereas with normal renal acidification, a negative value is observed during acidosis. Renal reabsorption of glucose, amino acids, and phosphate by the proximal tubule is not impaired. In children with distal RTA, the amount of bicarbonate excreted in the urine can be high as much as 15% of the filtered bicarbonate load; such severe "renal bicarbonate wasting" is more common in infants and young children, particularly in the weeks to months after initiation of alkali therapy when growth velocity has greatly increased. In older children and adult

Table 15–41. Causes of Proximal (Type 2) Renal Tubular Acidosis with Fanconi Syndrome

Primary: sporadic or familial
Familial systemic diseases: cystinosis, Lowe syndrome, hereditary fructose intolerance, galactosemia, Wilson disease
Vitamin D deficiency with low Ca, PO_4 and high parathyroid hormone, malabsorption syndromes
Drugs or toxins: acetazolamide, lead, cadmium
Other: medullary cystic disease, renal transplantation

patients with distal RTA, the magnitude of bicarbonaturia is less, approximately 1 to 3 mEq/kg/day.

Renal wasting of sodium and potassium are characteristic of untreated type 1 RTA; these abnormalities are corrected by alkali therapy in most but not all patients. The urinary excretion of calcium and renal clearance of phosphorus are increased, and urinary excretion of citrate is reduced; these abnormalities contribute to the occurrence of medullary nephrocalcinosis and recurrent nephrolithiasis in these patients. Sustained correction of acidosis tends to reverse these abnormalities, and although nephrocalcinosis and nephrolithiasis persist, stones may be passed less frequently.

Type 1 RTA may occur either alone or in association with a number of acquired or genetically transmitted systemic diseases (Table 15–42). In children, type 1 RTA most commonly occurs alone as either a sporadic or familial disorder. Autosomal dominant and autosomal recessive modes of transmission have been recognized; the latter has been associated with sensorineural hearing loss and nephrocalcinosis.

HYPERKALEMIC (TYPE 4) RENAL TUBULAR ACIDOSIS

In patients with hyperkalemic (type 4) RTA, most commonly those with chronic tubulointerstitial renal disease and moderate reduction in GFR, metabolic acidosis is associated with hyperkalemia and decreased renal clearance of potassium, and the severity of the acidosis and hyperkalemia is disproportionately great for the degree of renal insufficiency. Urine pH can decrease to less than 5.5 during acidosis, yet urinary excretion of NH_4^+ and, hence, of net acid are low. This reflects a suppression of renal ammonia production by the hyperkalemia in these patients. Proximal tubule function is not impaired.

The physiologic characteristics of type 4 RTA are those predicted to result from aldosterone deficiency or impairment in its renal effect. In the normal distal nephron, aldosterone is a major determinant of the secretion of both hydrogen ion and potassium; the resulting maintenance of a normal plasma potassium concentration enhances ammonia production and thus net acid excretion.

Clinical variants. Type 4 RTA occurs in a wide variety of clinical disorders, either with or without associated renal parenchymal disease (Table 15–43). The most common cause is tubulointerstitial renal disease, in which deficiency of aldosterone is caused by a deficiency of renin, so-called hyporeninemic hypoaldosteronism. Type 4 RTA and aldosterone deficiency also can occur in clinical conditions without renal parenchymal injury, as in infants with the salt-wasting form of congenital adrenal hyperplasia, 21-hydroxylase deficiency, or in patients with bilateral adrenal insufficiency. In some patients with type 4 RTA, there is evidence for renal resistance to aldosterone. In infants with congenital pseudohypoaldosteronism, failure to thrive, dehydration, hyponatremia, hyperkalemia, and hyperchloremic acidosis occur; plasma renin activity and urine and plasma aldosterone levels are greatly increased; and glucocorticoid hormone levels are normal.

DIAGNOSIS OF RENAL TUBULAR ACIDOSIS

Clinical features. Untreated children with RTA often have nonspecific symptoms, such as failure to thrive, polydipsia and polyuria, constipation, anorexia, vomiting, and listlessness. The presence of certain signs and symptoms suggest a particular type of RTA. Rickets and osteomalacia, often in association with hypophosphatemia and mild hypocalcemia, may be a prominent presenting feature in patients with Fanconi syndrome. Nephrocalcinosis is common in patients with type 1 RTA, but not in those with type 2 or type 4 RTA. Muscle weakness may be a prominent feature in patients with untreated hypokalemia who have either type 1 RTA or Fanconi syndrome.

Laboratory evaluation. The metabolic acidosis of patients with RTA is associated with hyperchloremia and thus with a normal plasma anion gap, calculated as serum concentrations of $[Na^+ - (Cl^- + HCO_3^-)]$ (normal range, 8 to 16 mEq/L). Other disorders that can cause metabolic acidosis with a normal anion gap are listed in

Table 15–42. Causes of Distal (Type 1) Renal Tubular Acidosis

Primary: sporadic or familial
Systemic diseases: sickle cell anemia, osteopetrosis
Autoimmune: Sjögren syndrome, chronic active hepatitis
Disorders causing nephrocalcinosis: hypercalciuria, primary hyperparathyroidism, vitamin D intoxication
Drugs or toxins: amphotericin B, lithium, analgesics
Other: pyelonephritis, obstructive uropathy, renal transplantation

Table 15–43. Clinical Spectrum of Hyperkalemic (Type 4) Renal Tubular Acidosis

Aldosterone deficiency
  Primary: Congenital adrenal hyperplasia, Addison disease
  Secondary: Tubulointerstitial renal disease with hyporeninemia, diabetes mellitus, obstructive uropathy, analgesic nephropathy

Aldosterone resistance
  Pseudohypoaldosteronism
  Tubulointerstitial renal disease
  Drugs: Spironolactone, amiloride

Uncertain pathogenesis   Chronic pyelonephritis, lupus nephritis, renal transplantation

Table 15–44. Differential Diagnosis
of Metabolic Acidosis

Normal Anion Gap	Increased Anion Gap
Gastrointestinal loss of HCO_3	Ketoacidosis
Diarrhea	Lactic acidosis
Small bowel or pancreatic	Uremic acidosis
drainage	Toxins
Ureterosigmoidostomy	Salicylate
Renal loss of HCO_3	Ethylene glycol
Renal tubular acidosis	Methanol
Diamox	Paraldehyde
Dilutional acidosis	Inborn errors of
Administration of NH_4Cl,	metabolism
arginine HCl	
Postrespiratory alkalosis	

Table 15–44. When metabolic acidosis is associated with the retention in plasma of the anions of endogenously produced or exogenously administered (nonchloride-containing) acids, the plasma anion gap is increased (Table 15–44).

To evaluate acid-base status, one should obtain an arterial or arterialized venous blood sample for measurement of blood pH, partial pressure of carbon dioxide (PCO_2), and total carbon dioxide concentration and, nearly simultaneously, a urine sample for measurement of pH and urine anion gap (see later). In healthy infants and young children, the normal values for blood PCO_2 and plasma bicarbonate and total carbon dioxide concentrations are lower than for those in healthy adults; the values increase with age. For measurement of urine pH, the sample should be taken promptly using a syringe to prevent loss of carbon dioxide, which can cause the pH to increase; pH should be measured using a pH meter.

Assessment of urine acidification. Urine pH reflects only the concentration of free H^+ in urine, which accounts for less than 1% of the total amount of H^+ excreted. Thus, urine pH by itself may not adequately reflect urine net acid excretion during acidosis. In normal individuals, the kidneys respond to chronic acidosis by substantially increasing the urinary excretion of ammonium. Because urinary NH_4^+ is not measured routinely in hospital laboratories, it is proposed that the urinary NH_4^+ concentration can be indirectly estimated by the urine anion gap, calculated as urine concentrations of $[Na^+] + [K^+] - [Cl^-]$. In nonacidotic healthy individuals, the urine anion gap is positive, approximately 30 to 35 mEq/L, and it becomes progressively more negative as the rate of NH_4^+ excretion increases during acidosis. In acidotic patients with type 1 or type 4 RTA, the anion gap remains inappropriately positive, consis-

tent with their failure to increase NH_4^+ excretion. In patients with proximal RTA, the urine anion gap would be predicted to be zero or positive, although negative values have been observed in children with proximal RTA. Thus, the diagnosis of RTA should be strongly considered in patients with persisting hyperchloremic metabolic acidosis in whom extrarenal causes of the acidosis have been excluded and in whom the urine anion gap is zero or positive; the urine pH typically is inappropriately high (>6). When the urine anion gap is negative, it can be inferred that the kidney is responding appropriately to the acidosis; thus, a nonrenal cause for the acidosis is more likely.

In patients with probable RTA and moderate metabolic acidosis (plasma total carbon dioxide concentration of approximately 18 mEq/L), and in whom urine pH is approximately 6.0 or greater, it is recommended that oral ammonium chloride be given to increase the severity of the acidosis in order to distinguish classic distal RTA from proximal or type 4 RTA. Before doing so, any existing ECF volume contraction or hypokalemia should be corrected. If with ammonium chloride, urine pH decreases to less than 5.5, the diagnosis of distal (type 1) RTA can be ruled out; if it does not, the diagnosis of type 1 RTA is likely. In patients with proximal RTA associated with Fanconi syndrome, the fractional renal clearance of phosphate, amino acids, glucose, and potassium are increased, and hypophosphatemia and hypokalemia typically occur.

The finding of hyperchloremic acidosis with hyperkalemia suggests type 4 RTA; urine pH may or may not be appropriately acidic (i.e., <5.5) during spontaneous acidosis; it should decrease to <5.5 after administration of ammonium chloride. The GFR may be mildly to moderately reduced. Evaluation of the status of renin-aldosterone activity helps to distinguish aldosterone deficiency from aldosterone-resistant states.

TREATMENT AND PROGNOSIS

Distal (Type 1) renal tubular acidosis. In some acidotic patients with type 1 RTA, hypokalemia can be severe enough to cause respiratory depression or muscle paralysis; if so, it should be corrected with intravenously administered potassium before or during correction of acidosis. In infants and children, sustained correction of acidosis can be achieved by oral administration of sodium bicarbonate or sodium citrate, 3 to 12 mEq/kg/d in 3 to 4 divided doses, until the plasma bicarbonate concentration becomes normal. In adult patients, 1 to 2 mEq/kg/d of alkali is usually sufficient. In patients who require potassium supplements to sustain normokalemia, if so, 20 to 50% of the alkali requirement can be given as potassium bicarbonate or potassium citrate. Sustained correction of acidosis in infants is associated with an increase in growth velocity; within 3 to 6 months, normal stature can be attained and maintained. Older children may require several years to attain normal height. With correction of acidosis, urinary calcium and phosphorus excretion decreases, and citrate excretion increases; nephrocalcinosis can be prevented by alkali therapy.

Proximal (Type 2) renal tubular acidosis. Correction of acidosis in patients with type 2 RTA requires administration of alkali in amounts ranging from 3 to 20 mEq/kg/d; alkali requirements must be determined empirically for each patient. In patients with type 2 RTA and Fanconi syndrome, correction of hypokalemia should be achieved by giving a substantial fraction, often 50% or more, of the alkali requirement as potassium bicarbonate or potassium citrate. In rare patients with isolated type 2 RTA, acidosis can be corrected by giving sodium bicarbonate alone. Supplemental oral phosphorus and sometimes magnesium and vitamin D may be required. When type 2 RTA is associated with Fanconi syndrome, treatment is directed where possible toward removal of those substances crucial to its causation, as in the case of hereditary fructose intolerance, galactosemia, Wilson disease, and tyrosinemia.

Hyperkalemic (Type 4) renal tubular acidosis. In patients with type 4 RTA who have tubulointerstitial renal disease and reduced GFR, administration of mineralocorticoid in either physiologic replacement doses (fludrocortisone, 0.10 to 0.15 mg/d) or superphysiologic amounts can increase net acid excretion and substantially ameliorate metabolic acidosis and hyperkalemia. Mineralocorticoid should be used cautiously, however, as it may exacerbate hypertension or increase the ECF volume in some patients. Restriction of dietary potassium, administration of furosemide, or administration of sodium bicarbonate, 1 to 2 mEq/kg/d, has also been shown to ameliorate acidosis and hyperkalemia. When type 4 RTA is due to deficiency of aldosterone, physiologic doses of mineralocorticoid should be administered; in patients with pseudohypoaldosteronism, administration of supplemental sodium chloride often suffices.

URINARY TRACT ANOMALIES

The overall incidence of structural genitourinary anomalies in the general population is approximately 4%, on the basis of autopsy studies. Many urinary tract anomalies are not symptomatic and remain undetected or are discovered accidentally. Most children with clinically significant urinary tract anomalies come to medical attention in one of the following ways: (1) an abnormal finding on a prenatal ultrasound, (2) detection of an abdominal or flank mass in the newborn period, (3) appearance of Potter syndrome at birth, (4) diagnosis of UTI, (5) detection of hypertension, or (6) development of renal insufficiency or failure. The most common, clinically significant anomalies of the urinary tract are listed in Table 15–45.

Table 15–45. Significant Congenital Anomalies of the Urinary Tract

Renal	Bladder
Agenesis	Vesicoureteral reflux
Hypoplasia	Ectopic ureterocele
Dysplasia	
Polycystic kidney disease	Urethral
	Posterior urethral
Ureteral	valves
Ureteropelvic junction	
obstruction	
Prune-belly syndrome	

Clinical Presentations of Urinary Tract Anomalies

This section discusses the clinical presentation of common urinary tract anomalies and the appropriate diagnostic evaluation and differential diagnoses for each.

ABNORMAL PRENATAL ULTRASOUND

Fetal ultrasonography has become a routine part of prenatal care and can identify urinary tract anomalies as early as 15 weeks postconception. The incidence of congenital urologic anomalies as detected by prenatal ultrasound ranges between 0.2 and 1.5%. Ultrasound examination of the fetal kidneys can determine their number, location, and size. The renal pelvis and calyces become discernible when they are dilated, and renal cysts are detectable as echolucent areas within the renal parenchyma.

Hydronephrosis, or dilatation of the renal pelvis and calyces, is the most common urinary tract abnormality found on prenatal ultrasound examination; it may be unilateral or bilateral. Of the causes of hydronephrosis listed in Table 15–46, the most common is obstruction of the ureteropelvic junction (UPJ). The obstruction usually is unilateral and incomplete; therefore, fetal urine output is adequate and oligohydramnios does not occur. Severe UPJ

Table 15–46. Abnormal Fetal Renal Ultrasound Findings and Their Causes

Hydronephrosis
Ureteropelvic junction obstruction
Posterior urethral valves
Duplex ureter with ureterocele
Transient, idiopathic
Renal cysts
Multicystic dysplasia
Dysplasia with cysts
Polycystic kidney disease

obstruction may lead to cystic changes within the affected kidneys, which are detectable on prenatal ultrasound. Postnatally, the diagnosis of UPJ obstruction is confirmed by a diuretic-augmented renal scan and/or an intravenous pyelogram.

Renal cysts detected prenatally, as with hydronephrosis, may be associated with many diseases, the most common of which are listed in Table 15–46. When cysts are large, they may be difficult to distinguish from severe hydronephrosis on prenatal ultrasound examination, whereas postnatal ultrasound examination, with its improved resolution, and radionuclide renal scans usually can distinguish between these two entities.

Oligohydramnios, which is a decrease in the volume of amniotic fluid, is a worrisome prenatal ultrasound finding. Because urine is the primary component of amniotic fluid, oligohydramnios often results from either renal dysfunction with decreased urine production or urinary tract obstruction. Renal dysfunction may be due to bilateral renal agenesis, bilateral multicystic dysplasia, or polycystic kidney disease. Obstructive causes of oligohydramnios are posterior urethral valves and bilateral obstruction of the ureteropelvic or ureterovesical junctions. In the past few years, attempts have been made to bypass the obstruction surgically in utero in an effort to relieve back-pressure on the developing kidneys and improve amniotic fluid volume, with varying success. Most patients with urinary tract anomalies detected by prenatal ultrasound, however, do not have oligohydramnios. Such patients usually are asymptomatic at birth and can safely undergo further diagnostic evaluation later in the newborn period.

POTTER SYNDROME

At birth, children with nonfunctioning or severely obstructed kidneys often have the classic signs and symptoms of Potter syndrome. Oligohydramnios, resulting from decreased urine output, causes compression of the fetus by the uterine walls and results in limb deformities and abnormal facial features termed *Potter facies* (epicanthal folds, low-set ears, flattened nose, and receding chin). Because amniotic fluid volume plays an important role in normal lung development, oligohydramnios also is associated with hypoplasia of the lungs. Pulmonary hypoplasia and respiratory failure are responsible for most of the deaths in newborns with renal failure and oligohydramnios.

The leading causes of Potter syndrome are bilateral renal agenesis; bilateral cystic, malformed kidneys (multicystic dysplasia); and bilateral obstructed kidneys. In evaluating newborn infants with this syndrome, one should first perform a renal ultrasound examination. Important features to note are the size of the kidneys and the presence of renal cysts, hydronephrosis, hydroureter, the size of the bladder, and the thickness of the bladder wall. With this information, the level of the obstruction, if present, usually can be localized. Evidence of obstruction necessitates urgent urologic consultation, and, if urethral obstruction is present, a bladder catheter should be placed. Renal function should be assessed immediately and repeatedly over time.

ABDOMINAL MASS

More than 50% of palpable abdominal masses in newborn infants are renal in origin. The vast majority of these are hydronephrotic or multicystic dysplastic kidneys. Noncongenital causes, such as renal vein thrombosis and tumors, account for fewer than 7% of renal masses.

Infants with a palpable abdominal mass should undergo renal ultrasound examination as soon as possible. When hydronephrosis is severe, the renal pelvis and calyces may be massively dilated and surrounded by only a thin rim of renal parenchyma. Patients with multicystic dysplasia have detectable cysts within the renal parenchyma; the cysts may be so large as to be indistinguishable from the dilated renal pelvis of a hydronephrotic kidney. A renal scan (DMSA) can be used to distinguish between these two entities. In multicystic dysplasia, the kidney is nonfunctional and will demonstrate no uptake of radioactive tracer, whereas in hydronephrosis, uptake of tracer will be visible in the rim of renal parenchyma surrounding the dilated pelvis.

The diagnosis of hydronephrosis, either unilateral or bilateral, should prompt a search for an obstructive malformation. The site of obstruction usually can be determined from the ultrasound study on the basis of the location of the dilatation and the size and appearance of the bladder. Obstruction of the UPJ most commonly causes unilateral hydronephrosis without dilatation of the ipsilateral ureter. Obstruction of the ureterovesical junction, either unilateral or bilateral, causes hydroureteronephrosis of the affected sides. Bladder outlet obstruction, as in male infants with posterior urethral valves, usually results in bilateral hydronephrosis with dilatation of both ureters and thickening of the bladder wall.

URINARY TRACT INFECTION

Both during and after the newborn period, infants with significant urinary tract anomalies often present with a urinary tract infection (UTI). The flow of urine is abnormal within cysts. Dilated, obstructed collecting systems or refluxing, incompletely emptying systems, predisposes patients to infection. Children with a documented UTI should undergo a renal ultrasound examination and a voiding cystourethrogram (VCUG) to determine whether anomalies, obstruction, or reflux are present. Boys should be evaluated after their first UTI, regardless of age, because UTIs in boys are highly associated with urinary tract anomalies. Urinary tract infections are more common in girls, particularly those aged 7 to 10 years, and less frequently associated with anomalies. Thus, it is recommended that girls older than 8 years with uncomplicated cystitis be evaluated radiographically after their second UTI, and girls younger than 8 years after their first infection. All children, regardless of age, with pyelonephritis or with cystitis caused by an unusual organism should undergo prompt evaluation with renal ultrasound; the VCUG should be performed when signs of the infection have resolved. Prophylactic antibiotics should be administered after completion of the therapeutic course until it is determined that vesicoureteral reflux (VUR) is not present.

HYPERTENSION

Although acquired renal disease accounts for most cases of hypertension in children (see earlier section, "Hypertension"), congenital urinary tract anomalies and their complications are responsible for a significant number. The most common congenital anomalies that cause hypertension are unilateral renal agenesis, VUR with kidney scarring, polycystic kidney disease, and multicystic dysplasia. The evaluation of renal causes of hypertension is discussed elsewhere.

CHRONIC RENAL INSUFFICIENCY

Unfortunately for many children, congenital anomalies may remain undetected until renal insufficiency becomes severe and symptoms of uremia develop. Congenital anomalies that can progress to end-stage renal failure include hypoplasia, dysplasia, polycystic kidney disease, VUR complicated by infection, and obstructive uropathies.

Specific Congenital Urinary Tract Anomalies

This section discusses in more detail the various congenital anomalies listed in Table 15–45. Normal development of the kidney requires the presence and interaction of two embryologic structures—the ureteric bud and the metanephrogenic blastema. Each structure exerts a developmental influence on the other. The ureteric bud ultimately becomes the trigone of the bladder, the ureter, the renal calyces and pelvis, and the collecting ducts, whereas the metanephros gives rise to the epithelial cells of the glomeruli, the proximal and distal tubules, and the loops of Henle. Absence of either of these embryologic structures or their failure to achieve the necessary contact with one another results in malformations of the kidney and/or the urinary tract.

RENAL ANOMALIES

Agenesis is defined as the failure of formation of the kidney; it may be unilateral or bilateral. Bilateral agenesis is incompatible with long-term extrauterine life, whereas unilateral agenesis is asymptomatic if the contralateral kidney is normal. This malformation arises when the ureteric bud, because of either its absence or malposition, fails to induce the metanephros.

The term *hypoplastic* designates a small kidney owing to a reduced number of otherwise normal nephrons; the remainder of the urinary tract is normal. When the ureteric bud has an abnormal origin, it contacts only a portion of the metanephros, and thus fewer nephrons develop; those present then become hypertrophied. Hypoplasia is clinically significant when both kidneys are affected. Patients with bilateral hypoplasia have polydipsia and polyuria during infancy, and inevitable progression to end-stage renal failure occurs by late childhood.

Dysplastic kidneys lack normally developed nephron structures. Strong evidence suggests that the abnormal development results from urinary tract obstruction in utero. More than 90% of dysplastic kidneys are associated with obstruction of the lower urinary tract, most commonly at the ureteropelvic junction, the posterior urethra, or the distal ureter due to an obstructing ureterocele. Dysplastic kidneys are characterized histologically by the presence of primitive ducts, metaplastic cartilage, and immature glomeruli. The extent of renal functional impairment reflects the degree of morphologic abnormalities and depends largely on the severity of the obstruction. The gross appearance of these kidneys is potentially quite varied and may be solid, cystic, small, large, reniform, or misshapen.

The most severe form of dysplasia, which results from atresia of the ipsilateral ureter, is termed *multicystic dysplasia*. These kidneys are large, contain macroscopic cysts, and usually are detected by prenatal ultrasound or as abdominal masses in the early newborn period. Approximately 30% of children with unilateral multicystic dysplastic kidneys have structural abnormalities of the contralateral kidney.

Polycystic kidney disease occurs as either an autosomal recessive (ARPKD) or an autosomal dominant (ADPKD) disease. The autosomal recessive form has previously been called *infantile polycystic kidney disease* because it commonly presents in the first year after birth. Babies presenting with ARPKD have extremely large kidneys with innumerable small (1- to 8-mm diameter) cysts of the collecting ducts. Many such infants tend to be critically ill owing to pulmonary hypoplasia, and most die within a few days of birth. Those with fewer cysts and, therefore, more functioning renal parenchyma present at a later age and have a better prognosis for survival, although many eventually progress to end-stage renal failure and require dialysis and transplantation. The outcome of patients with ARPKD is complicated by the associated liver disease characterized by periportal fibrosis and biliary duct dilatation. By contrast, ADPKD usually but not always remains asymptomatic until the fifth or sixth decade of life.

URETERAL ANOMALIES

Obstruction of the UPJ is the most common site of urinary tract obstruction in children. The obstruction may be caused by a segment of the ureter that lacks peristaltic activity, by muscular bands, or by aberrant vessels that cause external compression of the UPJ; unilateral cases predominate (75% of total). Complete UPJ obstruction is associated with severe renal dysplasia. Lesser degrees of obstruction result in hydronephrosis with a consequent increased risk of UTI and its sequelae. Treatment requires surgical removal of the obstructed segment and reanastomosis of the normal ends (pyeloplasty). The amount of function of the involved kidney should be determined by a renal radionucleotide scan before surgery, as an obstructed kidney with little or no function should probably be removed rather than repaired.

The *prune-belly syndrome* (Eagle-Barrett syndrome) consists of the triad of absent abdominal wall musculature, urinary tract anomalies, and cryptorchidism. The urologic anomalies range from mild, asymptomatic dilatation of the urinary tract to severe hydroureteronephrosis with renal dysplasia and renal failure; the dilatation almost always exists in the absence of obstruction. The diagnosis usually can be made at birth on the basis of the appearance of the abdominal wall. Evaluation of these children should include imaging of the urinary tract and assessment of renal function.

During normal micturition, contraction of the bladder wall musculature compresses the distal ends of the ureters, thereby preventing the passage of urine from the bladder into the ureters. Congenital *VUR* results from inadequate tunneling of the distal ureter through the bladder wall, due to either malposition or maldevelopment of the ureteric bud. Reflux can also develop in patients with obstruction of the bladder outlet in whom high intravesical pressures are generated by contraction of the bladder wall, as occurs with a neurogenic bladder and posterior urethral valves. Vesicoureteral reflux may range from mild to severe, as judged by the extent of reflux seen on a routine VCUG; the severity is routinely graded from 1 to 5 according to the system of the International Reflux Study Committee (Figure 15–9).

Reflux results in incomplete emptying of the bladder during voiding, which predisposes patients to infection. Furthermore, with more severe grades of reflux, urine may enter the renal collecting tubules under high pressure. Reflux of infected urine into the kidney is known to cause renal scarring; the evidence is compelling but still inconclusive as to whether reflux of sterile urine causes renal injury. In children with mild forms of reflux (grades 1 to 3) who have normal renal function and little or no renal scarring, it is recommended that prophylactic antibiotics be administered to prevent acute infection and prevent renal injury from occurring or progressing. The milder degrees of VUR tend to resolve as children age. Breakthrough infections due to noncompliance or the development of resistant organisms are common. In children with severe reflux (grades 4 and 5) or those with lesser

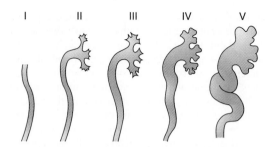

Figure 15–9. Grades of vesicoureteral reflux (International Classification): **I:** involving the ureter only; **II:** involving the ureter, pelvis, and calyces without dilatation; **III:** same level as II but with mild to moderate dilatation of ureter and pelvis; **IV:** same as III but with blunting of calyceal fornices and increased dilatation; **V:** increased dilatation and tortuosity of ureter and papillary impressions in calyces lost.

grades of reflux but decreased renal function, surgical correction of reflux is often necessary because the likelihood of spontaneous resolution of VUR is low. Surgical correction of reflux has not been shown to be superior to medical therapy in preventing progressive renal injury.

Complete *duplication* of the ureter occurs when two separate ureters each drain a different pole of a single kidney, and each ureter empties into the bladder. The ureter draining the lower pole frequently is malpositioned and consequently refluxes; the ureter draining the upper pole also is malpositioned and may be obstructed by a ureterocele, which is a cystic dilation of the distal end of the ureter, leading to hydronephrosis or dysplasia of the upper pole. Evaluation of a duplex system requires a renal ultrasound or intravenous pyelogram and a VCUG. The obstruction caused by a ureterocele is treated surgically.

URETHRAL ANOMALIES

Posterior urethral valves, which occur only in boys, obstruct the outflow of urine from the bladder. The obstructing tissue appears as a diaphragm with a slitlike orifice that is obliquely placed within the prostatic or posterior urethra; the embryologic defect responsible for urethral valves is unknown. Severe obstruction can cause dysplasia of both kidneys in utero, and the diagnosis is made in such severely affected children either prenatally or shortly after birth. Children with milder obstruction often are noticed to strain to urinate, to have a weak urinary stream, or to have frequent urinary tract infections.

The diagnosis of posterior urethral valves is made with a VCUG, which demonstrates that the posterior urethra is elongated and dilated from the bladder neck to the level of the valves, or by direct visualization under urethroscopy. The bladder wall is invariably thickened secondary to muscular hypertrophy. Half these bladders have trabeculations or diverticula, and approximately 60% of patients with urethral valves have secondary VUR.

Achievement of adequate urine drainage, either through a bladder catheter or vesicostomy, should be the immediate goal. Definitive therapy requires surgical ablation of the valves, which can be performed transurethrally with an endoscope, and reimplantation of the ureters.

RENAL INSUFFICIENCY

Acute Renal Failure

Acute renal failure (ARF) is a clinical syndrome characterized by a sudden decrease in renal function sufficient to cause retention of metabolic wastes. It is reflected by an increase in the serum concentrations of urea nitrogen and creatinine. When ARF is due to hypovolemia or shock, oliguria usually occurs; when it is due to toxic or inflammatory injury to the kidney, urine output may be decreased or may be normal (nonoliguric ARF). Acute renal failure that is caused by ischemic or toxic injury to the nephron is often referred to as *acute tubular necrosis (ATN)*.

Common causes of ARF in children are listed in Table 15–47. Acute renal failure can occur when there is inadequate perfusion of the kidneys, as with severe dehydration, hemorrhage, or shock (prerenal causes). If the circulating blood volume is promptly restored in such cases, oliguria and azotemia often can be quickly reversed. If hypoperfusion of the kidneys is prolonged, however, renal failure persists despite restoration of renal perfusion. Intrinsic renal causes of ARF are nephrotoxic or inflammatory injury or renovascular disorders, and the postrenal causes are obstructive lesions of the urinary tract. In newborn infants, the acute onset of renal failure can be due to ischemic or toxic injury to the kidney but also can be due to congenital renal abnormalities, such as multicystic dysplasia of the kidneys, bilateral renal agenesis, polycystic kidney disease, or obstructive lesions such as posterior urethral valves.

HISTORY

The history provides clues as to the underlying cause of ARF. A prerenal cause is suggested by a history of severe vomiting and diarrhea, hemorrhage, shock due to cardiac arrest, sepsis, or anaphylaxis. It also is suggested by hypovolemia due to severe nephrotic syndrome, diabetic ketoacidosis, or burns. Patients with renal concentrating defects, such as those with preexisting chronic renal insufficiency, polycystic kidney disease, or diabetes insipidus, are more susceptible to prerenal ARF.

An intrinsic renal cause of ARF is suggested by a history of exposure to nephrotoxins, such as aminoglycoside antibiotics, amphotericin B, radiocontrast agents, or drugs that can cause tubulointerstitial nephritis, such as the penicillins or nonsteroidal anti-inflammatory agents. The last group of drugs also can reduce renal blood flow in patients with cardiac dysfunction. A history of gross hematuria suggests acute glomerulonephritis; a history of bloody diarrhea, oliguria, and pallor suggests hemolytic uremic syndrome, which is discussed in detail later.

Table 15–47. Causes of Acute Renal Failure in Children

Prerenal	Intrinsic Renal	Postrenal
Hypovolemia	Nephrotoxins	Ureteral obstruction
Severe dehydration	Aminoglycosides, cephalosporins, amphotericin B	Calculi, clot, tumor
Hemorrhage	Radiocontrast agents	Ureteropelvic junction
Burns	Heavy metals	Ureterovesical junction
Diabetic ketoacidosis	Organic solvents, pesticides	Urethral obstruction
Hypotension/hypoperfusion	Myoglobin (crush syndrome)	Diverticulum, stricture
Shock (cardiogenic, septic, anaphylactic)	Parenchymal disorders	Ureterocele
Cardiac surgery	Acute glomerulonephritis	Hydrocolpos
Severe nephrotic syndrome, hepatic cirrhosis	Hemolytic uremic syndrome	Tumor
Hepatorenal syndrome	Systemic vasculitis (Henoch-Schönlein purpura, systemic lupus erythematosus, polyarteritis, Wegener granulomatosis)	
	Acute interstitial nephritis (bacterial, allergic)	
	Tubular obstruction (tumor lysis syndrome, uric acid, oxalic acid)	
	Acute tubular necrosis (prolonged ischemia)	
	Vascular disorders	
	Renal artery thrombosis or embolism	
	Renal vein thrombosis	
	Indomethacin (↓ renal blood flow)	

Obstructive disorders are suggested by a history of abdominal or flank pain, dysuria or UTI, poor urinary stream, passage of renal stones, prior administration of cancer chemotherapeutic agents, renal tubular acidosis, or instrumentation of the urinary tract.

PHYSICAL EXAMINATION

The physical examination may reflect the underlying cause of ARF and should focus initially on assessing the patient's state of hydration. Hypovolemia is revealed by sunken eyes, decreased skin turgor, tachycardia, and orthostatic hypotension; intravascular volume overload is revealed by periorbital or pedal edema, hypertension, or signs of congestive heart failure. A palpable flank mass or enlarged kidneys suggest hydronephrosis, polycystic kidney disease, or renal vein thrombosis; a palpable bladder suggests urethral obstruction.

LABORATORY EVALUATION

The following measurements are essential for evaluation of patients with ARF: complete blood cell count and determination of serum concentrations of sodium, potassium, chloride, total carbon dioxide content, urea nitrogen, creatinine, calcium, phosphorus, total protein, and albumin. Urine should be obtained for urinalysis and culture; evaluation of the urinary sediment can be particularly helpful (Table 15–48). The urine osmolality and concentrations of sodium and creatinine should also be measured; it is important that this be done before a diuretic agent is administered. In patients in whom acute glomerulonephritis is suspected, one should measure the ASO and anti-DNAse B titers, as well as serum complement and ANA levels (see earlier section, "Glomerulonephritis").

Oliguria is defined as a urine volume of <0.8 mL per 100 kcal/h in children, <1.0 mL/kg/h in infants, and <400 mL/d in adolescents and adults. In patients with oliguria, the chemical composition of the urine is a valuable aid in distinguishing prerenal azotemia from established intrinsic renal failure (Table 15–49); the former is potentially reversible if the patient's intravascular volume is restored promptly. In virtually all patients with unexplained ARF, one should perform a renal ultrasound study to rule out urinary tract obstruction. A chest radiograph and electrocardiogram (ECG) should be performed when volume overload and hyperkalemia, respectively, are present.

TREATMENT

The objectives of the initial management of patients with ARF are the assessment of intravascular volume status, treatment of life-threatening complications, and diagnosis of acute urinary tract obstruction. Diagnostic evaluation of the underlying cause of ARF should begin after initial stabilization of patients.

Initial measures. For patients with oliguria and signs of intravascular volume depletion, isotonic fluid (0.9% sodium chloride, Ringer lactate, or colloid), 10 to 40 mL/kg over 15 to 30 min, or blood, 10 mL/kg, should be given intravenously until skin turgor, pulse, blood pressure, and central venous pressure (if available) are normal. If the urine output increases and renal function improves, then prerenal azotemia is likely. If oliguria persists, furosemide, 1 to 2 mg/kg intravenously, or mannitol, 0.5 to 1 g/kg intravenously over 15 to 30 min, should be administered. If oliguria still persists, then established ARF is likely, and the patient's fluid intake should be restricted to insensible water loss, estimated at 35 mL per 100 kcal/d, plus other losses. If urine output increases with administration of diuretics (a positive response is urine output of 5 to 10 mL/kg over 1 to 3 h), ARF may be nonoliguric, and efforts to maintain a diuresis should be continued. Patients with ARF due to intrarenal obstruction by uric acid crystals (tumor lysis syndrome) may benefit from a sustained diuresis induced by mannitol, achieved by infusing a solution of 3% mannitol in 0.25% saline at a rate equal to that of urine output.

Specific treatments. Acute life-threatening complications of ARF that require immediate treatment are severe intravascular volume overload with congestive heart failure and pulmonary edema, severe hypertension, and severe hyperkalemia. Patients with severe intravascular volume overload require urgent dialysis. The treatment of severe hypertension is discussed later (see "Evaluation of Hypertensive Children"). Treatment of ARF includes the following:

Table 15–48. Urinary Sediment in Acute Renal Failure

No or scant abnormalities
   Prerenal or postrenal azotemia
   Hepatorenal syndrome

Red blood cells and casts
   Acute glomerulonephritis
   Hemolytic uremic syndrome
   Systemic vasculitis

White blood cells
   Pyelonephritis
   Interstitial nephritis (eosinophils)

Tubular epithelial cells casts, coarse granular casts, mild proteinuria, few red blood cells and white blood cells
   Acute tubular necrosis

Crystalluria
   Uric acid: tumor lysis syndrome
   Calcium oxalate: nephrolithiasis

Table 15–49. Laboratory Findings in Acute Renal Failure

Test	Prerenal	Intrinsic Renal	Postrenal
Ultrasound	Normal	Normal/increased size or echogenicity	Dilated pelvis, ureter, bladder
Urine osmolality (mOsm/kg)	>500	<350	Urinary indices not helpful
Urine/plasma creatinine	>14:1	<14:1	
Urine sodium (mEq/L)	<20	>30	
Fractional excretion of sodium (%)[1]	<1 >2.5 in neonates	>2 >2.5 in neonates	
Urinary sediment	Minimal findings Few granular casts	Trace to 2 + protein Few white blood cells, red blood cells Brown granular casts Tubular epithelial cells	Unremarkable; white blood cells with infection

[1] Fractional excretion of sodium (%) = $\dfrac{U_{Na}(mEq/L)}{U_{Creat}(mEq/L)} \times \dfrac{S_{Creat}(mg/dL)}{S_{Na}(mg/dL)} \times 100$

Energy and protein intake. To minimize catabolism of body protein which exacerbates azotemia, energy intake of 70 to 100 kcal/kg/d combined with protein intake of 0.7 to 1 g/kg/d should be provided, either orally or parenterally.

Electrolytes. Sodium and potassium should be restricted in patients with oliguria. In nonoliguric patients, urinary electrolyte and water losses should be replaced as necessary to maintain normal intravascular volume and serum electrolyte concentrations. Hyponatremia occurring during the oliguric phase of ARF is due to excessive administration of free water; in such cases, water intake should be reduced further, rather than administering additional sodium.

Hyperkalemia. Hyperkalemia is common and is due to release of potassium from cells as a result of catabolism, hemolysis, acidosis, and transfusion of blood products. If the serum potassium concentration is greater than 6.0 mEq/L and the ECG pattern is normal or reveals peaked T waves, sodium polystyrene sulfonate (Kayexalate) should be given to reduce the serum potassium concentration over a period of several hours and repeated as necessary. If more severe ECG changes are present or the potassium concentration is greater than 7.5 mEq/L, urgent additional therapy is required, as outlined in Table 15–13. If hyperkalemia persists or worsens despite these measures, acute dialysis is indicated.

Hypocalcemia. Treatment is indicated when tetany, either overt or latent, is present. Latent tetany may be demonstrated by eliciting the Chvostek sign (twitching of the muscles at the margin of the lips when the facial nerve is stimulated by tapping over the zygoma) or the Trousseau sign (carpal spasm induced when a blood pressure cuff is inflated to 20 mm Hg above systolic pressure for 3 min). Intravenous calcium should be given as a 10 mg/kg dose of elemental calcium over 5 to 10 min, as 10% calcium gluconate (94 mg elemental calcium per 10 mL ampul), 1 mL/kg per dose, or as 10% calcium chloride (270 mg elemental calcium per 10 mL ampul), 0.3 to 0.5 mL/kg/dose.

Hyperphosphatemia. Phosphorus-containing foods should be restricted. If the serum phosphorus level is greater than approximately 6 mg/dL, the phosphate-binding agent calcium carbonate, 2 to 3 g with each meal, or 3 times per day in patients without oral food intake, should be administered.

Metabolic acidosis. Severe metabolic acidosis (pH <7.1; plasma bicarbonate concentration, 12 to 15 mEq/L) should be treated with intravenous sodium bicarbonate, 1 to 3 mEq/kg per dose administered over 60 to 120 min. Care should be taken when administering alkali to patients who are both acidotic and hypocalcemic; tetany can be induced when systemic pH is rapidly increased because of increased binding of ionized calcium to albumin. In hypocalcemic patients, calcium should be given intravenously before giving alkali. Milder degrees of acidosis should be treated with sodium bicarbonate, 1 to 3 mEq/kg/d, either orally or intravenously.

Dialysis. Urgent dialysis, either peritoneal dialysis or hemodialysis, is required for children who do not respond to initial treatment of the preceding complications. Less urgent indications for dialysis are severe acidosis, hyponatremia, azotemia complicated by central nervous system depression or bleeding, and a serum urea nitrogen level >100 to 125 mg/dL.

OUTCOME

Children with ARF should be hospitalized. After initial stabilization, they require full evaluation to determine the cause of the ARF and treatment in consultation with a pediatric nephrologist. Frequent monitoring of blood pressure, cardiovascular status, and urine output, and meticulous fluid and electrolyte management are essential components of care. Children with ECF volume overload, hypertension, or electrolyte abnormalities should be admitted to a pediatric critical care unit; less ill patients may be managed on a pediatric ward.

Hemolytic Uremic Syndrome

The classic triad of ARF, microangiopathic hemolytic anemia, and thrombocytopenia characterizes hemolytic uremic syndrome (HUS). In children, HUS is the most common cause of ARF requiring acute dialysis. It is primarily a disease of childhood, but children of any age can be affected. Seasonal variation has been observed, with most cases occurring in late spring, summer, and early fall.

Two groups of patients may be distinguished on the basis of their presentation, either epidemic (typical or classic) or sporadic (atypical). In the former group, most patients have a gastrointestinal prodrome, characterized by abdominal pain, vomiting, and diarrhea with or without blood. In the latter group, patients have no prodrome at all. Familial and recurrent forms of the atypical variant have been described, with both types having high morbidity and mortality rates. Hemolytic uremic syndrome also has been associated with ingestion of drugs (cyclosporin, mitomycin, and oral contraceptives), postpartum, collagen vascular disease, malignant disease, and bone marrow and solid organ transplantation. Such secondary cases of HUS are seen more commonly in adult patients than they are in children (Table 15–50).

HISTOPATHOLOGY

The histopathologic lesion of HUS is characterized as thrombotic microangiopathy, with the major sites of involvement being the kidney, brain, skin, pancreas, heart, spleen, and adrenal. The picture of thrombotic microangiopathy is described as comprising (1) agglutinated

Table 15–50. Etiologic Classification of Hemolytic Uremic Syndrome

Idiopathic (atypical)
Infectious (typical): *Escherichia coli, Shigella dysenteriae*
    type I, *Campylobacter jejuni, Salmonella typhi,*
    Streptococcus pneumoniae
Hereditary: autosomal recessive, autosomal dominant
Recurrent: sporadic (atypical), posttransplantation
Associated with:
    Drugs: cyclosporine, oral contraceptives, mitomycin
Pregnancy
Radiation
Transplantation: bone marrow, kidney
Malignancy

platelets in arterioles and capillaries out of proportion to fibrin deposition, (2) endothelial swelling, and (3) minimal inflammatory infiltrate. These abnormalities of the microvasculature can be focal. Activation of platelets and the coagulation cascade occurs with deposition of platelets and fibrin-like material within the lumen of the glomeruli and, occasionally, the arterioles. In the glomeruli of the kidney, there is endothelial injury with detachment of the basement membrane and interposition of fluffy-appearing material similar to that in the capillary lumen. Three categories of renal histopathologic lesions have been defined: cortical necrosis, predominance of glomerular injury, and predominance of arteriolar injury. Data suggest that predominantly glomerular lesions are seen in typical cases and predominantly arteriolar lesions in atypical cases.

PATHOPHYSIOLOGY

The initial pathogenic event is thought to be injury to the endothelial cells of the renal microvasculature caused by bacterial toxins, with subsequent activation and aggregation of platelets. In many patients with classic HUS, gastrointestinal disease has been associated with *Escherichia coli* infection. For example, in an epidemic of HUS that occurred in a nursing home, infection with *E. coli* O157:H7 was found in 12 of 55 affected residents. This strain of *E. coli* has been shown to produce a specific toxin, known as verotoxin, which is directly toxic to endothelial cells *in vitro*. HUS has been associated with both gastrointestinal and respiratory infection due to other organisms, including *Shigella dysenteriae* type I, *Campylobacter jejuni, Salmonella typhi,* and *Streptococcus pneumoniae.* Evidence suggests that antibiotic treatment of children with *E. coli* O157:H7 infection is a risk factor in the development of the HUS.

Additional mechanisms that promote platelet activation and aggregation may contribute to the pathogenesis of HUS. In some patients with HUS, a deficiency of prostacyclin or of circulating von Willebrand factor multimers, both known to inhibit platelet aggregation, has been seen. However, whether these disturbances in platelet aggregation are primary or secondary to the endothelial injury is not clear.

CLINICAL FEATURES AND LABORATORY FINDINGS

After the typical gastrointestinal prodrome, most patients have hematuria and proteinuria with mild renal insufficiency, anemia, and thrombocytopenia. However, a number of patients have ARF with oliguria or anuria and severe azotemia. The anuria may last from a few days to several weeks. In a significant minority of patients, hypertension, due to either intrinsic renal disease or fluid overload, or both, develops.

The microangiopathic hemolytic anemia results primarily from physical destruction of red blood cells in the microcirculation and their subsequent removal from the circulation by the spleen. The degree of hemolysis varies from mild to severe and usually parallels the course of renal involvement. The peripheral blood smear reveals the presence of schistocytes, as well as Burr and target cells. The hemolytic process is associated with reticulocytosis, hemoglobinemia, reduced serum haptoglobin levels, and a negative Coombs test result. Jaundice may develop as a result of hemolysis and indirect hyperbilirubinemia. Intravascular clumping causes the thrombocytopenia and damaged platelets are removed from the circulation by the reticuloendothelial system. Occasionally, petechiae or purpura are noted on the skin. Leukocytosis is present, and evidence of a coagulopathy is typically absent.

Extrarenal and extrahematologic manifestations also can be seen in patients with HUS. Involvement of the central nervous system occurs in approximately one third of patients and ranges in severity from mild to severe. Irritability, personality changes, drowsiness, seizures, transient cortical blindness, hemiparesis, and coma are observed. Hypertension, electrolyte disturbances, or brain microthrombi may cause seizures. Cardiac involvement is rare in childhood and may be manifested by a cardiomyopathy, aneurysm, or myocarditis. A subset of patients can have severe disease of the gastrointestinal tract, which is due to injury of the gastrointestinal microvasculature, characterized by severe abdominal pain, sometimes associated with intussusception, perforation, frank necrosis, or stricture. Insulin-dependent diabetes mellitus may develop as a result of pancreatic dysfunction and can be transient or permanent. Other organ systems that may be involved during the course of HUS are the liver, with a transient elevation of enzymes, the skeletal muscle, and the eye.

TREATMENT

The degree of organ involvement and the severity of clinical manifestations usually guide therapy. Because children with typical HUS have an excellent prognosis, they can be managed conservatively with judicious transfusion of blood products to correct severe anemia and thrombocytopenia, treatment of hypertension, seizure control, and careful control of electrolyte and water disturbances. Either peritoneal dialysis or hemodialysis should be performed in patients with prolonged anuria who have severe azotemia, hyperkalemia, acidosis, or signs of severe intravascular volume overload such as pulmonary edema and hypertension. Such a comprehensive regimen of supportive therapy is primarily responsible for the decline in the mortality rates from 40 to 50% in the 1950s to the current rate of 5 to 10%.

Over the years, multiple therapeutic modalities have been used in an attempt to improve the clinical course. These include immunosuppressive agents, steroids, antiplatelet agents, anticoagulants, prostacyclin and plasma infusions, and plasmapheresis. Unfortunately, none of these therapies have been convincingly demonstrated to improve the outcome of this disorder. Therefore, it is recommended that patients with HUS be managed conservatively with supportive therapy.

OUTCOME

Important determinants of morbidity and mortality in children with HUS are the type of presentation, the severity and duration of renal involvement, and the severity of neurologic disease. Patients with a typical diarrheal prodrome have a good prognosis, whereas those with atypical presentations generally have a worse prognosis. The anuria associated with severe renal disease ranges in length from a few days to several weeks. Although in some studies prolonged anuria has been associated with a worse prognosis, most such patients eventually have complete resolution of disease and normalization of renal function. Nevertheless, a few patients have either irreversible renal failure during the acute episode or progressive renal insufficiency and end-stage renal failure months to years later. Such patients require chronic dialysis treatment and renal transplantation. In patients with seizures, hemiparesis, or coma during the acute illness, persistent neurologic involvement is rare.

Chronic Renal Failure

In patients with chronic renal failure, a slow deterioration of renal function is caused by a variety of renal and urologic diseases and results in a symptom complex involving multiple abnormalities of body composition and metabolism, hormonal regulation, and organ system functioning.

ETIOLOGY AND PATHOGENESIS

The more common causes of chronic renal failure in children are listed in Table 15–51. In infants and young

Table 15–51. Causes of Chronic Renal Failure in Children

	Percentage of Total
Glomerulonephritis	25
Urinary tract malformations	25
Reflux nephropathy and obstructive uropathy	
Renal hypoplasia/dysplasia	16
Cystic diseases	10
Medullary cystic disease and autosomal-recessive polycystic disease	
Cystinosis	4
Hemolytic uremic syndrome	3
Alport syndrome	3
Henoch-Schönlein syndrome	2
Other	12

children, congenital abnormalities of the kidneys and urinary tract and inherited diseases predominate, whereas in older children, various forms of glomerulonephritis are more common. In many of the conditions listed, renal failure is caused by the gradual destruction of renal parenchyma by an ongoing inflammatory, immunologic, or metabolic disease. In other conditions, however, after an initial insult to the kidneys, further gradual deterioration occurs despite the absence of an ongoing disease process. These conditions include such diverse entities as renal hypoplasia and dysplasia, surgically corrected renal reflux, and the slowly progressive renal failure that follows an episode of HUS. The common denominator in these conditions is a reduction in the number of nephrons, which is known to result in compensatory hypertrophy of the remaining nephrons. Studies in experimental animals have demonstrated that this hypertrophy response is mediated by an increase in intraglomerular plasma flow, hydrostatic pressure, and filtration rate and that this process eventually leads to glomerular scarring and obsolescence. The pathogenesis of this so-called hyperfiltration injury, and its significance in the progression of renal failure in humans, is incompletely defined and is the subject of continuing studies.

PATHOPHYSIOLOGY

As a consequence of nephron destruction in chronic renal failure and subsequent hypertrophy of the remaining nephrons, patients with mildly to moderately reduced GFR can maintain normal body fluid homeostasis. Although the amount of glomerular filtrate formed each day in these patients is greatly diminished, the tubules of surviving nephrons are sufficiently able to increase the fractional excretion of salt and water so that intake and output of these substances are balanced. This adaptive process, however, has limits. The ability of damaged kidneys to increase salt and water excretion in response to acute volume loads and to conserve salt and water in response to acute dehydration becomes progressively compromised as the GFR decreases.

CLINICAL FINDINGS

With kidney failure, there is retention in the body of a variety of substances that are normally excreted by the kidneys. These include urea nitrogen, creatinine, uric acid, potassium, phosphorus, hydrogen ions, sodium chloride, and water. The retention of these substances and a number of other, less–well-defined "uremic toxins" causes a variety of pathologic processes in the body, which include metabolic and hormonal abnormalities, decreased immune responsiveness, and organ-system dysfunction. In addition, blood concentrations of hormones normally synthesized and secreted by the kidneys, such as erythropoietin and $1,25(OH)_2D$, are decreased, and the level of the renal hormone renin may be increased.

Table 15–52. Clinical Manifestations of Chronic Renal Failure

Cardiovascular
Hypertension, pulmonary edema, pericarditis, cardiomyopathy
Nervous system
Drowsiness, obtundation, seizures, peripheral neuropathy
Gastrointestinal
Anorexia, nausea and vomiting, gastritis, colitis, malnutrition
Musculoskeletal
Rickets, osteomalacia, osteitis fibrosa, metastatic calcification, myopathy
Hematopoietic
Anemia, coagulation disorders
Metabolic
Acidosis with increased anion gap, glucose intolerance, hypertriglyceridemia
Hormonal
Increased parathyroid hormone, increased renin-angiotensin, increased prolactin and luteinizing hormone, decreased 1,25-dihydroxyvitamin D, decreased erythropoietin
Immunologic
Decreased cellular immunity

Some of the clinical and biochemical manifestations of the uremic state are listed in Table 15–52. The pathogenesis of many of these abnormalities is poorly defined but is thought to involve the action of as-yet unidentified uremic toxins. Some of the described abnormalities, such as decreased immune responsiveness, are of limited clinical significance, whereas others, such as peripheral neuropathy, occur only in patients with long-standing severe renal failure and are rarely seen in those who receive appropriate medical care, including the timely initiation of dialysis.

DIAGNOSIS

Although renal failure is readily diagnosed by a constellation of findings, including anemia, acidosis, and increased serum concentrations of creatinine and urea nitrogen, the cause of the renal failure and its duration are not always apparent. Findings that suggest chronicity are small kidney size, growth retardation, and renal osteodystrophy, although these are not invariably present in chronic disease. The definitive test, both to diagnose the underlying kidney disease and to determine its acuity or chronicity, is a renal biopsy.

TREATMENT

When there is no specific therapy for the underlying cause of renal failure, the management of chronic renal failure consists of instituting nonspecific measures that may retard the progression of renal failure and prevent or treat the complications of renal failure. The progression of renal failure may be retarded by aggressive treatment of hypertension and by dietary restriction of protein and, perhaps, phosphorus. Although hypertension can be a consequence of renal disease and renal failure in many patients, hypertension also can cause kidney damage, and effective control of blood pressure has been shown to retard the progression of renal failure in patients with a variety of renal diseases.

Restriction of dietary protein can decrease glomerular hydrostatic pressure and GFR and, in animals with reduced renal mass, has been shown to prevent compensatory hypertrophy and to slow the progression of renal failure. Although studies of the effects of protein restriction on the progression of renal failure in humans have been difficult to perform and have yielded uncertain results, most nephrologists prescribe protein restriction early in the course of renal failure. Malnutrition and, in children, growth retardation are possible complications of protein restriction.

The most important clinical manifestations of renal failure in children, which require prevention or treatment, are metabolic acidosis, disorders of calcium and phosphorus metabolism, renal osteodystrophy, hypertension, anemia, and nutritional and growth disturbances.

Metabolic acidosis. The acidosis of renal failure is caused by the inability of the kidneys to excrete the 1 to 3 mEq/kg of hydrogen ions that children generate daily. Acidosis can be a cause of the poor growth that is characteristic of children with renal failure. It is treated with sodium bicarbonate or sodium citrate, 1 to 3 mEq/kg/d.

Renal osteodystrophy. In severe renal failure, renal excretion of phosphorus is reduced, which results in hyperphosphatemia. Renal production of $1,25(OH)_2D$ is reduced as a result of both hyperphosphatemia and reduced renal mass and the consequence is decreased calcium absorption by the intestine and hypocalcemia. Hypocalcemia and hyperphosphatemia stimulate parathyroid hormone secretion and the development of secondary hyperparathyroidism, which leads to excessive resorption of bone (osteitis fibrosa). Other forms of bone disease have been described and characterized by impaired bone mineralization (osteomalacia and rickets), a combination of osteitis fibrosa and osteomalacia (mixed), and low turnover of bone, sometimes accompanied by aluminum deposition (aplastic). When the product of the calcium times the phosphorus concentration in serum exceeds 70, calcium phosphate may be deposited in soft tissues, such as blood vessels, viscera, and skin; the latter is manifested by pruritus.

These abnormalities are treated by restriction of dietary phosphorus, the use of drugs that bind phosphorus in the gut, such as calcium carbonate and sevelamer, and the administration of 1,25-dihydroxyvitamin D_3 (calcitriol).

Hypertension. Hypertension can be caused by salt and water retention and plasma volume expansion, by increased secretion of renin by the kidneys, and by less-well-understood mechanisms, such as overactivity of the sympathetic nervous system and decreased renal production of vasodilator prostaglandins and kinins. In advanced renal failure, salt and water retention is the most common mechanism. The diagnosis of volume-dependent hypertension is made when other signs of increased plasma volume are present, such as edema and cardiomegaly, whereas the diagnosis of renin-dependent hypertension depends on the finding of increased plasma renin activity.

Volume-dependent hypertension is best managed by dietary salt restriction and treatment with a thiazide diuretic or furosemide. Renin-dependent hypertension can be treated with a β blocker or, preferably, with more potent drugs affecting the renin-angiotensin system, specifically the angiotensin-converting enzyme inhibitors. Drugs commonly used to treat chronic hypertension in patients with renal failure are presented in the earlier section, "Evaluation of Hypertensive Children."

Anemia. The anemia of chronic renal failure is caused primarily by decreased renal production of erythropoietin, although RBC survival is shortened in uremic patients, presumably owing to the effect of a uremic toxin. The anemia is readily corrected by the parenteral administration of erythropoietin, initially given in a dose of 100 U/kg, 3 times a week. Coexisting iron deficiency must be treated before erythropoietin can be effective.

Nutrition and growth. Growth retardation is common in children with chronic renal failure, especially in those with congenital renal diseases. Causes of growth retardation include poor calorie intake, acidosis, renal osteodystrophy, and increased serum levels of growth hormone binding proteins. The most important of these is poor calorie intake, which is the result of anorexia, probably related to high serum concentrations of urea nitrogen or some other product of protein metabolism. The treatment involves protein restriction when the blood urea nitrogen concentration exceeds 80 mg/dL, although this value is arbitrary and protein restriction may be appropriately initiated at an earlier stage of renal failure to prevent hyperfiltration injury. Protein should not be restricted to less than the recommended dietary allowance for children. In infants and young children, protein restriction is best accomplished by substituting a low-protein formula, such as Similac PM60/40 (Ross Laboratories), which also has decreased concentrations of sodium, potassium, and phosphorus, for cow's milk.

Despite protein restriction and the maintenance of low blood urea nitrogen concentrations, calorie intake may be insufficient for growth. Added calories, in the form of carbohydrate or fat suspension, can be prescribed, and if children are unable or unwilling to take these orally, nasogastric or gastrostomy tube feeding are often undertaken. In children whose growth remains poor despite the provision of adequate calories and correction of acidosis and renal osteodystrophy, the administration of human recombinant growth hormone; 0.05 mg/kg/day, will usually stimulate normal growth.

REFERENCES

Evaluation of Renal Function

Geyer SJ: Urinalysis and urinary sediment in patients with renal disease. Clin Lab Med 1993;13:13.

Rose BD: *Clinical Physiology of Acid-Base and Electrolyte Disorders,* 4th ed. New York, McGraw-Hill, 1994.

Schwartz GJ, Brion LP, Spitzer A: The use of plasma creatinine concentration for estimating glomerular filtration rate in infants, children, and adolescents. Pediatr Clin North Am 1987; 34:571.

Disorders of Plasma Sodium and Potassium

Cogan MG: *Fluid and Electrolytes, Physiology and Pathophysiology,* 1st ed. Norwalk, Appleton & Lange, 1991.

Rose and Black's Clinical Problems in Nephrology, Boston, Little, Brown and Co., 1996.

Parenteral Fluid Therapy

American Academy of Pediatrics Provisional Committee on quality improvement, Subcommittee on acute gastroenteritis. Practice parameter: the management of acute gastroenteritis in young children. Pediatrics 1996;97:424

Avery ME, Snyder JD: Oral therapy for acute diarrhea: the underused simple solution. Curr Concepts 1990;323:891.

Hellerstein S: Fluid and electrolytes: clinical aspects. Pediatr Rev 1993; 14:103.

Evaluation of Hematuria

Benbassat J, Gergawi M, Offringa M, et al: Symptomless microhaematuria in schoolchildren: causes for variable management strategies. Quart J Med 1996;89:845.

Feld LG, Meyers KE, Kaplan BS, et al: Limited evaluation of microscopic hematuria in pediatrics. Pediatrics 1998;102:E42.

Matos V, van Melle G, Boulat O, et al: Urinary phosphate/creatinine, calcium/creatinine, and magnesium/creatinine ratios in a healthy pediatric population. J Pediatr 1997;131:252.

Stapleton FB: What is the appropriate evaluation and therapy for children with hypercalciuria and hematuria? Semin Nephrol 1998;18:359.

Vehaskari VM, Rapola J, Koskimies O, et al: Microscopic hematuria in school children: epidemiology and clinicopathologic evaluation. J Pediatr 1979;95:676.

Glomerulonephritis

Cole BR, Salinas Madrigal L: Acute proliferative glomerulonephritis and crescentic glomerulonephritis. In Holliday MA, et al (editors): *Pediatric Nephrology,* 3rd ed. Williams & Wilkins, 1994.

Donadio JV, et al: A controlled trial of fish oil in IGA nephropathy. N Engl J Med 1994;331:1194.

Milford DV: Glomerulonephritis in children. Brit J Hosp Med 1995;54:87.

Wyatt RJ, et al: IGA nephropathy: Long-term prognosis of pediatric patients. J Pediatr 1995;127:913.

Evaluation of Proteinuria

Dodge WF, et al: Proteinuria and hematuria in schoolchildren: epidemiology and early natural history. J Pediatr 1976;88:327.

Feld LG, et al: Evaluation of the child with asymptomatic proteinuria. Pediatr Rev 1984;5:248.

Loghman-Adham M: Evaluating proteinuria in children Am Fam Phys 1998; 58:1145, 1158. (published erratum appears in Am Fam Phys 1999;59:540).

Springberg P, Garrett L, Thompson A, et al: Fixed and reproducible orthostatic proteinuria: results of a 20 year follow-up study. Ann Intern Med 1982; 97:516.

Vehaskari VM: Orthostatic proteinuria. Arch Dis Child 1982; 57:729.

West CD: Asymptomatic hematuria and proteinuria in children: causes and appropriate diagnostic studies. J Pediatr 1976; 89:173.

Nephrotic Syndrome

Chesney RW: The idiopathic nephrotic syndrome. Curr Opin Pediatr 1999;11:158.

Grupe WE: Primary nephrotic syndrome in childhood. Adv Pediatr 1979;26:163.

International Study of Kidney Disease in Children: Nephrotic syndrome in children: Prediction of histopathology from clinical and laboratory characteristics at time of diagnosis. Kidney Int 1978;13:159.

Schnaper HW: Primary nephrotic syndrome of childhood. Curr Opin Pediatr 1996;8:14.

Trompeter RS: Immunosuppressive therapy in the nephrotic syndrome in children. Pediatr Nephrol 1989;3:194.

Tune BM, Mendoza SA: Treatment of the idiopathic nephrotic syndrome: regimens and outcomes in children and adults. J Am Soc Nephrol 1997;8:824.

Acute Renal Failure

Brady H, et al: Acute renal failure. In Brenner BM (editor): *Brenner and Rector's The Kidney*, 5th ed. Saunders, 1996.

Hemolytic Uremic Syndrome

Kaplan BS, Meyers KE, Schulman SL: The pathogenesis and treatment of hemolytic uremic syndrome. J Am Soc Nephrol 1998; 9:1126.

Small G, Watson AR, Evans JH, et al: Hemolytic uremic syndrome: defining the need for long-term follow-up. Clin Nephrol 1999; 52:352.

Trachtman H, Christen E: Pathogenesis, treatment, and therapeutic trials in hemolytic uremic syndrome. Curr Opin Pediatr 1999; 11:162.

Wong CS, Jelacic S, Habeeb RL, et al: The risk of the hemolytic-uremic syndrome after antibiotic treatment of *Escherichia coli* O157:H7 infections [see comments]. N Engl J Med 2000; 342:1930.

Chronic Renal Failure

Brenner BM, et al: Dietary protein intake and the progressive nature of kidney disease: the role of hemodynamically mediated glomerular injury in the pathogenesis of progressive glomerular sclerosis in aging, renal ablation, and intrinsic renal disease. N Engl J Med 1982;307:652.

Fine RN, et al for the Genentech Cooperative Study Group: Growth after recombinant human growth hormone treatment in children with chronic renal failure: report of a multicenter randomized double-blind placebo-controlled study. J Pediatr 1994; 124:374.

Wassner SJ: Conservative management of chronic renal insufficiency. In Holliday MA, et al (editors): *Pediatric Nephrology,* 3rd ed. Williams & Wilkins, 1994.

Evaluation of Hypertension

Loggie JMH (ed): *Pediatric and Adolescent Hypertension.* Blackwell 1992.

Update on the 1987 Task Force on High Blood Pressure in Children and Adolescents: a working group report from the National High Blood Pressure Education Program. Pediatrics 1996; 98:649.

Renal Tubular Acidosis

Portale AA: Renal tubular acidosis. In Holliday MA, et al (editors): *Pediatric Nephrology,* 3rd ed. Williams & Wilkins, 1994.

Congenital Anomalies of the Urinary Tract

Belman AB: A perspective on vesicoureteral reflux. Urol Clin North Am 1995;22:139.

Tripp BM, Homsy YL: Neonatal hydronephrosis: the controversy and the management. Pediatr Nephrol 1995;9:503.

Circulation

Michael M. Brook, MD, Phillip Moore, MD, & George F. Van Hare, MD

16

■ CARDIAC PHYSIOLOGY

The purpose of the circulation is to deliver oxygen to the tissues of the body to support their metabolic activities. To achieve this, the heart pumps blood, initiated by intrinsic electrical activity, through vessels to the lungs and body.

OXYGEN DELIVERY

Oxygen tissue delivery is determined by two main factors: the amount of oxygen carried by blood and the volume of blood the heart pumps to the body with each beat (stroke volume). Oxygen is carried by blood predominately bound to hemoglobin in red blood cells, although a small amount is dissolved. This means that the amount of oxygen in blood depends predominately on patients' hemoglobin concentrations and oxygen saturations. Cyanosis and anemia decrease oxygen delivery.

CARDIAC FUNCTION

The pump function of the heart is best determined by the cardiac output, which is the volume of blood (in liters) the heart pumps to the body per minute. Because of the variable size among the pediatric population, cardiac output typically is divided by the children's body surface area and reported as cardiac index (L/min/m²). Cardiac output equals stroke volume (L/beat) times heart rate (beats/min). Three factors determine stroke volume: preload, afterload, and contractility. Therefore, heart rate, preload, afterload, and contractility are the major determinants of cardiac function (Table 16–1).

Heart Rate

Although it would seem that an increase in heart rate should increase cardiac output, this usually is not the case because of adjustments in diastolic filling. Very fast or slow rates affect stroke volume through changes in preload and contractility. Because the duration of systole is relatively constant as heart rate changes, increases in heart rate diminish the time available for diastolic filling of the ventricle. At very fast heart rates, as seen during an episode of paroxysmal tachycardia, cardiac output may be reduced dramatically because of poor diastolic filling, which results in decreased preload. Mild bradycardia allows for increased diastolic filling, which improves stroke volume. The heart maintains a normal cardiac output, because the increase in stroke volume compensates for the decreased rate. As bradycardia becomes more severe, however, cardiac output is reduced as the decrease in rate overwhelms the limited increase in preload. Increasing heart rate has a direct effect on improving contractility acutely; however, chronic fast rates, such as those which occur in various forms of supraventricular tachycardia (SVT), can cause decreased contractile function leading to tachycardia-induced cardiomyopathy.

In addition to rate, cardiac rhythm plays a role in cardiac function. With atrioventricular dissociation, such as in second- or third-degree heart block, the normal atrial contribution to active filling of the ventricle is lost, adversely affecting preload and diminishing cardiac output. In junctional rhythm, if there is 1:1 retrograde conduction to the atrium, the atrium is always contracting against a closed atrioventricular valve, also leading to loss of the atrial contribution to active filling. Bundle branch block, ventricular pacing, and ventricular tachycardia all cause poorly organized ventricular contraction leading to decreased cardiac output.

Preload

In isolated strips of myocardium, preload refers to the amount of stretch applied to the muscle before contraction. Increased stretch results in increased force of contraction to a maximum; contraction then declines as stretch becomes more extreme. This relation is known as the Starling mechanism.

Precontraction myocardial stretch in the beating heart is best represented by the end-diastolic volume of the ventricle. Increased end-diastolic ventricular volume results in increased stretch on the ventricular myocytes, causing an increase in stroke volume. Unfortunately, there is no easy and accurate way to measure end-diastolic volume short of placing special catheters into the beating ventricle. There is, however, a nonlinear correlation between diastolic pressure and volume in the ventricle. This allows us to estimate ventricular diastolic volume, and therefore preload, from measurements of ventricular end-diastolic pressure, such as the mean central venous pressure (for the right ventricle) and the mean left atrial or

Table 16–1. Determinants of Left
Ventricular Output

Determinant	Clinical Measurement (in order of decreasing reliability)
Heart rate	Pulse Ventricular rate on ECG
Preload	End-diastolic volume End-diastolic pressure Mean left atrial pressure Mean pulmonary capillary wedge pressure
Afterload	Left ventricular end-systolic wall stress Systemic vascular resistance Mean aortic pressure Diastolic aortic pressure
Contractility	Slope of end-systolic pressure–volume relation Slope of velocity of shortening end-systolic wall stress Left ventricular ejection fraction Left ventricular % fractional shortening

ECG = electrocardiogram.

pulmonary arterial wedge pressure (for the left ventricle). All these pressures are easily and routinely monitored in critically ill children, particularly those recovering from cardiac surgery. Caution must be exercised in the interpretation of these pressures because of the nonlinearity of the ventricular end-diastolic pressure–volume relation. Compliance in the ventricle decreases with increasing stretch so that at higher end-diastolic pressures, large increases in pressure may be seen with little change in ventricular volume and, therefore, little change in actual preload. A rough indication of ventricular preload may be obtained by assessing organs or vessels "upstream" from the ventricle in question. Distended neck veins and an enlarged liver suggest elevated right ventricular preload, whereas pulmonary rales suggest pulmonary edema and elevated left ventricular preload.

If poor cardiac output is primarily due to inadequate preload resulting from reduced blood volume, such as with active bleeding or severe dehydration, dramatic increases in cardiac output are easily obtained by increasing preload, i.e., the infusion of blood, colloid, or crystalloid. If cardiac output is low for another reason, such as high afterload, low heart rate, or poor contractility, the preload usually is normal and often may be increased to compensate. Further increases in preload may result in limited and temporary increases in cardiac output, but optimal management should be directed to treatment of the primary problem, e.g., afterload reduction, pacing, or infusion of

inotropic agents. In fact, when preload is high as a compensatory mechanism, it often is the cause of many symptoms. For example, the compensatory increase in left atrial pressure that occurs with left ventricular failure may lead to pulmonary edema because of high pulmonary venous pressures, resulting in respiratory distress.

Afterload

Afterload refers to the resistance that isolated muscle works against during contraction, i.e., the force resisting shortening of the muscle. Although this force can be easily and accurately measured in isolated muscle, it is impossible to measure it directly in the beating heart. In the beating heart, the analogous concept is the resistance against which the ventricle contracts. For a given preload and intrinsic myocardial contractility, the cardiac output will decrease as the resistance or afterload increases. This resistance is provided by the semilunar valves, arteries, and capillary beds downstream and is influenced by the shape and thickness of the ventricle itself. The most accurate technique for estimating afterload is the measurement of systolic wall stress, which considers chamber size, thickness, and intraventricular pressure. This is somewhat time-intensive, however, as it requires simultaneous, continuous measurement of ventricular or arterial pressure with echocardiographic images of ventricular chamber size and thickness.

The practical clinical approach to evaluating afterload is to measure arterial blood pressure (P) and blood flow (Q) and to calculate mean vascular resistance ($R = \Delta P/Q$). This is an extreme oversimplification and limited estimate of afterload. Because mean vascular resistance is directly related to mean pressure and inversely related to mean flow, it assumes that the heart generates continuous, rather than pulsatile, flow. Even more problematic, mean vascular resistance reflects mainly the contribution of the peripheral vascular bed to afterload and ignores central vessel compliance, semilunar valve resistance, and ventricular size and shape. Despite these significant limitations, mean vascular resistance is a reasonable estimate of afterload in most patients. Exceptions include those patients with abnormalities of their proximal arterial tree (e.g., coarctation of the aorta, pulmonary artery banding, nondistensible conduit placement, and dilated aortic or pulmonary roots), semilunar valve stenosis, or significant ventricular dilation and/or hypertrophy (e.g., dilated cardiomyopathy, idiopathic hypertrophic subaortic stenosis [IHSS], and subaortic stenosis).

Increased afterload may result in significant impairment of cardiac function in children. Common examples include infants who are in shock and have severe aortic stenosis (AS) or coarctation or patients who have long-standing malignant hypertension. Often, even though increased afterload is not the primary cause of low cardiac output, it is a contributing factor. Compensatory mechanisms, such as endogenous catecholamine release, may increase systemic vascular resistance markedly. This elevation in afterload may be poorly tolerated by a ventricle with poor contractile function or mitral regurgitation. Careful use of afterload-reducing agents, such as nitroprusside, captopril, or prazosin, may improve cardiac output dramatically in these circumstances.

Contractility

Contractility refers to the inotropic state of the heart, or the intrinsic contractile characteristics of the myocardium not related to preload or afterload. Within a myocyte, this is determined by the activity of the contractile proteins actin and myosin. Contraction begins when an action potential depolarizes the myocyte by sequential influx of sodium and calcium. This results in intracellular calcium release from the sarcoplasmic reticulum, which binds to troponin causing a conformational change that interferes with the binding of troponin to actin. This allows the formation of cross-bridges between actin and the myosin head. The chemical energy of adenosine triphosphate rotates the myosin head, which displaces actin to the center of the sarcomere resulting in shortening of the myocyte. The amount of force developed by the contracting myocyte is, in part, dependent on the number of cross-bridges formed. The contractile state of the heart therefore depends on many factors, including the size and number of healthy myocytes, the availability of intra- and extracellular calcium, and the amount of circulating catecholamines.

For the beating heart, contractility is the potential for cardiac muscle to do work, i.e., eject blood. An increase in contractility results in greater shortening of the myocardium at a constant preload and afterload. The Starling curve is shifted up and leftward, so that for a given preload and afterload the ventricular output is increased (Figure 16–1). Unfortunately, neither in the laboratory nor at the bedside is an independent measure of myocardial contractility readily available.

Clinically, there is no reliable way to measure cardiac contractile state. The cardiac output should be assessed by physical examination and invasive techniques, such as cardiac output measurements by thermodilution technique or evaluation of the systemic arterial-venous O_2 saturation differential as indicated. Noninvasive measurement of left ventricular ejection fraction (the percentage of the left ventricular diastolic volume that is ejected) and subjective assessment of myocardial wall motion by echocardiography should be obtained.

The specific treatment of decreased cardiac contractility involves the use of inotropic agents. Digoxin is the most commonly prescribed digitalis preparation and the only liquid oral preparation available in the United States. For the acute management of contractile dysfunction, more

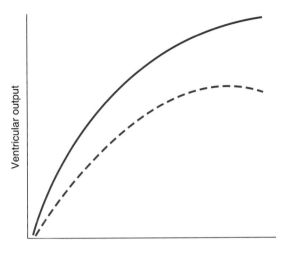

Figure 16–1. An increase in end-diastolic volume (preload) results in an increase in ventricular output. When contractility is increased **(solid line),** the output is greater at the same preload.

potent catecholamine agents, such as dopamine, dobutamine, isoproterenol, and epinephrine, are used more commonly. In addition, the phosphodiesterase inhibitors, such as amrinone and milrinone, can be used. All these agents have additional effects on the circulation, specifically with respect to heart rate and venous and/or arterial vessel tone. The most appropriate agent is chosen on the basis of the state of the children's preload, afterload, and heart rate (Table 16–2). In addition to inotropic support, patients with decreased contractility may benefit from direct alterations in preload, afterload, and heart rate.

■ CIRCULATION

To understand congenital heart disease fully, one must recognize fetal blood flow patterns in the central circulation and the changes in these flow patterns with birth. With very few exceptions, serious structural cardiac disease diagnosed in the newborn period is completely compatible with a relatively normal intrauterine existence. It is the transition to extrauterine life that makes the cardiac lesion hemodynamically significant. The best example of this principle is infants with pulmonary atresia (PA). While the infants are in utero, very little blood flow needs to be delivered to the lungs because oxygenation is provided by the placenta. With closure of the ductus arteriosus after birth, however, pulmonary blood flow may be inadequate to oxygenate infants, leading to a rapidly fatal condition if no intervention is undertaken.

Table 16–2. Properties of Inotropic Agents for the Acute Management of Decreased Cardiac Contractility

Agent	Contractility	Afterload	Heart Rate
Amrinone/milrinone	↑	↓↓	(↑)
Isoproterenol	↑	↓↓	↑↑↑
Dobutamine	↑↑	(↓)[1]	(↑)[1]
Dopamine	↑↑	↑↑[1]	↑↑[1]
Epinephrine	↑↑	↑↑	↑↑

[1] Effect very dose dependent.

FETAL CIRCULATION

In the normal fetus, as in the normal newborn, there are two atria, two ventricles, and two great vessels. The fetus, however, has additional structures: a patent foramen ovale, a patent ductus arteriosus (PDA), and a patent ductus venosus, as well as the placenta (Figure 16–2). The placenta serves as the site of gas exchange. Because pulmonary arteriolar vasoconstriction maintains high resistance in the pulmonary circuit, most right ventricu-

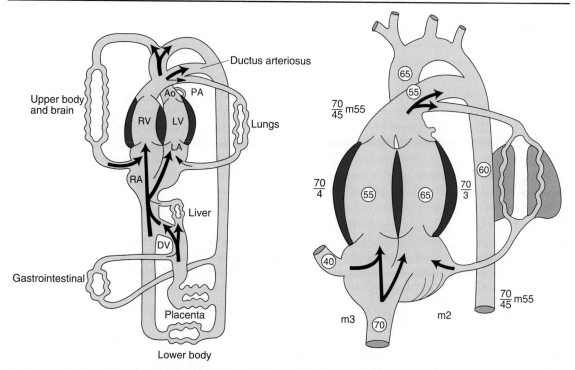

Figure 16–2. Diagrams of the fetal circulation. **Left:** Blood is oxygenated in the placenta and returns to the fetus through the umbilical vein. About half the umbilical venous blood passes through the liver, and the remainder bypasses the liver through the ductus venosus (DV) directly into the inferior vena cava. Inferior vena caval blood is distributed partly through the foramen ovale to the left atrium (LA) and partly through the tricuspid valve to the right ventricle (RV) **(left and right panels).** Superior vena caval blood passes almost exclusively into the right ventricle. Blood ejected from the right ventricle passes mainly through the ductus arteriosus to the descending aorta, and only a small amount enters the lungs. **Right:** Numbers in circles show oxygen saturations in cardiac chambers and great vessels. Numbers alongside are pressures (mm Hg). Ao = ascending aorta; LV = left ventricle; PA = pulmonary artery; RA = right atrium.

lar blood traverses the ductus arteriosus, rather than traversing the branch pulmonary arteries and lungs. The right ventricle, therefore, provides blood to the descending aorta and the placenta via the ductus. The left ventricle supplies the ascending aorta and the upper body, including the brain, and sends a small amount down the descending aorta to mix with right ventricular output. Therefore, there is a functional, but not absolute, separation in the systemic circulation in the fetus, with the right ventricle supplying the lower body and placenta and the left ventricle supplying the upper body.

Oxygenation occurs in the placenta, and blood of higher oxygen content passes from the placenta into the umbilical vein. Umbilical venous blood is distributed to both lobes of the liver, and about one-half bypasses the liver through the ductus venosus directly into the inferior vena cava. Portal venous blood is distributed almost completely to the right liver lobe.

Blood in the ascending aorta has a higher oxygen content than that in the descending aorta, and so the brain receives blood with a higher oxygen content than does the placenta. This separation in oxygen content is caused by the patterns of streaming in the right atrium. Blood from the superior vena cava, low in oxygen content, preferentially crosses the tricuspid valve and is sent by the right ventricle via the ductus to the descending aorta and placenta for reoxygenation. Blood from the inferior vena cava, higher in oxygen content because of the contribution from the placenta, preferentially crosses the foramen ovale to fill the left atrium and left ventricle and is sent predominantly to the upper body, brain, and coronary circulation.

TRANSITION TO EXTRAUTERINE CIRCULATION

A number of complex events occur with birth (Figure 16–3). Occlusion of the umbilical cord removes the low-resistance capillary bed from the systemic circulation. Breathing results in a marked decrease in pulmonary resistance. Two distinct mechanisms are responsible for this effect on the pulmonary vessels. Rhythmic physical expansion of the lungs releases a prostaglandin, probably prostacyclin (PGI_2). An increase in alveolar oxygen level stimulates production of nitric oxide, a powerful pulmonary vasodilator. The increased pulmonary blood flow returns to fill the left atrium, and this increased left atrial filling closes the foramen ovale, limiting and eventually eliminating flow from the inferior vena cava into the left atrium. Because blood that returns from the lungs is much more completely oxygenated than that which was provided by the placenta, arterial oxygen saturation increases. This increase in arterial oxygen saturation and, in particular, the loss of endogenous prostaglandins produced by the placenta eventually brings about closure of

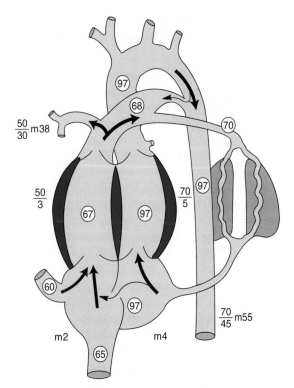

Figure 16–3. Neonatal circulation. Placenta has been removed. The foramen ovale has closed, and the ductus arteriosus has almost closed. Pulmonary arterial pressure has fallen from fetal levels, but it is still higher than adult levels. Numbers in circles show oxygen saturations in cardiac chambers and great vessels. Pressures (mm Hg) are shown alongside.

the ductus arteriosus and ductus venosus. Finally, the foramen ovale becomes nonpatent. Most of the transition from fetal to neonatal circulation takes place in the first several minutes after birth owing to changes in vascular resistance. Functional closure of the ductus arteriosus takes place within 10 to 15 h after birth, but anatomic closure occurs only after several days to 2 weeks. The foramen ovale typically remains patent with no flow through it for weeks or months and, in fact, may remain patent into adulthood in some individuals.

PULMONARY VASCULAR BED

Whereas the first breath is accompanied by a sudden and dramatic decrease in pulmonary vascular resistance, a further decrease in resistance occurs over the first several days of life, as pulmonary arterioles relax and subsequently lose much of the smooth muscle in the media. In normal infants, the pulmonary vascular bed resembles the adult pattern both in resistance and in histologic appearance by several weeks of age. In some individuals, however, this maturation of the pulmonary vascular bed may not occur or may occur over a long time course. Two factors may be responsible. First, alveolar hypoxemia maintains pulmonary vasoconstriction after birth, as in babies born at high altitude or with lung disease. Second, pulmonary hypertension may be responsible. An example is infants with a large ventricular septal defect (VSD). In such infants, the presence of the defect allows transmission of systemic left ventricular systolic pressure to the right ventricle and in turn to the pulmonary artery and peripheral vascular bed. This pulmonary hypertension interferes with the normal decrease in pulmonary vascular resistance described previously. In such patients, resistance may remain high until 1 to 2 months of age and does not decrease to normal levels while pulmonary arterial pressure remains elevated.

In any infants with congenital heart lesions comprising a large communication between the ventricles or aorta and pulmonary artery, pulmonary arterial pressure remains elevated. The normal disappearance of smooth muscle in the media does not occur, and this contributes to the maintenance of an increased pulmonary vascular resistance. If the cardiac defect is corrected, the pulmonary vessels lose the medial muscle layer and assume normal adult characteristics. If the pulmonary hypertension persists, secondary changes in the arterioles develop. Intimal proliferation, with migration of smooth muscle cells into the intima and then fibrosis, results in a progressive increase in pulmonary vascular resistance. These changes are permanent, and correction of the defect at this stage does not improve the pulmonary vascular resistance. For this reason, cardiac defects are repaired early. The intimal proliferative and fibrotic changes usually do not begin to develop before age 6 months, but they increase progressively, becoming severe as early as 9 to 12 months or as late as adolescence. The progressive increase in pulmonary vascular resistance results in a decrease of left-to-right shunt and subsequently in the development of a right-to-left shunt, with clinical cyanosis. Patients with high pulmonary blood flow but normal or only slightly elevated pressure, such as with a large atrial septal defect (ASD), undergo the normal decline in pulmonary vascular resistance after birth, but the intimal proliferative and fibrotic changes may occur, usually after adolescence.

■ CARDIAC ELECTRICAL ACTIVITY

Cardiac impulses are formed by cardiac cells that exhibit *pacemaker activity,* or *spontaneous automaticity.* In adults, such cells are found primarily in the sinus and atrioven-

tricular nodes and, to a lesser extent, in atrial muscle and the His-Purkinje (distal conducting) system. The sinus node develops quite early in gestation as a well-demarcated structure at the junction of the right atrium and superior vena cava.

Cardiac muscle cells have the ability to transmit electrical impulses to adjacent cells via *gap junctions,* specialized structures that make the cytosol of adjacent cardiac cells electrically continuous. An action potential that spreads down one cardiac cell will be transmitted easily to adjacent cardiac cells, leading to propagation throughout the heart. Instead of homogenous conduction in all directions, propagation is known to be more rapid along the long axis of cardiac cells than it is along the transverse axis. The velocity of impulse propagation in cardiac muscle depends on a number of factors, including fiber orientation; passive properties of cardiac muscle, such as membrane excitability threshold, resistance, and capacitance; and active properties related to the action potential. The most important of these factors is the rate of increase of phase 0 of the action potential, also known as dV/dT or maximum velocity (V_{max}). Conduction velocity is directly related to the magnitude of V_{max}, and factors that affect V_{max} also affect conduction velocity.

Phase 0 of the action potential occurs when the membrane potential is increased from its resting negative value to its excitability threshold (Figure 16–4). In cardiac muscle cells, or fast-response cells, this results in the opening of voltage-sensitive sodium channels, the rapid entry of positively charged sodium ions, and the further increase in the membrane potential toward 0 potential. The sodium channel is time dependent and inactivates, allowing other ionic mechanisms eventually to return the membrane potential to its resting potential. Antiarrhythmic agents, such as procainamide and quinidine, are thought to exert their effects by blocking fast sodium channels, thereby slowing the rate of increase of phase 0 and consequently decreasing conduction velocity.

In pacemaker, or slow-response, cells such as those found in the sinus and atrioventricular node, the upstroke of the action potential, and therefore the velocity of conduction, is much slower than in fast-response cells found elsewhere (see Figure 16–4). Phase 0 of the action potential is not mediated by the opening of fast sodium channels, but instead by the slow inward calcium current.

In normal sinus rhythm, the spread of cardiac excitation proceeds from the sinus node through the atrial muscle to excite both right and left atria. Excitation reaches the atrioventricular node by way of cell-to-cell intra-atrial conduction. The atrioventricular node gives rise to a bundle *(bundle of His)* that penetrates the central fibrous body and then divides to form the left and right bundle branches, made up of Purkinje cells. The atrioventricular node is made up of slow-response cells that are histologically similar to those found in the sinus node. The slower upstroke of the action potential in the atrioventricular node is asso-

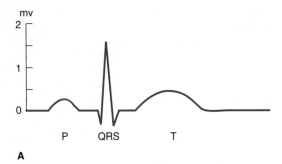

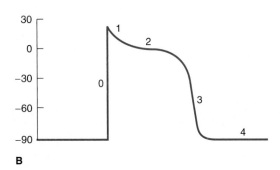

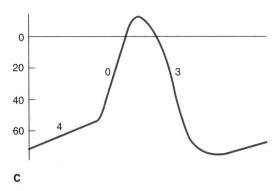

Figure 16–4. A: Typical electrocardiogram, lead II. **B:** Transmembrane potential of cardiac muscle cell. **C:** Transmembrane potential of pacemaker cell. (Reproduced with permission from Stanger P, Van Hare GF: Arrhythmias. Page 1441 in: Rudolph AM (editor): *Rudolph's Pediatrics*, 20th ed. Appleton & Lange, 1996.)

ciated with a lower conduction velocity than elsewhere in the heart, and the atrioventricular node is responsible for introducing a significant delay between atrial and ventricular contraction.

Nodal conduction time is age related. Little is known about conduction time in the node during fetal life. However, atrioventricular nodal conduction is normally quite short at birth (20 to 40 msec) but increases progressively with age to as long as 200 msec in adulthood. Conduction in the distal conducting system (His bundle and bundle branches), normally 20 msec at birth, increases to 40 to 50 msec in adulthood.

In addition to introducing a delay, the atrioventricular node also limits the number of atrial impulses that may conduct to the ventricles. This function is adaptive; arrhythmias, such as atrial flutter or fibrillation, occur with atrial rates as high as 500 to 600 beats per minute. Refractoriness in the atrioventricular node limits the resulting ventricular rate. Refractoriness is also age dependent. In late fetal life and in the newborn period, the atrioventricular node may conduct atrial rates as high as 300 beats per minute without block; however, with increasing age, atrioventricular block occurs at progressively slower atrial rates. Atrioventricular node refractoriness is also quite sensitive to autonomic influences.

The adult heart is well invested with nerve fibers, and both the sympathetic and parasympathetic nervous systems influence cardiac automaticity and conduction. Sympathetic fibers reach the sinus node, atrioventricular node, bundle branches, and atrial and ventricular myocardium, whereas vagal fibers are more limited in distribution, affecting mainly the atrial myocardium and the sinus and atrioventricular nodes. Innervation of the ventricles by the vagus nerve is limited, but vagal stimulation can lead to mild decreases in ventricular contractility.

Sympathetic stimulation leads to increased automaticity of both the sinus and atrioventricular nodes, shortening of refractory periods and conduction times through the atrioventricular node, and shortening of refractory periods in both atrial and ventricular myocardium. In short, sympathetic stimulation increases heart rate by increasing both the firing rate of the sinus node and the conduction rate of electricity through the heart. Sympathetic stimulation, of course, may have a host of other effects on the circulation, including increased contractility, changes in blood pressure, and effects on the coronary circulation. Vagal stimulation produces effects that, in general, are the opposite of those produced by sympathetic stimulation. Therefore, decreases in sinus and atrioventricular node automaticity and increases in atrioventricular node conduction time are demonstrable. Sympathetic and parasympathetic effects on the heart are age related and change during fetal and postnatal development. The two opposing influences may develop at different rates during fetal life. Heart rate is thought to be primarily under vagal control at the time of birth. In humans, sympathetic development is not complete at birth but is completed later.

■ DIAGNOSTIC TECHNIQUES

The evaluation of children with suspected heart disease involves the interpretation of many diagnostic studies, at each step forming and refining a list of possible diagnoses on the basis of the information available. In most patients, particularly infants, a probable diagnosis can be obtained before, or even without, obtaining a diagnostic study such as an echocardiogram or cardiac catheterization. Rapid determination of the physiologic process accounting for patients' symptoms is critical so that treatment can begin while a definitive diagnosis is being established.

CLINICAL ASSESSMENT

History

As in all children, a complete birth history is important. With respect to cardiac disease, prematurity and maternal rubella infection increase the risk of PDA and pulmonary artery stenosis. Medications used during pregnancy may act as teratogens. In the family history, siblings or other family members with congenital heart disease should be noted. If an immediate family member is affected, the risk of congenital heart disease increases from 0.8 to 2 to 3%. A history of sudden death, seizures, or arrhythmias may be important in diagnosing the long QT syndromes. The history of the present illness should investigate all possible cardiac symptoms, including failure to thrive, feeding difficulty, cyanosis, squatting, respiratory distress, sweating, pallor, chest pain, palpitations, dizziness, syncope, and exercise intolerance. Specific questions regarding feeding are often helpful, e.g., how much formula an infant consumes per feeding, how long the feeding takes, and what the causes are for slow feeding. Comparing the children's activity level to that of siblings and playmates is a good indicator of early fatigability.

Physical Examination

The approach to physical diagnosis of the cardiovascular system in children must, of course, be tailored to the age of the children as well as to the suspected cardiac problem. Percussion is rarely performed as part of the cardiac examination, particularly in children. Inspection, palpation, and auscultation are discussed later. Various strategies for auscultation may be used, depending on the age of the children. Although adolescents and older school-aged children usually are quite cooperative, younger children may not be. Infants several months of age or younger may be quieted with a pacifier or bottle or by nursing. In older infants, simple eye contact may quiet children for long enough to obtain at least an initial examination. Bright objects brought into the field of view may also help distract infants. Once children are old enough to recognize strangers, careful auscultation may become difficult or impossible. Some children may be quieted by partially redressing them, and others may become quiet when carried down the hall just out of view of their parents.

GENERAL EXAMINATION

Most important, an assessment of whether the children appear healthy or sick should be made, as this will modify the subsequent examination greatly. Children who appear acutely or chronically ill, of course, are approached with a much higher degree of suspicion. Identification of cyanosis is of great importance. Whereas peripheral cyanosis may be due to a cold room (especially in infants), central cyanosis suggests arterial deoxygenation, in turn suggesting cardiac or pulmonary disease, or both. The earliest signs of central cyanosis are in the perioral area. When one is in doubt about the presence of central cyanosis, pulse oximetry, should be obtained (see later). Estimation of oxygen saturation based on the intensity of cyanosis can be quite inaccurate. The intensity of cyanosis is determined by the concentration of desaturated hemoglobin, rather than by the actual oxygen saturation. Therefore, babies who are markedly polycythemic may appear quite cyanotic, despite relatively minor arterial desaturation, because of the high absolute concentration of desaturated hemoglobin. In contrast, infants with significant anemia appear relatively pink despite significant arterial desaturation. The latter situation is most common at 1 to 2 months of age, when normal physiologic anemia may occur. Infants that are somewhat cold, especially in the delivery room, may manifest impressive peripheral cyanosis that does not reflect central arterial desaturation. Arterial desaturation may be a sign of the following:

1. Right-to-left shunting of blood, as is seen in a variety of congenital heart lesions and in persistent fetal circulation

2. Transposition of the great vessels, with delivery of systemic venous blood directly to the aorta

3. Pulmonary venous desaturation due to alveolar hypoxia, as with pulmonary edema, pneumonia, or atelectasis with perfusion of unventilated alveoli

4. A combination of these factors

The degree of *respiratory distress* should be noted, as this can provide a clue to the cause of the problem. Respiratory distress should be distinguished from tachypnea. Distress implies increased work of breathing. This is manifested by increased accessory muscle use, resulting in retractions and nasal flaring, and attempts to increase intrathoracic pressure, causing grunting or sighing. In general, cardiac lesions with reduction in pulmonary blood flow present without significant respiratory distress, unless cyanosis is profound. Lesions with poor systemic output and acidosis, as well as those with increased pulmonary blood flow, present with respiratory distress. Finally, infants with primarily pulmonary disease, as well as those with superimposed pulmonary disease, have respiratory distress.

Careful assessment of the *pulses* and *peripheral perfusion* is crucial in infants with suspected heart disease. The femoral pulses are compared with an upper extremity pulse, usually the radial or brachial pulse, in assessing the possibility of aortic coarctation. Most experienced clinicians believe that such a careful comparison by palpation is more reliable than is the determination of four-limb blood pressures (see later). Conditions that cause a decreased pulse in all sites include any condition with decreased systemic blood flow, especially those lesions that depend on the patency of the ductus arteriosus for systemic flow, such as hypoplastic left ventricle.

Palpation. The precordium is palpated, noting location of the impulse, as well as the degree of precordial activity and the location of any thrills. An impulse from the left ventricle is normally palpated at the apex. An impulse along the left sternal border is due to the right ventricle and is abnormal except in newborns. A right ventricular or increased left ventricular impulse reflects increased volume or pressure load in the particular ventricle. In addition to being present precordially, a thrill may be felt at the suprasternal notch, where it usually indicates aortic or, occasionally, pulmonic valvar stenosis. The presence of a thrill is never normal, indicating severe turbulence of blood flow within the circulation.

The spleen tip may be palpable normally in infants but is otherwise not normally felt. The liver edge is palpated in most infants; it is sharp and normally felt as much as 2 cm below the right costal margin. An enlarged liver is a sign of congestive heart failure (CHF), and the liver edge may often be felt to extend to the left upper quadrant and to below the umbilicus. One should remember that pulmonary hyperinflation, as is seen in asthma and bronchiolitis, may push the liver down and make it appear enlarged when it is not. In this case, the edge is sharp and not felt to the left of the xiphoid process. Also, one should remember that in children with abnormal cardiac and abdominal situs, the liver may be entirely to the left or mainly at the midline.

Auscultation. A complete cardiac auscultatory examination includes use of both the bell (low frequency sounds) and diaphragm (high frequency sounds)of the stethoscope in each of the precordial areas. These areas typically are referred to as the aortic, pulmonic, tricuspid, and mitral areas; however, in children it is best to describe them by chest landmarks, because in many types of congenital heart disease the cardiac structures may not be positioned normally. Therefore, one listens at the upper right and left sternal borders (second intercostal space), along the lower left sternal border (third and fourth intercostal space), and at the apex and describes the position where the murmur or cardiac sound is maximal. One also listens for radiation of murmurs to both clavicles, axillae, and lung fields (pulmonary in origin) and to the carotid arteries (aortic in origin).

In children, although the sounds are louder than in adults, the heart rate is significantly faster, making accurate auscultation challenging. At each location, one should pay attention to each sound separately before moving. For example, one should concentrate on the first heart sound, ignoring all other sounds, then concentrate on the second heart sound, and so on. In this way, one may avoid missing more subtle findings in patients with prominent murmurs.

First heart sound. The first heart sound is caused by closure of the mitral and tricuspid valves (Figure 16–5). It is normally heard maximally at the apex, is of low frequency, and is usually single, although splitting is common. Splitting of S_1 may be differentiated from early systolic clicks by the low frequency of the sound, and the location nearer the apex. Variability of intensity of the first heart sound may be caused by atrioventricular dissociation due to complete atrioventricular block.

Second heart sound. The second heart sounds is caused by closure of the aortic and pulmonic valves (see Figure 16–5). The importance of accurately assessing the second heart sound cannot be overemphasized. Normally, in children and infants beyond several weeks of age, the sec-

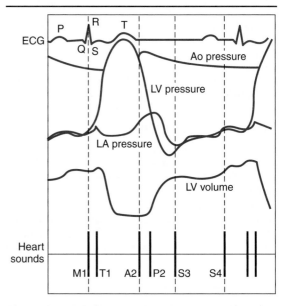

Figure 16–5. Timing of cardiac events. The changes of left atrial, left ventricular, and aortic pressure and left ventricular volume are related to the electrocardiogram (ECG) and to the heart sounds. The timing of the four heart sounds is represented by the vertical dashed lines. M1, T1–mitral, and tricuspid components of first sound; A2, P2–aortic, and pulmonary components of second sound; S3, S4–third, and fourth heart sounds.

ond heart sound is split with inspiration and narrow or single with expiration, and the aortic and pulmonic components are of about equal intensity and frequency. It is best heard at the base, and splitting is best evaluated at the upper left sternal border. Pulmonary hypertension causes earlier closure and accentuation of P_2, and so one may hear a loud and single second heart sound. Such a finding is of crucial importance, particularly in patients with correctable congenital heart defects, such as atrioventricular canal defect, as it involves the risk of progression to irreversible pulmonary vascular disease. In infants and children who have a normal arterial oxygen saturation, the loudness of the second heart sound often is more helpful than splitting, which can be masked by the fast heart rate. Pulmonic stenosis may cause delay and softening of P_2. Transposition of the great vessels may be associated with a single second heart sound at the upper left sternal border because of malposition of the semilunar valve. Splitting often is appreciated in such patients at the third intercostal space at the left sternal border, with a soft P_2 due to the posterior position of the pulmonic valve in transposition.

Third and fourth heart sounds. The third heart sound is caused by vibrations in the ventricle that occur in mid diastole at the end of rapid passive filling. These vibrations are due to an increased rate and volume of filling of the ventricle as occurs with a high cardiac output, mitral or tricuspid regurgitation, and ventricular dysfunction. In children, a third heart sound is often heard normally at the apex. Fourth heart sounds, caused by vibrations in the ventricle that occur during rapid atrial contraction, are not normally heard. A loud fourth heart sound suggests the presence of poor ventricular compliance, as might be present in dilated cardiomyopathy or CHF. Soft middiastolic murmurs often are mistaken for third or fourth heart sounds and are caused by increased flow across a normal tricuspid or mitral valve, as might occur in atrial or ventricular septal defects with a left-to-right shunt.

Clicks. Ejection and nonejection clicks may be appreciated. Ejection clicks occur early in systole, just after the first heart sound, and are thought to be caused by sudden tensing of the walls of the great vessel during ventricular ejection, rather than by actual valve movement. Aortic ejection clicks are heard best at the third left intercostal space, are of a slightly higher frequency than are first heart sounds, and do not vary with respiration. They are caused by valvar AS or by idiopathic aortic root dilatation. Pulmonic ejection clicks are heard best at the upper left sternal border, are quite high frequency, and become softer with inspiration. They are due to valvar pulmonic stenosis or to pulmonary root dilation. Nonejection clicks, also known as midsystolic clicks, occur well after the first heart sound, are heard best in upright or standing patients, are of medium frequency, and typically do not vary with respiration. They usually are due to mitral valve prolapse.

Murmurs. Murmurs, particularly nonpathologic ones, are a common occurrence in both neonates and children (see "Asymptomatic Murmur," later). The evaluation and description of murmurs involve assessment of several factors. The first is the *timing* of the murmur in the cardiac cycle as systolic, diastolic, or continuous (during both systole and diastole without interruption). The loudness of the murmur is described from grades 1 to 6: Grade 1 murmurs are clearly softer than the heart sounds; grade 2 murmurs are approximately as loud as the heart sounds; grade 3 murmurs are clearly louder than are the heart sounds; thrills are present with grade 4 murmurs; grade 5 murmurs can be heard with the edge of the stethoscope; and grade 6 murmurs can be heard with the stethoscope off the chest or with the naked ear. Grade 5 and 6 murmurs are very rare. The *frequency* of each murmur should be assessed. This may also be referred to as the "pitch" of the murmur. In general, the frequency will be determined by the difference in pressure between the two chambers creating the murmur. Therefore, in patients with small VSDs, a high-pitched murmur will be heard because of the difference between systemic pressure in the left ventricle and normal low pressure in the right ventricle. High frequency murmurs are heard loudest with the diaphragm piece of the stethoscope, low frequency murmurs with the bell. In addition, *form* or *shape* of the murmur (diamond-shaped or crescendo–decrescendo murmurs are termed *ejection murmurs*) and the relation to the first heart sound (beginning with the first heart sound, obscuring the first heart sound, or well separated from the first heart sound)should be described. In general, ejection murmurs are due to semilunar valve or vessel stenosis. Murmurs that start with the first heart sound but do not obscure it and are not of ejection quality are termed *long systolic,* or *decrescendo,* murmurs and are caused by atrioventricular valve insufficiency. Murmurs that obscure the first heart sound at the point when they are maximal are termed *holosystolic* murmurs, even if they end slightly before the second heart sound, and are usually caused by some form of ventricular septal defect.

Finally, the *position* and *radiation* of the murmur, defined as the origin of the murmur, should be noted. They usually are determined by the area in which the murmur is loudest. Some murmurs, however, are heard throughout the chest. In these cases, the area in which the frequency or pitch of the murmur is highest defines the origin, because high frequencies transmit less well than do low frequencies. Certain murmurs have classic patterns of radiation, such as valvar pulmonary stenosis (PS) or pulmonary artery stenosis to the axillae, and valvar or supravalvar AS to the carotids.

An example of a complete description of a murmur would be: "grade 2/6 medium-frequency, short systolic murmur at the lower left sternal border without radiation." This description is consistent with a small muscular ventricular septal defect.

Early diastolic decrescendo murmurs that start with A_2 or P_2 are caused by semilunar valve regurgitation. Mid-diastolic murmurs may be caused by atrioventricular valve stenosis or by increased flow across a nonstenotic atrioventricular valve, as might be heard in patients with left-to-right shunts.

Continuous murmurs are most commonly caused by a PDA or by some other condition in which shunting continues throughout the cardiac cycle, such as with a surgical aortopulmonary (AP) shunt or a pulmonary arteriovenous (AV) fistula. Continuous murmurs should be differentiated from the coexistence of separate systolic and diastolic murmurs, as can occur with an abnormal aortic or pulmonary valve that is both stenotic and regurgitant.

Blood pressures. Blood pressure should be routinely measured in all children, even when heart disease is not suspected (see screening procedures, Chap. 1). Auscultatory measurements in infants can be difficult, however systolic measurements can always be obtained by palpation. Using an appropriate-sized cuff for the children is essential for accuracy. Blood pressure measurement is most helpful for following changes in hemodynamic condition and for diagnosing coarctation of the aorta. The act of inflating a cuff in conscious infants (either manually or by machine) often is associated with agitation and straining on the part of the infants. Because nonsimultaneous measurements reflect different hemodynamic states, comparisons of upper and lower extremity pressures must be made carefully. One approach to increase the reliability of such comparisons is to use two automatic machines simultaneously on the upper and lower extremities and then to switch the machines and repeat the procedure. The difference between the two readings is averaged to correct for intermachine variation. Normally the leg has a slightly higher pressure than does the arm, because it is fed by a larger artery with a more rapid transmission of the fluid wave. An upper-to-lower-extremity difference of ≥10 mm Hg is considered significant. Children with mild-to-moderate coarctation of the aorta often are asymptomatic until they have hypertension in the arm during puberty. For children with suspected tamponade or other significant hemodynamic instability, the blood pressure measurement should include an assessment for an abnormal pulsus paradoxicus. A pulsus paradoxicus is an exaggeration of the normal decrease in blood pressure that occurs during inspiration. It is determined by the difference in systolic blood pressure during expiration and that during inspiration (with patients breathing normally). A value ≥ 10 to 15 mm Hg is considered abnormal.

LABORATORY ASSESSMENT

Radiography

The chest radiograph may provide subtle information concerning possible types of heart disease, but the most common use is for assessment of heart size and determination of pulmonary blood flow. Figure 16–6 shows the cardiac structures visible on a posteroanterior chest film. To determine heart size, the width of the cardiothymic silhouette is measured and compared with the width of the chest at its largest dimension. The ratio should be 0.65 or less. As true posteroanterior projections are unusual in infants, the measurement is made using an anteroposterior chest film. The most reliable measurements are from films on which a good inspiration was obtained, with the diaphragms seen at the ninth or tenth posterior rib margin. The heart may falsely appear enlarged if the film is taken on expiration. One should remember that the heart, thymus, and pericardial fluid may be seen as part of the cardiothymic silhouette. The degree of pulmonary vascularity should be noted as normal, increased, or decreased. In addition, the presence or absence of interstitial fluid, which is seen in pulmonary edema, should be noted.

The position of the cardiac apex on the cardiac silhouette should be evaluated; right ventricular enlargement causes an upturned apex, whereas left ventricular enlargement pushes the apex to the diaphragm. The size and distribution of pulmonary vasculature, particularly in cyanotic infants, can give clues to etiology. For example, patients with obstruction to pulmonary blood flow, as seen in tetralogy of Fallot (TOF) and related lesions, often

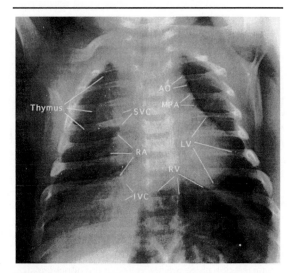

Figure 16–6. Posteroanterior (PA) chest x-ray of a normal heart. The superior vena cava (SVC) and right atrium (RA) form the main right heart border. The left heart border is comprised of the aorta (AO) and main pulmonary artery (MPA) superiorly, and the left ventricle (LV) inferiorly. The right ventricle (RV) comprises most of the diaphragmatic surface.

have a hypoplastic pulmonary vasculature, termed *black lung fields*. Patients with transposition complexes, however, have large pulmonary arteries, resulting in a picture of hypervascularity and white lung fields. The presence or absence of the pulmonary artery knob at the upper left heart border provides information regarding the position or size of the main pulmonary artery. Finally, the width of the mediastinum can provide information regarding great artery position and size. A narrow mediastinum, for example, often is seen in transposition of the great arteries because the great vessels are superimposed in the anteroposterior projection.

Electrocardiography

The interpretation of pediatric electrocardiograms (ECGs) is a large and complicated topic that is covered only superficially here. When interpreting an ECG, it is important to develop a stepwise, systematic approach, to ensure that all pertinent findings are seen. First, the rate should be determined as normal, fast, or slow. Second, the rhythm should be determined as regular or irregular: If the rhythm is irregular, does it display a repeating pattern or is it inconsistent? The association of P and QRS waves should be determined: Are they at the same rate? Is there a 1:1 relation, a 2, 3, or 4:1 relation, or no relation? Next, the P waves should be evaluated. In normal sinus rhythm, the P wave is upright in leads I, II, and III. Tall P waves in lead II indicate right atrial enlargement, whereas prolonged (wide) and biphasic P waves suggest left atrial enlargement. The PR interval should be measured and compared with normal values for age. The duration of the QRS and the QT interval also should be measured, and the QT corrected for heart rate. Machine interpretation of the interval should be confirmed, as errors are common. The QRS axis should be determined (Figure 16–7). The presence of

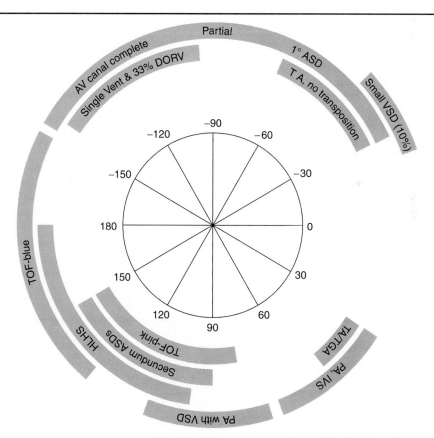

Figure 16–7. Typical frontal plane electrocardiogram axis in children with various congenital heart defects in the newborn period. 1 = primum; ASD = atrial septal defect; AV = atrioventricular; DORV = double-outlet right ventricle; HLHS = hypoplastic left heart syndrome; IVS = intact ventricular septum; PA = pulmonic atresia; TA = tricuspid atresia; TGA = transposition of the great arteries; TOF = tetralogy of Fallot; Vent = ventricle; VSD = ventricular septal defect.

normal septal Q waves in leads II, III, aVF, V5, and V6 should be sought. The precordial R- and S-wave amplitudes should be compared against normal values. Finally, the ST segments and T-wave pattern should be determined, particularly in the right precordial leads.

The utility of the ECG in the diagnosis of congenital heart disease is largely in the diagnosis of ventricular hypertrophy. Normal newborns have relative predominance of the right ventricle over the left ventricle. This predominance shifts to left ventricular predominance in the first year of life because of the decrease in pulmonary arterial pressure, and consequent decrease in right ventricular systolic pressure leads to a decrease in right ventricular muscle mass. All ECG interpretations in children must be made relative to the normal right or left ventricular predominance that exists at that particular age. Therefore, one never interprets a normal newborn ECG as showing "right ventricular hypertrophy, normal for age." Right ventricular hypertrophy at that age would require larger-than-normal right ventricular forces for a newborn. A rough idea of ventricular predominance may be determined by remembering that the right ventricle is oriented to the right, superior, and anterior, whereas the left ventricle is oriented to the left, inferior, and posterior. One chooses leads for examination that represent these orthogonal directions. Lead V5 is a good right-left lead, aVF is a good superior-inferior lead, and V2 is a good anteroposterior lead. One may then compare the forces present in these leads with normal standards for age to arrive at a judgment of relative ventricular predominance (Table 16–3). One may also examine the T-wave axis as an aid in diagnosing right ventricular hypertrophy, again remembering the normal shift that occurs with development. Normally, the T wave is upright in leads V1, V3R, and V4R for the first week after birth but inverts by 8-days and remains inverted until about 8 years of age. If it is upright between 8 days

and 8 years, right ventricular hypertrophy is likely. Finally, the axis may be an aid to diagnosis in newborns (Figure 16–7).

Unfortunately, with the exception of its use in the diagnosis of arrhythmias, the ECG rarely is diagnostic in the evaluation of the newborn with cardiac disease. Several points deserve emphasis, however. Although one might suppose that a lesion obstructing the left ventricle (e.g., aortic coarctation) would produce left ventricular hypertrophy, in the newborn such lesions are seen more often with right ventricular hypertrophy. This is most likely because in the intrauterine circulation, the right ventricle is responsible for a large amount of the combined ventricular output when the left ventricle is obstructed. The same often is true of lesions obstructing the right ventricle, which may be associated with left ventricular hypertrophy. The ECG picture varies a great deal within each of the diagnostic groups, and the ECG pattern may be completely normal in infants with serious disease, such as transposition or hypoplastic left side of the heart syndrome. In practice, the clinician uses the ECG as a confirmatory test to establish that heart disease is present and that the ECG fits the suspected diagnosis. An example is the pattern seen in infants with complete atrioventricular canal defects, who have an abnormally superior axis in the frontal plane (northwest axis). The physician should consider children with signs of a VSD, including a loud holosystolic murmur, signs of CHF, and little or no cyanosis at 1 month of age. If the ECG shows an abnormal superior axis, the diagnosis is probably atrioventricular canal defect rather than simple VSD.

Pulse Oximetry

Pulse oximetry provides an excellent method for assessing arterial oxygen saturation noninvasively by using a probe attached to the palm or foot of infants. Even though the

Table 16–3. Normal Electrocardiographic Voltages by Age (95th Percentile)

Age	V5		AVF		V2	
	R	S	R	S	R	S
0–24 h	18.0	24.0	*	*	28.1	33.8
1–7 d	19.3	16.2	10.5	3.1	31.1	34.1
8–30 d	27.0	12.3	12.4	3.8	29.0	25.7
1–3 mo	20.7	12.7	13.8	3.1	27.4	34.1
3–6 mo	25.5	15.4	18.5	3.4	28.6	26.5
6–12 mo	24.7	8.0	16.4	3.7	24.4	30.1
1–3 y	27.7	7.0	16.6	3.8	22.5	32.1
3–5 y	30.0	5.8	16.7	3.0	22.8	28.8
5–8 y	31.2	6.6	14.8	3.4	22.0	35.3
8–12 y	30.0	4.4	17.8	3.7	16.9	35.6
12–16 y	26.7	5.0	19.7	3.8	18.4	41.0

Reproduced with permission from Liebman J, et al (eds): *Pediatric Electrocardiography*. Baltimore, Williams & Wilkins, 1982.

measurement of arterial blood gas tension is always useful, pulse oximetry avoids a painful needle stick, which can cause agitation, struggling, and breath-holding, making such direct measurements somewhat unreliable. Measurements should always be made from the right hand and from a foot to provide information about ductus arteriosus flow patterns. For example, patients with severe aortic coarctation or interruption and a PDA providing flow from the pulmonary artery to the descending aorta have a much lower saturation in the feet than they do in the hands. In contrast, patients with transposition may have a much higher saturation in the feet than they do in the hands, because pulmonary arterial blood is highly saturated and passes from the pulmonary artery into the ductus and descending aorta. To avoid problems created by intermachine variability, it is helpful to use two machines simultaneously and then switch the leads. The final reading is the average difference between the upper and lower extremity readings.

Hyperoxic Test

The hyperoxic test is a method to help differentiate blood oxygen desaturation due to cardiac disease from that due to pulmonary disease. It does not distinguish this difference alone, however, and always should be interpreted in the context of all other data. Right-arm and lower-body measurements always should be made simultaneously to evaluate the pattern of ductus arteriosus shunting. Pulse oximetry is sufficient if the saturation measures less than 92 to 93%; otherwise, an arterial blood gas value should be obtained. Measurements are made at baseline conditions, ideally room air, and then after breathing 100% oxygen for approximately 5 min. Patients with pulmonary disease alone usually have an increase in partial pressure of oxygen (PO_2) >20 to 30 mm Hg or an increase in oxygen saturation >10%. Those with a fixed right-to-left shunt may have a small increase in oxygenation, but it usually is less than these amounts. The term *fixed right-to-left shunt* refers to lesions in which no increase is possible in either pulmonary blood flow or in mixing of systemic and pulmonary venous return. In such patients, therefore, pulmonary venous blood is already nearly completely oxygenated, and little additional oxygenation is possible. A good example is TOF, in which there is a high resistance to pulmonary flow because of PS and a right-to-left shunt through a VSD. Patients with large left-to-right shunts and systemic hypoxemia may have large increases in oxygenation because added inspired oxygen normalizes pulmonary venous saturation, which may be low because of pulmonary edema and the accompanying oxygen diffusion gradient. Patients with mixing of pulmonary and systemic venous return and no obstruction to pulmonary flow may also have a large increase in oxygen saturation because additional inspired oxygen may cause a large increase in pulmonary venous PO_2. In addition, oxygen may cause pulmonary vasodilation and a further increase in pulmonary blood flow. The best example of this phenomenon is total anomalous pulmonary venous return (TAPVR) without obstruction, in which there is a large amount of pulmonary flow, but cyanosis is present because of mixing that occurs in the right atrium. Supplemental inspired oxygen may increase arterial saturation somewhat. The same effect may be seen with the use of pulmonary vasodilators, such as prostaglandin E_1 (PGE_1).

A variant of this test involves repeating the measurements while making the children cry. This is particularly helpful at increasing differential saturation caused by right-to-left shunting through a PDA. If either the upper or lower body is predominantly supplied by ductal flow, the saturation usually will decrease, whereas the other saturation (that supplied by pulmonary venous blood) will remain stable.

Echocardiography

Cardiac ultrasonography is the definitive diagnostic procedure for the evaluation of infants with suspected cardiac disease. It is noninvasive and safe, can be done at the bedside of sick newborn infants, and can be used successfully in premature infants of all sizes. The resolution is sufficient to make complete anatomic diagnoses in even the smallest hearts. Doppler echocardiography and color Doppler flow mapping are now able to study flow patterns for the assessment of valve function and areas of shunting or obstruction. The quality of the diagnostic information is such that most infants who previously would have undergone cardiac catheterization now undergo cardiac surgery on the basis of the echocardiogram alone. There are two important issues to note concerning echocardiography. First, it is somewhat expensive; therefore, it should not be used in every infant with the slightest suspicion of cardiac disease. Patients should be referred for echocardiography based upon a complete cardiac evaluation, including physical examination, oxygen saturation measurement, and other modalities. Second, echocardiography must be guided by knowledge of infants' presenting signs and the results of the evaluation to date. Knowing patients' clinical statuses allows the experienced echocardiographer to have an appropriate differential diagnosis and ensure a complete and accurate examination. Otherwise, important and often subtle findings may be missed.

Echocardiography is also used to guide both interventional catheterization and surgical procedures. Many institutions routinely perform balloon atrial septostomy for D-transposition or other lesions under echocardiographic guidance rather than catheterization. In addition, the advent of transesophageal echocardiography allows evaluation of detailed anatomy in the operative suite and has decreased the incidence of postoperative residual defects substantially by allowing immediate assessment of the surgical repair.

Catheterization

The need for cardiac catheterization to diagnose cardiac defects has decreased dramatically, as the accuracy of ultrasound technology has allowed for more complete noninvasive initial evaluation. Certain features, however, remain beyond the scope of echocardiography, such as measurement of vascular pressures and accurate shunt flows. In addition, the peripheral pulmonary vasculature is best viewed by angiography. Finally, postoperative evaluation often includes catheterization because scarring can impair ultrasound examination. Therapeutic catheterization has become very successful at correcting or palliating several conditions previously amenable only to surgical therapy. Valvar aortic and pulmonary stenosis is best treated initially with balloon valvuloplasty performed in the catheterization laboratory. Closure of PDA in nonpremature infants is accomplished easily, with minimal expense and hospital stay, by using implantable coils. Closure of secundum ASDs with devices delivered percutaneously is becoming routine in some centers, making ASD repair an outpatient procedure. Closure of ventricular septal defects, although possible by catheter interventional techniques, remains experimental.

Catheterization can be performed safely at any age. In newborn infants, the umbilical vessels provide ready access to both venous and arterial circulation. When this route is unavailable, arterial access in infants is associated with increased risk of pulse loss. Currently, few patients require intubation and mechanical ventilation for catheterization. Patients with inferior and superior vena caval obstruction can be catheterized through the hepatic veins (transhepatic technique).

■ COMMON PROBLEMS

INFANTS WITH CYANOSIS

Cyanosis is a bluish discoloration of the skin and mucous membranes caused by deoxygenated or reduced hemoglobin (for a detailed discussion, see Chap. 4). It is crucial to determine rapidly the cause of cyanosis in a newborn, as it can be life threatening. Initial assessment should include evaluation of the extent and location of cyanosis (central versus peripheral), heart rate, presence and intensity of pulses, blood pressure, respiratory rate, and presence of respiratory distress. This evaluation, together with a few laboratory studies, can pinpoint the cause of the cyanosis (Figure 16–8). This discussion is focused upon the children with cyanosis due to cardiac disease. For a more complete discussion of the noncardiac causes of cyanosis see Chaps. 10 and 17.

Peripheral cyanosis refers to discoloration of the skin, particularly the extremities, whereas *central cyanosis* refers to involvement of the mucous membranes of the mouth and tongue. Skin color in newborns is very sensitive to changes in temperature and peripheral arterial or venous vasoconstriction. Isolated peripheral cyanosis is usually not associated with structural heart disease but can be caused by low cardiac output with decreased peripheral perfusion, as with sepsis, cardiomyopathy, hypocalcemia, or pneumopericardium. It can be caused by decreased peripheral perfusion with normal cardiac output (e.g., with hypoglycemia or hypothermia). In addition, abnormally high amounts of deoxygenated hemoglobin in the blood (e.g., with polycythemia or methemoglobinemia), may cause profound peripheral cyanosis.

Central cyanosis suggests hypoxia due to lung disease or structural heart disease resulting in some degree of right-to-left shunting. Differentiating between these two can be difficult. Any infants with significant central cyanosis and no respiratory distress have structural heart disease until proved otherwise. Severe polycythemia or methemoglobinemia can present this way, although it would be unusual. If infants have respiratory distress and tachypnea, with or without retractions, an arterial blood gas value should be obtained from either the right radial or temporal artery. Significant elevation in partial pressure of arterial carbon dioxide ($PaCO_2$) suggests lung disease, but if the $PaCO_2$ is normal or only mildly elevated, a hyperoxia test should be performed. Infants should be placed in 100% oxygen, and simultaneous blood gases drawn from both the right radial and pedal (or umbilical) arteries. If the PaO_2 is >150 mm Hg in the right radial (or temporal) arterial blood, structural heart disease is much less likely.

If the initial evaluation suggests that central cyanosis is due to structural heart disease, treatment with intravenous (IV) fluids (80 mL/kg/d) and prostaglandin E_1 (PGE_1; 0.05 µg/kg/min) should be initiated, as should consultation with a pediatric cardiologist. Prostaglandin E_1 is a potent vasodilator, and infants often need an IV fluid bolus of 10 to 20 mL/kg crystalloid at its initiation to maintain an adequate intravascular volume. In addition, because PGE_1 may cause apnea, intubation with mechanical ventilation may be necessary. Oxygen should be given in nontoxic doses (60% FiO_2) to minimize the effect of any associated lung disease; one should remember, however, oxygen will have little effect on cyanosis because of right-to-left shunting from structural heart disease. Metabolic acidosis should be corrected first with adequate fluid administration; if there is no response, IV sodium bicarbonate or another buffer should be given.

Once treatment has been initiated, a more definitive diagnosis of the type of congenital heart disease can be

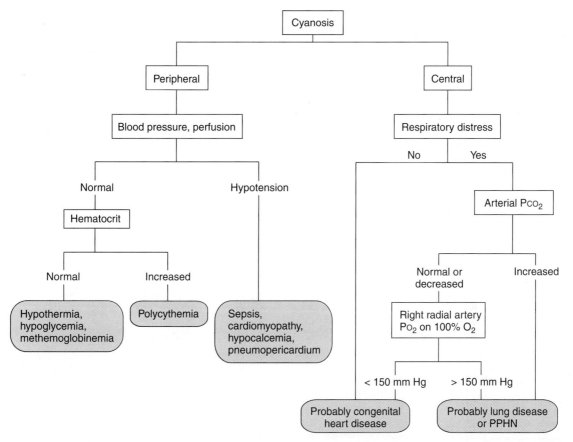

Figure 16–8. Algorithm showing evaluation of infants with cyanosis. Pco_2 = partial pressure of carbon dioxide; PPHN = persistent pulmonary hypertension of the newborn; Po_2 = partial pressure of oxygen.

made with further evaluation, including a chest radiograph and ECG (Figure 16–9). In general, infants who have cyanosis as their most prominent presenting feature for congenital heart disease fall into one of two groups: those with decreased pulmonary blood flow and those with normal or increased pulmonary blood flow.

Decreased Pulmonary Blood Flow

Pulmonary blood flow may be reduced in lesions associated with obstruction on the right side of the heart, such as atresia, hypoplasia, or stenosis of either the tricuspid valve, right ventricle, pulmonary valve, or pulmonary arteries. Infants with these lesions will all have decreased pulmonary blood flow on chest radiographs and obligatory right-to-left shunting across either the atrial or ventricular septum causing cyanosis. These lesions include TOF, critical valvar PS, pulmonary atresia with an intact ventricular septum (PA/IVS) or with a VSD (PA/VSD), tricuspid

atresia (TA), single ventricle physiology with associated subvalvar or valvar PS (SV with PS), and Ebstein anomaly (dysplastic tricuspid valve resulting in insufficiency, and subvalvar PS). Electrocardiogram findings can differentiate this group further. Infants with TOF, PS, or PA/VSD have findings of right ventricular hypertrophy and right axis deviation (>120°).

TETRALOGY OF FALLOT

Tetralogy of Fallot consists of four main features: PS, a large VSD, right ventricular hypertrophy, and dextroposition of the aorta so that it overrides the septal defect. The PS causes a systolic murmur that is easily audible over the left upper sternal border. Because of the large, unrestrictive VSD and the overriding aorta, there is significant right-to-left shunting through the ventricular septum, causing cyanosis. Patients may present late with hypercyanotic episodes, known as "tetralogy spells," in which vigorous crying results in increasing cyanosis because of reduced

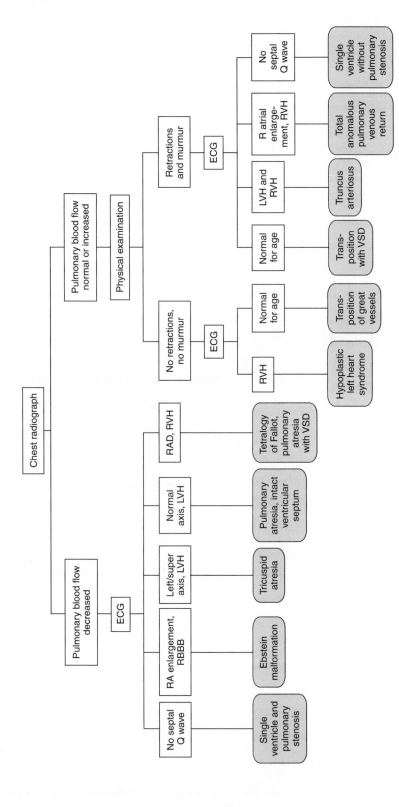

Figure 16–9. Algorithm of approach to specific diagnosis in infants with cyanotic congenital heart diseases. ECG = electrocardiogram; LVH = left ventricular hypertrophy; RAD = right axis deviation; RBBB = right bundle-branch block; RVH = right ventricular hypertrophy; VSD = ventricular septal defect.

pulmonary blood flow. Hypercyanotic spells are treated acutely with administration of oxygen, morphine for sedation, and phenylephrine to increase systemic vascular resistance. Pulmonary atresia with VSD is similar to TOF except that all pulmonary flow comes from either the ductus arteriosus or from aorta to pulmonary artery collateral vessels. Therefore, instead of a systolic PS murmur at the left upper sternal border, there may be a continuous murmur under the left clavicle or over the back because of continuous flow through the ductus arteriosus or collateral arterial circulation. The course of treatment is determined by the clinical status and the exact anatomy, particularly of the right ventricular outflow tract. Treatment options include a systemic-to-pulmonary shunt, balloon dilation of the pulmonary valve, and primary definitive repair.

PULMONARY VALVE STENOSIS AND ATRESIA

Infants with critical pulmonary valve stenosis have a systolic murmur over the left upper sternal border and may be profoundly cyanotic because of right-to-left shunting at the atrial level as the ductus arteriosus closes. Severe right ventricular hypertension, much greater than systemic levels, may result in tricuspid regurgitation. The treatment of choice is catheter balloon dilation of the stenotic valve. Infants may remain mildly cyanotic for several weeks after treatment because of slow regression of the severe right ventricular hypertrophy, which causes persistent right-to-left shunting through the foramen ovale.

An axis of 0 to 120° on the ECG with evidence of left ventricular hypertrophy suggests the diagnosis of PA/IVS. The right ventricle is hypoplastic with no egress, so the pressure commonly is suprasystemic, leading to tricuspid regurgitation, which may produce a high-pitched systolic murmur at the left lower sternal border. Cyanosis is due to right-to-left shunting through the atrial septum, and pulmonary blood flow is supplied by a PDA. Sinusoidal vessels may connect the right ventricle with the coronary arteries; this may limit the surgical options and ultimate prognosis. The initial treatment is to increase pulmonary blood flow with PGE_1; then, a surgical shunt from the systemic to pulmonary artery is performed.

TRICUSPID ATRESIA

In this lesion, the pulmonary blood flow is supplied either through a ventricular septal defect or a PDA. Tricuspid atresia often is associated with PS or a restrictive VSD, so pulmonary flow is obstructed. The exam is that of cyanosis with the high-pitched murmur of a small VSD at the lower sternal border, often with an associated thrill. The ECG in infants with TA and normally related great arteries shows a leftward superior axis (0 to −90) and left ventricular hypertrophy. Because these infants have no communication between their right atrium and right ventricle, all systemic venous blood crosses the atrial septum and mixes with pulmonary venous blood. The initial treatment is to increase pulmonary blood flow with prostaglandin infusion; then, an AP communication should be achieved surgically.

EBSTEIN ANOMALY

Ebstein anomaly should be suspected if the ECG shows right bundle branch block with right atrial enlargement. Up to 30% of patients will have delta waves suggestive of Wolff-Parkinson-White syndrome. The tricuspid valve is malformed, with displacement of the septal and posterior leaflets into the right ventricle. This results in tricuspid regurgitation, particularly in newborn infants with high pulmonary artery pressures. As pulmonary pressures decrease during the first week after birth, cyanosis and tricuspid regurgitation may resolve. Almost the entire right ventricle may be part of the right atrium ("atrialized"), resulting in severe tricuspid regurgitation. The displaced leaflet may obstruct the right ventricular outflow tract, further limiting pulmonary blood flow and increasing the right-to-left shunt across the atrial septum. These patients require a surgical systemic-to-pulmonary shunt to maintain adequate pulmonary blood flow.

Normal or Increased Pulmonary Blood Flow

The second group of infants with cyanotic congenital heart disease comprises those with normal to increased pulmonary blood flow. Pulmonary and systemic venous blood mixes within the heart chambers. These conditions include transposition of the great arteries, truncus arteriosus, TAPVR, hypoplastic left side of the heart syndrome, and single ventricle. They can be differentiated easily by physical examination and ECG findings (see Figure 16–9).

TRANSPOSITION OF THE GREAT ARTERIES

Infants with transposition of the great arteries, in which the aorta arises from the right ventricle and the pulmonary artery arises from the left ventricle, have a normal ECG for age and often no audible murmur. Because the desaturated systemic venous blood is delivered directly to the aorta, these infants can be profoundly cyanotic unless they have mixing of their saturated pulmonary venous blood through an ASD, VSD, or PDA. If there is considerable mixing, cyanosis may not be marked; if mixing is minimal, severe cyanosis occurs. In the immediate newborn period, PGE_1 may relieve cyanosis by opening the ductus. Emergency management of profoundly cyanotic infants with transposition of the great arteries involves tearing a hole in the atrial septum by performing a balloon atrial septostomy. The cardiologist may do this procedure either at the bedside with the use of ultrasound guidance or in the catheterization laboratory. Definitive treatment is a surgical switch of the pulmonary artery and aorta so that they arise from the correct ventricles.

TRUNCUS ARTERIOSUS COMMUNIS

In truncus arteriosus, there is no pulmonary valve. The pulmonary artery arises directly from the aorta (trunk) just above the aortic (truncal) valve, which straddles a large VSD. Complete mixing occurs in the proximal ascending aorta, causing cyanosis. The ECG typically shows biventricular hypertrophy, and there may be a loud systolic click on examination because of the large anterior abnormal aortic (truncal) valve. Definitive treatment for these patients is surgical correction, consisting of closure of the VSD and placement of an artificial pulmonary artery and valve between the right ventricle and the branch pulmonary arteries.

TOTAL ANOMALOUS PULMONARY VENOUS RETURN

Infants with TAPVR typically have right atrial enlargement and right ventricular hypertrophy on ECG. The chest radiograph characteristically shows a normal heart size with pulmonary edema, which is often severe. The pulmonary veins, instead of entering the left atrium normally, form a confluence behind the left atrium and drain to the right atrium. This may be via a vertical vein to the left innominate vein; to the superior vena cava, coronary sinus, or right atrium directly; or via a common pulmonary vein, which descends below the diaphragm and joins with the inferior vena cava via a portal vein and the ductus venosus. Complete mixing takes place in the right atrium with right-to-left shunting through the foramen ovale to fill the left ventricle and maintain an adequate cardiac output. If there is obstruction to the pulmonary venous return, as is almost always present with veins draining below the diaphragm, cyanosis is prominent because of both complete mixing and respiratory distress associated with pulmonary edema. If the hole in the atrial septum is restrictive, the left ventricle cannot fill and cardiac output will be compromised. Infants with this lesion can be mistaken for those with severe pulmonary hypertension of the newborn, since the presentation is similar. Echocardiography is generally performed before initiating extracorporeal support (ECMO) for this reason. Definitive treatment of TAPVR is surgical anastomosis of the pulmonary vein confluence directly to the left atrium. Total anomalous pulmonary venous return with obstruction remains one of the few cardiac surgical emergencies.

HYPOPLASTIC LEFT HEART SYNDROME

Hypoplastic left heart syndrome can also present with cyanosis if the ductus arteriosus remains open. Because there is obstruction at the mitral valve and hypoplastic left ventricle, all pulmonary venous blood shunts through the atrial septum to mix in the right atrium. Total systemic blood flow is derived through the ductus arteriosus from the pulmonary artery. If the ductus arteriosus is open, the patients will have normal pulses and a normal examination except for cyanosis. The ECG usually shows right ventricular hypertrophy with markedly decreased left-sided voltages, but occasionally can be normal. As the ductus closes, these infants have shock because systemic blood flow is reduced. Oxygen administration may result in ductus arteriosus constriction and therefore must be used with caution. Treatment options include a series of two or three palliative surgeries to create single ventricle physiology or heart transplantation.

SINGLE VENTRICLE

Infants with a single ventricle typically have an associated ASD as well as atrioventricular valve abnormalities; therefore, mixing occurs both at the atrial and ventricular levels. Electrocardiogram findings vary but always show an absence of the normal Q wave in the lateral chest leads (V6 and V7), indicating the absence of a ventricular septum. Infants may have associated valvar or subvalvar PS, causing reduced pulmonary flow, or no associated stenosis with markedly increased pulmonary flow. Initial treatment is determined by the amount of pulmonary blood flow. For infants with too much pulmonary blood flow, pulmonary artery band surgery is performed to reduce flow. For those with too little pulmonary blood flow, a shunt is placed from the aorta to the pulmonary artery to augment flow.

INFANTS WITH SHOCK

Shock is defined as the inability to generate sufficient cardiac output to meet tissue metabolic needs. In the face of inadequate output, the peripheral vasculature constricts to shunt blood to the crucial central organs. This results in a profound decrease in peripheral circulation. As cells convert to anaerobic metabolism, lactate is generated, resulting in acidemia. Profound acidemia can compromise cardiac output further, initiating a dangerous cycle that results in severe organ failure and, eventually, death.

When presented with infants in shock, the clinician should consider sepsis first and treat the infants accordingly until another cause becomes evident. Initial management should be directed toward the "ABCs," (*A*irway, *B*reathing, *C*irculation), including 100% oxygen administration, aggressive fluid management, and correction of acidosis (see Chap. 10). Cardiac involvement should be considered if appropriate fluid resuscitation does not result in improvement (Figure 16–10). *Hepatomegaly* suggests poor cardiac function associated with either primary cardiac disease or impaired cardiac function secondary to metabolic derangement. The liver in infants is an excellent general indicator of volume status and cardiac output. In general, shock in infants with sepsis is associated with profound intravascular volume depletion, caused by a combination of dehydration and vasodilatation, which requires large amounts of volume resuscitation. The car-

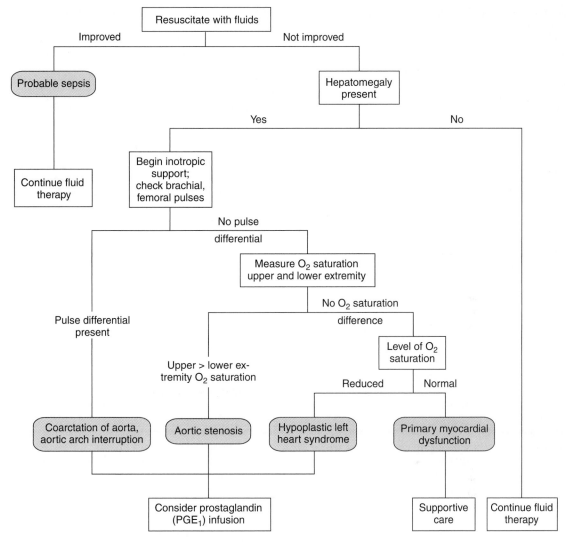

Figure 16–10. Algorithm of assessment and approach to infants with cardiogenic shock.

diac output in these infants initially is normal or increased. As a result, the liver usually is not palpable. An enlarged liver suggests volume overload or impaired cardiac function, often both. In this situation, a cardiac etiology of shock should be considered. As described earlier, severe acidemia can impair cardiac function. Therefore, hepatomegaly can develop in infants with profound acidemia associated with sepsis because of poor cardiac function. Even in these patients, however, hepatomegaly is an indication for inotropic support of cardiac function, as opposed to further volume resuscitation. *Cardiomegaly* also suggests cardiogenic shock, particularly in patients with myocarditis or cardiomy-

opathy, who often have a heart that appears to fill the entire chest.

LEFT HEART OBSTRUCTION

The most common cardiac cause of shock is *left heart obstruction* (see Figure 16–10). Infants with obstruction to left ventricular inflow or outflow can decompensate rapidly if systemic output is dependent on the right ventricle via the ductus arteriosus. As the ductus arteriosus closes, systemic blood flow is compromised and shock develops. The major clinical findings in these infants are *decreased or absent peripheral pulses,* either globally or in the lower extremities, and hepatomegaly. *Differential cyanosis* may be present, suggesting that the ductus arteriosus is partially patent and supporting the systemic output from the right ventricle via the pulmonary artery. Murmurs may be audible, which can be suggestive either of outflow obstruction (systolic murmur at the left sternal border) or of inflow obstruction (diastolic murmur at the apex). The ECG usually shows right ventricular hypertrophy with decreased left-sided forces because of the persistence of fetal right ventricular dominance. ST- and T-wave changes may occur in the left precordial leads.

Shock in infants due to left heart obstruction comprises a spectrum of diagnoses, from hypoplastic left side of the heart syndrome to simple coarctation of the aorta. All present with shock when the ductus arteriosus closes. After initiation of PGE$_1$, evaluation, including chest radiograph and ECG, can further delineate the specific diagnosis.

HYPOPLASTIC LEFT HEART SYNDROME

In this condition, there is severe stenosis of both the mitral and aortic valves, often with atresia of both valves and a very small left ventricle. The left ventricle has no effective output; therefore, all left atrial blood must cross the atrial septum and mix with systemic venous return, resulting in oxygen desaturation. The entire output, both systemic and pulmonary, is supplied by the right ventricle. If the ductus arteriosus is open, these patients have normal pulses and examination except for arterial O$_2$ desaturation. Physical examination is often unremarkable, but a third heart sound may be heard because of the high flow through the tricuspid valve. There is no differential in pulses or O$_2$ saturation between upper and lower extremities. The chest radiograph often is unremarkable but can show a relatively small heart with increased pulmonary vascularity. The ECG shows right ventricular hypertrophy with markedly decreased left-sided voltages. When the ductus arteriosus closes, systemic blood flow cannot be maintained and weak pulses with pallor develop; because of inadequate blood flow and oxygen to the tissues, metabolic acidosis results. Treatment options include a series of two or three palliative surgeries to create a single ventricle physiology or heart transplantation.

AORTIC STENOSIS

In AS, there is a variable degree of obstruction to left ventricular outflow. When the obstruction is moderate to severe, the ventricle is unable to provide adequate cardiac output through the dysplastic, usually monocuspid, valve. Physical examination often shows differential O$_2$ saturation, associated with ductal supply to the lower body, but does not show pulse differential if there is no aortic obstruction. Auscultation shows a systolic ejection murmur at the left sternal border, which can radiate to the neck, and there may be a thrill in the suprasternal notch. Chest radiograph may show cardiomegaly. The ECG usually shows right ventricular hypertrophy. Definitive treatment usually involves balloon valvuloplasty performed at cardiac catheterization. If this cannot be achieved, surgical relief of the obstruction is indicated.

AORTIC ARCH INTERRUPTION

This results when the normal left fourth fetal aortic arch abnormally regresses. Right-arm and head blood flows are provided by the left ventricle, whereas left-arm and lower-body flows depend entirely on the ductus arteriosus. Physical examination often reveals a systolic murmur at the left sternal border. Upper and lower body O$_2$ saturation differences usually are present, and pressure differences develop when the ductus arteriosus constricts. Chest radiograph may show a narrow upper mediastinum because the thymus often is absent. Aortic arch interruption frequently is associated with the DiGeorge syndrome of absent thymus and parathyroid glands. Hypocalcemia and immune deficiency may be important features. The ECG findings often are indistinguishable from those with other left side of the heart obstructions but can show normal or increased left forces, particularly after the immediate newborn period. Surgical correction of the interruption is required.

COARCTATION OF THE AORTA

This is the most common obstructive lesion of the left side of the heart. A ledge or ring of tissue is present just distal to the left subclavian artery opposite the ductus arteriosus. Patients may be asymptomatic, except for a higher upper body blood pressure when the obstruction is mild. Newborn infants are asymptomatic until the ductus closes but can have decreased lower body O$_2$ saturation, particularly when crying. As the ductus closes, the lower extremity pulses are decreased or absent. Auscultation often shows a systolic murmur at the upper right sternal border, because 40 to 60% of patients also have a bicuspid aortic valve. The chest radiograph of infants usually is normal until the ductus closes; however, if left ventricular failure develops, cardiomegaly occurs. The ECG usually shows right ventricular hypertrophy during infancy but may show biventricular hypertrophy. The standard treatment has been surgical resection of the narrowing, but balloon arterioplasty is also effective beyond the early newborn period.

MYOCARDIAL DYSFUNCTION

This is the second major cardiac cause of shock. Myocardial dysfunction has many causes; severe anemia and acidemia are two of the more common causes. Viral myocarditis and cardiomyopathy represent the major causes of cardiogenic shock in infants. Congenital coronary anomalies are rare causes of shock but should always be considered in the diagnosis. These infants have shock, poor peripheral pulses and perfusion, acidemia, pulmonary edema, severe cardiomegaly, and hepatomegaly. The presenting features are not substantially different from those of left side of the heart obstruction. The ECG may show a lack of ventricular hypertrophy and classically shows low voltages in the setting of myocarditis or severe biventricular hypertrophy in patients with hypertrophic cardiomyopathy (HCM). The ECG may show ST-T wave changes suggestive of ischemia or Q waves suggestive of prior infarct in patients with coronary abnormalities. Finally, children with prolonged abnormal tachycardia (e.g., as caused by supraventricular tachycardia) may have myocardial dysfunction. The ECG will be diagnostic and will show the abnormally fast heart rhythm.

TREATMENT

When cardiogenic shock is considered in infants, initial management should be directed toward supporting the cardiac output, correcting any metabolic defects, and opening the ductus arteriosus. An IV infusion of dopamine or dobutamine (5 to 10 µg/kg/min) or epinephrine (0.05 to 0.10 µg/kg/min) should be initiated, and the dose titrated to achieve an adequate cardiac output and blood pressure. Calcium should also be considered to increase the strength of cardiac contraction; this is of particular importance in preterm infants in whom hypocalcemia may occur. Sodium bicarbonate should be administered to correct any acidosis; anemia, if present, should be treated with packed red blood cells. PGE_1 should be administered (0.05 µg/kg/min) to maintain ductus arteriosus patency if left-sided obstruction is suspected. A pediatric cardiologist should be consulted. In infants with tachycardia-induced shock, treatment is directed at lowering the heart rate and/or converting the abnormal rhythm to sinus rhythm. This may be done with medications, conversion by overdrive pacing, or by direct current cardioversion.

INFANTS WITH RESPIRATORY DISTRESS

Two major cardiac pathophysiologies should be considered in infants who have respiratory distress. *Increased pulmonary arterial flow* causes transudation of fluid into the interstitium, thereby decreasing lung compliance and increasing the work of breathing. As a result, infants become tachypneic and dyspneic. As the course progresses, alveolar fluid may accumulate, further increasing the work of breathing and resulting in retractions. The main cardiac cause of increased pulmonary arterial flow in infants is a left-to-right shunt, either intracardiac or at the level of the great artery. *Pulmonary venous congestion,* an increase in pulmonary venous and capillary pressure, results in interstitial fluid accumulation and respiratory distress. Pulmonary venous congestion is due mainly to elevated left atrial pressure, either from poor cardiac function or from obstruction to left ventricular inflow (see "Infants with Shock," earlier).

In infants with respiratory distress, it can be difficult to distinguish cardiac disease from pulmonary disease. In both instances, tachypnea and retractions are usually present. Children with cardiac disease usually have a hyperactive, often visible, precordial impulse, indicating an increased volume load on the heart. The chest radiograph will not show focal infiltrates or atelectasis but usually shows cardiomegaly, with increased pulmonary arterial or venous markings. The ECG is helpful, in that most patients with respiratory distress of a cardiac cause have right ventricular hypertrophy. The causes of respiratory distress generally fall into three categories: arterial runoff into either the pulmonary or venous system, complete intracardiac mixing with no restriction to pulmonary blood flow, and obligate left-to-right shunting. An *obligate shunt* is defined as one that is not dependent on a decrease in pulmonary resistance (e.g., a communication between the left ventricle and right atrium, or between a systemic artery and vein).

TREATMENT

Initial treatment of respiratory distress is always supportive. The ABCs of initial resuscitation should always be followed (see Chap. 10). Oxygen should be administered, although it may not improve the pulmonary venous desaturation if pulmonary edema is marked. Diuretics will decrease interstitial pulmonary fluid, thus decreasing the work of breathing. When the distress is severe, mechanical ventilation should be considered. In addition to removing the work of breathing from the patients, positive pressure ventilation will also help to decrease alveolar edema. Inotropic agents, such as digoxin, may not be necessary in the acute setting but may improve symptoms if severe. In premature infants, the use of indomethacin to close a PDA should be considered. In severely symptomatic infants, IV inotropic agents, such as dopamine or dobutamine, may be indicated.

When cardiac disease is considered, initial evaluation of the arterial pulses can begin to distinguish various defects. Bounding pulses and a wide pulse pressure indicate a runoff from the arterial system, either into the pulmonary arteries, as occurs in truncus arteriosus, AP window, or large PDA, or into the venous system from an AV malformation (Figure 16–11). In atrioventricular canal defect, "single ventricle" defects, TAPVR, and intracardiac shunts there is no arterial runoff; therefore, the pulses are normal or decreased.

The arterial saturation distinguishes lesions that include a right-to-left, as well as left-to-right shunt, from those with a pure left-to-right shunt. Patients with bounding pulses and arterial desaturation most likely have truncus arteriosus. Infants with AP window, PDA, and AV malformation usually have normal arterial saturation. In patients with AV malformation, a bruit often is heard over the area of the malformation. Patients with TAPVR,

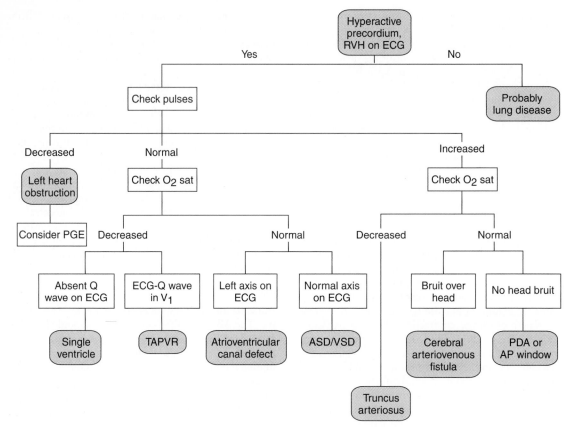

Figure 16–11. Algorithm showing approach in evaluating infants with respiratory distress due to cardiac disease. AP = aortopulmonary; ASD = atrial septal defect; ECG = electrocardiogram; PDA = patent ductus arteriosus; PGE = prostaglandin E; RVH = right ventricular hypertrophy; TAPVR = total anomalous pulmonary venous return.

complex heart disease, and "single ventricle" physiology have normal pulses and O₂ desaturation, whereas infants with atrioventricular canal or large atrial and ventricular defects usually are fully saturated.

Although the ECG usually shows right ventricular hypertrophy, it can be helpful in the differential diagnosis. A left or indeterminate axis is seen in atrioventricular septal defects, common in infants with Down syndrome but not with atrial or ventricular defects alone. Children with TAPVR often have a Q wave in the right chest leads indicative of severe right ventricular hypertrophy, whereas those with single ventricle often have an absence of Q waves throughout the precordium because of an absent or very abnormally placed ventricular septum.

TOTAL ANOMALOUS PULMONARY VENOUS RETURN

In TAPVR, the pulmonary veins do not enter the left atrium normally; rather, they form a confluence behind the left atrium and drain to the right atrium. Infants with

TAPVR and obstruction to pulmonary venous return have severe cyanosis (see "Infants with Cyanosis," earlier). Without obstruction, the presentation is respiratory distress with mild desaturation. There is a large increase in pulmonary blood flow, resulting in respiratory distress, and complete mixing, producing desaturation. The physical examination shows a hyperactive precordium with a widely split S2. The chest radiograph shows cardiomegaly and can show a "snowman" appearance. This characteristic picture is seen in TAPVR via a vertical vein and is caused by enlargement of the vertical vein and superior vena cava above the heart. The ECG typically shows right atrial enlargement and right ventricular hypertrophy. Definitive treatment is surgical anastomosis of the pulmonary vein confluence directly to the left atrium.

ATRIOVENTRICULAR CANAL DEFECT

This is a common cardiac defect, particularly in Down syndrome, being present in approximately 20% of these children. Atrioventricular canal defect forms as a result of failure of fusion of the endocardial cushions, structures normally responsible for separation of the common atrioventricular valve into tricuspid and mitral valves and for septation of the lower portion of the atria and upper posterior portion of the ventricles. As a result, children with this defect have a large common defect involving both the atria and ventricles. In addition, a single atrioventricular valve with five leaflets often is present. The combination of large atrial and ventricular defects results in a large left-to-right shunt and also can result in almost complete mixing of pulmonary and systemic venous blood. Physical examination shows a loud S1 caused by closure of the valve and can show a holosystolic murmur of atrioventricular valve insufficiency, commonly present in this lesion. Pulmonary hypertension often results, and the S2 also is increased. Chest radiograph shows cardiomegaly, often out of proportion to the degree of vascular markings. The ECG is often characteristic, with a "northwest" axis (180 to 270°). Biventricular hypertrophy often is present. Surgical correction is required and is performed at 3 to 6 months of age.

TRUNCUS ARTERIOSUS

In this defect, there is no pulmonary valve. The pulmonary artery arises directly from the aorta (trunk) just above the aortic (truncal) valve, which straddles a large VSD. Complete mixing occurs in the proximal ascending aorta causing cyanosis. Because pulmonary resistance is lower than systemic resistance, pulmonary flow is increased, causing respiratory distress. Children most commonly present in the first weeks postnatally. Physical examination shows a loud, single S2, often with an ejection click, and a continuous murmur due to flow through the pulmonary arteries. Systolic and diastolic murmur caused by stenosis and insufficiency of the common valve also may be heard. The pulses usually are bounding because of the large aortic runoff. The ECG typically shows biventricular hypertrophy. Definitive treatment for these patients is surgical correction consisting of closure of the ventricular septal defect and placement of an artificial pulmonary artery and valve between the right ventricle and the branch pulmonary arteries.

AORTOPULMONARY WINDOW AND ARTERIOVENOUS MALFORMATION

Other types of arterial communications, such as AP window and AV malformation, are uncommon. The AP window is a large communication between the ascending aorta and main pulmonary artery, just above the valve level. It usually occurs as an isolated defect. AV malformations are abnormal vessels that bypass the capillary bed, providing a very-low-resistance communication between the arterial and venous systems. They occur most commonly in the brain, liver, and skin. In both these lesions,

there is an increased pulmonary blood flow but no mixing; therefore, arterial O_2 saturation is normal. Physical examination shows bounding pulses from arterial runoff. In AV malformation, a bruit may be heard over the anterior fontanelle or the liver. Patients with AP window have a loud systolic murmur, which can be mistaken for a ventricular septal defect. In patients with AV malformation in the brain, the chest radiograph may show enlargement of the superior vena cava, whereas in AP window findings usually are not specific. The ECG will show right ventricular hypertrophy. Treatment of both lesions is surgical: AP windows can be corrected by closing the defect, whereas AV malformations require embolization of the abnormal vessels, which are often multiple.

SINGLE VENTRICLE

Patients with many different complex congenital defects can be grouped into what is termed *single ventricle physiology*. This includes lesions such as double-inlet left ventricle, in which both atrioventricular valves feed into the left ventricle, and double-outlet right ventricle, in which both the aorta and pulmonary artery arise from the right ventricle. In all these complex lesions, the physiology is that of a single atrium and ventricle, which results in complete mixing of pulmonary and systemic venous return. Systemic and pulmonary blood flows are determined by the relative resistances in these circulations. When there is no right-sided obstruction, the pulmonary flow is increased, often two to three times normal. Children with these abnormalities have respiratory distress as early as the first week after birth. Oxygen saturation is decreased because of complete mixing, often to 88 to 93% in room air. Physical examination can be deceptively normal. Some patients have dextrocardia, a clue to the severity of their disease. Likewise, the chest radiograph is not diagnostic but shows cardiomegaly. The ECG may show an ectopic atrial rhythm, or various degrees of atrioventricular block. There often is right ventricular or combined ventricular hypertrophy. For infants with increased pulmonary blood flow, a pulmonary arterial banding procedure is performed. For those with too little pulmonary blood flow, a shunt is placed from the aorta to the pulmonary artery to augment flow.

Large intracardiac shunts, such as a combination of a larger ASD and moderate or large VSD, can present with distress very early, within the first weeks. The systolic shunt of the VSD increases the diastolic shunt of the ASD to produce a rapid increase in pulmonary arterial flow. Finally, milder forms of left side of the heart obstruction can present with respiratory distress as a primary symptom. More commonly, poor perfusion is present (see earlier). Mild coarctation of the aorta and AS can result in elevated left atrial pressure and, thus, pulmonary venous pressure, resulting in pulmonary edema and distress.

ASYMPTOMATIC MURMURS

Innocent Murmurs

Asymptomatic murmurs in children are extremely common. The challenge for the pediatrician is to determine whether the murmur signifies cardiac disease and, if so, which evaluation and treatment are necessary. Innocent or "normal" murmurs occur in approximately 30 to 50% of children. They are heard most often in young school-aged children but are not infrequent in infants or adolescents. A heart murmur noted in the first 24 hours after birth carries a 1:12 risk of congenital heart disease; one heard first at 6 months, a 1:7 risk; and one heard first at 12 months, only a 1:50 risk. However, if a murmur detected at birth persists for 12 months, the risk of congenital heart disease is 3:5. Innocent murmurs usually can be recognized with the use of skilled auscultation and bedside maneuvers without the need for extensive and expensive diagnostic testing.

Innocent murmurs have several general characteristics that set them apart from murmurs associated with cardiac disease (Table 16–4). With the exception of the venous hum, which is continuous, innocent murmurs occur only in systole and tend to be short, peaking in the first half of systole. They usually are soft, rarely greater than a grade 2 (on a scale of 1 to 6) in intensity and tend to be well localized. Again with the exception of the venous hum, there are no innocent thrills. The most common innocent heart murmurs are described later.

STILL MURMUR

This vibratory, musical, medium-frequency, grade 1–2, systolic ejection murmur is localized midway between the left lower sternal border and the apex. It decreases in intensity with inspiration and upright position and increases with exercise, excitement, or fever. It is most commonly heard in children aged 2 to 7 years. It appears to originate in the left ventricle and may be related to vibrations of false chordae tendineae, although this remains controversial.

INNOCENT PULMONARY EJECTION MURMUR

This high-frequency, grade 1–2, crescendo–decrescendo systolic ejection murmur is well localized to the second left intercostal space along the sternal border. It is louder when patients are supine and is accentuated by exercise, excitement, and fever. The murmur usually disappears immediately with the Valsalva maneuver. This murmur is identical in quality with the murmur of an ASD, except that it is associated with a normal second heart sound. It is caused by relatively high velocity flow in the pulmonary artery and proximity of the pulmonary artery to the chest wall.

CERVICAL VENOUS HUM

This low-frequency, grade 1–2, continuous murmur is heard loudest at either the upper left or the right sternal border just above or below the clavicle. Because of its location and continuous nature, it often is mistaken for a PDA. It is loudest when patients are sitting and diminishes or disappears when patients are supine. The murmur usually can be accentuated by turning the patients' heads away from the side of the murmur and obliterated by pressing lightly over the jugular vein. It is caused by turbulent flow in the jugular veins.

SUPRACLAVICULAR ARTERIAL BRUIT

This grade 1–3, crescendo–decrescendo systolic murmur is heard best above the clavicles with radiation to the neck. The intensity is increased with exercise but not affected by posture or respiration. Compression of the subclavian artery against the first rib or hyperextension of the shoulders will diminish or abolish the murmur and can be used to differentiate it from the murmur of AS. It is thought

Table 16–4. Innocent Murmurs

Murmur	Location	Intensity	Quality	Other
Cervical venous hum	Right or left upper sternal border below clavicle	Grade 1–2 continuous	Low frequency	Diminishes with jugular vein compression
Peripheral pulmonic stenosis	Left upper sternal border with louder radiation to back or axilla	Grade 1–2 systolic ejection	Crescendo–decrescendo, low frequency	Newborn to age 4 mo
Pulmonary ejection	Left upper sternal border	Grade 1–3 systolic ejection	Crescendo–decrescendo, medium frequency	Decreases with Valsalva maneuver
Still	Midway between left lower sternal border and apex	Grade 1–2 systolic ejection	Vibratory, musical, low frequency	Decreases intensity with inspiration
Supraclavicular arterial bruit	Above right or left clavicle with radiation to neck	Grade 1–3 holosystolic	Crescendo–decrescendo, medium to high frequency	Decreases with shoulder hyperextension

to be caused by turbulent flow at the origin of the brachiocephalic vessels from the aorta.

PERIPHERAL PULMONIC STENOSIS

This is characterized by a grade 1–2, systolic ejection murmur heard best in the axilla or back and more softly over the left upper sternal border. It often is heard in newborn infants and disappears by several months of age. It is not caused by structural cardiac disease but by the normal reduction in diameter of the proximal branch pulmonary arteries arising from the pulmonary trunk during early infancy, resulting in turbulence of blood flow. Once identified, reexamination of infants at age 4 months is necessary to document resolution and ensure that the murmur is not due to pathologic pulmonary artery stenosis.

Pathologic Systolic Murmurs

In general, pathologic systolic murmurs tend to be louder, longer, and harsher than innocent murmurs and do not vary with respiration. Pathologic systolic murmurs are due to either a hole in the heart, such as a VSD or ASD; stenosis of the aortic or pulmonic valves or outflow tracts; stenosis of the pulmonary artery or aorta; or regurgitation of the mitral or tricuspid valves. Each abnormality has distinct features of the cardiac examination that distinguish it from the others (Table 16–5).

VENTRICULAR SEPTAL DEFECT

A VSD is a hole in the septum between the right and left ventricles; this results in a left-to-right shunt causing increased pulmonary blood flow, which can lead to cardiac failure. VSD is the most common congenital heart defect, occurring in 3/1000 live births and comprising 16% of all children with heart disease. Only 15% of VSDs are of a size sufficient to require diagnostic or therapeutic intervention; the remainder either close spontaneously or are so small that they have no hemodynamic effect. The murmur, due to turbulent blood flow through the defect, is medium- to high-frequency, is grade 2–4, occupies the whole of systole, and is loudest at the fourth intercostal space to the apex. Treatment for small VSDs is limited to antibiotic prophylaxis to minimize the small risk (0.7%/y) of bacterial endocarditis. Large VSDs should be closed surgically to prevent the development of pulmonary vascular disease.

ATRIAL SEPTAL DEFECT

An ASD is a hole in the septum between the right and left atrium. It results in a left-to-right shunt, causing right ventricular volume overload and increased pulmonary blood flow; this can lead to CHF and pulmonary hypertension but usually not until the second or third decade of life. Approximately 3 to 5% of children with significant heart disease have an ASD, making it the third most common

congenital heart defect. Most children are asymptomatic and present with a murmur at age 2 to 5 years. Small ASDs may close spontaneously, but this rarely occurs after the age of 2 years. Physical examination is remarkable for a medium- to high-frequency systolic ejection murmur heard loudest at the left upper sternal border because of the increased blood flow across the normal pulmonary valve. In addition, because of the increased pulmonary flow, the pulmonary valve takes longer to close, resulting in a widely split second heart sound. The widely split second heart sound differentiates an ASD from an innocent pulmonary ejection murmur. Small ASDs less than a few millimeters in diameter require no treatment and do not require antibiotic prophylaxis. Larger ASDs require surgical closure, but new catheter-directed closure techniques are being developed.

AORTIC STENOSIS

Aortic stenosis, a congenital abnormality of the aortic valve, consists of thickening and fusion of one or more of the valve leaflets, resulting in limited opening of the valve during systolic ejection. Neonates with severe, or "critical," AS present in shock (see "Infants with Shock," earlier). Infants and children usually are asymptomatic with a systolic murmur, most often at age 5 to 15 years. By the third decade, AS is the second most common congenital heart defect after VSD. Physical examination reveals a harsh, medium-frequency systolic ejection murmur at the second right intercostal space associated with an ejection click over the lower left sternal border; in addition, a thrill often is palpable in the suprasternal notch. The natural history of AS is to worsen over time; most children require treatment at some time during childhood or young adulthood. Treatment consists of either catheter balloon dilation or surgical repair. Antibiotic prophylaxis is needed both before and after treatment because, despite a good physiologic result from treatment, the valve remains abnormal and therefore at risk for endocarditis.

PULMONARY STENOSIS

Pulmonary stenosis is a congenital abnormality of the pulmonic valve consisting of thickening of the valve leaflets, resulting in limited opening of the valve during systolic ejection. It occurs in about 8% of children with congenital heart disease, making it the second most common lesion during childhood. Neonates with severe ("critical") PS have cyanosis, but most patients are asymptomatic as infants or preschool-aged children with a systolic murmur. Physical examination is significant for a harsh medium-frequency systolic ejection murmur at the second left intercostal space associated with an ejection click along the left sternal border. In contrast to AS, there is no suprasternal notch thrill, although in severe cases a thrill may be palpable over the left upper sternal border. Mild PS may not require treatment other than antibiotic

Table 16–5. Diagnostic Features of the Common Causes of Pathologic Murmurs in Children

Diagnosis	Chest Radiograph	Pulses	Electrocardiogram	Auscultation
Shunt lesions				
Ventricular septal defect	Increased pulmonary vascularity	Normal	LVH ± RVH, LAE	≥ Grade 3 holosystolic murmur LLSB, P2 normal to increased
Atrial septal defect	Increased pulmonary vascularity	Normal	Normal or RVH, RAE	Widely split S2, Grade 1–2 systolic ejection murmur ULSB, grade 1–2 mid-diastolic murmur LLSB
Atrioventricular canal defect	Increased pulmonary vascularity	Normal	RVH ± LVH, superior axis	≥ Grade 3 holosystolic murmur LLSB, P2 normal to increased
Patent ductus arteriosus	Increased pulmonary vascularity	Increased	LVH ± RVH, LAE	≥ Grade 2 continuous murmur ULSB, P2 normal to increased
Arteriovenous malformation	Increased pulmonary vascularity	Increased	LVH ± RVH	Grade 1–2 continuous murmur over area of shunt (head, liver)
Insufficiency				
Mitral insufficiency	Normal or pulmonary edema	Normal to increased	LVH, LAE	Grade 2–3 holosystolic murmur apex, grade 1 mid-diastolic murmur apex
Tricuspid insufficiency	Normal	Normal	RVH, RAE	Grade 2–3 holosystolic murmur LLSB
Intrinsic				
Myocarditis	Pulmonary edema	Decreased	ST & T abnormal, low voltage ± LVH	Soft sounds, S3 may be heard
Cardiomyopathy	Pulmonary edema	Decreased	ST & T abnormal, inferior axis, low voltage ± LVH	Soft sounds, S3 may be heard
Ischemia	Pulmonary edema	Decreased	ST & T abnormal, deep Q waves	Soft sounds, S3 may be heard
Obstruction				
Aortic stenosis	Pulmonary edema	Decreased	LVH ± ST abnormalities	≥ Grade 3 systolic ejection murmur URSB, ejection click
Pulmonary stenosis	Normal or decreased vascularity	Normal	RVH ± ST abnormalities, RAE	≥ Grade 3 systolic ejection murmur ULSB, ejection click
Coarctation of aorta	Pulmonary edema	Upper extremity > lower extremity	LVH	Grade 2–3 systolic murmur, possibly also in diastole paraspinally

LAE, RAE = left, right atrial enlargement; LVH, RVH = left, right ventricular hypertrophy; ULSB, LLSB = upper, lower left sternal border.

prophylaxis. However, the degree of stenosis may progress, so careful routine follow-up is required. Moderate or marked degrees of PS result in right ventricular hypertrophy on the ECG. The treatment of choice for moderate-to-severe PS is catheter balloon dilation.

VALVAR REGURGITATION

Isolated regurgitation of either the mitral or tricuspid valves is a rare cause of asymptomatic murmurs in children. The exception is tricuspid regurgitation in the newborn. The elevated pulmonary pressures can persist 24 to 48 h after birth and often cause tricuspid regurgitation despite a normal tricuspid valve. This murmur may be difficult to distinguish from a VSD murmur, as it is a medium-frequency holosystolic murmur heard loudest at the left lower sternal border. This murmur disappears during the first week after birth as pulmonary arterial pressure decreases.

MITRAL VALVE PROLAPSE

Mitral valve prolapse (MVP) is a condition in which the one or both of the mitral valve leaflets extend above the annulus of the mitral valve during systole. While MVP is fairly common in adults, it is much less so in children. It is caused by a primary abnormality of the mitral valve that results in a laxity. During systole, the laxity of the valve results in a saillike billowing of the valve into the atrium. This billowing is heard as a mid-systolic click. Mitral regurgitation is often present, resulting in the classic "click-murmur syndrome" of MVP. Most people with MVP remain asymptomatic, but some can have arrhythmias and chest pain, and a subset may be at increased risk for sudden death.

Pathologic Continuous and Diastolic Murmurs

With the exception of a venous hum, which can be made to disappear with maneuvers (see earlier), a continuous or diastolic murmur always should be considered pathologic until proved otherwise. A continuous murmur is most commonly due to a PDA, although continuous flow lesions, such as a fistulae (cerebral, hepatic, pulmonary, or coronary), AP window, or AP collateral circulation, may cause continuous murmurs. Diastolic murmurs are due either to aortic or pulmonic regurgitation or to mitral stenosis. Fortunately, these last three lesions are rare and usually associated with other cardiac defects.

PATENT DUCTUS ARTERIOSUS

Patent ductus arteriosus is a common lesion in children younger than 1 year (making it the sixth most common lesion in congenital heart disease). The PDAs are common in preterm infants; the more premature the infants, the greater the likelihood that ductus patency will persist after birth. If it is not necessary to close the ductus pharmacologically with indomethacin or surgically because of symptoms, it usually closes spontaneously within several weeks after birth. Ductus patency is the abnormal persistence of a normal fetal vessel that connects the main pulmonary artery with the descending aorta. After birth, it results in left-to-right shunting to the pulmonary arteries, which can cause cardiac failure, with enlargement of the left atrium and ventricle and pulmonary hypertension. In addition, a PDA carries a substantial risk of developing endocarditis. Symptoms are dependent on the size of the PDA, which determines the amount of the left-to-right shunt. Most children have small-to-moderate-sized PDAs and are asymptomatic with a murmur. Cardiac examination is significant for increased pulse volume and a continuous medium-to-low-frequency murmur heard loudest just inferior to the left clavicle. Treatment is closure, either by surgical ligation or a new catheter coil closure technique.

CHILDREN WITH RESPIRATORY DISTRESS AND CONGESTIVE HEART FAILURE

Congestive heart failure may be defined as inadequate contractile heart function for the specific hemodynamic needs. There may be normal requirements for flow but poor myocardial contractility (e.g., cardiomyopathy or coarctation), or flow requirements may be dramatically increased in the face of normal or even increased myocardial contractility (e.g., ventricular septal defect with large left-to-right shunt and increased pulmonary blood flow). The inadequacy of contractile function may be manifested as inadequate systemic output for metabolic needs, as in children with CHF caused by a large left-to-right shunt who do not grow and gain weight. Alternatively, it may be associated with adequate systemic output, but compensatory mechanisms may result in other clinical problems, such as an enlarged liver and tachypnea in children who have a large left-to-right shunt.

In practical terms, the signs and symptoms of cardiac failure in children include respiratory distress (tachypnea and/or retractions), increased cardiac activity (tachycardia and/or a hyperdynamic precordium), and cardiac enlargement (detected either by chest radiograph or echocardiogram). Two physiologic mechanisms can result in heart failure in children. The most common is a large left-to-right shunt, as with a large atrial or ventricular septal defect, atrioventricular canal defect, or PDA, causing markedly increased pulmonary blood flow and interstitial fluid accumulation. The large left-to-right shunt is a volume load for the atria and ventricles. To maintain an adequate cardiac output, the heart compensates by enlarging and by beating faster and with greater force, which leads to the cardiac enlargement and increased precordial activity. The second physiologic mechanism occurs when there is intrinsic myocardial dysfunction, as with myocarditis. Because of the dysfunction, cardiac output decreases and ventricular filling pressure increases, resulting in elevated left atrial and pulmonary vein pressures. This causes pulmonary edema, leading to respiratory distress. Because of the low cardiac output, the kidneys retain free water, which increases intravascular volume, causing cardiac dilation. The heart tries to maintain output by increasing heart rate.

The differential diagnosis of CHF in children includes a large left-to-right shunt (ASD, VSD, PDA, atrioventricular canal, or AV fistula), left-sided obstruction leading to myocardial dysfunction (severe coarctation or AS), or intrinsic myocardial dysfunction (myocarditis, cardiomyopathy, or infarct due to anomalous coronary artery). The evaluation should include a thorough physical examination, measurement of pulse oximetry, chest radiograph, and ECG. If the respiratory distress is marked, treatment must be initiated immediately. An echocardiogram should be performed to define the cause.

Infants usually present in CHF due to either a large shunt lesion or severe left-sided obstruction, particularly coarctation. Shunt lesions can be differentiated from obstructive lesions or intrinsic myocardial dysfunction on the appearance of the chest radiograph. Shunt lesions will have cardiomegaly with increased pulmonary artery size but minimal pulmonary edema, whereas obstructive or intrinsic dysfunction lesions will have cardiomegaly with predominately pulmonary edema. The specific physical and ECG findings of left-to-right shunt lesions and left-sided obstructive lesions in children are similar to those for infants (outlined earlier). Because coarctation is a common cause of heart failure in infants, careful evaluation of lower extremity pulses and blood pressure is a critical part of the physical examination.

Older children usually have CHF due to intrinsic myocardial dysfunction. The most common cause is viral myocarditis, however, other causes include dilated, restrictive, and hypertrophic cardiomyopathy, as well as chronic tachycardia. Presenting symptoms can often be subtle such as generalized fatigue or abdominal pain with nausea and vomiting due to hepatic and intestinal venous congestion. Cardiac examination in children with CHF due to intrinsic myocardial dysfunction is characterized by tachypnea, rales, tachycardia, hyperdynamic precordium, gallop rhythm heard loudest over the left lower sternal border or apex, and often systolic murmur at the apex due to mitral regurgitation. The liver is often enlarged and can be quite tender. There may be jugular venous distention. Peripheral edema and ascites are late manifestations and indicate very severe failure.

Myocarditis

Myocarditis is an active inflammation of the myocardium. This inflammation may result from many causes (Table 16–6). Tissue injury results from cytotoxic cell destruction and antibody complement-mediated destruction of myofibrils by the virus.

Many conditions causing myocarditis also may involve the pericardium and produce effusions and pericarditis. Inflammation and necrosis of cardiac muscle most frequently causes poor contractile function; this leads to cardiac dilation with an increase in left ventricular volume and mitral regurgitation. Left ventricular end-diastolic pressure increase is transmitted to the left atrium and pulmonary veins, resulting in pulmonary edema. Clinical findings include a soft third or fourth heart sound with displacement of the left ventricular impulse laterally, both indicating cardiomegaly. A systolic murmur of mitral regurgitation often is heard at the apex. Patients may complain of exercise intolerance, shortness of breath, or abdominal pain. If these symptoms occur in patients with current or recent evidence of an infectious or inflammatory process, myocarditis should be suspected. Less frequently, myocarditis may present primarily with arrhythmia, and the new onset of palpitations in patients with such evidence of infection or inflammation should also suggest myocarditis. A chest radiograph shows cardiomegaly with pulmonary edema. An ECG shows ST- and T-wave changes, often with low QRS voltages.

The most frequent cause of myocarditis is viral, and coxsackievirus A and B groups are most important. Myo-

Table 16–6. Most Frequent Causes of Myocarditis

Infectious	
Coxsackievirus B and A	Diphtheria
Influenza virus A and B	Typhoid fever
Echovirus	Lyme disease
Mumps virus	Rocky Mountain
Rubella	spotted fever
Rubeola	Chagas disease
HIV	(trypanosomiasis)
Infectious mononucleosis	Trichinosis
Varicella/zoster	Toxoplasmosis
Inflammatory	
Systemic lupus erythematosus	Ulcerative colitis
Scleroderma	Polymyositis
Acute rheumatic fever	Sarcoidosis
Kawasaki disease	
Toxic	
Doxorubicin (Adriamycin)	Acetazolamide
Sulfonamides	Amphotericin B
Cyclophosphamide	Scorpion bites
Neuromuscular	
Muscular dystrophies	Friedreich ataxia
Metabolic	
Beriberi	Hypothyroidism

carditis may follow a nonspecific prodrome that sometimes includes fever and an erythematous rash. Infants in the first year of life may be affected; in these patients, the disease may be fatal. Other viruses implicated in myocarditis include echovirus, influenza, and rubella. In many patients, however, a viral etiology of myocarditis is suspected, but no specific agent is isolated.

Other infectious etiologies, more rarely seen in North America, include typhoid fever, diphtheria, toxoplasmosis, and trichinosis. Of increasing importance is the myocarditis that sometimes occurs with Rocky Mountain spotted fever and Lyme disease. Specific therapy often is available for myocarditis caused by these agents.

The clinical course depends on the degree to which the myocardium is damaged. Some patients experience slow resolution of symptoms and cardiomegaly, which gradually improves over several months or even years. In others, chronic CHF develops. Infants may experience a rapidly progressive course, including severe CHF, cardiogenic shock, and death. There is no effective treatment for viral myocarditis; intensive support must be provided until the disease has run its course. Support includes positive pressure ventilation, diuretics, and inotropic agents. The use of IV immunoglobulins has been suggested but remains controversial. Mechanical myocardial support with a ventricular assist device and extracorporeal membrane oxygenation (ECMO) has been helpful in severe cases.

Myocarditis is rarely seen as the only manifestation of a more generalized inflammatory disease; more often, the disease may be diagnosed by the other inflammatory manifestations, including pericarditis. During acute rheumatic fever, acute cardiac decompensation may occur. In some patients, this is due to severe valvular dysfunction; in others, it is due to myocarditis with severe contractile dysfunction. The collagen vascular diseases may rarely be seen with major myocardial involvement, although pericardial involvement is more common. Examples include systemic lupus erythematosus and rheumatoid arthritis. Of great importance is the cardiac involvement in Kawasaki disease (see Chap. 8).

As in the viral forms, specific therapy is not available for myocarditis that occurs in association with systemic inflammatory disease. Although anti-inflammatory agents often are used, there is little or no evidence that they are effective in preventing or reversing myocarditis. This includes myocarditis in association with rheumatic fever. There is evidence that the administration of IV immunoglobulin early in the course of Kawasaki disease improves myocardial function and decreases the subsequent incidence of coronary arterial aneurysms.

Cardiomyopathy denotes damage to cardiac muscle in which no inflammatory process can be defined. It is associated with many storage diseases and has many causes (Table 16–7).

Table 16–7. Forms of Cardiomyopathy

Form (etiology)	Distinguishing Features

Dilated
  Idiopathic
  Doxorubicin toxicity
  Carnitine deficiency
  Sarcoidosis
  Amyloidosis
	Enlarged left ventricular chamber size, poor systolic function; ventricular arrhythmias common with severe cardiomyopathy

Restrictive
  Subendocardial
    fibroelastosis
  Gaucher disease
	Small left ventricular chamber size, diastolic dysfunction, pulmonary edema, atrial dilation and atrial arrhythmias common

Hypertrophic	Obstructive and nonobstructive forms; obstruction increases with exercise; may present with exercise-related chest pain or exercise intolerance; atrial or ventricular arrhythmias may be fatal, not related to degree of obstruction
Arrhythmogenic right ventricular dysplasia	Right ventricle dilated on echocardiogram; fatty infiltration on magnetic resonance imaging; ventricular arrhythmias are most prominent feature

Patients with *dilated cardiomyopathy* have signs of ventricular systolic (contractile) dysfunction and are found to have cardiac dilatation on chest radiography, which usually is mainly caused by left ventricular chamber enlargement. This enlargement occurs as a compensatory mechanism for poor cardiac contractile function. These patients may have signs of CHF, or they may be well compensated with little more than signs of cardiac enlargement. They may also manifest symptoms suggestive of arrhythmia, such as syncope or palpitations.

In most cases of dilated cardiomyopathy, no cause can be found; therefore, these are termed *idiopathic dilated cardiomyopathy.* In some cases, there may be a familial pattern. Rarely, there may be a familial carnitine deficiency or other abnormality of mitochondrial function. Infiltrative diseases, such as sarcoidosis and amyloidosis, which involve the myocardium in adults, are very unusual in children with dilated cardiomyopathy. In children receiving doxorubicin (Adriamycin) for cancer chemotherapy, the occurrence of dilated cardiomyopathy is related to the dose. Approximately 5% of patients have symptomatic cardiotoxicity after a cumulative dose of 500 mg/m^2; with higher doses, however, the incidence reaches 50%. The incidence of an identifiable cause of cardiomyopathy is extremely low, despite the use of techniques such as endomyocardial biopsy. Furthermore, even if a cause is found on the biopsy specimen, definitive treatment is unlikely to be available. Endomyocardial biopsies are performed to identify those rare cases for which treatment might be available, as well as to provide patients and families with a prognosis.

The clinical course of dilated cardiomyopathy is variable. Spontaneous resolution is not uncommon in younger children; in both older children and adults, however, progression is more common. Progressive development of CHF requires gradual intensification of medical management, including the use of afterload-reducing agents and beta blockers. Eventually, many such patients become candidates for cardiac transplantation. A particularly disturbing development in patients with dilated cardiomyopathy is the occurrence of syncope or documented ventricular arrhythmias. Repeated syncope in patients with dilated cardiomyopathy is an ominous sign and may signal the possibility of sudden death. Such patients are considered for cardiac transplantation even if their hemodynamic status is otherwise compensated. Finally, such patients may have mural thrombi that subsequently may embolize and cause strokes or other problems. This is a particular problem in patients with dilated cardiomyopathy in whom chronic atrial fibrillation has developed. Antiplatelet agents, such as aspirin or dipyridamole, should be used to prevent the development of mural thrombi. Anticoagulants, such as warfarin, should be used in patients in whom thrombi have already developed.

Restrictive cardiomyopathy differs from the dilated form in that there is no ventricular dilatation. Instead, the ventricle may be contracted and small, whereas the atria may be dilated because of the high ventricular diastolic pressures. Clinically, this often appears as cardiomegaly on the chest radiograph, despite the normal or small ventricular chamber sizes. There also may be evidence of passive congestion with pulmonary edema.

The main problem in restrictive cardiomyopathy is a dramatically reduced ventricular compliance, with an abnormally high pressure at normal ventricular volumes and therefore reduced ventricular diastolic filling. Although there may also be systolic dysfunction with reduced ejection fraction, the clinical picture is mainly that of diastolic dysfunction with pulmonary and hepatic congestion and atrial enlargement. Chronic atrial dilatation may lead to severe atrial arrhythmias, such as atrial flutter, which may be very poorly tolerated in such patients. Patients may have atrial thrombi and subsequent systemic embolization, as do patients with dilated cardiomyopathy.

In children, the principal cause of restrictive cardiomyopathy is endocardial fibroelastosis, a disease featuring deposition of dense fibrous tissue over the ventricular endocardium, particularly over the ventricular apex and mitral valve apparatus. A rare cause of restrictive cardiomyopathy in children is Gaucher disease, a deficiency of the enzyme glucocerebroside-β-glucosidase, which primarily affects the nervous system.

In the diagnosis of restrictive cardiomyopathy, it is important to rule out constrictive pericarditis, as this condition may also cause high venous pressures with atrial dilation and small ventricles. Patients with restrictive cardiomyopathy should not have significant pulsus paradoxicus, whereas most patients with constrictive pericarditis do. Echocardiographic indices of ventricular filling may also separate the two conditions. At cardiac catheterization, patients with constrictive pericarditis have similar elevations in right and left ventricular end-diastolic pressures, whereas patients with restrictive cardiomyopathy who have predominant involvement of the left ventricle usually have much higher left than right ventricular end-diastolic pressures.

The prognosis is poor for patients with extensive restrictive cardiomyopathy. No specific therapy is available, although there are reports of symptomatic improvement with the administration of calcium channel blocking agents, such as verapamil. Patients with this condition eventually may require referral for cardiac transplantation.

Hypertrophic cardiomyopathy refers to the condition of severe hypertrophy of the left ventricle, which is not secondary to a hemodynamic cause, such as hypertension or AS. In such patients, there may be concentric and symmetric hypertrophy of the ventricles or asymmetric septal hypertrophy, with the interventricular septum being thicker than the left ventricular free wall. The cause of HCM, known by several other names, including idiopathic hypertrophic subaortic stenosis (IHSS), is idiopathic although in some patients, a familial relationship has been noted, indicating genetic associations. When symmetric hypertrophy is present, metabolic diseases must be considered, such as glycogen storage disease type II (Pompe disease), carnitine deficiency, and pyruvate metabolism disorders. Extensive hypertrophy leads to a ventricle that is hypercontractile, with an abnormally high ejection fraction. This may cause dynamic subaortic obstruction, particularly if asymmetric septal hypertrophy is present. There may be evidence of diastolic dysfunction with atrial dilatation and higher than normal venous pressures. There often is a family history of HCM or sudden death. Histologically, the hypertrophied ventricular muscle is abnormal, with myocyte degeneration and myofibrillar disarray. In patients with Pompe disease, glycogen deposition is apparent in myocytes on light or electron microscopy.

Patients with HCM may have dyspnea on exertion, chest pain, dizziness, palpitations, or syncope. They may also experience sudden death as the first manifestation, although it is rare for a previously asymptomatic patients with HCM to die suddenly. Clinically, one may divide the condition into cases with left ventricular outflow obstruction and those without obstruction. When obstruction occurs, it is dynamic and related to the asymmetric septal hypertrophy, with dramatic narrowing of the left ventricular outflow tract during systole. Such narrowing is worsened with exercise, increased inotropic state, and dehydration. Dyspnea on exertion, chest pain, and exercise intolerance are most prominent in patients who have the obstructive form of HCM, as these symptoms are thought to be due to dynamic left ventricular obstruction. Arrhythmias that are unrelated to the degree of left ventricular obstruction may occur. These arrhythmias may be atrial or ventricular and are thought to be responsible for syncope and sudden death in these patients.

Clinically, one suspects HCM in patients with the preceding symptoms who also have a positive family history, particularly if the family history includes sudden death. The cardiac examination may suggest a problem, increased left ventricular impulse, loud ejection murmur, and paradoxical splitting of the second heart sound; however, HCM is difficult to diagnose on the basis of examination alone. The ECG usually shows evidence of left ventricular hypertrophy, often with additional left septal hypertrophy. There also is an increased incidence of the Wolff-Parkinson-White syndrome in this condition. The echocardiogram remains the best modality for establishing the diagnosis of HCM, as it demonstrates the ventricular and/or septal hypertrophy, atrial dilation, and the lack of another cause for hypertrophy.

In treating this condition, one must differentiate between the symptoms of obstruction and those of arrhythmia, as these two manifestations are, for the most part, unrelated to one another. Agents that increase the inotropic state, such as digoxin, are not usually necessary, as there is little or no systolic dysfunction. Furthermore, these agents may be contraindicated, as they may increase the outflow obstruction, which is dynamic and related to contraction. Diuretic agents, which decrease filling pressures, also may worsen obstruction. The two agents used effectively for patients with symptoms are propranolol, a beta-adrenergic blocker, and verapamil, a calcium channel blocker. Of the two, propranolol probably is used more often in children. Cardiac contractility may be reduced by both agents, thereby decreasing dynamic obstruction. Evidence indicates that these agents are effective in improving symptoms of HCM; unfortunately, however, they have not influenced the incidence of sudden death, which may be as high as 3 to 7% per year. Patients with syncope or dizziness are probably at higher risk of sudden death, and consideration in such patients should be given to the use of high-dose beta-blocking agents or amiodarone. In preliminary investigations, both have appeared to decrease the risk of death. Any patients with HCM must be restricted from vigorous exercise.

Arrhythmogenic right ventricular dysplasia is a rare cardiomyopathy occurring primarily in adults and, infrequently, in adolescents. It is characterized by fatty replacement of ventricular myocardium, limited to the right ventricular free wall. Although extensive fatty replacement may adversely affect cardiac function leading to hemodynamic derangements, the primary mode of presentation is of ventricular arrhythmias. Typically, these occur with exercise and may be responsible for sudden death. Management of such patients is directed at controlling the ventricular arrhythmia. In severe cases, surgical resection of the involved myocardium has been performed.

CHILDREN WITH CARDIAC STRIDOR-VASCULAR RINGS

Stridor is a common symptom of upper airway disease (see Chaps. 9 and 10), including croup and bronchomalacia (see Chap. 17). It also can be a symptom of heart disease, specifically vascular rings. A *vascular ring* is an aortic arch anomaly in which the esophagus and trachea are completely surrounded by vascular structures. Although this condition is rare compared with airway abnormalities, it nonetheless represents an important cause of stridor and feeding difficulties in infants. When vascular rings are diagnosed and treated, appropriately complete correction usually is possible.

In infants, the history associated with vascular rings is similar to that with tracheomalacia: "noisy breathing" since birth, which worsens during an upper respiratory infection or when children are agitated. Children can have difficulty feeding or have reflex apnea with feeding. In older children, a history of choking on food or difficulty in swallowing solids is common. A careful history reveals that these children often had respiratory symptoms early in life that were attributed to "bronchitis." In children with other heart disease and respiratory symptoms, these difficulties may be attributed to their heart disease. Rings that cause little compression can be asymptomatic and found incidentally when an imaging study is obtained for another reason.

Types of Vascular Rings

Vascular rings can be classified as complete (those that form a complete circle) and incomplete (those that form a "C" around the trachea and esophagus but still cause compression). Incomplete rings are more common but also more variable in the symptoms they produce.

The most frequent form of incomplete ring is the aberrant right subclavian artery. In this condition, the right subclavian artery does not arise as a branch of the first vessel from the arch (the innominate artery); instead, it arises as a branch from the normal aorta as it descends on the left. To reach the right arm, it must pass from the left descending aorta and behind the esophagus, occasionally causing some compression.

Pulmonary artery slings are very rare but more frequently symptomatic. In this condition, the left pulmonary artery does not arise normally; instead, it arises from the right pulmonary artery and then passes to the left lung between the esophagus and trachea. The most frequent symptoms are those of expiratory obstruction, with wheezing, because the site of obstruction is well below the thoracic inlet. Because compression is more severe to the right mainstem bronchus, asymmetric air trapping may occur. This may be a clue to the diagnosis. Pulmonary artery sling should be considered in the differential diagnosis of wheezing, particularly when it does not seem responsive to bronchodilators and especially when it is associated with persistent hyperinflation of the right lung.

The most common form of complete vascular ring is the double aortic arch (Figure 16–12). In this condition, the ascending aorta branches into an anterior (left) and posterior (right) branch. The posterior limb passes behind the trachea and esophagus. The two limbs join to re-form the descending aorta, to complete the ring. The carotid and subclavian arteries usually arise from both anterior and posterior limbs as four discrete vessels. Often, one of the two arches is dominant, and the other is substantially smaller.

The other common form of complete ring is the association of a right aortic arch with an aberrant retroesophageal left subclavian artery and a left-sided ductus or ligamentum arteriosum. This condition is similar to aberrant right subclavian artery.

A right aortic arch is common and often is associated with congenital heart disease, especially truncus arteriosus and TOF. Typically, the first vessel to arise is a left innominate artery; a right-sided ductus arteriosus originates from the base of the right subclavian artery. When the left subclavian artery arises aberrantly from the descending aorta and passes retroesophageally to the left arm, and when it gives rise to a left-sided ductus arteriosus, a complete vascular ring exists. This is because the trachea and esophagus are encircled by the ascending aorta to the right, the retroesophageal left subclavian artery behind, and the ligamentum arteriosum to the left, which passes to the pulmonary artery in front.

Diagnosis

If a vascular ring is considered, a barium swallow is the initial diagnostic procedure of choice. A posterior pulsatile indentation of the esophagus is the classic feature. Endoscopy shows similar features. Bronchoscopy shows an anterior pulsatile mass, representing the ascending aortic portion of the ring. Magnetic resonance imaging (MRI) provides a definitive diagnosis in most cases by clearly showing the anatomy of the head and neck vessels. Echocardiography can show the features of a vascular ring, particularly when a right aortic arch is present, but is not completely reliable. Angiography usually is not necessary, except in complex vascular anomalies. Barium swallow, followed by MRI, usually provides a definitive diagnosis for surgical correction. However, in patients with a ligamentum arteriosum (remnant of a ductus arteriosus), it may be difficult to demonstrate the lesion by any technique; the condition should be suspected in patients with symptoms of a vascular ring and the presence of an anomalous subclavian artery.

Treatment

In nearly all cases, surgery successfully eliminates the vascular ring. In the case of double aortic arch, the smaller of the two arches is divided, opening the ring. With pulmonary slings and aberrant right subclavian arteries, reimplantation is possible. With the right aortic arch, aberrant left subclavian artery, and left ligamentum arteriosum complex, simply dividing the ligamentum is all that is necessary.

Although surgery may successfully eliminate the ring, these patients often have severe bronchomalacia or tracheomalacia, which may be responsible for their continued respiratory symptoms. In some, these symptoms gradually improve with time and with growth of the trachea; in others, they remain a problem.

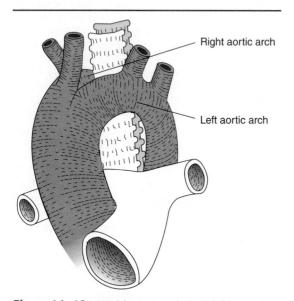

Right aortic arch

Left aortic arch

Figure 16–12. Double aortic arch. Arch bifurcates into left (anterior) and right (posterior) branches to encircle the trachea and esophagus. The two branches rejoin behind the esophagus to form a single descending aorta. (Reproduced with permission from Shuford WH, Sybers RG [editors]: *The Aortic Arch and Its Malformations.* Charles C Thomas, 1974.)

CHILDREN WITH PALPITATIONS AND ARRHYTHMIAS

Complaints of abnormalities of rhythm are common. They are often described as irregular beats, extra beats, "strange" or skipped beats, fast or "racing heart," or "jumping in the chest." Fortunately, most of these symptoms do not represent serious arrhythmias; however, potentially serious arrhythmias can present with mild symptoms initially. Determining the underlying diagnosis, as well as which children may need more thorough investigation, is often difficult without the presence of other associated findings.

The history often is nonspecific, but particular attention should be paid to a past history of syncope (see later) or light-headedness and chest pain. A complete family history of structural heart disease or of sudden death should be elicited. The association of the sensation with exercise, position, or food intake, particularly caffeine-containing substances, should be determined. In general, the findings of the physical examination are unremarkable, except for the arrhythmia. Diagnosis and treatment, therefore, become dependent on documentation of the rhythm.

Documenting an abnormal rhythm can be difficult, particularly when the symptoms are periodic and infrequent. An ECG should always be obtained. A sinus arrhythmia is a common, normal finding in children, as are occasional premature atrial contractions. Sinus arrhythmia is the normal variability of the heart rate associated with respiration. During inspiration, due to slightly decreased left ventricular filling, there can be a mild increase in the heart rate, which then slows during expiration. Preexcitation, when present, suggests reentrant tachycardia. More serious abnormalities, such as atrioventricular block, left ventricular hypertrophy, or a prolonged QT interval, warrant immediate referral to a pediatric cardiologist. The ECG, however, often is normal. If the suspected arrhythmia is frequent, occurring several times a day, then a 24-h Holter monitor recording is indicated. However, the episodes often occur less frequently, and the Holter monitor record is likely to be normal. In these instances, an event recorder is helpful. Patients carry an event recorder, which is placed on the chest when the arrhythmia is experienced, recording the rhythm. This allows capture of even infrequent events. Alternatively, a continuous memory loop recorder may be used, which is connected to patients at all times and which records a continuous loop of ECG data. When transient symptoms are experienced, patients press a button that stores the tracing for later analysis. With both types of recorder, the ECG data is transmitted over the phone to a monitoring center. For patients with extremely serious symptoms, which are also extremely infrequent, an implantable version of the looping recorder is available. Patients occasionally are asked to come to the emergency department or clinic as soon as they experience

symptoms, but this is reserved for those in whom diagnosis is very difficult, since it is quite unlikely to be successful in recording an episode. Exercise testing can be performed when symptoms are associated with exercise or to determine the severity of the arrhythmia for recommendations regarding athletic participation.

Premature Beats

The new onset of frequent premature beats often is the clue to underlying conditions, such as digoxin toxicity, other drug ingestions, myocarditis, hypoxia, hypokalemia, hypercarbia, or acidosis.

CAUSES

Supraventricular premature contractions. These are recognizable as narrow QRS beats that occur early. They may also have wide QRS complexes caused by bundle branch aberration. Those that originate in the atrium may be recognizable by finding a premature P wave superimposed on the previous T wave, deforming it. This sign may be subtle, however, and may require examination of multiple leads.

Ventricular premature complexes. These are recognizable as wide, often bizarre, early beats, usually without preceding P waves. The differentiation between ventricular contractions and aberrantly conducted supraventricular contractions is sometimes difficult or impossible from the surface ECG. Although traditionally premature ventricular beats may be differentiated from supraventricular beats by the presence of a full compensatory pause, this sign is somewhat unreliable. The identification of fusion beats, in which a sinus beat occurs simultaneously with a premature beat, thus creating an intermediate morphology, is very helpful and establishes the premature beat as ventricular in origin.

TREATMENT

In the absence of tachycardia, patients only occasionally require treatment for premature beats. Rare patients will be sufficiently symptomatic from single premature beats to warrant treatment for suppression of the premature beats. In the absence of such symptoms, supraventricular premature contractions virtually never require treatment. Asymptomatic ventricular premature contractions may require treatment in a few situations:

1. When they are multiform
2. When they occur in couplets or short runs of ventricular tachycardia
3. When they are seen in association with a recently converted ventricular tachycardia
4. When they exhibit the "R on T" phenomenon; i.e., they fall repeatedly on the early part of the T wave of the preceding beat.

Abnormal Tachycardia

Tachycardia in children is much more common than bradycardia. Tachycardia is classified by the duration of the QRS. A narrow QRS tachycardia is one in which the QRS duration is similar to that during normal sinus rhythm, or in the normal range for age if a baseline ECG is not available. A wide-QRS tachycardia is one in which the QRS duration is substantially longer than is the duration in normal sinus rhythm, or longer than the 95th percentile for age. Nearly all narrow QRS tachycardias in children are supraventricular in origin, and nearly all wide QRS tachycardias are ventricular in origin. Any form of narrow QRS tachycardia may manifest *aberration,* defined as widening of the QRS complex. Aberration usually is due to rate-dependent bundle branch block. The onset of aberration may be progressive; once established, aberration may persist until termination of the tachycardia. Because the QRS complex widening results from rate-dependent bundle branch block, it usually resembles a right or left bundle branch block pattern. Aberration with SVT often occurs at the onset of the tachycardia in the absence of preexisting bundle branch block, but sustained bundle branch aberration with SVT is rare in children.

Before discussing the various causes and mechanisms of tachycardia, it should be noted here that by far the most common diagnosis in children complaining of palpitation is normal sinus rhythm. In some patients, in the syndrome of "cardiac consciousness," children become acutely aware of their heart rate and rhythm and begin to worry about sensations they used to ignore. The concomitant anxiety may lead to more sinus tachycardia. In such patients, documentation of normal rhythm with reassurance is usually all that is necessary. Occasionally, patients will experience true "inappropriate sinus tachycardia," in which the heart rate is demonstrably higher than is expected for the level of activity. Often in such patients, sudden large swings in heart rate can occur with change in position and can be quite symptomatic. Some, but not all, such patients will respond to beta blocker therapy. The syndrome is as yet poorly understood and is rare in children. Finally, nearly everyone will display occasional premature atrial contractions or premature ventricular contractions on a 24-h Holter monitor. When patients are sensitive to these premature beats, they may complain of palpitation. Narrow QRS tachycardia is by far the most common major arrhythmia encountered in childhood. Most patients do not have underlying structural heart disease. Presentation can occur at any age. The arrhythmia can be an incidental finding or can present in infants with nonspecific symptoms, including irritability, sleep or feeding difficulty, lethargy, or even cardiovascular collapse. Older children are usually aware that their heart rate is fast, although some may have chest pain and/or dizziness as the major symptom. The rate of the tachycardia depends on both the age at presentation and the underlying etiology. The differential of narrow QRS tachycardia includes atrioventricular reentrant tachycardia (AVRT), atrioventricular node reentrant tachycardia (AVNRT), atrial ectopic tachycardia (AET), atrial flutter, and junctional tachycardia. Atrial fibrillation, common in older adults, is a rare cause of SVT in children. Of these, AVRT is most common.

Atrioventricular reentrant tachycardia refers to a narrow QRS tachycardia mediated by an accessory pathway. In patients with Wolff-Parkinson-White syndrome, this is a small strand of myocardium that bridges the atrioventricular groove and provides an alternant route for impulses to travel between the atrium and ventricle. In Wolff-Parkinson White syndrome, such pathways are capable of both antegrade (atrium to ventricle), as well as retrograde (ventricle to atrium), conduction. During sinus rhythm, antegrade conduction down the pathway fuses with antegrade conduction down the atrioventricular node to give rise to a widened QRS and a short PR interval. During AVRT, conduction is down the atrioventricular node in the antegrade direction and up the accessory pathway in the retrograde direction, giving rise to reentry and sustained tachycardia (Figure 16–13). P waves may be seen after the QRS but are often buried in the T wave. The tachycardia rate can be as high as 280 to 300 per

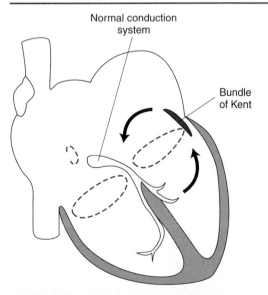

Figure 16–13. Diagram of reentrant circuit in Wolff-Parkinson-White syndrome. Impulses proceed down the normal conduction system to the ventricle and then retrograde up the bundle of Kent (accessory pathway) back to the atrium where they may then reenter the normal conduction system.

minute in infants (Figure 16–14) and 220 to 250 per minute in older children. The rhythm is extremely regular, such that a bedside monitor will read exactly the same rate consistently over several minutes. Patients who have an accessory pathway that functions in the retrograde direction only are said to have a "concealed accessory pathway." In these patients, the ECG is normal during normal sinus rhythm, with no sign of preexcitation. The mechanism of tachycardia is the same as with Wolff-Parkinson-White syndrome, as is the appearance of the ECG during tachycardia.

Atrioventricular node reentrant tachycardia is similar to AVRT in some ways. In this condition, there are thought to be two AV nodal pathways: a "fast" pathway and a "slow" pathway. Reentry occurs between these two pathways within the atrioventricular node. In the most common form, conduction proceeds antegrade down the "slow" pathway and retrograde up the "fast" pathway, giving rise to a continuous loop. In this arrhythmia, P waves are typically not easily seen during tachycardia, as they are superimposed on the QRS complex.

Atrial ectopic tachycardia (AET) is due to increased automaticity of atrial tissue outside the sinus node. It is distinguished from both AVRT and AVNRT by the relation of the P waves to the QRS complexes. In AET, the PR interval is normal-to-slightly prolonged and is much shorter than is the RP interval. The ECG will often show occasional AV block, or variability of rate, and the P-wave morphology will nearly always be different from that of the sinus. These findings can confirm the diagnosis. *Atrial flutter* is a reentrant tachycardia in which the entire reentrant circuit is located within the atrium. It can present with atrial rates as fast as 500 in young infants, but is usually seen with atrial rates of 300 in older children. The ventricular rate is typically a fraction of the atrial rate due to 2:1, 3:1, or 4:1 conduction, but in children the ventricular rate may be irregular due to variable AV conduction. *Atrial fibrillation* is very unusual in the absence of underlying congenital heart disease and shows an "irregularly irregular" rhythm. Often, no two R-R intervals are of the same length. *Junctional tachycardia* is extremely rare outside the immediate postoperative period, but there is a congenital form that presents with incessant tachycardia. It is recognized, but the narrow (normal) QRS complexes have a ventricular rate faster than that of the atrial rate and occasionally capture beats.

IMMEDIATE THERAPY FOR NARROW QRS TACHYCARDIA

For critically ill patients with any form of narrow-QRS tachycardia, synchronized DC cardioversion is indicated. The correct initial dose for cardioversion or defibrillation is 0.5 to 2 J/kg. Narrow QRS tachycardias should always be converted in synchronous mode, in which the shock is timed to fall on the next QRS complex, to avoid delivery on the T wave. Ventricular fibrillation should always be defibrillated in asynchronous mode. In general, with wide QRS tachycardias, an initial attempt using synchronous mode should be made. However, some forms of ventricular tachycardia appear almost sinusoidal, and the cardioverter-defibrillator may not sense R waves well. In these cases, the use of asynchronous mode may be necessary. For seriously ill patients in whom there may be signs of CHF but who have a measurable blood pressure and are conscious, the clinician must make a judgment about the stability of patients' hemodynamic status. If patients' conditions are judged unstable, they should undergo electrical cardioversion after placement of an IV line. Patients whose condition is more stable are managed with the use of vagal maneuvers, followed by pharmacologic therapy; electrical cardioversion is an option if these measures should fail.

In children with narrow complex tachycardia whose condition is stable, it is important to document both the rhythm and the attempts at conversion, because in many patients it may not recur and the rhythm during conversion or attempted conversion often is diagnostic. If patients are well, general vagal maneuvers can be attempted.

Carotid massage and orbital pressure should not be performed in children. The carotid sinus region is not easily located in infants. Orbital pressure may be dangerous because eye injury could occur. In infants, rectal stimulation (by taking the rectal temperature) frequently is effective. Gagging with a nasogastric tube occasionally is effective. The diving reflex may be elicited by placing a bag filled with ice over the face (and covering the ears) for 15 s. Older children may be coached to perform a standard Valsalva maneuver. These maneuvers should be performed with an IV line in place and should not be continued

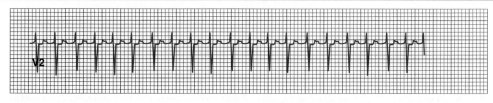

Figure 16–14. Narrow QRS tachycardia in an infant, aged 1 week, with atrioventricular reentrant tachycardia (AVRT). Notice the rapid rate (285 beats per minute), extreme regularity of the rhythm, and lack of obvious P waves.

longer than 5 min in seriously ill patients before one proceeds to other modalities. Although helpful, vagal maneuvers often are unsuccessful, and pharmacologic conversion is indicated.

Adenosine is valuable in the acute diagnosis and management of SVTs that involve the atrioventricular node as part of the reentrant circuit. This agent, when given rapidly by IV injection, induces a brief episode of complete atrioventricular block, thereby interrupting the reentrant circuit. The onset of effect is less than 1 min, the half-life in blood is less than 10 s, and the resulting atrioventricular blockade is therefore brief and self-limited. The successful conversion of AVRT with adenosine is evidence against other forms of tachycardia, such as atrial tachycardia, that do not involve the atrioventricular node as part of the reentrant circuit.

Although adenosine usually converts AVRT and AVNRT only, it can be extremely useful in the diagnosis of other types of narrow complex tachycardia. By inducing transient complete atrioventricular block, it slows the ventricular rate, allowing better determination of atrial rate and P-wave morphology. In atrial ectopic tachycardia, atrial flutter, and atrial fibrillation, adenosine induces ventricular slowing, but the atrial activation is unaffected (Figure 16–15), and the diagnosis may be made easily. Adenosine is given as a rapid IV bolus, beginning at 50 to 100 mg/kg and rapidly increasing until the desired effect—atrioventricular block—is achieved. Further increases in dosage are not indicated, or is repeated administration to convert the rhythm transiently without other pharmacologic treatment.

Verapamil has been used for conversion in the past but is rarely indicated today because of the severe hypotension that it may cause, especially in infants. In addition, asystolic cardiac arrests have been reported in infants younger than 6 months.

Digoxin is an effective agent for the treatment of most pediatric narrow QRS tachycardias. A disadvantage is the relatively long period necessary to digitalize patients safely.

One approach to IV digitalization is to give 10 mg/kg as a first IV dose, followed by a second dose 2 h later and a third dose at 6 to 12 h later. The dose should not be given if hypokalemia is present or if there is a suspicion of digoxin toxicity.

IMMEDIATE THERAPY FOR WIDE QRS TACHYCARDIA

Because most children with wide QRS tachycardia have ventricular tachycardia (Figure 16–16) rather than SVT with aberration, and because it is often nearly impossible to differentiate these possibilities firmly in children by using only a surface ECG, patients with wide QRS tachycardia are managed as if they had ventricular tachycardia. In practice, this means that electrical cardioversion is indicated in nearly all cases. In patients who are neither seriously nor critically ill, one may defer cardioversion while pharmacologic agents are administered. In this situation, procainamide would be a good choice because it is effective both for ventricular and supraventricular arrhythmias. Lidocaine may be used if there is certainty that the diagnosis is ventricular tachycardia. *Verapamil, however, should never be given to patients with wide QRS tachycardia.* If the diagnosis is actually ventricular tachycardia, and verapamil fails to convert the rhythm to sinus rhythm, the resulting hypotension in the face of continued tachycardia may be life-threatening.

Abnormal Bradycardia

CAUSES

Sinus bradycardia. Sinus bradycardia is recognized as a regular slow atrial rate with normal P waves and 1:1 conduction. Causes include hypoxia, acidosis, increased intracranial pressure, abdominal distension, and hypoglycemia. Drugs such as digoxin and propranolol may also cause significant sinus bradycardia. Mild slowing may be due to increased vagal tone or cardiac conditioning.

Atrioventricular block. *Complete atrioventricular block* may be congenital or surgically induced or may occur

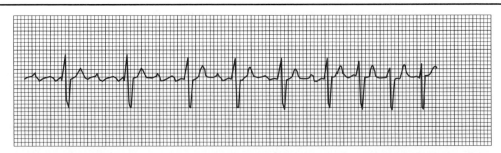

Figure 16–15. Diagnosis of atrial flutter by administration of adenosine. Adenosine-induced atrioventricular block slows the ventricular rate, allowing visualization of the characteristic "saw-tooth" pattern of atrial flutter. After metabolism of the adenosine and rapid ventricular response, the flutter is much less apparent.

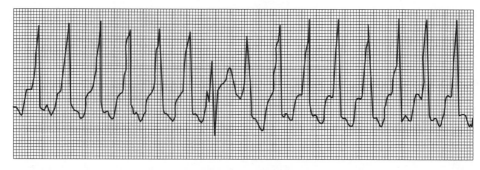

Figure 16–16. Ventricular tachycardia: Very wide QRS complexes are seen. A single capture beat is seen and occurs with a narrow QRS complex, proving the presence of ventricular tachycardia. (Reproduced with permission from Van Hare GF: Dysrhythmias. In: Grossman M, Dieckmann RA [editors]: *Pediatric Emergency Medicine. A Clinician's Reference.* Lippincott, 1991.)

suddenly because of myocarditis. It is recognized as atrioventricular dissociation, with regular RR intervals, regular PP intervals, an atrial rate greater than ventricular rate, and an absence of capture beats.

Second-degree atrioventricular block should be classified as Mobitz type 1 (Wenckebach) or Mobitz type 2. Wenckebach conduction is characterized by progressive PR interval prolongation followed by a blocked beat, followed by recovery of conduction. Type 2 block lacks this characteristic PR prolongation with shortening after the blocked beat. Type 1 generally has a better prognosis than does type 2 and responds to medication readily.

Other causes of bradycardia are sinus exit block, in which sinus P waves intermittently disappear owing to blockage of impulses leaving the region of the node, and frequent premature atrial contractions, which occur too early to be conducted to the ventricles and therefore slow the resulting ventricular rate.

TREATMENT

The hemodynamic effect of a slow heart rate depends on how different it is from patients' usual heart rate. Sudden decreases in rate may be poorly compensated by increases in stroke volume, particularly in those with preexisting poor cardiac function. Moderate bradycardia in normal children rarely requires treatment. Exceptions include the sudden occurrence of complete atrioventricular block or pacemaker failure. The urgency of treatment is dictated by the hemodynamic status. Underlying causes, such as hypoxia, should be corrected.

If treatment is indicated, initial treatment with atropine, followed by continuous isoproterenol infusion, will increase sinus rates, improve atrioventricular conduction, and may increase the rate of subsidiary pacemakers. After initial stabilization with medications, temporary transvenous pacing should be instituted, particularly in patients with very low ventricular rates (<30 per minute) or in

those with hemodynamic compromise. Subsequently, implantation of a permanent pacemaker may be necessary if bradycardia does not improve.

CHILDREN WITH SYNCOPE

Syncope is a sudden, brief loss of consciousness caused by diffuse transient impairment of cerebral function. The sudden loss of consciousness by definition is associated with loss of postural tone and falling, with a quick recovery of consciousness once in the supine position. The fall may cause physical trauma. If children cannot fall to the supine position, as when trapped upright in a school desk, recovery to consciousness may be delayed, and a tonic-clonic seizure may develop. Syncope is a common presenting symptom in older children and adolescents. Often patients have presyncope symptoms, including light-headedness, dizziness, weakness, pallor, cold sweat, or blurred vision. Although it most often is benign, syncope can be the presenting symptom for significant cardiac, neurologic, or metabolic disease and even the harbinger of sudden death (Table 16–8). Therefore, a careful evaluation to elucidate the cause is mandatory.

Noncardiac causes of syncope are extensive, and a detailed discussion is beyond the scope of this chapter. Seizure disorder is the most common. Psychogenic causes, such as breath-holding in toddlers and hyperventilation in teenagers, also occur frequently. Metabolic abnormalities, including hypoglycemia, electrolyte imbalance, and severe anemia, may cause syncope.

Evaluation of children with syncope begins with a careful, detailed history and physical examination. The history should describe events leading up to the episode, as well as the episode. This description should include the duration; observations during the episode, such as incontinence, vomiting, associated injuries, and tonic-clonic movements; and duration of the neurologic state during

Table 16–8. Causes of Syncope

Cardiac	Neurologic	Metabolic
Neurally mediated syncope	Seizures	Hypoglycemia
Bradyarrhythmia	Breathholding	Electrolyte
Sick sinus syndrome	Hyperventilation	abnormalities
Atrioventricular block		Severe anemia
Tachyarrhythmia		
Supraventricular		
Ventricular tachycardia		
Prolonged QT interval		
Hypertrophic cardiomyopathy		
Aortic stenosis		
Pulmonary hypertension		

the recovery. In addition, the family history is important, due to the occurrence of certain familial causes of sudden death such as the prolonged QT syndrome and HCM. If the history and physical examination findings suggest a neurologic cause, an electroencephalogram or a computed tomography (CT) or MRI scan of the brain might be indicated. If a metabolic cause is implicated, laboratory studies, including serum glucose and electrolyte levels and blood cell count, should be obtained. An ECG is mandatory in all patients with syncope, and a 24-h Holter monitor, echocardiogram, tilt-table test, and electrophysiology study might be necessary if the initial evaluation suggests a cardiac cause.

The most common cause of syncope in children is neurally mediated syncope. The classic example is the cadet who passes out while standing at attention for hours in the hot sun. This is benign except for the risk associated with falling during the episode. The mechanism is a sudden decrease in systemic venous return that results in less filling of the left ventricle and a decreased left ventricular end-diastolic volume. In response, increased contractility and stimulation of cardiac vagal fibers lead to reflex bradycardia, vasodilation, and hypotension, which in turn lead to transient hypoperfusion of the brain, causing syncope. Once the supine position is attained, perfusion to the brain is restored, as is normal systemic venous return, abolishing the transient reflex. There are three clinical types of neurally mediated syncope, identified on the basis of the predominate features: The first, vasodepressor, starts with and is dominated by hypotension; the second, cardioinhibitory, starts with and is dominated by

marked bradycardia; and the third, mixed response, is a mixture of both. Neurally mediated syncope is exacerbated by anything that predisposes to decreased systemic venous return (e.g., physical exhaustion, prolonged recumbency) or to peripheral vasodilation (e.g., exercise, hot weather, and emotional stress).

The diagnosis often can be made from a typical history, negative family history, normal physical examination findings, and lack of evidence for a neurologic, cardiac, or metabolic cause. If necessary, the definitive diagnosis is made with a positive tilt-test result. Patients lie supine on a table for 10 min while baseline heart rate and blood pressure are measured. Patients are then rapidly tilted to a nearly upright position (60 to 80°) while strapped to the table, with continuous monitoring of the blood pressure and heart rate. If the symptoms develop and are associated with hypotension and/or bradycardia, the diagnosis is clear. Treatment for a single episode should be conservative. For recurrent episodes, expansion of intravascular volume by increasing salt and water intake or treating with fluorocortisone (Florinef, 0.1 to 0.3 mg) may be adequate. Treatment with beta-adrenergic blockers, such as propranolol, atenolol, or pindolol, can be effective. In patients with a prominent vasodepressor response, the use of a new drug, midodrine may be effective. Midodrine is an alpha agonist and acts by increasing vasomotor tone and minimizing venous pooling in the lower extremities. In the cardioinhibitory type, if symptoms are severe, pacemaker implantation, particularly with devices that provide a so-called "rate-drop response" has been effective. With this type of pacemaker, a sudden deceleration in heart rate is sensed, and the response is dual chamber pacing at a much higher rate.

Other cardiac causes of syncope include arrhythmias and lesions that impair cardiac output. Either severe bradycardia, sick sinus syndrome or atrioventricular block, or supraventricular or ventricular tachycardia may cause syncope. All except SVT are extremely rare in children without congenital heart disease. Syncope may occur with SVT, although most children complain of chest discomfort, fatigue, weakness, or dizziness. However, patients with Wolff-Parkinson-White syndrome may be at risk for sudden death due to the occurrence of atrial fibrillation and rapid conduction to the ventricles. Prolonged QT syndrome must be considered, as it is associated with torsades de pointes, a form of polymorphous ventricular tachycardia that can lead to ventricular fibrillation and sudden death. QT prolongation may be associated with congenital deafness and autosomal-recessive inheritance (Jervell-Lange-Nielsen) or autosomal-dominant inheritance with deafness (Romano-Ward syndrome). Electrolyte abnormalities and some antiarrhythmic drugs (e.g., quinidine, procainamide, and amiodarone) can prolong the QT interval. Evaluation should include a 12-lead ECG with careful measurement of the corrected QT interval. Patients with HCM are also at risk for sudden death, and this risk appears unrelated to the severity of subaortic obstruction. Clues to the diagnosis of HCM, which would lead to echocardiographic diagnosis, include a prominent left ventricular impulse, loud murmur, or left ventricular hypertrophy on ECG. A 24 h Holter monitor or event recorder may be necessary to capture the abnormal rhythm, although when Wolff-Parkinson-White syndrome, prolonged QT syndrome, or HCM is diagnosed, treatment should be started without attempts to capture the symptomatic rhythm electrocardiographically. Treatment is directed at the specific type of arrhythmia and may include antiarrhythmic medications, radiofrequency ablation, cardiac pacemaker, or cardioverter-defibrillator implantation.

Transient decreased cardiac output due to left ventricular outflow tract obstruction may result in syncope, especially during or immediately after exercise. The inability to increase cardiac output leads to increased parasympathetic tone and systemic vasodilation by stimulating left ventricular baroreceptors. The lesion most frequently associated with syncope is HCM (see earlier). Severe fixed obstruction, such as severe AS, also may be responsible. Patients with severe pulmonary hypertension may have syncope associated with low output during a pulmonary hypertensive crisis. Rarely, children with dilated cardiomyopathy, anomalous left coronary artery, or a cardiac tumor have syncope. The cardiac examination will have an abnormality, which should be confirmed and defined with an echocardiogram. Treatment is directed at the specific cardiac abnormality.

CHILDREN WITH CHEST PAIN

Chest pain is a common complaint, particularly in school-aged children. Viral illness and emotional and physical stress, as well as trauma and cardiac disease, can all produce what is described as "chest pain." Noncardiac causes of chest pain are more common in children. Intermittent chest wall inflammation, also called costochondritis, is quite common. There often is a history of a preceding viral illness. The pain is sharp, very short in duration, easily localized by patients with a single finger, and associated with movement or exercise. In general, the children are well. The pain often can be reproduced by careful, firm palpation of the area in question. Laboratory examination is rarely indicated. Symptomatic pain treatment with anti-inflammatory medication usually is sufficient.

PULMONARY DISEASE

Pulmonary disease, such as pneumothorax, pneumonia, or pleural effusions, can present with chest pain. The pain often is unilateral, but smaller children cannot localize this. There usually is dyspnea, and blood oxygen desaturation often is present. Examination reveals decreased or absent breath sounds on the side involved. Chest radiograph confirms the diagnosis (see Chap. 8).

ESOPHAGEAL DISEASE

Esophageal disease, such as acute esophagitis, gastroesophageal reflux, or foreign body ingestion, can mimic the pain of pericarditis or ischemia. It is substernal but has a more burning quality, is associated with dysphagia, and often is relieved by antacids. Physical examination findings often are nonspecific. The diagnosis is suspected from the history. Direct esophageal examination or imaging confirms the underlying etiology.

When evaluating children with pain, one should determine the degree of acute illness. Chest pain can be grouped by the initial presentation: acute onset versus chronic and recurring.

Acute Onset

Children with acute-onset chest pain usually seek urgent relief from their pain. In these children, the etiology of their pain should be determined quickly, and treatment initiated. Acute-onset chest pain is by nature more severe than is chronic and recurring pain and is more likely to be caused by a serious medical illness. A focused history should be obtained, with specific attention to a history of trauma, viral illnesses, drug or toxin ingestions, and palpitations. The severity, location, and radiation of the pain; factors that exacerbate or relieve symptoms; and other symptoms should be determined. The position in which children prefer to lie should be noticed. Physical examination should focus on the degree of acute illness, skin color, respiratory effort, and peripheral pulses and perfusion. Auscultation should focus on the breath and heart sounds, with specific attention to unequal breath sounds or muffled heart sounds. Laboratory examination is directed by the results of examination.

PERICARDITIS

This represents an inflammation of the pericardial sac, with resultant fluid production and tension in the parietal pericardium. It can be caused by viral or bacterial illness and is associated with many autoimmune diseases. In children with pericarditis, pain is acute, substernal, and squeezing, and they are often quite ill. The description is similar to anginal pain. There often is a history of viral illness. The children prefer to lie very still, leaning forward, which relaxes the pericardium and decreases pain. Pressure on the chest, breathing, and movement exacerbate the pain. Examination can show thready peripheral pulses and a paradoxical pulse, indicating impending cardiac tamponade. Auscultation reveals tachycardia and distant heart sounds and sometimes a friction rub; this may not be heard with a large effusion. Echocardiography confirms the presence of an effusion. Initial treatment when signs of tamponade are present is emergent drainage. Other treatment is directed toward the underlying cause.

Related to pericarditis, the entity referred to as *pleurodynia* causes severe chest pain that is pleuritic in nature. Also termed *devil's grip,* it is thought to be due to pleuritis caused by infection with coxsackievirus. The syndrome is self-limited and is treated with nonsteroidal antiinflammatory agents. Another similar entity is called *Texidor's twinge,* a syndrome in which patients complain of a sudden severe and sharp pain, or "catch," and patients may even be doubled over in pain. It is brief and of no long-term significance. It is thought to be due to sudden restriction of pleural movement.

Chest Trauma

Chest trauma, particularly blunt trauma, can result in hemopericardium. The presentation and characteristics of this pain are similar to those of acute pericarditis, except that, in addition, chest wall tenderness usually is present at the site of trauma. These children should be quickly evaluated for signs of tamponade, undergo an echocardiogram for confirmation, and receive emergent pericardial drainage. They also should be evaluated for other mediastinal bleeding by CT scan after initial stabilization.

Myocardial Ischemia or Infarction

Fortunately, these are rare causes of pain in children. Most children at risk for myocardial ischemia have known underlying heart disease and are under the care of a pediatric cardiologist. Ischemic pain in children has two main causes: severe ventricular hypertrophy and coronary artery disease. Ischemia can develop in patients with *severe ventricular hypertrophy,* particularly of the left ventricle. With marked hypertrophy, the subendocardium is poorly perfused when the oxygen supply cannot meet demand, as during exercise. The history is typical for ischemia, except in very small children. Physical examination confirms the presence of the lesion. Initial treatment is directed at the underlying cause of hypertrophy or is directed at relieving symptoms when the cause is not apparent.

Coronary Artery Disease

Coronary artery disease is rare in children. Congenital anomalies of the coronary arteries, such as pulmonary origin of the left coronary artery (POLCA), more commonly present with CHF in the first year of life. Acquired coronary artery disease, such as the aneurysms seen in Kawasaki disease, can present with chest pain. In general, however, the diagnosis is known and treatment initiated before the development of disease. Ischemia may occur after recovery if thrombosis develops in an aneurysm, obstructing coronary flow.

Arrhythmias

Children with arrhythmias can have acute chest pain. This pain usually is not severe, and the children usually appear well. The pain is less localized and is associated with light-headedness and the sensation of palpitations or fast heart rate. Physical examination findings usually are unremarkable, except for the rhythm abnormality. The ECG confirms the diagnosis (see "Children with Palpitations and Arrhythmias," earlier).

Chronic and Recurrent Pain

Chronic, recurring chest pain is much more common than acute-onset pain. It usually is milder, and care is not sought until the pain has persisted for some time. The diagnosis can be difficult to establish because the children usually are seen when not experiencing pain. A thorough history, including potential emotional stressors, should be obtained. Major anxiety regarding severe underlying cardiac disease often is present. History should focus on trauma, viral illnesses, and the relation between the pain and movement, breathing, and daily activities, such as school or play. The periodicity, locality, radiation, if any, and severity of the pain should be determined. Physical examination should focus on signs of trauma, which can be subtle; symptoms of a viral, particularly upper respiratory, illness; and general state of the patients. One should always attempt to reproduce the pain by thoroughly and firmly palpating the chest or by placing the children in the position that reportedly produces the pain. Auscultation is directed primarily toward the intensity of the heart sounds and the presence of abnormal heart sounds or murmurs.

The most common cause of recurrent pain is not associated with any organic pathology. The terms *idiopathic, psychogenic,* and *growing pains* are used, although the term *psychogenic* should be avoided because of the negative connotation this gives to the family. The history often reveals an association between the pain and major stressful activities, such as schoolwork. It usually is not associated with either exercise or enjoyable activities. The pain is vague and localized as an oval over the entire chest. When challenged, the children cannot localize the pain. Most patients believe that the heart is the cause of their pain. Physical examination usually is normal but should be complete, even repeating some portions to reassure the patients and family that the heart is normal. Explanation of all the normal portions of the examination is helpful. Laboratory examination usually is not necessary. The situation should be explained thoroughly to the patients and family, without giving the impression that it is "all in their head."

Chest wall pain due to costochondritis is the next most common cause of recurrent pain (see discussion earlier).

INFECTIONS OF THE HEART

Pericarditis

Infections of the pericardium are discussed under "Children with Chest Pain," earlier.

Myocarditis

Disorders of the myocardium, including acute inflammatory conditions, termed *myocarditis,* and those without specific evidence of inflammation, termed *cardiomyopathy* are discussed under "Children with Cardiac Failure," earlier.

Infective Endocarditis

DEFINITION

The term *infective endocarditis* denotes a condition in which a bacterial or fungal infection involves the endocardial surface of the heart, most commonly the cardiac valves, or the endothelial surfaces of central vessels. Such infection may lead to destruction of the valves with resulting CHF, or it may lead to disseminated sepsis. In the preantibiotic era, this condition was almost uniformly fatal. Currently, despite the availability of antimicrobial agents effective against nearly all pathogens responsible for endocarditis, the disease carries a mortality rate of 15 to 20%. Therefore, the importance of prevention, as well as early diagnosis and institution of treatment, cannot be overstated.

PATHOPHYSIOLOGY

Whereas bacterial and fungal pathogens may cause endocarditis in any person, the patients at greatest risk are those with preexisting cardiac structural abnormalities. Because rheumatic heart disease has become rare in children, this group consists of children with congenital heart disease. Most forms of congenital heart disease are associated with an increased risk of endocarditis; however, this increased risk highest in those who have had placement of artificial tissue grafts.

The pathophysiology of the disease begins with the introduction of predisposing pathogens into the bloodstream. Although certain high-risk events, such as dental extractions and IV drug abuse, produce significant bacteremia, nearly all persons are thought to experience bacteremia occasionally, e.g., after tooth brushing and other activities. Once introduced into the bloodstream, the pathogen adheres to the endocardium. In general, the hemodynamic environment determines these sites, and areas of greatest turbulence are most often infected. For example, in patients with surgical shunts placed between the aorta and the pulmonary artery, infection develops in the pulmonary artery opposite the aortic jet. Such "jet lesions" are thought to be created by turbulent flow and to encourage the development of endocarditis. However, endocarditis has often been reported to involve nonturbulent areas of the endocardium, and invasive organisms can cause endocarditis even in patients whose hearts apparently are completely normal. The adherence of the pathogen to the endocardium leads to the deposition of plate-

lets and thrombin, which form a vegetation. The growth of this vegetation may be associated with progressive valve destruction, damage to the blood vessels, or the occurrence of embolization as pieces of the vegetation break off and travel to distant sites. The chronic presence of bacteria or fungi may lead to the development of immune complexes, which may in turn cause a serum-sickness–like reaction.

A great many pathogens have been found to cause endocarditis (Table 16–9). The viridans streptococci, which are normal mouth flora, have been the most common. However, reports have shown that *Staphyloccocus aureus* is increasing in frequency and now accounts for nearly as many cases in children. Other pathogens include the enterococci, the gram-negative enteric organisms, the pneumococci, *Staphyloccocus epidermidis,* and *Candida albicans.* In immune-compromised patients, more indolent, slow-growing pathogens may be involved.

DIAGNOSIS

In the past, infective endocarditis has been classified as either "acute" or "subacute" bacterial endocarditis. Although the classification is useful for remembering the different possible modes of presentation of the illness, few patients have either classic picture. More often, features of both presentations are present (Table 16–10).

Patients with an acute presentation have a short duration of illness, high fever, and signs of progressive CHF because of valve destruction. They may also manifest signs of serious embolization, which may include pulmonary embolus, stroke, hematuria, or peripheral emboli. Valve destruction may be so rapid that signs of cardiac failure are present. Patients with a subacute presentation have a long (often more than 2 weeks) duration of illness, low-grade or even absent fever, and signs of immune complex disease, such as glomerulonephritis, arthritis, and skin rash. Findings such as the presence of petechiae, Osler nodes (small digital nodules), Janeway lesions (hemorrhagic or purpuric skin lesions), and Roth spots (retinal hemorrhagic lesions) are helpful in making the diagnosis but are rarely seen in children. A new or changed cardiac murmur may be appreciated, but one must be careful: The presence of

Table 16–9. Organisms Most Frequently Isolated in Endocarditis

Viridans streptococci
Staphylococcus aureus
Enterococci
Streptococcus pneumoniae
Enteric gram-negative organisms (*Escherichia coli, Klebsiella* species, etc)
Candida albicans
Staphylococcus epidermidis

Table 16–10. Acute and Subacute Presentation of Endocarditis

Acute Presentation	Subacute Presentation
New murmur	New murmur
Cardiac decompensation	Little or no decompensation
Short duration of illness (<2 wk)	Longer duration of illness (>2 wk)
Major emboli	Splenomegaly
	Petechiae
	Osler nodes
	Janeway lesions
	Roth spots
	Splinter hemorrhages

fever often amplifies trivial cardiac murmurs in children. Signs of CHF usually are not part of the subacute presentation.

The diagnosis of infective endocarditis rests on clinical findings as well as on the results of blood cultures. Infective endocarditis produces a constant low-grade bacteremia, rather than episodic high-grade bacteremia. Therefore, multiple blood cultures are very helpful. One normally obtains four to six blood cultures, if possible, before the institution of therapy. When multiple cultures are positive for the same organism, endocarditis is more likely, whereas simple bacterial sepsis is less likely.

Echocardiography can be helpful in establishing the diagnosis in patients who have endocarditis but is not useful for ruling out the disease. This is because the prominent echocardiographic findings often are not present in patients who do have the disease. Diagnostic echocardiographic findings can include vegetations, dilatation of the aorta or pulmonary artery in patients with invasion of these vessels, and the presence of previously absent valvular regurgitation indicating valve destruction.

TREATMENT

The decisions that must be made in the treatment of endocarditis are complicated by two somewhat conflicting needs: the need to establish a microbiologic diagnosis and the need to institute therapy as quickly as possible to minimize valve destruction. The institution of broad-spectrum therapy before adequate blood cultures have been obtained may lead to uncertainty in the diagnosis and the possibility of prolonged unnecessary therapy with multiple toxic agents. In contrast, excessive delay in the institution of therapy to obtain cultures may lead to rapid valve destruction and progressive CHF or septic shock. In practice, one must consider both competing issues. In patients with a more "subacute" presentation, rapid valve destruction and sepsis are less likely, and 12 to 24 h for obtaining adequate cultures is reasonable. In patients with a more "acute" pre-

sentation, therapy should not be delayed, and as many cultures as is feasible should be rapidly obtained prior to starting therapy.

Initial therapy should include coverage for the viridans streptococci as well as for *Staph. aureus* and enterococcus. This is true both for patients with community-acquired infections, as well as for those who have undergone cardiac surgery. In the latter group, coverage for multiple-drug-resistant organisms (such as *Staph. epidermidis*) should be considered, as well as coverage for whatever locally prominent nosocomial pathogens are present in the hospital. Once the pathogen has been identified, more specific therapy may be substituted on the basis of the antibiotic sensitivities of the pathogen.

All patients being treated for infective endocarditis should receive daily repeated blood cultures, beginning 12 to 24 h after institution of therapy. Persistent positive cultures despite theoretically adequate antibiotics represent the potential for therapeutic failure. Therefore, higher doses of the antibiotic or additional agents may be necessary. Continued surveillance is vital for signs of emboli, for ECG changes that might indicate invasion of the cardiac conduction system, and for progression of cardiac valvular dysfunction.

Surgery for debridement or for valve replacement occasionally is necessary. The generally accepted indications for surgery include progressive CHF despite medical therapy, persistent infection despite theoretically adequate antimicrobial treatment, serious systemic embolization, infection involving a prosthetic cardiac valve, and, perhaps, the presence of fungal endocarditis. Timing of surgery will be dictated by the hemodynamic condition.

It is well established that relapse after successful treatment occurs, and, in the past, occurred more often after short courses of antibiotic therapy. Therefore, most patients should receive a prolonged course (commonly 4 to 6 weeks) of IV antimicrobial therapy. However, certain lower-risk patients with less virulent organisms can receive combination IV and oral courses.

PREVENTION

Most cases of infective endocarditis do not follow an identifiable invasive procedure or event. Therefore, the disease is by no means completely preventable. However, certain high-risk procedures have been identified, and one may perhaps lower the risk of the development of endocarditis if antibiotic prophylaxis is given in association with these events. Nearly all patients with congenital heart disease should receive antibiotic prophylaxis during these procedures. The exceptions include patients with isolated ASD and those who have had successful repairs of PDA, ASD, and simple VSD. The American Heart Association has proposed antibiotic regimens for prevention of bacterial endocarditis for these procedures (Table 16–11). The list of procedures for which prophylaxis is indicated is ex-

Table 16–11. Antibiotic Regimen for Prophylaxis of Bacterial Endocarditis in Children[1]

Procedure	Standard Regimen	For Penicillin-Allergic Individuals
Dental, oral, respiratory tract, or esophageal	Amoxicillin 50 mg/kg (max, 3.0 g) 1 h before procedure	Clindamycin 20 mg/kg or cephalexin or cefadroxil 50 mg/kg or azithromycin or clarithromycin 15 mg/kg 1 h before procedure
	Unable to Take Oral Medications	**For Penicillin-Allergic Individuals**
	Ampicillin 50 mg/kg IV or IM (max, 2.0 g) within 30 min before procedure	Clindamycin 20 mg/kg IV or cefazolin 25 mg/kg IV or IM within 30 min before procedure
Gastrointestinal, genitourinary (excluding esophageal) procedures or high-risk patients	Ampicillin 50 mg/kg plus gentamicin 1.5 mg/kg IV or IM 30 min before; amoxicillin 25 mg/kg orally or ampicillin 25 mg/kg IV or IM 6 h later	Vancomycin 20 mg/kg IV over 1–2 h plus gentamicin 1.5 mg/kg IV or IM, complete infusion/injection within 30 min of starting procedure

[1] Based on recommendations of the American Heart Association. JAMA 1997;277:1794.

tensive, but includes almost all dental procedures, including professional teeth cleaning, common airway procedures such as tonsillectomy and bronchoscopy (rigid or with biopsy), and most gastrointestinal and urinary procedures. Some common procedures for which prophylaxis is not indicated include circumcision, tympanostomy tube placement, and urinary catheterization.

EXERCISE AND SPORTS

Most children with congenital heart disease do not require specific physical activity restrictions. Children usually self-limit their activity to avoid overexertion. However, as children begin to participate in competitive sports, the pressure to perform can override these self-restrictions. Certain lesions, such as AS, carry an increased risk of decompensation with extensive physical activity and may require restriction. Even in these cases, however, most children with mild-to-moderate disease can participate in even intense physical activities after a thorough evaluation.

When evaluating children for possible participation in competitive athletics, a thorough history of activity tolerance should always be obtained. Specific questions should be asked about a family history of sudden death and early coronary artery disease. Blood pressure measurement and palpation of the radial and femoral pulses should be a part of the examination, since hypertension and coarctation can often go undiagnosed until well into adolescence and can affect activity tolerance. Any abnormalities should be fully investigated prior to clearance.

In general, types of physical activity can be divided into two groups comprising primarily static and primarily dynamic activity. Static activities represent those with a major isometric component or during which the Valsalva maneuver is common. Weight-lifting is an example of an activity that combines both Valsalva and isometric activity. Dynamic activities are those that involve more isotonic and aerobic activity, such as long-distance run-

ning. The distinction is important since static activity, particularly with the Valsalva maneuver, results in a large increase in blood pressure. Activities that are associated with a major risk of collision (e.g., football and martial arts), either with other participants or with other objects, need to be separated from those with minimal contact risk (e.g., running and swimming).

Although it is beyond the scope of this chapter to discuss specific recommendations in detail, a discussion is included of some general and certain specific situations with clear-cut guidelines. Most children with a physiologically corrected lesion (such as a VSD, ASD, or PDA) can be treated normally without restriction, including strenuous physical activity. Children with a shunt that is unoperated either have a hemodynamically insignificant shunt and can be treated normally, or have pulmonary vascular obstructive disease and will be severely limited in their exercise tolerance. Children with moderate or severe left-sided obstruction may need to avoid high levels of static activity. The combination of high blood pressure and significant obstruction can result in very high ventricular pressure. This may increase the risk for ischemia, arrhythmia, or ventricular dysfunction. Most children with right-sided obstruction have mild disease and can exercise normally; severe obstruction generally is corrected with excellent results. Cyanotic children have a decreased exercise capacity compared with healthy children. Exercise increases oxygen consumption, resulting in increased cyanosis. Also, the underlying lesion (even after palliation) is associated with a decreased ability to increase the heart rate with exercise. Therefore, although specific types of activity may not be contraindicated, competitive athletics are usually not appropriate due to their inability to sustain exercise. Finally, children with HCM have the same risks as those with left-sided obstructions, but also have the added risk of arrhythmia and sudden death, which may be mediated by catecholamines. Therefore, they can generally only exercise at low activity levels and are prohibited from competitive athletics.

Contact activities are generally discouraged in some patients. Children with Marfan's syndrome or other connective tissues diseases can rupture the aorta with the rapid deceleration of contact. Those that are on anticoagulation with warfarin (including most children with prosthetic valves and many children after Fontan procedure for single-ventricle physiology) are at increased risk for major bleeding with contact. Many other children are also on anti-platelet therapy, and exercise recommendations in these children are not clear-cut.

REFERENCES

Brook MM: Pediatric bacterial endocarditis. Treatment and prophylaxis. Pediatr Clin North Am 1999;46:275.

Committee on Rheumatic Fever, Endocarditis, and Kawasaki Disease: Prevention of bacterial endocarditis. Recommendations by the American Heart Association. JAMA 1990;277:1794.

Fyler DC, et al: Report of the New England Regional Cardiac Program. Pediatrics 1980;65(Suppl):375.

Gillette PC, Garson A, Jr (editors): *Pediatric Arrhythmias, Electrophysiology, and Pacing.* Philadelphia, W.B. Saunders, 1990.

Klaus MH, Fanaroff AA (editors): *Care of the High-Risk Neonate.* Philadelphia, W.B. Saunders, 1998.

Liebman J, et al (editors): *Pediatric Electrocardiography.* Baltimore, Williams & Wilkins, 1982.

Richards MR, et al: Frequency and significance of systolic cardiac murmurs in the first year of life. Pediatrics 1955;15:169.

Roberts NK, Gelband H (editors): *Cardiac Arrhythmias in the Neonate, Infant and Child.* Appleton-Century-Crofts, 1983.

Rudolph AM: *Congenital Diseases of the Heart.* Futura Publishing, 2001.

Shuford WH, Sybers RG (editors): *The Aortic Arch and Its Malformations.* Charles C Thomas, 1974.

Special Writing Group of the Committee on Rheumatic Fever, Endocarditis, and Kawasaki Disease of the Council on Cardiovascular Disease in the Young of the American Heart Association: guidelines for the diagnosis of rheumatic fever. Jones Criteria, 1992 update. JAMA 1992;268:2069.

Respiratory Diseases

Robert W. Wilmott, MD, Mark E. Dato, MD, PhD, & Barbara A. Chini, MD

The lungs represent a unique gas-exchanging interface between the host and the environment. The airways are a series of dichotomously branching tubes that connect to the alveolar space, which is a gas-exchanging interface with an area the size of a tennis court. Healthy 5-year-old children respire at least 5000 L of air per day. Because of the exposure to large amounts of inhaled microorganisms and antigens, the lungs have developed sophisticated host defense mechanisms. These exposures and host defense systems make the lungs susceptible to a wide variety of diseases.

This chapter will first describe the history, physical examination, and diagnostic procedures as they specifically relate to the evaluation of respiratory diseases. Then a discussion of the common problems that suggest a disorder of the respiratory system follows: noisy breathing, wheezing, chronic cough, acute and chronic respiratory distress, and disorders of respiratory control.

EVALUATION OF THE RESPIRATORY SYSTEM

History

A systematic medical history should be obtained, which includes information about the general medical history as well as the specifics of the chief complaint. Respiratory diseases are often affected by environmental factors, such as changes in temperature and exposure to noxious agents, such as cigarette smoke or wood-burning stoves. Therefore, the physician should specifically obtain a detailed description of the children's home when investigating a respiratory complaint. This includes the type of heating, condition of the home, proximity to urban or rural sources of potential allergens, and history of household pets, such as dogs, cats, and birds (budgerigars, parrots, or pigeons). The type of bedding used and the presence of soft furnishings or soft toys in the bedroom should be noted. The presence or absence of animal or vegetable fibers in feather pillows or soft furnishings, as well as the systems in use for air purification, air filtration, air conditioning, or humidification, should be recorded.

Pulmonary symptoms are often precipitated by trigger factors. Exercise is an important trigger factor for coughing and wheezing in children with asthma. Excitement, change in climate, or exposure to cold, dry air may also produce symptoms. Laughter may produce coughing or wheezing in children with asthma. Eating may bring on symptoms of respiratory disease if food is aspirated on swallowing or if the children have gastroesophageal reflux.

The composition of the household may provide clues; for example, the presence of other children at home or at day care may be important in terms of exposure to viral infections. If unusual infections are being considered, inquiries should be made about recent travel to unusual areas, exposure to exotic animals, and potential risk factors for HIV infections by the patients or parents.

Typical symptoms of respiratory disease are coughing, wheezing, chest tightness, sputum production, noisy breathing, fever, shortness of breath, stridor, cyanosis, and chest pain. The past medical history should be obtained. The birth history should specifically determine whether the pregnancy was normal and whether the delivery was premature. The feeding history also may be important, particularly in younger children. A history of current medications, as well as a history of any drug allergies, should be obtained.

The family history may suggest respiratory tract illnesses that have a genetic basis; for example, cystic fibrosis (CF) and α_1-antitrypsin deficiency are autosomal-recessive diseases. Other diseases, such as the immunodeficiency disorder, chronic granulomatous disease, are X-linked recessive conditions that may have serious pulmonary complications.

Important aspects of the social history include schooling and the children's performance at school. The structure of the family, the occupations of the parents, the coping strategies of the family, and the type of social support that the family has are important details.

The final part of the history is a review of organ systems, which is best performed systematically. In the interest of time, as well as relevance, this is often performed during the physical examination.

Physical Examination

One of the most important aspects of the physical examination, which is sometimes neglected in the enthusiasm to evaluate the organ systems, is the general examination. Patients should be examined for general health and the presence or absence of cyanosis, anemia, and tachypnea. The more serious pulmonary diseases, such as CF, are associated with failure to thrive, which may be evident on general appearance. However, it is important to measure children's height and weight, to obtain previous height and weight measurements if possible, and to plot these measurements on a percentile chart. Failure to thrive will then be seen as a crossing of the percentile chart in a downward direction (see Chap. 1 "Pediatric Health Supervision").

A very important physical sign to look for is the presence or absence of digital clubbing. Digital clubbing is present when the ends of the fingers are swollen with an increased amount of connective tissue under the base of the fingernail. This can be determined by visual inspection, palpation, or by looking for the absence of the normal diamond formed between the nail bases when two identical fingers are opposed; in North America, this is known as the Scamroth sign (Figure 17–1). The causes of digital clubbing are shown in Table 17–1.

Much can be learned by simple observation, especially in young children who may become uncooperative as the examination continues. The physician should observe the children for respiratory rate, rhythm, and effort. Use of accessory muscles of respiration indicates respiratory distress that may be associated with increased airway resistance due to asthma or decreased lung compliance due to interstitial fibrosis. Very high breathing rates are seen in children with decreased compliance of the respiratory system, fever, anemia, exertion, and metabolic acidosis. Anxiety can also cause hyperventilation. A slow respiratory rate can occur in children with central nervous system depression or metabolic alkalosis. Normal values for respiratory rate according to age are shown in Figure 17–2.

Abnormalities of the rhythm of breathing can be a normal finding in infants younger than 3 months, who often

Table 17–1. Causes of Digital Clubbing

Pulmonary
  Bronchiectasis
  Cystic fibrosis
  Immotile cilia syndrome
  Bronchiolitis obliterans
  Chronic lung infection
  Malignant tumors (primary or secondary)
  Interstitial fibrosis

Cardiac
  Cyanotic congenital heart disease
  Subacute bacterial endocarditis
  Chronic congestive heart failure

Hepatic
  Biliary cirrhosis
  Biliary atresia

Gastrointestinal
  Crohn disease
  Ulcerative colitis
  Chronic infective diarrhea
  Polyposis coil

Other
  Thyrotoxicosis

have respiratory pauses for up to 10 s. Children also may have cycles of increasing and decreasing tidal volume separated by apnea, so-called Cheyne-Stokes breathing, with congestive heart failure or increased intracranial pressure.

The signs of increased respiratory effort include subcostal retractions, intercostal retractions, supraclavicular retractions, movement of the trachea (a tracheal tug), use of the sternocleidomastoid muscles for respiration, and movements of the alae nasi. Movement of the chest wall should be evaluated visually. Normally, the chest wall and abdomen move outwardly during inspiration. Inward movement of the chest during inspiration characterizes paradoxical breathing. This occurs when the chest wall loses its stability, as seen in children with paralysis of intercostal muscles from a spinal cord lesion. This abnormality can be normal in young infants, who have a very flexible rib cage. Paradoxical breathing also may occur in patients with upper airway obstruction. Children with difficulty in breathing often have inspiratory in-drawing of the lower lateral chest, which eventually produces a depression called a Harrison groove. This is sometimes seen in children with severe asthma.

Inspection of the respiratory system should then focus on the upper airway. The nose should always be examined, and nasal patency should be evaluated. The turbinates are best examined with the use of an otoscope. Nasal polyps are commonly found in children with CF, and the tur-

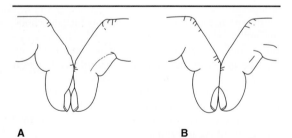

A   **B**

Figure 17–1. **A:** A normal child has a diamond-shaped window present between the nail bases when the fingers are opposed. **B:** The appearance of digital clubbing where the diamond-shaped window has been obliterated by the increased amount of soft tissue under the base of the nail. (Reproduced with permission from: Pulmonology. Page 502 in: Polin RA, Ditmar MF (editors): *Pediatric Secrets*, 2nd ed. Hanley & Belfus, 1997.)

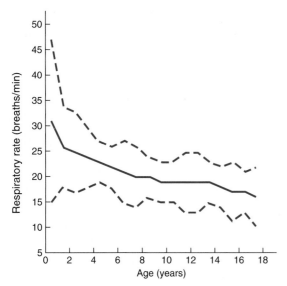

Figure 17–2. Mean values **(solid line)** ± 2 SD **(dashed lines)** of the normal respiratory rate at rest. There is no significant difference between the sexes, and the regression line represents data from both boys and girls. The respiratory rate decreases with age and shows the greatest normal variation during the first 2 years of life. (Data from Iliff A, Lee VA: Child Dev 1952;23:237; reproduced with permission from Pasterkamp H: The history and physical examination. In: Chernick V, Kendig EL (editors): *Disorders of the Respiratory Tract in Children.* Saunders, 1990.)

binates may appear boggy and bluish in children with allergies. The oropharynx should be inspected for the presence of cobblestoning from chronic sinusitis and for malformations, such as cleft palate. Examination of the oropharynx may reveal enlarged tonsils. The frontal, ethmoidal, and maxillary paranasal sinuses should be palpated for tenderness; transillumination of the sinuses in a darkened room may be attempted, but this approach is insensitive for the detection of reduced pneumatization. Young infants may have only rudimentary frontal sinuses.

Palpation usually commences with the cervical lymph nodes, followed by the trachea. A slight deviation of the trachea to the right is normal because of the presence of the descending aorta on the left side. Marked deviation to one side may signify atelectasis on that side or overexpansion of the other side, as seen with pneumothorax.

Percussion of the chest is best performed by tapping lightly with the middle finger (the plexor) of the dominant hand on the middle phalanx of the other hand's middle finger (the pleximeter). The pleximeter should be placed firmly (of course, the hand should be warm!), and percus-

sion should be gentle, with quick perpendicular movements. The anterior, lateral, and posterior surfaces of the chest should be examined by comparing symmetric sites between the right and left sides. Reduced resonance will be noted in the presence of consolidation or pleural effusion. Increased resonance will be present if there is replacement of lung by more air than normal, as seen with emphysema or pneumothorax.

Auscultation of the chest is performed by using the diaphragm of the stethoscope. The breath sounds should be evaluated; they should be equal and have a normal vesicular quality. Because of the smallness of the chest in young children, it is possible to hear tubular breath sounds in the periphery originating from the large airways; this is a normal finding. The quality and symmetry of the breath sounds also should be evaluated.

Adventitial respiratory sounds are best considered in two categories: crackles and wheezes. Crackles are nonmusical, interrupted lung sounds that can be classified as fine or coarse, depending on the duration and frequency of the sounds. Fine crackles that occur during late inspiration are common in interstitial pulmonary fibrosis and in the early stages of pulmonary edema. Coarse crackles may be heard in early inspiration and during expiration; they are often heard at the mouth. Coarse crackles are caused by increased airway secretions or pneumonic consolidation.

Wheezes are musical, continuous sounds that originate from narrowed airways. Widespread narrowing of the airways in asthma leads to multiple sources for these sounds and various pitches, or "polyphonic" wheezes. A fixed obstruction in a large airway, for example, an inhaled foreign body, produces a "monophonic" wheeze in a constant location that may be present on inhalation and exhalation. The intensity of expiratory wheezing is related to respiratory effort, and patients may need to cooperate with deep, forced inhalations and exhalations for wheezes to become evident. In younger children, it often helps to squeeze the upper part of the chest manually during exhalation to elicit a wheeze while holding the diaphragm of the stethoscope below the clavicle. This technique is called the way to "squeeze a wheeze."

Diagnostic Procedures

RADIOLOGY

Anteroposterior and lateral chest radiographs are valuable tools in evaluating children with suspected lung disease. Right and left lateral decubitus films are used to demonstrate the presence of an inhaled foreign body or to evaluate pleural effusions. Inspiratory and expiratory x-ray films to locate a foreign body are helpful in older patients who can cooperate, but they are not useful in younger children. Fluoroscopy of the diaphragm can be used to assess diaphragmatic motion and phrenic nerve

Table 17–2. Laboratory Tests to Distinguish Pleural Exudates from Pleural Transudates

	Exudate	Transudate
Protein	>2.5 g/dL	<2.6 g/dL
Pleural-plasma protein ratio	>50%	<50%
Lactic dehydrogenase	>200 IU	<200 IU
pH	<7.20	>7.20

function. Ultrasonography of the diaphragm has been used to evaluate these functions, but fluoroscopy is a more established method.

COMPUTED TOMOGRAPHY SCAN

High-resolution computed tomography (CT) is useful in evaluating the pulmonary interstitium for diseases such as idiopathic pulmonary fibrosis. Computed tomography scans are also useful to evaluate anatomic structures in the parenchyma, such as cysts and solid lesions, and mediastinal structures, such as vascular malformations, airway compression, and enlarged lymph nodes. Contrast enhancement may be helpful in diagnosing sequestrations and pulmonary arteriovenous fistulae.

BRONCHOSCOPY

Fiberoptic bronchoscopy has revolutionized pulmonary medicine. Although this technique was developed for use in adults, it is possible to examine young children if pediatric flexible bronchoscopes are used together with sedation and topical anesthesia or with general anesthesia. Direct visualization of the airways allows the diagnosis of congenital or acquired airway anomalies and airway obstruction by foreign bodies or mucous plugs. Mucous plugs can be treated effectively with lavage by using the suction channel of the instrument; foreign bodies are more easily removed with a rigid bronchoscope. Bronchoalveolar lavage is used to obtain bronchial secretions for microscopy and culture. Transbronchial biopsy and transbronchial needle aspiration are techniques that are more useful in adults than they are in children. The fiberoptic bronchoscope is also very useful for selective bronchography and difficult endotracheal intubations.

THORACENTESIS

Children with pleural effusions may have pneumonia, malignancy, tuberculosis, hypoproteinemia, or abnormal lymphatic drainage of the thorax. Fluid may be aspirated from the pleural space for diagnostic purposes or for relief of respiratory distress. The fluid is then examined with Gram stain, aerobic and anaerobic cultures, and measurement of glucose and protein levels, white and red blood cell counts, pH, and lactate dehydrogenase levels. These measurements allow the fluid to be classified as a transudate or an exudate (Table 17–2). Cytologic analysis should be performed on the pleural fluid if there is a possibility of a malignancy.

PULMONARY FUNCTION TESTS

Pulmonary function tests are extremely useful in the evaluation and management of pulmonary disease. They allow for the detection, characterization, and quantification of pathology; evaluation of responses to therapy; and objective follow-up of chronic diseases, such as asthma and CF. Pulmonary function tests measure vital capacity and expiratory flow by spirometry; lung volumes by body plethysmography; resistance, compliance, and diffusing capacity; maximal inspiratory and expiratory pressures; and maximal voluntary ventilation. The two main types of pulmonary function abnormality are restrictive and obstructive. In restrictive defects, lung volumes are reduced by fibrosis or by chest wall deformity. Obstructive diseases are characterized by airflow obstruction due to asthma, CF, or bronchopulmonary dysplasia (BPD) (Table 17–3). Special tests involving measurement of lung function before and after methacholine, histamine, or exercise can help in the evaluation of asthma.

These tests are noninvasive, but typically require cooperative patients who are 5 to 6 years of age. However, over the past decade, progress has been made in the area of infant pulmonary function testing. Various approaches have been tried, among others: the weighted spirometer, airway occlusion, expiratory volume-clamp, forced oscillation, negative pressure-induced deflation, and chest compression techniques. These methods require anything from sedation with chloral hydrate to general anesthesia. Once just a research tool, infant pulmonary function tests are becoming more standardized and reproducible, and therefore they have become more useful to the clinician. They offer a unique insight into the impact of acute and chronic pulmonary disease processes on lung growth.

The simplest device for evaluating pulmonary function is the peak flow meter, which measures the maximal velocity of gas generated at the mouth when patients (usually 5 years of age or older) exhale forcefully. Peak flow measurements are reduced in obstructive airways diseases, therefore they are helpful in the daily monitoring of asthma and adjustment of asthma medications. Unfortunately, peak flow measurements are very effort dependent and reflect primarily large and medium-sized airway function. Significant inflammation and obstruction can still exist in the small airways even when peak flow measurements are normal.

BLOOD GAS AND OXYGEN SATURATION MEASUREMENTS

Arterial blood gas measurements are used to assess acid-base balance, oxygenation, and carbon dioxide excretion. Carbon dioxide is retained and oxygenation is reduced in children with respiratory failure. Acid-base disturbances

Table 17–3A. Pulmonary Function Tests in Obstructive and Restrictive Lung Dysfunction

	Obstructive Lung Dysfunction	Restrictive Lung Dysfunction
FEV_1	↓	Normal or ↓ in proportion to ↓ lung vol
TLC	Normal or moderately ↑	↓
RV/TLC	↑	↑ or ↓ depending on whether VC or RV more affected
RV	↑ with ↑ airway obstruction	↓
FEV_1/FVC	↓	Normal or slight ↑
FVC or VC	Normal or ↓	↓

Table 17–3B. Definitions of Lung Volumes and Capacities

TLC	VC	IC	IRV
			TV
		FRC	ERV
	RV		RV

ERV = expiratory reserve volume; FEV = forced expiratory volume in 1 s; FRC = functional residual capacity; FVC = forced vital capacity; IC = inspiratory capacity; IRV = inspiratory reserve volume; RV = residual volume; TLC = total lung capacity; TV = tidal volume; VC = vital capacity.

can be classified into respiratory or metabolic causes of acidosis or alkalosis. The drawing of arterial blood gases has the disadvantage of being quite uncomfortable, which is a particular problem with children. An approximation of acid-base balance and carbon dioxide excretion can be obtained by drawing a venous blood gas. The arterial hemoglobin oxygen saturation can be measured by pulse oximetry with the use of a probe that measures the differential absorption of two wavelengths of red light by the capillary blood. The combination of a venous or capillary blood gas and oxygen saturation measurement by pulse oximetry is often sufficient to make clinical decisions.

SWEAT TEST

This test is used to diagnose cystic fibrosis with the finding of increased concentrations of chloride and sodium in the sweat. An experienced laboratory using pilocarpine iontophoresis as described by Gibson and Cooke must perform the test. The sweat is collected on a weighed filter paper or gauze for 30 min and then analyzed for chloride concentration. A value >60 mEq/L in a sample weighing at least 75 mg is diagnostic of CF, although the test should be repeated for confirmation. A value in the range 40 to 60 mEq/L is in the "gray zone," and the test should be repeated. Although the test is accurate, there are

many recognized causes of false-positive and false-negative sweat test results (Table 17–4).

EVALUATION OF NOISY BREATHING

Approach to Children with Noisy Breathing

Noisy breathing in infants and children is a common presenting complaint to the pediatrician. The sounds include snoring, stridor, and grunting and they are due to turbulent airflow caused by airway obstruction. The obstruction may exist anywhere between the nares and the distal tracheobronchial tree (Table 17–5). Noisy breathing may represent a benign self-limited problem, or it may be indicative of life-threatening airway obstruction. The

Table 17–4. Causes of False-Positive and False-Negative Sweat Test Results

False-Positive Results	False-Negative Results
Laboratory error	Laboratory error
Malnutrition	Peripheral edema
Renal diabetes insipidus	
Untreated adrenal insufficiency	
Untreated hypothyroidism	
Anorexia nervosa	
Familial cholestasis	
Celiac disease	
Fucosidosis	
Ectodermal dysplasia	
Hypogammaglobulinemia	
Hypoparathyroidism	
Type I glycogen storage disease	
Klinefelter syndrome	
Atopic dermatitis	
Mucopolysaccharidosis	
Pupillotonia-areflexia and segmental hypohidrosis	

Adapted with permission, from Ruddy RM, Scanlin TF: Abnormal sweat electrolytes in a case of celiac disease and a case of psychosocial failure to thrive. Clin Pediatr 1987;26:83.

Table 17–5. Causes of Noisy Breathing

Anatomic	Infectious
Choanal atresia	Croup
Subglottic stenosis	Epiglottitis
Laryngeal web	Retropharyngeal abscess
Vascular ring compression	Mononucleosis
Tracheoesophageal fistula	Upper respiratory infection
Craniofacial anomalies	
Micrognathia	Functional
Macroglossia	Laryngomalacia
Functional	Tracheomalacia
Foreign body	Gastroesophageal reflux
Congenital heart disease	Obstructive sleep apnea
Metabolic	Neurologic
Storage diseases	Encephalocele
	Cerebral palsy
Neoplasms	Vocal cord paralysis
Laryngeal neoplasms	Hypotonia/hyporeflexia
Papilloma	
Hemangioma	
Mediastinal tumors	
Hygroma	
Angiofibroma	
Neurofibroma	

physician therefore must have a logical and organized approach to the evaluation.

Pediatric patients are more susceptible to airway compromise because the airway is much smaller than it is in the adult. Therefore, a significant decrease in the cross-sectional area of the airway occurs from small increases in mucus production and swelling of the respiratory mucosa. This airway narrowing leads to a large increase in airway resistance. In addition, the pediatric airway is structurally more compliant and more readily collapses from the inspiratory pressure generated to overcome this increased airway resistance. This further narrows the airway and can lead to a downward cycle resulting in respiratory failure.

Since noisy breathing occurs with many different conditions that involve airway obstruction at many different areas, the evaluation of this problem can be quite challenging. The key to evaluation is to discern the level and severity of the obstruction. The history and physical examination may point to a specific etiology and location, but direct visualization of the obstruction is often required.

In the setting where there is acute onset of stridor and the potential for rapidly progressive airway obstruction (such as in epiglottis), immediate diagnosis and treatment is essential. (See Chap. 9, "Infectious Diseases," for more description of epiglottitis.) When there is little to no obvious obstruction, the evaluation can proceed with less urgency. This may allow the noisy breathing to resolve on its own, since the most common cause of noisy breath-

ing is upper airway congestion from a simple viral upper respiratory tract infection. Carefully chosen diagnostic tests are used systematically to ascertain the etiology of the noisy breathing. Referral of these patients to a pediatric subspecialist is often necessary for treatment of the airway anomalies.

History

Newborns and very young infants may have noisy breathing or stridor at birth. Changes in the quality of the cry or hoarseness, persistent coughing or other evidence of upper respiratory tract infection, and any periods of apnea or cyanosis should be noted. Alleviation of symptoms by positional change is also an important observation. Worsening of symptoms related to feedings is indicative of aspiration syndromes, which may be caused by laryngotracheal clefts or tracheoesophageal fistulae. A past history of intubation suggests the possibility of subglottic or tracheal stenosis. It is also important to note whether the abnormal sounds are persistent, or whether there are periods of alleviation. The quality of breath sounds during sleep, when the child's spontaneous tidal volume is lower, should be noted. A history of snoring while sleeping is suggestive of obstructive sleep apnea, commonly due to adenoidal or tonsillar hypertrophy. Functional abnormalities, such as laryngomalacia, improve during periods of calm or quiet breathing. Any associated abnormalities of swallowing should be ascertained. A history of foreign-body ingestion or aspiration should be explored in all children of toddler age with an acute onset of symptoms. *Even though a swallowed object may be lodged in the esophagus, it may apply pressure on the posterior wall of the trachea and partially obstruct it.* In school-aged children and adolescents, dyspnea or chest pain may be indicative of neoplastic growth in the mediastinum. Symptoms of gastroesophageal reflux should be sought, and any associated cough and its quality should be noted.

Physical Examination

The general appearance should be noted, and height, weight, and head circumference should be plotted on standard growth curves. The general appearance of the child should be noted for evidence of dysmorphic features suggestive of congenital syndromes. The examination of the head should include palpation of the cervical region for masses and inspection for evidence of midline dimples or tracts consistent with structural remnants. Inspection of the nasal passages is important for signs of obstruction. In all children, thorough examination of the oropharynx with notation of the mandibular structure, tongue size, palate integrity, and posterior pharyngeal contour is important. Elicitation of a gag reflex must also be carried out. Inspection of the chest for retractions, as well as degree of chest excursion, is important.

Auscultation can be most revealing when the phase of the respiratory cycle is correlated with aberrant breathing sounds. Stridor is indicative of upper airway obstruction and occurs during the inspiratory phase. Large airway noises commonly associated with tracheomalacia are heard in the expiratory phase; however, with severe obstruction, biphasic sounds are heard. Auscultation over the mouth and the lateral neck should be performed to differentiate upper airway noises from lower airway noises. In calm children, the examiner may purposely agitate patients to elicit abnormal breathing sounds and to check for augmentation of existing sounds with increased tidal volume. In infants, the breathing sounds should be evaluated in both a supine and a prone position, as supralaryngeal obstruction is usually worse when supine.

Palpation of the liver and spleen during the abdominal examination is useful for possible evidence of storage diseases, which may cause abnormal breathing sounds, secondary to infiltration of laryngeal structures. The presence of clubbing or cyanosis of the nail beds should be noted. A careful neurologic examination is important, and evidence of hypotonia or dysreflexia should be sought.

Diagnostic Evaluation

Anteroposterior and lateral chest radiographs should be obtained in all children requiring further evaluation for noisy breathing. Silhouettes of the heart and great vessels should be examined for proper size and orientation. Lung parenchymal disease may be secondary to aspiration, infection, or associated cardiac disease. Careful examination is necessary to detect tumors of the thorax, as compression of airway structures from tumors often results in noisy breathing.

Airway films in both the anteroposterior and lateral views are useful for evaluation of upper airway obstruction. These may be helpful in acute settings, such as croup or epiglottitis; however, normal airway films do not rule out all underlying pathologies.

Direct visualization of the respiratory tract is the most revealing investigation for noisy breathing. The flexible bronchoscope allows one to evaluate the nasal passages, laryngeal structures, and tracheobronchial tree. Dynamic compression is seen clearly with a flexible bronchoscope as compared to a rigid bronchoscopy, if patients are lightly sedated and breathing spontaneously. However, structures of the posterior larynx often require rigid bronchoscopy for complete evaluation.

A CT scan may be indicated when tumors of the head, neck, or mediastinum are considered. Choanal stenosis and atresia is best visualized by this technique. Vascular anomalies that may be causing external compression of the airway, such as aortic arch anomalies, innominate artery compression, and compression of the left or right main-stem bronchus by the pulmonary arteries, are best visualized by magnetic resonance imaging (MRI). The MRI scans should be obtained only after evidence of external compression has been demonstrated by bronchoscopy. Either MRI or CT may be used to evaluate the head of a neurologically abnormal child. Testing for metabolic diseases should be pursued when clinically indicated.

The use of a pediatric sleep laboratory may be helpful in evaluating children with noisy breathing. Neurologic, cardiac, and respiratory data are gathered and are used to measure the clinical severity of any obstruction and to help understand its etiology.

EVALUATION OF WHEEZING CHILDREN

Approach to Wheezing Children

Wheezing is a musical continuous respiratory sound that may be persistent or intermittent. Typically the sound is heard during expiration and is due to partial obstruction of the airways. Although wheezing is commonly caused by asthma, any disease process that narrows the airway can create a wheeze (Table 17–6).

The age of patients and timing of its onset may give important clues as to the etiology. Intermittent, generalized, and polyphonic (a combination of sounds of varying pitch) wheezing suggest asthma. If this same sound is heard in young infants with signs of upper respiratory tract infection who have never wheezed before, respiratory syncytial virus (RSV) bronchiolitis is more likely (see Chap. 9, "Infectious Disease"). A fixed obstruction in a large airway due to an inhaled foreign body produces a

Table 17–6. Differential Diagnosis of Wheezing

Infants and Children	Adolescents and Adults
Anaphylaxis	Anaphylaxis
Asthma	Angiotensin-converting
Bronchiolitis	enzyme inhibitors
Cardiovascular rings	Asthma
Congenital anomalies of	β-adrenergic receptor
the respiratory tract	blockers
Congestive heart failure	Chronic bronchitis
Cystic fibrosis	(smoking, substance
Extrinsic airway compression:	abuse)
lymph nodes, tumors,	Congestive heart failure
esophageal foreign bodies	Cystic fibrosis
Intraluminal obstruction:	Infections
foreign body	
Laryngeal wheezing or	
"factitious" asthma	
Paralysis of the recurrent	
laryngeal nerve	

monophonic (single-pitch) wheeze of sudden onset in a constant location. If a similar wheeze is found to be slowly progressive, it is more consistent with extrinsic compression of the airway from an enlarging lymph node or other intrathoracic mass.

Although wheezing is generally heard during respiratory disease, it may be generated voluntarily during an exaggerated forced expiratory maneuver in "factitious" asthma. In contrast, the absence of a wheeze does not necessarily guarantee that significant airway obstruction is not occurring. In fact, if the obstruction progresses to the point that little if any air is flowing, then the clinician must note the absence of wheezing sounds on auscultation in the face of increased work of breathing as a sign of severe respiratory distress.

In the following section on wheezing, clinical management of asthma will be discussed. The management of patients in acute respiratory distress from asthma is covered in Chap. 10, "Injuries and Emergencies."

Asthma

Asthma, the most common chronic lung disease in children, affects an estimated 4.8 million children. The death rate for children 19 years and younger increased by 78% between 1980 and 1993. Approximately 11 million school days are missed each year because of asthma-related illness. Approximately 80 to 90% of children who are affected by asthma have their first episode by 5 to 6 years of age. The prevalence of asthma has increased over the past 10 years, and African Americans are disproportionately affected. In general, asthma hospitalization rates have been the highest among African American patients (all ages) and children. Socioeconomic factors show that the poor are affected more than the affluent, and boys tend to be affected more than are girls up to the age of 10 years.

PATHOPHYSIOLOGY

Asthma, or *reactive airways disease (RAD),* is a chronic inflammatory disorder of the airways resulting in variable airflow obstruction that is usually reversible. The inflammation is associated with airway hyperresponsiveness. Children with asthma have recurrent symptoms of coughing, wheezing, and shortness of breath after exposure to "triggers" such as viral infections, allergens, strong fumes, cold air, and exercise.

Airway hyperresponsiveness is an invariable part of asthma, and the severity of disease correlates with the degree of hyperresponsiveness. Hyperresponsiveness can be measured in the laboratory with a pharmacologic challenge, such as methacholine or histamine, or with a physiologic challenge such as exercise. Possible mechanisms causing airway hyperreactivity include airway inflammation, abnormal autonomic regulation of airway caliber, changes in bronchial smooth muscle function, and loss of

bronchial epithelial integrity. The most important of these is airway inflammation. Pathologic studies have demonstrated the presence of inflammatory cells in the airways of patients with mild to severe asthma. Patients with asthma have altered cellular immunity and increased levels of inflammatory mediators, particularly in the airway. This has led to the use of anti-inflammatory drugs, such as systemic steroids, inhaled steroids, disodium cromoglycate, and nedocromil sodium; these drugs can reduce asthma symptoms by reducing airway hyperresponsiveness.

The mechanism of airflow obstruction has three components: bronchospasm, mucosal edema, and mucous plugging of the lumen. Bronchodilators effectively relieve bronchospasm, whereas anti-inflammatory drugs affect all three components.

Allergy is an important trigger factor in many children with asthma. There is a correlation between serum IgE level and the risk of sensitization to environmental allergens. School-aged children with asthma commonly have positive skin tests to inhaled allergens, such as house dust mites, cockroaches, molds, cat dander, and grass and tree pollen. Allergies are a less important factor in preschool children, in whom viral infections are the most common triggers. In the child with allergies, asthma may be associated with allergic rhinitis, conjunctivitis, or eczema.

CLINICAL FEATURES

Asthma is a dynamic disease, changing over time, which requires active management by both patients and health care providers. Clinical manifestations of asthma are the result of diffuse small airway obstruction and include wheezing, dyspnea, recurrent coughing, and accessory muscle use. Airway narrowing is due to bronchospasm and mucosal edema with subsequent plugging by thick, tenacious mucus. Air trapping occurs during the expiratory phase of respiration and results in a hyperinflated, barrel-shaped chest.

Numerous triggers stimulate the bronchospasm of asthma. Well-recognized triggers include viral infections, sinus infections, tobacco smoke, strong fumes, and allergens such as dust mites, animal hairs or fur, and cold air. Exercise-induced bronchospasm is seen in some children.

Classically, asthma has been divided into intrinsic and extrinsic types: Extrinsic asthma is IgE-mediated (allergic), whereas intrinsic asthma does not have an allergic etiology. This distinction is academically interesting; however, in the treatment of either type, the basic physiology of chronic inflammation and increased mucous production leading to airway hyperreactivity is the same. A key point in the clinical history is the history of recurrent exacerbations provoked by known triggers. The episodic nature of asthma should allow patients to have periods of normal breathing between attacks; a history of persistent noisy breathing should lead the physician to suspect other diagnoses. Symptoms can also occur predominantly at night and may be indicative of gastroesophageal reflux or exposure to allergens, such as house dust mites, in the child's bedroom. Eczematous skin rashes and seasonal rhinitis are common in children with asthma (the "atopic triad"). A family history of asthma is common. If one parent has reactive airways disease, the child has a 25% likelihood of having it as well. This risk doubles if both biologic parents have asthma.

DIAGNOSIS

The diagnosis of asthma is supported by (1) a history of recurrent symptoms, (2) reversible airflow obstruction demonstrated by spirometry, and (3) exclusion of other causes of wheezing. Polyphonic musical wheezing throughout the chest and evidence of atopy are key to the diagnosis, although wheezing has many other causes (Table 17–6). Spirometry showing a decrease in the forced expiratory volume in the first second (FEV_1) with a normal or decreased forced vital capacity (FVC) is consistent with airflow obstruction. Scooping on the expiratory flow volume loop further supports this diagnosis (Figure 17–3). Demonstration of reversibility of airflow obstruc-

tion by bronchodilators strongly supports the diagnosis of asthma.

Bronchial hyperresponsiveness may be demonstrated by pharmacologic challenge with histamine or methacholine or by exercise provocation. The methacholine bronchial provocation test has the greatest sensitivity and specificity, but it is time-consuming; this test probably is not required in most children with asthma, in whom a clinical diagnosis can be made confidently.

CLINICAL MANAGEMENT

Peak expiratory flow (PEF) rates, measured by handheld meters, can be helpful in managing asthma on an outpatient basis. These objective measurements can be communicated to the physician during periods of illness. A step-care plan based on patients' personal best flow rates is helpful in establishing a clear plan. Allergy testing may help to define suspected triggers (see Chap. 18 "Allergy: Mechanisms and Disease Processes"). The assessment of asthma severity (Table 17–7) is important for initial therapy and planning for stepped increases or decreases in future intervention.

The successful management of patients with reactive airways disease requires the following objectives:

- Education and establishment of a patient–clinician partnership
- Recognition and reduction of exposure to "triggers" of asthma symptoms
- Pharmacologic intervention to reduce airway inflammation in patients with persistent symptoms
- Active monitoring and management program
- Prompt intervention during exacerbations

Education and self-recognition. Asthma education gives patients an understanding of the logical approach to medications used in asthma. In addition, it allows clear communication of symptoms to the physician on an outpatient basis. Asthma is episodic, and recognition by patients of changing clinical status is helpful. The use of PEF meters gives patients the ability to monitor baseline flow rates and to detect any deterioration. It also allows objective changes to be communicated to the physician by telephone. Education should also provide a clear understanding of the goals of recommended therapy and establish the patient–provider relationship necessary for successful symptom control.

Pharmacologic approach. Pharmacologic reversal of chronic airway inflammation, airway obstruction, and airway hyperresponsiveness is the cornerstone of treatment. A stepwise approach to pharmacotherapy helps ensure optimal asthma therapy with minimal side effects. Initiation of a high level of therapy early on will establish prompt control, allowing for a stepdown in therapy sooner (Tables 17–8 and 17–9). Medications can be generalized broadly into two classes: long-term control medication

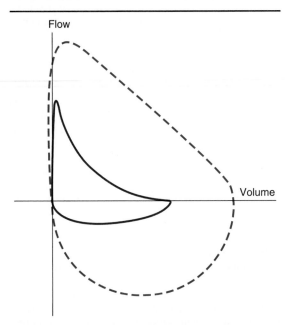

Figure 17–3. Flow-volume loop in a patient with intrathoracic airway obstruction because of small airways disease **(solid line)**. A normal flow-volume loop **(dashed lines)** is shown for comparison. The loop sags because of progressively increasing small airway obstruction at lower lung volumes. (Reproduced with permission from Evaluation of the airway. In: Myer CM, et al (editors): *The Pediatric Airway: An Interdisciplinary Approach.* Lippincott, 1995.)

Table 17–7. Classification of Asthma Severity[1]

	Symptoms	**Nighttime Symptoms**	**Lung Function**
Severe persistent	• Continual symptoms • Limited physical activity • Frequent exacerbations	Frequent	• FEV_1 or PEF $\leq$ 60% predicted
Moderate persistent	• Daily symptoms • Daily use of inhaled short-acting β_2-agonist • Exacerbations affect activity • Exacerbations $\geq$ 2 times a week; may last days	> 1 time a week	• FEV_1 or PEF > 60%–< 80% predicted
Mild persistent	• Symptoms > 2 times a week but < 1 time a day • Exacerbations may affect activity	> 2 times a month	• FEV_1 or PEF $\geq$ 80% predicted
Mild intermittent	• Symptoms $\leq$ 2 times a week • Asymptomatic and normal PEF between exacerbations • Exacerbations brief (from a few hours to a few days); intensity may vary	$\leq$ 2 times a month	• FEV_1 or PEF $\geq$ 80% predicted

[1] The presence of one of the features of severity is sufficient to place a patient in that category. An individual should be assigned to the most severe grade in which any feature occurs. The characteristics noted in this table are general and may overlap because asthma is highly variable. Furthermore, an individual's classification may change over time.

Modified from National Asthma Education Program: *Guidelines for the Diagnosis and Management of Asthma. Expert Panel Report 2.* U.S. Department of Health and Human Services, Public Health Services, National Institutes of Health, Bethesda, MD, 1997.

and quick-relief medication (Tables 17–10 and 17–11). The most effective medications for long-term therapy are those shown to have anti-inflammatory effects. Patients with persistent asthma may require a combination of both classes of medication. Because asthma is a state of chronic airway inflammation, the use of both steroidal and nonsteroidal anti-inflammatory agents is emphasized. Corticosteroids are the most effective anti-inflammatory drugs. They inhibit inflammatory cell migration and cytokine production; they also increase the response to β_2 agonists. Early use of these agents in asthma prevents progression of airway obstruction. In children with persistent asthma, corticosteroids are essential to control airway inflammation. Systemic corticosteroids have many adverse effects, including increased appetite, truncal obesity, glucose intolerance, mood alteration, hypertension, fluid retention, and cataract formation. Inhaled steroids have been shown to be extremely effective in persistent asthma. They should be the first-line medication in someone who has coughing or wheezing more than twice per week or has nocturnal symptoms more than twice per month. In general, they do not have systemic effects at low-to-medium doses (Table 17–12). However, controlled clinical studies of pediatric patients have demonstrated a reduction in growth velocity, which appears to be related to dose and duration of exposure to inhaled steroids. This

risk must be weighed against the remarkable efficacy of these agents. Oral thrush is another side effect of metered-dose inhaled steroids. The use of inhaled steroids has enabled previously systemic steroid-dependent children to be weaned from their treatment. Cromolyn sodium and nedocromil sodium are the best examples of non-steroidal anti-inflammatory agents. The mechanism of action of these drugs is poorly understood. The drugs are used prophylactically and inhibit both early- and late-phase allergic reactions. Four to 6 weeks of treatment are needed to determine the efficacy of these medications before treatment failure can be determined. Some patient's experience coughing when given these agents, particularly the dry powder formulations.

The β_2 adrenergic agonists have the ability to relax airway smooth muscle and have rapid onset of action. These drugs provide patients with immediate relief of symptoms; however, their limited duration of action may require repeated dosing. In addition, the β_2 agonists are associated with side effects, including dysrhythmias, tachycardias, hypokalemia, and systemic hypertension. They are administered by a metered-dose inhaler or nebulizer or are administered orally. Long-acting β_2 agonists are now available, but these agents should not be used on an acute basis, as their onset of action is delayed and repeated dosing may lead to toxicity with cardiac dysrhythmias.

Table 17–8. Stepwise Approach for Managing Infants and Young Children (5 Years of Age and Younger) with Acute or Chronic Asthma Symptoms

	Long-Term Control

Step 4
Severe
persistent
	• Daily anti-inflammatory medication
	    High-dose inhaled steroid[1] with spacer and face mask
	    If needed, add oral steroids (2 mg/kg/day); reduce to lowest daily or alternate-day dose that stabilizes
	       symptoms

Step 3
Moderate
persistent
	• Daily anti-inflammatory medication
	    Medium-dose inhaled steroid[1] with spacer and face mask
	    Once control is established, consider:
	       Lower medium-dose inhaled steroid[1] with spacer and face mask and nedocromil (1–2 puffs bid-qid)
	    OR
	       Lower medium-dose inhaled steroid[1] with spacer and face mask and theophylline (10 mg/kg/day up
	          to 16 mg/kg/day for children $\geq$ 1 year of age, to a serum concentration of 5–15 µg/mL)[2]

Step 2
Mild
persistent
	• Daily anti-inflammatory medication
	    Infants and young children usually begin with a trial of cromolyn (nebulizer is preferred, 1 ample
	       tid-qid; or MDI, 1–2 puffs tid-qid) or nedocromil (MDI only, 1–2 puffs bid-qid)
	    OR
	       Low-dose inhaled steroid[1] with spacer and face mask

Step 1 Mild intermittent	• No daily medication needed

All patients	**Quick-Relief**
	Bronchodilator as needed for symptoms: Short-acting inhaled β_2-agonist by nebulizer (0.05 mg/kg in
	    2–3 mL of saline) or inhaler with face mask and spacer (2–4 puffs; for exacerbations, repeat q 20 min for
	    up to 1 h).
	Asthma symptoms with viral respiratory infection, use short-acting inhaled β_2-agonist q 4 to 6 h up to 24 h
	    (longer with physician consult) but, in general, if repeated more than once every 6 weeks, consider
	    moving to next step up. Consider oral steroids if the exacerbation is moderate to severe or at the onset
	    of the infection if the patient has a history of severe exacerbations.

MDI = metered dose inhaler
[1] See Table 17–12 Estimated Comparative Daily Dosages for Inhaled Steroids.
[2] For children < 1 year of age: usual max mg/kg/day = 0.2 (age in weeks) + 5.
NOTES:

• The stepwise approach presents general guidelines to assist clinical decision making. Asthma is highly variable: clinicians should tailor medication plans to the needs of individual patients.

• **Gain control** as quickly as possible. Either start with aggressive therapy (e.g., add a course of oral steroids or a higher dose of inhaled steroids to the therapy that corresponds to the patient's initial step of severity); or start at the step that corresponds to the patient's initial severity and step up treatment, if necessary.

• **Step down.** Review treatment every 1 to 6 months. If control is sustained for at least 3 months, a gradual stepwise reduction in treatment may be possible.

• **Step up.** If control is not achieved, consider step up. Inadequate control is indicated by increased use of short-acting β_2-agonists on a daily basis OR more than 3 to 4 times in one day. But before stepping up: review patient inhaler technique, compliance, and environmental control (avoidance of allergens or other precipitating factors).

• A rescue course of oral steroids (prednisolone) may be needed at any time and step.

Modified from The National Asthma Education Program: *Guidelines for the Diagnosis and Management of Asthma. Expert Panel Report 2.* U.S. Department of Health and Human Services, Public Health Service, National Institutes of Health, Bethesda, MD, 1997.

The anticholinergic bronchodilators, such as ipratropium bromide, act by blocking vagal pathways and have minimal systemic absorption or side effects. Some evidence suggests that they effectively relieve bronchospasm from gastroesophageal reflux.

Methylxanthines, specifically theophylline, have mild-to-moderate bronchodilator activity and some anti-inflammatory activity and may augment respiratory muscle function. The intravenous administration of these (*text continues on page 708*)

Table 17–9. Stepwise Approach for Managing Asthma in Children Over 5 Years Old: Treatment

	Long-Term Control ***Preferred treatments are in bold print***
Step 4 Severe persistent	Daily medications: • Anti-inflammatory: inhaled steroid (high dose)[1] AND • Long-acting bronchodilator: either long-acting inhaled β_2-agonist (1–2 puffs q 12 h), sustained-release theophylline, or long-acting β_2-agonist tablets AND • Steroid tablets or syrup long term: make repeated attempts to reduce systemic steroid and maintain control with high-dose inhaled steroid
Step 3 Moderate persistent	Daily medication: • Either **Anti-inflammatory: inhaled steroid (medium dose)**[1] OR Inhaled steroid (low-to-medium dose)[1] and add a long-acting bronchodilator, especially for nighttime symptoms: either **long-acting inhaled β_2-agonist** (1–2 puffs q 12 h), sustained-release theophylline, or long-acting β_2-agonist tablets • If needed Anti-inflammatory: **inhaled steroids (medium-to-high dose)**[1] AND Long-acting bronchodilator, especially for night-time symptoms; either long-acting inhaled β_2-agonist, sustained-release theophylline, or long-acting β_2-agonist tablets
Step 2 Mild persistent	Daily medication: • **Anti-inflammatory**: either **inhaled steroid (low dose)**[1] or cromolyn (1–2 puffs tid-qid) or nedocromil (1–2 puffs bid-qid); (children usually begin with a trial of cromolyn or nedocromil) • Sustained-release theophylline to serum concentration of 5–15 µg/mL is an alternative, but not preferred, therapy. Zafirlukast or zileuton may also be considered for those ≥ 12 years old, although their position in therapy is not fully established
Step 1 Mild intermittent	• No daily medication needed
	Quick-Relief
All patients	Short-acting bronchodilator: inhaled β_2-agonist (2–4 puffs) as needed for symptoms. Intensity of treatment will depend on severity of exacerbation

[1] See Table 17–12 Estimated Comparative Daily Dosages for Inhaled Steroids.
NOTES:
• The stepwise approach presents general guidelines to assist clinical decision making. Asthma is highly variable: clinicians should tailor medication plans to the needs of individual patients.
• **Gain control** as quickly as possible. Either start with aggressive therapy (e.g., add a course of oral steroids or a higher dose of inhaled steroids to the therapy that corresponds to the patient's initial step of severity); or start at the step that corresponds to the patient's initial severity and step up treatment, if necessary.
• **Step down:** Review treatment every 1 to 6 months. Gradually decrease treatment to the least medication necessary to maintain control.
• **Step up:** If control is not maintained, consider step up. Inadequate control is indicated by increased use of short-acting β_2-agonists and in: step 1 when patient uses a short-acting β_2-agonist more than 2 times a week: steps 2 and 3 when patient uses short-acting β_2-agonist on a daily basis or more than 3 to 4 times in one day. But before stepping up: review patient inhaler technique, compliance, and environmental control (avoidance or allergens or other precipitating factors).
• A rescue course of oral steroids (prednisolone) may be needed at any time and at any step.
• Patients with exercise-induced bronchospasm should take two to four puffs of an inhaled β_2-agonist 15 to 20 min before exercise.

Modified from The National Asthma Education Program: *Guidelines for the Diagnosis and Management of Asthma. Expert Panel Report 2.* U.S. Department of Health and Human Services, Public Health Service, National Institute of Health, Bethesda, MD, 1997.

Table 17–10. Long-Term Control Medications

Name/Products	Indications/Mechanisms	Potential Adverse Effects	Therapeutic Issues
Corticosteroids (Glucocorticoids) *Inhaled:* Beclomethasone dipropionate Budesonide Flunisolide Fluticasone propionate Triamcinolone acetonide	*Indications* • Long-term prevention of symptoms; suppression, control, and reversal of inflammation. • Reduce need for oral corticosteroid. *Mechanisms* • Anti-inflammatory. Block late reaction to allergen and reduce airway hyper-responsiveness. Inhibit cytokine production, adhesion protein activation, and inflammatory cell migration and activation. • Reverse β_2-receptor down-regulation. Inhibit microvascular leakage.	• Cough, dysphonia, oral thrush (candidiasis).	• Spacer/holding chamber devices and mouth washing after inhalation decrease local side effects and systemic absorption. • The risks of uncontrolled asthma should be weighed against the limited risks of inhaled corticosteroids. The potential but small risk of adverse events is well balanced by their efficacy.
Systemic: Methylprednisolone Prednisolone Prednisone	*Indications* • For short-term (3–10 days) "burst": to gain prompt control of inadequately controlled persistent asthma. • For long-term prevention of symptoms in severe persistent asthma: suppression, control, and reversal of inflammation. *Mechanisms* • Same as inhaled.	• Short-term use: reversible, abnormalities in glucose metabolism, increased appetite, fluid retention, weight gain, mood alteration, hypertension, peptic ulcer, and rarely aseptic necrosis of femoral head. • Long-term use: adrenal axis suppression, growth suppression, dermal thinning, hypertension, diabetes, Cushing's syndrome, cataracts, muscle weakness, and—in rare instances—impaired immune function. • Consideration should be given to coexisting conditions that could be worsened by systemic corticosteroids, such as herpes virus infections, varicella, tuberculosis, hypertension, peptic ulcer, and strongyloides.	Use at lowest effective dose. For long-term use, alternate-day a.m. dosing produces least toxicity.

(continued)

Table 17–10. (Continued)

Name/Products	Indications/Mechanisms	Potential Adverse Effects	Therapeutic Issues
Cromolyn Sodium and Nedocromil	*Indications* • Long-term prevention of symptoms; may modify inflammation. • Preventive treatment prior to exposure to exercise or known allergen. *Mechanisms* • Anti-inflammatory. Block early and late reaction to allergen. Modulate chloride channel function. Stabilize mast cell membranes and inhibit activation and release of mediators from eosinophils and epithelial cells. • Inhibit acute response to exercise, cold dry air, and SO_2	15 to 20% of patients complain of an unpleasant taste from nedocromil.	• Therapeutic response to cromolyn and nedocromil often occurs within 2 weeks, but a 4- to 6-week trial may be needed to determine maximum benefit. • Safety is the primary advantage of these agents.
Long-Acting β₂-Agonists *Inhaled:* Salmeterol	*Indications* • Long-term prevention of symptoms, especially nocturnal symptoms; added to anti-inflammatory therapy. • Prevention of exercise-induced bronchospasm. • *Not to be used to treat acute symptoms or exacerbations.* *Mechanisms* • Bronchodilation. Smooth muscle relaxation following adenylate cyclase activation and increase in cyclic AMP producing functional antagonism of bronchoconstriction. • In vitro, inhibit mast cell mediator release, decrease vascular permeability, and increase mucociliary clearance.	• Tachycardia, skeletal muscle tremor, hypokalemia, prolongation of QT_c interval in overdose.	• Not to be used to treat acute symptoms or exacerbations. • Should not be used in place of anti-inflammatory therapy. • May provide more effective symptom control when added to standard doses of inhaled corticosteroid compared to increasing the corticosteroid dosage.
Oral: Albuterol, sustained-release			• Inhaled long-acting β₂-agonists are preferred because they are longer acting and have fewer systemic side effects than oral sustained-release agents.

Table 17–10. (*Continued*)

Name/Products	Indications/Mechanisms	Potential Adverse Effects	Therapeutic Issues
Methylxanthines Theophylline, sustained-release tablets and capsules	*Indications* • Long-term control and prevention of symptoms, especially nocturnal symptoms. *Mechanisms* • Bronchodilation. Smooth muscle relaxation from phosphodiesterase inhibition and possibly adenosine antagonism • May affect eosinophillic infiltration into bronchial mucosa as well as decrease T-lymphocyte numbers in epithelium. • Increase diaphragm contractility and mucociliary clearance.	• Dose-related acute toxicities include tachycardia, nausea, vomiting, tachyarrhythmias (SVT), central nervous system stimulation, headache, seizures, hematemesis, hyperglycemia, and hypokalemia. • Adverse effects at usual therapeutic doses include insomnia, gastric upset, aggravation of ulcer or reflux, increase in hyperactivity in some children, difficulty in urination in elderly males with prostatism.	• Maintain steady-state serum concentrations between 5 and 15 µg/mL. Routine serum concentration monitoring is essential due to significant toxicities, narrow therapeutic range, and individual differences in metabolic clearance. Absorption and metabolism may be affected by numerous factors, which can produce significant changes in steady-state serum theophylline concentrations. • Not generally recommended for exacerbations. There is minimal evidence for added benefit to optimal doses of inhaled β_2-agonists. Serum concentration monitoring is mandatory.
Leukotriene Modifiers Zafirlukast tablets	*Indications* • Long-term control and prevention of symptoms in mild persistent asthma for patients ≥ 12 years of age. *Mechanisms* • Leukotriene receptor antagonists; selective competitive inhibitor of LTC4 and LTE4 receptors.	• No specific adverse effects to date. High concentrations may develop in patients with liver impairment.	• Administration with meals decreases bioavailability; take at least 1 hour before or more than 2 hours after meals. • Inhibits the metabolism of warfarin and increases prothrombin time: it is a competitive inhibitor of the CYP2C9 hepatic microsomal isozymes.
Zileuton tablets	*Indications* • Long-term control and prevention of symptoms in mild persistent asthma for patients ≥ 12 years of age. *Mechanisms* • 5-lipoxygenase inhibitor.	• Elevation of liver enzymes has been reported. Limited case reports of reversible hepatitis and hyperbilirubinemia.	• Zileuton is a microsomal CYP3A4 enzyme inhibitor that can inhibit the metabolism of terfenadine, warfarin, and theophylline. Doses of these drugs should be monitored accordingly. • Monitor hepatic enzymes.

AMP = adenosine monophosphate; SVT = supraventricular tachycardia.

Modified from The National Asthma Education Program: *Guidelines for the Diagnosis and Management of Asthma. Expert Panel Report 2.* U.S. Department of Health and Human Services, Public Health Service, National Institutes of Health, Bethesda, MD, 1997.

Table 17–11. Quick-Relief Medications

Name/Products	Indications/Mechanisms	Potential Adverse Effects	Therapeutic Issues
Short-acting Inhaled β₂-Agonists Albuterol Bitolterol Pirbuterol Terbutaline	*Indications* • Relief of acute symptoms; quick-relief medication. • Preventive treatment prior to exercise for exercise-induced bronchospasm. *Mechanisms* • Bronchodilation. Smooth muscle relaxation following adenylate cyclase activation and increase in cyclic AMP producing functional antagonism of bronchoconstriction.	Tachycardia, skeletal muscle tremor, hypokalemia, increased lactic acid, headache, hyperglycemia. Inhaled route, in general, causes few systemic adverse effects. Patients with preexisting cardiovascular disease, especially the elderly, may have adverse cardiovascular reactions with inhaled therapy.	• Drugs of choice for acute bronchospasm. Inhaled route has faster onset, fewer adverse effects, and is more effective than systemic routes. The less β₂ selective agents (isoproterenol, metaproterenol, isoetharine, and epinephrine) are not recommended due to their potential for excessive cardiac stimulation, especially in high doses. Albuterol suspension is not recommended. • Regularly scheduled daily use is not generally recommended. • For patients frequently using β₂-agonist, anti-inflammatory medication should be initiated or intensified.
Anticholinergics Ipratropium bromide	*Indications* • Relief of acute bronchospasm. *Mechanisms* • Bronchodilation. Competitive inhibition of muscarinic cholinergic receptors. • Reduces intrinsic vagal tone to the airways. May block reflex bronchoconstriction secondary to irritants or to reflux esophagitis. • May decrease mucus gland secretion.	Drying of mouth and respiratory secretions, increased wheezing in some individuals, blurred vision if sprayed in eyes.	• Reverses only cholinergically mediated bronchospasm. Does not block exercise-induced bronchospasm. • May provide additive effects to β₂-agonist but has slower onset or action. • Is an alternative for patients with intolerance to β₂-agonists.
Corticosteroids **Systemic** Methylprednisolone Prednisolone Prednisone	*Indications* • For moderate-to-severe exacerbations to prevent progression of exacerbation, reverse inflammation, speed recovery, and reduce rate of relapse. *Mechanisms* • Anti-inflammatory.	Short-term produces reversible abnormalities in glucose metabolism, increased appetite, fluid retention, weight gain, mood alteration, hypertension, peptic ulcer, and rarely aseptic necrosis of femoral head. • Consideration should be given to coexisting conditions that could be worsened by systemic corticosteroids, such as herpes virus infections, varicella, tuberculosis, hypertension, peptic ulcer, and strongyloides.	• Short-term therapy should continue until patient achieves 80% PEF personal best or symptoms resolve. This usually require 3 to 10 days but may require longer. • There is no evidence that tapering the dose following improvement prevents relapse.

Modified from The National Asthma Education Program: *Guidelines for the Diagnosis and Management of Asthma. Expert Panel Report 2.* U.S. Department of Health and Human Services, Public Health Service, National Institutes of Health, Bethesda, MD, 1997.

Table 17–12. Estimated Comparative Daily Dosages for Inhaled Steroids

Inhaled Steroid	Low Dose	Medium Dose	High Dose
Adults and Children >12 years			
Beclomethasone dipropionate	168–504 µg	504–840 µg	> 840 µg
42 µg/puff	4–12 puffs, 42 µg	12–20 puffs, 42 µg	> 20 puffs, 42 µg
84 µg/puff	2–6 puffs, 84 µg	6–10 puffs, 84 µg	> 10 puffs, 84 µg
Budesonide DPI	200–400 µg	400–600 µg	> 600 µg
200 µg/dose	1–2 inhalations	2–3 inhalations	> 3 inhalations
Flunisolide	500–1000 µg	1000–2000 µg	> 2000 µg
250 µg/puff	2–4 puffs	4–8 puffs	> 8 puffs
Fluticasone	88–264 µg	264–660 µg	> 60 µg
MDI:			
44, 110, 220 µg/puff	2–6 puffs, 44 µg or 2 puffs, 110 µg	2–6 puffs, 110 µg	> 6 puffs, 110 µg or > 3 puffs, 220 µg
DPI:			
50, 100, 250 µg/dose	2–6 inhalations, 50 µg	3–6 inhalations, 100 µg	> 6 inhalations, 100 µg or > 2 inhalations, 250 µg
Triamcinolone acetonide	400–1000 µg	1000–2000 µg	> 2000 µg
100 µg/puff	4–10 puffs	10–20 puffs	> 20 puffs
Children ≤ 12 years			
Beclomethasone dipropionate	84–336 µg	336–672 µg	> 672 µg
42 µg/puff	2–8 puffs, 42 µg	8–16 puffs, 42 µg	> 16 puffs, 42 µg
84 µg/puff	1–4 puffs, 84 µg	4–8 puffs, 84 µg	> 8 puffs, 84 µg
Budesonide DPI	100–200 µg	200–400 mcg	> 400 µg
200 µg/dose		1–2 inhalations, 200 µg	> 2 inhalations, 200 µg
Flunisolide	500–750 µg	1000–1250 µg	> 1250 µg
250 µg/puff	2–3 puffs	4–5 puffs	> 5 puffs
Fluticasone	88–176 µg	176–440 µg	> 440 µg
MDI:			
44, 110, 220 µg/puff	2–4 puffs, 44 µg	4–10 puffs, 44 µg or 2–4 puffs, 110 µg	> 4 puffs, 110 µg or > 2 puffs, 220 µg
DPI:			
50, 100, 250 µg/dose	2–4 inhalations, 50 µg	2–4 inhalations, 100 µg	> 4 inhalations, 100 µg or > 2 inhalations, 250 µg
Triamcinolone acetonide	400–800 µg	800–1200 µg	> 1200 µg
100 µg/puff	4–8 puffs	8–12 puffs	> 12 puffs

Clinician judgment of patient response is essential to appropriate dosing. Once asthma is controlled, medication doses should be carefully titrated to the minimum dose required to maintain control, thus reducing the potential for adverse effects.

Data from *in vitro* and clinical trials suggest that different inhaled corticosteroid preparations are not equivalent on a per puff or microgram basis.

However, few data directly compare the preparations. The Expert Panel developed recommended dose ranges for different preparations based on available data.

Inhaled corticosteroid safety data suggest dose ranges for children equivalent to beclomethasone dipropionate 200–400 µg/day (low dose), 400–800 µg/day (medium dose), and > 800 µg/day (high dose).

Modified from The National Asthma Education Program: *Guidelines for the Diagnosis and Management of Asthma. Expert Panel Report 2.* U.S. Department of Health and Human Service, Public Health Service, National Institutes of Health, Bethesda, MD, 1997.

DPI = dry powder inhaler; MDI = metered dose inhaler.

drugs for acute exacerbations of asthma has become less common because of toxicity (affecting the cardiovascular system, central nervous system, and gastrointestinal tract) and questionable efficacy. In patients with moderate-to-severe asthma, the chronic use of slow-release preparations of theophylline may allow the physician to reduce the use of systemic steroids. Monitoring of blood levels is essential when using theophylline.

Leukotrienes are biochemical mediators that contract airway smooth muscle, attract inflammatory cells, increase vascular permeability, and increase mucus secretion. Leukotriene-modifying agents appear to improve lung function and decrease the need for β_2-agonists. These compounds have utility in patients with mild persistent asthma who are over 12 years of age (see Tables 17–9 and 17–10).

The overall management of children with asthma is based on the understanding of the disease process by the family and physician, the ability to measure deterioration in the children's status subjectively and objectively, and the appropriate use of medications to quell the ongoing chronic inflammation of the airways and provide acute bronchodilatation. It is also important to recognize asthma triggers and to avoid them. A step-care plan often enables children to control asthma independently and allows a method of communication between the physician and family during times of deterioration. Good communication between the physician and family typically leads to a better outcome, as well as a decrease in the frustration that this disease can present to families.

PROGNOSIS

Asthma is a chronic disease, and most children have persistent symptoms and persistent pulmonary function test abnormalities. In general, pulmonary function tracks throughout life according to earlier patterns; thus, patients who were mildly affected in the past will tend to have mild disease in the future. In general, lung volumes and flow rates increase through childhood until early adolescence, when they stabilize until the beginning of the aging process. This is the most probable explanation for the improvement seen in most children with asthma; however, even if the symptoms are minimal and pulmonary function tests are mildly affected, they still have an increased risk for the development of chronic obstructive pulmonary disease in adult life, and for the recurrence of symptoms. Approximately one-half of all children with asthma have a remission of their symptoms by early adulthood. The probability of resolution is less in children with severe persistent asthma; only 5% of these patients have prolonged remissions. Children who have asthma that begins before 2 years of age and have an allergic basis have a worse prognosis in terms of severity and persistence of symptoms than do children with asthma that begins later. Many children who have mild symptoms

in early childhood associated with viral respiratory tract infections become symptom-free in later childhood. Asthma tends to be more severe if children have other associated allergic diseases, such as eczema, or have a positive family history.

Other Causes of Wheezing

The differential diagnosis of wheezing is varied and must be considered each time, even though patients may have a past history of asthma (see Table 17–6). Acute anaphlaxis from allergens, such as a bee sting is discussed in Chap. 18, "Allergy: Mechanisms and Disease Processes."

Ingestion and inhalation of foreign bodies are common in children aged 1 to 3 years. Impaction of the foreign body in the airway results in persistent coughing, and a localized, unilateral wheeze is highly suspicious for this problem. A chest radiograph with asymmetric hyperinflation, secondary to a ball-valve effect, warrants immediate action. Inspiratory and expiratory chest films may accentuate the asymmetric hyperinflation and assist with making this diagnosis. In young infants who are unable to cooperate with voluntary inspiration and expiration, right and left lateral decubitus films may reveal hyperinflation because the mediastinum does not shift towards the affected lung field when it is dependent. Of course, the radiograph may be confirmatory if the object is radiopaque. In the United States, the most common inhaled foreign body is a peanut. Children who have inhaled foreign bodies can be asymptomatic until secondary infection ensues.

EVALUATION OF CHILDREN WITH CHRONIC COUGH

Approach to Children with a Chronic Cough

Children often have chronic or persistent coughing. The cough may be infrequent, or it may be debilitating and disruptive to both patients and families. The cough mechanism serves the dual purpose of protecting the tracheobronchial tree from the penetration of foreign substances and removal of endogenous materials with subsequent expectoration.

A *chronic cough* is defined as one that persists for 3 to 6 weeks; whereas recurrent coughing shows periods of intermittent resolution. The cough mechanism is dependent on the coordination of inspiratory and expiratory muscles, normal laryngeal function, intact irritant receptor reflex, and a functional diaphragm. Coughing may be voluntary or involuntary. The cough center is located in the pons, and voluntary input is supplied from the cerebral cortex.

Persistent coughing in infants should always be regarded as abnormal. Aggressive workup for anatomic abnormalities, functional abnormalities (such as gastro-esophageal reflux), congestive heart failure, or infectious diseases should be pursued. Involuntary coughing is the end result of stimulation of irritant receptors located in the upper and lower airways, including the sinuses, external ear, pleura, diaphragm, and pericardium; the highest concentrations are found at points of airway bifurcation, such as the carina. Stimulation may occur with allergies, infections, or the inhalation of noxious agents or foreign bodies in the aerodigestive tract. Ineffective coughing may also result in a persistent cough because of the inability of the cough to clear endogenous materials and persistent stimulation of irritant cough receptors. Voluntary coughing may become persistent in individuals with psychological problems.

History

Careful history taking is very important when examining children with a chronic cough. Precipitating factors should be sought, including association with feedings and position in young infants. The age at onset of symptoms is a valuable clue in considering congenital anomalies. The quality of the cough, as well as possible mucous production, should be ascertained. The quality of the cough can suggest the diagnosis. A dry, barking cough is classically seen in croup and epiglottitis. Paroxysmal coughing suggests the presence of an infectious disease, such as pertussis or *Chlamydia*.

Alleviating or exacerbating factors should be considered. Coughing after strenuous exercise is suggestive of exercise-induced bronchospasm. A cough that stops during sleep is suggestive of psychogenic causes. Coughing associated with seasonal variation may indicate allergic rhinitis. Children who are unaffected at school but have a persistent cough at home may have environmental allergies. Any treatments that seem to improve the cough are valuable diagnostically; these may include bronchodilator or antibiotic therapy.

Physical Examination

The general state of health and nutrition is important. Children with immunodeficiency states, CF, or chronic gastrointestinal disease typically have a chronically ill appearance. Careful examination of the oropharynx, external auditory canals, and nasal passages is also important. Examination of the chest for evidence of retractions or increased anteroposterior diameter may suggest obstructive diseases, such as asthma or bronchiolitis obliterans.

Auscultation may demonstrate a localized wheeze, as heard in foreign-body aspiration. Diffuse, polyphonic, musical wheezes are consistent with asthma or bronchiolitis. Coarse crackles are the result of mucopurulent plugging of small airways and can be associated with CF, bronchiectasis, or pneumonia. Fine end-inspiratory crackles suggest interstitial lung disease with pulmonary fibrosis or pulmonary edema. Careful palpation of the abdomen for hepatosplenomegaly is warranted; subdiaphragmatic abscess with resultant diaphragmatic irritation can cause a persistent cough. Examination of the extremities for digital clubbing should not be overlooked. Evidence of recurrent infections of the skin can be seen in immunodeficiency syndromes with neutrophil dysfunction.

Diagnostic Evaluation

All children with chronic or persistent cough warrant a chest radiograph. Gas trapping, peribronchial thickening, alveolar infiltrates, or cardiomegaly should be noted. Symmetry of the left and right hemithorax should be checked. Standard pulmonary function tests can be valuable in children able to participate, generally those older than 5 years. Pre- and post-bronchodilator studies may demonstrate reversible obstruction, as seen in asthma. Airway obstruction, either intrathoracic or extrathoracic, may be diagnosed by pulmonary function testing; the former might suggest airway compression from adenopathy or lymphoma.

Causes of Chronic or Recurrent Cough

There are many causes of chronic cough in children (Table 17–13), but most cases are associated with only a few possible causes. In cases of acute onset, the physician must be aggressive in the workup and diagnosis to provide alleviation of possible life-threatening events. An

Table 17–13. Causes of Chronic Cough

Infection	Inflammatory
Sinusitis	Asthma
Pneumonia	Allergic rhinitis
Pharyngitis	Cystic fibrosis
Laryngitis	Recurrent aspiration
Tracheobronchitis	
Pertussis	Chemical
Parapertussis	Smoke
Influenza	Strong fumes
Bronchiolitis	Hydrocarbon ingestion
Tuberculosis	
Immune deficiency	Congenital
	Laryngotracheomalacia
	Tracheoesophageal fistula
Neoplastic	Vascular ring
Lymphoma	Lobar sequestration
Mediastinal tumors	
	Miscellaneous
Trauma	Gastroesophageal reflux
Aspirated foreign body	Psychogenic
Foreign body in external	Congestive heart failure
auditory canal	

algorithm for the evaluation of an acute cough is provided in Figure 17–4. Children with acute onset of coughing may be at high risk for progressive airway obstruction and respiratory distress.

TRAUMA

A foreign-body aspiration can cause a cough of sudden onset that persists. A history of the aspiration is often not obtained in children. As described in the previous section, a monophonic wheeze in a constant location is suspicious for this problem. Interestingly, a foreign body in the external auditory canal can also stimulate irritant cough receptors and cause a reflex cough.

GASTROESOPHAGEAL REFLUX

Gastroesophageal reflux, with or without aspiration, causes a chronic cough by stimulation of esophageal receptors resulting in bronchoconstriction, as well as irritation of cough receptors in the hypopharynx or larynx. If the chest radiograph shows chronic parenchymal changes in children with chronic cough, recurrent aspiration should be considered.

CYSTIC FIBROSIS

Any children with unexplained chronic cough, with or without evidence of gastrointestinal malabsorption, should undergo a sweat chloride analysis.

SINUSITIS AND POSTNASAL DRIP

Irritation of receptors in the posterior pharynx by drainage of nasal secretions from chronic sinusitis is a common cause of a chronic cough. Sinusitis may also aggravate underlying reactive airways disease with resultant bronchoconstriction and exacerbation of cough. Parents often report an increase in coughing at night when their child is in the supine position. Overt nasal discharge may not be present. Careful examination of the posterior pharynx often will show tenacious mucus and a cobblestone appearance of the mucosa.

ASTHMA

Airway hyperreactivity with inflammation of the airways is an extremely common cause of chronic coughing. Cough-variant asthma, which is not associated with wheezing, is a

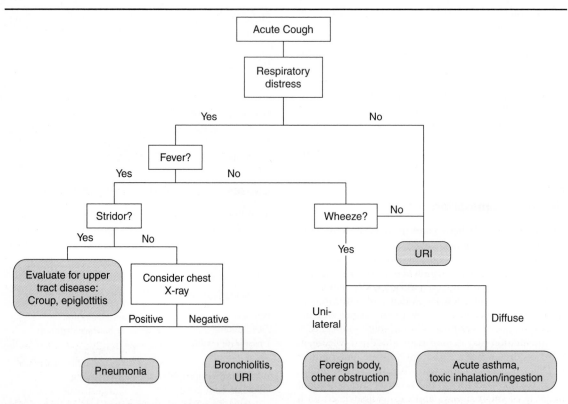

Figure 17–4. An algorithm for the evaluation of acute cough. URI = upper respiratory infection.

well-recognized entity in children; aggressive treatment often relieves the problem.

INFECTION

In early childhood, viral infections, such as respiratory syncytial virus (RSV), parainfluenza, adenovirus, and influenza, are common respiratory infections. Acute infection, resulting in pharyngitis, laryngitis, laryngotracheobronchitis (croup), bronchiolitis, and acute epiglottitis, is a common cause of acute cough. Pertussis or parapertussis should be considered in children with a paroxysmal cough. Diagnosis of pertussis may be made by fluorescent antibody testing of a per nasal swab; confirmation must be obtained by culture. *Mycoplasma pneumoniae* can cause a persistent cough in school-aged children that may last 8 to 10 weeks.

ENVIRONMENTAL TOXINS

Inhalation of cigarette smoke has been shown to cause an increase in otitis media in children, as well as an increased number and duration of upper respiratory infections. Chronic exposure to inhaled irritants should be sought in the history. Other environmental agents that may cause direct irritation of the airways are insecticides and industrial emissions.

CONGENITAL ANOMALIES

Congenital malformations of the airway, including tracheoesophageal fistulae, laryngotracheal clefts, and other anomalies that increase the risk of aspiration, can cause a persistent cough. Congenital anomalies of the lung parenchyma, including sequestration and cystic adenomatoid malformation, should be considered in the differential diagnosis. Vascular malformations and congenital heart disease can contribute to chronic cough through compressive effects on the airway or pulmonary edema.

CHILDREN WITH ACUTE RESPIRATORY DISTRESS

Approach to Children with Impending Respiratory Failure

ACUTE RESPIRATORY FAILURE

Acute respiratory failure describes any abnormality of the respiratory system that prevents or impairs the process of delivering oxygen to the pulmonary capillary bed or removing carbon dioxide from it. A conventional definition of acute respiratory failure is having a $PaCO_2$ >50 mm HG or a PaO_2 <50 mm Hg without any right-to-left intracardiac shunting.

Many acute respiratory diseases described in this chapter such as asthma, croup, and bronchiolitis can lead to acute respiratory failure. Respiratory failure can be defined as type I (hypoxia with normal or low $PaCO_2$) or type II (hypercapnea with or without hypoxemia). In infants, tachypnea is often the first sign of respiratory distress, followed by increased work of breathing and adventitial sounds such as stridor or wheezing. Expiratory grunting is a physical sign in infants and children that represents an effort to improve respiration by increasing positive end-expiratory pressure. Initially children will be anxious and restless, but as CO_2 retention develops this picture evolves into one of sleepiness, confusion, headache, and unresponsiveness. The presence of cyanosis is a late sign of respiratory failure; therefore arterial blood gas tensions should be measured whenever there is the possibility of serious respiratory impairment, even when there is no evidence of cyanosis.

TREATMENT OF ACUTE RESPIRATORY FAILURE

The treatment of respiratory failure depends on its cause. The overall goal is to maintain adequate oxygen delivery to the tissues and carbon dioxide removal from the tissues. The first step is to ensure airway patency and then to support breathing. This may lead to airway intubation or use of an oropharyngeal airway. Once the airway is established, the breath sounds and minute ventilation should be assessed. If they are reduced, it may be necessary to institute mechanical ventilation. Simultaneously, the degree of hypoxemia should be assessed by use of a pulse oximeter and, if reduced, supplemental oxygen should be provided. These treatments usually require that patients are admitted to the pediatric intensive care unit, although these interventions may be initiated in the emergency room or even in the field. Once admitted to the intensive care unit, many other clinical issues such as gastric distension from positive pressure ventilation, sedation of patients, and evaluation and treatment for infection will need to be addressed.

Causes of Acute Respiratory Distress

There are many causes of acute respiratory distress in children. Pneumonia is covered in Chap. 9, "Infectious Diseases," and asthma is discussed in this chapter and in Chap. 10, "Injuries and Emergencies." This section will discuss some other less common causes of acute respiratory distress: pleural effusions, pneumothorax, and pulmonary hemorrhage.

PLEURAL EFFUSIONS

Pleural effusions are abnormal collections of fluid in the pleural cavity. The pleural space is formed by the approximation of the parietal and visceral pleuras, which join at the hila of the lungs.

The pleura is composed histologically of a single layer of mesothelial cells, and the space between the visceral and parietal layers is 10 to 20 μm in width. Liter quantities of fluid may collect in this space, resulting in respiratory distress. Small quantities of fluid may exist in the pleural space and be clinically inapparent. In normal, healthy individuals, 0.1 to 0.2 mL/body weight (kg) of pleural fluid is contained between the parietal and visceral pleura. The pleura are supplied by systemic vessels and lymphatics. Hydrostatic and oncotic pressures maintain an equilibrium that is responsible for the normal circulation of pleural fluid, and disease states may alter these forces (Table 17–14).

Pleural effusions can be divided into transudates and exudates on the basis of chemical properties. Transudates are ultrafiltrates of serum with low levels of protein and markers such as lactate dehydrogenase (LDH). Conversely, exudates have high levels of protein and LDH. (See Table 17–2 for the chemical composition distinguishing transudates and exudates.)

Exudates are produced by disease states that cause inflammation of the pleura with subsequent disruption of its barrier filtration properties. Transudates are the result of changes in hydrostatic or oncotic pressures that cause accumulation of ultrafiltrate in the pleural space. In general, transudates are the result of systemic disease, whereas exudates are the result of inflammatory disease processes in the chest or adjacent organs of the upper abdomen. When exudates contain inflammatory cells and infectious agents, such as bacteria, an empyema results. Various causes of pulmonary effusions, both transudative and exudative, are shown in Table 17–15.

The medical history may contain symptoms that are highly suggestive of pleural effusion. In previously healthy children, there may be complaints of chest pain, shortness of breath, exercise intolerance, or a persistent irritating cough. Patients may find a position of comfort that relieves some or all of the symptoms. Fever may be present, depending on the etiology of the effusion. Exudative effusions, secondary to bacterial pneumonia, will often have increased coughing and sputum production. Pulmonary causes must be considered in patients with gastrointestinal complaints, especially upper quadrant abdominal pain. Trauma to the thoracic cage may result in pulmonary con-

Table 17–14. Pathophysiologic Mechanisms of Pleural Effusion

Increased hydrostatic pressure (systemic or venous hypertension)
Decreased oncotic pressure (hypoalbuminemia)
Decreased pleural space pressure (asthma, upper airway obstruction)
Increased microvascular permeability (infection)
Decreased lymphatic drainage (lymphangiectasia)
Movement of fluid from peritoneal space

Table 17–15. Causes of Pulmonary Effusions

Exudative	Transudative
Infectious	Congestive heart failure
Bacterial	
Viral	Neoplastic syndrome
Fungal	
Mycobacterial	Hypoalbuminemia
Gastrointestinal	Cirrhosis
Subdiaphragmatic abscess	Nephrotic syndrome
Pancreatitis	Protein-losing
Splenic infarct	enteropathy
	Chylothorax
Neoplastic	
Leukemia	Collagen vascular diseases
Lymphoma	
Neuroblastoma	Miscellaneous
Metastatic	Uremia
	Drug induced
Trauma	Radiation
Hemothorax	Pulmonary embolism
	Pulmonary contusion

tusion or disruption of the thoracic duct with secondary chylothorax. Unexplained joint pain or skin rashes may suggest autoimmune or collagen vascular disease.

The general appearance of the patients and overall nutritional status are important. The posture of the patients can be indicative of pleural irritation, as patients will splint the chest on the affected side. With larger effusions, percussion of the chest will reveal dullness in areas of fluid collection, and auscultation will reveal decreased breath sounds. Pleural effusion must be differentiated from parenchymal consolidation, which will also result in dullness to percussion and decreased breath sounds. This can be ascertained by attempting to elicit tactile vocal fremitus and egophony (signs of consolidation). Palpation of the trachea and cardiac impulse may show displacement of the mediastinum toward the contralateral side.

The diagnostic evaluation should include a chest radiograph. The minimum amount of fluid that can be visualized by a standard chest radiograph depends on the size of the child's thorax when upright. Blunting of the costophrenic angles, obliteration of the hemidiaphragms, and fluid tracking up the lateral margin of the chest should be identified. The position of the trachea and mediastinal structures should be noted. By placing patients in the lateral decubitus position, with the affected hemithorax down, as little as 50 mL of free-flowing effusion can be detected. The decubitus position may also be used to demonstrate a subpulmonic or subdiaphragmatic collection.

Thoracentesis, the withdrawal of fluid from the pleural space, is done for diagnostic or therapeutic indications. Occasionally, ultrasound guidance is necessary to accurately locate a loculated effusion. With massive effusions, tube thoracostomy is necessary.

Fluid analysis should include its gross appearance and its cytologic makeup. The fluid should also be submitted for biochemical analysis, including protein content, LDH, and pH. Microbiologic analysis should consist of culture for bacterial, fungal, and mycobacterial organisms. Other tests may be warranted depending on the suspected cause; for example, triglyceride analysis is needed if chylothorax is suspected.

Treatment is dependent on the accurate diagnosis of the cause of the effusion. Underlying infectious diseases should be appropriately treated. Repair of structures injured by trauma or previous surgery may require surgical intervention. Systemic diseases often require aggressive systemic management. Repeated or continued drainage of pleural effusions may be indicated when oxygenation and ventilation becomes compromised, whereas small effusions can be easily managed on an outpatient basis in the mildly symptomatic or asymptomatic individual.

PNEUMOTHORAX

Intrapleural accumulation of air is termed *pneumothorax*. The introduction of intrapleural air occurs from either direct penetration of the parietal pleura or penetration of the visceral pleura, secondary to alveolar rupture. Severe penetrating trauma may result in disruption of both the parietal and visceral pleura.

Pneumothoraces may be categorized as spontaneous or traumatic. Certain disease processes are associated with an increased risk of spontaneous pneumothorax (Table 17–16). Pneumothorax can also be divided into static and progressive forms. Progressive pneumothoraces result in tension pneumothorax that may be life threatening, secondary to compression of mediastinal structures and decreased cardiac output.

Blunt trauma to the chest wall may cause pneumothorax, secondary to rib fracture with parenchymal penetration. Shear forces may cause disruption of peripheral small airways with subsequent escape of gas. Common iatrogenic causes of traumatic pneumothoraces include thoracentesis, thoracotomy, central line placement, and tracheostomy. In general, disease processes that cause spontaneous pneumothoraces are associated with obstruc-

Table 17–16. Diseases Associated with Spontaneous Pneumothorax

Congenital bullae	Histiocytosis X
Congenital lobar emphysema	Malignancy
Cystic fibrosis	Pertussis
Marfan syndrome	Pulmonary abscess
Asthma	

tion of segmental or distal airways, resulting in a ball-valve effect with subsequent hyperinflation of the distal air space unit. Resultant forces on the overlying parenchyma are responsible for disrupting the pleura, leading to pneumothorax. Disruption of the visceral pleura can be seen in disorders such as histiocytosis X and metastatic disease. Congenital anomalies, such as congenital lobar emphysema, may result in spontaneous pneumothorax from overexpansion of the airway unit.

The onset of pneumothorax is acute with sudden onset of chest pain, progressive shortness of breath, tachypnea, and often shoulder pain on the ipsilateral side. Rapid hemodynamic deterioration in patients with suspected pneumothorax suggests a rapidly expanding pneumothorax or "tension pneumothorax" and requires immediate intervention. Any patients with rapid onset of respiratory distress, tachypnea, hypotension, and hypoxemia, in conjunction with absent or diminished breath sounds, require the introduction of a large-bore needle or chest tube into the affected side for immediate evacuation of air.

Physical findings in static or nonprogressive pneumothorax may include chest asymmetry, splinting of the thorax on the affected side, pleuritic pain on deep inspiration, and decreased or absent breath sounds on the affected side. Palpation of the trachea for deviation and the neck for subcutaneous air may be helpful.

The upright anteroposterior chest radiograph is extremely sensitive for the diagnosis of pneumothorax. It allows for the amount of intrapleural air and degree of mediastinal shift to be evaluated. In infants in whom an upright film is not feasible, a cross-table lateral film can be requested.

Treatment is based on the clinical status of patients and underlying etiology. Surgical intervention may be necessary for penetrating chest trauma or persistent air leak, secondary to blunt trauma. Small pneumothoraces in asymptomatic or mildly symptomatic patients usually resolve without treatment; these patients may benefit from the use of high FiO_2 to augment the reabsorption of intrapleural air. Large collections of intrapleural air (>25% of the volume on the affected side) usually need evacuation by needle or chest tube placement. Chest tube placement with continuous suction augments the re-expansion of the affected lung. Persistent air leak into the pleural space due to bronchopulmonary fistula formation is possible and necessitates medical or surgical pleurodesis. The end result of these procedures is adhesion of the parietal and visceral pleuras to seal the leak.

PULMONARY HEMORRHAGE

Pulmonary hemorrhage is usually suggested by a combination of hemoptysis with anemia and diffuse alveolar infiltrates on the chest radiograph. Sometimes it is difficult to distinguish hemoptysis from hematemesis. Clinical points of differentiation are listed in Table 17–17. The possible causes of pulmonary hemorrhage in children, listed in Table 17–18, should be kept in mind when obtaining the history and performing the physical examination. It is particularly important to ask about the possibility of foreign-body inhalation and to elicit symptoms that might suggest an underlying infection, such as a chronic cough, sputum production, or fever. Substance abuse or exposure to toxins may be relevant, and it is important to ask about overseas travel that might involve exposure to parasitic infections and tuberculosis. Individuals may have recently immigrated to the United States from Southeast Asia, where paragonimiasis is endemic; this is an important cause of pulmonary hypertension and hemoptysis that is otherwise asymptomatic. The nose and oropharynx should be examined carefully to ensure that the bleeding is from the lower respiratory tract and not from the upper airway. Sometimes nasopharyngoscopy or laryngoscopy is helpful.

A chest radiograph is usually obtained and may show diffuse alveolar infiltrates from diffuse pulmonary hemorrhage, atelectasis, or interstitial infiltrates. Localized air trapping would suggest airway obstruction, for example, by an inhaled foreign body.

Laboratory evaluation may include coagulation studies, hemoglobin measurement, arterial blood gas values, tuberculin test, sputum cultures, sputum cytology, examination of gastric aspirates for acid-fast bacilli or hemosiderin-laden macrophages, and an examination of stool for ova and parasites. In patients with renal involvement and hemoptysis, renal function should be assessed by measuring blood urea nitrogen and creatinine concentrations; the presence or absence of antiglomerular basement membrane antibodies should be determined as well. Renal biopsy may be needed to make the diagnosis of Goodpasture syndrome.

A CT scan of the chest is the best method to define the anatomy of any abnormal structures. Angiography is used

Table 17–18. Causes of Pulmonary Hemorrhage

Retained foreign body	Lung tumors
	Benign
Infection	Hamartoma
Bacterial	Malignant
Pneumonia	Carcinoma of the bronchus
Lung abscess	Bronchial adenoma
Bronchiectasis	
Tuberculosis	Pulmonary infarct
Fungal	Pulmonary embolism
Actinomycosis	Vaso-occlusive crisis
Aspergillosis	
Histoplasmosis	Cardiovascular
Coccidioidomycosis	Vascular
Parasitic	Arteriovenous
Hydatid disease	malformation
Strongyloides	Familial telangiectasia
Paragonimiasis	Pulmonary hemangioma
	Cardiac
Autoimmune	Mitral stenosis
Goodpasture	
syndrome	Trauma
Pulmonary	Crush injury
hemosiderosis	Penetrating injury
Wegener	Thoracic surgery
granulomatosis	
Collagen vascular	
disease	

to define congenital malformations, such as arteriovenous malformations or pulmonary telangiectasia.

Endoscopy is useful to identify the source of bleeding, to obtain samples for culture and acid-fast stains, and to obtain specimens for cytology. Bronchoscopy is also used for treatment in the case of inhaled foreign bodies or endobronchial lesions such as polyps. Treatment of pulmonary hemorrhage will vary according to the specific etiology.

CHILDREN WITH RECURRENT OR PERSISTENT PNEUMONIA

Approach to Children with Recurrent or Persistent Pneumonia

Evaluation of children with recurrent or persistent pneumonia requires a systematic approach to obtain the time course of both symptoms and radiographic changes. Pneumonia is an illness manifested clinically by fever, coughing, upper or lower respiratory symptoms, and dyspnea or tachypnea. Associated physical findings include dullness to percussion, coarse crackles, and decreased breath sounds; wheezing may or may not be present. This constellation of signs and symptoms, in conjunction with a chest radiograph showing an alveolar infiltrate, constitutes clinical evidence of pneumonia. A period of at least 1-month, and

Table 17–17. Differentiation of Hemoptysis from Hematemesis

	Hemoptysis	Hematemesis
Color	Bright red and trothy	Dark red or brown
pH	Alkaline	Acid
Consistency	May be mixed with sputum	May contain food particles
Symptoms	Preceded by gurgling noise; accompanied by coughing	Preceded by nausea; accompanied by retching

Reproduced with permission from Rosenstein BJ: Hemoptysis. Page 533 in: Hilman BC (editor): *Pediatric Respiratory Disease.* Saunders, 1993.

possibly a minimum of 3 months, has been proposed as the definition of persistence. Recurrent pneumonia is defined as two episodes of pneumonia during the same year or three episodes of pneumonia during any time period.

History

The first step in evaluating children with recurrent pneumonia is to review the history and radiographs carefully to determine whether they meet the criteria for recurrent pneumonia or whether they represent repeated evaluations of improperly treated or resolving pneumonia. Careful serial review of all available radiographs with a pediatric radiologist is very helpful. A detailed history should be taken to ascertain whether the children have had symptom-free periods between the suspected bouts of pneumonia and to establish the general baseline health of the children. Because recurrent pneumonia in children may be a manifestation of a more protean disease state, a careful review of systems, including the general nutritional status of children and any other recurrent infections, is important. Daytime and nighttime symptoms should be elicited, together with the history of attendance at day care and exposure to cigarette smoke. The children's medication history should be obtained, especially the chronic or recurrent use of antibiotics. In developing a differential diagnosis, it should be realized that pulmonary infections generally come from one of two possible sources: direct inoculation from the airways or hematogenous spread.

Because the physician relies on the chest radiograph to diagnose pneumonia, it is important to have an appreciation for the time scale of normal resolution of pneumonia in pediatric patients without complications. A community-acquired pneumonia, such as *Streptococcus pneumoniae*, usually shows radiographic resolution in 6 to 7 weeks. Severe RSV or adenoviral pneumonia may take as long as 12 to 15 months, depending on the severity of the initial infection. Therefore, careful longitudinal follow-up of these patients is necessary to make the diagnosis of recurrent or persistent pneumonia, as well as to appreciate improving symptoms or radiographs.

After recurrent or persistent pneumonia is diagnosed, a logical stepwise approach to understanding its etiology is necessary (Table 17–19). It is helpful to approach recurrent or persistent pneumonia by determining whether the pneumonia is unilobar or multilobar, as seen on the chest radiograph; the age of the children should also be considered. Recurrent pneumonia is often caused by aspiration syndromes, abnormal mucociliary clearance from obstruction or dysfunctional cilia, or congenital abnormalities of the cardiopulmonary system. Immunologic deficiencies also cause recurrent pulmonary infections. In the latter case, the history will reveal other evidence of immunologic dysfunction, including recurrent sinus disease, middle ear infection, failure to thrive, or recurrent skin infections.

Table 17–19. Differential Diagnosis of Persistent of Recurrent Pneumonia

	Unilobar	Multilobar
Aspiration syndromes		
Central nervous system abnormalities	+	+
Gastroesophageal reflux	+	+
Myopathies	+	+
Anatomic causes of aspiration		
Tracheoesophageal fistula	+	+
Laryngotracheal cleft	+	+
Cleft palate	+	+
Congenital anomalies		
Sequestration	+	
Bronchogenic cyst	+	
Cystic adenomatoid malformation	+	
Pulmonary hypoplasia	+	
Tracheal bronchus	+	
Heart disease		+
Mucociliary dysfunction		
Cystic fibrosis		+
Primary ciliary dyskinesia		+
Luminal obstruction		
Foreign body	+	
Bronchial stenosis	+	
Hilar adenopathy	+	
Vascular compression	+	
Immunodeficiency syndromes		+

In children with asthma or airway hyperreactivity, a recurrent pneumonia is often misdiagnosed on the basis of radiographic evidence of an increased density in the right middle lobe, referred to as right middle lobe syndrome. In this case, the asthma is exacerbated by intercurrent upper respiratory infections and mucous plugging, leading to fever, wheezing, crackles, and diminished breath sounds. Intraluminal obstruction due to inspissated mucus is seen in the take-off of the right middle lobe bronchus. Aggressive treatment of the underlying reactive airways disease, including chest physiotherapy and bronchodilator aerosols, with or without steroid therapy, often leads to resolution of the atelectasis. It is important to demonstrate normalization of the radiograph.

Causes of Unilobar Pneumonia

Single-lobe disease is indicative of three possible processes. The most common is a congenital structural abnormality, such as a bronchogenic cyst, a sequestered lobe, or congenital cystic adenomatoid malformation of the lung. The other causes of unilobar recurrent pneumonia are intraluminal or extraluminal obstruction. A history of acute choking or a witnessed episode of aspiration of a foreign body is most relevant. Extremely rare causes of intraluminal obstruction in childhood include bronchial adenomas and bronchial hamartomas. Any pathology causing extrinsic compression of the airway (extraluminal) can lead to recurrent pneumonia distal to the compression. These anomalies include vascular rings, congenital heart disease with enlargement of the atria or pulmonary arteries, and prior surgical repairs of congenital heart defects. Other extraluminal causes of obstruction include tumors of the mediastinum, such as lymphomas and neuroblastomas. Parahilar adenopathy from tuberculosis, histoplasmosis, coccidioidomycosis, or other infectious diseases is a common cause of extraluminal bronchial obstruction. Treatment of the underlying disease process usually results in resolution. Aspiration syndromes are generally thought to be multilobar processes; however, unilobar disease has been described in some children. A history of choking or feeding intolerance with increased respiratory distress after meals is helpful in discerning this problem.

PULMONARY SEQUESTRATION

Pulmonary sequestration refers to a segment of nonfunctioning, isolated pulmonary tissue with a systemic blood supply. There is neither pulmonary arterial blood supply nor communication with the tracheobronchial tree. The arterial blood supply usually arises from the thoracic or abdominal aorta. There are two types of sequestration: extralobar and intrapulmonary. Extralobar sequestrations are surrounded by their own pleural investment, whereas intrapulmonary sequestrations are located within a lobe, without a discrete separation. They have similar histologic structures. Intrapulmonary sequestration is much more common than is extralobar sequestration; both types occur predominantly in the left lower lobe in the posterior basal segment.

Many cases of intrapulmonary sequestration are asymptomatic or they present in adolescence, when detected on routine chest radiographs. Sometimes these lesions become infected and present as pneumonia or a pulmonary abscess. Extralobar sequestrations are usually detected in the first year of life because, in up to 50% of cases, they are associated with other congenital malformations, including diaphragmatic hernia, pulmonary vascular lesions, esophageal communications, and duplication of the colon. The diagnosis of sequestration is made by chest CT scan. If the diagnosis is unclear, a definitive diagnosis can be made by angiography to delineate the feeding vessel. Magnetic resonance imaging studies can also display the vessels clearly. An upper gastrointestinal series should be considered to rule out possible communication with the gastrointestinal tract.

Treatment involves surgical resection. Even if patients are asymptomatic, surgery should be recommended because of the risk of infection.

CYSTIC ADENOMATOID MALFORMATIONS

Cystic adenomatoid malformations occur when there is an overgrowth of the terminal bronchioles, causing an adenomatous appearance on histology. This malformation occurs early in fetal development, probably around 35 days gestation. The lesions have intracystic communications and are connected to the tracheobronchial tree. The cysts receive a blood supply from the bronchial circulation.

All lobes of the lung may be affected by cystic adenomatoid malformations, but usually only one lobe is involved. The most common presentation is with acute respiratory distress because the cysts expand and compress surrounding structures. Cystic adenomatoid malformation can also present on routine chest radiographs or as recurrent pneumonia.

Chest radiographic findings are variable and depend on the type of cyst. Typically, there are multiple air-filled cysts with depression of the ipsilateral diaphragm and mediastinal shift away from the lesion.

Cystic adenomatoid malformations can easily be confused with diaphragmatic hernias, because the air in a multiloculated cyst can mimic bowel in the thoracic cavity. Placement of a nasogastric tube and instillation of contrast medium will help distinguish the diaphragmatic hernia. A chest CT scan can help delineate the size and nature of the lesion, although it is not essential. Treatment involves surgical removal of the affected lobe.

BRONCHOGENIC CYSTS

Bronchogenic cysts represent islands of bronchial tissue left behind during the branching of the airways in early fetal development. If the bronchial tissue is separated from the airways early in gestation, the cyst tends to be placed in the mediastinum; if it occurs later in gestation, the cyst develops in the pulmonary parenchyma. The separation occurs before complete formation of the conducting airways (16 weeks gestation). Bronchogenic cysts are thin walled and have a ciliated columnar epithelial lining. The wall contains the histologic components of airways: smooth muscle, bronchial glands, cartilage, and nervous tissue. The cysts commonly contain serous or mucoid fluid.

Bronchogenic cysts are usually single, unilocular, and round; they average 2 to 10 cm in diameter. Most commonly, they are mediastinal and are located close to the carina; some are located between the trachea and esophagus. The cysts are often asymptomatic, but moderate-to-severe respiratory distress can occur with airway compression, and this is a common presentation in infancy. Pulmonary bronchogenic cysts develop later in gestation and are usually found in the lower lobes. These cysts often become infected.

Bronchogenic cysts can be diagnosed by chest radiograph and confirmed by a CT scan. Treatment usually involves surgical removal. Arguably, the status of these lesions could be followed by chest radiograph or CT scan. However, there is a small risk of malignant change, and the best approach is removal and histologic examination.

PULMONARY CYST

Congenital pulmonary cysts develop early in fetal life, at a time when the terminal airways have formed and alveolarization is occurring. No specific cause has been determined. These are characteristically thin-walled cysts lined by columnar epithelium.

Pulmonary cysts are usually singular and multilocular. They are usually >1 cm in diameter and affect just one lobe. They are peripherally located and usually communicate with the airways, so they are air-filled. Pulmonary cysts may present with respiratory distress because gas trapping can develop with inflation of the cyst and compression of the surrounding structures. Later in life, presentation with infection is more common.

The chest radiograph reveals a thin-walled, rounded, cystic lesion containing faint strands of lung tissue. If the cyst is large enough, there will be mediastinal shift and flattening of the ipsilateral diaphragm. Large pulmonary cysts and congenital lobar emphysema are difficult to distinguish on a chest radiograph but are readily differentiated by CT scan. Treatment involves surgical resection of the cyst.

Causes of Multilobar Pneumonia

Multilobar pneumonia is common with reflux and aspiration in young infants who are often in the supine position. When bilateral upper lobe infiltrates are noted on the chest radiograph of infants, a complete workup for aspiration should ensue. A thorough neurologic examination is essential. Myopathies or neuromuscular disorders and their associated esophageal dysmotility carry a high risk for aspiration. Aspiration syndromes can be diagnosed with the use of various tests including modified barium swallows, gastric-emptying scans, and pH probes. Direct visualization of the glottis by fiberoptic endoscopy is helpful in children with swallowing incoordination who may have intermittent aspiration according to food thickness. Signs and symptoms of gastroesophageal reflux should not be overlooked, as this condition is amenable to medical or surgical treatment. Congenital anomalies, such as laryngotracheal clefts, tracheoesophageal fistulas (whether undiagnosed or previously repaired), and esophageal webs or strictures, all lead to a higher incidence of aspiration. Congenital abnormalities of the upper airway, including laryngotracheal clefts, laryngomalacia, esophageal strictures, and webs, should be evaluated by bronchoscopy and esophagoscopy.

Dynamic anomalies of the airway may also lead to recurrent pneumonia, probably because of poor clearance of airway secretions and mucus. Laryngomalacia, tracheomalacia, and bronchomalacia may cause noisy breathing and recurrent pneumonia. Malacia of the trachea or the distal or mainstem bronchi is best visualized by flexible bronchoscopy with patients sedated and breathing spontaneously. Diseases such as CF are associated with abnormal mucociliary clearance, and any children with recurrent pneumonia should undergo a sweat chloride test. Environmental irritants often cause ciliary dysfunction with resultant mucous plugging. These irritants include secondhand cigarette smoke and strong fumes from solvents. Allergic pneumonitis, such as a hypersensitivity pneumonitis, is suspected when patients' symptoms seem to resolve when removed from the potential antigen exposure. Primary ciliary dyskinesia also results in poor airway clearance associated with recurrent sinus disease, bronchiectasis, and airway inflammation due to chronic infection. Functional studies of the cilia or electron microscopic examination of ciliary biopsy material can confirm this diagnosis (see immotile cilia syndrome).

Bronchiectasis may develop in children with recurrent pneumonia; therefore, a chest CT scan should be considered in children with recurrent pneumonia and signs of chronic pulmonary disease.

CYSTIC FIBROSIS

Cystic fibrosis is the most common lethal autosomal-recessive disease that affects the white population, with an incidence of approximately 1:3300. The incidence among African Americans is approximately 1:15,000, and among Native Americans, approximately 1:32,000. The disease affects three main organ systems: the lungs, with recurrent lower respiratory tract infections and progressive obstructive pulmonary disease; the gastrointestinal tract, with pancreatic exocrine insufficiency; and the sweat glands, with production of hypertonic sweat rich in sodium and chloride. Abnormal hyperviscous secretions characterize the disease and are probably responsible for the clinical manifestations.

Pathophysiology. The basic defect of CF is a mutation in a gene that is 250,000 base pairs long and resides on chromosome 7. This gene produces the CF transmembrane conductance regulator (CFTR) protein, which is an epithelial chloride channel. Mutations of the CFTR protein cause an abnormality of cyclic adenosine-monophosphate–regulated chloride conductance in epithelial cells. In 1989, the *CF* gene was identified and cloned, leading to a period of rapid and exciting advances in understanding the basic mechanisms underlying CF. In North America, approximately 75% of affected individuals with CF have a deletion of the amino acid phenylalanine at the 508 position of CFTR, designated ΔF508 on one or both chromosomes. Currently, there are more than 1000 known mutations of the *CF* gene. In CF, defective chloride transport occurs in epithelial cells of the respiratory, gastrointestinal, hepatobiliary, pancreatic, and reproductive tracts. The CFTR has regulatory effects on other chloride channels and also controls sodium reabsorption by epithelial cells. The net result of failure of CFTR function in respiratory epithelia is dehydrated, viscous secretions with reduced mucociliary clearance.

Clinical features. The primary organ systems affected by CF are the pulmonary, gastrointestinal, and reproductive systems (Table 17–20). Inspissated mucus in the airways of patients leads to recurrent infections of the lower respiratory tract with bacteria such as *Pseudomonas aeruginosa* and *Staphylococcus aureus.* These infections leads to chronic endobronchial inflammation with airflow obstruction. The airflow obstruction progresses, becoming worse with each intercurrent infection, although it usually responds to treatment with antibiotics. Over a period of years, there is progressive loss of lung function, eventually leading to severe airflow obstruction, ventilation perfusion mismatching, and hypoxemia. The hypoxemia, in turn, leads to increased pulmonary vascular resistance and pulmonary hypertension, so that most CF patients eventually die of respiratory failure complicated by right ventricular failure. Common pulmonary complications are bronchiectasis due to repeated bacterial infections of the airway that cause permanent weakening of the airway wall; atelectasis, particularly in young chil-

Table 17–20. Complications in Patients with Cystic Fibrosis

Pulmonary	**Gastrointestinal**
Recurrent infections	Pancreatic insufficiency
Atelectasis	Rectal prolapse
Pneumothorax	Intestinal obstruction
Hemoptysis	Failure to thrive
Respiratory acidosis	Cholecystitis
Pulmonary hypertension	Focal biliary cirrhosis
Respiratory failure	Portal hypertension
	Pancreatitis
Nose and throat	
Nasal polyps	**Endocrine**
Chronic sinusitis	Diabetes mellitus
Cardiac	**Reproductive**
Cor pulmonale	Azoospermia
	Decreased fertility in
Orthopedic	women
Hypertrophic pulmonary	
osteoarthropathy	**Metabolic**
	Hyponatremic, hypo-
	chloremic dehydration

dren who have smaller airways; and hemoptysis, which may be minor or, on occasion, massive. The latter problem occurs when an ulcerating airway lesion erodes a hypertrophied bronchial artery.

Gastrointestinal manifestations are caused by exocrine pancreatic insufficiency, which is thought to be the result of thick pancreatic secretions. Destruction of the exocrine portion of the pancreas leads to malabsorption of fat, carbohydrates, and proteins. This causes clinical symptoms of steatorrhea, diarrhea, and failure to thrive in infancy. Approximately 18% of infants affected by CF are born with an obstruction in the small intestine caused by thick inspissated meconium, termed *meconium ileus.* Men affected by CF are usually infertile because of obstruction of the vas deferens and obstructive azoospermia. Most probably, chronic inspissation of secretions in utero leads to fibrosis and obliteration of the vas deferens. In young women with CF, fertility rates are decreased to approximately 50% of normal; delayed menarche occurs in approximately 20% of patients.

Hypochloremic, hypernatremic dehydration with alkalosis occurs in very young infants with CF because of excessive loss of salt from sweat glands. It tends to occur in hot weather, particularly if oral intake of salt and water is decreased.

The *distal intestinal obstructive syndrome (DIOS),* formerly known as meconium ileus equivalent, can develop in patients with CF. This functional intestinal obstruction probably results from abnormal CFTR function in the mucous-secreting glands of the intestine. Patients with either abdominal distention or constipation must be evaluated promptly. Early intervention with mucolytic or osmotic agents is often successful and may obviate surgical intervention.

In approximately 15 to 20% of adolescents with CF, hepatobiliary disease, typically focal biliary cirrhosis, develops. This leads to intralobular cirrhosis with resultant portal hypertension, varices, and increased risk for gastrointestinal bleeding. Repeated and continued fibrosis of the pancreas, as well as a relative insulin resistance, results in diabetes mellitus in approximately 20% of adults with CF.

Diagnostic evaluation. The diagnosis of CF is based on the following criteria: the occurrence of at least one typical clinical symptom of CF, a positive family history, or a positive newborn screening test, combined with a positive sweat test result on two occasions; the finding of two CF mutations on analysis of the CF locus; or the finding of abnormal nasal potential difference measurements on two occasions. Nasal potential difference refers to the measurement of bioelectrical potentials in the nose using a perfusion method. The transepithelial potential difference is increased in CF because of the increased resorption of sodium ions from the lumen. (See Table 17–3 for causes of false-positive and false-negative sweat test results.)

In approximately 60% of patients with CF, the diagnosis is determined during the first 12 months after birth; in 85% of patients, the diagnosis is determined by the age of 5 years, and in 90 to 94%, by 10 years. Delayed diagnosis is due to wide variations in the clinical manifestations of CF, resulting in mild disease or misdiagnosis of the clinical presentation. Approximately 18% of affected newborns present with meconium ileus or rectal prolapse; any infant with these signs should undergo sweat testing when clinically stable. The diagnosis of CF should also be considered in newborns with prolonged neonatal jaundice, failure to thrive, or any pulmonary manifestation, such as wheezing, coughing, or tachypnea and retractions that cannot be explained clinically. Segmental or lobar atelectasis may be the presenting manifestation of pulmonary disease in affected infants. In older children, the diagnosis is often considered if there is recurrent wheezing, recurrent pneumonia, chronic cough, bronchiectasis, staphylococcal pneumonia, chronic recurrent pansinusitis, or nasal polyps. Nasal polyps occur in approximately 10 to 24% of children with CF, and more than 50% of adolescents. The presence of nasal polyps at any age requires investigation by sweat chloride analysis. Digital clubbing is almost always associated with cardiopulmonary or hepatic disease, and CF is an important cause of clubbing in children (see Table 17–1). Any patients with a positive culture for *P. aeruginosa* from sinuses, sputum, or epiglottic culture should be assumed to have CF until the diagnosis is disproved. Gastrointestinal symptoms include steatorrhea and malabsorption syndrome. Infants and children with failure to thrive or episodes of partial obstruction of the small or large intestine must also undergo a sweat test.

Clinical management. The treatment of CF is threefold:

- Treatment of recurrent, chronic endobronchial infections
- Clearance of hyperviscous secretions from the airway
- Pancreatic enzyme replacement with the subsequent alleviation of malabsorption

Augmentation of caloric intake by nutritional supplementation also benefits patients with CF.

Pulmonary management: Early pulmonary disease is manifested by endobronchial infection with **Staphylococcus aureus, Haemophilus influenzae,** and gramnegative bacilli, such as **Escherichia coli.** By adolescence, most patients with CF have become colonized with **P. aeruginosa.** Patients with CF have intermittent pulmonary exacerbations requiring the use of either oral or intravenous antibiotics on the basis of symptoms and culture results. At these times, they report an increased frequency of coughing with an increase in sputum quantity and tenacity. They often have dyspnea, decreased exercise tolerance, and decreased appetite. On physical examination, they may demonstrate an increased work of breathing with increased use of accessory muscles of respiration. Often, patients with more advanced CF are emaciated. Auscultation demonstrates coarse crackles either locally or globally; the crackles represent mucous plugging of small airways associated with chronic inflammation and increased production of hyperviscous mucus.

In young children, antibiotic coverage should include *H. influenzae,* as well as *S. aureus;* oral antibiotics, such as cephalexin, amoxicillin-clavulanate, cefprozil, and clarithromycin, are commonly prescribed. In children with known *Pseudomonas* colonization, anti-pseudomonal combinations of a β-lactam with an aminoglycoside are appropriate. Common choices are ceftazidime and tobramycin, or ticarcillin and tobramycin. Most of these antibiotics require intravenous administration. Newer, orally absorbed drugs in the quinolone class (such as ciprofloxacin) can be prescribed; however, *Pseudomonas* can quickly become resistant to their actions. Emergence of multidrug-resistant, Gram-negative organisms, such as *Burkholderia cepacia, Xanthomonas maltophilia,* and multidrug-resistant *P. aeruginosa* is a clinical problem. This most likely reflects the increasing use of antibiotics, as well as the increased survival of patients. In addition to antibiotic therapy, children with CF benefit from regular airway clearance therapy, which is often combined with aerosol delivery of dornase-α to reduce sputum viscosity.

Gastrointestinal management. Nutritional management is important in CF, as it seems to improve the overall prognosis and the resistance to pulmonary infections. The cornerstone of treatment is replacement of the missing exocrine pancreatic function by taking oral pancreatic supplements with food. This comes in the form of purified pancreatic enzymes (pancrelipase) prepared in microsphere or microtablet form and packaged in capsules. Children with CF will take several capsules with each meal and one or two capsules with each snack, so that enzymes are ingested just before food. A minority of patients with CF (about 15%) have preserved pancreatic function and do not require these enzyme supplements. Even with enzyme therapy, there may be ongoing mild steatorrhea, which tends to deplete fat-soluble vitamins. Therefore, the standard practice is to supplement vitamin intake with a multivitamin that includes vitamins A, D, E, and K. Children with CF have increased calorie requirements and may need as many as 30% more calories per kilogram. These increased requirements are met with calorie supplements. Children with mild disease can increase their caloric intake by consuming more snacks and larger meals than they normally consume. Children with more severe symptoms may require special supplement or even overnight enteral feeding through a nasogastric tube, gastrostomy, or jejunostomy. Increased salt losses should be addressed in hot weather, particularly if patients are going to exercise in high environmental temperatures.

Usually, it is sufficient to allow children with CF free access to table salt. They may also enjoy salty snacks, such as saltine crackers and pretzels. Some patients with high losses require treatment with sodium chloride tablets.

Prognosis. Even with optimal medical management, complications result from progression of the underlying disease (Table 17–20). Currently, the median age of survival in patients with CF is more than 31 years, and patients born today are expected to have life expectancies greater than 40 years. The current average life expectancy represents a doubling in the past 20 years. This is believed to be due to increased understanding of the pathophysiologic mechanisms associated with CF, use of antipseudomonal antibiotics, aggressive treatment of malabsorption, and improved methods for airway clearance.

The clinical expression of disease in CF is wide ranging. Many patients lead relatively normal lives, and many women have successfully borne children. General pediatricians and other physicians are becoming increasingly involved in the care and management of patients with CF, as the disease is common and the life expectancy is improving.

REFLUX AND ASPIRATION

Gastroesophageal reflux is defined as the movement of gastric contents into the esophagus due to a dysfunction of the lower esophageal sphincter, and aspiration is the introduction of foreign material into the tracheobronchial tree. The symptoms and signs of gastroesophageal reflux and aspiration are summarized in Table 17–21. Aspiration of foreign material may not be apparent clinically and occurs occasionally in healthy individuals, however, aspiration of a foreign body or large volumes of foreign material may be life-threatening. Aspiration during swallowing is often a chronic, repetitive process resulting in repeated lung injury, and chronic inflammation, of the airways and parenchyma.

Gastroesophageal reflux with or without aspiration can cause respiratory dysfunction by one of three mechanisms: (1) direct mechanical obstruction, that is, foreign-body or large-volume aspiration; (2) chronic aspiration pneumonitis; and (3) vagally mediated neuroreceptors. The latter line the esophagus and upper aerodigestive tract and

Table 17–22. Complications of Untreated Gastroesophageal Reflux

Common	Uncommon
Recurrent wheezing	Bronchiectasis
Recurrent pneumonia	Interstitial fibrosis
Obstructive lung disease	Restrictive lung disease

can cause reflex bronchospasm when subjected to low pH. Pulmonary complications due to gastroesophageal reflux and aspiration are significant (Table 17–22).

Various disorders leave patients at high risk for aspiration (Table 17–23). An increased incidence of gastroesophageal reflux is seen in obstructive lung diseases, including asthma, BPD, and CF. Hyperinflation of the lungs alters the configuration of the diaphragm and the function of the lower esophageal sphincter. Coughing and autogenic drainage techniques used by patients with chronic lung disease also increase the likelihood of gastroesophageal reflux.

Table 17–24 summarizes the diagnostic tests used to evaluate suspected gastroesophageal reflux and aspiration.

The diagnosis and management of gastroesophageal reflux is described in more detail in Chap. 12, "The Gastrointestinal Tract and Liver."

IMMOTILE CILIA SYNDROME

The immotile cilia syndrome is an inherited genetic disease with abnormalities of the ultrastructure of the respiratory cilia. The disease affects the ciliated epithelium in the paranasal sinuses, middle ear, and airway. Because the ultrastructural defect is also present in spermatozoa, males affected by this disease have abnormal spermatic mobility. Fifty percent of individuals with this disease have *situs inversus*.

The characteristic feature of this disease is discoordinate beating of the respiratory cilia, resulting in reduced

Table 17–21. Symptoms and Signs of Gastroesophageal Reflux and Aspiration

Emesis	Chronic recurrent wheezing
Apnea or bradycardia	Laryngospasm and stridor
Coughing or choking with feedings	Hoarseness
Feeding refusal	Failure to thrive

Table 17–23. Causes of Aspiration

Anatomic	Neuromuscular	Functional
Micrognathia	Immature swallow reflex	Gastro-esophageal reflux
Tracheoesophageal fistula	Seizure disorder	Achalasia
Laryngotracheal cleft	Vocal cord dysfunction or paralysis	
Cleft palate	Myopathies	
Esophageal stricture	Hydrocephalus	
Vascular ring	Dysphagia	

Table 17–24. Diagnostic Tests for Gastroesophageal Reflux and Aspiration

Test	Advantages	Disadvantages
Chest radiograph	Demonstrate lobar infiltrates: evaluates hyperinflation; may show bronchiectasis	Pathophysiology not elucidated
Upper gastrointestinal radiograph	Anatomic configuration of upper gastro-intestinal tract; evaluates patency of esophagus; can demonstrate aspiration	Approximately 50% sensitive for gastro-esophageal reflux; large amount of liquid used
Modified barium swallow	Examines swallow mechanism by fluoroscopy; small amount of liquid/paste used; patient in upright position	Increased radiation exposure; highly dependent on expertise of radiologist
Gastric emptying scan	Rate of gastric emptying evaluated; 75% sensitive for gastroesophageal reflux; delayed lung scan may detect aspiration	Specialized equipment needed; images dependent on prolonged patient immobilization; no anatomic information generated
pH probe	Considered "gold standard" for reflux; prolonged recording period with the patient in various positions: can establish association between clinical symptoms and pH data	Does not demonstrate aspiration; results dependent on scoring of raw data
Flexible endoscopic swallow study	Evaluation of upper airway structures: direct observation of swallow mechanism; direct visualization of laryngeal penetration by various food types; no radiation exposure	Does not evaluate reflux; success dependent on speech pathologist and the availability of an experienced endoscopist
Bronchoscopy with lavage for lipid-laden macrophages	Lipid-laden index sensitive for aspiration; lavage cultures revealing oral flora may be helpful	Invasive; highly dependent on pathologist for accurate assessment of specimen; low specificity

mucociliary clearance. Three well-recognized structural defects are usually inherited in an autosomal-recessive manner: (1) absent dyne in arms, (2) radial spoke defect, and (3) deletion of the central pair with translocation of a peripheral doublet (Fig. 17–5).

The clinical features of immolite cilia syndrome result from abnormal clearance of the mucous blanket from the respiratory tract. Characteristically, children with immotile cilia syndrome have recurrent otitis media and sinusitis with recurrent coughing and wheezing. They may have situs inversus, although this is not a diagnostic criterion. Infertility occurs in men, whereas fertility is usually normal in affected women.

Symptoms often start in infancy and are relatively mild. Most children with the immotile cilia syndrome have productive coughing with recurrent sinusitis and otitis media. Thirty percent have bronchiectasis, 20% have nasal polyps, and 20% have digital clubbing. Sputum cultures are positive for a variety of bacteria, including *H. influenzae, Staph. aureus,* and *Strep. viridans.*

The diagnosis is based on the clinical association of bronchiectasis, situs inversus, sinusitis, otitis media, and male infertility (Kartagener syndrome). The diagnosis is confirmed by electron microscopic examination of cili-ated epithelium obtained from the respiratory tract. This can be obtained in the outpatient setting by brushing the

nasal epithelium with a cytology brush, after administra-tion of a local anesthetic. Optimally, the cilia should be examined at two sites; therefore, a bronchial mucosal biopsy specimen is often obtained as well.

Treatment is symptomatic and involves controlling the recurrent infections with antibiotics, treating airway obstruction with bronchodilators, and improving mucocil-iary clearance with chest physical therapy. Surgical treat-ments are sometimes necessary for sinusitis, middle ear infections, and nasal polyps. In general, the prognosis is good.

OTHER CAUSES OF CHRONIC RESPIRATORY DISEASE

Bronchopulmonary Dysplasia

Bronchopulmonary dysplasia, one of the chronic lung dis-eases of infancy, is a relatively new disease. It has been rec-ognized only in the past 20 to 30 years as a consequence of our improved ability to treat infants of extreme prematu-rity with very low birth weights, as well as nonpremature infants who have had severe respiratory distress.

Most, but not all, infants with BPD have been prema-ture. BPD appears to be the result of the lung's response to initial injury and the lung's ability to repair and recover

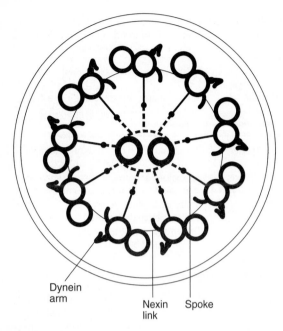

Dynein
arm

Nexin   Spoke
link

Figure 17–5. Diagram of the cross-section of a cilium. (Reproduced with permission from Eliasson R, et al: The immotile cilia syndrome. A congenital ciliary abnormality as an etiologic factor in chronic airway infections and male sterility. *N Engl J Med* 1977;297:1.)

from that injury. The initial insult, in the case of low-birth-weight infants, is pulmonary immaturity and injury resulting from necessary support measures, such as increased fraction of inspired oxygen (FiO_2), barotrauma from mechanical ventilation, resultant inflammation, and infections. Also, BPD is seen in children with chronic respiratory distress from meconium aspiration, congestive heart failure, severe neonatal pneumonia, diaphragmatic hernia with associated pulmonary hypoplasia, and pulmonary hemorrhage. The diagnosis of BPD depends on the clinical, radiographic, and histologic features (when available). More than 75% of cases involve premature infants with a birth weight of <1000 g; in addition, approximately 20% of ventilated newborns are affected with BPD. This represents approximately 3000 to 7000 affected infants in the United States each year. More common in boys than it is in girls, BPD is also more common in white infants than it is in African American infants. The incidence of BPD varies between medical centers, which is probably a reflection of variations in patient demographics, as well as variations in treatment.

The classic definition of BPD is chronic respiratory distress with tachypnea, increased work of breathing, air trapping, persistent oxygen requirement after 28 postnatal days, and consistent chest radiograph findings. The disease has been altered in recent years by changes in the approach to mechanical ventilation and therapeutic modalities. These include use of exogenous surfactant, nutritional support, improved ability to regulate and restrict fluids to the very low birth weight infant, and medical and surgical approaches to patent ductus arteriosus. Normal lung growth and development are disrupted by exposure to adverse environmental stimuli because of prematurity. The immature lung is most susceptible to oxidant- and pressure-related injury. Antioxidant levels are greatly reduced in premature infants as compared with full-term infants. The premature lung also appears to have immature repair mechanisms, the cellular regulation of which may be dysfunctional during the repair phase of lung injury.

PATHOPHYSIOLOGY

Most infants with BPD are premature. Soon after birth, the infant manifests respiratory distress with tachypnea, chest wall retractions, and nasal flaring often associated with cyanosis and grunting. Overall, there is greatly increased work of breathing. These infants require a high FiO_2 (often >60%) and often require ventilatory support. Hyperoxia causes injury to the epithelial and endothelial barriers, which leads to an increase in permeability of the alveolar capillary membrane. There is direct injury to type II pneumocytes, demonstrated by microscopic swelling. The combination of decreased surfactant production with protein leak into the alveolus leads to a decrease in lung compliance and worsening atelectasis. At the end of the first week, there is often a slight improvement, which usually heralds the proliferative or repair phase of BPD. Bronchoalveolar lavage studies of infants with BPD show an increase in the number of inflammatory cells. Various mediators, including leukotrienes, thromboxane, platelet-activating factor, and cytokines (e.g., interleukin-1), have been found in bronchoalveolar lavage samples, which supports the notion that inflammation of the airway causes the disease. With the institution of positive-pressure ventilation, damage to the lungs occurs by barotrauma. Compliance of the tracheobronchial tree is greater than that of the alveolar unit, leading to overdistention of the airways, distal gas trapping, and regional hyperinflation. Classic chest radiograph findings show areas of atelectasis mixed with areas of hyperinflation.

Features of BPD are summarized in Table 17–25. One functional abnormality is increased airway resistance. Older children with BPD show increased airway hyperreactivity to methacholine or cold-air challenge. Children with BPD have periods of clinical improvement and deterioration, usually with chronic hypercapnia and persistent oxygen requirements. Any cardiovascular lesion that leads to increased left-to-right shunting must be identified. Such lesions include patent ductus arteriosus, ventricular septal defects, and atrial septal defects. Other sources of

Table 17–25. Pathophysiologic Abnormalities in Bronchopulmonary Dysplasia

Pulmonary	Cardiovascular
Increased airway resistance	Pulmonary hypertension
Increased mucous production	Systemic hypertension
Increased airway hyperreactivity	Ventricular hypertrophy
Decreased compliance	Right heart failure
Decreased mucociliary clearance	Gastrointestinal
Pulmonary edema	Gastroesophageal reflux
Increased incidence of tracheobronchomalacia	Oral-motor hypersensitivity

lung injury need to be minimized, especially aspiration syndromes and gastroesophageal reflux.

Long-term abnormalities in BPD include pulmonary hypertension, right ventricular hypertrophy, and left ventricular hypertrophy, even in the absence of pulmonary or systemic hypertension. Large systemic-to-pulmonary collateral arteries, which increase pulmonary blood flow, are common findings at autopsy. Long-term airway intubation can lead to subglottic stenosis, inability to establish oral feedings, and increased incidence of pneumonia. Gastroesophageal reflux and electrolyte abnormalities secondary to diuretic therapy are common complications.

CLINICAL MANAGEMENT

The goals of clinical management are to treat hypoxemia, optimize ventilation with subsequent reduction in hypercarbia, minimize inflammation of the airways, and optimize somatic growth. Oxygen therapy is prescribed to keep arterial blood oxygen saturations between 92 and 95% while the infant is awake, asleep, and feeding. This has been shown to decrease the pulmonary vascular resistance and to optimize the growth of the child.

Chronic drug therapy for patients with BPD is aimed at bronchodilation, control of inflammation, and minimization of fluid retention. Bronchodilators used include the β_2-adrenergic agonists and the anticholinergic bronchodilator, ipratropium bromide. These improve lung compliance and airway resistance.

Steroidal and nonsteroidal anti-inflammatory agents are often used for more severe cases of BPD. Systemic steroids are the mainstays of treatment on both an acute and a chronic basis. The clinician has to measure carefully the risk and benefit of steroid use. Inhaled steroids have few systemic toxicities and could be a useful treatment however, there are few data on their efficacy in BPD.

Diuretic therapy is extremely effective in BPD. In the acute phase, loop diuretics are often prescribed to mini-

mize fluid retention. This may lead to hypokalemia and hyponatremia, and a hypochloremic metabolic alkalosis. Hypercalcuria can lead to nephrocalcinosis and decreased bone density.

The caloric requirements of infants with BPD are increased compared to the needs of children without chronic lung disease. The etiology of the increased caloric requirement is not fully understood; however, increased work of breathing accounts for some of this increase. Meeting the caloric requirement of children with BPD and optimizing weight gain and growth are essential to the long-term prognosis. Oral-motor dysfunction from delayed introduction of oral feedings often necessitates long-term placement of feeding tubes. The ability of infants to feed orally should be promoted by a team approach that involves speech pathology and occupational therapy.

PROGNOSIS

School-aged children with a history of BPD still have evidence of airflow obstruction and air trapping on pulmonary function tests. They also have a high incidence of airway hyperreactivity on methacholine challenge. Infants with chronic lung disease of infancy have an increased incidence of viral respiratory infections, as well as recurrent pneumonia in the first 2 years. Their pulmonary reserve is less, and their clinical deterioration with infections is usually more acute. The ability to promote the growth of infants with optimal nutrition provides the best long-term outcome for these children.

Restrictive Lung Disease

Diseases of the chest wall can cause an excessively stiff or small thoracic cage (reduced compliance) or one that is unstable and unable to generate sufficient inspiratory force (increased compliance or decreased respiratory muscle strength). The abnormalities that can cause restrictive or hypodynamic defects by affecting the chest wall include neuromuscular diseases, spinal deformities, chest wall deformities, trauma, obesity, and diaphragmatic deformities.

Neuromuscular diseases weaken the muscles of respiration and include muscular dystrophy, Guillain-Barré syndrome, poliomyelitis, and spinal cord injury. The earliest manifestations are easy development of respiratory fatigue. With increasing weakness, patients develop hypoventilation that tends to be particularly severe during sleep. This in turn leads to increased pulmonary vascular resistance, pulmonary hypertension, right ventricular hypertrophy, and the development of cor pulmonale. Many diseases characterized by respiratory muscle weakness are associated with kyphoscoliosis, which may compromise the respiratory muscle weakness even further. Sometimes there is difficulty in swallowing secretions, which may predispose to aspiration pneumonia. The major symptoms of respiratory muscle weakness are dyspnea, tachypnea, and, in severe cases with carbon dioxide retention, headaches. Patients feel anxious and may complain of being unable to sleep lying down. Physical signs include tachypnea, reduced thoracic excursions, paradoxical respiration, weight loss, and easy fatigue.

Assessment of respiratory muscle weakness includes pulmonary function tests, maximal inspiratory and expiratory pressures, maximal voluntary ventilation, and measurement of arterial blood gases. General supportive therapy includes physical therapy, optimal nutrition, and a pulmonary rehabilitation program based on exercise.

If respiratory failure, either acute or chronic, develops, ventilatory support should be considered. Whether this is appropriate will depend on the underlying condition and prognosis; consideration of the patient's and family's wishes and feelings is key. Acute deterioration can be precipitated by infection, general anesthesia, or a sudden deterioration in the underlying condition. If the precipitating cause is reversible, intubation and mechanical ventilation should be considered. Long-term ventilation will require a tracheotomy. We have had some success with negative pressure ventilation using either a cuirass or a poncho-style "raincoat" ventilator for this problem. Nasal mask ventilation or face-mask ventilation may be sufficient to support children in the early stages of respiratory failure from neuromuscular diseases. Details concerning the pathophysiology, diagnosis, and treatment of the neuromuscular diseases that cause respiratory failure are described in Chap. 20, "The Nervous System." A list of neuromuscular diseases that cause respiratory failure is presented in Table 17–26.

Severe abnormalities of the chest wall, such as depression of the sternum (pectus excavatum), can cause restrictive lung disease. Most cases of pectus excavatum do not lead to significant physiologic limitation of either respiratory or cardiac function. The most severe forms may become more pronounced with increasing age and lead to restrictive pulmonary disease. This defect is sometimes associated with mitral valve prolapse, Wolff-Parkinson-White conduction defects, or Marfan syndrome. The severe forms of pectus excavatum are unattractive, and surgical correction for cosmetic appearance is often appropriate. Surgical correction does not usually improve pulmonary function.

KYPHOSCOLIOSIS

Abnormal curvature of the spine due to kyphoscoliosis may be idiopathic. It can also be a secondary abnormality from myelomeningocele, neurofibromatosis, congenital vertebral anomalies, or neuromuscular diseases. Severe kyphoscoliosis causes a restrictive defect on pulmonary function testing. The results of pulmonary function tests are usually normal unless the scoliosis exceeds $60°$, and respiratory symptoms usually do not develop unless the angle exceeds $90°$. Severe kyphoscoliosis is associated with recurrent airway infections, atelectasis, and respiratory failure.

Treatment consists of prevention of the progression of the angle by bracing, spinal fusion, or insertion of paravertebral rods. Severe case of kyphospholiosis may require mechanical ventilation for respiratory support.

INTERSTITIAL DISEASES

Interstitial pulmonary diseases are characterized by restrictive defects on pulmonary function testing and a reticulonodular pattern of shadowing on the chest radiograph. The underlying pathologic feature of these diseases is inflammation of the alveolar septal tissue with fibrosis and an increased number of inflammatory cells, both in the septae and in the alveoli. Interstitial lung disease in children has a large number of known causes (Table 17–27).

Characteristically, children with interstitial lung disease have progressive dyspnea associated with coughing, tachypnea, poor weight gain, and exercise intolerance. Examination reveals digital clubbing and fine end-inspiratory crackles; wheezing may be present if airways disease is a feature. When pulmonary hypertension develops, there is an accentuated pulmonary second sound. Interstitial diseases are often progressive, depending on the underlying etiology.

Table 17–26. Neuromuscular Diseases that Cause Respiratory Failure Classified by Speed of Onset

Rapid	Moderately Fast	Slow
Spinal cord injury (C3–5)	Werdnig-Hoffman disease	Juvenile spinal muscular atrophy
Poliomyelitis	Pompe disease	Duchenne muscular dystrophy
Guillain-Barré syndrome	Myasthenia gravis	Becker muscular dystrophy
Drug toxicities	Congenital myotonic dystrophy	Congenital muscular dystrophy
Tick paralysis	Congenital muscular dystrophy	Chronic inflammatory demyelinating polyneuropathy
Botulism	Nemaline myopathy	(chronic Guillain-Barré syndrome)
Myasthenia gravis crisis	Fukuyama disease	Mitochondrial myopathy
Acute polymyositis		
Dermatomyositis		

Table 17–27. Causes of Interstitial Lung Disease in Children

Infectious or postinfectious	Environmental inhalants, toxic substances, foreign materials, or
Viral	antigenic dusts
Cytomegalic virus	Inorganic dusts
HIV	Silica
Respiratory syncytial virus	Asbestos
Adenovirus	Talcum powder
Influenza virus	Zinc stearate
Parainfluenza viruses	Organic dusts
Mycoplasma	Hypersensitivity pneumonitis
Measles	Bird-fancier's lung
Mycobacterial	Farmer's lung
Fungal	Fumes
Pneumocystis carinii[1]	Sulfuric acid
Aspergillus species	Hydrochloric acid
Bacterial	Gases
Mycobacteria	Chlorine
Legionella pneumophila	Ammonia
Bordetella pertussis	Nitrogen dioxide
Drug-induced disorders	Lymphoproliferative disorders
Antineoplastic drugs	Familial erythrophagocytic lymphohistiocytosis
Cyclophosphamide	Angioimmunoblastic lymphadenopathy
Nitroscureas (carmustine, lomustine)	Lymphoid interstitial pneumonitis
Azathioprine	Pseudolymphomas of the lung
Cytosine arabinoside	
6-Mercaptopurine	Metabolic
Vinblastine	Storage disorders
Bleomycin	Hermansky-Pudlak syndrome
Methotrexate	Pulmonary lipidosis
Miscellaneous drugs	Gaucher disease
Nitrofurantoin	Niemann-Pick disease
Penicillamine	Disorders of ion transport
Gold salts	Cystic fibrosis
Neoplastic diseases	Other
Leukemia	Cardiac failure
Hodgkin disease	Renal disease
Non-Hodgkin lymphoma	
Histiocytosis X	Degenerative disorders
Letterer-Siwe disease	Idiopathic pulmonary alveolar microlithiasis
Hand-Schüller-Christian disease	
Eosinophilic granuloma	Idiopathic
	Idiopathic pulmonary fibrosis
Neurocutaneous syndromes with interstitial lung disease	
Tuberous sclerosis	
Neurofibromatosis	
Ataxia-telangiectasia	

[1] *P. carinii*, previously considered a protozoan, is now classified as a fungus.

Adapted with permission from Hilman BC: Interstitial lung disease in children. Page 362 in: Hilman BC (editor): *Pediatric Respiratory Disease: Diagnosis and Treatment.* Saunders, 1993.

The diagnosis of interstitial lung disease is initially suspected from the chest radiograph and confirmed by chest CT scan. A high-resolution CT scan is most informative; it is more sensitive than regular CT scans for detecting the early stages of interstitial diseases. However, high-resolution CT has limitations in young children because of the motion artifact introduced by rapid respiratory movements. Sedation or general anesthesia may be necessary to obtain good images.

Pulmonary function tests show a restrictive pulmonary defect with a reduced carbon monoxide diffusion rate. Hypoxemia is characteristically present, especially with exercise. Lung biopsy is often necessary to confirm the general diagnosis of interstitial lung disease and to make a specific diagnosis.

Therapy of the idiopathic interstitial lung diseases is directed toward reducing the inflammatory processes in the pulmonary interstitium to prevent the progression to fibrosis. Immunosuppressive therapy may include corticosteroids and cytotoxic or immunosuppressive drugs, such as azathioprine, cyclophosphamide, and methotrexate. Supportive therapy includes supplemental oxygen and nutritional support. Patients in whom supportive therapy has failed and who are progressing to end-stage disease should be considered for lung transplantation.

Congenital Lobar Emphysema

Congenital lobar emphysema is the congenital overinflation of a pulmonary lobe; this most commonly affects the upper lobes, particularly the left upper lobe. Overinflation is usually caused by a ball-valve anomaly affecting the airway, so that the lobe inflates but does not deflate. The most commonly identified airway anomaly is segmental bronchomalacia, although folds of bronchial mucosa or polyps can produce similar lesions. In 50% of cases, no precise cause is found.

This is a relatively uncommon pulmonary malformation. It occurs more often in boys than girls, and 14 to 20% of cases are associated with congenital heart disease. The most common cardiac lesions are patent ductus arteriosus and ventricular septal defects. Some cases are associated with renal malformations or rib cage anomalies. One third of cases of congenital lobar emphysema present at birth, and half have presented by 4 weeks of age. The presentation is usually with moderate respiratory distress that worsens as the lobe inflates. Some cases are asymptomatic.

Physical examination shows hyperinflation of the affected hemithorax with reduced breath sounds over the affected lobe. The chest radiograph shows a large, hyperlucent lobe with indistinct markings. There is mediastinal shift away from the affected lobe and atelectasis of the normal ipsilateral lung. The diagnosis can be confirmed by CT scan. Treatment usually involves lobectomy. In some patients, however, who are asymptomatic or have mild symptoms, treatment may involve only observation.

Pulmonary Agenesis, Aplasia, and Hypoplasia

Pulmonary agenesis, aplasia, and hypoplasia represent a spectrum of lung malformations characterized by underdevelopment of the lung. In pulmonary agenesis, there is no development of the bronchial tree, pulmonary tissue, or pulmonary vasculature; in pulmonary aplasia, there is a rudimentary bronchial pouch. In pulmonary hypoplasia, which is the most common of these anomalies there is a decrease in the number and size of the airways, alveoli, and pulmonary vessels. These malformations are commonly associated with other congenital malformations. Pulmonary hypoplasia can occur as a complication of diaphragmatic hernia, oligohydramnios, or pleural effusion in utero.

Patients may remain asymptomatic or present with respiratory distress, according to the severity of hypoplasia. Common symptoms are tachypnea and cyanosis, and arterial blood gases may show hypoxia, hypercarbia, and acidosis.

The radiologic findings are small, underdeveloped lungs, unilaterally or bilaterally. The diaphragms may be elevated. In pulmonary agenesis or aplasia, there is a homogeneous density on the affected side with absence of a normally aerated lung. Often, there is herniation of normal lung from the other side that is best visualized on a lateral film, where it appears in the anterior mediastinum.

Chest CT scan will confirm the herniation of normal lung from the opposite side and will show the absence of pulmonary parenchyma and tracheobronchial tree. Bronchoscopy reveals the absence of the mainstem bronchus in the case of agenesis, or of one or more mainstem bronchi in the case of hypoplasia or aplasia. Angiography can be used to investigate the pulmonary blood supply to the affected side.

The treatment of pulmonary agenesis or hypoplasia is supportive. These patients appear to be at increased risk of infection, and broad-spectrum antibiotics should be used when they have respiratory infections. Chest physical therapy may help maintain clearance of respiratory secretions, and supplemental oxygen is necessary if patients have hypoxemia.

The prognosis of these abnormalities depends on the severity of the lesion and the associated anomalies.

ABNORMALITIES IN RESPIRATORY CONTROL

Central Hypoventilation Syndrome

Central hypoventilation syndrome (CHS) may be present at birth or soon afterward and results in severe hypoventilation or apnea. This disease is associated with a congenital defect in respiratory drive. In some cases, there is a history of injury to the central nervous system, and in others there is a genetic component. CHS is rare. There is no abnormality of the heart, lungs, or chest wall that would account for hypoventilation. Ventilation is often normal while awake but depressed when asleep; it can be abnormal even when awake during periods of infection or with exercise. Less severe forms of CHS are associated with a partial pressure of carbon dioxide (P_{CO_2}) of 45 to 50 mm Hg when awake, but with hypoventilation during sleep, the partial pressure of arterial carbon dioxide (Pa_{CO_2}) may increase to 80 to 90 mm Hg.

The cause of CHS is not well defined. There appears to be a defect of the central chemoreceptors located in the medulla of the brain, so there is apnea during nonrapid eye movement sleep when these chemoreceptors have an important role in maintaining respiratory drive. The diagnosis of CHS is often made clinically in infants who retains carbon dioxide and requires mechanical ventilation in the absence of cardiac, pulmonary, or neuromuscular disease. Tests of ventilatory responses to hypoxia and hypercapnia demonstrate a blunted response. Other evaluations include polysomnographic sleep studies and a CT or MRI scan of the brain.

Treatment in the first year of life relies on positive-pressure ventilation. This can be achieved with nasal or face-mask ventilation, but most infants require a tracheotomy and nighttime mechanical ventilation. After 1 year of age, children with CHS can be managed with phrenic nerve pacing in combination with nighttime mechanical ventilation. This allows for increased mobility and normal activities during the day. For pacing, bilateral phrenic nerve electrodes must be implanted. A tracheotomy is maintained because children with CHS often have difficulty maintaining a patent upper airway when asleep. Around-the-clock pacing is not recommended because of the risk of producing fibrosis of the phrenic nerves. Respiratory stimulants, such as theophylline and doxapram, are usually ineffective.

Other Causes of Abnormal Respiratory Control

Apnea of prematurity is described in Chap. 4, "The Perinatal Period." The pathophysiology of sudden infant death syndrome (SIDS) and acute life-threatening event (ALTE) are unknown. These syndromes are further discussed in Chap. 10, "Injuries and Emergencies."

REFERENCES

Davis PB, Drumm M, Konstan MW: Cystic fibrosis. Am J Respir Crit Care Med 1996;154:1229.

Farrell PA, Fiascone JM: Bronchopulmonary dysplasia in the 1990s: a review for the pediatrician. Curr Probl Pediatr 1997;27:129.

Gibson LE, Cooke RE: A test for concentration of electrolytes in sweat in cystic fibrosis of the pancreas utilizing pilocarpine by iontophoresis. Pediatrics 1959;23:545.

Hardie W, et al: Pneumococcal pleural empyemas in children. Clin Inf Dis 1996;22:1057.

Hulka GF, et al: Evaluation of the airway. Page 25 in: Meyer CM, III, et al (editors): *The Pediatric Airway: An Interdisciplinary Approach.* Lippincott, 1995.

National Asthma Education Program: *Guidelines for the Diagnosis and Management of Asthma. Expert Panel Report 2.* US Department of Health and Human Services, Public Health Service, Bethesda, MD, National Institutes of Health, 1997.

Orenstein SR: Gastroesophageal reflux. Pediatr Rev 1999;20:24.

Ramsey BW: Management of pulmonary disease in patients with cystic fibrosis. N Engl J Med 1996;335:179.

Richardson MA, Cotton RT: Anatomic abnormalities of the pediatric airway. Pediatr Clin North Am 1984;31:821.

Sahn SA: The pleura. Am Rev Respir Dis 1988;138:184.

Schidlow DV: Cough in children. J Asthma 1996;33:81.

Allergy: Mechanisms & Disease Processes

Richard S. Shames, MD

Allergy defines a disease or reaction caused by an immune response (usually IgE-mediated) to one or more environmental antigens, resulting in tissue inflammation and organ dysfunction. The terms *allergy* and *atopy* are often used interchangeably, although atopy more specifically refers to the inherited tendency to have a persistent IgE response to common, naturally occurring inhalant and ingested agents, known as *allergens*. Allergens possess *immunogenicity*—the ability to stimulate the production of antibody responses—and *reactivity*—the ability to react with preformed antibody. Common allergic conditions including allergic rhinitis, atopic dermatitis, and asthma, seen as isolated conditions or in combination, are frequently observed in pediatric practice. Other common allergic conditions include urticaria, angioedema and anaphylaxis, food hypersensitivity, and drug allergy. Asthma and atopic dermatitis are discussed in detail in Chaps. 17 and 11, respectively.

SIGNIFICANCE OF ALLERGIC DISEASE

Allergic disease affects 12 to 20% of the population worldwide. It is estimated that 40 million Americans have asthma or other allergic diseases. Allergic rhinitis, the most common allergic condition, has a prevalence of 10 to 12%, with a peak incidence in childhood and adolescence. Asthma affects 5 to 10% of children, and allergy is the predominant etiology in 80 to 90% of pediatric patients with asthma. The prevalence of atopic disease appears to be increasing over the past two decades, especially in industrialized countries. Complications of allergic rhinitis include sinus disease, eustachian tube dysfunction, worsening asthma, and impaired quality of life causing morbidity into the adult years. Allergic disease accounts for significant use of medical services; 9% of patient visits to a physician's office involve allergic diseases.

HYPERSENSITIVITY IMMUNE RESPONSES

Gel and Coombs devised a classification scheme to divide the mechanisms of immune responses to antigen into four distinct types of reactions to allow for clearer understanding of the immunopathogenesis of the disease (Figure 18–1). Allergy is classically defined by type I hypersensitivity, although types II, III, and IV hypersensitivity may also underlie some hypersensitivity reactions.

Type I

Anaphylactic or immediate hypersensitivity reactions occur after the binding of antigen to preformed IgE antibodies attached to the surface of the mast cell or basophil. These reactions result in the release of inflammatory mediators (see later, "Pathophysiology of the Type I Allergic Response") that produce the clinical symptoms of type I allergy that may include urticaria, angioedema, rhinitis, bronchospasm, and cardiovascular collapse. Type I IgE-mediated reactions include anaphylaxis, allergic rhinitis, allergic asthma, and IgE-mediated drug, food, and latex allergy.

Type II

Cytotoxic reactions involve the binding of either IgG or IgM antibody to antigens that are covalently bound to cell-membrane structures. Antigen-antibody binding activates the complement cascade and results in the destruction of the cell to which the antigen is bound. Examples of tissue injury by this mechanism include immune hemolytic anemia, Rh hemolytic disease in the newborn, and some types of drug allergy.

Type III

Immune-complex-mediated reactions occur when immune complexes are formed by the binding of antigens to antibodies. Complexes usually are cleared from the circulation by the phagocytic system. However, deposition of these complexes in tissues or in vascular endothelium can produce immune-complex-mediated tissue injury by leading to complement activation, anaphylatoxin generation, chemotaxis of polymorphonuclear leukocytes, phagocytosis, and tissue injury. Serum sickness, nephritis, and bacterial endocarditis are clinical examples of type-III-mediated diseases.

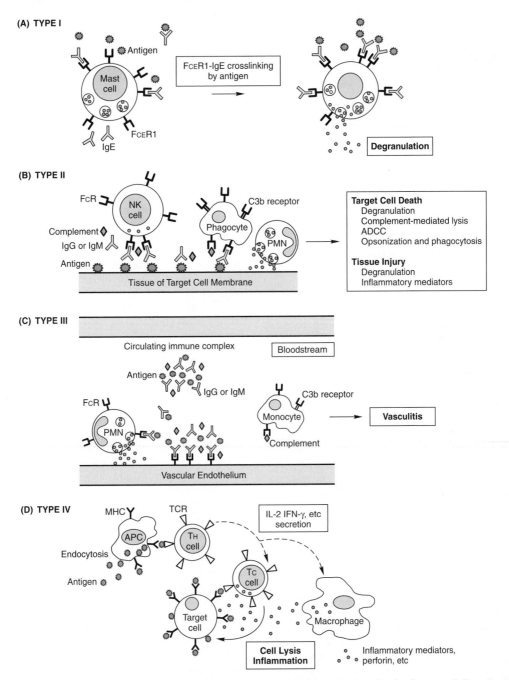

Figure 18–1. Gel and Coombs hypersensitivity immune responses I–IV are depicted in the diagram. **A:** Type I reaction. Mast cells and basophils bind IgE via high-affinity Fc receptors (Fcγ-RI). Antigen binding and cross-linking of Fcγ-RI IgE complexes induce cellular degranulation and release of inflammatory mediators. **B:** Type II reaction. IgG or IgM antibodies against tissue or cellular antigens induce complement activation, which result in cell death and tissue injury. **C:** Type III reaction. Circulating immune complexes composed of soluble antigen and IgG or IgM deposit on vascular endothelium of target organ tissues, activating the complement cascade and attracting inflammatory cells that induce local tissue injury and vasculitis. **D:** Type IV reaction. T-helper (TH) cell recognition of target cell antigen complexed to self MHC on antigen-presenting cells (APC) stimulates secretion of interleukin (IL) 2, interferon IFN-γ, and other lymphokines required for activation of tissue macrophages and cytotoxic T (Tc) cells. (Reproduced with permission from Shames RS: Hypersensitivity immune responses. In: Gluckman PD, Heyman MA (editors): *Pediatrics and Perinatology: The Scientific Basis,* 2nd ed, 1996.)

Type IV

Delayed hypersensitivity reactions are not mediated by antibodies, but rather are mediated primarily by T lymphocytes (cell-mediated immunity). Classic examples are the tuberculin skin test reactions and contact dermatitis.

ETIOLOGIC FACTORS

The development of allergy results from the interaction of genetic and environmental factors. Individuals who are genetically predisposed to the development of specific IgE responsiveness can develop clinical allergy with repeated exposure to the offending allergen.

GENETICS OF IMMUNE RESPONSE

The most important predisposing factor in the development of allergies is a family history of atopy, although no single specific genetic lesion has been identified as the etiologic factor. Family and twin studies indicate that total serum IgE concentration has a heritability of >50%. Additional genetic factors can modify the expression of allergic disease by influencing the regulation of IgE biosynthesis, control of specific immune responses, control of the release of endogenous mediators of inflammation, and regulation of overall immune responsiveness. Sibling pair studies suggest that at least 5 markers on chromosome 5q31.1 are linked with a gene modulating total serum IgE concentration. Evidence has been found for the linkage of 5q31.1 and the interleukin-4 (*IL-4*) gene (see later), suggesting that *IL-4* or a nearby gene in this chromosome locale regulates overall IgE production. Genetic polymorphism of the β_2-agonist receptor, IL-4 receptor, and enzymes of the leukotriene biosynthesis pathways that have been identified in patients may also influence susceptibility to allergic disease.

AGE, SEX, AND RACE

The onset of allergic disease peaks in childhood, although it may develop at any age. Most patients with a positive atopic family history develop signs of allergic disease before 10 years of age, suggesting a possible critical exposure period. Atopic dermatitis and food allergies usually begin in infancy or early childhood. Allergic rhinitis and asthma usually begin after infancy. In babies, gastrointestinal symptoms (colic) may herald the onset of allergy.

Before the age of 10 years, allergy occurs twice as often in males, whereas females appear to catch up during the teens and twenties. There are no specific racial patterns of allergic expression.

ENVIRONMENTAL FACTORS

Repeated exposure to environmental allergens is necessary to trigger the onset of clinical symptoms of allergy.

Exposure to nonallergic irritants such as viral agents, passive cigarette smoke, and indoor and outdoor airborne pollutants can influence the development and severity of allergic disease in susceptible children.

Allergens

Allergens are protein, glycoprotein, and/or carbohydrate materials of animal or vegetable origin of molecular weight 5000 to 60,000 Da. Inhalation of airborne substances, including house dust mites, animal danders, fungal spores, and plant pollens, can directly impact respiratory mucosa to trigger respiratory allergy in predisposed individuals. Exposure to stinging insect (Hymenoptera) venom, drugs, and food allergens can elicit respiratory, skin, gastrointestinal, and/or multisystem (anaphylactic) reactions. Latex is an increasingly important allergen that can cause type I (anaphylactic) and type IV (contact dermatitis) reactions in high-risk children with spina bifida and urogenital anomalies, cross-reacting food allergies, and in health care workers.

Improved immunochemical methods have led to the isolation and structural characterization of highly purified allergens. The specific properties that account for the allergenicity of these molecules are not known. Acarine mites (*Dermatophagoides* species) constitute the primary allergen in house dust. Its major antigenic determinant (Der p 1) is found in the proteinaceous membranes of mite fecal particles. The mite allergens become readily airborne and settle primarily on mattress surfaces, fabric-upholstered furniture, and floor carpeting. New radioimmunoassay techniques allow measurement of mite allergen content in house dust samples. The most important cat allergen (Fel d 1) is found in cat saliva and dander. Dog allergens are found among hair, dander, pelt, saliva, and serum proteins. Among pollen allergens, tree, weed, and grass species are important sources of seasonal respiratory allergy.

There appear to be at least 20 recognized latex allergens found in many common dipped or molded latex products, such as surgical gloves, balloons, catheters, and rubber toys. Latex proteins may induce hypersensitivity by mucocutaneous, intracutaneous, or aerosolized exposure.

Infection

Viral infection in particular may influence the development and exacerbation of allergy. Viral agents can damage epithelial cells and elicit inflammation, thus exposing nerve endings that control airway reactivity to increased stimulation and antigen absorption. Viral stimulation can also upregulate the expression of endothelial cell adhesion proteins (ICAM-1), which can trigger local inflammation and tissue damage. Respiratory syncytial virus (RSV), which can induce the development of viral-specific IgE, is a known risk factor for the development of asthma.

Air Pollutants

Exposure to indoor and outdoor air pollutants may aggravate existing disease in allergic patients. Some experts have attributed the increased incidence of allergic disease in urban populations to the increased exposure to airborne indoor pollutants (e.g., dust mites, household gases, and cockroaches). Passive exposure to cigarette smoke is considered a risk factor for the development of otitis media and upper and lower respiratory allergic disease. Tobacco polyphenols induce IgE responsiveness in animals, a finding that may underscore the in utero effects of smoke exposure in humans. Outdoor pollutants such as sulfur dioxide, emitted from the combustion of sulfur-containing fuels, can alter bronchial mucociliary clearance and impair pulmonary function in adolescents with asthma. Diesel exhaust particulate may trigger IgE responsiveness in susceptible patients.

MECHANISMS OF ALLERGY

Antibody Structure and Function

Immunoglobulins (antibodies) are proteins that combine specifically with antigens to mediate the humoral (antibody-mediated) immune response. Circulating immunoglobulins have unique specificity for one particular antigenic structure, as well as the diversity to encounter a broad range of antigenic materials. This diversity arises from complex DNA rearrangements and RNA processing within antibody-producing B cells. All immunoglobulin molecules share a four-chain polypeptide structure consisting of two heavy and two light chains. Each chain includes an amino-terminal portion containing the variable (V) region and a carboxy-terminal portion containing four or five constant (C) regions. V regions are highly variable structures that form the antigen-binding site, whereas the C domains are relatively invariant and mediate effector functions of the molecules. The five classes, or *isotypes*, of immunoglobulins are *IgG, IgA, IgM, IgD,* and *IgE* and are defined on the basis of differences in the C region of the heavy chains. Immunoglobulins serve a variety of secondary biologic roles, including complement fixation, transplacental passage, and facilitation of phagocytosis, all of which participate in host defense against disease.

The IgE molecule is a monomeric structure with a molecular weight of 190,000. IgE constitutes only 0.004% of the total serum immunoglobulins but binds with high affinity to mast cells and basophils via a site in the Fc region. IgE mediates the release of vasoactive, enzymatic, and chemotactic chemical mediators from activated mast cells and basophils that induce allergic inflammation (type I hypersensitivity, see Table 18–1). IgE participates in host defense against parasites.

Table 18–1. Mast Cell Mediators and Cytokines

Preformed secretory granule mediators
   Histamine
   Proteoglycans
   Serine proteases
   Carboxypeptidase A

Newly generated lipid-derived mediators
   Leukotriene B_4
   Leukotrienes C_4, D_4, and E_4 (SRS-A)
   Prostaglandin D_2
   Platelet-activating factor

Mast-cell-derived cytokines
   Mitogenic cytokines and/or growth factors
   Proinflammatory cytokines
   Immunomodulatory cytokines

IgE Synthesis and Regulation

The inappropriate and sustained production of IgE in response to environmental allergen defines type I allergic hypersensitivity. The synthesis of IgE by mature B cells is under the control of the cytokines interleukin (IL)-4 and IL-13 (Figure 18–2). IL-4 is the crucial factor for isotype-switching to IgE and is sufficient to initiate germ-line transcription of IgE. IL-13 has about 30% structural homology to IL-4 and shares many of the same activities on mononuclear cells and B lymphocytes. Compared with IL-13, IL-4 tends to be an earlier and more transient signal. Additional B-cell activation factors triggered through the binding of T-cell surface CD40 ligand to B-cell-membrane CD40 receptor are required for the expression of mature messenger RNA (mRNA) and subsequent IgE synthesis. In humans, a variety of secondary signals synergize with IL-4 to modulate IgE expression. IL-5 and IL-6 may upregulate the synthesis of IgE, whereas IFN-γ is inhibitory. Therefore, an imbalance favoring IL-4 over IFN-γ may induce IgE formation. Reduced IFN-γ at birth has been associated with clinical atopy at 12 months of age. A defect in IFN-γ secretion may be due to a posttranscriptional defect in secretion.

Role of T Cells in the Allergic Response

T cells play a central role in the induction of allergic inflammatory responses, both as a source of IL-4 and in delivery of secondary signals after interaction with B cells (Figure 18–3). Antigens, processed by antigen-presenting cells such as macrophages or by B cells directly, elicit the activation of CD4+ T-helper (TH) lymphocytes. The activated T-helper cells elaborate cytokines that direct B cells to synthesize IgE and that recruit and activate

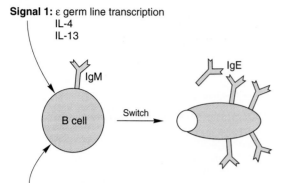

Signal 1: ε germ line transcription
         IL-4
         IL-13

Signal 2: B-cell activation and switch recombination
         CD40 engagement
         EBV infection
         Hormones (glucocorticoid)

Figure 18–2. Induction of IgE synthesis by B cells requires two signals. Interleukin (IL)-4 and IL-13 are the primary signals that influence isotype switching to IgE at the transcriptional level. Secondary signals that include the binding of CD40 ligand to its receptor trigger the activation of B cells required for mature expression of IgE. EBV infection and glucocorticoids may also act as secondary signals. IL-4–dependent IgE synthesis is inhibited by interferon-γ (IFN-γ) and stimulated by IL-5 and IL-6. (Modified with permission from Vercelli D, Geha RS: Control of immunoglobulin E synthesis. In: Middleton E, et al (editors): *Allergy: Principles and Practice,* 5th ed. Mosby-Year Book, Inc., 1998.)

inflammatory cells, such as eosinophils, neutrophils, and macrophages. Two primary TH-cell phenotypes are recognized based on their pattern of cytokine release (Figure 18–4). TH$_1$ cells elaborate IFN-γ and tumor necrosis factor β (TNF-β) but not IL-4 and IL-5 and have been found to participate in delayed hypersensitivity reactions (type IV). TH$_2$ cells secrete IL-4, IL-5, and IL-9 but not IFN-γ and TNF-β and have been implicated in allergic inflammatory responses. An imbalance of TH$_1$ and TH$_2$ cells favoring the development and proliferation of TH$_2$ cells appears to influence the development of allergic disease. IL-4 is crucial to isotype switch to IgE. IL-5 promotes maturation, activation, and chemotaxis of eosinophils, and IL-9 is a mast-cell and T-cell growth factor. Activated TH$_2$ cells and their characteristic cytokines have been demonstrated at sites of allergic inflammation in both skin and airway disease. The finding of allergen-specific T-cell lines that proliferate and secrete large amounts of IL-4 when exposed to relevant antigen in vitro further supports the existence of specific TH$_2$-like clones. What drives undifferentiated CD4 T- (e.g., TH$_0$) lymphocytes to become either TH$_1$ or TH$_2$ cells is not known, although the specific cytokine milieu

in which the TH-cell differentiation occurs appears to be important in determining the direction of differentiation. The presence of IL-4 appears to drive the differentiation of TH$_2$ cells, whereas the cytokine IL-12 appears to stimulate the differentiation of TH$_1$ cells.

Pathophysiology of the Type I Allergic Response

Type I immediate hypersensivity results from the activation of previously sensitized tissue mast cells and circulating basophils. *Sensitization* describes the binding of IgE to mast cells that results from early antigen exposure and synthesis of IgE by B cells. Repeated exposure to the offending allergen induces the expression of clinical allergy.

ALLERGIC SENSITIZATION

Allergen-specific IgE binds to high-affinity (Fcγ-RI) receptors on tissue mast cells and circulating basophils, as well as to low-affinity (Fcγ-RII) receptors on macrophages, eosinophils, and platelets, thus sensitizing these cells for future allergen encounters. Sensitization can be confirmed by in vivo immediate hypersensitivity skin test reactivity or by an in vitro radioallergosorbent test (RAST), even if clinical expression of disease is not apparent.

ALLERGEN STIMULATION OF MEDIATOR RELEASE

Upon reexposure to allergen, the sensitized individual can mount an accelerated hypersensitivity response. Mast cells, armed with antigen-specific IgE on their surfaces, can bind and cross-link allergen. Bridging of cell-bound IgE requires that two IgE molecules be linked by multivalent antigen. Binding and cross-linking of specific antigen induces a physical approximation of surface IgE receptors, triggering a sequence of biochemical events within the cell that results in the degranulation of mast cells and basophils.

MEDIATORS OF INFLAMMATION

Activation of mast cells and basophils triggers both release of preformed mediators (histamine, chemotactic factors, and enzymes) and synthesis and release of newly generated membrane-derived mediators [prostaglandins (PG)], leukotrienes, and platelet-activating factor (see Table 18–1). Histamine and the newly generated mediators bind to surface receptors on blood vessels, smooth muscle, and mucous glands, inducing vascular leakiness, smooth muscle constriction, and mucous secretion. Preformed chemotactic mediators, leukotrienes, and platelet-activating factor elicit the accumulation of inflammatory cells, including eosinophils, neutrophils, and mononuclear cells. Enzymes, including neutral proteases and acid hydrolases, participate in the chemical modification of intermediate compounds and in the formation of toxic oxygen

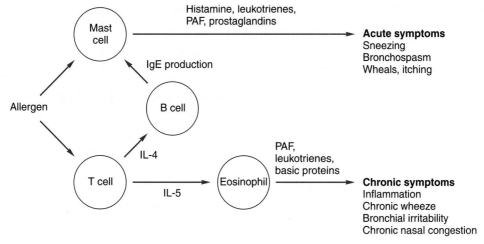

Figure 18–3. T lymphocytes play an important role in the induction of allergic inflammatory responses. Processed antigen presented to T-helper lymphocytes (CD4+) elicits the release of cytokines, including interleukin (IL)-4 and IL-5, which in turn induce IgE production by B lymphocytes and activation and recruitment of eosinophils, respectively. IgE-directed mast cell activation elicits the acute allergic response, whereas activated eosinophils in part mediate the chronic inflammatory state. PAF = platelet activating factor. (Reproduced with permission from Kay AB: "Helper" [CD+] T cells and eosinophils in allergy and asthma. Am Rev Respir Dis 1992;145[Suppl]:S22.)

metabolites. Mast cells, basophils, lymphocytes, and granulocytes also have the ability to synthesize and release proinflammatory cytokines, growth factors, and regulatory factors, which function in complex networks to precipitate and sustain the inflammatory response. Atopic individuals challenged intranasally with pollen allergen or with cold, dry air frequently demonstrate a biphasic pattern of mediator release, characterized by an initial early response

15 to 30 min after allergen exposure and a late, delayed response at 6 to 8 h, the latter of which does not require reexposure to allergen.

Early- and Late-Phase Responses

The *early-phase response (EPR),* or "classic" allergic reaction, in a sensitized individual occurs within minutes of

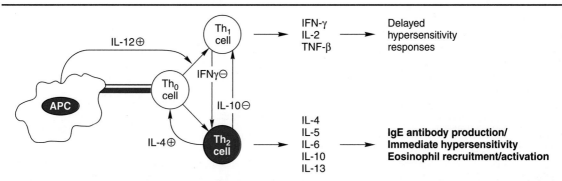

Figure 18–4. T-helper (TH) cell subsets. In allergic disease uncommitted TH_0 cells are programmed to become TH_1 or TH_2 cells after antigen presentation in the regional lymph nodes. TH_1 cells secrete IL-2, IFN-γ, and TNF-β, which induce delayed hypersensitivity responses (type IV hypersensitivity). TH_2 cells secrete IL-4, IL-5, IL-6, IL-10, and IL-13, which stimulate allergic inflammatory reactions (type I hypersensitivity). IFN-γ release by TH_1 cells inhibits the development of TH_2 cells, whereas IL-10 release by TH_2 cells is thought to inhibit the development of TH_1 cells. IL-12 and IL-4 stimulate the development of TH_1 cells and TH_2 cells, respectively.

antigen exposure and is marked by the release of vasoactive and bronchoconstrictor mediators including histamine, TAME esterase, leukotrienes, PGD_2, kinins, and kininogens. The *late-phase response (LPR),* which may either follow the EPR (dual response) or occur as an isolated event, begins 2 to 4 h after initial antigen exposure, reaches maximal activity at 6 to 12 h, and resolves within 12 to 24 h (Figure 18–5). The LPR, marked predominantly by an influx of eosinophils and mononuclear cells with recruitment of both monocytes and T cells, is thought to most closely mimic the chronic inflammation of clinical allergy. Mediators (except PGD_2) of the EPR reappear during the LPR in the absence of antigen rechallenge. Absence of PGD_2, an exclusive product of mast cell release, suggests that basophils are a potentially important source of mediators in the LPR. From such inflammatory cells, elaboration of cytokines and histamine-releasing factors may perpetuate the LPR, leading to a sustained hyperresponsiveness of the target tissue, e.g., bronchi, skin, or nasal mucosa. Products of activated eosinophils, such as major basic protein and eosinophil cationic protein, may be destructive to bronchial epithelial tissue and predispose to persistent airway reactivity. Epithelial damage is a feature of both atopic dermatitis and asthma. Pathophysiologic events of the LPR thus characterize a persistent inflammatory state.

Late-phase reactivity has been described in allergic rhinitis and conjunctivitis, asthma, food-sensitive atopic dermatitis, and anaphylaxis. Inflammatory changes in the airways are recognized as crucial attributes of chronic asthma and other allergic diseases. Therefore, therapeutic interventions that prevent or reverse inflammatory processes that characterize the LPR are most effective in the control of chronic and severe allergic disease (see later).

APPROACH TO PATIENTS WITH SUSPECTED ALLERGY

Fundamental to the evaluation of patients with suspected allergic disease is a thorough history and physical examination. Laboratory tests, particularly allergen-specific IgE skin or serum-specific-IgE (RAST) testing, confirm the diagnosis of allergy.

History

SYMPTOMS

Allergic rhinitis is characterized by paroxysmal sneezing; itching of the nose, eyes, palate, or oropharynx; nasal stuffiness; and rhinorrhea with or without postnasal drip. *Pruritus* (itching) results from the actions of histamine during the EPR and is the hallmark symptom of allergy.

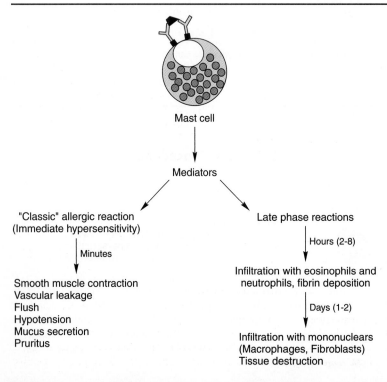

Figure 18–5. The early- and late-phase allergic response results from the activation of sensitized mast cells and release of inflammatory mediators. Chemical mediators act on blood vessels, smooth muscle, and mucous glands to initiate the classic allergic response. Late-phase reactions develop as a result of chemotactic activities of mediators. (Reproduced with permission from Oertel H, Kaliner MA: J Immunol 1981;127:1398.)

Sinusitis, serous otitis media, and eustachian tube dysfunction are frequent complications of underlying allergic disease. Asthma is indicated by chronic or recurrent cough, wheeze, dyspnea, and chest tightness, although cough may be the sole presentation in 5% of children with asthma. Atopic dermatitis is suggested by a recurring pruritic skin rash in a symmetric distribution with predilection for the extremities. Loss of well-being and irritability may accompany symptoms of allergic disease, although primary behavioral symptoms are not likely allergic in nature. Skin and respiratory diseases often coexist in atopic patients.

PATTERNS OF DISEASE

Allergic disease commonly begins in childhood. Symptom onset during early infancy suggests other etiologies (e.g., chronic lung disease and tracheoesophageal fistula), although infants may apparently be sensitized in utero or during breast feeding. Although allergic symptoms may be chronic and continuous, they are frequently episodic and can vary with seasonal exposure, location, and time of day. Symptoms commonly occur coincident with allergen exposure (e.g., housework, animal exposure, and foods), irritant exposure (e.g., perfumes, odors, and smoke), viral illness, ambient temperature change, or exercise.

ENVIRONMENTAL HISTORY

A careful environmental history should be elicited. Exposure to indoor pets; dust mites from stuffed toys, bedding, and bedroom carpeting; and mold may trigger allergic symptoms. Infants and young children attending day care and preschool have frequent exposures to viral illnesses, which are common nonallergic causes of upper and lower respiratory disease. Similarly, parental smoking can act as a nonallergic trigger for respiratory symptoms. Exposure to viral infection and environmental tobacco smoke can exacerbate allergy symptoms in atopic children.

PREVIOUS AND CURRENT THERAPY

A previous therapeutic response to allergen-avoidance measures, elimination diets, and pharmacotherapy can prompt a diagnosis of allergy. Discontinuing topical nasal vasoconstrictors after prolonged use may result in rebound congestion, known as rhinitis medicamentosa.

FAMILY HISTORY

Atopy in one or both parents or in siblings presents significant risk for development of allergic disease.

Physical Examination

A complete examination, emphasizing the skin and upper and lower respiratory systems, should be performed. Growth parameters in allergic disease are usually normal but may be impaired in chronic severe asthma. Impaired growth in the setting of chronic skin, nasal and/or airway disease should prompt an evaluation for immunodeficiency, cystic fibrosis (CF), or metabolic disease.

A horizontal nasal crease from frequent nasal itching or rubbing and allergic "shiners" due to bilateral infraorbital edema are characteristic signs of nasal allergy. Chronic nasal obstruction and mouth-breathing from allergic rhinitis may result in the appearance of an "adenoidal facies," characterized by long facies, narrow maxilla, flattened malar eminences, overbite, and a high-arched palate, which can lead to orthodontic problems.

Examination of the nose may reveal deformities from previous trauma, polyps, or septal deviation, suggesting structural etiologies of rhinitis. An internal examination by nasal speculum should *always* be performed. Pale, bluish, edematous nasal turbinates are characteristic of allergic rhinitis, but seen in only about 50% of cases. Nasal polyps are infrequently found in children with allergic rhinitis and may indicate aspirin-sensitive asthma or CF. Clear and watery nasal secretions suggest allergy, whereas chronic or recurrent mucopurulent secretions may indicate rhinosinusitis, ciliary defects, or immunodeficiency.

Tearing, scleral or conjunctival injection, and periorbital swelling suggest allergic conjunctivitis. Persistence of middle ear fluid (serous otitis media) and hearing impairment may suggest eustachian-tube dysfunction as a result of chronic nasal obstruction.

Acute or chronic patchy skin lesions involving the face and extensor surfaces of the extremities suggest atopic dermatitis (*eczema*) in infants and children. Later in older children and adults, the lesions show a flexural pattern of distribution, with predilection for the antecubital and popliteal areas and the neck. The skin lesions of atopic dermatitis are frequently infected with *Staphylococcus aureus*.

Signs of acute asthma include wheezing, a prolonged expiratory phase of respiration, and respiratory distress. Since asthma may be episodic, children with chronic asthma will frequently have a normal examination.

Laboratory Procedures

Specific diagnostic tests may be used to confirm a history and examination suggestive of clinical allergy.

ANTIGEN-SPECIFIC IGE

In vivo skin testing and in vitro RAST can be performed to look for the presence of antigen-specific IgE. The identification of specific environmental allergens is essential for directing specific avoidance measures and for consideration of immunotherapy.

Skin testing is the primary tool used by most allergist-immunologists for the evaluation of antigen-specific IgE. Improved characterization of allergen immunochemistry and standardization of testing devices have rendered testing increasingly sensitive. Skin testing is simple, inexpensive, and may be rapidly performed. The correlation of positive skin tests with the history of relevant exposure is necessary to determine the importance of specific allergens for individual patients.

Percutaneous or intradermal administration of dilute concentrations of specific antigens elicits a wheal and flare response within 15 to 30 min (positive skin test) in sensitized individuals. Skin test reactions whose wheal diameter is at least 3 mm larger than a negative control are usually considered as positive. Skin testing cannot reliably be performed on patients taking antihistamine drugs, which suppress skin test reactivity, or on patients with extensive eczema.

Positive skin test reactions to airborne allergens, combined with a history and examination suggestive of allergy, strongly incriminate the allergen as a cause of the symptoms. Negative skin tests with a history that does not suggest allergy favor a nonallergic etiology. Skin testing to food allergens is less reliable than it is for inhalant allergens because only 40 to 50% of positive skin test reactions for food allergens correlate with double-blind placebo-controlled oral food challenge. Negative skin test reactions to food allergens generally exclude suspected hypersensitivity to specific foods. Skin testing with insect venoms is an obligate confirmation of clinical hypersensitivity.

Radioallergobsorbent testing provides quantitative in vitro assay of allergen-specific IgE (Figure 18–6). The patient's serum is reacted initially with antigen bound to a solid phase material and then labeled with a radioactive or enzyme-linked anti-IgE antibody. RAST has a 70 to 80% correlation with skin testing to pollens, dust mites, and animal danders. Because of its decreased sensitivity and specificity and increased cost, RAST is not considered the diagnostic test of choice for allergy except for patients on chronic antihistamine therapy, in patients with severe dermatitis, and in patients with prior severe anaphylaxis.

TOTAL SERUM IgE LEVEL

Although increased IgE levels occur in many patients with atopic diseases, its usefulness as a diagnostic test is limited by its reduced sensitivity. IgE levels >200 IU/mL suggest allergy, whereas values <20 IU/mL make allergy unlikely. Frequently, however, patients with or without allergy have intermediate levels of total serum IgE. Serum IgE levels also vary with age and are more frequently elevated in patients with asthma and atopic dermatitis than they are in those patients with allergic rhinitis. The presence of IgE in cord serum is a predictor of the subsequent development of atopy. Patients with immunodeficiency syndromes, neoplasm, and parasitic disease can also have marked elevations of serum IgE concentration.

TOTAL EOSINOPHIL COUNT

Although eosinophils play an important role in the inflammatory response of allergic disease, it is primarily a tissue-dwelling cell. Eosinophils are present 100-fold more frequently in the marrow and tissues than they are in the peripheral blood. Circulating cells reflect only trafficking between sites of production and function. Peripheral eosinophilia is therefore of limited value in the diagnosis of allergic disease.

NASAL CYTOLOGY

Nasal secretions of patients with suspected allergic rhinitis can be examined for evidence of inflammatory cells. Specimens from allergic patients usually show high numbers of eosinophils, basophils, and neutrophils, whereas secretions of nonatopic patients demonstrate few inflammatory cells. The degree of nasal eosinophilia is related to the extent of allergic exposure and symptoms. Specimens may be obtained from blown secretions or by nasal scraping with a plastic curette from the medial third of the inferior turbinate. Specimens stained with Wright or Hansel stain

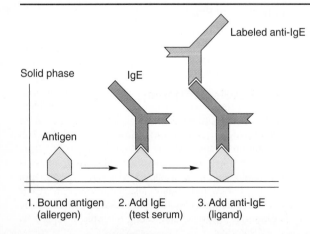

Figure 18–6. Radioallergosorbent testing (RAST) provides a quantitative in vitro measure of antigen-specific IgE. Patient serum is reacted with solid-phase-bound antigen and labeled with a radioactive or enzyme-linked anti-IgE.

have 70% sensitivity and 94% specificity for the diagnosis of allergic rhinitis.

LUNG FUNCTION TESTING

Pulmonary function testing (spirometry) and broncho-provocation are discussed in Chap. 17. Spirometry and peak expiratory flow monitoring can be utilized in asthmatic children to determine the extent of airway obstruction. Spirometry is helpful for diagnosing asthma, monitoring severity, and evaluating patient response to treatment. For children with atypical signs and symptoms of asthma, bronchoprovocation to methacholine or histamine can be used to demonstrate bronchial hyperresponsiveness that can establish a diagnosis of asthma. Bronchial hyperresponsiveness may also be demonstrated in patients with seasonal allergic rhinitis, in individuals after a viral respiratory infection, and in children with CF.

SINUS EVALUATION

Acute and chronic sinusitis are common complications of allergic airway disease. Approximately 70% of patients with chronic sinusitis have underlying allergy. In some patients with chronic asthma and sinusitis, asthma relief occurs only after treatment of the sinus disease. Sinus CT scans have generally replaced plain radiographs as the diagnostic method of choice for patients with suspected sinusitis. Radiographic or CT evidence of air-fluid levels, opacification, and thickening of sinus membrane tissue (>6-mm thickness) are associated with sinus infection. A single Waters view x-ray can be used to screen for acute maxillary and frontal sinusitis. Flexible nasopharyngoscopy (*rhinoscopy*) permits direct visualization of the upper airway and may be useful in the evaluation of persistent nasal obstruction, epistaxis, and laryngeal symptoms.

OTHER TESTS

Gastrointestinal studies, including stool pH, ova, and parasite studies; esophageal pH monitoring; and endoscopy can exclude diagnoses that mimic gastrointestinal allergy (e.g., malabsorption, parasitosis, reflux, or structural lesions). Recurrent sinopulmonary infection, chronic rhinitis and otitis media can prompt evaluation for immunodeficiency, ciliary dyskinesia syndrome, and CF. Quantitative immunoglobulins with functional testing of antibody responses to protein and polysaccharide antigens can be ordered to exclude humoral (antibody) immunodeficiency (see Chap. 7). Persistent nasal obstruction and sleep apnea should prompt evaluation for tonsillar or adenoidal hypertrophy. The presence of a foreign body in the nasal passage can cause chronic unilateral purulent drainage.

BASIC APPROACHES TO THERAPY

The general therapeutic approach to patients with allergic disease includes patient education, environmental control of relevant allergens, pharmacologic management, and immunotherapy.

Patient Education

The clinician should strive for a partnership with patients and their families in the management of allergic disease. Teaching the basic elements of allergic disease, the role of environmental allergens, and the mechanisms, appropriate use, and adverse effects of drug therapy represents a critical aspect of patient management. Thoughtful and specific educational strategies permit patients to acquire the skills (self-management) and confidence (self-efficacy) essential for successful management of their disease. Education should be continuous from the point of initial diagnosis.

Environmental Control

Effective environmental control strategies can be implemented following the identification of relevant allergens by history and skin testing. Avoidance of the indoor allergens dust mite, cockroach, animal danders, and molds and avoidance of seasonal outdoor pollens to the extent possible can reduce allergen exposure levels, thus reducing symptoms and medication requirements for allergic individuals. Controlled studies have demonstrated that dust mite control measures (which include the use of airtight encasements for mattresses, box springs, and pillows; removal of bedroom floor carpeting; regular hot water laundering of bedding sheets; and dehumidification of indoor environments) can produce significant clinical improvement in mite-allergic patients.

For many animal-sensitive patients, removal of the family pet can be an effective, although emotionally difficult measure. The family should at least be implored to restrict the family pet from the child's room and, if possible, the entire house. Some studies have shown that weekly bathing of a cat may remove considerable amounts of allergen and result in clinical improvement. The use of air conditioning in the car and the home and restricting outdoor activity on high–pollen-count days may prove helpful for pollen-allergic children. Elimination of cigarette smoke, gas stoves, strong detergents, and perfumes in the home can benefit allergic children as well.

Pharmacologic Therapy

SYMPTOMATIC TREATMENTS

Antihistamines, the first-line treatment for mild seasonal or periodic allergic rhinitis and/or conjunctivitis, can relieve nasal itching, sneezing, and rhinorrhea. Because they do not act on vascular structures, antihistamines are less effective for the control of nasal congestion. These agents act by competitively inhibiting the binding of histamine to H_1 receptor sites.

Conventional (first-generation) antihistamines cause varying degrees of sedation and performance impairment. Generally patients who use these medications regularly become tolerant to the sedating effects. Newer (second-generation) antihistamines (fexofenadine, cetirizine, and loratadine) are generally nonsedating (or low sedating) at effective doses. Both cetirizine and loratadine are currently available for use in young children.

α-adrenergic agents constitute a class of *sympathomimetics* that induce vasoconstriction by stimulation of α-adrenergic receptors. Oral sympathomimetics (pseudoephedrine) can therefore reduce nasal congestion and mucosal edema and are often used in conjunction with antihistamines for the treatment of acute and chronic allergic rhinitis and nasal obstruction. Topical nasal vasoconstrictor sprays have limited usefulness in patients with chronic allergic rhinitis because overuse can lead to rhinitis medicamentosa.

PROPHYLACTIC AND ANTI-INFLAMMATORY AGENTS

Topical cromolyn sodium sprays and aerosols can be used to prevent and treat allergic rhinitis, conjunctivitis, and asthma. Cromolyn blocks early- and late-phase reactions in sensitized allergen-challenged patients. While cromolyn is an exceptionally safe drug, it cannot reverse or terminate an allergic response once it has started and therefore must be used regularly and frequently as a preventative treatment to be most effective.

As the most effective and potent anti-inflammatory agents available, *corticosteroids* have become indispensable therapy in the management of chronic allergic disease. Topical dermatologic, nasal, and pulmonary preparations in the form of skin creams, ointments, and aerosols are highly potent, locally active, and rapidly metabolized drugs with rare systemic effects at therapeutic doses. Nasal and pulmonary preparations have been found to rarely cause growth suppression in susceptible children and, therefore, growth should be carefully monitored for any children taking topical steroids for asthma and/or allergic rhinitis. Oral corticosteroids are reserved for short-term use in patients with extremely severe and intolerable nasal allergy and as rescue therapy for patients with severe acute asthma exacerbations. Long-term use of oral corticosteroids is reserved for children with severe recalcitrant asthma.

Corticosteroids impair arachidonic acid metabolism, limit the generation of inflammatory cytokines and mediators, and prevent directed migration and activation of inflammatory cells. These agents also upregulate β-receptors, rendering β-stimulatory agents more effective. Corticosteroids block late-phase, but not early-phase, reactions in sensitized allergen-challenged individuals.

Aqueous nasal steroid sprays are highly effective as maintenance treatment of moderate-to-severe seasonal or perennial allergic rhinitis. No significant adverse long-term effects have been demonstrated, although the potential for mucosal atrophy and septal perforation exists with prolonged improper use of the nasal inhaler. Several nasal steroid sprays have now been approved for use in children as young as 3 years.

IMMUNOTHERAPY

Allergen immunotherapy (desensitization or hyposensitization; "allergy shots") denotes the repeated subcutaneous administration of increasing quantities of allergen extract in sensitized patients to reduce the threshold for the development of clinical symptoms. Although this therapy has been used for more than 80 years, controlled studies to document its effectiveness have been available for only 20 to 30 years. Proper use of immunotherapy requires an accurate assessment of individual sensitivity by skin testing and symptom correlation with allergen exposure. Effective treatment of patients with allergic rhinitis and/or allergic asthma requires the long-term administration of high doses of allergen (6 to 12 μg of allergen per injection at maintenance dosing for 3 to 5 years). Optimally, these extracts should be standardized using the most modern techniques. The use of low-dose immunotherapy or administration by sublingual or oral route is of no proven value.

The use of immunotherapy is adjunctive to the pharmacologic and environmental management of patients with allergic rhinitis and/or allergic asthma. Immunotherapy is generally recommended for patients who cannot avoid relevant allergens and have had a suboptimal response to, or poor tolerance of, pharmacotherapy. Immunotherapy is the primary treatment for insect sting (Hymenoptera) anaphylaxis. Treatment with immunotherapy is not indicated for management of atopic dermatitis, urticaria, or food allergies.

Hymenoptera venom immunotherapy has demonstrated considerable effectiveness in preventing subsequent sting anaphylaxis. Treatment of allergic rhinitis patients with dust mite, cat, ragweed, grass, and tree pollen immunotherapy has also been demonstrated to reduce symptoms and medication use in these patients. In asthma patients, immunotherapy appears to be most effective when administered to patients with relevant and unavoidable allergic triggers, including cat, house dust mite, grass, and tree pollen. Its effectiveness has been difficult to assess from the literature, in part because of differing methodologies and the presence of confounding nonallergic asthma triggers.

The mechanism of action of immunotherapy has not been precisely defined. Evidence suggests that long-term allergen immunotherapy can downregulate TH_2-cell responses and diminish the production and release of cytokines that initiate and sustain allergic responses. Levels of antigen-specific IgE increase initially but then diminish so that the observed seasonal increase in pollen-specific IgE is blunted. Patients who receive immunotherapy also develop increased levels of antigen-specific IgG (blocking antibodies), which are thought to preclude IgE-mediated responses but do not correlate with clinical improvement.

Allergen immunotherapy should be performed under the supervision of specially trained physicians (usually allergist-immunologists). Immunotherapy is generally safe and well tolerated. Erythema and swelling at the injection site are frequently observed but these reactions are normally transient and spontaneously resolving. Two to three percent of patients may develop systemic reactions, including generalized hives, angioedema, bronchospasm, and anaphylaxis. The early recognition and aggressive treatment of systemic reactions is essential. For this reason, patients should normally be observed for 20–30 min in a physician's office following the injection. No adverse long-term effects from immunotherapy have been described. In fact, patients who become pregnant while receiving immunotherapy may continue receiving injections if they are at maintenance doses.

ROLE OF THE ALLERGIST-IMMUNOLOGIST

The allergist-immunologist is a specialist with expertise in diseases of hypersensitivity, immune-mediated disorders, and immunological deficiency diseases (see Chap. 7). These physicians have primary boards in pediatrics or internal medicine and subspecialty training in allergy and clinical immunology. Diseases of immediate hypersensitivity that are commonly seen in conjunction with an allergist-immunologist are subsequently reviewed and summarized in Table 18–2.

DISEASES OF IMMEDIATE HYPERSENSITIVITY

Allergic Rhinitis and Conjunctivitis

Respiratory allergy involving nasal and conjunctival mucous membranes (allergic rhinitis and conjunctivitis) represents a hypersensitivity response to primarily airborne allergens. Children with chronic moderate-to-severe rhinitis and nasal obstruction are the most frequent source of referral to the allergist-immunologist. With a prevalence of 10 to 12%, allergic rhinitis ranks as the most common of allergic diseases. Allergic rhinitis most often presents in early childhood or adolescence.

The condition may be seasonal or perennial, as defined by the predominant pattern of reactivity and allergen exposure. Most seasonal allergies are caused by pollens from local tree, grass, or weed species. Perennial allergens such as those from dust mites, cockroaches, animal proteins, and molds are primarily found in the indoor environment.

A diagnosis of allergic rhinitis is suggested by nasal and/or eye symptoms that are more frequent than expected for age, persist without an interval between acute episodes, and are not caused by viral infections. Patients can have profuse watery rhinorrhea, paroxysmal sneezing, nasal obstruction, nasal and palatal itching, and conjunctivitis, in association with relevant allergen exposures. A family history of atopy is usually present. "Allergic shiners" (darkened infraorbital edema), nasal mucosal swelling, middle ear effusions, and ocular injection and tearing support historical findings. Allergic rhinitis often coexists with atopic dermatitis and asthma in children.

The differential diagnosis in patients with perennial rhinitis and nasal obstruction includes anatomic obstruction (septal deviation or spurs, nasal polyposis, tonsillar and adenoidal hypertrophy, or foreign body), sinusitis, vasomotor (nonallergic) rhinitis, rhinitis medicamentosa, and drug effects. Vasomotor rhinitis is an entity of nasal mucosal hyperirritability, characterized by nasal congestion and postnasal drainage in the absence of skin test reactivity. Pregnancy, oral contraceptive agents, and tricyclic antidepressants may produce nasal congestion. Hypothyroidism, nasal mastocytosis, and nasopharyngeal tumors are extremely rare causes of chronic rhinitis in children. Persistent nasal congestion, chronic or recurrent purulent nasal secretions, headache, recurrent otitis media, and cough may suggest a complicating sinusitis (see later).

Patients with allergic rhinitis or conjunctivitis may demonstrate large numbers of eosinophils in nasal secretions or conjunctival scrapings. Immediate skin test reactivity to a panel of relevant allergens can be performed to identify antigens responsible for disease.

The treatment of patients with allergic rhinitis and/or conjunctivitis should include patient education, avoidance of relevant allergen and irritant triggers, and pharmacotherapy and/or immunotherapy. Antihistamines and decongestants may be used to reduce symptoms of mild-to-moderate seasonal or episodic allergic rhinitis. Treatment of chronic or moderate-to-severe allergic rhinitis should focus on anti-inflammatory therapies, such as nasal or ocular cromolyn or nasal steroid aerosols. Immunotherapy is indicated for patients with clinically relevant skin test reactivity who cannot avoid relevant allergen exposure and have inadequate response to environmental control and pharmacotherapy.

Sinusitis

Acute sinusitis usually presents with facial pain, headache, fever, and purulent nasal secretions of less than 3-weeks duration. Chronic sinusitis should be considered
(*text continues on page 742*)

Table 18–2. Clinical Evaluation of Allergic Disorders

Disease	Symptoms/History	Signs	Diagnostic Tests	Treatment
Allergic rhinitis	• Recurrent or chronic pattern of watery rhinorrhea, paroxysmal sneezing, nasal stuffiness, nasal/palatal itching • Seasonal or parennial pattern • Family history of atopy • Personal history of asthma, atopic dermatitis	Allergic shiners Mouth breathing Nasal crease Nasal mucosal edema Conjunctivitis	• Nasal smear for eosinophils (suggestive) • Skin testing to aeroallergens	• Avoidance/environmental control • Antihistamines/decongestants • Nasal cromolyn • Nasal corticosteroids • Allergen immunotherapy
Sinusitis	• Acute: facial pain, headaches, fever, purulent nasal secretions • Chronic: nasal discharge, cough, halitosis, nasal obstruction	Inflamed nasal turbinates Purulent rhinorrhea "Cobblestone" features Recurrent/chronic otitis	• Waters x-ray (screening) • Sinus CT scan	• Antibiotics • Analgesics • Antihistamines/decongestants • Nasal corticosteroids • Surgery
Food allergy (immediate-type)	• Immediate response to food intake (within 2 h) • Mouth/perioral itching, nausea, abdominal cramping, diarrhea; urticaria, angioedema; atopic dermatitis; anaphylaxis; rhinitis/asthma (rare)	Hives Angioedema Eczema	• Skin testing to select foods (screening) • Food elimination/challenge	• Elimination of specific foods • Epinephrine kit prn

Anaphylaxis	• Immediate reaction to inciting agent • Upper/lower airway obstruction, urticaria/angioedema, nausea, abdominal pain, diarrhea, cardiovascular instability/collapse	Pruritus Skin erythema Hives Swelling Stridor/wheeze Hypotension/shock	• Skin, in vitro testing to suspected food, drug, latex, insect venom allergens	• Acute event: epinephrine IV fluids oxygen ±IV/IM antihistamines ±Aerosolized bronchodilators ±Endotracheal intubation/tracheostomy • Avoidance • Epinephrine prn
Insect sting reaction	• Systemic reaction including upper/lower airway obstruction, cardiovascular instability/collapse	See anaphylaxis (above)	• Skin testing to Hymenoptera venoms or fire ant	• See anaphylaxis (above)
Urticaria/angioedema	• Multiple hives • Lips, tongue, pharyngeal, periorbital, genital swelling	Hives Localized swelling	• Skin, in vitro testing to suspected allergens (food, drug) • Ice cube test (cold urticaria) ± Complete blood cell count, erythrocyte sedimentation rate, chem panel, LFTs, CXR, stool O&P (chronic urticaria)	• Avoidance of offending agent if known; treatment of underlying disease • H₁ antagonists • H₁ + H₂ antagonists
Hereditary angioedema	• Angioedema of the upper airway, GI tract		• C4 level (screening) • C1 inhibitor/function	• Androgens • Anabolic steroids
Drug allergy (immediate hypersensitivity)	• Urticaria/angioedema, upper/lower airway obstruction, cardiovascular instability/collapse, gastrointestinal symptoms	Hives Localized swelling Stridor/wheeze Hypotension/shock	• Skin testing to β-lactams (major and minor determinants) and other selected agents	• Acute event (see anaphylaxis) • Avoidance; use of alternative agent • Desensitization

CT = computed tomography; CXR = chest x-ray; GI = gastrointestinal; H₁, H₂ = histamine; LFTs = liver function tests; O&P = ova and parasites.

in the presence of protracted symptoms of upper respiratory tract infection, allergic rhinitis unresponsive to therapy, worsening asthma, or chronic cough. Children with chronic sinusitis generally have greater than 3 months of persistent nasal congestion, nasal secretions, cough, halitosis, and/or recurrent otitis media. Infraorbital edema, inflamed nasal turbinates, with purulent rhinorrhea, and pharyngeal lymphoid hyperplasia ("cobblestone" features) may also be suggestive of chronic sinusitis (see Chap. 9, section on sinusitis). Factors contributing to the development of sinusitis include swelling of sinus ostia, mucociliary abnormalities, mucus overproduction, and immunodeficiency (especially IgA deficiency). The resulting accumulation of secretions in the sinus cavities leads to bacterial proliferation and subsequent infection.

Allergic Asthma

Asthma is discussed in Chap. 17. It is the most common chronic illness of childhood—a leading cause of pediatric hospitalization—and seriously affects the quality of life for children and their families. Despite an increased understanding of the pathophysiology of the disease, as well as the availability of new treatments, the morbidity and mortality of asthma have been increasing since the early 1980s, especially in poor, urban-dwelling, minority children. Important factors contributing to this trend are underdiagnosis and undertreatment. Acute exacerbations from asthma, resulting in emergency department care and hospitalization, are largely preventable, if diagnosis and treatment are comprehensive and ongoing.

There has been increased recognition of the importance of airway inflammation in patients with even mild asthma. Inflammation induced by chronic allergen exposure is associated with airway hyperresponsiveness and bronchial obstruction that lead to the persistence of cough, wheeze, breathlessness, and chest tightness in asthmatic children. Approximately 80 to 90% of children over the age of 2 years with asthma have associated allergy. The frequency and intensity of skin test reactivity to allergen has been correlated with asthma severity. Studies have demonstrated that allergen exposure in early life can influence the age of onset and severity of asthma.

Patients with chronic persistent asthma are advised to obtain evaluation by an allergist-immunologist to document sensitization to relevant allergens and to provide specific strategies for controlling or eliminating allergen exposures. Patient education, control of environmental triggers, objective monitoring of airway function through peak flow monitoring and spirometry, use of chronic anti-inflammatory pharmacotherapy, use of an emergency asthma action plan, and regular follow-up care are the essential tools in the successful management of these patients.

Atopic Dermatitis

Atopic dermatitis (allergic eczema) is discussed in Chap. 11. An inflammatory skin condition with onset in early childhood, atopic dermatitis is characterized by a chronic or relapsing pruritic dermatitis with typical morphology and distribution. Atopic dermatitis (with allergic rhinitis and asthma) is considered part of the triad of atopic conditions. Approximately two thirds of children with atopic dermatitis have a positive family history for atopy; in 50 to 80% of children, allergic rhinitis or asthma develops. Both elevated serum total IgE levels and positive immediate skin test reactivity to food and environmental allergens are characteristic of these patients. Studies have confirmed an important role for food allergy in 30 to 40% of young children with moderate-or-severe atopic dermatitis. Both immediate and late-phase reactions have been observed in patients with food-sensitive atopic dermatitis following double-blind placebo-controlled oral food challenge. Therefore, an allergy evaluation is advised for children who experience moderate-to-severe atopic dermatitis.

Food Allergy

Although food allergy may encompass a broad spectrum of immunologic mechanisms, type I immediate hypersensitivity is the most common and best understood process. IgE-mediated hypersensitivity to food allergens may be an underlying etiology in atopic dermatitis (see earlier), urticaria and angioedema, and anaphylaxis. Allergic gastroenteropathy (eosinophilic gastroenteropathy), characterized by multiple IgE food sensitivities associated with local gastrointestinal tract pathology, is an uncommon condition associated with food allergy in infants. These children can present with vomiting, diarrhea, bloating and weight loss, peripheral and intestinal eosinophilia, and gut loss of fluid, protein, and blood. Immunologic mechanisms other than type I hypersensitivity reactions can cause other food allergic conditions including milk-protein-induced enteropathies, gluten-sensitive enteropathy (GSE, celiac disease), and dermatitis herpetiformis (pruritic skin condition associated with GSE). Food allergy should be distinguished from food intolerance (e.g., dyes, flavorings, and toxins), food aversion, structural abnormalities of the gastrointestinal tract, enzyme deficiencies, inflammatory bowel disease, ulcer disease, gastrointestinal infection, and pharmacologic or adverse effects of foods or medications that may mimic symptoms of allergy but do not result from immunologic pathologies.

IgE-mediated sensitization develops when food macromolecules pass through the gastrointestinal epithelium, interact with the mucosal immune system, and access the general circulation. That food allergy is more common in infants and young children is thought to reflect an immaturity of the gastrointestinal epithelial barrier and insufficient levels of protective secretory IgA that predispose infants to sensitization and allergy. Sensitized children can develop a spectrum of food-induced reaction from mild itching and discomfort to life-threatening systemic anaphylaxis often within minutes of exposure. In some susceptible children, systemic anaphylaxis may be provoked when food ingestion is followed by vigorous exercise.

In infants and young children, milk, eggs, peanuts, soy, fish, and wheat are responsible for approximately 90% of food allergies. In addition to these foods, allergy to tree nut and shellfish can develop in older children and adolescents.

Typical symptoms that occur shortly after exposure to foods in children with a family or previous personal history of atopy can suggest the diagnosis of food allergy. The preparation of the food (e.g., raw or cooked), amount consumed (e.g., dose), and use of concurrent medications may influence the expression of food allergy; a suspected food may fail to induce an allergic reaction consistently. A 10- to 14-day diet record may be useful for establishing a cluster of suspected foods when the diagnosis is unclear. Immediate hypersensitivity skin testing to food antigens suspected of causing allergy can be of benefit in identifying relevant food allergens. When compared to gold-standard double-blind, placebo-controlled oral food challenges, negative skin tests to foods are usually more reliable (>95% negative predictive value) at excluding specific IgE-mediated food hypersensitivity than are positive tests in diagnosing food allergy (40 to 50% positive predictive value). Radioallergosorbent (in vitro) tests have lower sensitivity and lower specificity when compared to skin testing in diagnosing food allergy.

A strict 3- to 4-week elimination of suspected allergenic foods, as determined by history and skin testing, should be instituted to look for resolution of symptoms. Elimination diets followed by the return of suspect foods to the diet can be applied when symptoms are not life-threatening, such as in urticaria, atopic dermatitis, gastrointestinal allergy, and rhinitis. The empiric long-term initiation of severe elimination diets should be avoided, as malnutrition and vitamin deficiencies may result.

Patients diagnosed with severe food allergy must avoid exposure to those specific foods. Patients and families must therefore be instructed to scrutinize ingredient labels, to recognize technical and scientific nomenclature, and to be especially vigilant when eating meals away from home.

Patients with life-threatening food allergy must be prescribed self-injectable epinephrine and should be in-structed as to its indications and procedure for use as inadvertent ingestion of foods that are known to be allergenic is common. The use of prophylactic drugs and desensitization therapy have no current role in treating patients with food allergy. Children with milk, egg, and soy allergies will most often lose their allergy by age 3 years. However, peanut, tree nut, and shellfish allergies tend to be life-long.

Anaphylaxis

Anaphylaxis denotes a generalized, multisystem, immediate, life-threatening IgE-mediated hypersensitivity reaction triggered by the sudden, massive release of bioactive mediators from sensitized mast cells. Patients with anaphylaxis experience a rapid onset of itching, discomfort, and generalized urticaria (hives) that can progress to upper and lower airway obstruction (rhinitis and bronchospasm), angioedema, gastrointestinal symptoms (vomiting, diarrhea), and cardiovascular instability or collapse (hypotension, shock) following exposure to an inciting agent. Involvement of some or all of these target organs may occur. Allergens that elicit anaphylaxis most commonly include foods, drugs, latex, and stinging insect venoms. While many foods have been reported to induce anaphylaxis, the most frequently involved are peanuts, nuts, fish, and egg whites. Penicillins and cephalosporins are the most common drugs to elicit anaphylaxis, although a large number of antimicrobials, chemotherapeutic agents, and vaccines can induce anaphylaxis less commonly. Anaphylaxis to latex has been increasingly recognized in children with spina bifida and urogenital anomalies, with allergy to foods that share immunologic reactivity with latex (e.g., banana, avocado, kiwi, and chestnut), in health care workers, in rubber industry workers, and in patients with prior intraoperative anaphylaxis. Anaphylactic-like (anaphylactoid) reactions to radiographic dyes, aspirin and nonsteroidal anti-inflammatory drugs, opiate analgesics, intravenous immune globulin, and exercise mimic the symptoms of true anaphylaxis but do not involve type I IgE-mediated hypersensitivity mechanisms. A syndrome of recurrent idiopathic anaphylaxis has been described primarily in adults.

Anaphylaxis is a clinical diagnosis based on its constellation of symptoms closely following an inciting event or exposure. Antigen-specific IgE in vitro or skin testing may be performed for suspected food, venom, latex, and drug exposures several weeks after the initial anaphylactic event. Such testing can help to identify allergens that must be strictly avoided to minimize the risk of future recurrences of anaphylaxis.

Anaphylaxis is a life-threatening emergency that must be promptly recognized and treated. Patients should receive an injection of 0.01 mg/kg epinephrine (1 : 1000 dilution) subcutaneously that can be followed by repeated injections every 15 to 30 min as indicated. Patients should be advised to use autoinjectable epinephrine prior to transport to an emergency facility. Intravenous access should be secured for administration of antihistamines, fluids, and possibly vasopressors. Supplemental oxygen should be given; endotracheal intubation or emergent tracheostomy may be needed for severe life-threatening airway obstruction. Intramuscular or intravenous anti-histamines (diphenhydramine, 1 to 2 mg/kg) should be administered for urticaria, angioedema, and gastro-intesinal reactions. Aerosolized albuterol may be given to treat bronchospasm. Systemic corticosteroids may be use-ful for prevention of late-phase anaphylaxis. Patients who experience anaphylaxis should be observed for 8 to 24 h in an emergency room or hospitalized setting, discharged on 24 to 48 h of oral corticosteroids, and prescribed an autoinjectable epinephrine. Patients experiencing ana-phylaxis should obtain consultation with an allergist-immunologist to assist with identifying the etiology of the event, and to provide important education to min-imize the risk of future recurrences.

Insect Sting Reactions

Allergic reactions to stinging insect (Hymenoptera) venom and to the bites of fire ants (found in the South-ern United States) can be potentially life-threatening. In North America, Hymenoptera stings are mainly due to apidae (honeybee) and the vespidae (yellow jackets, yellow hornets, bald-faced hornets, and paper wasps). Venom proteins tend to show cross-reactivity within the vespid family, although there is little cross-reactivity between the apidae and the vespidae. The use of specific venom anti-gens has replaced the use of whole body extracts for diagnostic skin testing and desensitization. Whole-body extracts from fire ants contain most relevant allergens and are still used for the diagnosis and treatment of allergic reactions to fire ants.

Systemic cutaneous reactions (generalized hives) may be the sole manifestation of systemic insect sting re-action in 60% of children. Respiratory symptoms occur in 50% of patients; hypotension is uncommon. Chil-dren who develop urticaria alone following insect stings have a 10 to 20% risk of anaphylaxis with subsequent stings. Anaphylaxis involving the cardiorespiratory sys-tems carries a 50 to 60% risk of recurrence with sub-sequent stings.

Insect sting hypersensitivity is diagnosed based on his-tory and confirmed by evidence of skin test reactivity to venom-specific IgE. Children with only local reactions or systemic urticaria alone do not require skin testing and subsequent desensitization since the risk of anaphylaxis

on re-sting is low. Patients with a history of multisystem anaphylaxis following insect sting, however, should be referred to an allergist-immunologist for skin testing to a complete set of venoms to confirm the diagnosis and to determine the specific venom hypersensitivity. Skin test-ing to venoms is more sensitive and specific than RAST, which is not recommended for diagnostic use.

Patients who demonstrate positive skin test reactivity should be placed on venom immunotherapy. Immuno-therapy is 97 to 99% effective in protecting against ana-phylaxis with any subsequent stings.

Patients who develop localized itching, swelling, and discomfort following insect sting may be treated with ice packs, rest, oral antihistamines, and analgesics. A brief tapering course of systemic steroids can be given for re-actions involving the head and neck. Patients with a his-tory of stinging insect anaphylaxis should avoid high-risk situations and should be prescribed an autoinjectable epi-nephrine kit with careful instruction regarding its indi-cations and proper use.

Urticaria

Urticaria (hives) affects 20% of individuals during their lifetime. *Acute urticaria* is common in children and is fre-quently caused by IgE-mediated hypersensitivity to foods, drugs, latex, and stinging insect venom. *Chronic urticaria,* with lesions extending beyond 6 weeks, is less common in children than it is in adults, is rarely associated with a spe-cific allergic etiology, and is often idiopathic.

Urticarial lesions appear as raised areas of erythema and edema involving the superficial dermis. The lesions may be single or multiple, are intensely pruritic, and usu-ally resolve spontaneously within 24 to 48 h. A careful medical and environmental exposure history can often reveal the etiology in acute urticaria. A physical examina-tion is performed to rule out other skin conditions such as vasculitis, fungal infection (tinea corporis), scabies, and cutaneous mastocytosis (urticaria pigmentosa). In addition to allergic causes, urticaria may be triggered by cold exposure, pressure, and rarely by sunlight (solar urticaria), water (aquagenic urticaria), and vibratory stimuli. Cold urticaria induced by local skin cooling can be confirmed by applying an ice cube to patients' fore-arms for 5 min and observing for localized urticaria 10 min after skin rewarming. Pressure urticaria may be iso-lated or seen in conjunction with other forms of urticaria. Cholinergic urticaria, a condition characterized by the appearance of distinctive small punctate wheals with prominent surrounding erythema, usually appears after exercise, heat, or emotional stress. Aspirin and nons-teroidal anti-inflammatory drugs may induce acute or chronic urticaria by non–IgE-mediated mechanisms.

Urticaria is best treated by the identification and elim-ination of specific underlying triggers. Factors that may aggravate urticaria such as aspirin and nonsteroidal inflammatory drugs and hot baths should generally be avoided. Histamine (H_1)-receptor antagonists are first-line therapy for acute or chronic urticaria. For patients who fail to respond to H_1 blockers, treatment with combined H_1 and H_2 antagonists may be attempted. Epinephrine injections should be used when pharyngeal or laryngeal edema is present. Brief bursts of oral corticosteroids can be used in severe episodes of acute urticaria, but long-term use should generally be avoided in children with chronic urticaria.

Angioedema

Angioedema, a condition defined by localized well-demarcated areas of tense, nonpitting subcutaneous edema, can be isolated or seen in conjunction with acute urticaria. Angioedema frequently involves the lips, tongue, oropharynx, and periorbital and genital regions.

Hereditary angioedema (HAE), an autosomal-dominant inherited disorder with typical onset in childhood, presents as recurrent episodes of edema of the extremities and bowel, which can be triggered by surgery, physical trauma, and emotional stress. Life-threatening episodes involving the upper airway may cause acute obstruction and asphyxiation. Two forms of HAE have been described. Most patients (85%) have low levels of C1-inhibitor protein, a compound that stabilizes the initial complex in the classic complement pathway. Deficient levels of C1-inhibitor protein promote autoactivation of the complement system. Fifteen percent of patients with HAE have normal (or elevated) levels of C1 inhibitor, but the existing protein is nonfunctional. C4 levels are decreased between attacks and are frequently undetectable during episodes. C2 levels are frequently decreased during attacks as well. The diagnosis of HAE can be confirmed by the finding of deficient levels or function of the C1-inhibitor protein and by a reduced C4 level. Acquired C1-inhibitor deficiency is a rare condition that can be associated with lymphoproliferative or connective tissue diseases such as systemic lupus erythematosus.

HAE is treated effectively in most patients by administration of androgens or anabolic steroids that probably augment synthesis of C1-inhibitor protein. These drugs markedly diminish the frequency and severity of attacks. Patients with HAE tend to respond poorly to drugs used to treat episodic angioedema such as antihistamines, epinephrine, and glucocorticoids.

Drug Allergy

Drug allergy may involve any of the Gel and Coombs immunologic mechanisms. Large-molecular-weight compounds (e.g., heteroantisera) are complete antigens that directly induce an immune response, whereas small-molecular-weight compounds (e.g., penicillin and its metabolites) must bind to carrier proteins or cell surfaces *(haptenation)* to become immunogenic. Almost all pharmacologic agents have been reported to induce hypersensitivity, although the most common drugs known to cause IgE-mediated hypersensitivity are antibiotics. Drug allergy may involve single or multiple target organs. The clinical presentation, propensities of certain drugs to induce allergy, and the temporal relation of the reaction to drug exposure assist in identifying the likely agent and immunopathologic mechanism. Immunodiagnostic testing, including immediate or delayed hypersensitivity skin testing, may be useful in confirming a suspected reaction.

β-LACTAM HYPERSENSITIVITY

Drug allergy due to β-lactam antibiotics (e.g., penicillins and cephalosporins) may occur by types I, II, or III Gel and Coombs immunologic mechanisms. β-lactam antibiotics are the most frequent class of drugs that cause type I IgE-mediated hypersensitivity. Allergic reactions occur in up to 10% of treatments with penicillin; anaphylactic reactions occur in 0.01%, and fatal reactions in about 1 per 50,000 treatment courses. Following its administration, penicillin is metabolized to biochemically active compounds that combine with plasma proteins to become immunogenic. The most abundant metabolite, penicilloyl, is known as the "major determinant" because it accounts for 95% of protein-bound drug metabolites. The three other penicillin metabolites (penicillin, penicilloic acid, and penillic acid) are generated in smaller amounts and are termed collectively the *minor determinants.* Identification and characterization of these immunogenic metabolites have made possible the use of immediate hypersensitivity skin testing reagents to prospectively identify patients at risk for life-threatening anaphylaxis. Children with a previous allergic reaction with β-lactam use who present an immediate and absolute need for penicillin therapy should be referred to an allergist-immunologist to perform skin testing to assess the risk of type I hypersensitivity. If these children demonstrate absence of immediate hypersensitivity skin test reactivity to major and minor determinants, they have less than a 1% risk of a subsequent anaphylaxis when challenged with penicillin. Positive skin test reaction to any of the penicillin determinants carries approximately a 70% risk of systemic reactions if the drug is administered subsequently. Children with positive skin test reactivity can undergo penicillin desensitization in order to minimize the risk of allergic reaction when given the drug. Patients with prior adverse reactions to β-lactam antibiotics that are consistent with the spectrum of immediate hypersensitivity events should be considered for alternative antibiotics.

REFERENCES

Barnes PJ: Pathophysiology of Allergic Inflammation, Page 356 in: Middleton E, et al (editors): *Allergy: Principles and Practice,* 5th ed. Mosby-Year Book, Inc., 1998.

Bochner BS: Cellular adhesion and its antagonism. J Allergy Clin Immunol 1997;100:581.

Charlesworth EN: Urticaria and angioedema: a clinical spectrum. Annals Allergy, Asthma Immunol 1996;76:484.

Costa JJ, Weller PF, Galli SJ: The cells of the allergic response. JAMA 1997;278(22):1815.

deShazo RD, Kemp SF: Allergic reactions to drugs and biologic agents. JAMA 1997;278(22):1895.

Eigenmann PA, et al: Prevalence of IgE-mediated food allergy among children with atopic dermatitis. Pediatrics 1998;01:463.

Leung DY: Molecular basis of allergic diseases. Molec Genet Metab 1998;63:157.

Naclerio RM, Solomon W: Rhinitis and inhalant allergens. JAMA 1997;278:1842.

Nicklas RA, et al: The diagnosis and management of anaphylaxis. Joint Task Force on Practice Parameters, American Academy of Allergy, Asthma and Immunology, and the Joint Council of Allergy, Asthma and Immunology. J Allergy Clin Immunol 1998;101:S465.

Norman P: Immunotherapy: Past and present. J Allergy Clin Immunol 1998;102:1.

Platts-Mills TA, al: Indoor allergens and asthma: report of the third international workshop. J Allergy Clin Immunol 1997; 100:S1.

Portnoy JM, et al: Stinging insect hypersensitivity: a practice parameter. J Allergy Clin Immunol 1999;103:963.

Sampson HA: Immediate Reactions to Food in Infants and Children. In: Metcalfe DD, Sampson HA, Simon RA (editors): *Food Allergy: Adverse Reactions to Foods and Food Additives,* 2nd ed. Science, 1997.

Slavin RG: Nasal polyps and sinusitis. JAMA 1997;278(22):1849.

Tovey E, Marks G: Methods and effectiveness of environmental control. J Allergy Clin Immunol 1999;103(2, Part 1):179.

Vercelli D, Geha RS: Control of immunoglobulin E synthesis. Page 72 in: Middleton E, et al (editors): *Allergy: Principles and Practice,* 5th ed. Mosby-Year Book, Inc., 1998.

Endocrinology

Stephen M. Rosenthal, MD, & Stephen E. Gitelman, MD

This chapter focuses on an approach to the evaluation and management of the most common pediatric endocrine disorders. In general, the diagnosis and management of specific disorders are presented within the context of broader discussions of common clinical presentations. When possible, algorithms are utilized to emphasize a logical clinical approach to these problems.

SHORT STATURE

Short stature may be defined as a height that is 2.5 SD or greater below the mean for age, or a height that is 2.5 SD or greater below the expected mean based on the child's midparental height (Table 19–1). In the latter case, a specialized chart is used to determine the appropriateness of the child's height in relation to that of the parents. Suboptimal growth, however, may be present without absolute short stature (e.g., an unexplained change in height from 1 SD above to 1 SD below the mean). This may become apparent when serial growth points or rates of growth over time are plotted on a linear growth chart or height velocity chart, respectively. A *subnormal growth rate* is defined as a height velocity less than the third percentile for age, or less than 4 cm per year at any time between 5 years of age and the onset of puberty. Growth charts for absolute height, height velocity, and comparison of absolute height with midparental height are widely available. It should be remembered, however, that the most commonly available growth charts have been derived from primarily white populations and may not be applicable to all ethnic groups.

Differential Diagnosis

The differential diagnosis of short stature is extensive and includes both nonendocrine and endocrine causes (Table 19–2). Short stature most often represents a normal variant (see later) or is a consequence of chronic, nonendocrine disease. An altered growth potential may also be seen with intrauterine growth retardation and in a large number of genetic syndromes. Hormonal causes of short stature are relatively less common.

NORMAL VARIANTS

The most common causes of short stature in the United States, **familial short stature** (i.e., short parents) and **constitutional growth delay**, are both normal variants. The hallmarks of constitutional delay in growth are summarized in Table 19–3. Such children are normal-sized at birth but then cross percentiles downward (on a cross-sectional growth curve) falling below the mean for absolute height and growth velocity during the first 2 to 3 years of life. These children exhibit a similar, although often less pronounced, pattern with respect to weight growth. Head growth, however, remains normal. This growth pattern appears to be an exaggeration of the normal shifting along growth curves that may occur during the first 2 years after birth. Subsequent height velocity is normal, although the timing of the onset of puberty and its associated linear growth spurt are often delayed. Children with constitutional growth delay typically achieve an adult height in the normal to low-normal range for their genetic potential. With the exception of a delayed bone age (an index for skeletal maturation), laboratory evaluations are unremarkable. The family history often reveals a similar pattern of delayed growth during early childhood or adolescence in one of the parents.

CHRONIC NONENDOCRINE DISEASE

Chronic nonendocrine disease is often associated with short stature (see Table 19–2). Occasionally, poor growth may be the first presenting sign. Abnormal metabolic demands or malnutrition are thought to contribute to growth failure in these situations.

HORMONAL CAUSES

Although children with short stature are often referred to an endocrinologist for evaluation, hormonal causes of growth failure are relatively rare. These include hypothyroidism of any etiology, growth hormone (GH) deficiency, glucocorticoid excess (whether from exogenous or endogenous sources), and poorly controlled diabetes mellitus. Hypothyroidism, hypercortisolism, and diabetes mellitus are discussed in subsequent sections of this chapter.

Growth hormone deficiency. The common clinical features of GH deficiency are summarized in Table 19–4. Children with congenital GH deficiency are of normal size at birth. However, after approximately 6 months of life, when linear growth becomes GH dependent, growth fail-

Table 19–1. Definition of Subnormal Growth

Height ≥ 2.5 SD below mean for age, OR
Height ≥ 2.5 SD below mean for that expected based on the midparental height, OR
Height velocity less than 3rd percentile for age, or <4 cm/year at anytime between 5 years of age and the onset of puberty

ure becomes apparent. Patients with GH deficiency have short stature associated with a pudgy, immature, doll-like appearance. Growth hormone also plays a significant role in glucose homeostasis through its effects on fat metabolism (lipolysis). Therefore, GH deficiency may be associ-

Table 19–2. Differential Diagnosis of Short Stature

Normal variants
Familial short stature
Constitutional growth delay
Chronic nonendocrine disease
Renal
Renal tubular acidosis
Chronic renal failure
Gastrointestinal
Inflammatory bowel disease
Malabsorption syndromes
Chronic liver disease
Cardiac
Congestive heart failure
Cyanotic heart disease
Pulmonary
Severe asthma
Cystic fibrosis
Hematologic
Hemoglobinopathies
Skeletal
Rickets
Osteochondrodystrophies
Pseudohypoparathyroidism
Pseudopseudohypoparathyroidism
Hormonal causes (see specific sections below):
Hypothyroidism
Growth hormone deficiency
Hypercortisolism
Poorly controlled diabetes mellitis
Other causes
Genetic/chromosomal syndromes (examples)
Turner syndrome, Down syndrome
Russell Silver syndrome, Prader-Willi syndrome
Primary skeletal dysplasias
Intrauterine growth retardation
Malnutrition

Table 19–3. Clinical Features of Constitutional Delay in Growth

Normal size at birth
Height velocity subnormal during first few years, then normalizes
Delayed adolescence
Delayed skeletal maturation
Final height normal to low-normal range for family
Family history often positive for constitutional delay

ated with severe hypoglycemia in addition to short stature, particularly in infancy. Uncomplicated GH deficiency is associated with a normal head circumference and normal intelligence.

The clinical characteristics of GH deficiency result from abnormalities of any of the components of the physiologic growth hormone axis. The secretion of GH from the anterior pituitary gland is regulated principally by the hypothalamic stimulatory factor GH-releasing hormone (GH-RH) and by the hypothalamic inhibitory factor somatostatin. Growth hormone secretion is influenced by a wide range of physiologic and metabolic processes, which are summarized in Table 19–5. In many cases, these processes exert their effects on GH secretion by influencing hypothalamic GH-RH or somatostatin. Growth hormone mediates its growth-promoting effects primarily through the generation and subsequent local and circulating action of insulin-like growth factors (IGFs), peptides that play a role in the growth and differentiation of a wide variety of tissues. The biologic effects of IGFs, which are mediated through specific cell-surface receptors, may be modified either positively or negatively by IGF-binding proteins.

Abnormalities that result in disruption of the GH physiologic axis are listed in Table 19–6. Most patients with GH deficiency (80 to 90%) are GH-RH deficient and are capable of secreting GH in response to exogenous GH-RH. A deficiency of GH may be isolated or

Table 19–4. Common Clinical Features of Congenital Growth Hormone Deficiency

Normal size at birth
Growth failure at or after 6 months of age, when linear growth becomes GH dependent
Excessive adiposity
Hypoglycemia in 10–20% of patients
Normal head circumference and normal intelligence in uncomplicated GH deficiency

GH = growth hormone.

Table 19–5. Factors that Influence Growth Hormone Secretion

Potentiating Factors	Inhibiting Factors
Exercise	Obesity
Sleep (stage III, IV)	Hyperglycemia
Stress	Hypothyroidism
Hypoglycemia	Glucocorticoid excess
Sex steroids	Increased β-adrenergic tone
Increased α-adrenergic tone	Psychosocial deprivation

associated with other hypothalamic and pituitary hormone abnormalities. It also may be associated with a wide variety of conditions, including breech delivery, midline developmental defect syndromes, intracranial tumors, infections, central nervous system (CNS) irradiation, and CNS trauma. Significant emotional deprivation may additionally be associated with transient GH deficiency.

OTHER CAUSES

Other causes of short stature include intrauterine growth retardation, malnutrition, and a large number of genetic and dysmorphic syndromes, including those associated with primary skeletal abnormalities. Short stature is seen in virtually all patients with Turner syndrome (gonadal dysgenesis), Down syndrome, Russell-Silver syndrome, and Prader-Willi syndrome, and in a variety of other conditions with or without associated chromosomal abnormalities. Primary skeletal abnormalities are often associated with abnormal body proportions, which become apparent with measurement of arm span and sitting height.

Table 19–6. Differential Diagnosis of Growth Hormone Deficiency

GH deficiency (80–90% are GH-RH deficient)
Isolated: idiopathic or genetic
Multiple hypothalamic and pituitary hormone deficiencies
Idiopathic, genetic
Associated with breech delivery or traumatic delivery
Associated with midline developmental defect syndromes
Intracranial tumors, infections, infiltrative or hemorrhagic processes
CNS irradiation, CNS trauma
Transient GH deficiency
Emotional deprivation
Abnormalities in GH signaling, IGF generation, or IGF signaling
Structurally abnormal GH

CNS = central nervous system; GH = growth hormone; IGF = insulin-like growth factor; RH = releasing hormone.

Evaluation

Components of the evaluation of children with short stature are given in Table 19–7. A thorough history, physical examination, and review of growth points and curves over time provide etiologic clues that are as important as the laboratory evaluation. The extent and direction of subsequent laboratory testing is guided by information obtained in the initial clinical assessment. The history should focus particular attention on perinatal events, growth patterns, a history of family-related or emotional problems, and final adult heights of family members. In addition to careful measurements of height (on a wall-mounted device), weight, and head circumference, particular attention should be given to body proportions, the presence or absence of dysmorphic features, and the genital and neurologic examinations.

An algorithm for the evaluation of short stature and/or subnormal height velocity is presented in Fig. 19–1. It is first important to determine whether chronic nonendocrine disease, malnutrition, or poorly controlled diabetes—each of which may be associated with suboptimal growth—is present. In the absence of these conditions, the evaluation is based on assessment of body proportions, height velocity, birth weight and gestational age, bone age (as a measurement of skeletal maturation), karyotype, and relative obesity.

Abnormal body proportions are often apparent by measurement of the sitting height and arm span (the latter normally closely approximates the standing height) and usually indicate a primary skeletal abnormality or disease and/or irradiation of the spine. For a discussion of the approach to children with disproportionate

Table 19–7. Evaluation of Children with Short Stature

Examination of growth charts
History and physical examination
Laboratory studies
Radiographic studies
Bone age
MRI if indicated by CNS symptoms or demonstration of hypothalamic/pituitary abnormality
Blood tests
General: CBC, ESR, chemistries
Hormonal: Free T$_4$, TSH, IGF-I, IGF-BP-3
Consider provocative GH testing
Consider evaluation of hypercortisolemia
Consider karyotype analysis

BD = binding protein; CBC = complete blood cell count; CNS = central nervous system; ESR = erythrocyte sedimentation rate; IGF = insulin-like growth factor; MRI = magnetic resonance imaging; T$_4$ = thyroxine; TSH = thyroid-stimulating hormone.

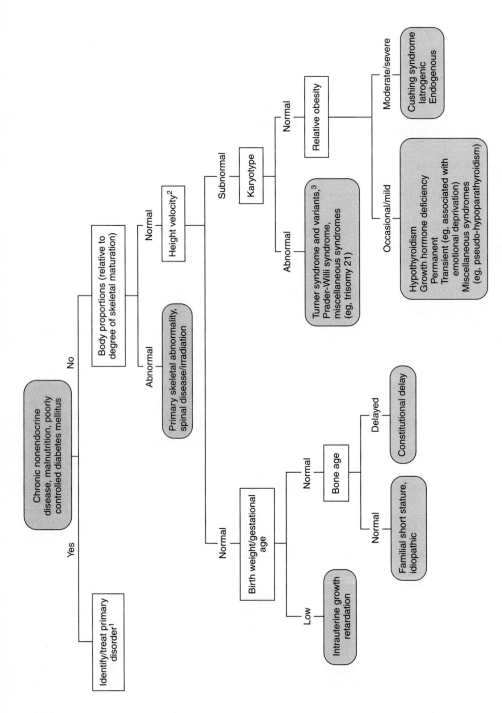

Figure 19–1. Approach to children with short stature (height >2.5 SD below the mean for chronologic age). [1]As short stature may be a primary manifestation of chronic nonendocrine disease before other signs or symptoms are apparent (e.g., certain gastrointestinal or renal disorders), generalized screening tests (e.g., complete blood cell count, or routine serum chemistries) are often considered useful to identify otherwise subtle chronic disease. [2]Height velocity in children with familial short stature is usually normal after 2 to 3 years of age. Height velocity in children with constitutional delay is usually normal after 3 to 4 years of age. [3]Girls with Turner syndrome may have some degree of intrauterine growth retardation and, in late childhood, may have abnormally immature body proportions secondary to greater retardation in growth of the legs. Height velocity is usually normal before 3 years of age and decelerates thereafter.

short stature, see Chap. 5, "An Approach to Clinical Genetics."

In children with short stature associated with normal body proportions, it is essential to evaluate the height velocity, preferably by serial measurements using the same wall-mounted device over a period of at least 4 to 6 months. In the absence of a history of intrauterine growth retardation, a normal height velocity will usually lead to a diagnosis of idiopathic short stature, familial short stature, or constitutional delay. Of note, height velocity in children with familial short stature or constitutional delay usually is subnormal before 3 to 4 years of age and normal thereafter. A delayed bone age distinguishes constitutional delay from familial or idiopathic short stature, although it is not uncommon for children to have a combination of familial short stature and constitutional delay.

Subnormal height velocity in children with normally proportioned short stature will often lead to a diagnosis of an endocrine disorder or one of a number of genetic syndromes. A karyotype analysis will identify girls with Turner syndrome and its variants, as well as a variety of other syndromes associated with short stature. In patients with subnormal height velocity and a normal karyotype, the presence and degree of obesity are often useful diagnostic indicators. Occasional or mild obesity in this context occurs in hypothyroidism, GH deficiency (permanent and transient forms), and miscellaneous syndromes (e.g., pseudohypoparathyroidism).

The diagnosis of GH deficiency is often difficult to make with a single blood test in view of the pulsatile nature of GH secretion. Levels of IGF-I and IGF binding protein-3 may serve as useful screening tests. If GH deficiency is suspected from the initial evaluation, standard provocative tests of GH secretion should be carried out. Moderate to severe obesity in patients with subnormal height velocity warrants an investigation for possible Cushing syndrome, including iatrogenic and endogenous causes (see section, "Endocrine Causes of Obesity" later).

Treatment

Appropriate treatment of short stature is directed at the specific etiology of the growth failure. Children with classic GH deficiency are treated with exogenous growth hormone. Commercial availability of recombinant human GH has led to many studies addressing its potential usefulness in non–GH-deficient short stature. Growth hormone may augment final height in girls with Turner syndrome and may be of benefit in other types of non–GH-deficient short stature, including children with chronic renal insufficiency. Growth hormone has been recently approved for use in children with Prader-Willi syndrome. There is some evidence that GH may also be of modest benefit to some children with idiopathic short

stature. The long-term risks and benefits of GH treatment in non–GH-deficient short stature are still being defined. In children whose GH deficiency is a result of inadequate GH-releasing hormone, short-term studies have demonstrated that treatment with GH-RH can induce GH secretion and improve growth rate.

ABNORMALITIES OF PUBERTY

Normal Physiology and Development

Puberty, the transitional period between the juvenile state and adulthood, is characterized by the attainment of secondary sex characteristics and, ultimately, reproductive capability. An overview of key pubertal events and their hormonal control is discussed below. Physical, cognitive, and psychological changes that characterize adolescence are discussed in more depth in Chap. 2, "Adolescence."

The physical changes that occur during puberty result from a marked increase in plasma gonadal sex steroid concentrations, which in turn result from pulsatile pituitary secretion of gonadotropins [luteinizing hormone (LH) and follicle-stimulating hormone (FSH)]. Gonadotropin secretion is a consequence of synchronous, pulsatile release of gonadotropin-releasing hormone (GnRH) from neurons in the medial basal hypothalamus.

Puberty is not a sudden event, but rather reflects a gradual maturation of the activity of the hypothalamic-pituitary-gonadal axis (Table 19–8). The hypothalamic-pituitary portal circulation is functional before the end of the first trimester of gestation, and the morphogenesis of the hypothalamic-pituitary gonadotropin unit is complete by midgestation. Subsequently, a characteristic pattern of activity emerges. Fetal gonadotropin secretion becomes pulsatile by midgestation and is initially unrestrained. At term, gonadotropin secretion is reduced to low levels, presumably secondary to the maturation of sex steroid negative feedback and other mechanisms. Shortly after birth, the GnRH neurosecretory neurons (referred to as a "pulse generator") are again highly active, concurrent with the withdrawal of maternal and placental sex steroids from the fetal environment. Late infancy and childhood are characterized by marked inhibition of pulsatile GnRH secretion. This restraint of the GnRH pulse generator is a consequence of both a highly sensitive sex steroid negative feedback mechanism and an as yet poorly defined CNS inhibitory mechanism. After a quiescent period of approximately 10 years, the GnRH pulse generator is disinhibited, ultimately leading to the attainment of clinical puberty. The hypothalamic-pituitary-gonadal axis is functionally intact in the prepubertal child as well as in the fetus. The CNS inhibitory mechanism is considered to be the rate-limiting factor controlling the onset of puberty.

Although temporally related to the maturation of the hypothalamic-pituitary-gonadal axis, *adrenarche* is an

Table 19–8. Ontogeny of the Hypothalamic-Pituitary Gonadotropin-Gonadal Unit

Fetus	**Late prepubertal/early pubertal period**
• GnRH detected in human fetal brain by 4.5 week gestation	• Disinhibition of GnRH pulse generator secondary to
• Hypothalamic/pituitary portal circulation intact by 11.5 week gestation	Decreased sensitivity of sex steroid negative feedback
• Morphogenesis of hypothalamic/pituitary gonadotropin unit complete by midgestation	Decreased effectiveness or a modification of CNS inhibitory mechanism
• GnRH/gonadotropin secretion	• Increased amplitude and frequency of GnRH pulses
Pulsatile at least by midgestation	• Increased amplitude and frequency of gonadotropin pulses; initially most prominent with sleep
Initially unrestrained	• Increased secretion of gonadal sex steroids
Decreases to low levels at term, presumably secondary to sex steroid negative feedback and other mechanisms	**Puberty**
Early infancy	• Progressive development of secondary sex characteristics
• GnRH pulse generator highly functional by second week	• Spermatogenesis in males
• Transient rise in gonadal sex steroids to midpubertal levels	• Development of estrogen-induced positive feedback mechanism and LH surge in females
Late infancy/childhood	• Ovulation in females
• Inhibition of GnRH pulse generator secondary to:	
Highly sensitive sex steroid negative feedback mechanism	
• Intrinsic CNS inhibitory mechanism	

CNS = central nervous system; GnRH = gonadotropin-releasing hormone; LH = luteinizing hormone.

independent developmental process that is clinically typified by mild androgenic effects such as a change in body odor and the appearance of pubic hair and acne. Adrenarche represents a poorly understood maturational process in the zona reticularis of the adrenal cortex, which results in enhanced secretion of the androgen dehydroepiandrosterone (DHEA) and its sulfated form [DHEA(S)]. An increase in circulating adrenal androgens begins at 5 to 6 years of age, and, approximately, 1 to 2 years later, clinical adrenarche is manifest.

The normal age of onset of secondary sexual characteristics (defined as 2.5 SD on either side of the mean or where approximately 99% of the population falls), is 6 to 13 years in girls and 9 to 14 years in boys. A study of American children demonstrated that 6% of African-American girls developed glandular breast tissue by 6 years of age, while 5% of white girls demonstrated breast development by 7 years of age. This study also showed that pubic hair development began in 10% of African-American girls by 6 years of age and in 2.8% of white girls by 7 years of age. Completion of secondary sexual development occurs an average of 4.2 years after its start for girls and 3.5 years for boys.

In the male, puberty begins with testicular enlargement (≥2.5 cm in maximum diameter) followed by the development of sexual hair and phallic enlargement (see Chap. 2, "Adolescence"). The growth spurt occurs during midpuberty; growth continues until there is full maturation and fusion of the growth centers in the long bones and spine. Laboratory evidence of puberty includes an increase in circulating testosterone to concentrations of >50 ng/dL associated with evidence of pulsatile gonadotropin secretion and a pubertal level increase in LH after an intravenous injection of synthetic GnRH.

In approximately 90% of girls, breast enlargement is the initial sign of secondary sexual development. Ten percent of girls demonstrate sexual hair as their initial secondary sexual characteristic. For girls, the growth spurt occurs early in puberty. Menarche is achieved near the end of puberty and is normally followed within 1 to 2 years by completion of linear growth. Laboratory evidence of puberty in girls includes a circulating estradiol level of >10 pg/mL associated with pulsatile gonadotropin secretion and a pubertal gonadotropin response to synthetic GnRH similar to that described earlier for boys.

Pubertal Delay

DEFINITION AND DIFFERENTIAL DIAGNOSIS

Delayed puberty may be defined, in boys, as the absence of testicular enlargement (above prepubertal size) by 14 years of age, and in girls, the absence of any breast development by 13 years of age. The differential diagnosis of delayed puberty comprises three major categories: constitutional delay in growth, hypogonadotropic hypogonadism, and hypergonadotropic hypogonadism (Table 19–9).

Constitutional delay in growth, the most common cause of delayed puberty, is a normal variant (see earlier, "Short Stature"). Such patients often have a family history of delayed puberty and have a delayed bone age but do not have evidence of endocrinopathy or other organic disease.

Table 19–9. Causes of Delayed Puberty

Constitutional delay in growth—normal variant
Hypogonadotropic hypogonadism—defect at level of hypothalamus/pituitary
- Isolated gonadotropin deficiency
  Kallmann syndrome
  In association with other syndromes that may include cleft palate, congenital deafness, X-linked form of congenital adrenal hypoplasia (can be associated with glycerol kinase deficiency and muscular dystrophy), Prader-Willi syndrome, Laurence-Moon-Biedl syndrome
- Multiple hypothalamic/pituitary hormone deficiencies
  Idiopathic
  CNS disorders: tumors (involving primarily third ventricular area), infection, trauma, other invasive disease, irradiation, congenital malformations
- Functional gonadotropin deficiency:
  chronic systemic disease and malnutrition, hypothyroidism, hypercortisolism, hyperprolactinemia, diabetes mellitus, anorexia nervosa, some female athletes and ballet dancers, marijuana use
Hypergonadotropic hypogonadism—defect at level of the gonads
- Primary testicular failure
  Klinefelter syndrome and its variants, anorchia and cryptorchidism, XY gonadal dysgenesis, Noonan syndrome, other causes
- Primary ovarian failure
  Turner syndrome and its variants, XX gonadal dysgenesis, other causes

---

CNS = central nervous system.

Hypogonadotropic hypogonadism may result from a variety of CNS disorders. A defect at the level of the hypothalamus or pituitary results in deficient GnRH or gonadotropin secretion, as measured by low basal LH and FSH values and the absence of an appropriate LH response to exogenous GnRH. Gonadotropin deficiency can be isolated, such as in Kallmann syndrome, or it may occur in association with multiple hypothalamic and pituitary hormone deficiencies. Kallmann syndrome is associated with anosmia or hyposmia and is transmitted in an X-linked or autosomal dominant fashion with variable penetrance. In addition to microphallus and undescended testes, this syndrome may be associated with renal aplasia and with skeletal and ocular anomalies. Causes of hypogonadotropic hypogonadism often associated with multiple hypothalamic and pituitary abnormalities include idiopathic, CNS tumors (primarily third ventricular), CNS infection, trauma, cranial irradiation, and congenital midline defect syndromes. A functional gonadotropin deficiency may occur in association with chronic systemic disease and malnutrition, hypothyroidism, hypercortisolism, hyperprolactinemia, diabetes mellitus, anorexia nervosa, and marijuana

use. It also may occur in some female athletes and ballet dancers. In general, weight loss to less than 80% of ideal weight may result in functional gonadotropin deficiency.

Hypergonadotropic hypogonadism indicates a defect at the level of the gonads, with serum concentrations of the gonadotropins, particularly FSH, elevated in children older than 10 years. Primary testicular failure is associated with Klinefelter syndrome (the XXY form of seminiferous tubule dysgenesis), XY gonadal dysgenesis, anorchia (associated with apparent testicular regression after fetal male differentiation), and cryptorchidism. It may also be seen after chemotherapy or local irradiation. Primary ovarian failure is most commonly found in patients with Turner syndrome (45X or in association with structural abnormalities of the X chromosome and mosaicism) and, less commonly, in XX gonadal dysgenesis. It may also occur in association with autoimmune disease.

EVALUATION

An algorithm for evaluating delayed puberty is presented in Figure 19–2. As part of the initial evaluation, basal gonadotropin levels (LH, FSH) should be measured. If these are elevated, patients have hypergonadotropic hypogonadism (primary ovarian or testicular failure). A karyotype analysis should then be performed to distinguish Turner or Klinefelter syndrome from other causes of primary hypogonadism associated with a normal chromosomal pattern. If basal plasma gonadotropin levels are low or normal, patients have either constitutional delay or hypogonadotropic hypogonadism. The demonstration of a pubertal LH response to an injection of synthetic GnRH will identify patients with constitutional delay; however, many patients with constitutional delay, when initially examined, will have a prepubertal LH response to GnRH indistinguishable from that seen in patients with hypogonadotropic hypogonadism. If hypogonadotropic hypogonadism is strongly suspected based on the history or physical examination, further evaluation to identify a specific associated etiology should be undertaken. Unless other clinical findings point to CNS abnormalities associated with hypogonadotropic hypogonadism or to a functional cause of gonadotropin deficiency, only prolonged clinical observation will distinguish constitutional delay from hypogonadotropic hypogonadism. Sexual maturation will become apparent on follow-up examinations in those with constitutional delay. Although the bone age is invariably delayed in all causes of delayed puberty and, therefore, is not diagnostically useful, the bone age may nevertheless be useful to determine the severity of the pubertal delay.

TREATMENT

Short-term hormonal therapy may be useful in constitutionally delayed adolescents, whereas long-term therapy is indicated in hypergonadotropic or hypogonadotropic hypogonadism. In addition to reassurance and observation,

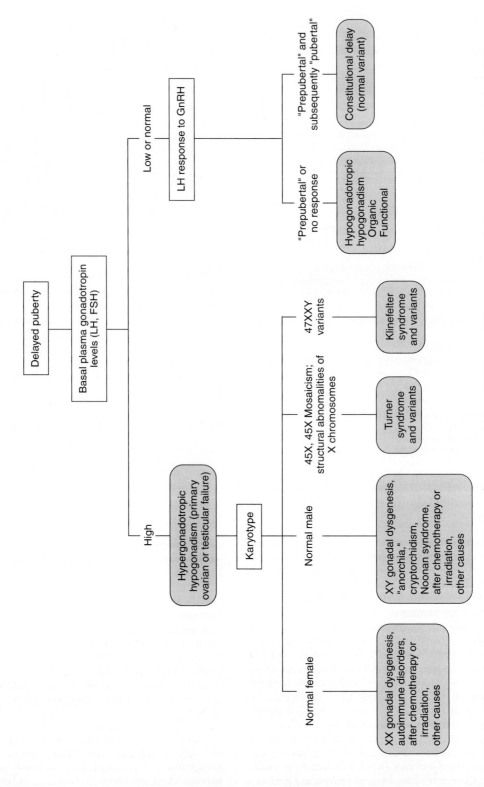

Figure 19–2. Approach to patients with delayed puberty. FSH = follicle-stimulating hormone; GnRH = gonadotropin-releasing hormone; LH = luteinizing hormone.

some adolescents with constitutional delay may benefit from a short course of testosterone enanthate (TE) for boys or conjugated estrogen or ethinyl estradiol for girls. Long-term hormonal therapy for boys with hyper- or hypogonadotropic hypogonadism includes monthly or semi-monthly injections of TE. Long-term hormonal therapy for girls includes the use of estrogen and progestin cycling in doses that sustain full development of secondary sexual characteristics, result in adequate withdrawal bleeding, and prevent osteoporosis.

Sexual Precocity

DEFINITION AND DIFFERENTIAL DIAGNOSIS

Sexual precocity is usually defined as the development of secondary sexual characteristics before 6 to 7 years of age in girls and before 9 years of age in boys. The differential diagnosis of precocious sexual development is extensive but conceptually straightforward. As sexual precocity results from an increase in circulating sex steroids, etiologic considerations may be divided into exogenous and endogenous sources for these steroids. Exogenous sources include estrogen-containing creams, birth control pills, and anabolic steroids. Endogenous sources include the gonads and the adrenal cortex, either of which may inappropriately secrete sex steroids as the result of a primary process intrinsic to these tissues or secondary to a circulating stimulating factor.

Endogenous feminizing sexual precocity in girls. The differential diagnosis for endogenous causes of feminizing sexual precocity in girls is summarized in Table 19–10. The most common form of early sexual development in girls is premature thelarche. *Premature thelarche* is the appearance of unilateral or bilateral breast tissue between infancy and early childhood. This condition is benign and is often associated with single or multiple ovarian follicular cysts. There are no other signs of puberty, such as increased growth velocity, vaginal mucosal thickening, or the appearance of pubic hair. These patients require close follow-up, with observation for other signs of sexual precocity. A pelvic ultrasound study may be considered to evaluate the ovaries, as well as uterine size and contour. No treatment is required.

Other primary ovarian processes include large ovarian cysts, which may be seen with McCune-Albright syndrome, and rare tumors. *McCune-Albright syndrome* is characterized by a clinical triad of irregularly shaped café-au-lait spots (Coast of Maine lesions), polyostotic fibrous dysplasia of long bones and skull, and sexual precocity (primary ovarian cysts). It may also be associated with other endocrine abnormalities.

Secondary ovarian processes occur in idiopathic true precocious puberty (the most common etiology of precocious puberty, especially in girls), CNS disease or injury, and after late treatment of congenital virilizing adrenal

Table 19–10. Sexual Precocity in Females: Endogenous Causes

Ovary
- Primary processes
  Premature thelarche/follicular ovarian cysts
  McCune-Albright syndrome: ovarian cysts associated with abnormal skin pigmentation and polyostotic fibrous dysplasia
  Tumors: granulosa or theca cell tumors, gonadoblastoma, lipoid tumors, ovarian carcinomas
- Secondary processes: precocious puberty
  Idiopathic
  CNS disease or injury: hamartoma of the tuber cinereum, tumors, subarachnoid cysts, congenital malformations, other invasive disease, infection, irradiation, severe trauma
  After late treatment of congenital virilizing adrenal hyperplasia

Adrenal gland
- Neoplasm

CNS = central nervous system.

hyperplasia (CVAH). Adrenal neoplasms are rarely the source of precocious feminization. In girls, ectopic secretion of human chorionic gonadotropin (hCG) will not by itself cause puberty.

Endogenous virilizing sexual precocity in girls. The endogenous causes of virilization in girls are summarized in Table 19–11. Primary adrenal processes include premature adrenarche, congenital virilizing adrenal hyperplasia (CVAH), and virilizing adrenal neoplasms. Premature adrenarche is the most common cause of premature pubic hair development, or pubarche. This is a benign condition without significant growth acceleration; no

Table 19–11. Endogenous Causes of Virilization in Females

Adrenal cortex
- Primary processes
  Premature adrenarche
  Congenital virilizing adrenal hyperplasia
    21-OH deficiency (P450$_{c21}$)
    11-OH deficiency (P450$_{c11}$)
    3β-Hydroxysteroid dehydrogenase deficiency
  Virilizing adrenal neoplasm
- Secondary process
  Cushing disease

Ovary
  Virilizing ovarian neoplasm

OH = hydroxylase.

other signs of pubertal changes are seen. It is caused by early maturation of the adrenocortical zona reticularis, resulting in mild-to-modest elevations of the principal adrenal androgens, DHEA and DHEA(S). Excessive corticotropin (ACTH) stimulation of the adrenal cortex in Cushing disease may result in virilization in addition to signs of glucocorticoid excess. Virilization may also result from ovarian neoplasms.

Endogenous sexual precocity in boys. The differential diagnosis for endogenous causes of sexual precocity in boys is summarized in Table 19–12. Primary adrenal processes include premature adrenarche, CVAH, and virilizing adrenal neoplasms. As noted previously, Cushing disease may result in virilization from increased adrenal androgens. Primary testicular processes are rare and include Leydig cell tumors, familial Leydig cell hyperplasia, and McCune-Albright syndrome. Secondary testicular processes resulting in sexual precocity include premature reactivation of the hypothalamic-pituitary-gonadal axis (true precocious puberty) and ectopic hCG-secreting tumors.

Endogenous feminization in male adolescents (gynecomastia) is associated with elevated estradiol-testosterone

ratios. This form of gynecomastia is common and is discussed further in Chap. 2, "Adolescence." Gynecomastia may also be seen in patients with Klinefelter syndrome and in those with partial androgen resistance.

EVALUATION OF CHILDREN WITH SEXUAL PRECOCITY

Evaluation of girls with precocious feminization. To evaluate precocious feminization in girls (Figure 19–3), one must first consider the possibility of an exogenous source of estrogens. A thorough history, physical examination, and review of growth data are essential to defining the clinical severity and rate of progression of the sexual precocity. The physical examination should especially focus on identifying the degree of breast development, the presence or absence of estrogen effects on the vaginal mucosa, and any concomitant androgen effects. A bone age examination is also useful. If the degree of feminizing sexual precocity is mild and the bone age is not advanced, patients most likely have premature thelarche, as discussed earlier, and require only observation. If the sexual precocity has progressed rapidly and the bone age is advanced, it would then be appropriate to carry out a GnRH stimulation test. A prepubertal response to GnRH indicates a primary ovarian process (e.g., large ovarian cyst or tumor) or, rarely, a feminizing adrenal neoplasm; imaging studies can be used for confirmation. A pubertal response to GnRH indicates precocious puberty and should be followed by a cranial magnetic resonance imaging (MRI) study to determine whether there is evidence of CNS disease, injury, or malformation.

Evaluation of girls with precocious virilization. To evaluate precocious virilization in girls (Figure 19–4), it is again important to begin by considering an exogenous source of androgens. In the absence of an exogenous source, the androgens causing precocious or excessive virilization are derived either from the adrenal cortex or from the ovaries. A bone age study should be obtained. If the bone age is not advanced, patients most likely have premature adrenarche (discussed earlier). Although usually associated with a nonadvanced bone age, girls with premature adrenarche can also have an advanced bone age. Girls with virilization and an advanced bone age should have an ACTH stimulation test during which plasma levels of androgens [DHEA, DHEA(S), androstenedione, and testosterone] and cortisol and its precursors (in particular, 17-OH-progesterone and 11-deoxycortisol) are measured just before and 60 min after an intravenous injection of ACTH. As indicated in the algorithm, the ACTH test results can be used to diagnose a variety of primary virilizing adrenal disorders. Markedly elevated DHEA(S) or testosterone levels before ACTH stimulation suggest the possibilities of a virilizing adrenal or ovarian neoplasm, respectively.

Evaluation of boys with precocious virilization. An algorithm for evaluation of virilizing sexual precocity in

Table 19–12. Sexual Precocity in Males: Endogenous Causes

Adrenal cortex
- Primary processes
  Premature adrenarche
  CVAH
     21-OH deficiency (P450$_{c21}$)
     11-OH deficiency (P450$_{c11}$)
  Virilizing adrenal neoplasm
- Secondary process
  Cushing disease

Testis
- Primary processes
  Leydig cell tumor
  Familial Leydig cell hyperplasia
  McCune-Albright syndrome
- Secondary process
  Precocious puberty
  Idiopathic
  CNS disease or injury: hamartoma of the tuber cinereum, tumors, subarachnoid cysts, congenital malformations, other invasive disease, infection, irradiation, severe trauma
  After late treatment of CVAH
  Ectopic hCG-secreting tumors

CNS = central nervous system; CVAH = congenital virilizing adrenal hyperplasia; hCG = human chorionic gonadotropin; OH = hydroxylase.

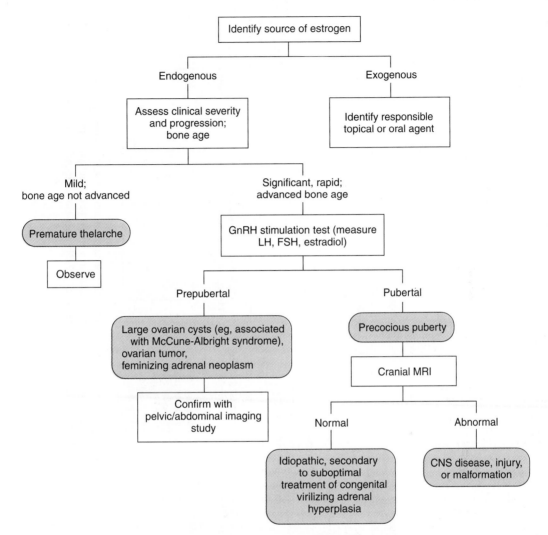

Figure 19–3. Approach to the evaluation of girls with feminizing sexual precocity. CNS = central nervous system; FSH = follicle-stimulating hormone; GnRH = gonadotropin-releasing hormone; LH = luteinizing hormone; MRI = magnetic resonance imaging.

boys is presented in Figure 19–5. If an exogenous source of androgens has been excluded, it would then be appropriate to proceed with an evaluation based on the testicular size. If the testes are enlarged, a GnRH stimulation test should be carried out. A pubertal response to GnRH indicates precocious puberty, and a cranial MRI study should be performed, as noted for girls with precocious puberty. If one or both testes are enlarged but the response to GnRH is prepubertal, patients either have a primary testicular process (e.g., familial Leydig cell hyperplasia, McCune-Albright syndrome, or Leydig cell tumor) or have an ectopic hCG-

secreting tumor. If the testes are not enlarged, a bone age study should be obtained. If the bone age is not advanced, patients most likely have premature adrenarche, which can be confirmed by measurement of DHEA and DHEA(S) levels. This benign condition requires observation only. As noted earlier, patients with premature adrenarche also may have a bone age that is significantly advanced. If the bone age is advanced, an ACTH stimulation test should be performed, as previously described, which will distinguish a variety of primary adrenal disorders.

(text continues on page 760)

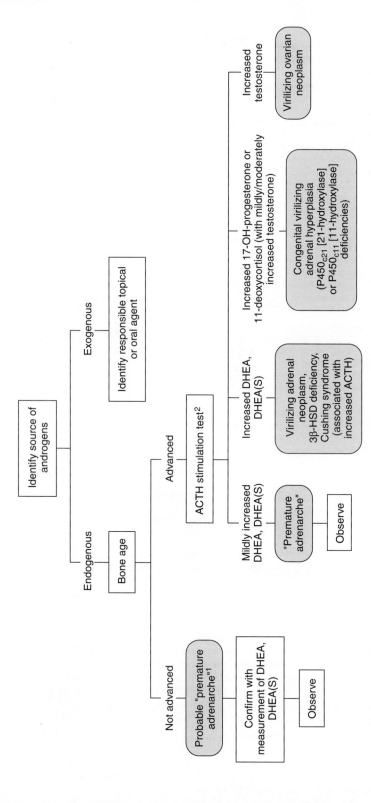

Figure 19–4. Approach to the evaluation of girls with virilizing sexual precocity. [1]Patients with premature adrenarche may have bone ages that range from not advanced to significantly advanced. [2]Adrenocorticotropic hormone (ACTH) test: Measures androgens—dehydroepiandrosterone (DHEA), DHEA sulfate [DHEA(S)], androstenedione, and testosterone—cortisol, and cortisol precursors—17-OH-progesterone and 11-deoxycortisol. 3β-HSD = 3β-hydroxysteroid dehydrogenase deficiency.

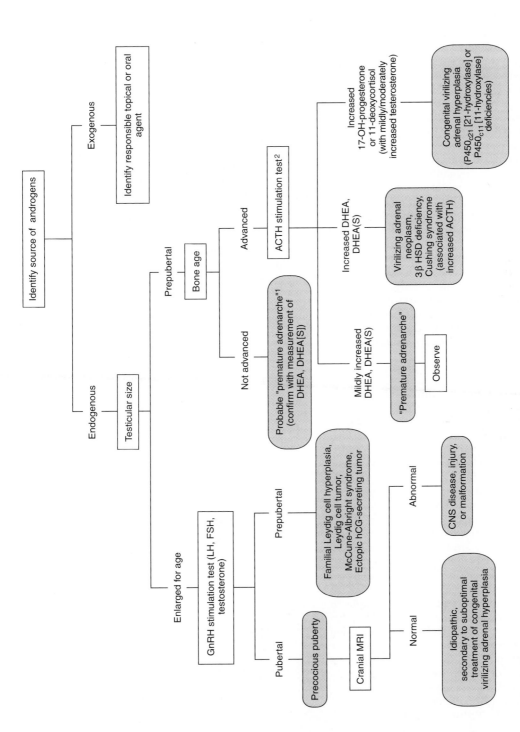

Figure 19–5. Approach to the evaluation of boys with virilizing sexual precocity. [1]Patients with premature adrenarche may have bone ages that range from not advanced to significantly advanced. [2]Adrenocorticotropic hormone (ACTH) test: Measures androgens—dehydroepiandrosterone (DHEA), DHEA sulfate [DHEA(S)], androstenedione, and testosterone—cortisol, and cortisol precursors—17-OH-progesterone and 11-deoxycortisol. CNS = central nervous system; MRI = magnetic resonance imaging; 3β HSD = 3β hydroxysteroid dehydrogenase deficiency.

TREATMENT OF SEXUAL PRECOCITY

The appropriate therapy for sexual precocity is directed toward the specific etiology. Treatment of idiopathic central precocious puberty is aimed at prevention of early epiphyseal fusion and adult short stature, as well as preventing premature menses in girls. The current approach for treatment of true precocious puberty is the use of a long-acting GnRH agonist. Gonadotropin-releasing hormone agonists desensitize the pituitary to endogenous GnRH stimulation, resulting in decreased gonadotropin secretion and, ultimately, decreased gonadal sex steroid secretion. These analogues are currently administered daily by subcutaneous or intranasal routes, or monthly in a depot form. Studies indicate that after such treatment, the normal pubertal process resumes, both hormonally and clinically. Long-term side effects of these agonists are still being evaluated. Medroxyprogesterone acetate, which has direct inhibitory effects on gonadal steroidogenesis, is useful in the rare disorders of familial Leydig cell hyperplasia and McCune-Albright syndrome. Testolactone, an aromatase inhibitor that blocks the conversion of androgen to estrogen, and ketoconazole, an inhibitor of several steps in both adrenal and gonadal steroidogenesis, have been used in nontumor primary gonadal causes of sexual precocity.

ENDOCRINE CAUSES OF OBESITY

Pediatric obesity is occurring with increased frequency in the United States and places many children at increased risk for significant immediate and future health problems. Most cases of pediatric obesity are caused by a combination of environmental and genetic factors, rather than an underlying organic disorder. Endocrine causes of obesity include Cushing syndrome, hypothyroidism, and GH deficiency. Typical exogenous obesity in children and adolescents is usually associated with a normal or above-average height velocity and stature. In contrast, endocrine causes of obesity are virtually always associated with subnormal height velocity and often short stature. Rarely, severe obesity may be caused by abnormalities in the regulation of appetite. Such entities include deficiency of leptin (a secreted peptide from adipocytes that mediates satiety in the hypothalamus), an abnormality of the leptin receptor, and/or an abnormality of the melanocortin-4 receptor. It is likely that additional genetic abnormalities of appetite regulation resulting in obesity will be discovered. While most obese patients do not have primary defects in leptin or leptin signaling, such patients often have elevated leptin levels indicating some degree of acquired leptin resistance.

An overall approach to children who are obese is provided in Chap. 1, "Pediatric Health Supervision." The clinical presentation, diagnosis, and management of hypothyroidism and GH deficiency are discussed elsewhere in this chapter. A discussion of Cushing syndrome follows.

Cushing Syndrome

DIFFERENTIAL DIAGNOSIS

Cushing syndrome results from exogenous or endogenous glucocorticoid excess. The differential diagnosis of Cushing syndrome is summarized in Table 19–13. Exogenous or iatrogenic glucocorticoid excess may occur in patients with adrenal insufficiency who receive overtreatment and in patients with a variety of disorders treated chronically with pharmacologic doses of glucocorticoids. Prolonged use of topical glucocorticoids may also result in Cushing syndrome.

Endogenous hypercortisolism is either ACTH dependent or ACTH independent. Of the ACTH-dependent causes, a pituitary adenoma (usually a microadenoma) is most common. In this condition, referred to as *Cushing disease,* individual ACTH levels may be only minimally or moderately elevated. However, these patients have loss of diurnal variation in ACTH secretion and thus, over the course of 24 h, have an overall increase in ACTH secretion. A less common ACTH-dependent cause of endogenous hypercortisolism is ectopic ACTH production, associated with oat cell carcinoma, carcinoid tumors, pancreatic islet cell tumors, neuroblastoma, pheochromocytomas, and other neoplasms. ACTH-independent causes result from increased glucocorticoid production in disorders of primary adrenocortical hyperfunction, including adenomas, carcinomas, and primary macronodular hyperplasia. Ectopic ACTH syndrome and ACTH-independent syndromes are less common than Cushing disease. Ectopic production of corticotropin-releasing hormone (CRH) is a rare cause of Cushing syndrome.

CLINICAL APPROACH

The characteristic clinical features of Cushing syndrome, arising from any etiology, are summarized in Table 19–14. Marked impairment of linear growth, often with some degree of truncal obesity, is one of the most important clinical signs of Cushing syndrome in the pediatric population and may be present long before other features commonly associated with this syndrome are noted.

Table 19–13. Differential Diagnosis of Cushing Syndrome

Exogenous/iatrogenic glucocorticoid excess
Endogenous hypercortisolism
ACTH-dependent
Pituitary ACTH-secreting adenoma (Cushing disease)
Ectopic ACTH production
Ectopic corticotropin-releasing hormone production
ACTH-independent
Primary adrenal hyperfunction

ACTH = adrenocorticotropic hormone.

Table 19–14. Clinical Features
of Cushing Syndrome

Growth: impaired linear growth; retardation of skeletal
  maturation
Habitus: "buffalo hump"; truncal obesity
Facies: rounding, plethora
Skin: thin; wide striae
Endocrine: some degree of insulin resistance and
  hyperglycemia
Other: weakness, fatigue; depression; hypertension

When hypercortisolism is suspected, iatrogenic causes must first be ruled out. An organized laboratory evaluation should subsequently be undertaken to document excessive cortisol levels, establish the etiology, and determine the appropriate treatment (Table 19–15). Hypercortisolism is first established by obtaining a 24-h urine collection for 17-hydroxycorticosteroids (17-OHCS) and free cortisol excretion. Urinary creatinine levels and total urinary volume should be measured to determine the adequacy of the collection. Baseline values of 17-OHCS or urinary free cortisol that exceed 2.5 SD above the mean for age-matched controls likely indicate hypercortisolism. A single, overnight dose of dexamethasone at 11:00 PM with subsequent measurement of plasma cortisol concentration at 8:00 AM has also been useful to distinguish patients with mild hypercortisolism (as may be seen in exogenous obesity, depression, or stress) from patients with true Cushing syndrome. With true Cushing syndrome, plasma cortisol will not suppress to <5 μg/dL during this test. One study indicates that a single, midnight serum cortisol value effectively distinguishes Cushing syndrome from pseudo-Cushing states (PCS). In this study, a midnight serum cortisol of >7.5 μg/dL correctly identified

Table 19–15. Laboratory Evaluation
of Hypercortisolism

- 24-h urine for 17-OHCS, free cortisol, creatinine
- Baseline AM, PM serum cortisol, ACTH (multiple samples) concentrations, including midnight sample
- Dexamethasone suppression test
- Overnight (limited value), OR
- Standard low- and high-dose test (more informative)
- Peripheral CRH stimulation test
- Consider bilateral inferior petrosal sinus sampling, pre-CRH and post-CRH, with simultaneous peripheral ACTH sampling
- MRI of hypothalamic and pituitary areas or of chest and abdomen

ACTH = adrenocorticotropic hormone; CRH = corticotropin-releasing hormone; MRI = magnetic resonance imaging; 17-OHCS = 17-hydroxycorticosteroids.

225 of 234 patients with Cushing syndrome and all patients with PCS. The sensitivity of this test (96%) was greater than that obtained for any other measure of serum or urine cortisol in making the correct diagnosis. The distinction between ACTH-independent and ACTH-dependent Cushing syndrome usually is straightforward, as plasma ACTH levels are low in the former and normal or elevated in the latter.

The principal challenge in the differential diagnosis of Cushing syndrome is differentiating Cushing disease (pituitary overproduction of ACTH) from ectopic ACTH production. For approximately 20 years, the standard approach has been to carry out a low- and high-dose dexamethasone suppression test. This test begins with a 2-day baseline period during which 24-hour urine collections are obtained for 17-OHCS, free cortisol, and creatinine; plasma is serially sampled in the morning and afternoon for cortisol and ACTH concentrations to determine whether the normal pattern of diurnal variation is present. Subsequently, low-dose dexamethasone (5 μg/kg every 6 h for 2 days) and then high-dose dexamethasone (20 μg/kg every 6 h for 2 days) are administered. Daily urine collection and plasma cortisol and ACTH sampling continue until 6 h after the last dose of dexamethasone. As with the overnight dexamethasone test, individuals with mild hypercortisolism secondary to exogenous obesity, depression, or stress suppress ACTH and cortisol levels with low-dose dexamethasone. Patients with pituitary adenomas may show some degree of suppression with low-dose dexamethasone and usually suppress significantly (>50%) with high-dose dexamethasone. In contrast, patients with ectopic ACTH production usually do not suppress with either low- or high-dose dexamethasone.

Unfortunately, the low- and high-dose dexamethasone suppression test does not always accurately distinguish Cushing disease from ectopic ACTH production. Of note, approximately 20% of patients with Cushing disease do not suppress with high-dose dexamethasone, whereas an equivalent percentage of patients with ectopic ACTH production suppress under similar conditions. Peripheral corticotropin-releasing hormone administration with measurement of plasma ACTH concentration in serial samples may help to distinguish some patients with pituitary adenomas from those with ectopic ACTH production. An MRI of the hypothalamic and pituitary areas should be obtained if Cushing disease is suspected, whereas chest and abdominal imaging studies should be obtained if ectopic ACTH production is a likely consideration.

TREATMENT

The treatment of choice for an ACTH-secreting pituitary adenoma is transphenoidal adenomectomy. Occasionally, findings on surgical exploration of the pituitary will be negative even when all laboratory studies indicate pituitary disease. Therapeutic options include repeated pituitary exploration, bilateral adrenalectomy, pituitary irradiation, and use of pharmacologic agents that directly impair cortisol synthesis and secretion.

APPROACH TO CHILDREN WITH AMBIGUOUS GENITALIA

Normal Sexual Differentiation

Although most infants are easily identifiable as male or female, some have ambiguous genitalia. The evaluation of children with ambiguous genitalia is founded on an understanding of the normal sexual differentiation process. Sexual differentiation occurs at three anatomic levels: gonads, genital ducts, and external genitalia. The fetus has the primordia of both male and female genital ducts; under normal circumstances, the bipotential fetal gonads become either testes or ovaries, and the bipotential external genitalia become those of either a normal male or female infant (Figure 19–6).

Sexual differentiation follows an orderly sequence that begins at approximately the sixth week of fetal life and is completed by the twelfth week (Table 19–16). The bipotential gonads in the male or female infant are initially indistinguishable. Under the influence of the testis-determining factor (TDF), the gonads begin testicular

Table 19–16. Sexual Differentiation

Gonad
- Bipotential
- Testicular differentiation at 6th–7th week of fetal life, SRY-dependent
- Ovarian differentiation occurs in the absence of SRY

Genital ducts
- Fetus has primordia of both male and female ducts by 7th week of gestation
- Male (wolffian) ducts: epididymis, vas deferens, seminal vesicles, ejaculatory ducts; testosterone-dependent
- Female (müllerian) ducts: fallopian tubes, uterus, cervix, upper third of vagina; develop in the absence of AMH

External genitalia
- Bipotential
- Differentiation occurs between 8th–12th week of fetal life
- Normal masculinization is DHT-dependent
- Inherent tendency to feminize with androgen deficiency or unresponsiveness

AMH = antimüllerian hormone; DHT = dihydrotestosterone; SRY = sex-determining region Y.

differentiation by 43 to 50 days of gestation. The TDF has been identified as a gene near the pseudoautosomal region of the Y chromosome. (*Pseudoautosomal* refers to a small region of homology between the X and Y chromosomes that allows pairing of the sex chromosomes during meiosis.) This gene, which encodes a DNA-binding protein, has been termed *sex-determining region Y (SRY)*. The SRY gene product is thought to function as a switch mechanism, initiating a cascade of events involving genes on the autosomes as well as on the X chromosome that ultimately results in testicular differentiation. Strong evidence that SRY is the TDF comes from studies in which transgenic female mice carrying and expressing the SRY gene develop as male mice. Thus, if SRY is present, the bipotential gonads become testes, with differentiation of Leydig cells, Sertoli cells, and, later, spermatogonia. In the absence of SRY, the bipotential gonads become ovaries.

Differentiation of the genital ducts is a direct consequence of gonadal differentiation. As noted earlier, the developing fetus has the primordia of both male and female genital ducts. If testes are present, testosterone from Leydig cells cause the male (or wolffian) ducts to develop into the epididymis, vas deferens, seminal vesicles, and ejaculatory ducts. Antimüllerian hormone (AMH), a dimeric glycoprotein secreted by Sertoli cells, prevents differentiation of the ipsilateral female (or müllerian) ducts into the fallopian tubes, uterus, cervix, and the upper third of the vagina. In the absence of testosterone and AMH (i.e., if an ovary or a nonfunctional testis is present), the male genital ducts involute, and the female genital ducts continue to develop.

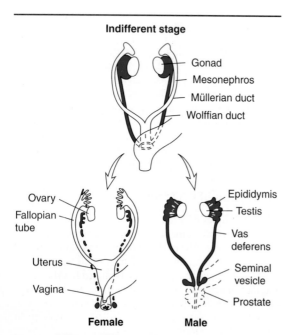

Indifferent stage

Gonad
Mesonephros
Müllerian duct
Wolffian duct

Ovary
Fallopian tube
Uterus
Vagina
Female

Epididymis
Testis
Vas deferens
Seminal vesicle
Prostate
Male

Figure 19–6. The differentiation of the internal genital ducts in males and females. (Reproduced with permission from Wilson JD, Foster DW [editors]: *Williams Textbook of Endocrinology.* Saunders, 1992, p 873.)

Differentiation of the bipotential external genitalia occurs between the eighth and twelfth weeks of gestation. Masculinization of the external genitalia and urogenital sinus results from the action of the androgen dihydrotestosterone (DHT). Testosterone is converted to DHT in the target tissues by the enzyme 5α-reductase. In the complete absence of DHT or of a normally functioning androgen receptor, the bipotential external genitalia feminize. If the DHT concentration or androgen receptor function is partially deficient in an otherwise normal male fetus, the external genitalia appear as intermediate between those of a male and female fetus, and thus ambiguous. Conversely, if inappropriately elevated androgen levels (which can be converted to DHT in the target tissues) are present in the developing female fetus, the external genitalia masculinize to varying degrees. There is, however, a critical period for androgen action on the external genitalia. After approximately the twelfth week of gestation, fusion of the labioscrotal folds to form a scrotum does not occur, no matter how intense the androgen stimulation. Phallic growth, however, does continue in response to androgen stimulation after the twelfth fetal week.

Differential Diagnosis of Ambiguous Genitalia

Infants with ambiguous external genitalia may generally be grouped into one of three categories: female pseudohermaphroditism, male pseudohermaphroditism, and true hermaphroditism.

Female Pseudohermaphrodites

Female pseudohermaphrodites are individuals with a 46XX karyotype, normal ovaries, and normal female genital ducts but with ambiguous external genitalia. Ambiguous external genitalia in these individuals is either a consequence of inappropriate androgen stimulation or is associated with non–androgen-induced structural malformations of the intestine and urinary tract. If the pseudohermaphroditism results from excess androgens, the source is either fetal or maternal. Fetal sources are essentially limited to the adrenal cortex and usually ensue from one of three virilizing forms of congenital adrenal hyperplasia (see later). These include, most commonly, a deficiency of $P450_{c21}$ 21-hydroxylase with or without salt loss and, less often, a deficiency of $P450_{c11}$ (11-hydroxylase) or 3β-hydroxysteroid dehydrogenase (3β-HSD or 3β-OL). Rarely, female pseudohermaphroditism results from fetal and placental aromatase deficiency, in which the placenta is unable to aromatize androgens to estrogens. This defect leads to an accumulation of androgens in the fetal and maternal circulations, resulting in virilization of the fetus' external genitalia and temporary virilization in the mother (which regresses after the pregnancy). Potential maternal sources include androgens or synthetic progestins with androgenic activity transferred from the maternal circulation.

Unclassified forms of abnormal sexual development also occur in females and are associated with absence or anomalous development of the uterus, fallopian tubes, and vagina. A uterus is present in all other instances of female pseudohermaphroditism previously noted.

Male Pseudohermaphrodites

Male pseudohermaphrodites are individuals with a 46XY karyotype (rarely, XO/XY mosaicism) whose gonads are testes but who have ambiguous external genitalia. Ambiguity of the external genitalia in these individuals results from deficient DHT or response to androgens. DHT deficiency may arise from several causes, including testicular unresponsiveness to hCG/LH, an inborn error in testosterone biosynthesis, deficient 5α-reductase activity, and various forms of dysgenetic testes. Deficient androgen responsiveness results from androgen receptor or postreceptor defects. In these individuals, male genital duct development is variable.

Unclassified forms of male pseudohermaphroditism also exist. Hypospadias occurs as an isolated finding in 1/700 male newborns and usually does not appear to be associated with either androgen deficiency or unresponsiveness. Rarely, ambiguous external genitalia can occur in XY male newborns without obvious explanation in association with multiple congenital anomalies.

True Hermaphrodites

True hermaphroditism is a condition in which individuals have both ovarian and testicular tissue and usually have ambiguous external genitalia. Some degree of uterine development is present in all cases. Most true hermaphrodites have a 46XX karyotype, and a minority have either 46XY or sex chromosome mosaicism or chimerism. If all forms of male and female pseudohermaphroditism have been excluded in the work-up of ambiguous genitalia, true hermaphroditism should be evaluated by histologic examination of the gonadal tissue.

Evaluation of Children with Ambiguous Genitalia

An approach to the evaluation of infants with ambiguous genitalia is summarized in Figure 19–7. A number of clinical clues assist in narrowing the differential diagnosis. The presence of palpable gonads in the external genitalia or inguinal area indicates the presence of testes (or, rarely, an ovotestis) and thus a karyotype that most likely will be 46XY. Another useful point is that, with the possible exception of patients with dysgenetic testes, all other patients with male pseudohermaphroditism produce antimüllerian hormone and thus will not have a uterus. Therefore, if no gonads are palpated and a pelvic ultrasound study reveals a uterus, these infants

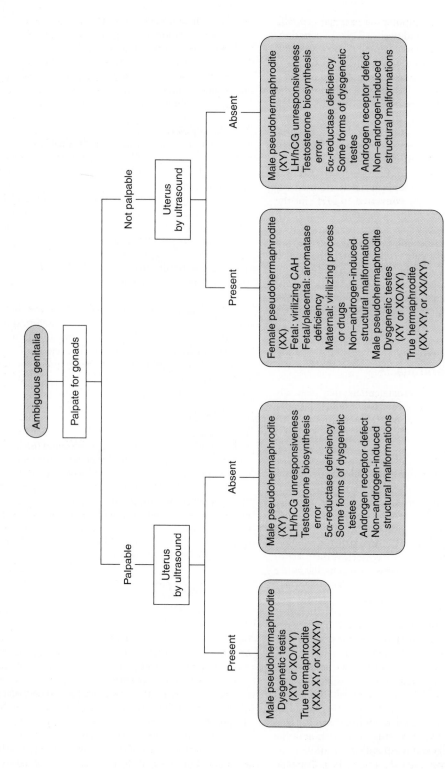

Figure 19–7. An approach to the initial evaluation of infants with ambiguous genitalia. A karyotype and Barr body test should also be performed. Additional studies are guided by initial grouping and other clinical features. CAH = congenital adrenal hyperplasia; hCG = human chorionic gonadotropin; LH = luteinizing hormone.

probably have female pseudohermaphroditism. While awaiting the results of karyotyping, one can perform the Barr body analysis of cells from the buccal mucosa on the first postnatal day. This will reveal a sex chromatin body corresponding to a partially inactivated X chromosome in 20 to 30% of the nuclei of 46XX interphase cells (or cells in which two or more X chromosomes are present). In normal 46XY male infants, the sex chromatin body is absent. Using this approach, the clinician can determine relatively quickly whether the infants are male or female pseudohermaphrodite. For example, individuals with ambiguous genitalia who have no palpable gonads, have a uterus by ultrasound, and have a positive Barr body analysis most likely are female pseudohermaphrodites, which is most commonly secondary to deficiency of P450$_{c21}$.

Management of Children with Ambiguous Genitalia

The birth of a child with ambiguous genitalia may not only represent a medical emergency, particularly if there is underlying congenital adrenal hyperplasia with associated adrenal insufficiency, but also an immediate psychosocial emergency. The usual first question asked by parents and family of a newborn is the child's sex. If the gender is not readily identifiable, this presents immediate difficulties for the family. The family must cope not only with the notion of having a child with a physical malformation, but also with the question of what to tell other relatives and friends. What health care providers communicate to the parents in the first few hours of life can have a crucial effect on the parents' future relationship with the child.

The parents should be allowed to see the infant's genitalia with the physician so that they can understand the problem and ask questions. It is helpful to describe the problem as either "overdevelopment" or "under-development," rather than "something in between." Parents should be reassured that urgent investigations will establish the child to be definitely male or female. They should be advised to postpone giving the child a name and not to complete the birth certificate until a final decision has been made regarding the child's sex of rearing.

If it is established that the infant is a female pseudo-hermaphrodite, hormonal studies to evaluate whether excess androgens are present can be carried out, with results available often within 1 week. Determining the particular cause of male pseudohermaphroditism often requires a longer period, particularly if one embarks on a trial of testosterone treatment to determine androgen responsiveness.

Management issues in the infant with ambiguous genitalia are complex, involving not only diagnostic considerations, but also an assessment of which sex for rearing is most compatible with a well-adjusted life and sexual adequacy. Female pseudohermaphrodites who have in-born errors of cortisol and aldosterone biosynthesis can be treated with hormonal replacement and with surgical repair of the external genitalia. Female pseudohermaphro-dites usually are fertile. In contrast, virtually all patients with male pseudohermaphroditism are infertile. Issues surrounding surgical repair of the external genitalia are complex. Some health care providers advocate deferring consideration of potential surgery in some instances until the affected child is old enough to participate in this decision.

THYROID GLAND

The thyroid gland produces the thyroid hormones thyroxine (T_4) and triiodothyronine (T_3), which regulate the rate of metabolism in virtually all tissues. These hormones mediate the rate of growth and development, oxygen consumption and heat production, neural development, erythropoiesis, respiratory drive, skeletal maturation, and many other processes.

Physiology and Assessment of Function

The thyroid gland forms as an invagination of endoderm at the base of the tongue during the first trimester of pregnancy and then descends along the midline to its final position anterior to the second to fourth tracheal cartilage rings. Integration of the thyroid axis proceeds during the second to third trimesters and results in a classic negative feedback loop between hypothalamus, pituitary, and thyroid gland (Figure 19–8).

Thyroid function may be evaluated through a series of different laboratory studies. Unlike many hormones, thyroxine (T_4) exists at a relatively constant level in the blood, and may be measured reliably at any time of day. T_4 is primarily bound to serum proteins such as thyroid binding globulin, with <0.1% existing as free hormone. The level of total T_4 changes dramatically from the newborn period until adulthood, primarily as the level of binding proteins change, and one must be careful to use age-matched normative data in assessing any T_4 level (Table 19–17). An indirect estimate of free T_4 (which attempts to correct for deviations in thyroid-binding proteins) can be obtained by multiplying the total T_4 by the T_3 resin uptake (a measure of the ratio of bound to free hormone). This product is referred to as the free thyroxine index (FTI). However, many laboratories now offer only a free T_4 measurement, which is more constant over time, and in general has simplified the evaluation of thyroid hormone levels. With such an assay, one no longer needs to be concerned with variations in binding proteins such as thyroxine-binding globulin. A simultaneous TSH level will help the clinician assess the thyroid hormone axis (see Figure 19–8). The current assay is quite sensitive: elevations in TSH indicate inadequate T_4 production by the thyroid gland, and suppression of TSH suggests overproduction of T_4. In most

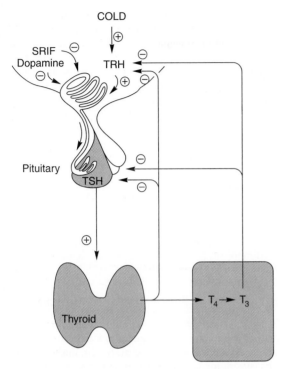

Figure 19–8. Feedback control of the thyroid gland. Plus sign indicates positive feedback, and minus sign indicates negative feedback. SRIF = somatostatin; T_3 = triiodothyronine; T_4 = thyroxine; TRH = thyroid-releasing hormone; TSH = thyroid-stimulating hormone. [Reproduced and adapted with permission from Fisher DA: in Kaplan SA (editor): *Clinical Pediatric Endocrinology*, 2d ed. Saunders, 1990, p 90.]

laboratories, TSH normal ranges also change over time, with values up to 8 μU/mL considered normal in the first year of life, and then decreasing to lower ranges thereafter. In rare situations, one may need to measure triiodothyronine (T_3), the bioactive form of thyroid hormone, or reverse triiodothyronine (rT_3), an inactive thyroid hormone metabolite. T_3 is formed primarily via peripheral metabolism of T_4 and is usually maintained in the normal range, even with profound hypothyroidism. There are also instances of hyperthyroidism in which T_4 is normal, but T_3 is elevated. Low T_3 and increased reverse T_3 are seen in the sick euthyroid syndrome where severe illness causes abnormalities in the thyroid hormone levels in the absence of intrinsic thyroid disease. Thyroid autoantibodies help determine the cause for underlying thyroid dysfunction, with thyroglobulin and thyroperoxidase antibodies often present in Hashimoto thyroiditis, and thyroid-

stimulating immunoglobulin found in Graves disease (discussed later). Imaging studies, either ultrasound or nuclear medicine scans with ^{123}I or ^{99m}Tc-pertechnetate, are used to delineate problems with thyroid gland structure and function.

Clinical Presentations of Thyroid Problems

Problems with thyroid gland hypo- or hyperfunction are relatively common and may occur at any time of life. The signs and symptoms of **hyperthyroidism** and **hypothyroidism** may arise insidiously and are often nonspecific (Tables 19–18 and 19–19). Potential causes of hypo- and hyperthyroidism are listed in Tables 19–20 and 19–21.

Hypothyroidism in the newborn period usually comes to medical attention after routine neonatal screening, at which time the child may be asymptomatic. Perturbations in thyroid hormone secretion later in life may be detected through clinical symptoms but often present with enlargement of the entire thyroid gland, termed *goiter,* or with single isolated masses within the gland. These problems are discussed in the sections that follow.

Hypothyroidism in the Neonate

A defect in the thyroid axis is one of the most common inborn errors of metabolism, with a frequency of 1/4000. Potential signs and symptoms of thyroid hormone deficiency are listed in Table 19–18. However, even the most astute clinician has trouble detecting an affected infant early in life, as many of the findings are nonspecific and subtle, and the infant may be asymptomatic early in life.

Despite mild or even no initial symptoms, the consequence of delayed treatment of congenital hypothyroidism is permanent mental retardation. As a result, most industrialized countries have instituted a neonatal screening program with the goal of detecting problems and initiating thyroid hormone replacement in infants early in life so as to prevent neurologic deficits. Blood is collected on a piece of filter paper at 24 h of age or later and sent to a central laboratory. In many North American laboratories, the screening strategy begins with a T_4 measurement. If this is in the lowest tenth percentile for the day, a thyroid-stimulating hormone (TSH) assay is subsequently performed. Some laboratories now start with a TSH assay, reporting an absolute value >20 μU/mL as abnormal. The physician is notified and then further diagnostic evaluation is pursued. This approach is designed to detect those infants with a defect in the thyroid gland itself, that is, primary hypothyroidism, but not those with a defect in the pituitary or hypothalamus (secondary and tertiary levels, respectively). These latter defects are much rarer, occurring in about 1 in 100,000 infants. In addition, sec-

Table 19–17. Normal Range for Serum Thyroxine (T_4) Concentrations in Infancy and Childhood

	Free T_4 ng/dL range	Total T_4 µg/dL mean and (Range)	TSH µU/mL
Cord blood		10.2 (7.4–13)	
1–3 Days	2.2–5.3	17.2 (11.8–22.6)	1–39
1–2 Weeks		13.2 (9.8–16.6)	
2–4 Weeks	0.9–2.3	11.0 (7.0–15)	1.7–9.1
1–4 Months	0.9–2.3 (until 6 months)	10.3 (7.2–14.4)	1.7–9.1 (until 6 months)
4–12 Months	0.8–2.1 (until 2 years)	11.0 (7.8–16.5)	0.8–8.2 (until 2 years)
1–5 Years	0.8–2.1 (2–7 years)	10.5 (7.3–15)	0.7–5.7 (2–7 years)
5–10 Years	0.8–2.1	9.3 (6.4–13.3)	0.7–5.7
10–15 Years	0.8–2.1	8.1 (5.6–11.7)	0.7–5.7
Adult	0.9–2.5	8.4 (4.3–12.5)	0.4–4.2

Reprinted with permission from Nelson JC, Clark SJ, Borut DL, et al. J Pediatr 123:899–905, 1993.

ondary and tertiary hypothyroidism usually occurs in conjunction with other CNS anomalies or midline defects. Therefore, the physician should already have been alerted to the potential of thyroid hormone deficiency in these children.

Table 19–18. Signs and Symptoms Associated with Hypothyroidism

In the Neonate
Lethargy
Hypotonia
Constipation
Umbilical hernia
Prolonged jaundice
Characteristic facies with enlarged, protruding tongue
Hoarse cry
Feeding problems
Enlarged fontanelles
Hypothermia

In the Child and Adolescent
Decreased height velocity
Increased weight gain
Cold intolerance
Constipation
Deteriorating school performance
Goiter
Delayed adolescence
Galactorrhea
Scaling skin, hair loss
Puffiness
Delayed dentition
Delayed relaxation phase of reflexes
Lethargy

Approach to an abnormal neonatal screen. An approach to the infants with an abnormal newborn thyroid screen is outlined in Figure 19–9. One should see the child as soon as possible to perform a complete history and physical examination and to repeat the T_4 and TSH assays to verify a diagnosis of hypothyroidism. If the screening test was done when the child was younger than 24 h of age, a false-positive result may occur because of the physiologic neonatal TSH surge. Early hospital discharges of newborns now account for up to 5 false-positive results for every true case of congenital hypothyroidism.

The history may suggest the etiology of the abnormal screening result. If the mother has a history of autoimmune thyroiditis, maternal IgG directed against the thyroid gland could have crossed the placenta and disrupted neonatal thyroid hormone production. In addition, if the mother has Graves disease, thionamides (such as propylthiouracil) used to block thyroid hormone synthesis, may cross the placenta and block neonatal thyroid hormone production. Finally, a family history of recurrent hypothyroidism may suggest either

Table 19–19. Signs and Symptoms of Hyperthyroidism

Diaphoresis	Increased systolic blood
Emotional lability	pressure, with widened
Fatigue	pulse pressure
Goiter	Tachycardia
Heat intolerance	Proptosis
Increased appetite	Lid lag
Weight loss	Tremor
Acceleration in growth rate	Restlessness
Frequent stools	

Table 19–20. Causes of Hypothyroidism

Congenital
  Dysgenesis
    Hypoplasia or aplasia ectopic
  In-born errors in thyroid hormone synthesis or action
    (resistance syndrome)
  Maternal ingestion of goitrogens or drugs
  Maternal antibodies crossing placenta
  Hypothalamic/pituitary deficiency

Acquired
  Chronic lymphocytic thyroiditis (Hashimoto)
  Endemic goiter, usually secondary to iodine deficiency
  Exposure to goitrogenic agents
  Hypothalamic/pituitary deficiency
  Iatrogenic, following radiation, surgery, or antithyroid
    drugs

Table 19–21. Causes of Hyperthyroidism in Children

TSH Independent
  Graves disease (diffuse toxic goiter)
  Hyperfunctioning adenoma (toxic adenoma) or carcinoma
  Toxic multinodular goiter
  McCune-Albright syndrome (Gsα-activating mutation)
  TSH receptor activating mutation
  Destruction, acute phase
    Subacute thyroiditis, Hashimoto thyroiditis

TSH-dependent
  TSH producing pituitary adenoma

Exogenous thyroxine

TSH = thyroid-stimulating hormone.

an autoantibody-mediated process or an inborn error in thyroid hormone synthesis, transmitted as an autosomal recessive trait.

All infants with abnormal thyroid function tests on follow-up should undergo an imaging study, if possible, with either ultrasonography or radionucleotide imaging. If no gland is visualized by ultrasonography, or if the gland is ectopic (superior to its expected location), the children will have permanent primary hypothyroidism

and will need to receive therapy for life. A normal-appearing gland in the usual location may indicate the presence of a TSH receptor defect, a TSH-receptor-blocking antibody (which may be detectable by an additional serum study and would constitute a transient defect), or a defect in thyroid hormone synthesis, either as a permanent inherited enzymatic defect or as a transient defect from exogenous drugs. Because a reliable ultrasound study is dependent on the experience of the

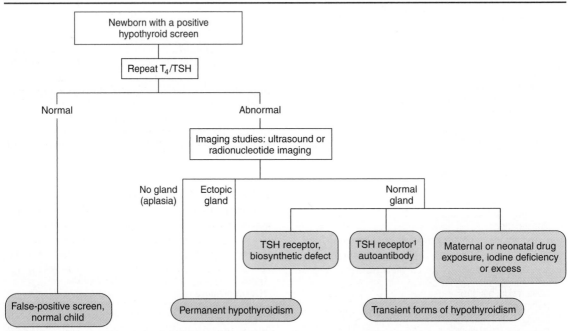

Figure 19–9. Approach to newborns with a positive screening test for hypothyroidism.[1] May also cause permanent hypothyroidism. T_4 = thyroxine; TSH = thyroid-stimulating hormone.

sonographer, many clinicians prefer to use a radionuclide scan for such evaluations. Furthermore, sonography provides only anatomic information about the thyroid gland, whereas a scan with either ^{123}I or technetium may reveal additional insight into gland function.

A bone age obtained from the distal femur and proximal tibia may be helpful in the management of neonates. The degree of impairment in skeletal maturation has been correlated with severity of congenital hypothyroidism and with eventual neurologic outcome.

Treatment of congenital hypothyroidism. Thyroid hormone replacement therapy should begin as soon as the diagnosis of hypothyroidism has been confirmed. It has been estimated that if congenital hypothyroidism is untreated, such infants may lose up to 5 IQ points monthly during the first year of life. Thus, their initial evaluation should be completed within 2 to 5 days, and treatment should not be delayed if the ancillary studies, such as thyroid imaging, cannot be immediately obtained.

The goal of therapy is to normalize serum T_4 concentrations as rapidly as possible. To ensure adequate replacement, the T_4 level is maintained in the upper half of the normal range. The initial dose is 10 to 15 μg/kg/day. With such therapy, growth and development of these infants is normalized. Long-term neurologic assessment suggests that aggressive and early thyroxine replacement results in normal outcomes, even in those infants with the most severe forms of congenital hypothyroidism. Infants who are thought to have a transient form of hypothyroidism usually receive treatment for 3 to 4 years to ensure normal neurologic development. At the end of that time, the children are given a trial period of several weeks without thyroid hormone replacement. If their TSH and T_4 levels remain within the normal range, they are considered to have had a transient condition.

Thyroid Mass

Up to 5% of school-aged children have enlargement of their thyroid glands. In the initial evaluation, the principal issue is to determine whether the neck mass is actually part of the thyroid gland or potentially one of many other neck structures. Possibilities include lymph nodes or branchial cleft cyst if the mass is lateral. Midline masses include an ectopic thyroid gland that failed to migrate far enough inferiorly to its proper location. Another possibility is a thyroglossal duct cyst, a fluid-filled remnant of the tract along which the thyroid gland descended from the base of the tongue. Both an ectopic gland and thyroglossal duct cyst will rise upon swallowing. With an ectopic gland, a normal thyroid gland will not be detected inferiorly. The distinction between gland and cyst can be made definitively with an imaging study, again by either ultrasonography or a radionuclide scan.

The thyroid mass should be characterized as either symmetric enlargement of the gland, termed *goiter,* or a separate nodule or nodules within the gland. These possibilities are discussed in the following section.

Goiter. There are several possible causes for a goiter. The differential diagnosis can be significantly narrowed by performing a thorough history, physical examination, and laboratory assessment of the patient's thyroid status (Fig. 19–10). Patients may be euthyroid or have the signs and symptoms of hyper- or hypothyoidism (see signs and symptoms in Tables 19–18 and 19–19). Thyroid function tests should be obtained in all patients with thyroid gland enlargement.

Euthyroid goiter. Patients with clinical and biochemical evidence of euthyroidism have two primary etiologies for goiter. *Hashimoto thyroiditis,* or *chronic lymphocytic thyroiditis,* is an autoimmune disorder in which the gland is infiltrated by lymphocytes. These patients often have autoantibodies directed against thyroglobulin and thyroid hormone peroxidase (previously referred to as antimicrosomal antibody). There is a female predominance with autoimmune thyroid disorders, as well as a higher incidence in the Asian population. Patients may have either euthyroidism or hypothyroidism (see later). The second possibility is simple colloid goiter, also known as nontoxic goiter. It may present in similar fashion to Hashimoto thyroiditis but is always associated with normal thyroid function tests, and there is no evidence of the autoantibodies associated with Hashimoto thyroiditis. Although the thyroid gland usually is symmetrically enlarged in both these conditions, some patients may have solid or cystic nodules (see later).

Goiter with hypothyroidism. These individuals may have either compensated primary hypothyroidism, in which T_4 concentration is normal but TSH level is elevated, or frank hypothyroidism, in which the elevated TSH is unable to maintain T_4 concentration in the normal range. Most of these patients have Hashimoto thyroiditis. Other considerations include mild cases of inborn errors in thyroid hormone biosynthesis, treatment with drugs that block thyroid hormone biosynthesis, or dietary ingestion of substances that also cause such a phenomenon (termed *goitrogens*). Worldwide, iodine deficiency is one of the most common reasons for such a presentation. However, iodine supplementation makes this consideration extremely rare in the United States. An unusual pattern may also be encountered with thyroid hormone resistance, secondary to a defect in the thyroid hormone receptor. Such patients appear clinically hypothyroid, with an elevation in both T_4 and TSH.

Goiter with hyperthyroidism. If patients have a goiter and signs and symptoms of hyperthyroidism, then the diagnosis is usually *Graves disease.* This autoimmune disorder results from autoantibodies directed against the TSH receptor, termed *thyroid-stimulating immunoglobulins*

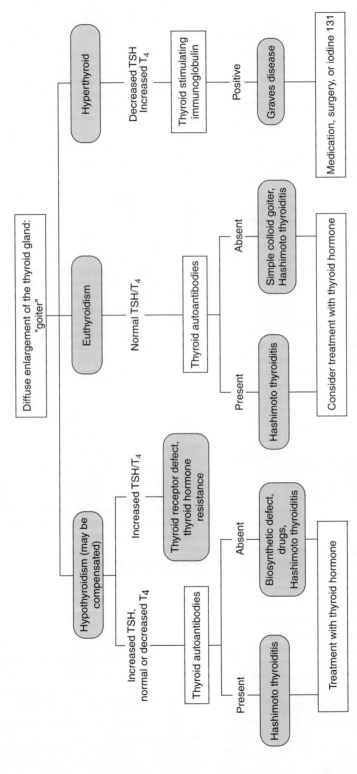

Figure 19–10. Approach to patients with goiters. Note that serum autoantibodies do not detect all patients with an underlying diagnosis of Hashimoto thyroiditis; therefore, a negative autoantibody study does not rule out this condition. The autoantibodies present with Hashimoto thyroiditis also may be detected in Graves disease, but patients with this disorder frequently have thyroid stimulating immunoglobulin as well. T_4 = thyroxine; TSH = thyroid-stimulating hormone.

(TSI), resulting in autonomous production of thyroxine. Thus, T_4 levels are elevated, and TSH is suppressed. These patients may also have a mixture of thyroglobulin and peroxisomal autoantibodies as well, and Hashimoto and Graves disease are thought to represent opposite ends of a spectrum of autoimmune thyroiditis. Rarely, individuals with Hashimoto thyroiditis may present with hyperthyroidism, usually in the early stages of the illness, when autoimmune destruction results in release of preformed thyroid hormone into the circulation. The clinical course and autoantibody pattern help to distinguish this entity from Graves disease.

Treatment of goiter. Treatment for hypothyroidism and goiter is thyroxine, and the gland will slowly shrink in size over time as TSH is suppressed. The recommended initial thyroxine dose is 100 $\mu g/m^2$/day, given once daily. The T ½ (thyroxine half-life) is 5 to 7 days, and laboratory studies should be repeated after 4 to 6 weeks to assess the therapy and adjust the medication dose as needed. Patients with euthyroid goiter may also receive treatment in attempts to shrink the size of the gland, if it is of cosmetic concern to patients. Individuals with a hyperthyroid goiter should receive agents to suppress thyroid hormone synthesis, such as methimazole. Children with moderate to severe symptoms may require additional agents, such as β-adrenergic blockers. Alternatively, they may elect to have surgical correction with subtotal thyroidectomy or ablation by ingestion of radionuclide (^{131}I).

Painful thyroid gland. The previously mentioned conditions are associated with a painless goiter. However, if patients have a painful thyroid gland, the diagnosis may be acute suppurative thyroiditis. The gland may be infected with staphylococci or with mixed aerobic and anaerobic organisms. The white blood cell count and erythrocyte sedimentation rate are elevated, but thyroid function test results often are normal. Treatment includes salicylates, antibiotics, and, occasionally, surgical drainage. Subacute thyroiditis is rare in childhood and is a self-limited illness often associated with an upper respiratory tract infection. Typically, the thyroid gland is enlarged and tender, and patients initially have hyperthyroidism from leakage of preformed thyroid hormone into the circulation from the damaged gland.

Solitary thyroid nodule. A solitary thyroid nodule found in a child has a much greater risk for malignancy than those found in adults, with the incidence of cancer ranging from 20–40% for children with thyroid nodules. Thus, one must exercise great care in the evaluation of such individuals. Important risk factors from the history include a prior history of radiation exposure to the neck; a family history of thyroid cancer, which may be suggestive of a multiple endocrine neoplasia syndrome and medullary thyroid cancer (marked by elevated calcitonin

levels); and a rapidly growing neck mass. Physical findings suggestive of malignant disease include a single, hard nodule, with fixation to surrounding tissues; compressive symptoms, such as hoarseness or dysphagia; and, as the thyroid cancer metastasizes locally, adenopathy.

The differential diagnosis of a solitary thyroid nodule includes thyroid follicular adenoma, cystadenoma, and a functioning adenoma. Multiple follicular nodules are often seen with Hashimoto's thyroiditis. These patients often have euthyroid goiter, although individuals may have hypo- or hyperthyroidism and positive autoantibodies from autoimmune thyroiditis rather than from malignant disease. Imaging studies are most helpful in evaluation of these patients. Ultrasonography is useful in defining the number of nodules present, the size of each nodule, and whether the mass is solid or cystic. Cystic lesions generally are considered benign, although they may contain some solid elements from a degenerating carcinoma.

Radionuclide scanning with ^{123}I or ^{99m}Tc (pertechnetate) provides additional insight into the nature of the lesion: Functional nodules that demonstrate increased concentration of radionuclide (referred to as "warm" or "hot") usually are benign, but patients may require surgical excision of the nodule if there is resultant hyperthyroidism. By contrast, cold nodules are more typically malignant. Thus, individuals with a nodule that is solid by ultrasound and hypofunctioning by radionuclide scanning would be at high risk for a malignant disease and would warrant aggressive evaluation. Such patients are referred to a surgeon for open excisional biopsy of the lesion. In some centers, fine-needle aspiration in an outpatient setting is used for the initial evaluation of a thyroid nodule, although the use of such an approach in pediatrics remains controversial. Individuals with a suspicious fine-needle biopsy result proceed to open surgical resection of the nodule. Patients with benign-appearing tissue obtained by fine-needle biopsy may be given a trial of daily thyroid hormone treatment in attempts to suppress nodule growth.

HYPOGLYCEMIA

Hypoglycemia is an endocrine emergency. Although absolute hypoglycemia or a significant and rapid decrease in blood glucose concentration may be associated with clinically evident seizure activity, permanent CNS damage may occur during hypoglycemia even in the absence of overt symptoms. Thus, appropriate evaluation and management of hypoglycemia are of crucial importance.

Definition

Although the precise definition of hypoglycemia is somewhat controversial, hypoglycemia is generally agreed to be present when the blood glucose concentration is 40 mg/dL or less. Maintenance of euglycemia in infants normally requires glucose production (derived from dietary intake and metabolic processes) of 5 to 7 mg/kg/min. In contrast, older children and adults normally require a glucose production rate of 1 to 2 mg/kg/min.

Glucose Regulation

At any time, the blood glucose concentration is a reflection of glucose production and use. Glucose production depends on three factors: (1) adequate substrate for gluconeogenesis and for glycogen breakdown; (2) enzyme activities for gluconeogenesis, glycogenolysis, and other metabolic processes that enter into these pathways; and (3) normal function of insulin and the counter-insulin hormones, which exert their effects on blood glucose principally by regulating the previously noted enzyme activities. Glycogen stores can provide children with adequate glucose for 8 to 12 h, after which glucose homeostasis becomes dependent on gluconeogenesis. The principal substrates for gluconeogenesis are amino acids (from muscle breakdown or from transamination of amino acid precursors), lactate (from glycolysis), and glycerol and acetyl-CoA (from lipolysis).

The primary hormones that regulate blood glucose concentrations are insulin and the counter-insulin hormones glucagon, epinephrine, cortisol, and growth hormone. The principal mechanisms by which these hormones regulate blood glucose are summarized in Table 19–22. Insulin is an anabolic peptide produced by the pancreatic β cells. The principal target tissues for insulin action are adipose tissue and muscle, where insulin promotes glucose uptake and storage, promotes amino acid uptake and protein synthesis, and decreases use of fat stores for energy. In the liver, insulin inhibits glycogen breakdown and promotes glycogen synthesis by inhibiting adenyl cyclase activity and, therefore, cyclic adenosine monophosphate (cAMP) generation. In addition, insulin has been shown to inhibit transcription of phosphoenolpyruvate carboxykinase (PEPCK), the rate-limiting enzyme in gluconeogenesis.

Both epinephrine and glucagon increase blood glucose concentrations principally by promoting glycogen breakdown. Epinephrine and glucagon activate adenyl cyclase, leading to an increase in cAMP, which ultimately promotes glycogen breakdown by activating the enzyme phosphorylase and inhibits glycogen synthesis by inactivating the enzyme glycogen synthetase. Cyclic adenosine monophosphate also upregulates the rate-limiting enzyme in hepatic gluconeogenesis, PEPCK. In addition, epinephrine and glucagon promote lipolysis, ultimately generating glycerol and acetyl-CoA, which are substrates for gluconeogenesis. Cortisol increases glucose production by increasing the activity of gluconeogenic enzymes and by increasing amino acid substrates for gluconeogenesis through protein breakdown. Growth hormone increases glucose production principally by increasing lipolysis.

Differential Diagnosis of Hypoglycemia

The differential diagnosis of hypoglycemia may be divided conceptually into two general classes: ketotic and nonketotic. Table 19–23 lists conditions associated with both types of hypoglycemia. The frequency of ketotic versus nonketotic forms of hypoglycemia varies with age. Causes of hypoglycemia by age are also discussed in the following section.

KETOTIC HYPOGLYCEMIA

Ketosis results from lipolysis, with β oxidation of free fatty acids and accumulation of acetyl-CoA. Essentially every cause of hypoglycemia is associated with ketosis unless the process of ketone generation is inhibited or the pathway for generating ketones is defective. Ketotic forms of hypoglycemia include decreased substrate (inadequate gluconeogenic substrate and inadequate dietary intake), transient and nontransient abnormalities of gluconeogenesis, some forms of glycogen storage disease, deficiencies of one or more of the counter-insulin hormones,

Table 19–22. Hormonal Regulation of Blood Glucose

Hormone	Actions
Insulin	Glucose uptake by cells; glycogen synthesis and storage
Glucagon	Glycogen breakdown; lipolysis and gluconeogenesis
Epinephrine	Glycogen breakdown; lipolysis and gluconeogenesis
Cortisol	Gluconeogenesis
Growth hormone	Lipolysis and gluconeogenesis

Table 19–23. Differential Diagnosis of Hypoglycemia

Ketotic
Decreased substrate
Transient and nontransient abnormalities of gluconeogenesis
Some forms of glycogen storage disease (excluding glucose-6-phosphatase deficiency)
Deficiency of counterinsulin hormone(s)
Other abnormalities of amino acid and carbohydrate metabolism (e.g., defects in metabolism of branched-chain amino acids, galactose, and fructose)
Nonketotic
Hyperinsulinism
Fatty acid oxidation abnormalities, with or without associated carnitine deficiency
Glucose-6-phosphatase deficiency (glycogen storage disease type I)

and abnormalities in amino acid metabolism or carbohydrate metabolism that limit conversion of metabolites to substrates that can enter the gluconeogenic pathway. All these forms of hypoglycemia may be associated with ketosis, as insulin is suppressed and stress-induced lipolysis occurs.

Nonketotic Hypoglycemia

The principal cause of nonketotic hypoglycemia is hyperinsulinism. The high concentrations of insulin lead to an accelerated rate of glucose use, decreased hepatic glucose production, and general suppression of the ketogenic pathway. Less common causes result from specific defects in the ability to produce ketones, such as abnormalities of fatty acid oxidation. This includes deficiency of carnitine, which plays a role in translocation of free fatty acids from the cytosol to the mitochondria, where β oxidation occurs.

Infants with Hypoglycemia

In infants with transient hypoglycemia, ketotic forms predominate and are associated with prematurity, intrauterine growth retardation, asphyxia, sepsis, starvation, and maternal ingestion of propranolol. Such stressed infants may have depleted glycogen stores and a transient defect in gluconeogenesis but have an intact lipolytic and ketogenic pathway. Ingestion of ethanol, salicylates, and acetaminophen also may be associated with transient ketotic hypoglycemia. Transient neonatal hypoglycemia may be nonketotic when associated with transient hyperinsulinism in infants of diabetic mothers or with erythroblastosis fetalis, or in association with maternal ingestion of oral hypoglycemic drugs.

Among the nontransient forms of hypoglycemia from birth to 1 year of age, nonketotic forms predominate. *Hyperinsulinism,* the most common cause of persistent, nonketotic hypoglycemia in newborns appears to result principally from a process often referred to as nesidioblastosis. In this condition, hyperinsulinism was initially thought to arise from a diffuse proliferation of endocrine cells budding off from the exocrine ducts. However, another study indicates that the histologic pattern of nesidioblastosis is not a pathologic entity, as it may occur in age-matched infants without hypoglycemia. Nontransient hyperinsulinism in most infants is thought to be secondary to abnormalities in the regulation of insulin secretion. A variety of genetic forms of congenital hyperinsulinism have been recently identified. These include mutations in the pancreatic β-cell sulfonylurea receptor (SUR) and the pancreatic islet inward rectifier K$^+$ channel, Kir 6.2, encoded by adjacent genes on chromosome 11p. Both SUR and Kir 6.2 form subunits of the pancreatic β-cell K$_{ATP}$ channel, which plays a critical role in regulating insulin secretion. Autosomal recessive mutations in SUR or Kir 6.2 generally result in diffuse hyperinsulinism while the presence of an abnormal paternal

SUR gene with somatic loss of maternal 11p15 is associated with focal adenomatosis. Loss of heterozygosity in maternally derived genes in chromosome 11p15 may also contribute to the hyperinsulinism seen in patients with Beckwith-Wiedemann syndrome. Additional genetic forms of hyperinsulinism of infancy include activating mutations of glucokinase (thought to be the pancreatis β-cell glucose sensor) and gain-of-function mutations of glutamate dehydrogenase. The latter cause both hyperinsulinism and hyperammonemia.

Nontransient ketotic forms of hypoglycemia in the neonate or young infant include counter-insulin hormone deficiencies, some forms of glycogen storage disease, gluconeogenesis abnormalities, and abnormalities in the metabolism of galactose, fructose, and branched-chain amino acids.

Children with Hypoglycemia

In children from about 18 months of age through mid-childhood, hypoglycemia is most often ketotic. Such children usually do not have an obvious abnormality in glycogen breakdown or gluconeogenesis or a deficiency of the counter-insulin hormones. Plasma alanine concentrations, however, may be decreased in such children, possibly reflecting decreased efflux of amino acids from skeletal muscle. Hypoglycemia in these children most often occurs when fasting is sustained for 8 to 16 h and frequently is associated with an intercurrent illness. This condition often resolves spontaneously as children approach the peripubertal years. In late childhood, nonketotic hypoglycemia again predominates, with hyperinsulinism (often associated with multiple endocrine neoplasia) the most common cause.

Clinical Approach to Children with Hypoglycemia

History and Physical Examination

Useful diagnostic clues in the evaluation of hypoglycemia can be found in the history, physical examination findings, and treatment course. A history of intrauterine growth retardation, prematurity, or maternal drug use, should be sought. The physical examination should include a search for midline defects such as cleft lip or palate and optic nerve abnormalities (may be associated with hypopituitarism), ambiguous genitalia (may be associated with cortisol deficiency), omphalocele, macroglossia, visceromegaly (Beckwith-Wiedemann syndrome), microphallus and undescended testes (may be associated with multiple hypothalamic/pituitary abnormalities), and hepatomegaly (may be associated with glycogen storage disease and other metabolic disorders).

Laboratory Evaluation and Initial Management

The initial laboratory evaluation of hypoglycemia is outlined in Table 19–24. A diagnostic algorithm for

Table 19–24. Laboratory Evaluation
of Hypoglycemia

Urine
Ketones
Organic acids
Reducing substances
Plasma[1]
Ketones
Insulin [insulin (μU/mL): glucose (mg/dL) ratio should not exceed 0.3]
Growth hormone
Cortisol
Glucagon
Lactate
Electrolytes (to measure anion gap)
Organic acids
Alanine

[1] Samples should be drawn when hypoglycemia is present (glucose ≤ 40 mg/dL).

infants with hypoglycemia is presented in Figure 19–11. It is desirable to obtain both urine and plasma samples before administering glucose (0.5 to 1 g/kg intravenous bolus as 10 or 25% dextrose in water, followed by a glucose infusion). The urine sample should be analyzed for ketones, organic acids, and reducing substances (e.g., galactose and fructose). Ketones may not always be present in the urine during acute hypoglycemia associated with one of the ketotic causes. The plasma sample should be analyzed for glucose, ketones, insulin, GH, cortisol, glucagon, lactate, electrolytes (to determine whether there is an abnormally high anion gap), organic acids, and alanine concentrations. Of crucial importance, the glucose sample must be placed in a tube with sodium fluoride or another inhibitor of enzymes involved in glucose metabolism. Otherwise, if analysis is delayed, the glucose concentration in the sample will decrease at a rate of 5 to 10 mg/dL/h at room temperature. Moreover, the previously noted blood tests are most useful when the simultaneous blood glucose is 40 mg/dL or less. Therefore, if hypoglycemia is suspected, it may be prudent to determine the blood glucose concentration by Chemstrip at the bedside initially and then to proceed with the evaluation as outlined previously, including a laboratory blood glucose determination, if indicated.

Of particular diagnostic importance in the diagnostic work-up are the glucose requirements to maintain euglycemia and the glucose response to an injection of glucagon (0.1 mg/kg intramuscularly, up to 1 mg). Glucose requirements of 15 mg/kg/min or greater are virtually diagnostic of hyperinsulinism. In addition, a major glycemic response to glucagon during hypoglycemia probably will lead to a diagnosis of hyperinsulinism.

Management

Appropriate management of hypoglycemia requires proper treatment of the underlying disorder. The optimal management of nontransient hyperinsulinism is somewhat controversial. Medical management often includes a low-leucine diet (leucine is an insulin secretogague in most individuals) and oral diazoxide therapy, which inhibits insulin secretion. Side effects of diazoxide increase when the dose exceeds 10–15 mg/kg/day and include fluid retention, decreased white blood cell count, thrombocytopenia, hyperuricemia, hypertrichosis, and soft tissue facial abnormalities with prolonged use. If medical management is unsuccessful, subtotal pancreatectomy (85 to 95%) is often undertaken. Hypoglycemia may persist even after 95% pancreatectomy, whereas pancreatic exocrine insufficiency and diabetes may also occur. Somatostatin analogues and calcium channel blockers, which suppress insulin secretion, have been used with some success in patients with hyperinsulinism. In view of recent studies which indicate that a significant percentage of infants with congenital hyperinsulinism may have focal adenomatosis which may be curable by surgery, the use of biochemical tests (e.g., intravenous tolbutamide) in conjunction with selective catherization of the pancreatic veins may be of great importance in the identification of such patients.

CHILDREN WITH POLYURIA

Polyuria, which must be distinguished from urinary frequency, is one of the principal presenting signs of two endocrine disorders: diabetes mellitus and diabetes insipidus. Polyuria may result from an osmotic agent (e.g., hyperglycemia in diabetes mellitus), a deficiency or impaired responsiveness to antidiuretic hormone (ADH), or excessive water intake (primary polydipsia).

Because deficiency or impaired responsiveness to ADH constitutes the principal component of the differential diagnosis of polyuria, it is important to review the principles of ADH physiology. Antidiuretic hormone, in concert with an intact thirst mechanism, maintains plasma osmolality in the normal range of 280 to 290 mosmol/kg.

Arginine vasopressin (AVP) is the principal ADH in humans. This nonapeptide is produced in the supraoptic and paraventricular nuclei of the hypothalamus. Axons from these neurons terminate in the posterior pituitary gland, where they secrete AVP. The principal action of AVP in regulating water balance is to increase permeability to water in the renal collecting tubules and thus enhance its absorption.

Arginine vasopressin secretion is regulated principally by changes in plasma osmolality and in effective circulating volume. Osmoreceptors in the hypothalamus stimulate the secretion of AVP when plasma osmolality increases by as little as 1%. In healthy individuals, AVP levels are

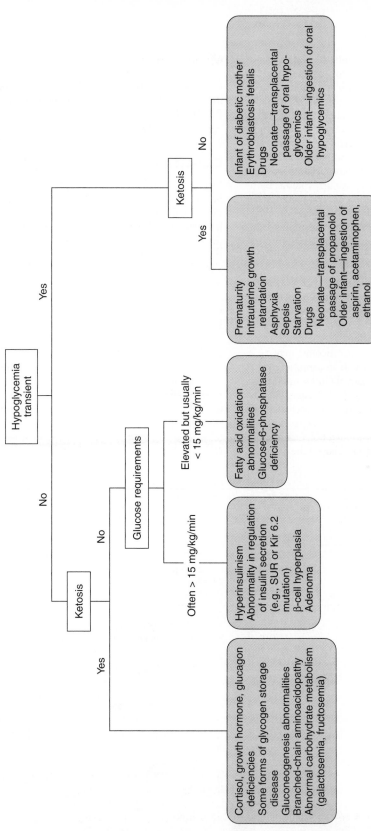

Figure 19–11. An approach to the evaluation of hypoglycemia in infants. Kir 6.2 = pancreatic islet inward rectifier K⁺ channel; SUR = sulfonyl urea receptor.

normally low and do not increase until the plasma osmolality exceeds 280 mosmol/kg. Arginine vasopressin secretion is also regulated by changes in blood volume. Baroreceptors in the systemic venous circulation, right side of the heart, and left atrium ("low pressure" areas), as well as in the systemic arterial systems of the carotid sinus and aortic arch ("high pressure" areas), transmit information to the hypothalamus via the vagus and glossopharyngeal nerves, respectively. These baroreceptors become activated when stretched by increases in intravascular volume. Baroreceptor activity leads to inhibition of AVP secretion. In addition, many other factors affect AVP secretion. Arginine vasopressin is stimulated by pain, stress, and drugs such as β-adrenergic agents, morphine, and barbiturates. It is inhibited by α-adrenergic agents, ethanol, and phenytoin.

An algorithm for evaluating children with polyuria is given in Figure 19–12. It is important to first determine whether an osmotic agent, such as glucose, is present in the urine. The finding of glycosuria suggests the diagnosis of diabetes mellitus (see later), although some medications (e.g., pharmacologic doses of glucocorticoids) may cause glucose intolerance and glycosuria. If an osmotic agent is not present in the urine, the impact of fluid restriction on urinary output and concentration should be assessed (discussed later). Decreased urinary output and increased urinary concentration after fluid restriction suggest the diagnosis of primary polydipsia. Continued polyuria without an increase in urinary concentration leads to the diagnosis

of diabetes insipidus. An antidiuretic response to exogenous ADH suggests ADH deficiency, or central diabetes insipidus, whereas lack of an antidiuretic response indicates nephrogenic diabetes insipidus. Diabetes mellitus (DM) and diabetes insipidus (DI) are discussed in more depth in the following section.

Diabetes Insipidus

Deficiency of AVP or impaired responsiveness of the kidney to AVP results in DI, characterized by polyuria, polydipsia, and defective urinary concentrating ability. Hypernatremia usually does not occur if patients have an intact thirst mechanism, adequate access to fluids, and no additional ongoing fluid losses, such as from diarrhea. Infants with DI, in addition to polyuria and polydipsia, may be irritable and have fever of unknown origin, growth failure secondary to inadequate caloric intake, and hydronephrosis. Older children may also have nocturia and enuresis. Diabetes insipidus may not be apparent in patients with concurrent untreated glucocorticoid deficiency, because cortisol is required to generate a normal free water loss.

Diabetes insipidus results from a wide range of abnormalities. These are listed in Table 19–25. Arginine vasopressin deficiency (*central DI*) is most commonly acquired but rarely can occur as a familial, autosomal dominant disorder. Acquired forms of DI may be idiopathic or may occur in association with tumors, trauma, neurosurgery, infection, granulomas, histiocytosis, and vascular and

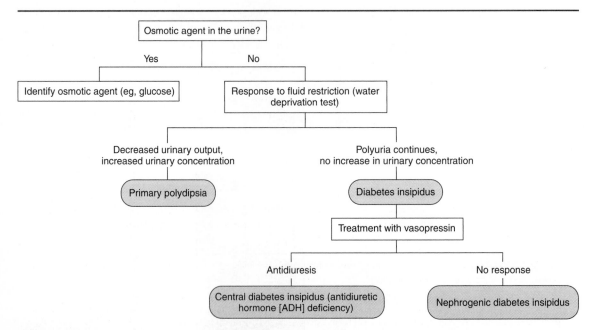

Figure 19–12. Approach to the evaluation of children with polyuria.

Table 19–25. Etiologies of Diabetes Insipidus

Arginine vasopressin deficiency: Central diabetes insipidus
- Acquired: CNS diseases: tumors, trauma, neurosurgery, infection, granulomas, histiocytosis, vascular and autoimmune diseases
- Familial autosomal dominant

Impaired arginine vasopressin responsiveness: Nephrogenic diabetes insipidus
- Familial X-linked
- Acquired: Some forms of primary renal disease, obstructive uropathy
- Metabolic: hypokalemia, hypercalcemia, sickle-cell disease
- Drug-induced (e.g., lithium, demeclocycline)
- Secondary to prolonged polyuria of any cause

CNS = central nervous system.

autoimmune diseases of the hypothalamus and pituitary. Impaired AVP responsiveness (*nephrogenic DI*), may be familial or acquired. Familial nephrogenic DI (X-linked) results from either a defect in the ADH receptor or a post-receptor signaling pathway defect. Acquired nephrogenic DI occurs with some forms of primary renal disease, obstructive uropathy, hypokalemia, hypercalcemia, and sickle-cell disease. It may also be induced by drugs such as lithium and demeclocycline. Prolonged polyuria of any cause can result in some degree of nephrogenic DI secondary to a reduction of tonicity in the renal medullary interstitium and a subsequent decrease in the gradient necessary to concentrate the urine.

A modified 7-h water deprivation test is useful to distinguish patients with DI from those with normal urinary concentrating ability. After unrestricted fluid intake the night before the test, patients are given a normal breakfast. Patients urinate (the urine is discarded), and a 7-h fast is begun. During the first hour, plasma and urine osmolality are measured. After 6 h, patients again urinate and discard the urine. After 7 h, plasma and urine osmolality are measured again. If the initial urine-plasma osmolality ratio is greater than 1.5, normal concentrating ability is demonstrated, and it is unnecessary to continue the test. After 7 h, normal function is indicated by a urine-plasma osmolality ratio greater than 1.5, an increase from the beginning of the fast in the urine-plasma osmolality ratio of 1 or greater, or a final urine osmolality greater than 450 mosmol/kg. In small children, weight, as well as serum and urine osmolality, should be monitored periodically during the water deprivation test to avoid excessive water loss.

If DI is suspected, a baseline plasma sample should be obtained for a radioimmunoassay for AVP. Arginine vasopressin or a synthetic analogue should then be administered to distinguish AVP deficiency from AVP un-

responsiveness. Aqueous AVP or 1-deamino-8D-arginine vasopressin (DDAVP) may be administered.

The drug of choice in most patients with AVP deficiency, DDAVP (subcutaneous, intranasal, or oral forms), has a longer duration of action than does AVP. Hydrochlorothiazide, alone or in combination with the K+-sparing diuretic amiloride, is the principal treatment for nephrogenic DI.

If DI is associated with significant hypernatremia from free water loss, the free water deficit should be replenished slowly. Rapid correction can result in swelling of cells, cerebral edema, and seizures. It is recommended that plasma sodium be brought down by 10 to 12 mEq/L/day. The free water deficit may be calculated by the following formula:

$$(0.6) \times (\text{body wt. in kg}) \times \left(1 - \frac{140}{\text{plasma Na}^+ \text{ mEq/L}}\right)$$

If patients have mild hypernatremia, hypotonic NaCl intravenous solutions or oral fluids may be used as initial therapy. If hypernatremia is severe, initial therapy should include normal saline solutions to minimize the risk of iatrogenic cerebral swelling.

Diabetes Mellitus

One of the most common reasons for polyuria is the presence of a nonresorbable solute, usually glucose. When serum glucose concentration exceeds 180 mg/dL, the filtered glucose level exceeds the capacity of the renal tubule to reabsorb the solute fully and an obligate diuresis of glucose and water will occur. Thus, the principal complaint with new onset of diabetes mellitus (DM) is polyuria with concomitant polydipsia.

DEFINITION

The criteria established for the diagnosis of diabetes mellitus relate to the degree of derangement in carbohydrate metabolism. In the absence of frank hyperglycemia with metabolic decompensation, the presence of any of the following findings on two separate testing occasions establishes a diagnosis of DM: a random serum glucose concentration of more than 200 mg/dL, a fasting glucose concentration of more than 125 mg/dL, or an abnormal oral glucose tolerance test (Table 19–26).

ETIOLOGIC CLASSIFICATION

Hyperglycemia is caused by a variety of different processes, and DM refers to a heterogeneous group of disorders. As one approaches patients with newly diagnosed diabetes, it is helpful to consider the possible mechanisms of patients' carbohydrate metabolism derangement. The types of DM are now classified by the underlying cause, rather than by

Table 19–26. Criteria for Diagnosis of Diabetes[1]

Random plasma glucose >200, OR
Fasting plasma glucose >125 on two occasions OR
Oral glucose tolerance test (1.75 g/kg glucose, to maximum of 75 g)
2 h plasma glucose >200
One intervening value >200

[1]Unless there is unequivocal hyperglycemia with acute metabolic decompensation (such as diabetic), ketoacidosis then any one of the above criteria must be repeated on a subsequent day to confirm the diagnosis. All glucose concentrations expressed as mg/dL.

the traditional treatment-based classification of insulin-dependent DM (IDDM) versus non-insulin dependent DM (NIDDM) (Table 19–27). Most cases fall into one of two groups: type 1 DM, with β-cell destruction resulting in a state of insulin deficiency, or type 2 DM, a condition marked predominantly by insulin resistance with a relative decrease in insulin secretion. Table 19–28 lists common distinguishing features between these two disease types. The etiologic subtypes of diabetes are discussed in further detail in the following sections.

Type 1 diabetes mellitus. For most children, the derangement in carbohydrate metabolism is the result of type 1 DM. This process follows the autoimmune destruction of the pancreatic β cell, often occurring slowly over

Table 19–27. Etiologic Classification of Diabetes Mellitus

Type 1 diabetes (β-cell destruction, leading to absolute insulin deficiency)
Immune mediated
Idiopathic
Type 2 diabetes (predominantly insulin resistance with relative insulin deficiency)
Other specific types
Genetic defects of β-cell function
Genetic defects in insulin action
Disease of the exocrine pancreas
Endocrinopathies
Drug or chemical-induced
Infections
Uncommon forms of immune-mediated diabetes
Other genetic syndromes sometimes associated with diabetes
Neonatal diabetes
Gestational diabetes mellitus

Modified with permission from American Diabetes Association: Clinical Practice Recommendations. *Diabetes Care* 22(Suppl 1): S7, 1999.

many years. Type 1 DM appears to be a complex, multigenetic process, with greatest risk conferred by genes in the class II region of the human leukocyte, locus A (HLA). Nonetheless, the genetic risk is quite low, as first-degree relatives of an individual with type 1 DM have approximately a 5% chance of acquiring the disease. There appears to be a synergy between an underlying genetic risk and environmental exposures. The actual environmental triggers are unknown but are postulated to include viruses or toxins. Pancreatic destruction can be tracked by detection of autoantibodies directed against the β cell as early as 10 or more years before the clinical presence of disease. These markers include autoantibodies such as islet cell autoantibody (ICA), and antibodies directed against insulin, glutamate decarboxylase, and tyrosine phosphotase (also known as IA-2), all of which are now available commercially. As β-cell destruction proceeds, one may detect abnormal metabolic function with an intravenous glucose tolerance test before clinical symptoms become prominent. Overt clinical evidence for diabetes is not apparent until 80 to 90% of the β-cell mass has been destroyed. As a result of insulin insufficiency, patients often present with polyuria and polydipsia, in addition to a thin-body habitus and weight loss despite polyphagia.

Although previously considered to be predominantly a disorder of juvenile onset, type 1 DM is now known to occur in adults of any age and should be considered in those with lean-body habitus who require insulin rather than oral agents to achieve metabolic control.

Type 2 diabetes mellitus. Type 2 DM had previously been considered to be solely an adult-onset form of DM. However, it is now diagnosed with increasing frequency in children, especially adolescents. Currently type 2 DM comprises 20% or more of many pediatric diabetes practices. Up to 50% of new diabetes presentations in 10–19 year olds are now from type 2 DM.

The cause of this form of the disease is not well delineated but results from either a defect in peripheral insulin action or insulin secretion. It is considered primarily a disorder of insulin resistance, rather than insulin deficiency. These patients therefore may have elevated insulin levels and readily measurable C-peptide levels, reflecting processing of pro-insulin to insulin. There is a much stronger risk for genetic transmission of this disorder than there is with type 1 DM. The classic patient is obese and, on physical examination, may have acanthosis nigricans, a velvety hyperpigmented overgrowth of skin noted in the skin folds that is associated with insulin resistance. However, such a rash is not always apparent. Additional risk factors for type 2 DM include non-white ethnicity, puberty (which increases insulin resistance), a history of either over-growth or growth retardation in utero, and the presence of syndromes associated with insulin resistance such as syndrome X or polycystic ovarian syndrome (Table 19–29). Individuals with a condition referred to as impaired glucose tolerance where carbohydrate meta-

Table 19–28. Common Distinguishing Features of Type 1 and Type 2 Diabetes Mellitus

	Type 1	Type 2
Pathophysiology	Insulin deficient autoantibody positive insulin level, C-peptide: decreased or –	Insulin resistant, autoantibody negative insulin, C-peptide: often elevated
Presentation	Ketosis prone	Usually without ketosis or mild
Onset	Frequently <18 years	Most common in adults, risk increases with age but seen with increasing frequency in adolescents
Body habitus	Thin	Obese, often with acanthosis nigricans
Family history	Negative in 90%	Often positive
Prevalence in United States	1.7 million	15 million

bolism is not entirely normal but frank DM is not present, are also at increased risk for developing type 2 DM. By definition, such individuals have a fasting glucose ≥110 but <126 mg/dL, or a 2-h glucose of ≥140 but <200 mg/dL on an oral glucose tolerance test. A significant percentage of these individuals will progress to type 2 DM over time.

Other specific etiologic types of diabetes mellitus. This category consists of a miscellaneous collection of disorders associated with DM that do not fall within the two primary groupings (see Table 19–27). *Maturity onset diabetes of the young (MODY)* is perhaps the best characterized genetic form of DM and accounts for 2 to 5% of all types of diabetes. Age of onset is usually less than 25 years of age, and the individuals are often not obese. These are autosomal dominant disorders that can usually be shown to have affected multiple past generations. At least 6 different genetic loci have been described to date and include mutations in glucokinase and several different transcription factors that influence insulin transcription and/or β-cell development.

Diabetes is also associated with mitochondrial DNA defects. Many of these patients also have sensorineural hearing loss. Genetic defects in insulin action are rare

Table 19–29. Risk Factors For Type 2 Diabetes Mellitus In Children

Family history of type 2 diabetes mellitus
Obesity
Ethnicity
Puberty
History of large for gestational age or intrauterine growth retardation
Pattern of evolving syndrome X (hypertension, hyperlipidemia, insulin resistance, and atherosclerosis) or polycystic ovarian syndrome
History of impaired glucose tolerance

causes of DM. Structural abnormalities of the insulin molecule are very unusual. Insulin resistance syndromes are more commonly related to defects in either the insulin receptor or in the post-receptor signaling cascade. The lipodystrophy syndromes are associated with severe insulin resistance and either complete absence of subcutaneous fat or partial absence localized to distinct body areas.

Any process that causes diffuse injury to the exocrine pancreas can also lead to diabetes. Examples include pancreatitis, trauma, infection, pancreatectomy, neoplasia, iron overload syndromes, and chronic obstruction of ductal flow, such as from calculi or inspissated secretions in cystic fibrosis.

Various endocrinopathies may cause DM. Growth hormone, cortisol, glucagon, and epinephrine are counter-regulatory hormones that antagonize the effects of insulin. Thus, endogenous overproduction of such hormones, or exogenous use, may unmask DM, especially in children who already harbor some underlying risk. Diabetes mellitus may resolve as the underlying endocrinopathy is treated.

Exposure to various drugs can also lead to the development of DM, either by impairing insulin secretion and/or inhibiting insulin action. Treatment with one or more of such agents, in combination with a significant stress and/or an underlying predisposition to DM, may result in DM. Such patients are often encountered following organ transplantation or during treatment of illnesses such as cancer or asthma (with exposure to agents such as FK-506, cyclosporin, glucocorticoids, diuretics, β agonists).

An increased incidence of DM is also noted among children with many different genetic syndromes, although diabetes is usually not the primary manifestation.

CLINICAL PRESENTATION AND ACUTE MANAGEMENT

An understanding of insulin action helps explain how patients with DM present and, in some instances, this understanding allows clinicians to distinguish type 1 from

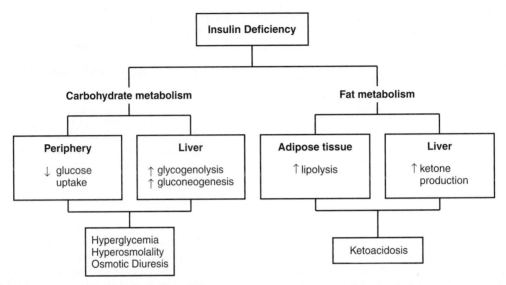

Figure 19–13. Acute presentations for diabetes mellitus. Diabetic ketoacidosis results from more marked insulin deficiency, with derangements in both carbohydrate and fat metabolism. Individuals may present with less profound insulin deficiency, with a defect in only carbohydrate metabolism (as is often seen with type 2 diabetes mellitus or early onset type 1).

type 2 diabetes (Figure 19–13). Insulin is an anabolic agent, enhancing energy storage in the form of glycogen, adipose tissue, and protein. The effects of insulin on fat metabolism are much more sensitive than its effect on carbohydrate metabolism. Thus, with a relative deficiency of insulin, there is a breakdown of glycogen stores with release of further glucose into the circulation, increased gluconeogenesis, and diminished glucose uptake into cells. This scenario is observed in both types 1 and 2 diabetes. The subsequent hyperglycemia results in the classic symptoms of polyuria and polydipsia. The failure to use carbohydrate leads to a net catabolic state and subsequent weight loss. Patients often complain of fatigue and weakness, which may in part be the result of breakdown of muscle protein to provide amino acids as substrate for gluconeogenesis. Elevation in serum osmolality will also lead to lethargy, with many patients becoming stuporous and entering coma at levels of 340 mosmol or higher.

Diabetic ketoacidosis

Pathophysiology. The combination of profound insulin deficiency and increased levels of counterregulatory hormones initiates lipolysis, using fat as an alternative fuel source. The liver processes the fatty acids into ketone bodies. The resultant diabetic ketoacidosis (DKA) often differentiates patients with type 1 DM from those with type 2. Nonetheless, some patients with type 2 DM may develop DKA, although it is usually not as severe as that seen with type 1 DM. Patients with type 2 DM often

make enough insulin to limit onset of lipolysis but not enough to normalize carbohydrate metabolism.

Laboratory and clinical features. The laboratory findings in DKA are given in Table 19–30. These include a serum pH that may decrease below 7.25 and bicarbonate that may decrease below 15 meq/L in more severe cases, and an increased anion gap from accumulation of ketoacids. Electrolyte abnormalities (Na+ and K+) are also quite common (see later). Clinical features of DKA are presented in Table 19–31. Ketoacidosis will be reflected by respirations that are deep and labored (Kussmaul respirations), reflecting the patient's attempt to correct the underlying metabolic acidosis with respiratory compensation. The fruity odor of acetone may be discernible on the patient's breath. Ketoacidosis also exacerbates the ongoing dehydration induced from hyperglycemia and osmotic diuresis: The ketones often result in nausea and vomiting, which further limit oral intake.

Treatment. The treatment of DKA involves aggressive reversal of the cascade of events that have conspired against patients (Table 19–32).

ABCs and hydration: The first line of therapy is to protect the airway and maintain respiration and circulation. Patients may, on rare occasion, require intubation and ventilation. In the comatose patient, one may also need to insert a nasogastric tube to prevent emesis and subsequent aspiration. Next, the patient's state of dehydration is assessed. The patient with DKA may have as much

Table 19–30. Laboratory Findings
in Diabetic Ketoacidosis

- Hyperosmolality, hyperglycemia (>200 mg/dL)
- Lipemia, ketonemia, acidosis pH <7.25, bicarbonate <15 mEq/L
- Hyponatremia
  Na depressed 1.6 mEq/L for every 100 mg/dL glucose
  Artifact from lipemia
- Potassium: total body depletion
- Blood urea nitrogen/creatinine elevated from dehydration
- Leukocytosis

as 10 to 15% dehydration. Recent weights from a previous clinic visit are invaluable in this assessment. The initial goal of the fluid resuscitation is to restore circulation, usually with a 10 to 20 mL/kg bolus of normal saline or Ringer lactate. The patient's fluids can then be changed over to 0.5 normal saline, with the goal to replace the calculated fluid deficit evenly over the next 48 h. One may calculate the rate of fluid replacement by the following formula:

- Maintenance fluids at the rate of 1500 mL/m²/day
- Deficit replacement (minus initial bolus as part of this correction)
- Ongoing losses (such as emesis)

Urinary losses usually are not replaced, because the maintenance fluid replacement accounts for some urinary loss, and additional replacement often leads to overhydration. Urinary losses should decrease steadily as insulin replacement is initiated and serum glucose falls (see insulin section later). The fluid status of the patient needs to be reassessed frequently and readjusted as deemed necessary by the clinical course: Poor peripheral perfusion with prolonged capillary refill time may necessitate administration of additional boluses of normal saline. Urinary output is not necessarily a reliable indicator of hydration status, because ongoing glycosuria may lead to continuing polyuria. Fluid replacement in excess of 4 L/m²/day may

Table 19–31. Clinical Features
of Diabetic Ketoacidosis

- Weight loss, fatigue, weakness
- Polyuria, polydipsia, polyphagia; dehydration
- Difficulty breathing
  Kussmaul respirations
  Acetone breath
- Gastrointestinal complaints
- Lethargy progressing to obtundation

Table 19–32. Diabetic Ketoacidosis:
Goals of Therapy

Maintain airway and breathing; restore circulation
Institute insulin to correct hyperglycemia and clear ketones
Correct metabolic abnormalities
Determine cause of DKA; rule out infection
Look out for complications, especially cerebral edema

DKA = diabetic ketoacidosis.

be associated with cerebral edema, and infusion of more than this amount is not recommended unless necessary to maintain perfusion.

Insulin: Diabetic ketoacidosis results from relative or absolute insulin deficiency. To reverse the condition, insulin therapy needs to be started as soon as possible after the diagnosis has been established, preferably as the initial fluid bolus is given. Most patients respond appropriately to an intravenous bolus of 0.1 U/kg of regular insulin, followed by a continuous infusion of 0.1 U/kg/h. Subcutaneous insulin administration is much less effective in patients with dehydration as its slower onset of action is exaggerated further by poor peripheral perfusion. The goal of insulin therapy is to reduce the serum glucose concentration at a rate of about 75 to 100 mg/dL/h to avoid dramatic shifts in serum osmolality. As the serum glucose concentration approaches 250 mg/dL, intravenous fluid should be changed to 5% dextrose to maintain glucose levels at 150 to 300 mg/dL. The insulin infusion should be continued until the ketoacidosis resolves, which is often longer than the time it takes for the serum glucose concentration to normalize.

Associated metabolic derangements: During the course of rehydration and insulin infusion, other associated metabolic derangements should be corrected. Patients with DKA often have hyponatremia. Although they may have significant sodium deficits from urinary loss, the hyponatremia is also caused by an influx of water from the intracellular space in order to maintain serum osmolality in the face of hyperglycemia. An artifactually low serum Na⁺ may also be seen from the associated hyperlipidemia. Serum levels of sodium should slowly increase as deficits are replaced with intravenous sodium infusion and ongoing insulin therapy results in decreasing serum levels of glucose and inhibition of lipolysis.

In addition, many patients have profound potassium deficits, although the serum potassium concentrations may be high, normal, or low. Intracellular potassium is exchanged for extracellular hydrogen ion during states of metabolic acidosis. Insulin treatment will drive potassium back into the cell thus potentially causing a precipitous drop in patients' serum potassium concentrations as the treatment for DKA proceeds. If patients are urinating and the potassium concentration is 5 meq/L or lower, then one needs to begin aggressively replacing the potassium deficit at 40 mEq/L. This supplementation may be done with KCl alone or in part with K-acetate (which is converted to bicarbonate), or with K-phosphate (which may help with phosphate repletion). Patients may require potassium replacement at up to 0.5 mEq/kg/h to avoid profound hypokalemia. However, this should be administered only while the patient's status is followed on a cardiac monitor. Aggressive phosphate replacement may precipitate hypocalcemia; therefore, one may not want to initiate such replacement unless the serum level of phosphate has decreased to less than 2 mEq/L. Hypo- and hyperkalemia may be associated with life-threatening cardiac arrhythmias; thus, one must monitor serum electrolytes frequently during DKA treatment.

The metabolic acidosis of individuals with DKA is also of concern and results from both the ketoacidosis that arises from the underlying insulin deficiency and the lactic acidosis associated with osmotic diuresis and dehydration. Both components should steadily improve with rehydration and insulin therapy. Failure to do so may reflect a need for further insulin or inadequate fluid replacement. The acid-base status is readily evaluated with serial blood gas and electrolyte measurements, noting both the serum level of bicarbonate and anion gap. Sodium bicarbonate administration is rarely indicated for the treatment of DKA and, in prospective randomized trials, has not improved the outcome. Several important considerations limit the utility of sodium bicarbonate in the treatment of DKA. First, rather than helping to normalize pH, it may cause a paradoxical decrease in the pH of the cerebrospinal fluid. Although bicarbonate itself cannot cross the blood-brain barrier, it is converted in the circulation to carbon dioxide and then diffuses across the blood-brain barrier. This, in turn, lowers the pH of the cerebrospinal fluid and may exacerbate mental obtundation. Second, with a shift in serum pH from acidosis toward alkalosis, one may precipitate hypokalemia. As mentioned earlier, individuals with DKA have a net deficit of total body potassium, but their serum levels often are in the normal-to-high range as potassium shifts from the intracellular to the extracellular space in exchange for hydrogen ions. However, with normalization or overcorrection of acidosis with sodium bicarbonate, the shift of these ions is reversed: H^+ ions move from the intracellular back to the extracellular space, and K^+ ions shift from the extracellular to the intracellular space. Life-threatening cardiac arrhythmias may result from the hypokalemia. Third, the change in pH toward alkalosis may increase the patient's risk for hypocalcemia as the pH change will result in a dissociation of hydrogen ions from albumin, serving to decrease the free calcium concentration. Fourth, one must consider the effects of sodium bicarbonate on the oxygen dissociation curve: Oxygen is off-loaded from hemoglobin

much more readily at an acidic pH; thus, normalization or overcorrection of serum pH may impair oxygen delivery to the tissues. Finally, a retrospective analysis showed that children with DKA treated with sodium bicarbonate were 4 times more likely to develop cerebral edema. For all these reasons, unless patients have a pH <7.0 and are unresponsive to the initial measures previously described, and the metabolic acidosis appears to be compromising cardiovascular function, sodium bicarbonate therapy should not be given. If indicated, one may use 1 to 2 mEq/kg intravenously over 2 h, discontinuing therapy when the pH increases to >7.1 or the serum bicarbonate level is >10 mEq/L.

Identifying and addressing inciting factors: As the aforementioned issues are attended to, one also must consider why such a presentation has occurred. It may be the initial diagnosis with type I DM. An underlying stress, such as an infection, may have precipitated the episode of DKA. Therefore, one needs to examine patients carefully for evidence of infection and consider appropriate laboratory tests, such as urinalysis or chest radiograph and determine if antibiotics should be initiated. The white blood cell count may not be helpful initially in guiding the work-up because it is often nonspecifically elevated secondary to the stress of DKA. Noncompliance with insulin therapy should be considered in any patient with known diabetes.

Recurrent DKA is a particularly difficult problem that requires ongoing evaluation and management by a diabetic specialist and their support team. In such situations, one needs to consider simplifying the insulin regimen, and assuring careful adult direct supervision of all insulin injections in the outpatient setting.

Cerebral edema: The most worrisome complication encountered in the treatment of DKA is cerebral edema. Cerebral edema is rare, affecting ~1% of those with DKA, but as many as 50% who develop this condition either die or suffer from significant permanent neurologic deficits. Although excessive fluid, rapid decrease in serum glucose concentration and osmolality, and use of sodium bicarbonate have all been considered as possible causes, none has been definitively linked with this complication.

Younger patients appear to be at highest risk, particularly those younger than 5 years of age and those presenting with their initial episode of DKA. Signs and symptoms of cerebral edema may include headache, behavioral changes, incontinence, temperature dysregulation, seizure, pupillary changes (asymmetry or fixed, dilated pupils), and hypertension with bradycardia. The symptoms often develop in the first 5 to 12 h of treatment, as patients are improving. Patients' statuses should be evaluated at least hourly for changes in the neurologic examination during treatment of DKA. If cerebral edema is suspected, then one must act quickly and aggressively to prevent central, downward herniation of the brain:

Mannitol, fluid restriction, elevation of the head of the bed, intubation with hyperventilation, and immediate consultation with a neurosurgeon may all be indicated.

Hyperglycemia without ketoacidosis. Individuals with hyperglycemia but without ketoacidosis may not need intensive treatment with an insulin drip. These patients may either have type 1 diabetes with early presentation or a type 2 pattern of diabetes. One will need to consider the features outlined in Table 19–28, determine serum acid-base status, and consider measurement of urinary ketones, serum C-peptide or insulin levels, and autoantibodies to distinguish between the types of diabetes. In those suspected of having type 1 DM, or in type 2 patients with blood glucose concentrations in excess of 600 mg/dL or those receiving glucocorticoids, insulin often is the initial treatment of choice. Individuals with serum glucose values >600 mg/dL without significant ketoacidosis have a condition referred to as a nonketotic hyperosmolar state and often have altered mental status or coma. They may have profound fluid deficits, exceeding those found with DKA and leading to lactic acidosis. The absence of ketones may result from residual endogenous insulin production, although others postulate that this is secondary to lower levels of counterregulatory hormones or inhibition of lipolysis by hyperosmolality. Patients with lower blood glucose concentrations and a pattern more suggestive of type 2 DM may respond to an oral agent (discussed in the following section).

OUTPATIENT MANAGEMENT

Type 1 Diabetes Mellitus

Goals of therapy. The treatment goals for children with type 1 DM are outlined in Table 19–33. Important management components for achieving these goals are derived from the Diabetes Control and Complications Trial (DCCT). Patient, family and provider expectations are given in Table 19–34. Children should be followed by a pediatric diabetes team consisting of a nurse practitioner/certified diabetes educator, social worker or other mental health professional, registered dietitian, as well as a pediatric endocrinologist. The family should receive ongoing diabetes education, so that they are empowered

Table 19–33. Goals for Management of Children with Type 1 Diabetes Mellitus

Stabilize blood glucose within target range
Avoid acute metabolic decompensation (DKA, severe hypoglycemia)
Insure normal growth and development (physical and emotional)
Prevent long-term complications

DKA = diabetic ketoacidosis.

Table 19–34. Diabetes Outpatient Management

Family and patient expectations

Monitor glucose levels before each meal, at bedtime, occasionally during the night, and when symptomatic

Maintain written log books

Follow meal plan, with attention to carbohydrate intake

When out of honeymoon, administer 3 or more insulin injections per day, make adjustments for exercise, variation in intake

Provider expectations

Health care visit at least every 3 to 4 months, with HbA$_{1C}$ more frequent if not meeting goals

Regular access to a diabetes team, with ongoing education diabetologist, nurse educator, dietitian, counselor

Frequent telephone contact with family between visits, review of glucose logs, adjust regimen as needed, available for sick-day management

Screen for long-term complications, begin when patient has had diabetes mellitus for 5 years AND is in puberty, assess with yearly retinal exam, urinary microalbumin

with self-management skills. Visits with a health care professional are ideally scheduled at 3 to 4 month intervals, at which time a glycosylated hemoglobin or hemoglobin A$_{1C}$ (HbA$_{1C}$) is obtained (reflecting a 3-month average of blood glucose control). Visits may need to be more frequent in those with new-onset disease or in those unable to achieve target goals or with other problems related to DM. Blood glucose should be monitored routinely before each meal and at bedtime, occasionally in the middle of the night, and whenever the child is symptomatic. The family should maintain a written record of glucose levels, insulin doses, and variation in daily routine, and these records should be reviewed by the provider at regular intervals between clinic visits to reassess and adjust the daily regimen as needed.

There is no consensus among pediatric diabetologists on specific target ranges for glucose control during childhood. Some advocate similar ranges as used for adults, although children appear to be at higher risk for hypoglycemia and may have a lower risk for long-term complications prior to puberty. For the child under age 6, recurrent hypoglycemia carries a higher risk for permanent neurocognitive deficits, and thus many suggest a looser target range, with avoidance of hypoglycemia as the primary goal. Thus, many aim for target ranges between 100 to 200 mg/dL or even looser, especially in the affected toddler. For the prepubertal school-age child, one can assume a tighter target range than that in toddlers. The benefits of tight control for the pubertal adolescent have been established by the DCCT, and one should proceed with target ranges of 80 to 180 mg/dL, with glucose levels in the lower half of this range expected before meals and in the upper half postprandially. Ideally, the HbA_{1C} for the child above age 6 years should be within 1 to 2 percentage points of high normal for the assay that is used, with somewhat looser goals for the preschooler. A HbA_{1C} in the normal or nearly normal range is not always reassuring, as recurrent hypoglycemia will depress the overall average.

Therapeutic goals need to be individualized for each family. Above all, pediatricians need to foster healthy habits in daily diabetes management that will remain with the child for life. Thus, even if the target ranges are somewhat looser than they are in adults, the daily process of diabetes management should remain the same.

Insulin therapy. For patients whose DKA has been resolved with a continuous intravenous insulin infusion, one must convert patients to a subcutaneous insulin regimen in preparation for outpatient management. The pharmacokinetics of the most frequently used types of insulin are shown in Table 19–35. Because subcutaneous regular insulin has a delayed onset of action, it must be given 30 min before discontinuation of the intravenous insulin, which has an action limited to minutes.

Traditionally, patients have been placed on a regimen of sliding scale regular insulin around the clock for one or more days and then converted to a regimen that incorporates a longer-acting insulin, such as neutral protamine Hagedorn (NPH). However, one may directly institute an outpatient regimen using a combination of short- and long-acting insulins, often a combination of Lis-pro or regular and NPH insulins. The dose is initially derived empirically: Many children will require ~1 U/kg/day, but toddlers may need as little as 0.25 to 0.5 U/kg/day and adolescents may require ≥1.5 U/kg/day. The simplest initial regimen that approaches physiologic glucose control is administration of short- and intermediate- or long-acting insulins such as regular and NPH insulin before breakfast and before dinner (Figure 19–14A). Patients usually require more insulin during

Table 19–35. Pharmacokinetics of Different Human Insulin Preparations

	Onset	Peak	Duration
Lis-pro	5–15 min	30–90 min	3–4 h
Regular	30–60 min	2–4 h	5–8 h
NPH	1–2 h	4–8 h	10–18 h
Lente	1–3 h	4–10 h	12–20 h
Ultralente	2–6 h	8–14 h	18–30 h
Glargine	Few h		24 h

The timing of insulin action varies according to many different variables, including size of the dose; age and weight of the child; site of injection; and activity level. The specific action profiles of these insulin preparations must be derived for each individual.

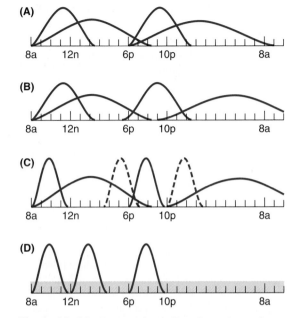

Figure 19–14. Commonly used insulin regimens for patients with type 1 diabetes mellitus. **A:** Standard split-mixed regimen, with short-acting and intermediate-acting insulins (in this case regular and NPH) given before breakfast and dinner. **B:** A 3-shot regimen, with the NPH moved to bedtime to prevent nocturnal hypoglycemia while providing better coverage through to breakfast, and minimizing effects from the dawn phenomenon. **C:** A 4-shot regimen commonly employed by school-aged children, with no injections during school. Lis-pro has been substituted for the regular insulin at breakfast and dinner. An extra injection of lis-pro may be needed in the midafternoon to cover snacks and to minimize hyperglycemia before dinner, as well as with bedtime NPH to cover that snack (denoted by dashed lines). **D:** An insulin regimen referred to as "the poor man's pump", in which ultralente administered at breakfast and dinner covers basal insulin needs (represented by the shaded area), and lis-pro at meals provides bolus coverage for carbohydrate intake and correction of glucose levels above target range. Alternatively, one can substitute a single evening injection of glargine to provide comparable basal insulin coverage provide by the ultralente. (Reprinted with permission from Gitelman SE, Diabetes mellitus, in *Rudoph's Pediatrics*, 21st ed, in press).

the day than they do at night, primarily to cover the carbohydrate that is ingested during the day. Therefore, two thirds of the total dose is commonly given in the morning. In addition, two thirds of the total insulin dose often is given as the longer-acting NPH. In the evening, the dose is often split evenly between the short- and long-acting insulins.

Blood glucose concentrations are monitored with a glucometer before each meal and at bedtime to evaluate the action of insulin at each interval. The morning (fasting) blood glucose level reflects the action of the pre-dinner NPH dose; the pre-lunch glucose concentration documents the morning regular insulin dose effect; the pre-dinner glucose concentration determines the efficacy of the morning NPH dose; and the bedtime reading reflects the response to the dinnertime regular insulin. If a consistent pattern is seen for several days in a row, then one should consider a 10% change in dose for the insulin covering that particular interval. A preset amount of insulin is used to cover the given carbohydrate intake at each meal (see nutrition section), and a sliding scale is determined for patients so that higher blood sugar readings can be compensated for with additional insulin. The size of these doses varies according to age and size of the child, but often is in the range of 0.5 to 1 U for each 15 g of carbohydrate ingested and 0.5 to 1 U for each 50 mg/dL that the blood glucose is elevated above target range.

Individuals may be initially resistant to insulin for the first several days after recovery from DKA, and their insulin needs may decrease significantly thereafter. This change may reflect increased physical activity or different dietary habits after leaving the hospital. In patients newly diagnosed with diabetes, this may represent their entrance into a remission or honeymoon phase of diabetes. At the time of initial diagnosis, many patients still have 10 to 20% of β-cell function. As blood glucose concentrations are reduced with initial insulin therapy, endogenous insulin secretion will resume for some time. However, this usually is for no more than 1 to 2 years. During this period, individuals may find that it is relatively easy to maintain blood sugar control, while exogenous insulin supplements ongoing endogenous insulin secretion.

As the honeymoon period wanes, patients may find that their previous insulin dose does not consistently correct their blood sugar concentrations. Whereas they may have been able to go to bed in the past with an elevated blood sugar level and awaken to find that it had normalized without supplemental exogenous insulin, they now note that their blood sugar levels remain elevated. Their dose of insulin supplementation may need to be increased to compensate for decreased endogenous insulin secretion.

Patients may become limited by the twice daily administration of insulin, particularly with insulin coverage at night. If they eat dinner at 6 PM, then the pre-dinner NPH dose will peak 4 to 8 h later, sometime between 10 PM and 2 AM. At this time, the NPH peak is not matched with carbohydrate absorption, and patients are at risk for nocturnal hypoglycemia. These patients may awaken with elevated blood sugar concentrations in the morning as a result of a Somogyi reaction, in which counterregulatory hormones have been secreted to compensate for the previous hypoglycemia. Alternatively, blood sugar levels naturally tend to increase between 4 and 8 AM, as cortisol and growth hormone levels increase. This process is known as the dawn phenomenon. In addition, the pre-dinner NPH effect is waning by this time; thus, the individual may simply be running out of insulin. To distinguish between these possibilities for patients with morning hyperglycemia, one may need to check the blood glucose concentration in the early morning hours. Nonetheless, one may need to not only increase the nighttime NPH dose, but also split the pre-dinner injection, giving regular insulin to cover dinner carbohydrate absorption and moving the NPH component to bedtime, at 10 to 11 PM (see Fig. 19–14B). Many school-aged children are reluctant to administer insulin at school; therefore, one of the most common regimens for these patients is to continue receiving 3 injections per day, with regular and NPH insulins before breakfast, regular at dinner, and NPH at bedtime.

Some patients can achieve tighter blood glucose control and more dietary flexibility with more frequent injections of regular insulin during the day. These patients will move to an injection of regular insulin before each meal with NPH at bedtime. A faster-acting insulin analogue, named lis-pro, is now often used in place of regular insulin in many of the regimens alluded to above. Regular insulin has a significant delay in its onset of action because it first associates into a larger crystal and must dissociate into a monomeric form to become biologically active. Lis-pro, so named because of the reversal of two amino acids of the β chain, is less likely to remain in a larger aggregate and therefore possesses significantly faster pharmacokinetics. Hence, this form of insulin is better designed to deal with postprandial carbohydrate absorption, which peaks 1 to 2 h after ingestion. Lis-pro can also be injected after the meal, when one is sure that the meal has been consumed, which may be particularly helpful for management of toddlers with DM. Because of its short duration of action, additional injections may be necessary, and it must be used in conjunction with a longer-acting insulin, such as NPH or ultralente.

One can also use an even longer-acting basal insulin, such as ultralente, in combination with a short-acting insulin (regular or Lis-Pro) before food ingestion (see Fig. 19–14D). This regimen has been referred to as the "poor man's pump," and has the most dietary flexibility, as the basal insulin coverage allows one to eat meals late, or even skip meals, without having to adjust the insulin regimen. Ultralente has some peak effect, and is often dosed twice per day. A new insulin analogue, glargine, appears to have more of a true basal effect, with no significant peak and a duration of 24 hours.

One increasingly popular option for DM management is the use of an insulin pump. This external device infuses short-acting insulin, usually lis-pro, continuously throughout the day via an indwelling subcutaneous catheter. One pre-programs the pump to deliver a continuous basal rate of insulin, which may change at various times throughout the day (such as for coverage of the dawn phenomenon). The pump wearer enters the doses of bolus insulin needed to cover food intake and to correct high blood glucose values. The pump cannot sense blood glucose concentrations and release an appropriate amount of insulin, i.e., it is not a closed-loop system, and therefore constitutes nothing more than a sophisticated insulin delivery device. Advantages of the pump include improved metabolic control, with reduced erratic swings in glucose, improved coverage of the dawn phenomenon, less tendency toward hypoglycemia, and increased flexibility and independence. Disadvantages of the pump include the stigma that may be associated from wearing a device that is readily viewed by others, possible skin infections at the catheter site, the need for set changes every 3 days, and the possibility of DKA if the pump should malfunction or, more commonly, if the infusion site becomes dislodged.

Nutrition and activity. Blood sugar concentration is affected not only by insulin, but also by food intake and exercise. Consistency in blood sugar readings is related to a reproducible pattern of food intake and exercise each day. Traditionally, individuals with diabetes have been taught to use an exchange system, with monitoring of protein, fat, and carbohydrate intake at each meal. Current recommendations are for patients with diabetes to follow a meal plan similar to that recommended generally for all individuals, with approximately 60% of caloric intake coming from carbohydrates and the remainder derived from an equal distribution between protein and fat. The carbohydrate intake often is divided evenly among the 3 daily meals but may be altered according to patients' eating habits. Furthermore, attention is now focused solely on total carbohydrate intake, and there is no attempt to subdivide carbohydrate intake into exchanges of fruit, dairy, and bread, for example. Thus, patients' diets or meal plans consist of a known total quantity of carbohydrates at each meal, and the specific components of the meal are left to the discretion of the individual. This approach lends more freedom to food selection. With more experience, individuals can alter their insulin dose to compensate for greater or lesser carbohydrate intake and may therefore eat according to appetite and food availability, rather than be tied to a rigid meal plan. In the past, the pharmacokinetics of regular insulin have made it necessary for many patients to have small carbohydrate snacks between meals and at bedtime; this may not be as important with the more discrete action of lis-pro insulin.

Physical activity will also affect blood sugar levels and often enhances sensitivity to a particular insulin dose.

These effects may occur during the exercise itself or may linger for hours after the event. One may compensate for such effects by either decreasing the dose of insulin or increasing carbohydrate intake before or during the activity, or by some combination of the two.

Sick days. Families must receive anticipatory guidance for DM management during acute illnesses. With adherence to the guidelines and ready telephone access to a health care provider, most hospital readmissions for DM can be averted (Table 19–36). Illness, even a mild upper respiratory infection, or stress may greatly increase insulin resistance and the tendency toward DKA. Insulin doses may need to be increased by 10 to 25% or more to compensate for the increased production of counter-regulatory hormones. If blood glucose remains >240 mg/dL over a 4 to 6 h interval or if there are gastrointestinal symptoms, then urinary ketones should be monitored. If ketones are moderate or large, then the family should be in contact with their physician for further guidance on insulin dosing. The family will need to monitor blood glucose and urinary ketones at 2- to 4-h intervals, and short-acting insulin doses may need to be repeated at 2- to 4- h intervals to treat hyperglycemia and curtail further ketoacidosis. Clear fluids should be encouraged to maintain hydration status and help clear ketones. With glucose levels >240 mg/dL, one should use sugar-free solutions. As glucose levels fall, one will need to introduce sugar-containing liquids.

If patients are vomiting, then one will need to distinguish DKA from a primary gastrointestinal process, most often gastroenteritis. One common mistake is to omit insulin in the absence of enteral intake. However, even if glucoses are not elevated, patients must continue to take

Table 19–36. Sick-Day Management

Stress of illness can increase insulin needs
Hyperglycemia or diabetic ketoacidosis may develop
If glucose concentrations >240 mg/dL × 2 or gastrointestinal symptoms, check for urine ketones
Call for advice if ketones moderately or markedly increased
May need to increase insulin doses ≥10–20%, and dose insulin more frequently
If vomiting
Maintain hydration, glucose concentration
<240 mg/dL, give glucose-containing fluids
>240 mg/dL, give glucose-free fluids
Consider use of an antiemetic
Never omit insulin
may need to reduce long-acting insulin by half to two thirds or use only short-acting at 2–4 h intervals

insulin to cover their basal needs and to avoid DKA. The insulin dosing can be adjusted in several different ways for such a scenario. One can elect to give small doses of short-acting insulin at 2- to 4-h intervals, using a sliding scale to adjust for variation in intake and glucose level. Alternatively, one can give one-half to two-thirds of the usual intermediate or long-acting insulin to provide basal needs and give additional doses of short-acting insulin as needed. One will need to pay close attention to hydration status and encourage small frequent sips, preferably of an electrolyte-containing solution. Promethazine hydrochloride suppositories, or other antiemetics, may be particularly helpful for those with recurrent vomiting, enabling continued outpatient management. The principal drawback to their use is the risk for sedation, but the benefits of such agents greatly outweigh the risks and may save unnecessary emergency room visits or hospitalizations. In exploring the cause of vomiting, one must always consider the possibilities that the current insulin has lost its potency and the family may need to use a new bottle, preceding insulin injections may have been omitted, or there is a serious underlying problem unrelated to DM such as appendicitis.

Hypoglycemia. One of the major limitations in diabetes therapy is the risk for hypoglycemia. Because exogenous insulin is not delivered in a closed-loop feedback system, the inevitable mismatches between administered insulin, carbohydrate availability, and exercise will result in hypoglycemia. The signs and symptoms of hypoglycemia are given in (Table 19–37). Mild-to-moderate episodes of hypoglycemia are associated with autonomic nervous system activation and result in neurogenic signs and symptoms. More profound decreases in serum glucose result in neuroglycopenia, with signs and symptoms secondary to cerebral dysfunction from lack of substrate availability.

The first line of treatment for hypoglycemia is oral ingestion of a simple carbohydrate, such as juice or glucose tablets (Table 19–38). These items need to be readily available for children throughout all daily situations. The

Table 19–37. Signs and Symptoms of Hypoglycemia

Neurogenic	Neuroglycopenic
Shakiness	Weakness
Palpitations	Confusion
Nervousness, anxiety	Difficulty in speaking
Diaphoresis	Incoordination
Hunger	Personality change
Tingling	Sleepiness, loss of consciousness
	Seizure

Table 19–38. Management of Hypoglycemia

Have simple carbohydrates available at all times
Verify signs and symptoms with a glucometer reading
Follow the rule of "fifteens"
    Take 15 g simple carbohydrate
    Recheck plasma glucose concentration in 15 min
    Repeat cycle if glucose concentration is not above
        100 mg/dL
For severe hypoglycemia
    Consider use of oral glucose if conscious
    May require intramuscular glucagon injection

amount of carbohydrate that needs to be ingested to treat hypoglycemia varies and must be individualized. Families should follow "the rule of fifteens" (see Table 19–38). As a rough guide, 15 g will raise the blood glucose of an adult approximately 50 mg/dL. Smaller children may require less simple carbohydrate for hypoglycemia correction, and those with more profound hypoglycemia may require greater amounts of carbohydrate for recovery. With moderate or severe hypoglycemia, children may require assistance to appropriately treat hypoglycemia. For the combative subject, or one who is not fully alert or conscious, treatment consists of an intramuscular glucagon injection. Although larger doses are often used, children under age 6 years (<30 kg) will exhibit a brisk response to 0.3 mg, and 0.5 mg will suffice for older children and adults.

Type 2 diabetes mellitus. Patients with new-onset type 2 DM often have hyperglycemia without ketoacidosis and are usually not acutely ill. Hospitalization may not be necessary. Possible outpatient treatment options are outlined in Table 19–39. For mild hyperglycemia (glucose levels <200 mg/dL and HbA_{1C} <8), one may first offer lifestyle changes, with elimination of simple carbohydrates and reduced fat intake coupled with increased

Table 19–39. Treatment of Type 2 Diabetes Mellitus

Lifestyle modifications
    Dietary changes
    Increased exercise

Pharmacotherapy
    Increase insulin concentration
        Sulfonylurea
        Exogenous insulin
    Decrease insulin resistance
        Metformin
        Thiazolidinediones
    Inhibit carbohydrate absorption
        α-Glucosidase inhibitors

exercise. For persisting or more significant hyperglycemia, one will need to initiate medial therapy. In the past, the only choices were sulfonylureas, which enhance endogenous insulin secretion, or exogenous insulin. The problems with these choices are a tendency to gain further weight and the risk for hypoglycemia. There now are means to attack the underlying insulin resistance in these patients with the use of either metformin (a biguanide) or thiazolidinediones. Both classes of drugs help improve lipid profiles, a concern in this patient population, without the risk of hypoglycemia. Metformin is favored over thiazolidinediones because patients tend to lose a modest amount of weight with the former, and the latter has been associated with hepatic injury. An alternate choice is an alpha-glucosidase inhibitor, which blocks absorption of complex carbohydrates, but which may lead to problems associated with the subsequent malabsorption (cramping, bloating, and loose stools). Patients who remain hyperglycemic on one medication will need to be placed on additional medications until metabolic control is achieved, in much the same way that one approaches asthma or hypertension.

NATURAL HISTORY AND LONG-TERM ISSUES

After 5 or more years, individuals with diabetes may have complications resulting from diseases that are microvascular (manifest as retinopathy, neuropathy, and nephropathy) and macrovascular (atherosclerosis). Diabetes is currently the leading cause of blindness, end-stage renal disease, and nontraumatic limb amputation for adults in the United States, and is a significant risk factor for myocardial infarction and stroke. The DCCT has confirmed the long-held suspicion that better blood glucose control lessens the risk for development of such complications. Better glucose control reduces the risk of development of microvascular complications in patients who have never had such findings and slows the progression in those with long-standing diabetes in whom complications have already developed. This study was conducted primarily in an adult population; approximately 10% of the study population were adolescents. It remains controversial as to how to apply such findings to younger children because signs of end-organ damage are rarely detected in prepubertal individuals, regardless of the duration of their diabetes. However, preliminary studies suggest that prepubertal blood glucose control may alter the rate at which complications develop during adult years. Nevertheless, one must exercise caution in how tightly one attempts to control blood sugar levels in children. Children appear to be at greater risk for development of hypoglycemia than are adults, perhaps because of less predictable daily schedules, with more variable exercise and diet. Furthermore, children younger than 6 years of age with diabetes who have experienced recurrent hypoglycemia are at increased risk for neurocognitive deficits.

Therefore, one may need to accept less stringent control of blood sugar levels in toddlers to avoid the risks of hypoglycemia, but to expect tighter control as these children approach adulthood.

Screening for complications should begin when children have had diabetes for 5 years and have entered puberty. Studies should include a yearly dilated retinal examination to screen for retinopathy and a urine test to screen for microalbuminuria, which is an early sign of nephropathy.

FUTURE DEVELOPMENTS

"Cures" for type 1 DM have proved elusive over the years. Investigators continue to pursue alternate means of insulin delivery, including implantable pumps, which deliver insulin directly into the portal system, and inhaled insulin. These remain temporizing measures, until a closed-loop system has been devised. Transplantation of pancreas tissue or β cells is currently possible but requires ongoing immunosuppression to inhibit graft rejection by the recipient. The resultant side effects render this approach unacceptable, except in those individuals who require an additional organ transplant, such as in the case of renal failure. Newer, more selective agents may allow suppression of organ graft rejection without global immunosuppression. Current research efforts are also directed at means of bypassing the immune system, such as transplanting β cells in a semipermeable membrane. With such a system, glucose can diffuse across the membrane to the β cells and secreted insulin can diffuse out into the circulation, but lymphocytes and larger molecules, such as antibodies and cytokines, cannot directly contact and destroy the cells.

Development of an "artificial" pancreas has also met numerous roadblocks. Such a device will need to function as a closed-loop system, in which it senses blood glucose and delivers an appropriate amount of insulin to maintain glucose levels in a normal range. Although the technology currently exists for insulin delivery, as with insulin pumps, the ability to detect glucose accurately has proved to be a more difficult task. Ongoing efforts are directed at development of invasive sensors that rest within a blood vessel or subcutaneous tissues and noninvasive monitoring, such as transcutaneous infrared devices. Several prototypes have been approved by the FDA and are used in limited fashion.

Investigators are also seeking ways to screen for and prevent the development of type 1 DM. Many agents have been used in an attempt to prolong the honeymoon phase, but none have proved reliable, as it appears that too much β cell damage may have been incurred by that time. The presence of islet cell autoantibodies and an abnormal intravenous glucose tolerance test result are sensitive indicators for those in whom diabetes will likely develop in the future. Trials are underway to determine whether treatment with insulin will induce tolerance and help prevent diabetes in these individuals.

Additional studies are being performed to determine if nicotinamide will protect the β cell from autoimmune destruction and if early infant feeding with an elemental formula decreases the future risk for type 1 DM.

HYPONATREMIA

The causes and diagnostic aspects of hyponatremia are considered in Chap. 15, "Kidneys and Electrolytes." Hyponatremia is a prominent manifestation of adrenal insufficiency. The features of adrenal insufficiency are presented in the following section.

Adrenal Insufficiency

ANATOMY AND PHYSIOLOGY

The adrenal glands, once referred to as suprarenal glands, are so named for their location just above the kidney. The adrenal gland consists of an outer cortex, in which steroid hormones are produced, and an inner medulla, which produces catecholamines (Figure 19–15). The cells of the adrenal cortex originate from mesoderm, whereas the medulla arises from ectoderm.

To understand the mechanism for salt loss with adrenal insufficiency, one must first understand the normal physiology of steroid hormone production within the adrenal cortex. The cortex may be further subdivided into three layers histologically, each of which produces a distinct class of steroid hormones. The production of these hormones is mediated by different factors (Table 19–40).

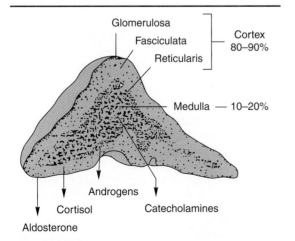

Figure 19–15. Anatomic zones and secretions of the adrenal gland. (Reproduced with permission from Guyton AC: *Textbook of Medical Physiology*. Saunders, 1986.)

The glomerulosa is the outermost cortical layer in which mineralocorticoids are produced. Aldosterone is the end product of this pathway. Aldosterone acts on the kidney at the distal tubule, where it augments sodium reabsorption and potassium and hydrogen secretion, thereby expanding vascular volume and maintaining blood pressure. The production of aldosterone is mediated principally by the renin-angiotensin system. Diminished blood pressure and sodium depletion stimulate release of renin from the juxtaglomerular apparatus in the kidney. Renin then acts enzymatically on angiotensinogen to convert it to angiotensin I. This product is, in turn, converted to angiotensin II by converting enzyme, a protein synthesized in the lungs and vasculature. Angiotensin II subsequently acts at two different levels to maintain blood pressure: First, it acts directly on the vasculature as a potent vasoconstrictor. Second, it stimulates synthesis and secretion of aldosterone, in turn promoting sodium retention and expansion of vascular volume.

The middle layer of the adrenal cortex, the fasciculata, is the site of glucocorticoid production. The end product of this pathway is cortisol. Cortisol influences a number of basic physiologic processes essential to survival, including maintenance of vascular tone and integrity, maintenance of serum glucose levels, and clearance of free water. Cortisol production is mediated directly by ACTH release from the pituitary gland, which in turn is stimulated indirectly by corticotropin-releasing factor (CRF) from the hypothalamus. The release of CRF and ACTH is modulated by cortisol in a classic negative feedback loop. Glucocorticoids are known to inhibit both pituitary ACTH and hypothalamic CRF. The ACTH also exerts a short negative feedback effect on CRF release. Cortisol and ACTH are produced in a pulsatile manner, with diurnal variation: Peak concentrations are achieved in the early morning, and lower values are noted in the afternoon and evening. The adrenal gland produces 6 to 9 mg/m²/day of cortisol; however, under stress this may increase to 3 to 15 times this amount. Cortisol circulates principally attached to binding proteins, of which transcortin (also known as corticosteroid-binding globulin) is the main such factor.

The innermost layer of the adrenal cortex, the reticularis, is where the adrenal androgens DHEA, DHEA(S), and androstenedione are produced. These are weak androgens that have only limited clinical effects on virilization. In the peripheral tissues, they are converted to testosterone and dihydrotestosterone, resulting in pubic and axillary hair growth, body odor, and acne. A central factor from the hypothalamus and pituitary gland has been postulated to regulate adrenal androgen production, but no such factor has been identified to date.

DIFFERENTIAL DIAGNOSIS AND CLINICAL PRESENTATION OF ADRENAL INSUFFICIENCY

Adrenal insufficiency may result either from a problem in the adrenal gland itself, termed a *primary defect*, or

Table 19–40. Steroid Hormone Production within the Adrenal Cortex

Zone	Type of Steroid	End Product	Regulator of Production
Glomerulosa	Mineralocorticoid	Aldosterone	Renin/angiotensin
Fasciculata	Glucocorticoid	Cortisol	Corticotropin-releasing factor
			Adrenocorticotropic hormone
Reticularis	Androgens	Dehydroepiandrosterone, androstenedione DHEA-S	Unknown

from a problem in the pituitary gland or hypothalamus (a secondary or tertiary defect, respectively). Possible causes of a primary defect are shown in Table 19–41. Primary etiologies associated with salt losing are given in Table 19–42.

Congenital adrenal hyperplasia. The most common cause of primary adrenal insufficiency is congenital adrenal hyperplasia (CAH) (see earlier section, "Approach to children with Ambiguous Genitalia."), which is secondary to an enzymatic defect in the biosynthesis of cortisol (Figure 19–16). These are autosomal recessive defects and have been described at every possible step of steroid hormone production except at the initial step, P450 scc. The effect on steroidogenesis may be predicted from inspection of the pathway, with some enzymatic defects affecting both glucocorticoid and mineralocorticoid synthesis (such as 21-OH defi-

ciency), some having an isolated effect on glucocorticoid synthesis (such as 11-β hydroxylase deficiency) or mineralocorticoid synthesis (aldosterone synthase deficiency), and some having an effect on neither but affecting androgen production (17-β hydroxysteroid dehydrogenase deficiency). The heterogenous collection of disorders affecting glucocorticoid production is referred to as CAH because the defect leads to increased secretion of ACTH, which in turn results in hypertrophy of the adrenal gland.

21-hydroxylase deficiency. 21-OH deficiency is the most common form of CAH, accounting for approximately 95% of cases in the United States. The clinical presentation depends on the severity of the enzymatic block. The most severe deficiency, in which no 21-OH activity is present, occurs early in life with salt-wasting crisis. This condition is relatively common, occurring in approximately 1/12,000 individuals. Because 21-OH is involved in both aldosterone and cortisol production, individuals with absence of this enzyme lack the ability to synthesize either hormone. Transfer of maternal steroid hormones across the placenta helps to maintain the neonate for the first 5 days to 2 weeks of life. These patients then manifest their hormone deficiency with nonspecific gastrointestinal symptoms, such as nausea and vomiting, and finally progress to dehydration and shock. Biochemical findings include metabolic acidosis with hyponatremia, hyperkalemia, and hypoglycemia.

Table 19–41. Causes of Adrenal Insufficiency

Primary
  Congenital adrenal hyperplasia
  Autoimmune adrenalitis—may be component of
    polyglandular syndromes
  Congenital adrenal hypoplasia or aplasia
  Infection
    Tuberculosis, fungal
    AIDS, opportunistic infections
    Hemorrhage secondary to sepsis (meningococcus,
      others)
  Trauma
  Adrenoleukodystrophy
  Metastatic disease
  Infiltration
    Sarcoidosis, hemochromatosis
  ACTH unresponsiveness

Secondary
  Withdrawal from glucocorticoid therapy
  Isolated CRF or ACTH deficiency
  Hypothalamic defect or hypopituitarism—may be from
    developmental defect, tumor, infiltrative lesion, radiation

ACTH = adrenocorticotropic hormone; CRF = corticotropin-releasing factor.

Table 19–42. Causes of Salt-Losing Primary Adrenal Insufficiency

Salt-losing forms of congenital adrenal hyperplasia (includes
    mineralocorticoid and glucocorticoid deficiencies)
Isolated defects of aldosterone synthesis and responsiveness
Destructive lesions of the adrenal cortex
    Autoimmune
    Fulminant infection
    Hemorrhage
    Peroxisomal disorders (including adrenoleukodystrophy)
    Tumor metastases

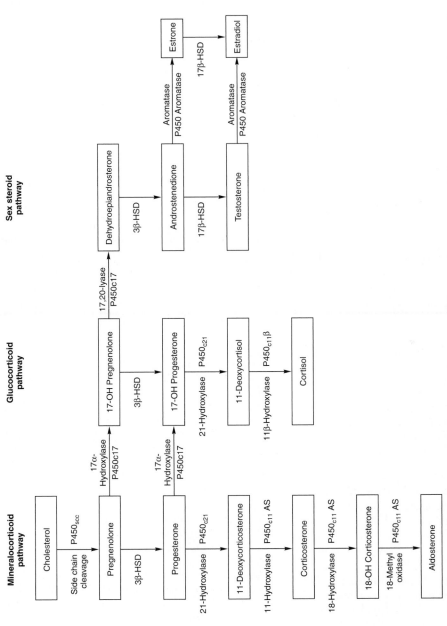

Figure 19–16. Biosynthetic pathways of adrenal steroid production. The diagram is laid out according to the layers of the adrenal cortex, with the outermost layer, glomerulosa, shown on the left (site of aldosterone production); the fasciculata layer (site of cortisol production) is in the middle; and the innermost reticularis layer (site of androgen production) is on the right. These enzymatic reactions occur primarily in the gonads, not in the adrenal cortex. The enzymatic activity is shown on the left or above each arrow, whereas the actual enzyme is shown on the right or below each arrow. Different enzymatic steps are often mediated by a single enzyme. 3β-HSD = 3β-hydroxysteroid dehydrogenase; P450$_{c11}$ AS = P450$_{c11}$ aldosterone synthetase; 17β-HSD = 17β-hydroxysteroid dehydrogenase. (Reproduced and adapted with permission from Miller WL: Molecular biology of steroid hormone synthesis. Endocrine Rev 1988;9:295.)

Another manifestation of this enzymatic defect results from an accumulation of steroid hormone precursors in the glucocorticoid and mineralocorticoid pathways. These precursors are then diverted into the sex steroid pathway and result in overproduction of testosterone. Female infants are virilized, and the condition therefore may be detected before the onset of salt loss by virtue of the physical examination. In male infants, however, the condition may not be detected (unless there is a prior family history of this disorder). A subtle clue on physical examination may be the presence of hyperpigmentation, most notable over the labioscrotal folds and in other skin creases. This finding is the result of overproduction of melanocyte-stimulating hormone, which is secreted in conjunction with ACTH.

The specific diagnosis of CAH is confirmed by measurement of the steroid hormone intermediate immediately preceding the enzymatic block, such as 17-hydroxy progesterone (17-OHP) in the case of 21-OH deficiency. The levels of this steroid intermediate are mildly elevated in normal infants for the first 24 h after birth and are even more elevated in premature infants. In equivocal cases, an ACTH stimulation test will confirm the diagnosis: One obtains baseline levels of cortisol and steroid hormone precursors, including 17-OHP, then gives an intravenous bolus of ACTH and measures the steroid hormone levels 60 min later. If 21-OH deficiency is present, a hyper-responsiveness of 17-OHP is noted. A nomogram to verify this diagnosis has been established for baseline and ACTH-stimulated 17-OHP values.

Initial treatment of CAH requires stress dose glucocorticoid replacement along with dextrose, normal saline, and aldosterone replacement (see later). When stable, treatment may be continued with oral glucocorticoid, mineralocorticoid, and sodium chloride.

Most cases of 21-OH deficiency that present in the newborn period are associated with salt loss, at least to some degree. Milder forms of 21-OH deficiency may manifest as ambiguous genitalia without salt loss in the neonatal period or with premature pubarche during childhood; such cases are referred to as simple virilizers. Even milder cases of 21-OH deficiency have been described as presenting later in life with hirsutism and menstrual irregularities; these individuals are considered to have nonclassic CAH. Such variant forms of 21-OH deficiency occur quite commonly, affecting about 1/1000 individuals.

Other causes of primary adrenal insufficiency. Other disorders that may cause primary adrenal insufficiency are listed in Table 19–41 and are referred to collectively as *Addison disease*. In the past, tuberculosis was the most common cause of adrenal insufficiency, but now autoimmune adrenalitis is the most commonly diagnosed etiology. The inciting antigens appear to be the steroidogenic enzymes themselves. This condition may be associated with other endocrinopathies; when occurring in conjunction with thyroiditis or diabetes mellitus, it is referred to as *Schmidt syndrome*. More extensive multiorgan involvement may be noted with autoimmune polyglandular syndromes, one of which also involves chronic mucocutaneous candidiasis. There may be an underlying developmental defect in adrenal gland formation, resulting in congenital adrenal aplasia or hypoplasia. This is transmitted in autosomal recessive or X-linked fashion: The latter is associated with a contiguous gene syndrome, in which a gene affecting adrenal development is deleted along with genes causing Duchenne muscular dystrophy and glycerol kinase deficiency. Congenital lipoid adrenal hyperplasia may have a similar clinical presentation but entails grossly enlarged adrenal glands in which cholesterol cannot be shuttled into the mitochondria for subsequent metabolism. The adrenal gland may also be destroyed by massive adrenal hemorrhage during a traumatic delivery and during sepsis with meningococcus (*Waterhouse-Friderichsen syndrome*), as well as by other organisms. In addition, the adrenal gland may be damaged by various agents in the stages of AIDS. Adrenoleukodystrophy is an X-linked disorder of very-long-chain fatty acid metabolism characterized by CNS white matter disease in association with adrenal insufficiency. The neurologic disorders may either precede or follow adrenal defects, depending on the nature of the genetic lesion. Finally, infiltration from metastatic cancer, sarcoid, or hemochromatosis can also lead to adrenal insufficiency.

The aforementioned disorders are all associated with defects of both mineralocorticoid and glucocorticoid deficiency. With sudden absence of the steroid hormones, patients may have adrenal crisis, in similar fashion to neonates with salt-losing CAH. More insidious onset of hormonal insufficiency will be initially associated with milder symptoms, including malaise, weakness, dizziness with orthostatic hypotension, nonspecific gastrointestinal complaints, and hyperpigmentation (Table 19–43). A superimposed stressful event, such as an infection, may in turn precipitate an acute adrenal crisis.

Table 19–43. Signs and Symptoms of Adrenal Insufficiency

Lethargy, weakness
Anorexia
Nonspecific gastrointestinal complaints; nausea and vomiting
Postural hypotension
Salt craving
Hyperpigmentation (primary)
Dehydration
Hyponatremia, hyperkalemia, hypoglycemia, metabolic acidosis

An isolated defect in cortisol production, without mineralocorticoid deficiency, may also present with hyponatremia, although this does not result from salt loss. Rather, glucocorticoid deficiency results in an inability of the kidneys to clear free water thought to be secondary to inappropriate secretion of ADH. Isolated cortisol deficiency usually occurs with defects in either CRF or ACTH production. Although an isolated defect in this particular axis may occur, it usually is associated with a lesion that affects other hormonal axes, such as a CNS tumor, infiltrative or granulomatous lesion, and destruction radiation therapy. The most common reason for an isolated defect in this axis is previous chronic treatment with glucocorticoids at supraphysiologic levels. Exposure to more than the equivalent of 20 mg/m²/day of cortisol for more than 10 days may lead to suppression of the adrenal axis at the hypothalamic levels, and it may take 6 months or longer to recover from such suppression. Finally, a rare mutation of the ACTH receptor may be associated with isolated cortisol deficiency and is referred to as ACTH unresponsiveness.

DIAGNOSIS OF ADRENAL INSUFFICIENCY

The diagnosis of adrenal insufficiency may be established by monitoring endogenous secretion of cortisol or by evaluating the response to provocative stimuli. With the diurnal and pulsatile nature of cortisol secretion, it is difficult to establish adrenal insufficiency on the basis of a single blood test result. However, a morning cortisol level of less than 5 μg/dL is very suspicious for adrenal insufficiency, especially if coupled with an elevated ACTH value. To evaluate cortisol secretion over time, it often is helpful to measure a 24-h urine collection for 17-OHCS, with normal being 3 ± 1 mg/m²/day. The ACTH stimulation test (as described in the section, "Congenital adrenal hyperplasia") is often used to evaluate adrenal function, with a stimulated cortisol value greater than 20 μg/dL considered a normal response. Various other provocative stimuli have been used to evaluate the entire CRF-ACTH-adrenal axis, including metyrapone (a compound that blocks the final enzymatic step in cortisol production), response to insulin-induced hypoglycemia, and the CRF stimulation test.

TREATMENT OF ADRENAL INSUFFICIENCY

To treat adrenal insufficiency, one must replace the missing steroid hormones at physiologic doses. Cortisol production has been estimated at 6 to 9 mg/m²/day of cortisol. Such an amount is adequate for parenteral supplementation, but one often needs to use slightly greater amounts (approximately 10 to 15/m²/day) for enteral replacement. There are a number of different preparations that one can select (Table 19–44). Some agents have combined glucocorticoid and mineralocorticoid actions, whereas others have isolated glucocorticoid effects. These medications have vastly different potencies in their

Table 19–44. Relative Potency of Various Steroids (Relative to Hydrocortisone)

	Glucocorticoid	Mineralocorticoid
Hydrocortisone	1	1
Prednisone	4	1
Dexamethasone	25	0
Betamethasone	20	0
Aldosterone	0.2	400
9α-Fluorocortisol	8	400

glucocorticoid-like activity. In children, the replacement doses often are so small and require such fine incremental changes that the least potent glucocorticoids (usually hydrocortisone) are used. This enables one to minimize overtreatment, with the attendant problems of Cushing syndrome, including growth suppression.

During times of stress, such as a febrile illness or a surgical procedure, an individual with a normal adrenal axis will produce 3 to 15 times the basal amount of cortisol. Patients with adrenal insufficiency must mimic this stress response at such times, administering 3 times their usual dose of glucocorticoid to avoid adrenal crisis. If patients are vomiting and unable to take medications enterally, then they must receive parenteral glucocorticoid treatment. Families must be instructed on the use of intramuscular hydrocortisone: Patients receive a single injection of 50 mg/m² and then are brought to the emergency department for further management. In the emergency department, the physician must quickly assess patients' cardiovascular statuses (blood pressure, heart rate, and perfusion) and glucose and electrolyte levels. Patients may require ongoing support with parenteral glucocorticoid treatment (50 mg/m²/day of hydrocortisone, divided into doses every 6 h), normal saline, and dextrose intravenous fluids. When the stress has passed, and patients have been afebrile for 24 h, the usual maintenance regimen may be quickly reinstated.

For mineralocorticoid replacement, one uses 9α-fluorocortisol at doses of 0.05 to 0.2 mg/day. Blood pressure, electrolyte levels, and plasma renin activity are monitored to determine whether the dose is adequate. Unlike glucocorticoids, the mineralocorticoid replacement does not need to be altered in the face of stress; aldosterone secretion does not change acutely in such settings. These patients also need additional sodium chloride in their diet. Neonates usually have a salt-restricted diet, with limited sodium in their formula; however, in this instance they may need up to 1 to 3 g of added salt per day. Older children may be able to adjust their salt intake spontaneously, either choosing salty food items or using additional table salt in their foods to maintain an appropriate balance.

Syndrome of Inappropriate Antidiuretic Hormone

Syndrome of inappropriate antidiuretic hormone (SIADH) is characterized by an inability to dilute urine maximally in the face of hyponatremia and volume overload (Table 19–45). In this condition, secretion of ADH persists despite a hypotonic plasma. This results in water retention and hyponatremia, which is primarily dilutional but also in part is due to a volume expansion-induced natriuresis. The causes of SIADH are outlined in Table 19–46. Most commonly, excessive ADH secretion is associated with CNS diseases, including tumors, trauma, and infection. Less frequently, inflammatory lung disease may cause SIADH, apparently by decreasing the normal baroreceptor-mediated inhibition of ADH secretion. The SIADH is also associated with pharmacologic agents that potentiate ADH secretion or action. Ectopic ADH secretion is rare in children and may be associated with carcinoma of the lung and pancreas, thymoma, hepatoma, lymphoma, or carcinoid tumors.

Therapy for SIADH includes treatment of the underlying disorder and fluid restriction. Replacement of lost body sodium also may be necessary but usually can be achieved through normal dietary salt intake. Severe hyponatremia (plasma sodium <120 to 125 mEq/L) may be associated with CNS abnormalities, such as seizures, and may require treatment with hypertonic intravenous sodium chloride solution (3%). Concurrent use of a diuretic, such as furosemide, may be indicated when volume expansion is severe. The sodium deficit is calculated by the following equation:

$$\text{Sodium deficit} = (0.6) \times (\text{body weight in kilograms}) \times (\text{normal plasma sodium} - \text{observed plasma sodium}).$$

However, the plasma sodium concentration should not be corrected too quickly. Overzealous treatment may result in CNS damage, including central pontine myelinolysis. It is generally recommended that plasma sodium

Table 19–45. Features of Syndrome of Inappropriate Antidiuretic Hormone (SIADH) Secretion

Persistent secretion of ADH despite hypotonic plasma
Inability to maximally dilute the urine in face of hyponatremia and volume overload
Laboratory
Plasma: hyponatremia (plasma Na <135 mEq/L); hypoosmolality (plasma osmolality <280 mosmol/kg)
Urine: less than maximally dilute (urine osmolality >100 mosmol/kg); persistent sodium excretion (urine Na generally >20 mEq/L)

Table 19–46. Causes of Syndrome of Inappropriate Antidiuretic Hormone Secretion

ADH from posterior pituitary
• CNS disease (e.g., tumors, trauma, infection)
• Lung inflammatory disease
• Drugs that stimulate ADH release
Ectopic ADH production
• Carcinoma of lung and pancreas
• Thymoma
• Hepatoma
• Lymphoma
• Carcinoid tumors

ADH = antidiuretic hormone; CNS = central nervous system.

be corrected to a "safe" level of approximately 125 mEq/L at a rate no greater than 0.5 to 1 mmol/L/h. Thereafter, plasma sodium concentration can be corrected gradually over several days. Chronic SIADH is treated with fluid restriction and may require supplementation with a diuretic or an agent such as demeclocycline, which impairs the responsiveness of the renal tubule to AVP.

REFERENCES

Short Stature

Drug and Therapeutics Committee, Lawson Wilkins Pediatric Endocrine Society: guidelines for the use of growth hormone in children with short stature. J Pediatr 1995;127:857.

Hintz RL, et al (Genentech Collaborative Group): Effect of growth hormone treatment on adult height of children with idiopathic short stature. N Engl J Med 1999;340:502.

Oberfield SE: Growth hormone in normal short children—a plea for reason. N Engl J Med 1999;340:557.

Rosenfeld RG, et al: Growth hormone therapy of Turner's syndrome: beneficial effect on adult height. J Pediatr 1998;132:319.

Tanner J: The diagnosis and treatment of endocrine disorders. In Kappy MS, et al (editors): *Wilkins The Diagnosis and Treatment of Endocrine Disorders in Childhood and Adolescence.* Thomas, 1994.

Abnormalities of Puberty

Ehrhardt AA, Meyer-Bahlburg HF: Psychosocial aspects of precocious puberty. Horm Res 1994;41(Suppl 2):30.

Grumbach MM, Styne DM: Puberty: Ontogeny, neuroendocrinology, physiology, and disorders. In Wilson JD, et al (eds): *Williams Textbook of Endocrinology.* Saunders, 1998.

Herman-Giddens ME, et al: Secondary sexual characteristics and menses in young girls seen in office practice: a study from the Pediatric Research in Office Settings Network. Pediatrics 1997; 99:505.

Kaplowitz PB, Oberfield SE: Reexamination of the age limit for defining values when puberty is precocious in girls in the United States: implications for evaluation and treatment (Drug and

Therapeutics and Executive Committees of the Lawson Wilkins Pediatric Endocrine Society). Pediatrics 1999;104:936.

Werber E, et al: Six year results of spironolactone and testolactone treatment of familial male-limited precocious puberty with addition of deslorelin after central puberty onset. J Clin Endocrinol Metab 1999;84:175.

Obesity

Kalra SP, et al: Interacting appetite-regulating pathways in the hypothalamic regulation of body weight. Endocr Rev 1999;20:68.

Troiano RP, Flegal KM: Overweight children and adolescents: description, epidemiology, and demographics. Pediatrics 1998; 101:497.

Cushing Syndrome

Papanicolaou DA, et al: A single midnight serum cortisol measurement distinguishes Cushing's syndrome from pseudo-Cushing states. J Clin Endocrinol Metab 1998;83:1163.

Tsigos C, Chrousos GP: Differential diagnosis and management of Cushing's syndrome. Annu Rev Med 19996;47:443.

Sexual Differentiation

Federman DD, Donahoe PK: Ambiguous genitalia: etiology, diagnosis, and therapy. Adv Endocrinol Metab 1995;6:91.

Goodfellow PN, Lovell-Badge R: SRY and sex determination in mammals. Annu Rev Genet 1993;27:71.

Grumbach MM, Conte FA: Disorders of sex differentiation. In Wilson JD, et al (editors): *Williams Textbook of Endocrinology.* Saunders, 1998.

Thyroid Gland

Burrow GN, et al: Maternal and fetal thyroid function. N Engl J Med 1994;331:1072.

Dayan CM, Daniels GH: Chronic autoimmune thyroiditis. N Engl J Med 1996;335:99.

Fisher DA: Management of congenital hypothyroidism. J Clin Endocrinol Metab 1991;72:523.

Foley TP, Jr: Goiter in adolescents. *Endocrinol Metab Clin North Am* 1993;22:593.

Nelson JC, Clark SJ, Borut DL, et al: Age-related changes in serum free thyroxine during childhood and adolescence. J Pediatr 1993;123:899.

Ridgeway EC: Clinician's evaluation of a solitary thyroid nodule. J Clin Endocrinol Metab 1992;74:231.

Hypoglycemia

Fernandes J, Berger R: Hypoglycaemia: principles of diagnosis and treatment in children. Baillieres Clin Endocrinol Metab 1993; 7:591.

Grimberg A, et al: Dysregulation of insulin secretion in children with congenital hyperinsulinism due to sulfonylurea receptor mutations. Diabetes 2001;50:322.

Hawdon JM, et al: Prevention and management of neonatal hypoglycaemia. Arch Dis Child Fetal Neonatal Ed 1994;70:F60.

Schwitzgebel VM, Gitelman SE: Neonatal hyperinsulinism. Clin Perinatol 1998;25:1015.

Thomas PM, et al: Mutations in the sulfonylurea receptor gene in familial persistent hyperinsulinemic hypoglycemia of infancy. Science 1995;268:426.

Antidiuretic Hormone Physiology

Frasier SD, et al: A water deprivation test for the diagnosis of diabetes insipidus in children. Am J Dis Child 1967;114:157.

Kovacs L, Robertson GL: Syndrome of inappropriate antidiuresis. Endocrinol Metab Clin North Am 1992;21:859.

Robertson GL: Diabetes insipidus. Endocrinol Metab Clin North Am 1995;24:549.

Robinson AG, Verbalis JG: Diabetes insipidus. Curr Ther Endocrinol Metab 1997;6:1.

Diabetes Mellitus

Atkinson MA, Maclaren NK: The pathogenesis of insulin-dependent diabetes mellitus. N Engl J Med 1994;331:1428.

Burge MR, Schade DS: Insulins. Endocrinol Metab Clin North Am 1997;26:575.

Diabetes Control and Complications Research Group: Diabetes Control and Complications Trial (DCCT): The effect of intensive treatment of diabetes on the development and progression of long-term complications in adolescents with insulin-dependent diabetes mellitus. J Pediatr 1994;125:177.

Kahn CR, Weir GC [editors]: *Joslin's Diabetes Mellitus,* 13th ed. Philadelphia, Lea & Febiger, 1994.

Kaufman FR: Diabetes in children and adolescents: Areas of controversy. Med Clin North Am 1998;82:721.

Medical Management of Type 1 Diabetes, 3d ed. Alexandra, Va, American Diabetes Association, 1998.

Plotnick L, Henderson R: *Clinical Management of the Child and Teenager with Diabetes.* Baltimore, Johns Hopkins University Press, 1998.

Rosenbloom RL, Joe JR, Young RS, Winter WE: Emerging epidemic of type 2 diabetes in youth. Diabetes Care 1999;22:345.

Santiago JV: Insulin therapy in the last decade. Diabetes Care 1993; 16(Suppl 3):143.

Siperstein MD: Diabetic ketoacidosis and hyperosmolar coma. Endocrinol Metab Clin North Am 1992;21:415.

Adrenal Insufficiency

Grinspoon SK, Biller BMK: Laboratory assessment of adrenal insufficiency. J Clin Endocrinol Metab 1994;79:923.

Miller WL: Genetics, diagnosis, and management of 21-hydroxylase deficiency. J Clin Endocrinol Metab 1994;78:241.

New MI, et al: The adrenal hyperplasias. Page 1881 in: Scriver C, et al (editors): *The Metabolic Basis of Inherited Disease.* New York, McGraw-Hill, 1989.

Oelkers W: Adrenal insufficiency. N Engl J Med 1996;335:1206.

The Nervous System

20

Francis J. DiMario Jr., MD

OVERVIEW AND ORGANIZATION

This chapter will present a practical approach to pediatric neurology. Despite a wide variety of neurologic complaints that can present to the practitioner, the cause of these complaints can often be identified after obtaining a careful history and examination. Specific neurologic history and examination techniques useful in delineating specific diagnostic entities will be emphasized. This chapter will cover the most common pediatric neurologic problems, except for infectious diseases affecting the nervous system. To learn more about this topic, the reader is referred to Chap. 9, "Infectious Diseases."

NEUROLOGIC HISTORY AND EXAMINATION

The ability to obtain a careful, succinct, and pertinent history of the present illness is a fundamental skill every practitioner must possess. In young patients, this requires developing a nonthreatening rapport from the outset. Because of their age, many pediatric patients are unable to clearly articulate the specific problems they are experiencing but must transmit that information in nonverbal ways. Nonetheless, careful questioning of even young children can sometimes elicit information necessary in making an accurate diagnosis. The clinician should not hesitate to ask children even as young as 2 or 3 years of age what they perceive their problem to be. Similarly, the clinical examination relies heavily on astute and skillful directed observation of the children in spontaneous activity or engaged in specific activities that demonstrate the relevant information desired. A detailed examination of the various functions of the nervous system is often obtained in a piecemeal but carefully orchestrated fashion.

Patients' evaluation begins with the careful delineation of the chief complaint. Recording the events that occurred around the time when the problem was first identified and detailing when the problem is more apparent and when it is less evident are important. It should be determined whether the problem appears to be static, variable in severity, or is getting progressively worse. A developmental history can be obtained using any number of available screening tools. When parents have a hard time remembering the exact age the children passed certain developmental milestones, one could inquire about the developmental skills of the children at certain events in their lives, such as birthdays, holidays, and vacations. A past history of similar problems for the children or other family members should be sought. Sometimes further information can be obtained by asking family members about specific types of complaints or behaviors as opposed to disease names, which are often not well recalled. A comprehensive family history can be easily recorded by using a simple pedigree diagram. A general review of systems, revealing such things as the impact of concurrent medications, recent illnesses or trauma, and integrity of the family dynamics are all-important aspects to explore and may offer clues to the diagnosis.

The majority of the neurologic examination of young children is simple observation with some direction at different junctures. Engaging the children relatively quickly in an effort to gain some degree of trust and allay fear will maximize the information that can be obtained. This is particularly true of toddlers and preschool-aged children. Allowing them to play with some small office toys, play catch, or draw, write, or copy onto a piece of paper is very helpful in assessing their cognitive understanding and hand–eye coordination and serves as a benchmark for serial comparisons. This can be done while obtaining the history from the parents.

The physical examination should include a general assessment of the patients, as well as a more focused neurologic examination according to the complaint. Vital signs and growth parameters (especially head circumference) should be obtained in each patient and plotted against expected norms. It should be noted whether the children appear to be dysmorphic or have facial characteristics of their parents. The skin should be inspected, looking in particular for neurocutaneous markers. When examining the extremities, loosely shaking the arms and legs will obtain a quick assessment of tone and recoil. As a routine procedure, one should gently percuss the spine from bottom to top looking for tenderness. This should be done particularly in patients with back pain or gait disturbance and can be a helpful clue in detecting an underlying occult dysraphism or intraspinal processes.

Neurologic examination of children should incorporate some assessment of their cognitive ability, general level of alertness, and understanding of language (both speech and nonverbal communication). While formal mental status testing is not often performed in children, by 4 years

796

of age most children can recite their name and address and, with some prompting, may give more detailed information with regard to their phone number and friends. Older children can be asked to repeat words or phrases, identify primary colors, and follow a sequence of three instructions. School-aged children should be able to spell specific words forwards and then backwards. These questions give an assessment of concentration, attention, and cognitive ability. Asking children at the end of a visit about the words they were asked to remember can give you an idea of memory and recall. The quality and articulation, as well as the grammatical construct of children's speech, offers a sense of their coherence and age-appropriate language skill. Their curiosity for surroundings and degree of impulsivity will help assess their visual and auditory attention.

The cranial nerve examination can be directed even in young age groups. Visual tracking and visual fields can be assessed grossly with confrontational testing methods. This is accomplished by facing the children, directly eye to eye, and slowly bringing a hand puppet or other object into the peripheral field until they are distracted toward the side of the stimulus. Obvious deficits can be readily identified, but more subtle ones will require formal visual field testing. Observing for ocular movement in all directions and for the presence of nystagmus in a direction of gaze or at rest is important. The red reflex of the optic fundi, as well as pupillary reactivity and consensual response to direct light, can be easily seen using an ophthalmoscope. It is helpful to give the children a flashlight to hold and shine against an opposite wall while examining the fundi. This simple method distracts attention from the examiner and focuses the children's eyes on a distant point when assessing for convergence and strabismus. A complete facial nerve motor assessment can be done during the interview process and examination by looking for forehead wrinkling, eyelid closure, mouth movement, and facial symmetry. The assessment of hearing is accomplished by rubbing one ear with your hand and whispering in the other ear. Another simple bedside testing method is by simultaneously placing your hands next to each ear and then rubbing fingers together on alternating sides. The children are then asked to identify which side the noise is on. The oropharynx should be examined for movement of the soft palate and tongue position, bulk, and presence or absence of fasciculations.

Examination of muscle tone and strength involves observing for symmetry of muscle bulk, limb deformity, or length discrepancies. Formal strength measurement is not always feasible, but a functional assessment can be made. For example, engaging children in a game of catch and then having them run after the ball can assess motor performance. Lower leg strength can be assessed if the children can walk on their tiptoes and heels. Children can be asked to climb up on furniture or ambulatory children can be asked to lie on the floor on their stomach or

back and quickly rise. Gowers maneuver can assess weakness or abnormal tone if it is a concern (Figure 20–1). A positive Gowers sign is indicated by the children's need to use the arms to climb up the body or to pull on a nearby object to arise from the floor; it is an indication of proximal muscle weakness in the hip girdle. While this sign is not specific for any particular muscle disorder, it does suggest the need to further assess muscle strength and function. Another good manual method of assessing proximal muscle strength is to suspend patients with one's arms under their axillae. If the children slip through one's hands, this indicates shoulder girdle weakness.

Reflex testing should be performed routinely and is readily obtainable in all children. A simple assessment of whether the reflexes are present, absent, or extremely brisk is helpful. Testing for plantar responses should be done; the first movement of the great toe is the most important

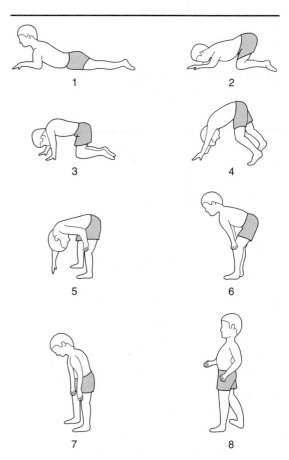

Figure 20–1. The Gowers maneuver: Observe as child "climbs-up" the legs and trunk to stand. (Reproduced with permission from Dubowitz V: *Muscle Disorders in Childhood.* 2d ed. Saunders, 1995.)

assessment of this response. Typically, a flexor response is normal. An extensor response is acceptable in infants up to the age of 6 to 9 months. Its significance should always be interpreted in light of other pertinent findings because it is rarely found in isolation when central nervous system pathology is present.

Watching children's postural stability when seated alone and unsupported is part of the initial assessment of cerebellar function. Wavering movements of the head or trunk are suggestive of cerebellar dysfunction. Observing for ataxic limb movements when the children reach for an object in front and above their shoulder level provides another clue. Another test of cerebellar function is rapidly tapping the index finger onto the thumb. This can be done by children as young as 3 years of age.

The approach to the neurologic examination of infants is somewhat different. In addition to the observations described earlier, more physical manipulation is needed to elicit appropriate information. As babies mature from newborn through infancy, primitive reflex responses are replaced by protective reflexes and then finally by voluntary responses (Table 20–1). Identification of aberration in the sequence of development of motor status may indicate an underlying nervous system dysfunction. Children who begin to regress and lose development skills should be examined for reemergence of postural and/or primitive responses. This is the hallmark of progressive neurodegenerative diseases, which require immediate investigation.

PAROXYSMAL EVENTS IN CHILDHOOD

Some of the most common and interesting neurologic problems in children are the paroxysmal phenomena. By definition, a paroxysmal event is episodic in nature, variable in duration, and fairly stereotypic in character. It is most important for the practitioner to determine whether the event is a seizure. Epileptic events are associated with abnormalities in the brain electroencephalogram (EEG) recording, which correspond to and cause the episodic event. It may not at first be possible to differentiate between epileptic and nonepileptic phenomena. The key to making a diagnosis is by detailed history. The age of children when the events began, the existence of specific precipitants of the spells, their periodicity and frequency, recognition of a preceding warning or aura, and their duration need to be determined. In addition, it is important to decide if the same stereotypic event occurs each time or if there are different types of events.

It is unusual that a practitioner actually observes the phenomenon. However, with the greater availability of video cameras, parents often will bring a recording of an event they have witnessed. It can be invaluable to actually see what the parents are describing.

Although several classifications of nonepileptic paroxysmal events are available, it is useful to consider the following groups: Those associated with altered mental status or occurring during sleep and those occurring while awake or with no altered mental status (Tables 20–2, 20–3 and Figure 20–2).

Nonepileptic Events Associated with an Alteration in Consciousness or Sleep

BREATH-HOLDING SPELLS

Breath-holding spells in childhood are relatively common nonepileptic events associated with a disturbance in mental status. Despite the term, these events are not actually breath-holding but occur rather in full exhalation. The diagnosis is readily made by obtaining a very specific history of the event. Typically, children first become upset and begin to cry. This is followed by an immediate or gradually developing state of noiselessness with either marked pallor or cyanosis, followed by decreased consciousness. The children's tone may progress to an opisthotonic posture and myoclonic jerks may be exhibited. As many as 15% of children with severe breath-holding spells develop a generalized convulsion during the terminal phase of the spell. The children then suddenly gasp, with full inspiration and improvement in color and consciousness returns fairly rapidly. Although the children may appear dazed briefly, they typically are back to normal activity within a few minutes. These spells are sometimes misdiagnosed as epilepsy, but the stereotypical sequence of color change followed by loss of consciousness distinguishes breath-holding events from seizures. The breath-holding spells are considered severe when consciousness is lost. Children who have color change and noiselessness but do not lose consciousness are described as having "simple" breath-holding spells. Breath-holding spells are also defined by the skin color during a spell. Pallid breath-holding spells usually begin with a few whimpers followed by sudden pallor and noiselessness and then loss of consciousness. Cyanotic breath-holding spells are characterized by a more protracted period of crying, accompanied by deepening cyanosis before loss of consciousness occurs.

In the majority of children, breath-holding spells first develop around 12 months of age and can increase in frequency to one or more per week over the second year of life. The frequency gradually declines, with approximately one-half of affected children experiencing resolution of the events by 36 to 42 months of age. On occasion, children may continue to have these spells up to 7 years of age. A strong family history is often obtained; in more than one-third of families there is a history compatible with an autosomal dominant pattern with reduced penetrance. While serious sequelae have not been observed routinely, up to 17% of children with pallid spells may develop syncopal episodes in adolescence. A dysregulation of autonomic maturation has been postulated as the underlying physio-

Table 20–1. Evolution of Primitive, Postural, and Protective Reflexes

Reflex	Stimulus	Response	Ages Present
Palmar grasp	Place finger into palm	Hand grasps finger promptly and persistently	~26 weeks–7 months
Plantar grasp	Place thumb onto ball of foot	Toes grasp thumb promptly and persistently	~26 weeks–7 months
Babinski sign	Stroke dorsum of foot from lateral surface over ball of foot toward great toe	Extension of great toe with extension and fanning of toes	~26 weeks–8 months
Moro	Sudden drop of head from 30° supine upright to horizontal	Extension of arms followed by adduction over chest	~30 weeks–5 months
Rooting	Touch corners of mouth and midpoints of each lip	Rotation and lip pursing toward site of stimulus	~34 weeks–4 months
Placing	Touch dorsum of foot on table edge	Raises foot and places it on table	~34 weeks–5 months
Gallant	Suspend prone with one hand under chest and draw thumb of opposite hand from scapulae inferiorly adjacent to spine	Truncal incurvature toward side of stimulus	~34 weeks–5 months
Asymmetric tonic neck	In supine position turn head from neutral to side position	Nonobligate extension of the ipsilateral arm into direction the face is turned toward with simultaneous flexion of opposite arm	1–5 months
Crossed adductor	While infant is seated, place palm over inner thigh of one leg and tap dorsum of hand	Hip adduction observed in both legs	1–8 months
Neck righting	In supine position turn head from neutral to side position	Contralateral shoulder and arm rotation across chest toward direction the face is turned	3–5 months
Landau posture	Suspend prone with one hand under chest observe prone posture	Inverted "U" Bobs head up horizontal Head remains horizontal Head and back arch past horizontal	Birth 0–2 months 4–6 months 6 months
Lateral propping	In supported seated position facing away from examiner, briskly tip infant toward alternate sides, observe arms	Arm extends out in support of trunk at side being moved downward	5–7 months
Parachute	Suspend prone with hands around chest and move briskly toward table surface, observe arms	Arms extend out in protective position	7 months–2 years
Blink to threat	Quickly flick fingers into direction of eyes	Automatic blink	10 months

logic mechanism. A relation between iron deficiency and provocation of spells has been suggested but not proved.

SYNCOPE

Orthostatic syncope may occur with sudden changes in posture. A hot environment, frequently associated with mild dehydration, or a sudden surprise or fear are common precipitants. These events are seen more often among adolescents than among younger children. There is a rapid loss of postural tone following the patients' sensation of "visual gray-out." Patients should be able to describe a gradual constriction of their visual fields and the sensation of collapse. The history of attempts to protect themselves while falling and a prompt resolution upon lying prone are consistent with orthostatic syncope. Other causes of syncope are discussed in Chap. 16, "Circulation."

Table 20–2. Paroxysmal Nonepileptic Events of Childhood Associated with Alterations in Consciousness or Sleep

Severe breath-holding spells
Cyanotic
Pallid
Syncope
Gastroesophageal reflux
Nasopharyngeal reflux
Physiologic sleep myoclonus
Sleep-related motor activity
Parasomnias
Night terrors (pavor nocturnus)
Somnambulism
Bruxism
Enuresis
Nightmares
Narcolepsy
Cataplexy
Sleep paralysis
Hypnogogic hallucinations
Apnea
Obstructive
Central (Ondine curse)
Somatoform disorder
Munchausen syndrome
Munchausen syndrome by proxy

Table 20–3. Paroxysmal Nonepileptic Events of Childhood without Alterations in Consciousness or Sleep

Simple breath-holding spells
Movement disorders
Tics
Myoclonus
Tremor
Shuddering spells and hyperexplexia
Stereotypies and self-stimulatory behaviors
Head banging
Chorea
Ballism
Athetosis
Dystonia
Headaches
Migraine
Migraine variants
Paroxysmal vertigo
Paroxysmal torticollis
Cyclic vomiting
Hemiplegic migraine
Ophthalmoplegic migraine
"Alice in Wonderland"
Tension and muscle contraction
Increased intracranial pressure
Somatoform disorder
Sandifer syndrome
Masturbation
Temper tantrums
Rage attacks
Alternating hemiplegia
Munchausen syndrome

SLEEP-RELATED EVENTS

There are a number of sleep-related phenomena that are responsible for paroxysmal nonepileptic events in children. The history verifies that these events occur exclusively during sleep. In addition to a detailed description of the event, it is particularly useful to determine when it occurs in relation to the start of sleep. Sleep disorders can be characterized as abnormally short sleep (insomnia), disturbed sleep (parasomnia), and excessive sleep (hypersomnia).

Seventy percent of infants develop the ability to sleep "through the night" by 3 months of age, 85% of infants by 6 months, and 95% by the end of the first year. *Sleeping through the night* is referred to as settling. A more complete description of normal sleep is described in Chap. 1, "Normal and Abnormal Development in the Infant and Child." A number of environmental factors can interrupt normal achievement of settling, including family stresses, intercurrent illness, drug effects, and changes in sleeping quarters. Approximately 50% of infants aged 6 to 12 months will experience multiple awakenings after settling has been established.

The basic stages of sleep are divided into REM (rapid eye movement) sleep and non-REM sleep. To appreciate the clinical phenomena associated with each sleep stage, it is helpful to understand some of the basic physiologic changes that occur (Table 20–4). Non-REM sleep has four discrete stages characterized by alterations on EEG recordings. These are characterized by a gradual transition from near-wakefulness (stage I) to slow wave activity across a greater proportion of recorded sleep time (stage IV). Respiration and pulse during non-REM sleep are characterized as slow and regular. There are very few eye movements during non-REM sleep, and they are typically slow and dysconjugate. This stage is accompanied by normal muscle tone. As sleep state transitions from non-REM stage I through IV, body activity gradually diminishes. Dreams are experienced in the REM sleep stage. It is accompanied by rapid irregular respirations and pulse rate; eye movements are characteristically rapid and conjugate, and muscle tone is generally flaccid.

Sleep follows a typical maturation pattern with age. Although adults normally enter sleep in non-REM stage I, the onset of sleep in the neonate is typically in REM sleep followed by frequent cycling between non-REM and REM

(*text continues on page 803*)

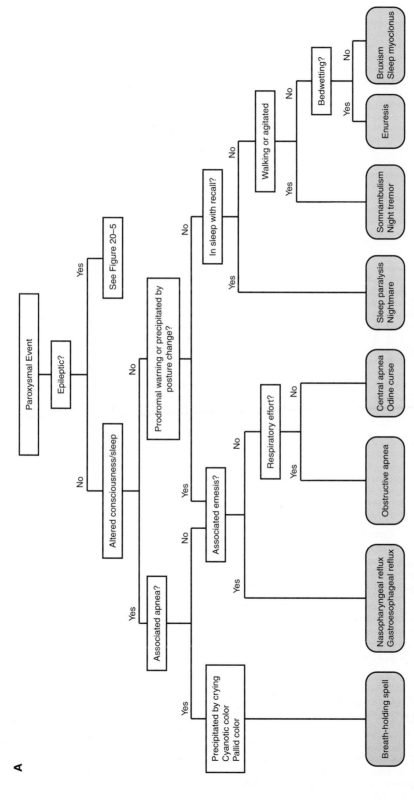

Figure 20–2. **A:** Decision algorithm for nonepileptic paroxysmal events with altered consciousness or sleep.

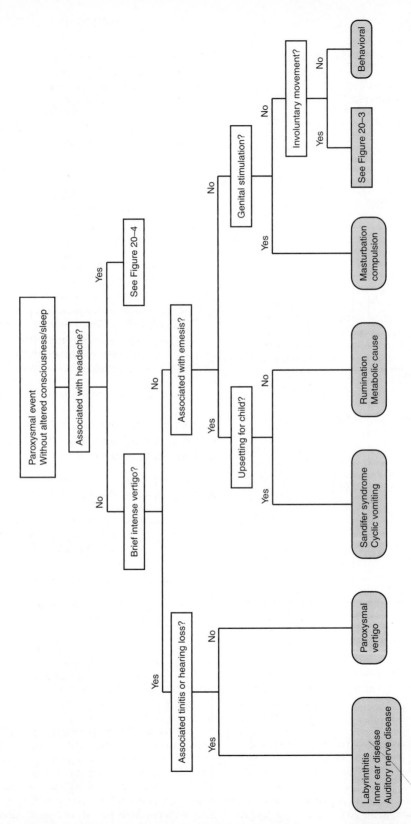

Figure 20–2. (*Continued*) **B:** Decision algorithm for nonepileptic paroxysmal events without altered consciousness or sleep.

Table 20–4. Physiologic Markers of Sleep

	Non-REM[1] (stages I–IV)	REM[1]
Respiration	Slow and regular	Rapid and irregular
Pulse rate	Regular sinus rhythm	Rapid rhythm
Eye movements	None–slow dysconjugate	Rapid conjugate
Axial muscle tone	Normal	Flaccid

[1] REM = rapid eye movement.

sleep. The REM sleep stage declines in total amount from 8 or 9 h per day in the neonate to only 1 or 2 h in the adolescent. It is not until the latter half of the first year that distinct stages (I to IV) develop in the non-REM sleep phase. The REM cycle recurs every 50 or 60 min in infants and then gradually increases in the cycle length to about every 100 min by adolescence. Most sleep-related phenomena are related to the intrastage transitions of normal sleep and normal physiologic movements associated with sleep cycles.

Myoclonic jerks and night terrors. Myoclonic movements are common during sleep in infants. These quick fragmentary jerks of the limbs or face, lasting seconds, are normal movements associated with transitions within non-REM sleep stages. In toddlers and early school-age children, night terrors (pavor nocturnus) are associated with transition from non-REM to REM sleep stage. This is one of several *parasomnias* appreciated in childhood; (see Chap. 3, Developmental-Behavioral Pediatrics).

Hypersomnias. A common complaint, particularly during adolescence, is that of excessive daytime sleepiness. Although adolescents normally have increased sleep requirements, additional history may direct the physician to consider the diagnosis of narcolepsy. **Narcolepsy** typically presents after the age of 11 years. It is an uncommon disturbance with an incidence of about 0.03 to 0.05% with a slightly higher incidence in families with narcoleptic patients. This disorder is characterized by frequent daytime microsleeps. Similar to the sleep pattern of neonates, these patients often enter sleep with REM activity. They rapidly pass into a dream state and are often plagued by physiologic changes during wakefulness that are normally associated with dream activity, such as sudden loss of muscle tone. As a result of this paroxysmal and instantaneous onset of muscle paralysis, patients may suddenly drop to the ground. These attacks are typically provoked by sudden emotions or surprise and are known as cataplectic attacks. Another symptom associated with the quick transition into REM sleep includes hypnagogic

hallucinations. These are frightening and vivid nightmare hallucinations that occur just prior to the start of sleep. Narcoleptic patients may also have sleep paralysis upon awaking. This is produced because patients "awaken" to mental awareness before fully recovering from the physiologic flaccid muscle tone characteristic of normal REM sleep. Narcolepsy is a life-long disorder, but the condition can be managed with treatment aimed at ameliorating specific symptoms (e.g., stimulants for excessive sleepiness).

Sleep apnea is another uncommon problem that produces excessive daytime sleepiness. It should be considered in children with signs and symptoms of upper airway obstruction. Coexistent nasopharyngeal, oropharyngeal, or laryngopharngeal dysfunction or deformity may be predisposing anatomic factors, as well as thoracic rib cage deformity (such as achondroplasia). Excessive obesity (such as Prader-Willi syndrome) is an additional predisposing condition. Children with bulbar dysfunction may subsequently develop lower cranial nerve paresis, and this may result in orolaryngopharngeal weakness with airway obstruction. This can be seen with progressive brainstem compression in children with Arnold-Chiari malformation. Patients with neuromuscular disorders affecting bulbar musculature may develop hypoventilation due to airway obstruction and inadequate inspiration.

Paroxysmal Nonepileptic Events Not Associated with Alterations of Consciousness or Sleep

Paroxysmal nonepileptic events in childhood not associated with an alteration in consciousness or sleep include a range of involuntary movements disorders (see Table 20–3); it is helpful to define the movement as rapid or quick versus slow or prolonged (Figure 20–3). The body segment involved in the movements should be determined. Fairly slow, prolonged, and sustained movements are called *athetosis;* slow irregular episodic movements are termed *dystonia.*

Rapid or quick movements should be further characterized as stereotyped (same in quality and location each time) or nonstereotyped. Nonstereotyped rapid movements, with an amplitude of several centimeters or more of limb displacement, are referred to as ballistic-type movements. Choreiform movements are those typically involving only a few millimeters of excursion. In some patients, there is an overlap along a continuum between the two movement disorders.

If the rapid movements are stereotyped, it should be ascertained whether the movement itself is rhythmic. Rhythmic movement or to-fro oscillation is most consistent with tremor. Nonrhythmic movements are classified as myoclonic (simple, sudden, and single movements) or tics (complex movements that incorporate a more elaborate body posture or organization).

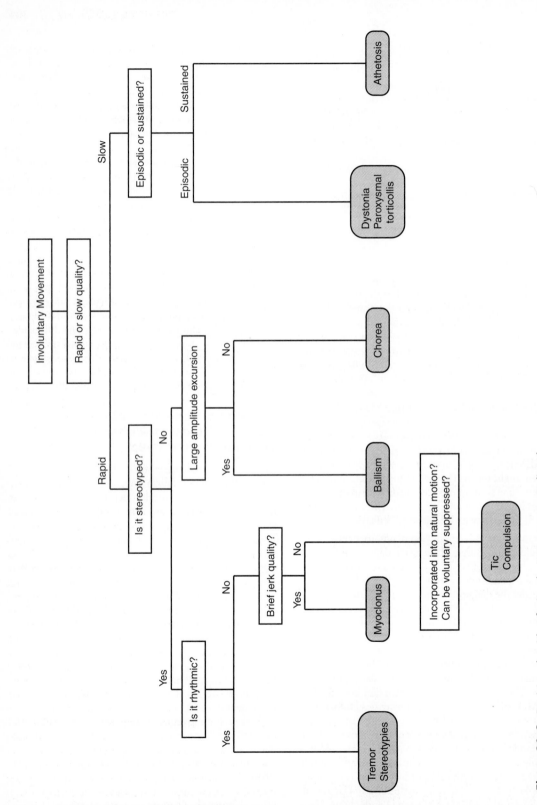

Figure 20–3. Decision algorithm for involuntary movement disorders.

Tics

Tics are probably the most common involuntary movements observed in children. Many children are unaware of the movement until it is brought to their attention by a parent or teacher. When they are intense and frequent, the children may be able to voluntarily suppress them, but they experience a sense of relief when they are ultimately expressed again. Thus, tic movements may be limited during school hours, but exacerbate when the children arrive home. Tics can be a motor, vocal, or sensory phenomena. Common motor tics incorporate eye blinking, facial grimacing, head and neck craning, arm twitching, shoulder shrugging, or lip lapping. More complicated motor behaviors include obsessive-compulsive behaviors such as skipping or engaging in a ritual set of behaviors. Vocal tics are usually variations of squeaking, chirping, coughing, or sniffing. Sensory tics, in contrast, are more difficult for patients to describe but often involve an unusual or uncomfortable sensation such as tingling or itching or having clothing not feel quite right.

Tics are generally transient, with a duration of less than 1 year. Transient tics are usually simple and most often involve single motor behaviors. Typically, there are no other associated morbid features or long-term sequelae. When tics endure for longer than 1 year, a chronic tic disorder should be suspected. These children often develop multiple motor tics that are not incapacitating and wax and wane in frequency and severity. Most tics disappear with sleep and are exacerbated by stress or anxiety. If the children experience multiple motor and vocal tics, a diagnosis of Tourette syndrome should be considered (Table 20–5). Less frequent phenomena associated with Tourette syndrome include the repetition of obscenities (coprolalia), the repetition of another person's spoken word (echolalia), and the repetition of one's own words (palilalia). Other associated comorbid features can include attention-deficit hyperactivity disorder, learning disabilities, and obsessive-compulsive disorder. Treatment is directed at symptoms and is recommended only if the tics become incapacitating from a physical, emotional, or

Table 20–5. Diagnostic Criteria
for Tourette Syndrome

- Presence of both multiple motor and vocal tics during illness.
- Tics present intermittently over 1-year duration.
- Tics with evolving complexity and waxing and waning character.
- Onset prior to age 18 years.
- Occurrence not exclusively during psychoactive drug use or known central nervous system (CNS) disease.

social perspective. Attention to comorbid diagnoses and occasionally family therapy can be of value.

Myoclonus

Myoclonus is a simple nonrhythmic stereotyped movement disorder that is uncommon in childhood. However, a form of physiologic myoclonus is common in infants and children as they enter non-REM sleep. Hiccups are another well-known physiologic form of myoclonus. Pathologic forms of myoclonus are encountered in a number of degenerative processes and can be secondary to intercurrent diseases. Infants and children with hypoxic brain injuries may develop myoclonic movements shortly after sustaining the event. These movements are most frequent over the face and proximal limbs and may persist with variable frequency and severity. Epileptic myoclonic movements can be associated with atypical and typical absence seizures. When they occur with atypical absence seizures, they may be associated with progressive encephalopathy with cognitive impairment and other mixed-seizure types. An unusual familial syndrome of sudden startle responses occurring in both childhood and infancy is termed *hyperexplexia*. This myoclonus, or exaggerated startle response, is typically provoked by a sudden sound or tactile stimulus and can cause the children to fall from a standing position. It is often enhanced by anxiety or lack of sleep and is variable in its frequency. In infancy and childhood the children's motor tone appears more rigid or stiff. With increasing age, jerking during sleep becomes a fairly prominent component.

Stereotypies and Tremor

Tremors and stereotypies are the most common stereotyped and rhythmic movement disorders. Stereotypies are habit-type movements, sometimes complex in nature, often seen in children with autism. However, perfectly normal children with appropriate language development may also engage in stereotypies. These vary in complexity from simple twirling or flapping behavior to more rhythmic soothing movements such as rocking or head banging. Tremors are oscillatory, to-fro movements of variable amplitude and frequency. Characteristically, tremors are exacerbated by postures or actions against gravity, such as sitting, standing, or reaching. Shuddering spells are a common infantile form of tremor. These occur at about 6 months of age, are usually abrupt, and typically appear as a sudden shivering movement while the children are seated. There is no associated loss of awareness and the children behave as if an "ice cube was dropped down their back." The movements are very quick, lasting only a few seconds, and may be fairly frequent during the day. Tremors or similar phenomenon may be encountered in family members. Some medications can precipitate involuntary tremors; common among those are stimulant medications, caffeine, nicotine, bronchodilators, and valproic acid.

CHOREA AND BALLISMUS

Chorea and ballismus are much less common movement problems in childhood. A helpful clinical maneuver to elicit subtle choreiform movement is to utilize the "milk maid" sign. This is done by having the children grasp the extended index finger of the examiner and by feeling for the contraction and release of the children's hand while having them attempt to maintain a steady grip. An additional maneuver to elicit chorea is to ask the children to extend the arms above the head, assuming "a ballet" posture with the palms of the hands upward. Subtle involuntary proximal arm movements are more readily observed in this position, and the children may have difficulty in maintaining this pose.

An important cause of acute chorea and ballismus in childhood is Sydenham chorea. This occurs after an acute infection with group A *Streptococcus*. The chorea is often accompanied by some personality or emotional change, detected by the parents. Prominent ballistic movements can accompany chorea, dependent on the extent of central nervous system involvement. Antibody and inflammatory mediators produce irritation of extrapyramidal nuclei (caudate) and are responsible for precipitating the involuntary movements. The presence of Sydenham's chorea should prompt investigation for potential associated cardiac involvement. Less frequent causes of chorea include systemic lupus erythematosus, hyperthyroidism, and Wilson's disease.

ATHETOSIS

Athetosis is a slow and sustained movement disorder best recognized as facial grimacing, a writhing posture, and an undulating extremity or truncal torsion. It has been described as appearing as if the children are trying to swim through molasses. Athetosis usually occurs in association with choreiform movements and is frequently a manifestation of an underlying static encephalopathy, such as cerebral palsy. Other causes of athetosis include drug-induced movement disorders such as those occurring with certain anticonvulsants (phenytoin), antidepressants, and neuroleptics, as well as metabolic and genetic disorders (e.g., Lesch-Nyhan syndrome).

DYSTONIA

Dystonia is an episodic movement disorder precipitated by the simultaneous contraction of agonist and antagonist muscle groups within the same limb or segment of the body; it is often painful and sometimes involves a torsional quality. Idiopathic focal dystonias involve discrete segments of the body and includes blepharospasm (eye blinking), writer's cramp, and torticollis. Acute idiosyncratic drug reactions can precipitate dystonic reactions in children. These often present as an oculogyric crisis, focal torticollis, or opisthotonic posture. Common precipitants include neuroleptic medication such as dopamine antagonists and phenothiazines. A particular form of dystonia referable to the posterior neck muscles, resulting in hyperflexion of the neck, is referred to as *retrocollis*. This can be acquired from inferior cerebellar tonsillar compression secondary to posterior fossa abnormalities such as Arnold-Chiari malformation or cervical skeletal dysplasia. A childhood migraine variant can be manifested as episodic torticollis in young children. Dystonia syndromes may have a genetic basis, and dystonia may be a prominent feature of some neurodegenerative disorders (e.g., Niemann-Pick type C).

Headaches

The most common paroxysmal phenomenon in childhood is headache. Epidemiologic studies suggest that approximately 40% of children will experience a headache by 7 years of age with 1.5% having a true migraine headache by that age. These figures increase to 75% of children having headaches and over 5% experiencing true migraine attacks by 15 years of age. Headaches may present as acute recurrent events, may be chronic and progressive in nature, or chronic and nonprogressive (Figure 20–4).

It should first be determined whether the headache is associated with raised intracranial pressure or an associated systemic illness. Several sequential questions can help to categorize headaches. One should ask whether there is a single type of headache or multiple types. Even young children under age 3 or 4 years will be able to identify if there are different types of headache. The quality of the pain should be ascertained; a pounding or throbbing quality is most often associated with vascular or migraine-type headache. Young children may be able to qualify their headache pain by demonstration if they cannot describe it. For example, young children may squeeze a finger rhythmically to mimic a throbbing pain versus squeezing continuously to indicate a pressure-type of pain. Events that help reduce or exacerbate headache should be determined. A common feature of migraine-type headaches is their improvement with sleep. Whereas most other headaches improve with rest or diminished activity level, true sleep is not usually a necessary palliative feature. Identifying whether the pain radiates in a generalized fashion or if it is localized to one region is helpful. When children point to an area with the index finger, the practitioner should examine for more local causes of pain, such as adenopathy, neck injury, or scalp and skull lesions. Using the open palm to generally identify the area of pain is often associated with muscle contraction or vascular-type headache.

Grading the severity of the pain allows the practitioner to follow the effectiveness of interventions. Grading the pain on a scale of 0 to 10 in older children or assessing the functional disability induced by the headache (e.g., lies down and will not play or watch television) is

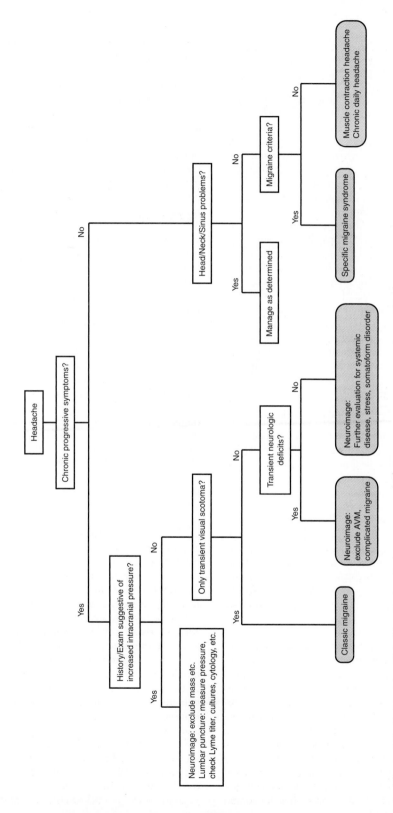

Figure 20–4. Decision algorithm for headache assessment.

useful. Associated signs and symptoms such as anorexia, nausea, vomiting, and pallor can help identify true migraine headache events, particularly in young children and toddlers. The timing of each individual headache, as well as its progression or course, will help clarify its nature. Headaches with associated vomiting, which consistently awaken patients from sleep, worsen in the morning, aggravate by postural change, and increase in severity, are likely to be associated with increased intracranial pressure. Headaches secondary to increased intracranial pressure ultimately produce changes in mental status or focal neurologic signs particularly if they evolve over a relatively short period of days to weeks.

The examination should be aimed at identifying signs of raised intracranial pressure (i.e., papilledema, visual loss, sixth cranial nerve palsy, and meningismus), as well as evidence of local processes, systemic disease, and additional focal neurologic deficits. Auscultation should include the skull and neck for bruits. Palpation of a "jaw click" during opening and closing of the mouth suggests that headaches may be due to abnormal closure of the temporomandibular joint. Brain imaging should be reserved for patients with focal examination findings, history and examination features suggestive of raised intracranial pressure, or progressive symptoms.

Common etiologic mechanisms for headaches in children include systemic disease, cranial inflammation, muscle contraction, and vascular headaches, especially migraine. Intracranial mass lesions can produce traction and displacement of intracranial structures, resulting in meningeal irritation and headache. Fortunately, this not a common cause of headache in childhood.

MIGRAINE

The diagnosis of migraine is usually based on a history of recurrent headaches separated by pain-free intervals. The headache is usually unilateral, throbbing in quality, and relieved by sleep. Additional features that help to identify the syndrome are anorexia, gastrointestinal upset, neurologic aura, photophobia, phonophobia, and a positive family history. In young children the presence of pallor is quite common. Migraine headaches are classified into several types. The *classic* variety is initiated by a visual obscuration or scotoma, followed by hemicranial throbbing pain. In the *common* migraine, headaches are similar but not accompanied by visual changes. *Complicated* migraine includes those varieties with neurologic deficits, such as hemiplegic migraine. In children, a special migraine category exists that includes variants such as paroxysmal vertigo and paroxysmal torticollis.

The pathophysiology of migraine had been thought to be initiated by an electrical stimulus resulting changes in vascular tone, based on regional changes in blood flow and the throbbing nature of the headache. Other mechanisms, however, have been suggested, such as a thalamic origin

and a chemical hypothesis involving serotonin among other neurotransmitters and neuromodulators.

Benign paroxysmal vertigo is a migraine variant occurring in children up to age 3 to 4 years.

Characteristically, the onset is abrupt and it presents with sudden fear, fright, nausea, and pallor. There is no loss of awareness, and the children typically cling to the parents unable to stand or walk steadily. Careful observation may reveal jerk nystagmus of the eyes. These episodes last from 20 to 30 seconds to a few minutes and may occur as frequently as several per week. After early childhood, they evolve into more readily identifiable migraine headaches. *Benign paroxysmal torticollis* is a less common migraine variant observed in young infants and toddlers. During these abrupt episodic events, the infant's head is turned to one side and any attempt to straighten the head is resisted. There is often associated pallor, vomiting, and apathy. There is no loss of awareness, but an unsteady gait or unstable truncal posture is often noted. These events last from several hours to days and occur once or twice a month. Over time, these episodes eventually evolve into more typical migraine headaches.

MANAGEMENT OF HEADACHE

Initial treatment of headaches is directed at removing exposure to anything that provokes events. A headache diary should be kept and should include associated phenomenon, palliative and provocative features, functional impairment, as well as duration and frequency. One should try to identify whether there is an element of secondary gain afforded to the children by the complaint of headache. Migraine headaches can be helped by acute symptomatic therapies (Table 20–6). These include analgesic, anti-inflammatory, and antiemetic medications. The use of combination medications in children over 10 or 12 years of age, such as butalbital/aspirin/caffeine or butalbital/acetaminophen/caffeine, for definitive migraine attacks are helpful. Ergot compounds and serotonin receptor agonists can also be effective, but they have as yet been approved by the Federal Drug Administration for use in children. If the frequency of headaches interferes with the children's activities more than several times each month, chronic preventative medication should be considered in addition to acute symptomatic treatments for each headache event. The choice of chronic preventive agents is dependent on the age of the children and their symptoms and tolerance (Table 20–7). Other treatments include various anticonvulsants, neurotransmitter modulators, vascular receptor blockers, and anti-inflammatory agents.

It is worth reemphasizing that neuroimaging is not always necessary when evaluating children with headaches. Evidence of raised intracranial pressure, focal neurologic deficits, or specific concurrent systemic illnesses should direct a specific radiological investigation. However, if neuroimaging is not performed, frequent follow-up is advised to clarify the headache course and allay parental anxiety. It is useful to have an open discussion regarding the likelihood of an underlying brain tumor as the cause for the particular child's headache syndrome. Since most parents have already thought about this possibility, if there is no evidence for this, it is important to directly state it is not the cause of the headache. When signs of raised intracranial pressure are evident or symptoms are suggestive, neuroimaging with computed tomography (CT) to rule out mass, hemorrhage, and hydrocephalus is appropriate. Magnetic resonance imaging (MRI) provides better definition of the central nervous system, but it is usually not as readily available in acute circumstances. When signs of raised intracranial pressure are evident (i.e., papilledema, sixth cranial nerve palsies, etc.) and neuroimaging is normal, a lumbar puncture is indicated to measure opening pressure and to examine cerebrospinal fluid.

PSEUDOTUMOR CEREBRI

Increased intracranial pressure in the absence of an identifiable cause is referred to as *pseudotumor cerebri*, or *benign intracranial hypertension*. This diagnosis is based on appropriate signs and symptoms, normal neuroimaging procedures, and measurement of raised intracranial pressure by lumbar puncture. The cerebrospinal fluid should be analyzed for evidence of infection, neoplasia, and inflam-

Table 20–6A. Acute Pharmacologic Analgesic Agents for Migraine Headaches[1]

Drug	Dosage	Formulation	Potential Side Effects
Acetaminophen (Tylenol)	10–15 mg/kg/dose q4h	Tablets: 80, 325, 500 mg; syrup: 160 mg/tsp	Gastritis, hepatic dysfunction
Ibuprofen (Motrin)	5–10 mg/kg/dose q6h	Tablets: 200, 400, 600, 800 mg; syrup: 100 mg/tsp	Gastritis, thrombocytopenia
Naproxen sodium (Naprosyn)	10–20 mg/kg/day twice daily	Tablets: 250, 275 mg	Gastritis, thrombocytopenia
Combination preparations			
Butalbital, aspirin/acetaminophen, caffeine (Fioricet, Fiorinal, Esgic)	1–2 tablets bid/tid/qid	Tablets	Sedation, hallucinations, gastric upset
Isometheptane, acetaminophen, dichloralphenazone (Midrin)	1–2 capsules, repeat hourly, ≤5 capsules per dose	Tablets	Dizziness, rash, contraindicated with glaucoma

[1] Modified with permission from Lewis DL: Page 102 in: Rothner AD: *Headaches in Children and Adolescents.* Semin Pediatr Neurol 1995; 2(2): 102.

Table 20–6B. Acute Pharmacologic Antiemetic Agents for Migraine Headaches[1]

Drug	Dosage	Formulation	Potential Side Effects
Promethazine (Phenergan)	0.25–0.5 mg/kg/dose q4–6h	Tablets: 12.5, 25, 50 mg; syrup: 6.25, 12.5 mg/tsp; suppository: 12.5, 25, 50 mg	Sedation, hallucinations, dry mouth, constipation, dystonia
Trimethobenzamide (Tigan)	15–20 mg/kg/day divided tid; max 250 mg tid	Tablets: 100, 250 mg; suppository: 100, 200 mg	Sedation, Reye syndrome, seizures, dry mouth, constipation, dystonia
Prochlorperazine (Thorazine)	0.4 mg/kg/day tid/qid	Tablets: 10, 15 mg; syrup: 5 mg/tsp; suppository: 2.5, 5.25 mg	Sedation, hallucinations, dry mouth, constipation, dystonia
Metoclopramide (Reglan)	0.1–2.0 mg/kg/dose Repeat 6–8 h	Tablets: 5, 10 mg; syrup: 5 mg/tsp	Sedation, hallucinations, dry mouth, constipation, dystonia
Hydroxyzine (Atarax)	2 mg/kg/day bid/tid; up to 10–25 mg bid/tid	Tablets: 25, 50 mg; syrup: 10 mg/tsp	Sedation, hallucination, dry mouth, constipation, dystonia

[1] Modified with permission from Lewis DL: Page 102 in: Rothner AD: *Headaches in Children and Adolescents.* Semin Pediatr Neurol 1995; 2(2): 102.

Table 20-6C. Acute 5-HT Receptor Agonists for Migraine Headaches[1]

Drug	Onset of Action	Bioavail Half-Life	Efficacy (Approximate)	Rebound (12–24 h)	Side Effects	Adverse Effects
Sumatriptan (Imitrex 1993)	PO: 1–3 h; SC: 15 min–1 h; IN: 15–60 min	10–15%; 2 h	PO: 65% @ 2 h; SQ: 70% @ 2 h; IN: 65% @ 2 h	30–40% adults; 6–10% children	Nausea, tingling, dizziness, chest tightness/heaviness, panic, metallic taste (IN)	Myocardial infarction, coronary spasm, ventricular arrhythmia
Zolmitriptan (Zomig 1997)	PO: 1–3 h; SC: ?; IN: ?	60–70%; 3 h	PO: 75% @ 2 h	20–35% adults	Same	Probably similar to above
Naratriptan (Amerge 1998)	PO: 1–3 h; SC: ?; IN: ?	65–75%; 6 h	PO: 80% @ 4 h; PO: 60–70% @ 4 h equal to placebo (children)	15–30% adults; not reported in children	Same	Probably similar to above
Dihydroergotamine (DHE-45)	IM: 30 min; IV: 2–11 min; SC: 15–45 min; IN: 30–90 min	60–70%; 4–6 h	IM: 70% @ 1 h	10% adults	Nausea, vomiting, diarrhea, leg cramps, abdominal pain	Coronary spasm, peripheral arterial spasm

[1] Not approved for use in children under 17 years. IN = intranasal; IV = intravenous; PO = oral; SC = subcutaneous.
Reproduced from Matthew NT: Serotonin 1D agonists and other agents in acute migraine. Neurol Clin N Am 1997;15(1):61.

Table 20–7. Chronic Preventative Agents for Migraine Headaches[1]

Drug	Dosage	Available Form	Potential Side Effects
Cyproheptadine (Periactin)	0.25–1.5 mg/kg/day bid/tid	Tablets: 4 mg; syrup: 2 mg/tsp	Sedation, weight gain
Beta receptor blockers			
Propranolol (Inderal)	0.6–1.5 mg/kg/day q8h	Tablets: 10, 20, 40, 60, 80 mg; LA capsule: 60, 80, 120, 160 mg	Asthma, congestive heart failure, COPD, peripheral vascular disease, cardiac conduction defects, brittle diabetes
Metoprolol	0.8–1.5 mg/kg/day	Tablets: 50, 100 mg	Tiredness, cold extremities, vivid dreams, depression
Anticonvulsants			
Carbamazepine (Tegretol)	5–20 mg/kg/day bid/tid	Tablets: 100, 200 mg; syrup: 100 mg/tsp	Bone marrow suppression, hepatotoxicity
Valproic acid (Depakote)	20–40 mg/kg/day tid/qid	Tablets: 250, 500 mg; syrup: 250 mg/tsp; sprinkles: 125 mg	Bone marrow suppression, hepatotoxicity
Phenytoin (Dilantin)	3–7 mg/kg/day bid/tid	Tablets: 50, 100 mg; liquid: 125 mg/tsp	Bone marrow suppression, hepatotoxicity
Antidepressants			
Amitriptyline (Elavil)	0.1–2 mg/kg at bedtime	Tablets: 25, 50	Narrow angle glaucoma, urinary retention, cardiac arrhythmia, renal or liver disease
Calcium channel blockers			
Verapamil (Calan)	3–5 mg/kg/day bid	Tablets: 40, 80 mg; SR: 80, 120, 240 mg	Constipation, bradycardia, atrioventricular conduction defects
Nonsteroidal anti-inflammatory agents			
Naproxen sodium	10–20 mg/kg/day bid	Tablets: 250, 500 mg	Peptic ulcer disease, hypersensitivity reactions, platelet dysfunction

[1] COPD = chronic obstructive pulmonary disease.

Modified with permission from Lewis DL. Page 102 in: Rothner AD: *Headaches in children and adolescents.* Semin Pediatr Neurol 1995;2(2):102.

matory disease. While most childhood cases are idiopathic, obesity in older children and adolescents may be a factor. Other identifiable causes of suspected pseudotumor cerebri include Lyme infection of the central nervous system, dural sinus thromboses, central nervous system leukemia and lymphoma, and use of certain medications (e.g., steroids, birth control pills, tetracycline, and hypervitaminosis A). Several other metabolic and toxic disorders and infectious and parainfectious disorders have also been associated with this syndrome (Table 20–8). Treatment is aimed at lowering intracranial pressure by removing cerebrospinal fluid by lumbar puncture and decreasing the

Table 20–8. Etiology of Pseudotumor Cerebri

Idiopathic	Dural sinus thrombosis
Obesity	Chronic otitis media
Corticosteroid therapy and withdrawal	Guillian-Barré syndrome Unrecognized chronic
Tetracycline	meningitis
Oral contraceptives	Pregnancy
Hypervitaminosis A	Hyperthyroidism
Hypovitaminosis A	Collagen vascular disease

cerebrospinal fluid production by administration of aceta-zolamide, furosemide, and/or steroids. The prevention of visual loss is the ultimate goal of intervention. If there is no response to medical therapy, surgical decompression procedures, such as optic nerve sheath fenestration or lumbar-to-peritoneal shunting procedure, may be necessary.

Seizures and Epilepsy

A seizure is a sudden transient event due to abnormal brain neuronal electrical functioning. Epilepsy is the tendency to have recurrent seizures. Acute causes of seizures that are reversible are not considered to be epilepsy, but may result in brain injury, which can lead to epilepsy. Seizures manifest clinically in a variety of ways depending upon the region of the brain involved with the abnormal electrical discharge. The most common manifestations are motor behaviors (rhythmic jerking) with or without alteration in mental status. Occasionally children are found following the seizure in a postictal state, when the cause of the decrease in mental status may not be readily appreciated. Patients may also have a variety of episodic motor behaviors or other paroxysmal phenomenon that may be confused with nonepileptic events. Some patients may experience their seizures as autonomic changes, psychic phenomenon, or special sensory changes. A careful and detailed history should distinguish between these diagnostic possibilities.

If it is determined that the event was likely to be a seizure, the next important step is to determine the type of seizure, especially if an acute underlying reversible cause can be found. The clinician should determine whether there was associated fever, inflammatory disease or overt infection, or a history of recent head trauma, toxic ingestions, or symptoms suggestive of raised intracranial pressure. An underlying metabolic disturbance should be sought if there are additional supportive symptoms, such as food intolerance, growth failure, rash, unusual odors, etc. (see Chap. 6, "A Clinical Approach to Inborn Errors of Metabolism"). The most important metabolic measure to determine in all children with acute seizures is plasma glucose concentration.

It should also be determined if this was the first seizure or it was one of a number of recurrent events that might diagnose the children as having epilepsy. The history should elicit information about perinatal difficulties, developmental abnormalities, and head trauma. A review of systems should focus on intercurrent systemic illnesses and progressive neurologic symptoms. A family history for epilepsy, inherited diseases, or other potentially relevant medical problems in siblings and immediate family members should be obtained.

The physical examination should center around identifying evidence of systemic disease, intracranial infection, signs of trauma or toxic ingestion, and neurocutaneous

disorders. The neurologic examination should assess evidence of raised intracranial pressure or focal neurologic deficits. The laboratory evaluation is designed to differentiate potential etiologies suggested by the history and physical examination. A more specific evaluation should be based on the children's age, the specific history, and examination. For example, in the infant–toddler age range, looking for underlying metabolic disease states, brain dysgenesis, as well as intracranial infections, is more likely to yield positive findings than it does in adolescents. The acute evaluation should seek to identify all correctable causes of seizures. Although obtaining an EEG after the first seizure is reasonable, it would be most prudent after a recurrence. Unfortunately, the EEG will rarely confirm a diagnosis of epilepsy but may help assess future risk of recurrence.

Once it has been decided that the children have experienced a seizure from a nonreversible cause, the seizure should be further characterized based on the clinical description of the witnessed event. Seizures are categorized as either generalized or partial. Generalized seizures occur when abnormal neuronal electrical activity emanates from the entire brain simultaneously, as opposed to from only one hemisphere (or region of a hemisphere) in partial seizures.

Primary generalized epilepsy does not have an identifiable cause, i.e., it is idiopathic. Secondary generalized epilepsy has a recent or remote known (or suspected) cause for the seizures. Each of the generalized motor seizures has characteristic features that differentiate them from one another. The distinction between a myoclonic seizure and a clonic seizure is one of duration. Myoclonic seizures are body jerks that last milliseconds in duration, whereas the jerks seen with clonic seizures are slower, lasting a second or more and usually occur in a series. Atonic seizures are those in which the patients lose postural tone and might drop completely to the floor, although the change in body posture may be as little as a simple head nod. Tonic seizures cause the patients to maintain a stiffened posture either in flexion or in extension. Tonic–clonic convulsions (i.e., grand mal seizures) are those in which the patients first experience a brief tonic event followed by a series of clonic convulsive movements.

Partial seizures may be either simple or complex. In simple partial seizures, consciousness is preserved as opposed to complex partial seizures, in which there is an alteration but not necessarily total loss of consciousness. Both simple partial seizures and complex partial seizures can develop into a generalized convulsion.

It is important for the practitioner to distinguish between absence (i.e., petit mal seizure) and complex partial seizures. Parents may describe both absence and complex partial seizures as "staring spells" or "phase outs." Further history, however, can help differentiate between the two conditions (Table 20–9). Complex partial seizures

Table 20–9. Clinical Distinction between Absence and Complex Partial Seizures

	Complex Partial Seizures	Absence Seizures
Auras	+	–
Automatism	+	–
Duration	Long (30 s–min)	Short (seconds)
Frequency	Infrequent–variable	Numerous per day
Postictal state	+	–
Hyperventilation	–	+

are more likely to be accompanied by a neurologic aura, consist of more dramatic automatic behavioral mannerisms, and are usually longer in duration (i.e., 20 to 30 s) with postictal clouding of consciousness. In comparison, absence seizures do not have an aura, are not usually accompanied by extensive automatic behavior aside from subtle eye blinking, usually last only a few seconds (5 to 10 s), and are fairly frequent throughout the day without postictal alteration in consciousness. A useful office maneuver is to have the children hyperventilate for a 2- to 3-min interval. Absence seizures will often be triggered by hyperventilation and can confirm the clinical phenomenon of staring behavior. It would be rare for complex partial seizures to be precipitated in this manner. The patient's EEG should readily help to differentiate between these two conditions.

When the seizure type has been better clarified, it is then important to consider whether the children have epilepsy. This can be determined only by obtaining a history of, or directly observing recurrent epileptic seizures. If the children have epilepsy, an underlying epileptic syndrome should then be considered. An epileptic syndrome is characterized by a group of commonly occurring symptoms and signs that include age of onset, seizure types, associated clinical features such as mental retardation, and specific EEG patterns (Figure 20–5). By identifying whether the seizures are part of an epileptic syndrome, one is better able to prognosticate outcome and determine the treatment that is most appropriate (Table 20–10).

FEBRILE SEIZURES

The most common epileptic syndrome presenting to pediatric practitioners is that of febrile seizures. Simple febrile seizures are usually less than 15 min in duration and occur before 5 years of age in otherwise healthy normal children. They are usually generalized tonic–clonic convulsions but may be partial seizures. They are associated with fever in the absence of infections of the central nervous system. Typically, the EEG is normal and the prognosis is excellent. The initial evaluation is directed at identifying intercurrent infections and excluding meningitis or encephalitis. This may require a lumbar puncture for cerebrospinal fluid examination and culture, especially in young infants or children in whom clinical signs are thought to be less reliable. Treatment is aimed at the underlying cause of the fever and reducing body temperature with antipyretics. Anticonvulsant therapy is not generally indicated. Intermittent diazepam at the onset of subsequent febrile illnesses or administration of daily prophylactic phenobarbital has been used in instances where conservative approaches fail to reassure the family.

Certain factors predispose children with febrile seizures to recurrences. Up to 30% of children who have experienced one febrile seizure will have a recurrence. The lower the degree of fever (i.e., <101°F or 38.3°C) at the time of seizure the more likely the recurrence risk. The younger the children (especially under age 12 months) at onset, the higher the recurrence risk. The likelihood of idiopathic epilepsy is increased if there is a family history of epilepsy, if the children are neurologically or developmentally abnormal, and if they have experienced complex febrile seizures. *Febrile seizures* are defined as complex if they are focal rather than generalized, have a duration of longer than 15 min, and recur more than once over a 24-h period.

OTHER EPILEPTIC SYNDROMES

Other syndromes with seizures include West syndrome, which is characterized by early-onset infantile spasms with a hypsarrhythmia pattern on EEG and poor prognosis. Benign rolandic epilepsy is a condition associated with childhood focal motor seizures with or without secondary generalization during sleep and an EEG demonstrating centrotemporal (rolandic) spike discharges; this has an excellent long-term prognosis (see Table 20–10).

MANAGEMENT OF SEIZURES

Deciding to institute or withhold antiepileptic treatment often depends upon defining and weighing the relative risks and benefits of therapy for the individual patients. The practitioner and family should consider the potential risk of therapeutic toxicity and cognitive and behavioral effects of therapy, as well as the potential psychosocial and economic costs of therapy. These considerations are compared to the risk of recurrence and the risks that the seizures pose to the individuals. Assessment of the risk for physical injury, psychosocial impact, and/or alteration in daily life activity must be weighed in contrast to the benefits of treatment.

The recurrence risk for children with a first unprovoked seizure varies from 25 to 70%. The highest risk categories include children who have an associated potential etiology such as cerebral palsy and head trauma with contusion, those with epileptiform activity on EEG, and

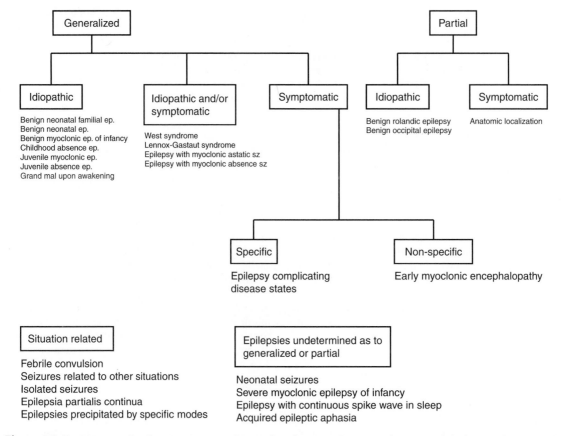

Figure 20–5. Diagram of epileptic seizure syndrome classifications. (From Dreifuss FE et al. Epilepsia 1985;26:268.)

those with seizures occurring during sleep. Recurrences are also more likely in those with mixed-seizure types, certain abnormal EEG patterns, and/or the presence of an identified specific seizure syndrome. The duration of the initial seizure does not influence the likelihood of recurrence. Approximately 50% of children will have their recurrence within 6 months after the first seizure and 80% within the following 2 years. In general, antiepileptic drug treatment is not routinely started after the first seizure unless circumstances predict a high likelihood of recurrence. If patients have already had a prior unprovoked seizure and are now experiencing a recurrence, there would be an approximately 70 to 80% risk of another seizure in the next 2 years. After weighing individual circumstances, most practitioners would then begin antiepileptic drug treatment after the second unprovoked seizure.

The specific antiepileptic drug treatment is dependent upon both seizure type and seizure syndrome. Drugs of first choice are usually administered as monotherapy. Combination multidrug therapies are usually reserved for children with seizure disorders that are intractable or difficult to manage (Table 20–11). Withdrawal of antiepileptic drug therapy typically is considered only 1 to 2 years after remission of seizure activity. In general, approximately 50% of seizures recur within the first 6 months after withdrawal of medication and 80% within the first year.

STATUS EPILEPTICUS

Status epilepticus (SE) is defined as prolonged or recurrent seizure activity without return to normal consciousness
(*text continues on page 818*)

Table 20–10. Selected Seizure Syndromes

Syndrome	Age of Onset	EEG Pattern	Associated Clinical Features	Possible Treatments
Febrile convulsions	3 months–5 years	Normal interictal	Normal development, generalized convulsions lasting ≤15 min, fever >38°C in absence of CNS infection	Antipyretics, phenobarbital, valproate, intermittent diazepam
West syndrome	2 months–2 years	Hypsarrhythmia (random high voltage slow-waves and spikes)	Sudden truncal flexor spasm with arm and head extension/adduction ("Morolike"), occasional truncal extensor spasm; occur in clusters typically upon awakening or entering sleep. Poor prognosis for neurodevelopmental outcome; commonly associated with tuberous sclerosis, Down syndrome, brain injury/malformation	ACTH gel injections, oral corticosteroids, clonazepam, valproate, topiramate, ketogenic diet, vigabatrin
Lennox-Gastaut syndrome	Any age >2 years	Atypical slow spike-wave (1–2.5 Hz) bursts, diffusely slowed background with high voltage spikes	Mixed-seizure pattern with atonic, myoclonic, atypical absence, and generalized tonic–clonic convulsions; sleep-associated tonic seizures evolve over time; heterogeneous causes with associated cognitive impairment	Clonazepam, valproate, felbamate, ketogenic diet, topiramate, lamotrigine, tiagabine, vigabatrin
Absence ("petit mal")	3–12 years	3 cps spike-wave generalized discharges ictally	Sudden onset starring with/without facial automatisms (blinking, head nod, etc.) numerous per day; provoked with hyperventilation; no postictal period or awareness of events.	Ethosuximide, valproate, lamotrigine, ketogenic diet
Juvenile myoclonic epilepsy	10–15 years	Interictal "fast spike-wave" 4–6 Hz polyspike discharges	Mixed-seizure pattern with combinations of myoclonic, absence, and generalized tonic–clonic convulsions; myoclonic seizures typical upon awakening; lifelong propensity for seizures.	Valproate, ethosuximide, lamotrigine, ketogenic diet
Benign rolandic epilepsy	5–15 years	Interictal spike discharges in the centro-temporal (rolandic) regions bilaterally independently, augmented with sleep, background normal	Partial or generalized convulsions in sleep; rarely occur during wakefulness; boys > girls, high concordance of abnormal EEG in first-degree relatives	Carbamazepine, phenytoin, phenobarbital, valproate

ACTH = adrenocorticotrophic hormone; CNS = central nervous system; EEG = electroencephalogram.

Table 20–11. Commonly Used Antiepileptic Drugs[1]

AEDs	Maintenance Dose	Starting Dose	Half-Life (H)	Therapeutic Range	Common Side Effects	Serious Idiosyncratic Side Effects
		Established drugs				
Carbamazepine (Tegretol, Carbitrol)	10–20 mg/kg/day	5–10 mg/kg/day	8–25	8–12 µg/mL	Diplopia, lethargy, blurred vision, ataxia	Rashes, hepatic dysfunction, pancreatitis, aplastic anemia, leukopenia
Ethosuximide (Zarontin)	12–40 mg/kg/day, most children require 15–20 mg/kg/day	<6 years: 10 mg/kg/day; >6 years: 250 mg/day	25–40	40–100 µg/mL	Gastrointestinal distress, hiccoughs, lethargy	Rashes, leukopenia, pancytopenia, systemic lupus erythematosus
Phenobarbital	<1 year: 3–5 mg/kg/day; >1 year: 2–4 mg/kg/day; teenagers, adults: 2–3 mg/kg/day	Same as maintenance	40–70	15–40 µg/mL	Irritability, hyper-activity, lethargy	Rashes
Phenytoin (Dilantin)	5 mg/kg/day (may need higher doses in children <5–6 years)	Same as maintenance	Dependent on concentration	10–20 µg/mL	Lethargy, dizziness, ataxia, gingival hypertrophy, hirsutism	Rashes, hepatic dysfunction, lymphadenopathy, blood dyscrasias
Primidone (Mysoline)	12–25 mg/kg/day	<6 years: 50 mg qhs; <12 years: 100 mg qhs; >12 years: 150 mg qhs	5–8	5–12 µg/mL (Phenobarbital 15–40 µg/mL)[1]	Irritability, hyper-activity, lethargy, nausea	Rashes
Valproic acid (Depakene, Divalproex sodium, Depakote)	15–60 mg/kg/day tid/qid	15 mg/kg/day; increase by 10–15 mg/kg/d every 2 weeks	4–14	50–150 µg/mL	Lethargy, weight gain or loss, hair loss, tremor	Hepatic dysfunction, pancreatitis, anemia, thrombo-cytopenia

Newer antiepileptic drugs

Drug	Maintenance dose	Titration	Half-life (h)	Therapeutic range	Side effects	Idiosyncratic reactions
Gabapentin (Neurontin)	20–50 mg/kg/day	10 mg/kg/day increase by 5–10 mg/kg q 3–7 day	5–8	Not established	Lethargy, dizziness	Rashes
Lamotrigine (Lamictal)	5–15 mg/kg/day; w/H-inducers: 10–15 mg/kg/day; w/VPA: 5 mg/kg/day	12.5–25 mg/day; w/VPA increase slowly	15–60	Not established	Rash, lethargy, dizziness	Rashes
Tiagabine (Gabatril)	0.5–1.0 mg/kg/day; w/H-inducers: 0.7–1.5 mg/kg/day; w/o H-inducers: 0.3–0.4 mg/kg/day	0.1 mg/kg/day; increase weekly by 0.1 mg/kg/day	3–8	Not established	Lethargy, confusion, mental dullness, poor concentration	None known
Topiramate (Topamax)	5–10 mg/kg/day	1–2 mg/kg/day; increase weekly by 1 mg/kg/d	12–30	Not established	Irritability, hyperactivity, mental dullness, kidney stones, weight loss	None known
Felbamate (Felbatol)	30–45 mg/kg/day	15 mg/kg/day; increase in 10 mg increments to 60 mg/kg/day	13–24	Not established	Anorexia, insomnia, somnolence	Aplastic anemia, hepatotoxicity

[1] Phenobarbital is a metabolite of primidone, and plasma concentration of phenobarbital may be used to determine therapeutic range.

AED = antiepileptic drugs; qhs = given at the hour of sleep; H-inducers = hepatic enzyme inducers of the cytochrome P450 system.

Adapted with permission from Holmes GL: *Diagnosis and Management of Seizures in Children.* Philadelphia, WB Saunders Co., 1987; and Pellock JM: New antiepileptic drugs in childhood epilepsy. Semin Pediatr Neurol 1997;4:1.

over at least a 30-min period. Children, for the most part, tolerate SE well if attendant medical complications do not occur. Most morbidity and mortality from SE is related to the underlying etiology of SE (such as meningitis and encephalitis and asphyxia). Treatment always begins by supporting the children's airway, breathing, and circulation (Table 20–12). Measurement of serum glucose level and administration of intravenous glucose, oxygen supplementation, and intravenous fluid therapy should be

Table 20–12. Treatment Approach for Status Epilepticus

1. Airway, breathing, circulation
2. Stat laboratory (serum glucose, electrolytes, pH, antiepileptic drug levels; other directed labs)
3. Glucose and oxygen administration
4. Intravenous hydration with 5% dextrose/normal saline
5. Attention to possible underlying acidosis and precipitants
6. Drugs
   Lorazepam: 0.05 mg/kg to 0.2 mg/kg IV, up to 3 doses at 5- to 10-min intervals
   OR
   Diazepam: 0.25 mg/kg to 0.5 mg/kg IV, up to 3 doses at 5- to 10-min intervals to a maximum of 10 mg
   AND
   Phenytoin: 15 mg/kg to 20 mg/kg IV
   - slowly, not more than 1 mg/kg/min
   - IV normal saline
   - monitor blood pressure, electrocardiogram
   OR
   Fosphenytoin: 15 to 20 mg/kg PE (phenytoin equivalent) IV/IM
   If barbiturates needed, intubate
   Phenobarbital: 10 mg/kg to 20 mg/kg IV
   - Monitor blood pressure and respirations
7. Correct metabolic disturbances. Assess underlying etiology, i.e., CNS infection, sepsis, intracranial structural lesion, toxic ingestion, and other organ failure
8. Consider short-acting forms of anesthesia or other drugs
   - Paraldehyde: 0.3 mL/kg mix with equal amounts of oil-pr
   - Pentobarbital: 4–7 mg/kg loading dose, then 1–10 mg/kg/h infusion
   - Midazolam: 0.2 mg/kg loading dose, then 0.1–2.0 mg/kg/h infusion
   - Propofol: 3–5 mg/kg–loading dose, then 1–15 mg/kg/h infusion
   - Valproate sodium: 15–60 mg/kg/d over ≥1 h IV
   - General anesthesia

Reprinted with permission from Bleck TP: Management approaches to prolonged seizures and status epilepticus. *Epilepsia* 1999;40(suppl 1):S59.
Note: Slightly lower doses of some of the drugs have been used (see Table 10–10).

initiated promptly. Assessment for possible underlying etiological precipitants should be sought. Drug therapy usually begins with the administration of a fast-acting benzodiazepine such as lorazepam or diazepam. If the seizures are unresponsive to repeated doses (up to 3 doses over 10 to 15 min), concurrent administration of intravenous fosphenytoin is suggested. Metabolic parameters, blood pressure, and electrocardiogram (ECG) should be repeatedly monitored. If the administration of fosphenytoin is not successful in stopping the SE, the addition of a second drug such as phenobarbital, valproate, or midazolam should be considered. The management of SE is further discussed in Chap. 10, "Injuries and Emergencies." The decision whether to maintain long-term treatment with antiepileptic drugs can be made after further evaluation. Children whose first seizures present as SE do not necessarily have a higher recurrence risk for future seizures than do those children who do not present with SE. They do, however, have a higher likelihood of SE when recurrences do occur.

ALTERATIONS IN MENTAL DEVELOPMENT

Primary care practitioners will commonly evaluate children with developmental delays. It is important to first distinguish whether development is progressing, but at a slowed pace, or if development has stopped and the children are regressing. This may only be evident on longitudinal follow-up. The clinician should determine whether the delay is restricted to one domain, multiple domains, or affects global development. The use of screening tools such as the Denver Developmental Screening Test (DDST) or other instruments can be helpful in identifying those children at risk. The evaluation of children with developmental delays is discussed in Chap. 1, "Pediatric Health Supervision." When the delay appears to be static and restricted to the motor domain, the diagnosis of cerebral palsy should be considered. However, developmental regression or loss of skills is serious and referral to appropriate specialists will be necessary to clarify the underlying condition.

Progressive Encephalopathy

With progressive developmental delay, it is important to consider whether the children have evidence of central and/or peripheral nervous system disease alone, or if it is associated with multisystem involvement. It should be determined that appropriate newborn screening tests have been performed and a history for risk factors of AIDS should be obtained. It is important to identify treatable disorders such as hypothyroidism, phenylketonuria (PKU), and galactosemia. During the general examination, it is important to make note of any rashes or neurocutaneous markers. Careful inspection of the hair for fragility or brittleness can indicate the presence of Menkes disease. Abnormal blood vessels in the bulbar conjunctiva may identify ataxia-telangiectasia. The examination should include evaluation for joint and spine deformity, facial coarsening, and the presence of organomegaly to identify storage disorders.

Neurodegenerative and neurometabolic disorders are typically classified on the basis of the clinical features, including neuroanatomic dysfunction, symptoms of acute intoxication or energy deficiency, age at onset, pace of neurologic deterioration, and specific unique physical characteristics or signs. Disorders are classified into those that affect primarily the central or peripheral nervous system. Central nervous system disorders are divided into those affecting either the cortical gray matter, subcortical gray matter including the cerebellum, and/or the white matter. The central nervous system disorders may or may not incorporate evidence of peripheral nervous system dysfunction. Symptoms of intoxication or energy deficiency are usually the result of an accumulation of toxic compounds or an impaired production or utilization of energy-producing metabolites. These disorders tend to have acute and catastrophic presentations but can be insidious, depending upon the underlying disease. Storage diseases may be associated with organomegaly, skeletal deformity, corneal opacity, or connective tissue and skin changes. The specific organs involved depend on the particular disorder.

The pace of deterioration also helps to differentiate these disorders. Acute encephalopathies generally present early in life with recurrent vomiting, lethargy, poor feeding, dehydration, or seizures. Respiratory compromise and rapid alteration in mental status, progressing to coma, will subsequently occur. This presentation is more often due to small molecule intoxication such as amino acid/organic acid and simple sugar disorders. Chronic encephalopathies with insidious and progressive development of signs and symptoms tend to present in late infancy and older children. These commonly produce progressive development of motor signs such as spasticity and ataxia in concert with dementia, visual impairment, and hearing loss at later stages (see Chap. 6, "A Clinical Approach to Inborn Errors of Metabolism").

ACUTE ALTERATIONS IN MENTAL STATUS

Although changes in mental status or consciousness are usually readily perceived by parents and caretakers, the description of what is different about the children is often imprecise. Acute encephalopathy is the sudden change in children's state of consciousness, awareness, cognition, and interaction. Children generally fall into one of two categories of acute encephalopathy; they may be agitated and confused or lethargic and less aware (Figure 20–6). An inability to respond may not necessarily be associated with a lack of awareness. This may occur in certain neuromuscular paralytic disorders and in central nervous system brainstem injury in which preservation of consciousness occurs in the face of paralysis ("locked-in syndromes").

When evaluating agitated or confused children, other signs of nervous system excitability are often noted. These may include tremor, myoclonic movements, or a continuous fidgeting type of behavior. There may be accompanying visual or auditory hallucinations that may occur suddenly during the examination. Whereas hallucinations usually suggest a psychiatric disorder, this diagnosis is more likely if the hallucinations are recurrent and occur in the absence of other signs of nervous system excitability. The history should pay careful attention to circumstances immediately around the time that the children began exhibiting the change in mental status. The history should identify all household medications or toxic substances available to the children. A family history should explore the occurrence of similar acute alterations of mental status, as well as that of migraine or epilepsy. The examination should be directed toward excluding central nervous system infection, signs of trauma, and/or evidence of systemic disease. Special attention to vital signs, breathing patterns, eye movement, and pupillary function are particularly helpful in assessing for potential toxidromes. The fundoscopic examination should assess the presence of papilledema, suggesting raised intracranial pressure. Focal neurologic deficits should prompt an evaluation for focal lesions, such as an intracranial mass. Nonconvulsive seizures should be considered. The presence of fever in agitated and confused children, particularly when seen with a focal or generalized seizure, should prompt an evaluation for encephalitis or meningoencephalitis.

When children are in a diminished state of consciousness with lethargy, the immediate concern is that the findings are due to a progressive encephalopathy that will quickly result in coma. Although the etiologies of depressed levels of consciousness and of agitation or delirium are similar, some important differences should be noted. Perhaps the most important difference is the increased possibility of an intracranial mass lesion and/or increased intracranial pressure in lethargic patients.

Patients in Coma

Patients are considered to be in coma when both arousability and level of awareness for the surroundings is diminished. Anatomically, coma is produced by 1 of 3 mechanisms: a process that affects the cortex of both hemispheres simultaneously; involvement of the brainstem regions specifically controlling the reticular activating systems; or a unilateral hemisphere lesion producing a shift of midline structures and interrupting brainstem activating systems. A careful history of the events leading up to the

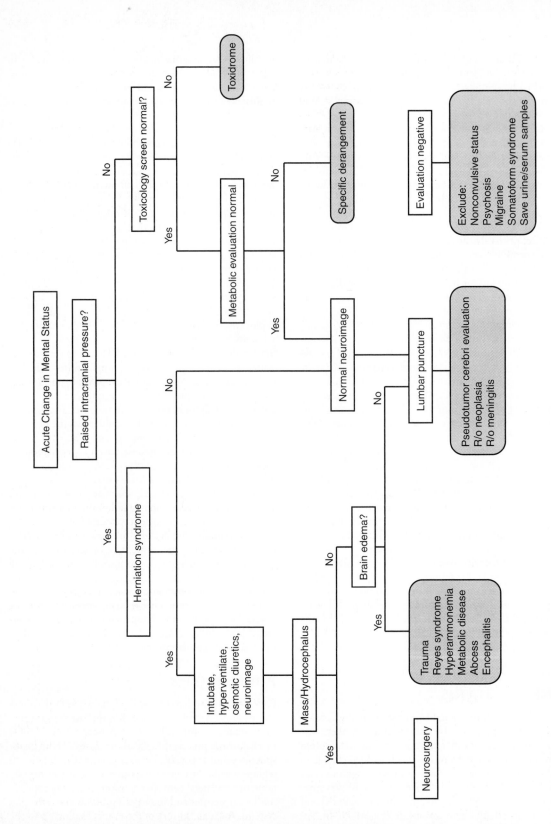

Figure 20–6. Decision algorithm for assessment of acute changes in mental status.

time the children had a change in mental status is imperative. A sudden onset of coma suggests etiologies such as stroke, hemorrhage, seizures, and toxins. A subacute onset is more likely with brain tumors, hydrocephalus, chronic subdural hematomas, and metabolic disorders.

Examination of children with diminished level of consciousness and lethargy or with agitation and/or delirium is similar. The vital signs should be assessed immediately and monitored. Signs of increased intracranial pressure (see later) may be noted including hypertension and papilledema. Evidence of trauma, such as retinal hemorrhage, hemotympanum, Battle's sign (ecchymoses over the mastoid area occurring with basilar skull fractures), and cerebrospinal fluid leak, should be specifically sought.

Serial examinations of children with diminished responsiveness and/or coma is critical to determine whether the encephalopathy is progressive. The Glasgow coma scale is used to grade the severity of coma (see Table 10-27, Chap. 10, "Accidents and Poisoning"). This scale assesses eye opening and motor and verbal responses by assigning a point scale depending on the level of responsiveness. This can provide a general sense of the severity of coma, as well as document if patients' conditions are changing over time.

In addition to monitoring the level of consciousness, the examination should include assessment of the respiratory pattern, pupillary reflexes, extraocular movements, and motor response to a painful stimulus. Cheyne-Stokes breathing, an alternating pattern of hyperventilation and apnea, occurs with bilateral cortical or thalamus and upper midbrain dysfunction. Midposition pupils without direct or consensual response to light indicates midbrain dysfunction and usually represents irreversible brainstem damage. The pupillary light reflex is usually normal in coma resulting from diffuse metabolic disorders. Asymmetry of the pupils (anisocoria) >1 mm with an asymmetric light reflex indicates a focal midbrain or third cranial nerve dysfunction and can herald uncal herniation syndrome (see later). The doll's eye maneuver assesses brainstem function above the pontomedullary junction. This test is performed by rotating the head back and forth while the eyes are open. The eyes will move with full conjugate gaze if the brainstem is intact. If they remain fixed, a stronger stimulus, the caloric test, should be attempted to test the brainstem. If the tympanic membrane is intact, the caloric test is performed by holding the patient's head at 30° of elevation and injecting cold water into one of the ear canals. The caloric test assesses the vestibular portion of the eighth cranial nerve and the oculovestibular reflex. Both eyes will tonically deviate toward the side of the cold water if the midbrain and pons are intact. The motor system is tested by using a painful stimulus to determine whether there is purposeful withdrawal, posturing, or no response at all. Posturing may be decorticate or decerebrate; in decorticate posturing, flexion of the upper and extension of the lower extremities indicates thalamic damage; with decerebrate posturing, extension of all suggests midbrain dysfunction. No response occurs with pontomedullary dysfunction.

These findings on neurologic examination can be categorized by the characteristic pattern of responses that correspond to different levels of brain functioning. The early diencephalic stage represents an intact brainstem but a nonfunctioning cerebral hemisphere. The late diencephalic stage involves the loss of thalamic function, while the midbrain stage indicates damage to the midbrain and rostral structures. The pontomedullary stage represents complete brainstem dysfunction (Table 20-13).

The conditions commonly affecting the cerebral hemispheres bilaterally include diffuse metabolic disturbances, central nervous system infections, and hydrocephalus. Regardless of whether patients are agitated or lethargic, the possibility of the initial presentation of an underlying neurometabolic or degenerative disease must be considered when children have acute encephalopathy.

Raised Intracranial Pressure

Although there are many causes of increased intracranial pressure, the most important include acute infections such

Table 20–13. Brain Herniation Syndromes

Herniation Syndrome	Key Clinical Signs
Transentorial central herniation	
Diencephalic stage	• Cheyne-Stokes respiration • Small reactive pupils • Intact ocular movements
Midbrain stage	• Hyperventilation • Mid-position non-reactive pupils • Dysconjugate ocular movements • Decerebrate posture
Medullary stage	• Gasping irregular respiration • Dilated non-reactive pupils • Fixed ocular movements • Flaccid motor tone
Uncal herniation	• Progressive third nerve dysfunction (dilated pupil, ptosis, diminished ocular movement) • Contralateral hemiparesis
Upward herniation	• Sudden cardiorespiratory dysfunction • Preserved pupil reactivity and oculomotor function

as meningitis and encephalitis, obstructive hydrocephalus, and intracranial mass (e.g., hemorrhage or tumor). Increased intracranial pressure in children usually first presents with severe headache. However, the headache is soon accompanied by a progressive constellation of signs and symptoms, such as focal neurologic findings or altered mental status with lethargy progressing to coma.

Helpful signs in infants are a bulging anterior fontanelle and the sun-setting sign (the eyes look downward due to pressure on the upgaze center in the midbrain tectum). The Cushing triad of hypertension, bradycardia, and apnea associated with raised intracranial pressure is usually observed in older children. Papilledema, cranial nerve palsies, and progressive increased muscle tone with hyperreflexia eventually appear. If the pressure is allowed to increase, particularly in children in whom the skull sutures are fused, rostral-caudal herniation syndromes will ultimately occur (see Table 20–13). If the increase in intracranial pressure is evenly distributed throughout the intracranial compartment, symmetric clinical findings are observed as a portion of the cerebrum is pushed through the tentorium, eventually exerting pressure on the brainstem. The clinical features of transtentorial central herniation syndromes resemble those other forms of coma, typically beginning in the early diencephalic stage and gradually progressing to the late diencephalic, midbrain, and, finally, pontomedullary stages of coma. It is therefore important to characterize changes in respiratory pattern, motor posture, and oculomotor responses to monitor the rostral-caudal progression of symptoms (see earlier section).

When the mass effect on the brain is distributed unevenly, the clinical findings will be asymmetrical. The uncal herniation syndrome is the result of herniation of the temporal lobe medially and inferiorly into the subtentorial compartment. This produces ipsilateral third cranial nerve dysfunction with pupillary dilatation, ptosis, paresis of ocular movement, and contralateral hemiparesis. Upward herniation syndromes arise from focal lesions in the subtentorial compartment, usually within the cerebellum. This syndrome typically produces a sudden cardiorespiratory disturbance without a recognized change in pupillary reactivity or oculomotor function, indicating disturbance of the midbrain or pontomedullary areas of the brainstem.

When the history and physical findings suggest raised intracranial pressure, immediate neuroimaging of the brain with CT scanning or MRI is essential. In the absence of a discernible mass or hydrocephalus on neuroimaging, a lumbar puncture to obtain cerebrospinal fluid for culture and analysis is appropriate. Measurement of the opening pressure is important to identify the level of intracranial pressure. Analysis of cerebrospinal fluid for the presence of malignancy by cytology, viral and bacterial cultures, Lyme disease antigens, cryptococcal antigen, and other infectious and inflammatory etiologies should be considered. In the absence of an identifiable etiology, a diagnosis of pseudotumor cerebri can be made (Table 20–8; see earlier section).

WEAKNESS, HYPOTONIA, AND HYPERTONIA

Weakness is evidenced by loss of, or inability to perform, some type of motor skill. This may be localized to a segment of the body or have a generalized distribution. It may result from problems of the upper or lower motor unit (Table 20–14). Muscle tone, the resistance of the muscles and joints to passive range of movement at rest, is an important part of the evaluation of the motor system. Tone is determined not only by muscle and connective tissues themselves, but by all aspects of muscle function including muscle stretch receptors, neuromuscular junctions, and the peripheral and central nervous system. *Hypotonia* is the diminished resistance to passive range of movement or muscle stretch and is one manifestation of dysfunction in the motor system. Although hypotonia can be associated with some degree of weakness, it is non-specific and in some situations, such as cerebellar disorders, hypotonia is present with normal motor strength. *Hypertonia* is the increase in resistance to passive range of motion, often described as a "clasp-knife" feeling. Both hypotonia and hypertonia may have an axial (midline trunk) or appendicular (extremities) distribution.

Approach to Children with Weakness

Classifying problems of the motor system as acute, chronic and insidious, or variable during the day helps to differentiate between various neuromuscular disorders. A history from the mother of in utero movements of the fetus during pregnancy is important, because lack of movement may suggest that the problem was present before birth. Associated symptoms such as muscle cramps or pain should be noted because they suggest a metabolic

Table 20–14. Upper and Lower Motor Neuron Components

Upper motor neuron (UMN)	Descending motor tracts (pyramidal, extrapyramidal, cerebellar outflow, etc.)
	Fiber tracts in transit from cerebrum, cerebellum, through brainstem into spinal cord until synapse with LMN
Lower motor neuron (LMN)	Anterior horn cell
	Peripheral nerves
	Neuromuscular junction
	Muscle

or inflammatory disorder rather then a structural muscle problem. The history should also elicit the presence of other neurologic problems such as diplopia, dysarrthria, and dysphagia. Other aspects of the history, such as encephalopathy, cardiac disease, contractures, fever, and rash, may help to identify specific syndromes and metabolic diseases. The identification of other family members with similar problems is essential for determining inheritable causes of motor dysfunction (Figure 20–7A).

Neonates or infants may manifest weakness in a variety of ways: by a poor suck or incomplete seal of the lips around the nipple during feeding, a feeble cry, respiratory distress, or lack of spontaneous body movements. Particular attention should be directed at facial movements because they may identify certain specific disorders; facial movements are decreased in Möbius' syndrome and myopathies. Muscle diseases tend to affect facial muscles as well as skeletal muscles and therefore the face will have less expression compared to children with motor neuron disease. A delay in acquisition of motor milestones in infants and toddlers may herald possible underlying weakness. In toddlers and older children, attention to gait and posture, as well as comparison of overall motor activity with that of peers, may help identify subtler forms of weakness.

A functional assessment of strength can be readily undertaken in cooperative children. A commonly used grading system rates muscle strength on a scale of 0 to 5 (Table 20–15). Determining the distribution of the weakness as focal, multifocal, or diffuse in location may provide important clues to diagnosis. Diffuse muscular weakness should be further categorized as involving predominantly proximal (hips and shoulder girdles) versus distal (hands and feet) muscle groups. Proximal distribution of weakness is usually myopathic in origin, while selective weakness that involves segments of a limb is more often neuropathic in origin. The Gowers maneuver should be performed in any children with suspected weakness (see Fig. 20–1). This maneuver, as previously described in this chapter, readily identifies proximal muscle weakness, particularly in the pelvic girdle region. A positive Gowers test does not imply a specific muscle disease or etiology.

The examination should exclude concurrent systemic illness, as well as dysmorphic syndromes, skeletal dysplasia, and other congenital malformations. Associated cerebral dysfunction (i.e., encephalopathy), mental retardation, and/or seizure disorder indicate brain involvement. The spine should be examined for evidence of occult dysraphism. A simple and effective means of identifying intraspinal lesions in children with gait disturbances or lower extremity weakness is to elicit focal tenderness by percussing the spine.

The neurologic examination should determine whether there is upper motor unit versus lower motor unit dysfunction (Table 20–16). The upper motor unit includes the motor tracts descending from the brain through the spinal cord to their synapses with anterior horn cells. The lower motor unit encompasses the anterior horn cell, peripheral nerve, neuromuscular junction, and muscle. One can usually determine clinically whether the weakness results from disorders of the upper versus the lower motor unit. Although strength is decreased with both, more profound weakness is usually evident in lower motor unit disorders. Hypotonia may be noted in both categories and is therefore not specific. However, hypertonia occurs exclusively with upper motor unit disease. Increased reflexes are noted in upper motor unit disorders even in the presence of hypotonia. Decreased or absent reflexes are observed only in lower motor unit diseases. The presence of fasciculations, which are small involuntary muscle twitches occurring at the sites of denervated muscle, denotes disorders affecting anterior horn cells. The Babinski sign, or extensor plantar response, can be elicited only in upper motor unit disease.

Patients' muscles should be palpated to assess whether muscle bulk is diminished symmetrically or in focal patterns. Muscle atrophy results with both upper and lower motor unit disease but occurs earlier in the course and is more prominent in lower motor unit disease. The presence of muscle tenderness should also be noted.

Some combinations of clinical findings suggest localization to the upper motor neuron (Table 20–17). Children may demonstrate paresis that incorporates half of the body (hemiplegia), may affect legs to a greater degree than arms (diplegia), or involve one, two, three, or four extremities (monoplegia, paraplegia, triplegia, or quadriplegia). Paraplegia refers to weakness involving the legs exclusively. Each of these patterns may be associated with brisk reflexes and positive Babinski signs and suggest involvement of pyramidal tracks. The presence of involuntary movements along with "lead-pipe" rigidity in muscle tone suggests involvement of the basal ganglia. Cerebellar disease affects coordination and is identifiable by the presence of slurred speech and difficulty with eye movement, as well as truncal and limb unsteadiness or ataxia. Brainstem diseases will produce abnormal eye movements in addition to disturbances of pharyngeal and tongue movement. Spinal cord involvement produces weakness that is generally bilateral and asymmetric in distribution. In addition, incontinence, hyperreflexia, positive Babinski signs, and sensory loss to a discrete trunk level are commonly observed. There may be associated back pain as well.

Lower motor unit lesions primarily affect the anterior horn cells and produce focal atrophy and fasciculation of the muscles, combined with diminished reflexes (Table 20–18). If a nerve root or plexus is involved, multifocal motor and sensory disturbances may be found, as well as associated pain radiating from the spine along the nerve roots. When the peripheral nerves are involved, there

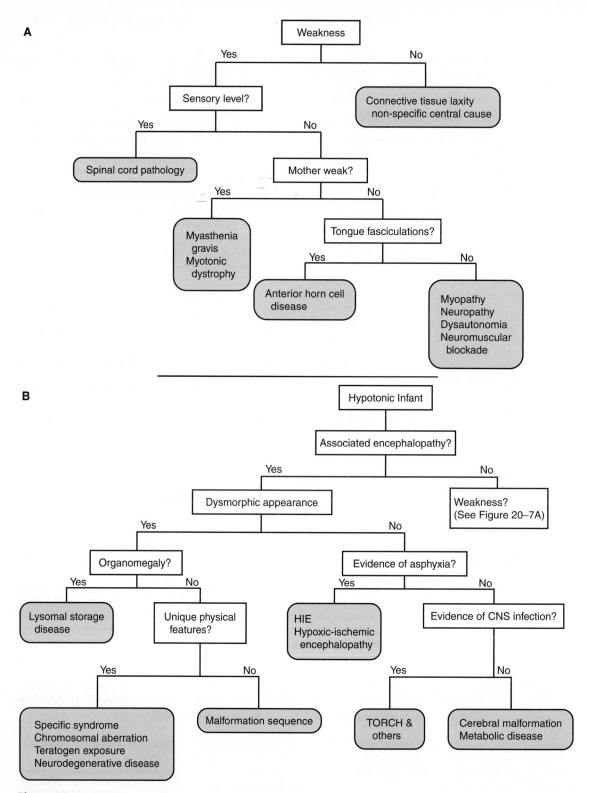

Figure 20–7. **A:** Decision algorithm for evaluation of children with weakness. **B:** Decision algorithm for evaluation of hypotonic infants.

Table 20–15. Muscle Strength Grading

Grade	Strength
0	No detectable muscle movements
1	Only trace muscle movements detected, no active movement of the body part
2	Active movement of the body part when gravity is eliminated
3	Active movement against gravity
4	Active movement against gravity with some minor resistance
5	Active movement against gravity with full resistance, normal muscle strength

is focal motor weakness and focal sensory disturbances along the distribution of the affected nerves. This process can affect multiple nerves equally (polyneuropathy) or individual nerves in isolation (mononeuropathy) and in combination (mononeuropathy multiplex).

Depending on the extent and distribution of the lower motor unit disorder, there may be weakness and diminished reflexes. In neuromuscular junction disease (such as myasthenia gravis), however, reflexes and sensation are preserved. Evanescent cranial nerve deficits, in association with ptosis or facial weakness, may become manifest. Neuromuscular junction diseases are associated with weakness that shows diurnal variations, or that is exacerbated by prolonged activity. Muscle disease generally produces weakness in the proximal musculature with certain exceptions (i.e., myotonic dystrophy). The reflexes are typically decreased in myopathies, usually in proportion to the degree of weakness.

Hypotonic Infants

The detection of hypotonia requires some experience because the findings are somewhat subjective and normally change with age. One can observe whether the head lifts with the body or remains hyperextended when pulled to a sitting position; the presence of head lag in older infants suggests significant hypotonia. Infants should also flex back at the knees and elbow against traction. This response should be present in infants after 33 to 34 weeks gestation and increases as the infant ages. The vertical suspension maneuver is performed by holding infants under the axilla and lifting them vertically into the air. Most infants will have enough shoulder girdle tone to resist "slipping through" the examiner's hands. When held in a prone horizontal position, infants should intermittently attempt to maintain erect head posture. The extent and ability of infants to maintain the head in an upright position are normally dependent upon age. If infants remain draped over the hand in an upside down U position, significant hypotonia is present. Indirect signs of hypotonia and hypoactivity in infants include flattening of the skull (plagiocephally), localized alopecia, pectus excavatum, and a frog-leg posture.

To differentiate between the various causes of hypotonia, it must be determined whether it is due to an upper or lower motor unit dysfunction, or is part of a general systemic disease, connective tissue process, or genetic syndrome (see Figure 20–7B). Important signs of cerebral causes for hypotonia include the presence of encephalopathy (e.g., diminished awareness of environment, seizures, visual inattention, and excessive startle), dysmorphic appearance, organ malformations, abnormal primitive and postural responses, and brisk tendon reflexes. Down and Prader-Willi syndrome are both well known for the associated generalized hypotonia. Evidence of significant cerebral dysfunction can be found by testing for various postural reflexes; this will also help determine the developmental age of infants (see Table 20–1).

Generalized hypotonia is usually the result of a central nervous system process. This could result from metabolic disorders, including hypoxia, hypoglycemia, and medications (such as phenobarbital, other sedatives, and magnesium sulfate). So called "central hypotonia" may be accomplished by mild motor incoordination (dyspraxia), speech and adaptive functioning delays, and learning problems, but without structural brain or peripheral nervous system abnormality. In addition to other findings

Table 20–16. Neuroanatomic Clinical Examination Correlation

	Strength	Tone	Reflexes	Atrophy	Fasciculations	Babinski Response
UMN	↓	↑↑	↑↑	+	0	++
LMN	↓↓	↓↓	↓↓	++	++	0
Cerebellum	0	↓	↓	0	0	0
Basal ganglia	0	↑	0	0	0	0

LMN = lower motor neuron; UMN = upper motor neuron.
Decreased = ↓; increased = ↑; present = +; absent = 0.

Table 20–17. Upper Motor Neuron Lesions—Clinical Examination Correlations

Upper motor neuron lesions
- Cerebral cortex
  - Hemiplegia, diplegia, quadriplegia, monoplegia
  - Brisk reflexes and positive Babinski
- Basal ganglia
  - Rigidity (lead pipe)
  - Involuntary movements
- Cerebellum
  - Ataxia (truncal, limb)
  - Incoordination (speech, eye movement)
- Brainstem
  - Oculomotor dysfunction
  - Bulbar dysfunction
- Spinal cord
  - Usually bilateral/asymmetric
  - Sensory disturbance
- Incontinence
- Back pain
- Brisk reflexes and positive Babinski

Table 20–18. Lower Motor Neuron Lesions—Clinical Examination Correlations

Lower motor neuron lesions
- Anterior horn cell
  - Fibrillation/fasciculation
  - Atrophy
  - Diminished reflexes
- Nerve root/plexus
  - 1° multifocal motor change
  - 1° multifocal sensory change
  - Radicular pain
  - Diminished reflexes
- Nerve
  - Focal motor change
  - Focal sensory change
  - Diminished reflexes
- Neuromuscular junction
  - Cranial nerve palsies
  - Spares reflexes/sensation
- Muscle
  - Proximal greater than distal distribution
  - Reflexes proportional to weakness

of central nervous system involvement, the proximal muscles are generally weaker than are the distal muscles, the hypotonia is more prominent than the weakness, and the reflexes are normal or increased. Reflexes may be slightly depressed in hypotonia associated with cerebellar disorders, but muscle strength and motor functional ability may be entirely normal. Other signs of cerebellar disease, such as ataxia, are also usually evident. In older children, connective tissue diseases may result in muscle weakness that presents with hypotonia.

Hypotonia affecting a specific area is usually the result of a disorder of the lower motor unit. Other signs that suggest lower motor unit disease include lack of spontaneous movement, absent or diminished reflexes, absence of facial expression, and muscle fasciculations.

Cerebral Palsy

One of the most common disorders associated with weakness is cerebral palsy. It has been estimated that the prevalence of cerebral palsy is approximately 2 in 1000 children at 7 years of age. This disorder, in which involvement of the upper motor unit produces primary motor impairment, is often referred to as a static encephalopathy. *Cerebral palsy* is not a single disease but rather a term that describes a constellation of clinical findings of chronic nonprogressive motor impairment secondary to diverse causes. The diagnosis is usually made by 2 years of age.

The clinical manifestations include abnormal motor tone, posture, and movement. However, these may be accompanied by a variety of additional disabilities including cognitive impairment, special sensory disturbances, and emotional and behavioral problems. Although cerebral palsy is a nonprogressive disorder, the clinical manifestations evolve as the children get older. The diagnosis is usually suspected when primitive reflexes persist and the infants do not attain expected developmental motor milestones; this is usually accompanied by hypertonia, or less frequently, hypotonia. The persistence or asymmetry of the Moro reflex or delay in acquiring protective reflexes such as the parachute reflex and lateral propping response are clues to motor dysfunction. In addition, the development of early hand preference (before age 2 years) is suggestive of a subtle hemiparesis.

The cause of cerebral palsy for the majority of children is unknown, but both prenatal and postnatal factors contribute. Extreme prematurity and associated cerebral insults increase the risk of long-term cerebral injury and resultant cerebral palsy. Underlying intrinsic brain malformation, genetic disease, superimposed central nervous system infection, and hypoxic ischemic injury to the brain are all potential causes. Premature infants with intraventricular hemorrhage have a higher likelihood of neurologic sequelae, particularly if severe or intraparenchymal in location. Any white matter injury with or without intraventricular hemorrhage, which results in periventricular leukomalacia, is also at high risk for inducing cerebral palsy.

The classification of cerebral palsy typically rests on the pattern of motor impairment. The vast majority of children have spastic motor tone (65%) resulting in hemiplegia, diplegia, or quadriplegia (Table 20–19). Dyskinetic syndromes (20%) manifest with a combination of spasticity with dystonia, choreoathetosis, or hypotonia as the predominant motor findings. A smaller fraction (2.5%) will have an almost pure ataxic syndrome, and the remainder of children have mixed pictures (12.5%) without a clear predominance.

Children with hemiplegia and quadriplegia are particularly likely to have associated learning disabilities, mental retardation, and seizure disorders. Visual deficits and speech disturbances may also accompany the motor impairments to varying degrees. Auditory deficits are less common particularly as bilirubin toxicity (kernicterus) has become less prevalent.

Common issues faced by patients with cerebral palsy include growth and feeding difficulties, drooling, incontinence, and transport and mobility problems, as well as overall societal prejudice and difficulties with integration into the educational system. The goals of therapy should be tailored to meet the needs of the individual children. Enhancing parent–child interactions and fostering appropriate bonding and nurturing is paramount. Functional impairments should be assessed, and realistic goals and expectations should be established; these should be reassessed as the child gets older. Integration into the school system and the development and implementation of educational and vocational programs should be reevaluated periodically.

Medical therapy incorporates a balance of various physiotherapies and infant stimulation programs. Antispasticity management incorporates both medication (benzodiazapines, baclofen, and botulinum toxin injections) and surgical interventions. Attention to maintaining optimal orthopaedic integrity such as minimizing scoliosis, preventing hip dislocation, and optimizing positioning, are important. Orthotics and equipment for transportation, seating, and ambulation are all critical. When spasticity is impairing patients' quality of life, neurosurgical intervention should be considered. This includes procedures such as selective dorsal rhizotomy and the insertion of intrathecal baclofen pump devices. The primary care provider should serve as coordinator for the multidisciplinary care of children with cerebral palsy.

Spinal Dysraphism

Malformations of the spinal cord frequently result in flaccid weakness of the lower extremities, often evident at birth. With the advent of prenatal screening, many neural tube defects are now being identified before birth. Ingestion by women of at least 0.4 mg of folic acid daily, prior to conception and through the first several weeks of pregnancy, has been effective in preventing neural tube defects in infants. The risk for neural tube defects is greater in the offspring of women who have an already affected child. These women also benefit from folate supplementation, but higher doses may be required. Embryological failures of induction occurring in the first 3 to 6 weeks of gestation result in a spectrum of dorsal neural tube defects Table 20–20.

Malformations occurring at this stage of fetal development include myelomeningocele, encephalocele, anencephaly, corpus collosum abnormalities, and Arnold-Chiari and Dandy-Walker malformations. Holoprosencephaly (dysmorphogenesis of the midface and failure of division of the forebrain into cerebral hemispheres, resulting in hypotelorism, cyclopia, proboscis, and anomalies of brain development) may occur in conjunction with chromosome 13 and 18 abnormalities. Other nervous system malformations are the result of failures of migration and proliferation that occur later in gestation (second to sixth gestational month).

Myelomeningocele, the most overt form of spinal dysraphism, is due to failure of the neural tube to close during development. This results in a defect in neural tissue (i.e., spinal cord) and overlying tissues including meninges, vertebrae, connective tissue, and skin. Ninety percent of spinal dysraphic lesions are located in the thoracolumbar region. Associated malformations of other organs are found in 20 to 30% of affected children.

Myelomeningoceles cause flaccid paraplegia at the functional level of the lesion and below; complete sensory loss occurs in the same distribution. Bowel and bladder incontinence is usually also present, but this depends on the level of the lesion. Ambulation is preserved if hip flexor function is retained (Table 20–21).

In the Arnold-Chiari II malformation sequence, the contents of the posterior fossa and the hindbrain are displaced caudally. This results in downward herniation of the inferior cerebellar tonsils and the inferior medulla and fourth ventricle into the upper cervical spinal cord. In approximately 80% of these patients, there is an associated obstructive hydrocephalus, most commonly at the level of the aqueduct of Sylvius. There may be an accompanying

Table 20–19. Classification of Cerebral Palsy

Spastic	Dyskinetic
Hemiplegia	Dystonic
Diplegia	Choreoathetotic
Quadriplegia	Hypotonic
Monoplegia	Ataxic
Triplegia	Mixed

Table 20–20. Malformations of the Central
Nervous System

Failures of induction (3–6 weeks gestation)
Dorsal neural tube: Dysraphism
- Cranioschisis
   Encephalocele
   Anencephaly
   Myelomeningocele
- Corpus callosum
   Lipoma
   Agenesis
- Arnold-Chiari (types 1–4)
- Dandy-Walker
Ventral neural tube: Diverticulation/segmentation
- Holoprosencephaly
   Lobar
   Alobar
   Septooptic dysplasia
- Anophthalmia
- Aventricular Cerebrum

**Failures of migration and proliferation (2–6 months
   gestation)**
Failure of sulcation/convolution
- Lissencephaly
- Polymicrogyria
- Schizencephaly
- Heterotopia
Disorders of size
- Microcephaly
   Hydranencephaly
- Macrocephaly
   Hydrocephaly
   Megalencephaly
   Somatic overgrowth
Abnormalities of tract formation
Destructive lesions

bony abnormality at the base of the skull and/or upper cervical vertebrae. The Arnold-Chiari malformation may produce vocal cord paresis, dysphagia, and oculomotor dysfunction. If there is associated cerebral dysgenesis, cognitive impairment may be anticipated.

Patients with spinal dysraphism require long-term multidisciplinary management, often with orthopedic interventions, to maintain spine, hip, and lower extremity integrity. Functional ambulation may be accomplished by the use of braces and appliances. Urologic management utilizing intermittent bladder catheterization and hygiene is aimed at preventing the development of hydronephrosis complicated by urinary tract infections. It is necessary to observe closely for the development of seizures, which occur in approximately 25% of patients. Also, the onset of symptomatic hydrocephalus may necessitate ventriculoperitoneal shunting procedures. Associated learning disabilities should be addressed. Specific questioning for symptoms of Arnold-Chiari malformation such as apnea and/or bulbar pharyngeal motor dysfunction due to cervical-medullary cord compression should be part of the periodic evaluation.

Ten percent of neural tube defects only involve the meninges and are called meningoceles. In these lesions, the thecal sac with cerebrospinal fluid herniates through the defect without involving neural tissue. Occult spinal dysraphism is an important clinical entity; all newborn infants should be evaluated for this lesion. It is a form of neural tube defect that is less overt and may be asymptomatic, particularly in infancy and early childhood. Congenital lesions, such as tufts of hair, skin tags, small sinus tracts, or small subcutaneous masses or hemangiomas overlying the spine or paraspinal region, should prompt further evaluation when they are above the gluteal cleft. These may be associated with intraspinal lipomas or bony spicules, with resultant diastematomyelia or other dysraphism. Although these children may be asymptomatic

Table 20–21. Myelomeningocele: Functional Neurologic Assessment

Dysraphic Level	Sensation Level	Most Distal Muscle Function	Sphincter Function	Reflexes Present
T1–11	Variable over upper abdomen/chest	Arms	–	Biceps/triceps
T12–L1	Lower abdomen/groin	Weak hip flexion	–	Biceps/triceps
L2	Anterior upper thigh	Strong hip flexion	–	Biceps/triceps
L3	Anterior thigh/knee	Knee extension	–	Weak knee jerk
L4	Medial leg	Knee flexion/hip adduction	–	Knee jerk
L5	Lateral leg	Foot dorsiflexion/eversion	–	Weak ankle jerk
S1	Sole of foot	Plantar flexion	–	Ankle jerk
S2	Posterior leg/thigh	Toe flexion	+/–	Anal wink
S3	Middle buttock	Buttocks	+	Anal wink
S4–5	Medial buttock	Buttocks	+	Anal wink

in early life, symptoms may manifest with growth and lengthening of the axial skeleton. As a result of these intraspinal lesions, the spinal cord is tethered in place and over time traction develops on the spinal cord and nerve roots. This eventually produces orthopaedic deformities such as progressive clubfoot deformity, pes cavus, scoliosis, and discrepancies of limb size. There may be associated incontinence, frequent urinary tract infections, as well as leg weakness and gait disturbances. In the newborn, high resolution ultrasound of the spine may be adequate to identify underlying dysgenesis; however, MRI is a more precise method of evaluation.

Transverse Myelitis

Transverse myelitis is a rapidly evolving inflammatory condition of the spinal cord that may occur at all ages. The incidence is about four cases per million of the population per year. The diagnosis is usually suspected when there is a sudden onset of weakness in the legs. Generally, this is accompanied by back pain and sensory disturbances below the level of the lesion. Bladder and bowel dysfunction may be associated. After the initial presentation symptoms and signs usually develop rapidly over 2 to 8 h, but progression may occur gradually over 1 to 3 days.

This condition has a seasonal incidence, with a peak between April and August. Causes include inflammatory, paraneoplastic, autoimmune, postinfectious and postvaccinal, demyelinating, and ischemic diseases. A history of a preceding upper respiratory infection or other nonspecific viral illness is obtained in about 35 to 45% of patients. Approximately 10 to 15% are associated with spinal cord ischemia and a small number are associated with multiple sclerosis. About 25% of cases are deemed to be idiopathic. The association of optic neuritis with acute transverse myelitis is known as Devic disease.

Because the spinal cord may be affected asymmetrically, there may be partial signs of cord dysfunction at the level of the lesion. These include segmental anterior horn cell weakness, ascending contralateral pain and temperature loss, ipsilateral motor paresis, and ipsilateral vibration and proprioception loss (Brown-Sequard syndrome). Approximately 20% of lesions occur in the cervical region with 75% occurring in the thoracic cord and the remainder in the lumbosacral area.

The diagnosis rests upon recognizing the clinical syndrome associated with evidence of spinal cord swelling on imaging studies. MRI may also demonstrate hyperintensity on T2 sequences. Cerebrospinal fluid analysis may demonstrate pleocytosis and elevated protein concentrations in 50% of patients. The treatment is supportive although intravenous methylprednisolone 0.5 to 2.0 mg/kg/day has been tried in some cases. Prognosis for recovery is best for children who have had a gradual progression of their symptoms and in whom improvement is noted by the first to second week after the onset. A gradual improvement may be evident over subsequent months with approximately 40% attaining complete recovery.

Anterior Horn Cell Disorders

The lower motor unit comprises the anterior horn cells of the ventral spinal cord gray matter, the peripheral nerve, the neuromuscular junction and the muscle. Weakness caused by anterior horn cell disease is flaccid in quality, and the reflexes are typically absent. While the weakness may affect only localized muscle groups such as a single limb, it can also be generalized. One of the hallmarks of anterior horn cell disease is the sparing of facial musculature.

Chronic degenerative diseases of the anterior horn cell include the spinal muscular atrophies. These conditions are autosomal recessive but can rarely be autosomal dominant or X-linked in inheritance. Spinal muscular atrophies have now been identified as having genetic defects on chromosome 5q13. There is an incompletely characterized interaction between genes coding for the survival motor neuron gene and associated proteins. Presumably this results in premature death of anterior horn cells.

The hallmark clinical feature of spinal muscular atrophy type I (Werdnig-Hoffmann disease) is profound weakness, apparent before 6 months of age. This lack of spontaneous movement is associated with hypotonia and hyporeflexia. The presence of tongue fasciculations and preserved movement of the face, distal hands, and feet classically characterize this disorder. A bell-shaped chest and paradoxical abdominal breathing are noted. These infants never attain the ability to sit and their life expectancy is generally less than 2 years. Spinal muscular atrophy type II (intermediate Werdnig-Hoffmann disease) has a later onset at 6 to 18 months of life. Although these infants manifest features clinically similar to type I, it is not until after they have attained the ability to sit that their disorder becomes apparent. They typically do not attain the ability to stand or walk, and their prognosis is much more variable. Spinal muscular atrophy type III, or juvenile spinal muscular atrophy (Kugelberg-Welander), has a less severe clinical presentation. It does not usually manifest until after children walk and are of variable severity. The life span of these patients is near normal in the absence of intervening medical complications. Respiratory complications and scoliosis typically complicate the course of these patients. The appearance of hepatomegaly and cardiomegaly in conjunction with anterior horn cell disease should prompt consideration of glycogen storage disorders.

Acute anterior horn cell disease is most commonly the result of an infection. Acute infectious motor neuron disease is most commonly due to the poliomyelitis virus, but other enteroviruses, such as echovirus, coxsackie, and enterovirus 71, may be responsible. An initial generalized viral illness characterized by vomiting and diarrhea or occasionally by cough and fever is followed by the development of progressive weakness. The weakness may be segmental and asymmetric or more generalized. As this is a motor neuron disease, children develop a flaccid paralysis, hypotonia, and hyporeflexia, but sensation is preserved. Cerebrospinal fluid analysis generally demonstrates a pleocytosis. The prognosis is guarded with considerable variability in recovery of motor function. Although not common, involvement of the medullary region or cervical spine may be life-threatening, because swallowing and respiration may be affected.

Nerve Root and Plexus Disorders

The most common nerve plexus and root disorder presenting to the pediatrician is a brachial plexus palsy secondary to trauma incurred during the birth process. The incidence is 0.5 to 2 infants per 1000 live births. It is thought to be due to mechanical traction injury on the plexus due to extreme lateral flexion and extension of the neck during delivery. A similar injury may result rarely from in utero compression. Features associated with a higher incidence of brachial plexus injury include maternal gestational diabetes, prior macrosomic infants, prior infants with birth-related brachial plexus palsy, maternal obesity, infants born with midforceps assistance, and prolonged failure to progress due to shoulder dystocia.

The brachial plexus extends from cervical root 5 to thoracic root 1. Complete brachial plexus palsy occurs in only about 20% of affected infants. This produces a flaccid arm and diminished or absent reflexes and is often associated with a fractured clavicle. Most commonly (in 70 to 75%), the upper plexus extending from cervical root 5 through cervical root 7 is affected, resulting in Erb palsy. The infant's arm assumes an internally rotated flexed wrist posture and is referred to as the *waiter's tip* position. Weakness of the proximal arm and shoulder girdle results in "winging" of the scapula, shoulder adduction with internal rotation, and an extended elbow and pronated forearm. Diminished sensation to pinprick may be evident over the lateral shoulder. There may be associated diaphragmatic paralysis, stridor, and tongue weakness. The full extent of the injury becomes evident at about 2 weeks after birth. Rarely, bilateral involvement of the brachial plexus may occur.

Lower brachial plexus palsy involves cervical root 8 and thoracic root 1 and is referred to as *Klumpke palsy*. Weakness of the distal arm and hand results in a claw hand deformity in association with ipsilateral Horner's syndrome (ptosis, miosis, enophthalmos, and diminished facial sweating) due to interruption of sympathetic fibers at the thoracic root level. Complete recovery occurs in most infants with partial palsies, but about 10 to 15% will have variable degrees of residual weakness. The condition is managed by placing the arm in a sling to prevent further stretching of the nerve roots. Assessment for underlying clavicle fracture and diaphragmatic paralysis is important. If there is evidence of leg weakness, the possibility of associated cervical cord traction injury should be evaluated by MRI. Evaluation over 3 to 6 months will help to determine the long-term outcome; if recovery has not occurred during this period, root avulsion is likely and the prospect for improvement is poor. Electromyogram (EMG) and nerve conductor velocity (NCV) tests will confirm the extent of the injury. Many infants will continue to improve over the first year of life. Neurosurgical repair can be considered in select instances.

A less common affliction of the brachial plexus is brachial neuritis, a painful inflammatory syndrome of the arm and shoulder associated with weakness and ultimately muscle atrophy. It is often preceded by a nonspecific viral illness or immunization. Spontaneous resolution begins in 3 to 4 weeks; the majority recovers fully over 1 to 2 years.

Peripheral Neuropathies

In peripheral neuropathies strength and/or sensation are impaired by disturbance of motor efferent and sensory afferent neuromuscular transmission secondary to axonal injury or demyelination or both. The causes of neuropathy include toxins, infectious-inflammatory diseases, traumatic injuries, and chronic hereditary disorders. Weakness may be confined to a body segment, have a focal nerve distribution, or be more generalized. The weakness is usually eventually accompanied by sensory disturbance.

The most common cause of acute generalized paralysis is Guillain-Barré syndrome (GBS), an acute inflammatory demyelinating polyneuropathy. The incidence of this condition is approximately 1 to 2 cases per 100,000 population per year. It usually presents 1 to 2 weeks after an antecedent upper respiratory infection, gastrointestinal illness, or vaccinations and is associated with *Campylobacter jejuni,* enterovirus, HIV, Lyme disease, and Epstein-Barr virus infections. Parents often complain that their children gradually demonstrate "less energy." As constitutional symptoms from the initial illness begin to wane, mild progressive neurologic symptoms ensue. Usually there are complaints of paresthesias or painful "pins and needles" sensations in the soles of the feet. Another common complaint is pain in the back of the thighs. Guillain-Barré syndrome is classically associated with ascending paralysis, first noted as leg weakness, followed by progressive weakness in the trunk and arms. Mild facial weakness is also common. During the first week of the illness, limb weakness may be mild and reflexes are diminished. Weakness can be readily demonstrated by asking the children to walk on the toes and heels or to squat. The paresis progresses and areflexia develops. Dysphagia and shortness of breath may quickly follow if innervation to respiratory muscles and pharyngeal musculature is affected (Table 20–22). The clinical features supporting the diag-

Table 20–22. Guillian-Barré Syndrome: Diagnostic Features

Required features:
- Progressive weakness in more than one limb
- Areflexia or hyporeflexia in distal legs and hyporeflexia elsewhere

Supportive features:
- Progression of symptoms over days to weeks
- Relative symmetry
- Mild sensory disturbances
- Facial nerve palsies
- Autonomic dysfunction
- Absence of fever with antecedent illness
- Elevated CSF protein with fewer than 10 WBCs/mm³
- Electrodiagnostic evidence

Features casting doubt on diagnosis:
- Discrete sensory level
- Marked asymmetry of motor findings
- Severe bowel/bladder dysfunction from onset
- >50 WBCs/mm³ in CSF
- >2.5 g/L protein in CSF

Exclusionary features:
- Botulism, myasthenia, poliomyelitis, diphtheria, porphyria, heavy metal or hexacarbon poisoning, tick paralysis
- Pure sensory syndrome

CSF = cerebrospinal fluid; WBC = white blood cells.

Reprinted with permission from Asbury AK, Cornblath DR: *Assessment of current diagnostic criteria for the diagnosis of Guillain-Barré syndrome.* Ann Neurol 1990;27(suppl):S21.

nosis of Guillain-Barré syndrome include relative symmetry of signs and symptoms, mild sensory disturbances, facial paresis, and a gradual ascending weakness. The laboratory evaluation includes cerebrospinal fluid analysis that shows elevation in protein concentration and minimal pleocytosis. It is important to exclude the presence of spinal cord disease in any patient who develops weakness in the legs. This should be evaluated by determining if a sensory disturbance level can be detected and whether signs of bowel or bladder dysfunction are present.

Treatment of Guillain-Barré syndrome includes supportive measures and the use of intravenous gamma globulin or plasmapharesis. The course is somewhat variable, but complete respiratory paralysis may develop, requiring mechanical ventilation. The symptoms usually increase over the first 2 weeks of the illness, followed by a plateau phase and then gradual recovery after the third to fourth week (Table 20–23). Most children recover completely, but 15 to 20% may have variable degrees of residual weakness.

Guillain-Barré syndrome does not generally recur. Repeated bouts of demyelinating polyneuropathy that are evident on neurophysiologic studies (EMG/NCV), suggest the diagnosis of chronic inflammatory demyelinating polyneuropathy (CIDP). This is a chronic disorder characterized by relapses and remittances. The condition is treated with steroids.

The hereditary motor and sensory neuropathies (HMSN) encompass several genetic diseases, which may have an autosomal dominant or autosomal recessive pattern of inheritance (Table 20–24). Many cases however, are sporadic or not defined. Disorders in this group are

Table 20–23. Guillian-Barré Syndrome: Clinical Course

Time	Symptoms	Exam	Lab
2 weeks prior	Antecedent respiratory or gastro-intestinal illness, vaccine	Systemic or constitutional symptoms	Nonspecific
1 week prior	None	Normal	Normal
Week #1	Fine paresthesias Pain in thighs	Mild facial and extremity weakness, ↓ reflexes	↓ VC and MIF; CSF, normal; NCV ↓
Week #2	Weakness and paresthesias progress, dysphagia/shortness of breath	Generalized weakness, arreflexia, nonambulating	↓↓ VC and MIF; CSF, ↑ protein NCV, ↓↓
Week #3	Plateau phase	Exam constant	↓↓ VC and MIF; CSF, ↑↑ protein NCV, ↓↓
Week #4	Gradual recovery: walk, 25 days w/Rx; walk, 60 days w/o Rx	Exam evolves: 15% completely recovered, remainder gradually improve	

CSF = cerebrospinal fluid; MIF = maximal inspiratory force; NCV = nerve conduction velocities; VC = vital capacity; ↓ = slowed or decreased; ↑ = elevated or increased.

Table 20–24. Hereditary Motor and Sensory Neuropathies (HMSN) and Hereditary Sensory and Autonomic Neuropathies (HSAN)

Designation	Inheritance Pattern	Clinical Characteristics
HMSN I (CMT disease)	Autosomal dominant • CMT 1a–17p11 duplication • CMT 1b–point mutations (MPZ and PMP22 genes) • CMT 1c–? Autosomal recessive • Linkage to 11q23, 8q13, 5q23 X-Linked • Deletion Xq13.1	Pathology: predominantly demyelination with onion bulb formation Onset: early childhood-adolescence Exam: distal leg wasting and weakness with pes cavus/hammer toes/"stork legs"; gradual loss of position/vibration sensation with loss of ankle then knee reflexes
HMSN II (CMT disease)	Autosomal dominant • Linkage to 1p35, 3q13, 7p14 Autosomal recessive	Pathology: predominantly axonal degeneration Onset: late childhood–adulthood Exam: similar to type 1 but milder weakness and more prominent sensory loss
HMSN III (Dejerine-Sottas disease; hypomyelinating disease)	Autosomal recessive • Point mutations (MPZ and PMP22 genes)	Pathology: hypomyelination myelination. Onset: infancy Exam: hypotonia, motor delays, proximal weakness with distal wasting legs > arms and arreflexia. Enlarged palpable nerves.
HMSN IV–VII (Refsum disease, and others)	Autosomal dominant Autosomal recessive	Heterogeneous group of neuropathies with combinations of clinical findings including: spastic paraplegia, retinitis pigmentosa, and pigmentary retinopathy
HSAN I	Autosomal dominant • Linkage to 9q22.1	Pathology: myelinated fiber degeneration Onset: adolescence–adulthood Exam: shooting pains in legs with eventual foot ulcers with diminished touch sensation and arreflexia in legs
HSAN II–V (Riley-Day syndrome and others)	Autosomal recessive	Pathology: central autonomic nervous system degeneration with peripheral nerve fiber loss Onset: infancy Exam: hypotonia, motor delays, breath-holding spells, diminished tears, diffuse weakness, difficulty with suck/swallow, reflux, smooth tongue, and arreflexia with autonomic instability
Friedreich ataxia (spinocerebellar degeneration)	Autosomal recessive • 9q13 GAA triplet repeat, point mutations	Pathology: dorsal root ganglion, peripheral nerve, posterior column, and cerebellar degeneration; axonal loss/secondary demyelination, degeneration of spinocerebellar/corticospinal tracts. Frataxin deficiency Onset: childhood with progression through adolescence Exam: proprioceptive/vibratory loss, ataxia, progressive weakness/atrophy legs and hands, kyphoscoliosis, pes cavus, hammer toes, arreflexia, cardiomyopathy, and diabetes mellitus

CMT = Charcot-Marie-Tooth; GAA = guanine, adenosine, adenosine; HMSN = hereditary motor and sensory neuropathies; HSAN = hereditary sensory and autonomic neuropathies.

known by various eponyms such as Charcot-Marie-Tooth disease (HMSN types I, II), Dejerine-Sottas disease (HMSN type III), and Refsum disease (HMSN type IV). They are defined primarily by electrophysiologic studies identifying demyelination (slowed conduction velocities) or axonal loss (diminished action potential amplitudes).

Hereditary motor and sensory neuropathies types I and II (Charcot-Marie-Tooth disease) are the most common disorders in this group. These have an autosomal dominant inheritance. The gene for HMSN type 1 has been identified on chromosome 1 and 17. Children may first have pes cavus deformity or minor gait disturbances, including subtle weakness in the feet. An additional complaint is pain or a pressure sensation that their "shoes are too tight." A prominent high arch is noted in the foot as the children get older, because of an imbalance between the weak intrinsic muscles of the plantar surface and the relatively stronger dorsiflexor muscles. Hammertoes may also be noted. The clumsiness and awkward running style of these children often brings them to medical attention. The examination reveals an inability to walk on the heels, due to peroneal weakness. The diagnosis relies on the family history that reveals a similar distribution of weakness in either parent. Nerve conduction and EMG studies provide electrophysiologic evidence for demyelination and/or axonal loss.

Weakness in the hands and a definitive sensory loss eventually become evident. The other hereditary motor and sensory neuropathies may have other clinical features such as ataxia, deafness, tremor, and retinitis pigmentosa. Specific genetic testing is available for several of these disorders (see Table 20–24).

Diseases of the Neuromuscular Junction

The hallmark of neuromuscular junction disease is muscle fatigue. These disorders typically present with facial and ocular weakness with or without proximal muscle weakness. However, even in the presence of weakness, the tendon reflexes are usually present, although they may be diminished. The most widely recognized disorder is myasthenia gravis. This is a sporadic disease caused by autoantibodies directed against the acetylcholine receptor at the motor endplate. As a result of blockade and destruction of this receptor, postsynaptic neurochemical transmission cannot occur and muscle contraction is not produced. Myasthenic syndromes usually involve either oculomotor or facial and bulbar weakness. A common presentation is ptosis with associated diplopia that worsens in a particular direction of gaze. This is accompanied by variable degrees of strabismus (noncomitant strabismus). The weakness can be accentuated or incurred by repetitive muscle action. A simple office maneuver to demonstrate oculomotor weakness or ptosis is to have the children stare upward for a prolonged period, after which

ocular motility and lid position are reassessed. Similarly, repeated hand grasp can induce weakness in the hands. The diagnosis is confirmed by observing the reversal of muscular weakness after an intravenous injection of edrophonium chloride (Tensilon). This inhibits the enzyme cholinesterase, allowing a transient increase in acetylcholine at the neuromuscular junction and a greater degree of neuromuscular transmission. An EMG study can also confirm a generalized disorder by repetitively stimulating the muscle at various locations and identifying a decremental physiologic response in neuromuscular transmission. Since this is an autoimmune disease, antibodies directed at the acetylcholine receptor as well as other autoantibodies can be measured (e.g., ANA and anti-thyroglobulin).

Other forms of myasthenia include two clinical presentations in the neonatal period. Neonatal myasthenia presents as transient neuromuscular weakness in newborn infants because of transplacental transfer of autoantibodies from a mother with myasthenia gravis. If weakness does not develop within the first 5 to 7 days after birth, it is unlikely to do so later. However, in affected infants, antibodies may not decrease significantly for several months after birth, and symptoms may persist. Several congenital forms of myasthenia have now been identified. The primary mechanism in some of these newborns is also the presence of autoantibodies, but these may not be evident early in their course. Ptosis is the most common presenting symptom, with swallowing difficulties and truncal weakness occurring later. Physiologic abnormalities of the neuromuscular junction receptor and ion channels produce other forms of myasthenia syndromes not caused by circulating autoantibodies. The hallmark of all of these myasthenic syndromes is muscle fatigue.

Infant botulism is now an uncommon cause of acute neuromuscular weakness. It is a result of exotoxin production by *Clostridium botulinum*, bacteria found in the infant's gastrointestinal tract. This toxin blocks presynaptic acetylcholine release, resulting in a failure of neuromuscular transmission. As in other myasthenic syndromes, this produces a flaccid paralysis but with a more global and rapid progression. The clinical hallmark of botulism is the descending progression of weakness. Infants lose the ability to suck and swallow soon after developing facial paresis. This progresses to include weakness of the respiratory musculature as well as that of trunk and limb muscles. The pupils become dilated and poorly reactive to light as a result of the presynaptic parasympathetic blockade. While toxin and bacteria can be isolated from stool specimens, EMG and nerve conduction studies can confirm the diagnosis electrophysiologically. Treatment is supportive and recovery is usually complete.

Other causes of acute neuromuscular junction blockade include tick paralysis, organophosphate poisoning, and aminoglycoside administration.

Muscular Diseases

MYOPATHIES

The majority of primary myopathies present with proximal muscular weakness. This is generally recognized by parents as an awkward gait, toe walking, and general clumsiness (Table 20–25A). Of the genetically determined myopathies, Duchenne and Becker muscular dystrophies are the most common. These are X-linked disorders (Xp21) that have genetic defects of the dystrophin gene in common. In Duchenne muscular dystrophies minimal to no dystrophin is produced, whereas in Becker muscular dystrophies, dystrophin production is reduced. Both disorders are characterized by pseudohypertrophy of muscles, especially in the calves. Weakness is most prominent in the pelvic girdle, resulting in lordosis of the spine, a waddling type of gait, and a positive Gowers sign. The shoulder girdle musculature is also eventually affected. There is progressive degeneration of muscle producing elevations of plasma creatine phosphokinase concentrations, frequently to levels 10 to 50 times the norm. In boys with the Duchenne phenotype, the clinical course is one of progressive decline. There is gradual decline in ambulation over the first 5 to 10 years of life, and most boys lose their ability to walk by age 12. Deterioration of respiratory musculature, progressive neuromuscular scoliosis, and symptomatic cardiomyopathy dominate the clinical picture until death. The Becker phenotype, however, has a milder effect on muscle function. As a result, boys often maintain their ability to ambulate independently well into the second and third decades of life. Mutation analysis is now available as a diagnostic test. It is also useful as a means of identifying asymptomatic female carriers and for prenatal fetal detection.

Other genetically determined progressive myopathies of childhood can be identified by the pattern of weakness and mode of inheritance. Facioscapulohumeral (FSH) syndromes are seen in children who develop insidious and progressive weakness of the shoulder girdle and face during the second decade of life. While dystrophic muscle may be evident on biopsy, elements of both neuropathy and inflammation can also be identified on nerve pathology specimens. This is an autosomal dominant disorder in which the gene is located on the long arm of chromosome 4 (4q35). While there is an elevation in creatine phosphokinase, this is generally of a milder degree than that seen in the other muscular dystrophies. The course is somewhat variable, with a normal life expectancy. Important, however, is the development of retinal vascular disease by adulthood in a majority of patients.

A less precise diagnostic category of muscular dystrophy is referred to as limb-girdle dystrophy. These are usually inherited in an autosomal recessive manner, but they encompass more than one disease entity. The diagnosis is often established in patients in whom no other specific myopathy can be determined. Patients develop either shoulder girdle or pelvic girdle weakness as a predominant site of proximal weakness. Facial weakness and diminished tendon reflexes may also be noted. Creatine phosphokinase enzyme levels are generally less elevated than they are in the Duchenne or Becker dystrophies.

MYOTONIA

Unique among the myopathies is myotonic dystrophy, because it primarily involves distal limb weakness. There is a gradual development of facial weakness as the patient ages. It may be diagnosed in the newborn period when infants have congenital contractures, hypotonia, and secondary asphyxia. When the practitioner encounters infants with extensive congenital contractures, the examination of the parents is paramount. Mothers are typically carriers of the disease, but may not be aware of any problems. They characteristically will have hollowed temporalis muscles and a transverse smile due to atrophy and weakness of facial musculature. In addition, they have myotonic contractions that can be elicited by shaking their hands and noting their difficulty in relaxing the hand grasp. Myotonic contractions can also be elicited by percussing a muscle, such as the thenar eminence, which will produce a protracted contraction. In children with myotonic dystrophy, gastroesophageal reflux may be a significant clinical problem. Over time other problems such as diabetes mellitus, early cataracts, cardiac arrhythmia, and cardiomyopathy may develop.

Myotonic dystrophy is an autosomal dominant disorder with the responsible gene identified on chromosome 19. The disease is produced by an unstable triplet repeat (CAG), which progressively lengthens as the gene is passed from generation to generation. This mechanism accounts for the increase in clinical severity from one generation to the next (anticipation). The muscle myotonia may be responsive to muscle-membrane-stabilizing drugs such as quinidine, phenytoin, and carbamazepine. Myotonia usually develops in adolescence and adulthood.

MUSCLE PAINS AND CRAMPS

A common complaint of preadolescent children is muscle pains. While these usually occur when children are at rest or settling down for the night, occasionally they are evident at other times of the day. It is important to try to distinguish between nonspecific diffuse leg pain and more specific muscle cramps, leg stiffness, and spasms. Cramps are painful, and continual muscle contractions occur in normal children, especially after vigorous exercise. When they occur at rest or awaken children from sleep, motor neuron disease or neuropathy should be considered. Cramps occurring during prolonged exercise may indicate muscle energy failure that can be associated with metabolic myopathies. Muscle stiffness and spasms are

Table 20–25A. Muscular Dystrophies

Designation	Inheritance Pattern	Clinical Characteristics
Duchenne muscular dystrophy	X-Linked • Deletions/duplications Xp21	Pathology: absent muscle dystrophin with degenerating fibers and connective tissue Onset: early childhood Exam: pseudohypertrophic calves, progressive weakness, waddling gait, some intellectual impairment, nonambulatory by 12 years, develops joint contractures, scoliosis, cardiomyopathy, and respiratory failure in late adolescence
Becker muscular dystrophy	X-Linked • Deletion Xp21	Pathology: deficient or defective muscle dystrophin with degenerating fibers and connective tissue Onset: late childhood-adolescence Exam: muscle cramps after exercise, pseudohypertrophic calves, progressive weakness, waddling gait, remain ambulatory well into adulthood, may develop joint contractures, scoliosis, cardiomyopathy
Emery-Dreifuss muscular dystrophy	X-Linked • Deletions/duplications Xp28	Rigid spine syndrome: childhood presentation with neck and back stiffness; atrophy and weakness of shoulder and/or pelvic girdles associated with elbow contractures, without muscle pseudohypertrophy; prominent cardiac arrhythmia and cognitive impairments; absence of nuclear membrane protein emerin
Limb-girdle muscular dystrophy	Autosomal dominant (LGMD1) • Linkage to 5q22, 1q11, 21q22 Autosomal recessive (LGMD2) • Linkage to 15q15, 17q21, 4q12, 13q12, 5q33 X-Linked • Deletion Xp28	Heterogeneous group of disorders affecting either shoulder or pelvic girdles predominantly; variable onset from childhood through adulthood; associated with specific muscle structural tramsmembrane sarcoglycan protein deficiencies
Facioscapulohumeral dystrophy	Autosomal dominant • Deletion 4q35	Variable onset age; congenital to adulthood; prominent facial weakness with incomplete eye closure, inability to puff cheeks, minimal facial expression, and scapular winging; CK may be normal; limb weakness may be asymmetric; associated with neurosensory hearing loss and retinal detachments
Myotonic dystrophy	Autosomal dominant • Linkage to 19q13, CTG triplet repeat	Congenital presentation with contractures, hypotonia, ptosis, poor swallowing, tented upper lip and secondary asphyxia; multisystem disorder (reflux, endocrinopathy, cardiac arrhythmia, cataracts, cognitive impairment) variable expression, distal weakness with myotonia
Congenital muscular dystrophy	Autosomal recessive	Pathology: dystrophic muscle and deficient extracellular matrix protein merosin; proximal > distal weakness with generalized hypotonia and contractures; clinical course is stable without deterioration, some with cognitive impairments
Fukuyama CMD	Autosomal recessive	As above with prominent CNS migration anomalies and mental retardation

CK = creatine phosphokinase; CMD = congenital muscular dystrophy; CNS = central nervous system; LGMD = limb-girdle muscular dystrophy.

prolonged contractions of muscle that may or may not produce pain and can signify myotonic contractions or dystonia. Systemic disorders such as hypocalcemia, hypomagnesemia, thyroid disease, mitochondrial disorders, and specific muscle enzyme disturbances of glycogen storage, lipid storage, potassium metabolism, and adenosine triphosphate (ATP) metabolism are all potential causes of muscle spasms.

INFLAMMATORY MYOPATHIES

The inflammatory myopathies are a heterogeneous group of disorders associated with muscle pain and acute weakness (see Table 20–25B). They are most commonly associated with intercurrent viral illnesses, particularly influenza. The pain usually begins in the distal muscles such as the calves, but may be present in any group such as the quadriceps, hamstrings, and shoulder girdles. Creatine phosphokinase enzyme concentrations are typically elevated during the course of the disease. The associated weakness is usually transient and is only rarely debilitat-

ing. A transient form of myositis is associated with intercurrent illness and should be differentiated from the more chronic inflammatory myopathies. While muscle tenderness on palpation is present in both types, focal muscle swelling and warmth with erythema are observed in the more chronic varieties. Dermatomyositis often develops insidiously and usually has its onset in the early school-aged child. There may be symptoms of malaise, low-grade fever, and fatigue. Muscle weakness is proximal in distribution and associated with tenderness and swelling. Periorbital edema (heliotrope) and skin changes, including edema, erythema, and Gottron papules (usually noted over extensor surfaces of the hands and knuckles), eventually become evident. The course of the disease is one of increasing debilitation. The diagnosis is determined by muscle biopsy demonstrating classic perivascular atrophy and inflammation. Treatment with steroids and immunosuppressive agents is usually palliative. Relapses are common if the treatment is not prolonged (see Chap. 8, "Rheumatic Diseases").

Table 20–25B. Myopathies

Designation	Inheritance Pattern	Clinical Characteristics
Congenital myopathies • NM • CCM • CNM • FTD • Others	• Autosomal recessive, autosomal dominant, X-linked • Autosomal dominant • Autosomal recessive, autosomal dominant • Sporadic, autosomal dominant	Pathology: characteristic morphologic features for each type; nemaline rods in NM, centrally placed cylinders in CCM, centrally located nuclei in CNM, and disparate myofiber sizes in FTD Onset: congenital, severe, childhood and adult, moderate to mild. Exam: hypotonic infants, most with nonprogressive weakness rarely can be progressive with respiratory failure and death in CCM and CNM; clinical features nonspecific: high arch pallate, narrow facies, kyphoscoliosis, hip dislocation, and extraocular muscle involvement in CNM
Metabolic myopathies • Mitochondrial myopathies • Defects in fatty acid oxidation • Defects in glycogenolysis • Defects in glycolysis • Others	• mtDNA, nDNA • Autosomal recessive • Autosomal recessive • Autosomal recessive	Clinically heterogeneous disorders that are enzyme specific and often affect multisystems; present with acute, recurrent, or chronic progressive weakness, encephalopathy, and other systemic symptoms often precipitated by exercise, fasting, and/or acute illness
Inflammatory myopathies • Polymyositis/dermatomyositis • Myositis associated with collagen vascular diseases, granulomatous diseases and others • Myositis associated with infection: viral, HIV, parasites, bacteria, and fungus	• Sporadic	Clinical features specific to each etiologic entity; common to all is muscle pain associated with elevated CK enzyme and muscle pathology demonstrating inflammation with etiology-specific characteristics

CCM = central core myopathy; CK = creatine phosphokinase; CNM = centronuclear; FTD = fiber-type disproportion; mtDNA = mitochondrial DNA; nDNA = nuclear DNA; NM = nemaline myopathy.

GAIT DISTURBANCES

Disturbances of gait and stance may be the first indications of a neurologic problem in childhood. A stride is divided into the stance phase (first 60%) and the swing phase (latter 40%). The stride is defined from the moment the foot first makes contact in front of the patients. The stance phase extends from shifting of the weight over the lead foot as the children move forward, until the second foot is planted forward. The swing phase begins at the so-called "toe off" point, when the initial foot leaves contact with the ground. All parts of the motor system are required and must be well integrated to achieve a smooth and functional gait. The cerebral cortex, pyramidal and extrapyramidal systems, cerebellum, brainstem, spinal cord, peripheral nerves, neuromuscular junctions, muscles and special sensory inputs from visual and proprioceptive sensors, as well as skeletal integrity, all impact the ability to ambulate.

The gait should be observed when the children are undressed enough to allow visualization of the spine, hips, and pelvis, as well as the legs and arms. Joint mobility, as well the presence of scoliosis should be evaluated. The Rhomberg test is performed by observing for truncal sway or loss of position when the children stand with feet together, the arms held to the side, and the eyes closed. If unsteadiness is ameliorated when the eyes are opened, proprioceptive deficits are likely. The children's movement while walking should be symmetric and freely flowing. A spastic hemiplegia is likely when there is scuffing of the foot and flexion of the ipsilateral elbow and knee. A spastic diplegic gait is associated with toe walking and flexion at the hips and knees that resembles a crouching position. Crossing or "scissoring" of the legs when the children are held in vertical suspension by support under the axillae indicates the presence of increased hip abductor tone. A lurching or lunging quality of the gait that does not concern the children suggests a cerebellar disturbance. The incoordination often involves the arms and trunk when seated. Unilateral cerebellar disturbances usually, but not always, produce lurching toward the side of the lesion. Diseases that affect the extrapyramidal system typically produce a shuffling gait with a stooped posture. Bradykinesia with a characteristic festinating quality to the gait (a series of very small steps) may be noted before a normal walking stride is attained. Weakness of the dorsiflexors of the feet and toes causes foot drop, and the children will walk as though stepping over an imaginary barrier. This so-called "steppage" gait is often characteristic of distal muscle weakness or a peripheral neuropathy such as Charcot-Marie-Tooth disease. If the weakness is confined to the hip girdle, the pelvis will be unstable, resulting in accentuation of lumbar lordosis and a waddling gait. This gait, recognized by the marked shifting of weight from side-to-side with the pelvis moving up and down, is observed with primary myopathies such as muscular dystrophy. An antalgic gait or limp favors one leg and is characteristic of pain on ambulation. A wide variety of gait disturbances may accompany conversion reactions.

Ataxia

Ataxia is a disturbance characterized by incoordination (Table 20–26) and is usually not associated with weakness. While this is most commonly due to cerebellar dysfunction, other causes exist. It is important to differentiate ataxia from both weakness and vertigo. Children experiencing vertigo are quite upset with the symptom, prefer not to move, or appear frightened and seek comfort. Ataxic children do not appear to be perturbed by the degree of difficulty they often have. They are not appreciably weak and continue to attempt to climb, run, and arise from the lying position with little hesitation. The examiner and parent are usually more concerned about the children falling than are the children. The children become frustrated,

Table 20–26. Causes of Ataxia

Acute
 Ingestion (anticonvulsants, alcohol, sedatives, etc.)
 Infectious/postinfectious acute cerebellar ataxia (varicella, enteroviruses, Epstein-Barr virus, etc.)
 Acute disseminated encephalomyelitis
 Guillian-Barré syndrome
 Trauma
 Cerebellar stroke (hemorrhage, thrombosis)
 Vasculitis
 Conversion reaction

Recurrent
 Basilar artery migraine
 Vasculitis
 Paraneoplastic (neuroblastoma, carcinoma)
 Metabolic disease (hypoglycemia, Hartnup syndrome, pyruvate decarboxylase deficiency, mitochondrial disorders, etc.)
 Postictal state

Chronic progressive
 Posterior fossa tumor (hemangioblastoma, astrocytoma, medulloblastoma, ependymoma}
 Degenerative disease (ataxia-telangiectasia, spinocerebellar degeneration, neuronal ceroid lipofuscinosis, etc.)
 Chiari malformation
 Hydrocephalus
 Storage disorders/metabolic diseases (sialidosis, vitamin E deficiency, urea cycle disorders, etc.)

Chronic static
 Cerebral palsy
 Cerebellar malformation (aplasia, dysplasia, Dandy-Walker malformation, etc.)

however, with the inability to perform smoothly coordinated activities. It is important to determine whether the symptoms are acute, chronic, progressive, or recurrent in nature, because these features may help to identify the etiology (Figure 20–8). A family history of a similar disability suggests a hereditary disorder.

On examination, the gait and stance are wide-based, lurching, and staggering in quality. Truncal posture against gravity is sometimes wavering (titubation). Subtler signs of incoordination can be detected by observing directed movements against gravity. The children's hands may not find their target precisely when asked to reach for an object. Eye movements can also display an ataxic quality with a need to repeatedly fix and refix on a visual target. Similarly, the voice may be slurred and the timber diminished.

Acute cerebellar ataxia in young children are most often postinfectious or the result of a toxic ingestion. Common antecedent illnesses include chickenpox, enteroviruses, infectious mononucleosis, and influenza, but other viral infections may be responsible. Meningismus and vomiting can at times be significant, but symptoms suggestive of raised intracranial pressure such as lethargy, diplopia, or papilledema should not be present. If an appropriate antecedent illness is identified, further investigation is usually not necessary. Cerebrospinal fluid analysis is usually normal except for a mild pleocytosis. Neuroimaging studies such as CT scanning or MRI are noncontributory. The exclusion of a toxic ingestion is important, particularly in toddlers. A careful history of the availability of household medications and pesticides should be obtained. Specific screening may be needed to exclude toxins such as anticonvulsants, antihistamines, sedative hypnotics, and alcohol.

Acute ataxia has been observed as an unusual initial presentation of Guillian-Barré syndrome. The children subsequently develop the typical features of generalized weakness and hyporeflexia or arreflexia. The Miller-Fisher variant of Guillian-Barré syndrome is characterized by acute ataxia and cranial neuropathies affecting eye movements that appear before any weakness is noted. Rarely bacterial meningitis and/or encephalitis may present with acute ataxia; the children usually appear acutely ill and demonstrate meningeal irritation.

If the ataxia is episodic and recurrent, the differential diagnosis includes migraine attacks, seizure disorders, and other rare conditions. Young children with migraine may not yet complain of headache, but manifest gait instability or incoordination. There is often associated pallor and a family history of migraine. Postictal ataxia is not uncommon in children with epilepsy. This may transpire when the seizure has occurred during sleep and the ataxia is evident upon awakening. Intermittent ataxia may present as the primary manifestation in several metabolic disorders, such as Hartnup disease (tryptophan dysmetabolism) and abnormalities of pyruvate metabolism.

Analysis of urine or plasma obtained during the acute event for organic acids, amino acids, and pyruvate cycle components may elucidate the diagnoses. When ataxia is coupled with chaotic eye movements and with myoclonus, the syndrome of opsoclonus-myoclonus (dancing eyes-dancing feet syndrome) should be considered. This syndrome occurs with occult neuroblastoma; the urine should therefore be examined for catecholamine metabolites. In this syndrome, the tumor is often in the mediastinum rather than in the paraspinal region of the abdomen or in the adrenal glands.

If the ataxia is chronic, it is important to determine whether it is progressive and associated with other symptoms. Static ataxia usually represents a form of cerebral palsy. This diagnosis is supported by findings of hyperreflexia and cerebellar dysfunction. Chronic progressive ataxia is most commonly the result of a hereditary disorder that involves degeneration of both the cerebellum and other descending motor and ascending sensory tracts. When progressive ataxia is accompanied by scoliosis, particularly before puberty, Friedreich ataxia should be considered (see Table 20–24). In these patients, reflexes are reduced and light touch and position senses are diminished. Approximately 30 to 40% of patients have concomitant diabetes mellitus and cardiomyopathy. The pes cavus deformity develops with age. This disorder may be sporadic or inherited as a dominant or recessive trait and is confirmed by identifying a triplet repeat (CAG) on chromosome 9.

Ataxia-telangiectasia (Louis-Bar syndrome) is a genetic disorder that presents with chronic progressive ataxia in children. These children first manifest clumsiness and subtle truncal sway or instability when standing upright. As the disease progresses, truncal ataxia and ataxic limb movements become more evident and bulbar scleral telangiectases become apparent. Frequent sinopulmonary infections and immunodeficiency are other features of the syndrome. Laboratory findings include decreased plasma immunoglobulin levels (IgA, IgG, and IgE) and elevated embryonic tissue protein levels (carcinoembryonic antigen and alpha-fetoprotein). Other rare hereditary ataxia syndromes, including spinocerebellar degeneration, are beyond the scope of this discussion (see Table 20–26).

Primary brain tumors can present with the gradual onset of progressive ataxia. Central nervous system tumor is the second most common malignancy in childhood and the most common solid tumor in childhood (Table 20–27). Ataxia usually results from tumors located within the posterior fossa, the most common being cerebellar astrocytomas, ependymomas, medulloblastomas, and brainstem gliomas. The development of symptoms with primary central nervous system tumors in the posterior fossa may be insidious. Acute presentations may be the result of hemorrhage into the tumor, or obstructive hydrocephalus leading to an acute increase in intracranial

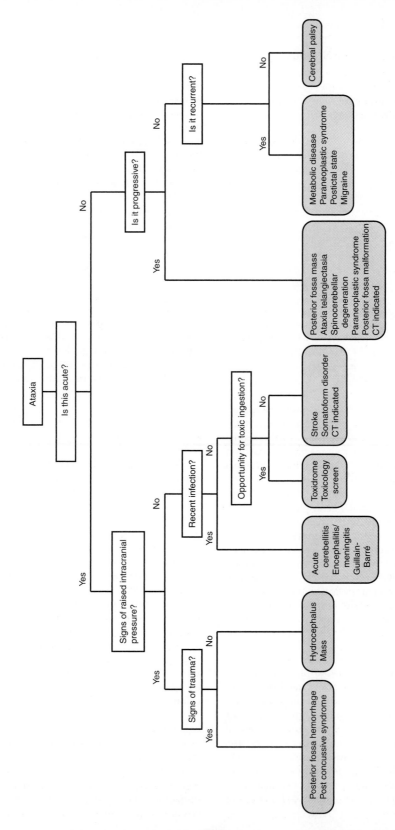

Figure 20–8. Decision algorithm for evaluation of children with ataxia.

Table 20–27. Primary Central Nervous
System Tumors

Descending order of frequency (%)
Astrocytoma (pilocytic, low-grade) (25)
Medulloblastoma (23)
Cerebellar astrocytoma (12)
Astrocytoma (anaplastic, high-grade) (11)
Brainstem glioma (9)
Ependymoma (8)
Unclassified (7)
Oligodendroglioma (2)
Mixed glioma (1)
Cerebellar glioblastoma (1)
Choroid plexus papilloma (0.3)
Meningioma (0.2)
Ganglioneuroma (0.1)
Others: teratoma, subependymal giant cell astrocytoma, pineocytoma, pinealoblastoma, craniopharyngioma, germinoma, ganglioglioma, etc.

Modified with permission from Duffner PK, Cohen ME, et al: Survival in children with brain tumors: SEER program., 1973–1980. Neurol 1986;36; 597.

pressure. Posterior fossa tumors should always be considered in children with progressive ataxia, particularly when associated with headache and vomiting. Other cranial nerve abnormalities and upper motor unit dysfunction (hyperreflexia, hypertonia, and positive Babinski signs) are commonly associated.

Brain malformations that may be associated with chronic ataxia include cerebellar hemisphere hypoplasia, vermis aplasia, and Arnold-Chiari malformations. Arnold-Chiari malformations, which include inferior cerebellar displacement into the cervical spinal canal, may also produce cervical medullary junction compression, which manifests as lower cranial neuropathies. Oculomotor function, swallowing, and respiratory function may be affected. Surgical decompression of the posterior fossa may be necessary to relieve these symptoms.

Hemiparesis

Hemiparesis may present acutely, or the onset may be insidious and subtle. The presence of hand preference in infants under 2 years of age should suggest the possibility of hemiparesis in the nondominant hand. Other possible presentations include delay in the acquisition of motor milestones, asymmetry of somatic growth and size, and awkwardness in gait. The physical examination should assess the presence of atrophy and quality of movement, tone, and functional strength and should determine whether the problem is a result of upper or lower motor dysfunction.

Nonprogressive weakness or asymmetry of motor movement evident at an early age suggests a diagnosis of cerebral palsy. Infants with congenital hemiparesis may not be recognized until there is failure in attaining motor milestones. The etiology should be evaluated by neuro-imaging with MRI or CT scans. A structural lesion, such as brain dysgenesis, brain infarction, or periventricular leukomalacia, can usually be identified.

The incidence of periventricular and intraventricular hemorrhage of newborns, which was extremely high, has currently decreased to approximately 20 to 25% of all premature infants. The highest risk groups are infants born at 28 to 32 weeks gestation, those with very low birth weights, and infants with circulatory or respiratory failure, infection, and coagulopathy. Intraventricular hemorrhages are graded on the basis of the degree of hemorrhage and associated ventricular dilatation. In grade 1, hemorrhage is isolated to the region of the germinal matrix. Grade 2 includes those with extension of hemorrhage into the ventricle, but with no dilatation. Hemorrhages that fill more than 50% of the ventricle or dilate the ventricular system are classified as grade 3; grade 4 refers to those with intraparenchymal hemorrhage. Parenchymal hemorrhages are more often due to venous obstruction and hemorrhagic infarction, rather than to extension of an intraventricular hemorrhage. The higher the grade of the hemorrhage, the greater is the risk for long-term sequelae, which occur in almost 75% of infants who have suffered grade 3 and 4 hemorrhages.

Periventricular leukomalacia (PVL) may be observed in association with intraventricular hemorrhage or as an isolated lesion. Pathologically this represents necrotic white brain matter adjacent to the ventricular walls. On ultrasound examination it presents initially as small cystic foci of damaged white matter that coalesce to form white matter cavities (cystic PVL). Eventually ventriculomegaly results from white matter volume loss with adjacent "scarring." These lesions are usually the result of hypoxia and ischemia. There is now some evidence for an inflammatory-mediated tissue destruction, triggered by perinatal inflammation or infection. Intraventricular hemorrhage may result from a combination of mechanical and physiologic factors, including fluctuations in intracerebral blood pressure and perfusion, alterations in serum osmolality and viscosity, abnormalities in coagulation, and extreme variability in intravascular volume.

Acute hemiparesis in children is likely to be due an ischemic or hemorrhagic stroke and should prompt immediate referral for further evaluation (Table 20–28). It may, however, be a postictal phenomenon of an unwitnessed or unrecognized seizure. Postictal paresis (Todd paresis) typically resolves within 24 h, provided no additional focal seizures occur. (The more common causes of acute cerebral infarction are shown in Table 20–28.)

Table 20–28. Causes of Acute Hemiplegia

Stroke
  Thrombotic
    Hemoglobinopathies
    Thrombocytosis
    ITP, TTP, HUS
    Hypercoaguable states
    Hyperosmolar states
    Homocystinuria
    Hyperlipidemia
    Vascular dissection
    Vasculopathy/vasculitis
    Trauma
    Vasoconstricting drugs (ergots, cocaine, etc.)
    Dehydration
    Sinus thrombosis
  Hemorrhagic
    Coagulopathy (hemophilia, DIC, etc.)
    Thrombocytopenia
    Vascular malformation
    CNS neoplasm
    Trauma
    Anticoagulant drugs (aspirin, coumadin, etc.)
  Embolic
    Congenital heart disease
    Intracardiac tumor
    Cardiac valvular disease
    Carotid dissection
    Cardiomyopathy
Complicated migraine
Mitochondrial encephalomyopathy lactic acidosis and
  stroke-like episodes (MELAS)
Postictal Todd paralysis
Alternating hemiplegia
Acute disseminated encephalomyelitis
Multiple sclerosis
Hypertensive encephalopathy
Transient ischemic attack
Uremia

CNS = central nervous system; DIC = disseminated intravascular coagulation; HUS = hemolytic uremia syndrome; ITP = idiopathic thrombocytopenic purpura; TTP = thrombotic thrombocytopenic purpura.

Neuroimaging is indicated to define the location, extent, and type of stroke.

Chronic progressive hemiparesis may be difficult to recognize particularly when it occurs over months or years. A history of functional loss of skills and careful documentation of serial examinations will facilitate identification of the problem. Unlike acute hemiparesis, chronic hemiparesis is more often associated with progressive mass lesions and/or neurodegenerative conditions. Neuroimaging by MRI or CT is indicated. Important causes are vascular malformations, cerebral hemisphere tumors, inflammatory or hemorrhagic collection (i.e., abscess or subdural hematoma), and demyelinating disorders. Sturge-Weber syndrome is a readily recognized neurocutaneous disorder that often presents with progressive hemiparesis contralateral to the facial port wine stain (see later).

Paraplegia

Paraparesis implies weakness and paraplegia (paralysis) in the legs without arm involvement. Acute paraplegia usually manifests as flaccid paralysis of the legs and may be associated with back pain, bowel and/or bladder incontinence, and a discrete "level" of sensory loss (spinal shock). When this evolves acutely over a several hours, evaluation for spinal cord injury due to compression and/or inflammatory disease is important (see discussion on transverse myelitis earlier). Conditions associated with a high risk for spinal cord compression are connective tissue disorders and ligamentous laxity, as in Marfan syndrome, Ehlers-Danlos syndrome, and Down syndrome. Children with these conditions are at risk for subluxation and cervical medullary junction compression owing to the laxity of anchoring ligaments of the atlantoaxial joint. Spinal cord compression may also be associated with cervicovertebral anomalies—storage disorders involving vertebrae and skeletal dysplasias. Trauma to the spine may also result in acute paraplegia or paraparesis. This may initially present with only minimal gait disturbance, or a sensation of the legs "giving out" while walking. Subsequently other clinical evidence of upper motor unit signs such as hypertonicity, increased reflexes, and Babinski sign develop after several hours to days. Determining the level of sensory function best identifies the inferior level of injury. Administration of intravenous methylprednisolone may improve the ultimate outcome of acute paraplegia.

When fever and general systemic illness is associated with the acute onset of back pain and paraplegia, an epidural abscess must be excluded. Corroborating signs of meningitis such as headache, vomiting, stiff neck, spine rigidity, and exquisite tenderness to percussion of the spine over the level of the abscess may also be noted. Evaluation of the spine with MRI and institution of appropriate antibiotic therapy and steroids in conjunction with neurosurgical drainage will be necessary.

Primary tumors of the spine may also present with progressive paraparesis (Table 20–29). This is often associated with gradually increasing back or chest pain, increasing gait disturbance, and bowel and bladder dysfunction. Any children with back pain and gait disturbance should be evaluated for an intraspinal lesion. The most common histologic types of spinal cord tumors are astrocytoma, neuroblastoma, and ependymoma. Metastatic lesions from other malignancies are also possible.

Vascular malformations, developmental lesions (e.g., syrinx and cyst) and benign intraspinal tumors, particularly

Table 20–29. Spinal Cord Tumors

Intramedullary
  Astrocytoma
  Ependymoma
  Oligodendroglioma
  Hemangioblastoma

Extramedullary
  Neurofibroma
  Dermoid
  Epidermoid
  Teratoma
  Lipoma
  Meningioma
  Metastatic

neurofibromatosis types II and I, can also produce progressive paraparesis. Intraspinal schwannoma or neurofibroma may develop from nerve roots exiting the spinal cord within the paraspinal regions and cause compression.

CRANIAL NERVE ABNORMALITIES

Cranial nerves are the peripheral nerves emanating from the brainstem that serve both sensory and motor functions for the eyes, face, throat, and neck. Three cranial nerves serve special sensory functions only (cranial nerves I, II, and VIII), five cranial nerves serve purely motor functions (cranial nerves III, IV, VI, XI, and XII), and four cranial nerves serve both sensory and motor functions (cranial nerves V, VII, IX, and X). Because of its compact anatomy, lesions of the brainstem often affect several cranial nerves simultaneously. The hallmark of brainstem dysfunction is the presence of cranial nerve abnormalities ipsilateral to the lesion (the exception is cranial nerve IV) with motor paresis contralateral to the lesion. The cranial nerves penetrate the dura at various sites as they exit the subarachnoid space and course through cranial foramina. They are subject to inflammatory disorders and traumatic injury along their paths. Inflammatory and infectious processes usually affect cranial nerves in the inferior portion of the brainstem. The sixth cranial nerve is particularly vulnerable to increases in intracranial pressure, which can produce bilateral sixth nerve palsies from compression of the nerve against bony prominences. Similarly, the optic nerves are affected by increases in intracranial pressure because of a subarachnoid sleeve extending around each nerve as it pierces the posterior portion of the globe. Increases in intracranial pressure are readily transmitted through this subarachnoid sleeve, forcing the optic nerve head to swell. This swelling is recognized as papilledema on fundoscopic examination.

Visual Disturbances

Visual disturbances in children are not common, but routine clinical assessment of vision should be a part of the general examination at all ages. Visual loss may be congenital or acquired. (Examination of the visual system and visual loss are discussed in detail in Chap. 21, "Ophthalmology.")

Strabismus

Strabismus or abnormalities of ocular alignment are common in childhood. When this misalignment is latent, and evident only under fatigue, it is termed *heterophoria.* When the strabismus is constantly evident it is termed *heterotropia.* The degree of misalignment can be constant despite varying directions of gaze (comitant). If the degree of strabismus is variable when redirecting gaze the strabismus is noncomitant and suggests ophthalmoplegia (paralytic strabismus). An inward deviation of eyes is termed *esotropia* and an outward deviation is termed *exotropia.* If the strabismus is significant enough to cause the children to fixate continually with only one eye, there is the potential for the development of permanent visual loss in the nonfixating eye (amblyopia). The most important aspect of misalignment to be determined by the practitioner is whether or not it represents a comitant or a noncomitant strabismus. Noncomitant strabismus needs to be evaluated further to determine the underlying cause of the paralysis (see Chap. 21, "Ophthalmology").

Nystagmus

Nystagmus is an involuntary oscillatory movement of the eyes. When the oscillations are equal in speed and in amplitude they are termed *pendular.* Oscillations of unequal speed (a slow and a fast phase in opposite directions) are known as jerk nystagmus. Other ocular oscillatory movements can be defined that relate to disordered brainstem control mechanisms. For the pediatric practitioner it is important to be able to differentiate physiologic nystagmus from congenital and acquired nystagmus.

Physiologic nystagmus is observed upon extremes of gaze. It is usually pendular, but as the muscles fatigue with continued gaze it may become more jerky in quality. It quickly diminishes if gaze is redirected slightly more toward the midline. Congenital nystagmus may not necessarily be noticed until later. The delay in recognition is due to the gradual development of visual fixation in newborns, and the associated null point, i.e., the point where both eyes are aligned. The nystagmus is suppressed when gazing in a specific direction, but when the children look away from the null point, the nystagmus reappears. It is usually horizontal and can be jerky or pendular in quality (see also Chap. 21, "Ophthalmology").

Facial Weakness

Facial weakness may result from disorders affecting the central nervous system or from involvement of the pathways extending from the facial nerve nuclei within the brainstem to the peripheral facial musculature. Facial weakness is recognized by an asymmetry of facial movement or expression. The examination reveals widening of the palpebral fissure on the affected side, loss of the normal nasolabial fold, and a diminished ability to puff the cheeks and purse the lips. The presence of forehead wrinkling and eyebrow raising is an important finding in differentiating between central and peripheral involvement. The upper but not the lower portion of the face has bilateral innervation at the level of the midbrain. Therefore, when a unilateral hemispheric lesion produces paresis of the face, the forehead still moves due to preservation of innervation from the opposite hemisphere. Disorders affecting the facial nerve nuclei, peripheral facial nerves, or the neuromuscular junction at the facial muscles result in loss of forehead and lower facial movement on the same side of the lesion. Depending on the specific site along the course of the facial nerve that is affected, other signs and symptoms including hyperacusis, alteration of taste, and disturbances in lacrimation may be associated.

Congenital facial weakness (particularly when bilateral) is usually the result of perinatal asphyxia. There may be an associated encephalopathy with disturbance in facial expression as well as bulbar functioning. Congenital absence of various cranial nerve nuclei, including the facial nerves (Möbius syndrome), results in bilateral facial weakness in conjunction with other cranial neuropathies, usually those concerned with ocular movement. Facial weakness may occur as part of other syndromes such as congenital myotonic dystrophy, primary myopathies, and congenital myasthenic syndrome. The facial nerve may be damaged during delivery from trauma of forceps extraction, or by pressure of the face on the sacral promontory during delivery. The nerve is usually damaged in its' extracranial location within the facial canal and usually recovers spontaneously unless it is completely severed. A condition that should be differentiated from facial palsy in newborn infants is neonatal facial asymmetry or "asymmetric crying facies." This is due to an isolated absence or weakness of the depressor anguli orsi muscle at one of the angles of the mouth. When the child cries one corner of the mouth fails to move downward. The remainder of the face, however, has full expression and movement.

BELL PALSY

Bell palsy, or acute idiopathic paralysis of the face, can be caused by postinfectious or autoimmune disease. Following a nonspecific viral illness, children may complain of facial tingling or pain in the jaw or ear region for several days prior to the weakness of the face. Usually facial weakness develops rapidly over a few hours. Parents often complain of their children's faces "pulling to one side." This pulling is the result of normal facial muscle contracting against unopposed contralateral facial weakness. There may be difficulty in speaking, dribbling of liquids from the mouth, and an inability to completely close the eye on the affected side. Taste and lacrimation may be impaired, and there may be hyperacusis on the affected side. The examination should be directed to excluding involvement of other cranial nerves and the motor system. If the facial palsy is accompanied by more generalized weakness, the Guillian-Barré syndrome or myasthenia gravis should be considered. Lyme disease may also present with facial palsy. Examination of the cerebrospinal fluid is not usually necessary in the evaluation of Bell palsy unless the presence of meningitis is suspected. Neuroimaging should be considered only when additional neurological deficits are evident. Treatment for Bell palsy is directed toward symptomatic relief and protecting the eye during sleep. The use of oral corticosteroids, tapered over a 7- to 10-day period, may be helpful to speed recovery. The vast majority of children experience spontaneous and complete recovery within 2 to 4 weeks.

Hearing Loss

Even infants who are deaf at birth will make sounds over the first 2 to 3 months of life but have a waning of vocalizations thereafter. In older children with impaired hearing, speech development may be delayed or misarticulated. While speech and language are related, they are a distinct phenomenon. Language refers to the more global use of symbols to represent ideas as a means of expression. Speech is but one modality of expressive language. Language and speech are both dependent upon the reception of sound (the ear and auditory pathways), the processing of sound and information (the brain and auditory cortex), and the mechanics of expression (verbal, gestural, and written).

If hearing impairment is suspected, the examination should be directed at defining the extent and degree of sound perception and the understanding and utilization of symbolic language. The examiner can test hearing threshold by simply rubbing the fingers together next to each ear and noting alerting response and turning of the head toward the side of the stimulus. Older children can be tested by whispering into one ear while masking sound in the opposite ear (rubbing the ear with the hand) and then asking what was said. More formal testing of hearing may need to be done to identify partial degrees of hearing loss.

NEUROCUTANEOUS DISORDERS

The neurocutaneous diseases have in common the presence of cutaneous markers and the potential for underlying neurologic dysfunction and multiorgan involvement. It is necessary to determine whether a particular cutaneous marker is an isolated finding or represents part of a more generalized process. The skin, hair, nails, and nervous system (central and peripheral) are all derivatives of ectodermal tissue. When the normally ordered developmental sequences of cells and tissues are disturbed, disordered growth results. These disturbances in tissue organization and growth results in what we recognize as hamartomas (an abnormal proliferation of normal tissue elements), heterotopias (abnormal location of normal tissue elements), and nevi (birthmarks characterized by localized overgrowths of skin elements). As a group, the neurocutaneous syndromes have distinctive and sometimes overlapping features. These diseases are also discussed in Chap. 11, "Skin."

Neurofibromatosis

TYPE I

Neurofibromatosis type 1 (NF-1) is a common disorder with a prevalence of approximately 1 in 3000. The hallmark of NF-1 is multiple café-au-lait spots. These are typically present over the trunk within the first few weeks after birth and may increase in number and size over the following several years. Café-au-lait spots usually have fairly homogenous pigmentation. They are discreet and do not merge with surrounding skin tone at the margins. While they initially may be small (millimeters in size), they enlarge and pigmentation deepens with increasing age. The development of freckling (multiple 1- to 2-mm spots) in the axillary or inguinal regions typically begins to develop before puberty. A diagnosis of NF-1 is established when two or more definitive clinical criteria are identified (Table 20–30). Most children will not experience significant physical or neurologic compromise, although up to 30 to 40% have an associated learning

Table 20–30. Diagnostic Criteria for Neurofibromatosis Type-1 (NF-1)

Definitive diagnosis based on a patient having 2 or more of the following:

• Six or more café-au-lait spots
    0.5 cm or larger in prepubertal children
    1.5 cm or larger in postpubertal patients
• Two or more neurofibromas of any type *or*
    One or more plexiform neuromas
• Axillary or inguinal freckling
• Optic glioma
• Two or more iris Lisch nodules
• A distinctive bony lesion (dysplasia of sphenoid wing or long bone)
• A first-degree relative with definite NF-1

Reprinted with permission from NIH Consensus development conference: Neurofibromatosis: Conference statement. Arch Neurol 1988;45:575.

disability. Approximately 10 to 15% of children with NF-1 develop an optic nerve glioma. Many of these lesions are asymptomatic but have the potential to produce insidious and progressive visual loss. Acute or gradual changes in visual ability, ocular alignment, or nystagmus are important clinical clues to diagnosis. Yearly ophthalmologic examinations are recommended for children under age 8 years. Periodic blood pressure measurements and examination of the spine for scoliosis should be done at each health care visit. Many children have macrocephaly in addition to relative short stature. Precocious puberty can also develop with or without evidence of hypothalamic dysfunction. This may also be the initial manifestation of a hypothalamic glioma or extension of an optic chiasm tumor. Most patients will eventually develop cutaneous and subcutaneous neurofibromas. These are benign peripheral nerve tumors that can present significant cosmetic problems. More serious consequences can arise if the growth of paraspinal "dumbbell" neurofibromas enlarge and compress the spinal cord or produce progressive scoliosis. No routine laboratory tests or radiological examinations are indicated for patients with NF-1. These examinations are reserved for patients with specific signs and symptoms requiring further evaluation. The gene for NF-1 has been localized to chromosome 17. This is an autosomal dominant disorder with approximately 50% of patients having a spontaneous mutation. In children with identified NF-1, other family members should also be evaluated for the disorder. While genetic testing is now currently available, it is not yet 100% sensitive, and the diagnosis still rests upon clinical criteria.

TYPE II

Neurofibromatosis type II (NF-2) is much less common than type I, occurring in approximately 1 per 20,000 population. This is also an autosomal dominant disorder with the gene identified on chromosome 22. While this disorder may also produce cutaneous neurofibromas these are relatively few and café-au-lait spots are typically absent. The diagnosis rests primarily on the development of auditory nerve tumors (vestibular schwannoma or acoustic neuroma; Table 20–31). These are typically bilateral and produce gradual and progressive hearing loss. If children have a parent with NF-2, surveillance neuroimaging with MRI by age 16 years old is required to exclude the early development of acoustic neuromas. These, however, may not become radiologically evident until early adulthood (age 30 years). Additional intracranial and intraspinal lesions (meningiomas, gliomas, and schwannomas), as well as ocular findings (juvenile posterior subcapsular cataracts), complete the clinical picture.

Tuberous Sclerosis Complex

Tuberous sclerosis complex (TSC) is a neurocutaneous disorder primarily identified by distinctive and multiple

Table 20–31. Diagnostic Criteria
for Neurofibromatosis Type-2 (NF-2)

Definitive diagnosis based on a patient confirmed to have the following:
• Bilateral vestibular schwannomas
   or
• Family history of NF-2
   plus
     Unilateral vestibular schwannoma *or*
     Any two of the following: meningioma, glioma, schwannoma, or juvenile posterior subcapsular lenticular opacities/juvenile cortical cataract

NIH Consensus development conference: Neurofibromatosis: Conference statement. Arch Neurol 1988;45:575.

Table 20–32. Diagnostic Criteria for Tuberous Sclerosis Complex (TSC)[1]

Major features
• Facial angiofibromas or forehead plaque
• Nontraumatic ungual or periungual fibroma
• Hypomelanotic macules (3 or more)
• Shagreen patch
• Multiple retinal hamartomas
• Cortical tuber
• Subependymal nodule
• Subependymal giant cell astrocytoma
• Cardiac rhabdomyoma, single or multiple
• Lymphangiomatosis
• Renal angiomyolipoma
 	
Minor features
• Multiple, randomly distributed dental enamel pits
• Hamartomatous rectal polyps
• Bone cysts
• Cerebral white matter radial migration lines
• Gingival fibromas
• Nonrenal hamartoma
• Retinal achromic patch
• "Confetti" skin lesions
• Multiple renal cysts
 	
Definite TSC:
   Either two major features *or* one major feature plus two minor features
 	
Probable TSC:
   One major *plus* one minor feature
 	
Possible TSC:
   Either one major feature *or* two or more minor features

[1] Reprinted with permission from Roach ES, et al: Consensus Statement: Diagnostic criteria for tuberous sclerosis complex. J Child Neurol 1998;13:624.

hypopigmented macules (Table 20–32). While these are recognized in more than 90% of patients with TSC, they are neither specific nor diagnostic for the condition. Patients usually first come to medical attention because of seizures, often presenting with infantile spasms. Careful examination of the skin may uncover hypopigmented lesions; use of a Wood lamp may help to define these lesions. The diagnostic evaluation includes neuroimaging of the head by CT scanning or MRI to detect subependymal nodules with calcifications as well as cortical and subcortical tubers. The brain lesions are evident in neonates but become better circumscribed with age. Language delay and autism are other common presentations, so all children with these complaints should be carefully examined for the presence of neurocutaneous markers suggestive of TSC. Other neurocutaneous markers of TSC, such as facial angiomas and shagreen patches develop with increasing age. Facial angiofibromas are papullar eruptions over the malar eminences and nasolabial folds. These may first become evident as a "malar flush" in preschool children and gradually evolve into the more recognizable papular appearance during preadolescence and adolescence. Connective tissue nevi over the flanks are known as shagreen patches; they may also be evident in preschool children and gradually increase in size during puberty

Tuberous sclerosis complex is a multisystem disease. The diagnosis rests upon identification of specific major and minor clinical criteria (see Table 20–32). Since some manifestations of the disorder become evident in later ages, continued surveillance for the possible development of renal disease (cysts and angiomyolipomas), as well as potentially progressive central nervous system tumors (subependymal giant cell astrocytoma), is required. The renal disease can lead to significant renal compromise with the development of renal failure, hypertension, or renal hemorrhage. A unique feature of TSC is the association with cardiac tumors known as rhabdomyomas. These tumors may be first identified prenatally by ultrasonography, and they usually gradually regress over time without intervention. Occasionally, they produce cardiac arrhythmia as well as outflow obstruction, requiring specific interventions.

Tuberous sclerosis complex is an autosomal dominant disorder with up to 60% of patients having a spontaneous mutation. Two gene loci located on chromosomes 9q and 16q have been identified, which produce the TSC. Diagnostic genetic testing, however, is not yet available, and diagnosis relies on identifying specific clinical features.

Sturge-Weber Syndrome

Sturge-Weber syndrome (encephalofacial angiomatosis) is a sporadic disease with some recognized familial cases

Table 20–33. Diagnostic Criteria
for Sturge-Weber Syndrome[1]

Facial port wine stain *or* glaucoma
and
Clinical or radiological evidence of a leptomeningeal angioma
• Hemiparesis
• Hemiatrophy (cerebrum or body)
• Convulsions
• Visual field deficit
• Mental retardation
• Computed tomography or magnetic resonance imaging evidence of leptomeningeal angioma

[1] Modified with permission from Bodensteiner JB, Roach ES: *Sturge-Weber Syndrome.* Mt Freedom Press, 1999.

and is characterized by vascular nevi (port wine stains) over the face (Table 20–33). The nevi are usually unilateral but can be bilateral in the distribution of the trigeminal nerve, extending variably from forehead over the maxilla and jaw. The importance of the port wine stain is its potential association with intracranial and intraocular vascular abnormalities. Glaucoma may occur in the ipsilateral eye in as many as 50% of patients. Additionally leptomeningeal angiomatosis may involve the ipsilateral hemisphere of the brain. The extent of the intracranial angiomatosis has been noted to correlate with the size of the facial stain. The further the port wine stain extends from the forehead inferiorly over the face, the greater is the extension of hemispheric involvement from the occiput anteriorly toward the frontal lobe. The affected hemisphere undergoes gradual atrophy with the development of subcortical laminar calcification. Patients may experience partial seizures due to cortical injury. The epilepsy may become intractable and require partial or total hemispherectomy to control or eliminate seizures. Laser ablation of the facial stain is also possible in selected patients for cosmetic purposes.

Von Hippel-Lindau Disease

Von Hippel-Lindau disease (VHL) is a rare autosomal dominant disorder caused by a gene abnormality on chromosome 3p25. Most patients present with progressive cerebellar signs due to the development of cystic hemangioblastomas in the cerebellum. Sudden retinal detachment and visual loss may occur as a result of hemorrhage from a retinal hemangioblastoma. The vascular tumors may occur in the brainstem and spinal cord producing symptoms referable to their location. Cysts may also develop in the pancreas, kidneys, and epididymis, and renal cell carcinoma and adrenal pheochromocytoma occur in adults. Patients with this disorder require routine surveillance with imaging of the abdomen and central nervous system through adulthood to detect the development of malignancy. Genetic testing is currently available, but only informative in approximately 70% of identified patients.

Ataxia-Telangiectasia

Ataxia-telangiectasia (Louis-Bar Syndrome) is an autosomal recessive neurocutaneous disorder; the clinical hallmark is the development of telangiectatic vessels over the bulbar sclera. Over time similar telangiectasias may appear over the face and the helices of the ear. The disorder is further characterized by progressive neurologic deterioration affecting the cerebellum and, ultimately, the spinal cord, and immunological disturbance. This disorder is further described in the section, "Gait Disturbances" and in Chap. 7, "Immunologic Disorders."

REFERENCES

Asbury AK, Cornblath DR: Assessment of current diagnostic criteria for the diagnosis of Guillain-Barré syndrome. Ann Neurol 1990;27(suppl):S21.

Bleck TP: Management approaches to prolonged seizures and status epilepticus. Epilepsia 1999;40(suppl 1):S59.

Bodensteiner JB, Roach ES: *Sturge-Weber Syndrome.* Mt Freedom Press, 1999.

Commission on Classification and Terminology of the International League Against Epilepsy: Proposal for Revised Classification of Epilepsies and Epileptic Syndromes. Epilepsia 1989;30:389.

DiMario FJ: Breath-holding spells in children. Curr Concepts Pediatr Nov–Dec, 1999.

Duffner PK, Cohen ME, et al: Survival in children with brain tumors: SEER Program, 1973–1980. Neurol 1986;36:597.

Dunn DW, Epstein LG: *Decision Making in Child Neurology.* B.C. Deckers Inc., 1987.

Fenichel GM: *Clinical Pediatric Neurology: A Signs and Symptoms Approach,* 3d ed. W.B. Saunders Co., 1999.

Holmes GL: *Diagnosis and Management of Seizures in Children.* W.B. Saunders Co., 1987.

Jennett B, Bond M: Assessment of outcome after severe brain damage. Lancet 1975;1:480.

Mattew NT: Serotonin 1D agonists and other agents in acute migraine. Neurol Clin North Am 1997;15(1):61.

NIH Consensus development conference: Neurofibromatosis: Conference statement. Arch Neurol 1988;45:575.

Pellock JM: New antiepileptic drugs in childhood epilepsy. Semin Pediatr Neurol 1997;4:1.

Raimondi AJ, Hirschauer J: Head injury in the infant and toddler. Coma Scoring and Outcome Scale. J Childs Brain 1984;11:12.

Roach ES, et. al: Consensus Statement: Diagnostic Criteria for Tuberous Sclerosis Complex. J Child Neurol 1998;13:624.

Rothner AD: Headaches in children and adolescents. Semin Pediatr Neurol 1995;2(2):102.

Swaiman KF, Ashwal S: *Pediatric Neurology, Principles & Practice,* 3d ed. Mosby, 1999.

Volpe JJ: *Neurology of the Newborn,* 3d ed. W.B. Saunders Co., 1995.

Ophthalmology

Ronald V. Keech, MD

The primary care health practitioner should be skilled in basic pediatric eye examination techniques and should be knowledgeable regarding the appropriate management of ocular disorders in children. Ocular abnormalities are common in the pediatric age group. Between 2 and 6% of the population is affected by amblyopia or strabismus. By the time they reach 16 years of age, approximately 20% of children have refractive errors that require correction. One in 1650 live births will have a congenital ocular anomaly, and 50% of these are major eye malformations resulting in severe visual impairment.

Early recognition of ocular abnormalities is important in order to provide appropriate treatment and prevent permanent visual impairment or other systemic problems. Amblyopia resulting from cataracts, strabismus, or refractive errors is less responsive to treatment as the visual system matures. Failure to detect the signs and symptoms of retinoblastoma can lead to blindness and, possibly, death. Finally, a normal visual system facilitates early childhood development, motor coordination, and academic achievement.

This chapter begins with a brief overview of visual system development and its clinical relevance. Basic examination techniques used for the assessment of specific ocular signs or symptoms and for routine screening evaluations are discussed. The clinical presentations, differential diagnoses, and management of important pediatric ocular disorders are subsequently reviewed.

VISUAL SYSTEM DEVELOPMENT

The ocular sensory and motor pathways are a dynamic biological system that develops from conception through the first decade of life. The eye is first recognized as an outgrowth of the forebrain around 21 days of gestation. The eye and orbit are formed from elements of the ectoderm, mesenchyme, and mesoderm. Although well differentiated at birth, significant postnatal development of the eye is necessary before the visual system can function optimally. The average length of the eye at birth is 17 mm or about 70% of the adult size. Approximately 50% of the total postnatal eye growth occur in the first year of life and 95% occur by 3 years of age.

Postnatal maturation of the visual system is well understood. The ocular motor system matures more rapidly than the sensory system. Slowed saccadic eye movements (rapid eye movements when changing fixation from one point to another), the lack of pursuit movement (following eye movements when fixating on a moving target), and variable eye alignment are normal findings in the newborn. By 6 months of age, however, all of these ocular motor parameters are similar to adult responses. Normal ocular alignment, stereoacuity, accommodation, and convergence movements are demonstrated in most infants between 3 and 6 months of age. In contrast, the sensory elements of the visual system from the retinal photoreceptors to the cortical neurons require several years to reach maturity. Full-term infants progress from about 20/400 visual acuity with almost no clinically apparent vision at birth to 20/200 and the ability to visually fixate briefly on an object by about 8 weeks of life. At 3 to 4 months of age, the average child has roughly 20/100 vision and is actively fixating on and following small moving objects with their eyes. Research suggests that children may reach the equivalent of 20/20 visual acuity between 6 and 24 months of age. Using standard clinical tests, however, it is common to find a normal eye to have a visual acuity of less than 20/20 in the first 5 years of life.

EXAMINATION TECHNIQUES

The optimal management of pediatric ocular disorders begins with an accurate and thorough examination of the visual system. While visual screening tools are often suggested as a substitute for all or part of an eye examination, no current screening technique has proved to be as accurate or as useful for children of all ages as traditional examination methods. In this section, basic eye examination techniques useful for visual screening as well as for the evaluation of specific visual disorders are described in detail. Practice of these skills coupled with exposure to pediatric visual abnormalities will help to provide a solid framework for the diagnosis and management of pediatric ocular disease.

A thorough assessment of the visual system includes an evaluation of visual acuity, eyelids and orbit, ocular motility, anterior segment of the eye (cornea, anterior chamber, iris, crystalline lens), and posterior segment of the eye (vitreous, retina, and optic disc) (Figure 21–1). Table 21–1 provides guidelines regarding the timing and content of routine ocular and vision screening in children using the basic examination techniques described in this section.

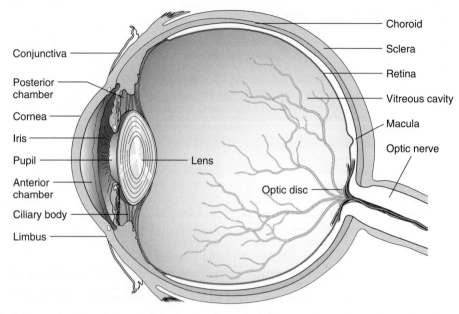

Conjunctiva
Posterior chamber
Cornea
Iris
Pupil
Anterior chamber
Ciliary body
Limbus
Lens
Choroid
Sclera
Retina
Vitreous cavity
Macula
Optic nerve
Optic disc

Figure 21–1. Anatomy of the human eye.

A useful approach for pediatric patients is to divide the examination into three parts (Table 21–2). Each part consists of several tests that are described in detail in Table 21–3. The first part consists chiefly of an assessment of visual acuity. In general, if a child is 3 years or older, an attempt should be made to determine visual acuity using optotype charts. If the child has not yet learned the alphabet, then charts with numbers, tumbling *E*, or with picture symbols can be used. This test should be performed relatively quickly in order to maintain the child's interest. Occluder patches placed over the untested eye provide the best assurance that the child is not peeking. Commercially available vision testing machines are accurate for assessing visual acuity in older children and may be used as an alternative to the standard optotype charts. If the child is too young to do optotype testing, an indirect estimate of the acuity can be made using binocular and monocular fixa-tion and following techniques while the child is fixating on a small toy. A young child with poor vision in one eye will often object to covering the normal-sighted eye or will display poor fixation and following movements of the abnormal eye.

The fixation and following test is also useful for assessing ocular motility. Ocular movements (ductions) are evaluated by moving the fixation target in the different gaze positions. The ocular alignment is assessed by performing an alternate cover test while fixation is maintained on a target. Any movement of the uncovered eye in order to pick up fixation during the test is strongly suggestive of strabismus (see "Strabismus" later).

The second part of the pediatric ocular examination consists of an evaluation of the eyelids and orbit, anterior segment, and pupils using a penlight. A careful inspection is important to detect abnormalities such as asym-

Table 21–1. Suggested Guidelines for Routine Eye and Vision Screening

Infancy	2–4 years	School age
Newborn and every well baby check: red reflex, external exam; by 6 months: include pupils, fixation preference, and corneal light reflex	At least one examination during this period to include optotype measurement of visual acuity, ocular motility, pupils, external exam, and direct ophthalmoscopy of the retina	During every routine physical examination ocular screening should include optotype measurement of visual acuity, ocular motility, pupils, external exam, and direct ophthalmoscopy of the retina

Table 21–2. Basic Pediatric Vision Examination

Part one (using a near-fixation target)	Part two (using a penlight)	Part three (using a direct ophthalmoscope)
Binocular fix and follow Monocular fix and follow Alternate cover test Add optotype visual acuity if 3 years or older	External examination Pupil light response Corneal light reflex	External examination Pupil light response Red reflex/retina

metry of the eyelids, proptosis, corneal cloudiness, or pupil anomalies. During this step, the corneal light reflex test should also be performed. Although it is not as accurate as an alternate cover test, the corneal light reflex test may be the only assessment of ocular alignment possible in a young child. Asymmetry of the light reflex will be found if there is a strabismus.

The last part of the examination is the assessment of the red reflex in a young child, or a detailed view of the ocular fundus in an older child with the direct ophthalmoscope. The red reflex is usually performed on one eye at a time. The absence of the red reflex suggests a media opacity. Another useful technique is to perform the test on both eyes simultaneously to compare the reflexes of both eyes. Asymmetric reflexes may be caused by a unilateral media opacity, an asymmetric refractive error, or strabismus. During this part of the examination the direct ophthalmoscope can also be used to provide a magnified view of the anterior segment of the eye and to assess the pupil responses.

Several other methods of screening for visual disorders in children have been considered as possible alternatives to a standard ocular examination, including protocols for visual acuity testing, stereoacuity testing, and photoscreening techniques. Photoscreening is the visual screening method currently undergoing the most research. It is based on the premise that most amblyopia-inducing conditions will result in an abnormality of the corneal light reflex or ocular red reflex that can be detected by a photograph. While photoscreening has been shown to be effective in some studies, there are a number of issues that require further research before it should be endorsed as a substitute for a standard ocular examination.

The indications for referring patients for a complete ophthalmological examination are listed in Table 21–3. They include abnormal visual fixation responses or a visual acuity below normal for the patient's age, abnormalities of ocular motility or ocular alignment, abnormal red reflex or retinal pathology on direct ophthalmoscopy, abnormal pupil responses, and abnormalities of the eyelids, orbit, or anterior segment. Other indications for a complete eye evaluation are a family history of a heritable ocular disorder, such as congenital cataracts or retinoblastoma; a suspected systemic disorder with ocular manifestations, such as neurofibromatosis or juvenile rheumatoid arthritis; suspected child abuse; and prematurity.

IMPORTANT PRESENTATIONS OF OCULAR DISORDERS IN CHILDREN

There are several important clinical manifestations of pediatric ocular disorders. The primary care health practitioner should be well versed in the diagnosis and management of the more common ocular clinical presentations such as a red eye or blurry vision. Other presentations, such as leukocoria (white pupil) or a cloudy cornea, occur less frequently but are important because of the increased risk of serious visual or systemic complications. This section covers the clinical presentations of the more common and serious ocular disorders of childhood and includes a discussion of the characteristics of each condition, the differential diagnosis, and basic management strategies.

Ocular Problems in the First Year of Life

Infantile ocular abnormalities constitute a unique group of disorders that rarely present in older children. Most of these conditions are closely associated with an embryological malformation, a problem during the birth process, or a disruption in the early postnatal visual development. Two other ocular entities that often present in infancy are visual impairment and strabismus. They are discussed in separate sections.

CONGENITAL OCULAR ANOMALIES

Congenital anomalies of the eye are uncommon but have a significant impact. More than 50% of congenital ocular anomalies detected in infancy result in permanent visual impairment. Approximately one third of childhood blindness in the United States is due to a congenital anomaly. The congenital ocular anomalies most likely to be encountered by the primary care physician include microphthalmos, persistent pupillary membrane, ocular coloboma, and congenital cataract. Congenital cataracts

Table 21–3. Pediatric Vision Tests

Optotype Visual Acuity	
Purpose:	Evaluate visual acuity
Technique:	Use an optotype chart appropriate for the child's age. Cover one eye and test one or two symbols on each line. After one line is missed, go to the next larger optotype and test the entire line. Matching optotypes on a distance chart with a near card is useful when the child is not verbal.
Referral indications:	If visual acuity is <20/40 by age 3 or <20/30 by age 5 years
Fixation and Following	
Purpose:	Evaluate visual acuity and ocular motility
Technique:	
Visual acuity	Hold a small toy (i.e., finger puppet) approximately 18 in. away and directly in front of the child. Move the target slowly about 6–8 in. off center from side to side and up and down. The younger the child, the slower the target should be moved. Test both eyes, then cover one eye at a time with your thumb and repeat.
Ocular motility	Evaluate the ocular alignment by alternately covering one eye, then the other while the child is fixating straight ahead on a toy.
Referral indications:	Poor fixation for age in one or both eyes, inability to move one or both eyes 30° from center horizontally or vertically, or any reproducible eye movement during alternate cover test.
External Examination and Pupil Assessment	
Purpose:	Evaluate eyelids, orbit, anterior segment of the eye, and pupil light reflex
Technique:	
Anterior segment	Use a penlight placed temporal to the visual axis. Magnifying loupes are helpful. A direct ophthalmoscope also works well and provides a magnified view.
Pupils	Obtain fixation on a distant target. Bring the light in temporal or inferior to the visual axis and test each pupil for a response. Follow with a swinging flash light test to assess for a relative afferent defect.
Referral indications:	Any abnormalities of the ocular adnexa, anterior segment, or pupil responses.
Corneal Light Reflex	
Purpose:	Evaluate for strabismus
Technique:	Have the child look directly at a penlight placed approximately 3 ft away in a dimly lit room. Identify the light reflex reflected from the cornea. Compare the location in relation to the pupil in each eye. The light reflex is usually very slightly nasal to the center of the pupil.
Referral indications:	Any asymmetric reflex
Red Reflex Test	
Purpose:	Evaluate anterior and posterior segment, refractive errors, and strabismus
Technique:	Perform in a dimly lit room using a direct ophthalmoscope with a halogen bulb. Set to a +1 or +2 lens power and perform at arm's length with the child fixating on the light. Test one eye using small aperture, then both eyes using the larger aperture. In the older child, direct ophthalmoscopy of the fundus should be performed.
Referral indications:	Any abnormality of one or both light reflexes, or any abnormality noted by direct ophthalmoscopy.

usually present as leukocoria and will be discussed in that section.

Microphthalmos is a general term describing a smaller than normal eye. One or both eyes may be affected. Microphthamic eyes are often visually impaired and have an increased risk of glaucoma, high hypermetropia (far-sightedness), and other ocular malformations. Numerous possible etiologies and associated conditions have been reported. Inheritance as a single gene mutation has been documented in autosomal dominant, autosomal recessive, and x-linked recessive forms. The most common infectious causes include congenital rubella and congenital varicella. Maternal exposure to alcohol and thalidomide during pregnancy are known causes of microphthalmos. A number of complex congenital disorders such as trisomy 22, ectodermal dysplasia, and CHARGE syndrome have also been associated with microphthalmos. Ocular anomalies most frequently associated with microphthalmos include ocular coloboma, cataract, or persistent hyperplasia of the primary vitreous (PHPV).

A horizontal corneal diameter of less than 9 mm in newborns or 11 mm in adults suggests the diagnosis of microphthalmos, although microcornea may rarely occur in a normal-sized eye. The diagnosis can be confirmed by measuring the anterior-to-posterior length of the eye with ocular ultrasonography. A diagnosis of microphthalmos requires a thorough ocular and systemic evaluation to rule out other associated disorders.

Persistent pupillary membrane results from a lack of regression of normal fetal iris structures. Between 12 and 24 weeks of gestation, a vascularized membrane is formed over the anterior surface of the iris and then becomes atrophic. Partial atrophy of the membrane may result in distortion of the iris and pupil, with iris strands crossing the pupil. Occasionally, there may be a lens opacity where the iris strands attach to the anterior lens surface. Most persistent pupillary membranes do not affect vision. On rare occasions, a significant refractive error due to lens-induced astigmatism or vision impairment from a lens opacity may occur. If a lens opacity is present, or if the pupil is distorted, the patient should be evaluated by an ophthalmologist.

Ocular coloboma is a segmental absence of ocular tissue, usually involving the iris, lens zonules, retina, optic nerve, or a combination of any of these structures (see Figure 21–1). Typical ocular colobomas are congenital anomalies caused by the incomplete closure of the ocular fetal fissure, which occurs along the inferior nasal quadrant of the eye. Iris colobomas are usually recognized at birth. Retinal and optic nerve colobomas are more difficult to detect. They may present clinically as an impairment of vision or a leukocoria in the involved eye. Ocular colobomas are commonly inherited as an autosomal-dominant trait with variable penetrance and expressivity. They are also associated with chromosomal anomalies such as trisomy 13 and other genetic conditions, such as Aicardi syndrome. Management should include a thorough ocular and systemic evaluation for other possible congenital anomalies.

NEONATAL CONJUNCTIVITIS

Conjunctivitis in infants less than 4 weeks of age is an important condition with potentially serious ocular and systemic consequences (see also the conjunctivitis section in Chap. 9, "Infectious Diseases"). Blindness may occur as a result of corneal opacification or as a corneal perforation with the development of endophthalmitis. Infection with herpes simplex virus can lead to devastating neurological impairment. Prompt recognition of the characteristics of neonatal conjunctivitis in association with laboratory confirmation is necessary in order to provide optimal management and resolution (Table 21–4). Standard diagnostic techniques include Gram and Giemsa stains, cultures for bacteria, *Chlamydia,* and herpes and antigen or DNA analysis for chlamydia and herpes.

The frequency of neonatal conjunctivitis varies from 0.14 to 18.9% depending on the population studied and the availability of newborn ocular prophylaxis. The incidence in the United States is relatively low. However, when prenatal care is lacking, the incidence of maternal infection and neonatal conjunctivitis rises. The use of prophylactic antimicrobial agents significantly decreases the occurrence of neonatal conjunctivitis and is either recom-

Table 21–4. Neonatal Conjunctivitis

Etiology	Onset After Birth	Clinical Characteristics	Laboratory Diagnosis and Management
Chemical	3–36 h	Mild injection, watery discharge	Observation
Bacterial	1–7 days	Variable injection and lid edema, purulent discharge; especially severe with *Neisseria* or *Pseudomonas*	Gram stain, Giemsa stain and cultures, treat mild cases with a broad spectrum topical antibiotic, severe cases, especially *Neisseria*, require the addition of systemic antibiotics
Chlamydial	5–14 days	Usually mild injection, but can be severe, watery to purulent discharge, pseudomembranes, chronic course, associated pneumonia	Giemsa stain, cultures, enzyme immunoassay, direct fluorescent antibody assay, treatment with oral erythromycin
Viral	1–14 days	Watery discharge, variable injection and lid edema, associated keratitis is common	Giemsa stain, cultures, antigen, or DNA assay, treatment with topical and systemic antivirals

mended or mandated in most states. Silver nitrate 1%, tetracycline ointment 1%, or erythromycin ointment 0.05% has all been shown to reduce the incidence of this condition.

The clinical presentation of neonatal conjunctivitis varies depending upon the severity and the type of infection. Diffuse unilateral or bilateral redness due to injection of the conjunctival vessels is the hallmark. Other common findings include edema of the conjunctiva and discharge. Less common but more serious findings include keratitis (inflammation of the cornea) and orbital cellulitis. The most important causes for neonatal conjunctivitis are chemical toxicity and infectious conjunctivitis due to *Chlamydia,* bacteria such as *Neisseria gonorrhea,* or viruses such as herpes simplex.

Chemical toxicity from silver nitrate is common. It usually presents as a mild injection of the conjunctiva with minimal discharge occurring within a few hours after instillation of the agent. If this diagnosis is suspected, a laboratory evaluation is not necessary unless there is an increase in the severity of the clinical signs, persistence of redness, or purulence. This condition improves on its own within 2 to 3 days and does not require specific treatment. Chemical conjunctivitis is less common than it was in the past with the increased use of erythromycin and tetracycline as a prophylactic antimicrobial agent.

Bacterial conjunctivitis in the newborn may be due to a variety of organisms. The time of onset after birth and the severity of the clinical signs depend upon the virulence of the organism. Gonococcus, *Pseudomonas,* or *Haemophilus* may present within a few days after birth as a hyperacute conjunctivitis characterized by severe redness, swelling of the conjunctiva and eyelids, and copious purulent drainage. Other bacteria may present several days after birth with mild redness and minimal discharge. Gram stain and cultures are essential for establishing the diagnosis. Topical antimicrobial agents, such as polymyxin B/trimethoprim or ofloxacin, are usually effective for most bacterial conjunctivitis. Suspected or proven gonoccocal conjunctivitis requires systemic therapy with penicillin. If a penicillinase-producing organism is suspected, a third-generation cephalosporin is recommended.

Chlamydia is the most frequent cause for infectious conjunctivitis in the newborn in industrialized countries. It is most common in young indigent mothers who receive inadequate prenatal care. About 30 to 40% of newborns of infected mothers develop conjunctivitis. The classic presentation for chlamydia conjunctivitis is an onset from 5 to 14 days after birth with gradually worsening signs and symptoms. Mild or moderate conjunctival erythema and edema and mucopurulent drainage are usually present. Occasionally, severe swelling and discharge may occur. If left untreated, chlamydia conjunctivitis runs a 6- to 12-week course and may result in mild scarring of the conjunctiva and cornea. Untreated or topically (rather than systemically) treated chlamydia conjunctivitis is frequently followed by an afebrile pneumonitis that usually presents between 2 and 20 months of age. Giemsa stains of conjunctival scrapings demonstrate intracytoplasmic inclusion bodies in the epithelial cells. Enzyme immunoassay or direct fluorescent antibody assays are useful in making this diagnosis. The recommended treatment is a 14-day course of oral erthryomycin.

Herpes simplex is the most important cause of viral conjunctivitis in the newborn. Neonatal herpes conjunctivitis is usually due to type 2 herpes simplex transmitted from an active infection in the birth canal. It presents in the first 2 weeks of life with moderate injection, edema, and nonpurulent discharge. Corneal clouding with dendritic or geographic corneal ulcers may occur. Vesicular lesions of the skin are sometimes present and may precede the eye involvement. The typical findings on Giemsa stain include lymphocytes, plasma cells, and multinucleated giant cells. The recommended treatment for infants with suspected or proven ocular herpes includes systemic and topical antiviral agents.

NASOLACRIMAL DUCT OBSTRUCTION (CONGENITAL DACRYOSTENOSIS)

Nasolacrimal duct obstruction or congenital dacryostenosis is the most common infantile ocular disorder, affecting 6 to 33% of all newborns. It is usually due to an incomplete opening of the distal end of the nasolacrimal duct as it enters the nasal cavity. In most cases it is self-limiting or responds to nonsurgical management. Congenital dacryostenosis is characterized by tearing and mucopurulent drainage. The periorbital skin may become excoriated due to the excessive moisture. The conjunctiva is usually not injected. Occasionally, the nasolacrimal duct may become swollen secondary to an acute infection (dacryocystitis) or to obstruction of the distal and proximal end of the duct (dacryocystocele). Although congenital nasolacrimal duct obstruction is a common cause of tearing in infants, other possible etiologies should always be considered. Irritation from a conjunctival or corneal foreign body results in tearing and light sensitivity. In this case, there is usually an acute onset of symptoms. Tearing is also one of the common signs of congenital glaucoma. Additional signs include light sensitivity and enlargement of the eye.

The treatment of congenital dacryostenosis depends upon the severity of the symptoms and the age of the patient. Since most cases resolve spontaneously, observation for the first few months of life is reasonable. A dacryocystocele or a breakdown of the eyelid skin may require earlier intervention. Excessive purulent drainage can be treated with a short course of topical antibiotics, although the infection will recur as long as the duct remains obstructed. Downward massage of the tissues over the duct (at the nasal corner of the eye) significantly improves the chances for eliminating the obstruction. Children over 6 months of age who remain obstructed despite massage are likely to benefit from referral to a pediatric ophthalmologist for nasolacrimal duct probing.

RETINOPATHY OF PREMATURITY

Retinopathy of prematurity (ROP) is a disorder of the retina characterized by incomplete vascularization, neovascularization, and fibrovascular proliferation, which may result in a retinal detachment and blindness. Formerly known as retrolental fibroplasia, ROP occurs almost exclusively in premature infants. The incidence and severity of the disorder is directly correlated with the immaturity of the newborn. Infants with a gestational age of less than 27 weeks or who weigh less than 750 g at birth have a 10 to 15% chance of developing severe disease. In the past, supplemental oxygen was thought to be a contributing factor to the development of ROP. Currently, the role of supplemental oxygen is not clear, with some studies even suggesting that insufficient oxygen may increase the severity of the disorder.

Retinopathy of prematurity is characterized by an acute phase that begins approximately 4 to 6 weeks after birth and lasts 4 to 6 months. Depending upon the severity of the acute phase, the retina and vitreous undergo a scarring phase that can vary from minimal pigment changes in the peripheral retina to a complete retinal detachment with total loss of vision. Acute ROP is classified into five different stages. The stage and the extent of peripheral retinal involvement determine the severity of the disease (Figure 21–2). Plus disease refers to dilation and tortuosity of the posterior pole blood vessels and is another important sign that is present in severe cases.

Rare hereditary retinovascular disorders such as familial exudative vitreoretinopathy and metabolic conditions such as protein C deficiency may cause retinal changes that can be confused with ROP. The diagnosis of ROP, however, is usually not difficult to establish when there is a history of extreme prematurity. Severe ROP with a total retinal detachment is included in the differential diagnosis of leukocoria.

Retinopathy of prematurity is initially managed by identifying and closely following infants at risk for the disorder. Screening guidelines, adapted from the 1997 recommendations of the American Academy of Pediatrics and the American Academy of Ophthalmology, are listed in Table 21–5. Infants with an incompletely vascularized retina or mild ROP require frequent follow-up examinations. If the ROP progresses to "threshold disease," cryotherapy or laser photocoagulation of the retina may be indicated. Infants with threshold ROP have a significantly greater chance for a good visual outcome with treatment.

Premature infants with or without ROP have an increased risk of developing other ocular disorders such as myopia, astigmatism, and strabismus compared with normal full-term infants. For this reason, all premature infants should undergo periodic ophthalmologic evaluation during the first few years of life.

CLOUDY CORNEA

A cloudy cornea in infants is an uncommon but serious vision-threatening ocular condition that may have important systemic implications. The differential diagnosis for a cloudy cornea in infancy includes infectious causes, congenital anomalies of the eye, congenital glaucoma, corneal dystrophies, systemic conditions with corneal manifestations, and birth trauma (Table 21–6).

Infectious keratitis in infants may be caused by a number of different organisms. Important infectious causes include syphilis, gonorrhea, rubella, and herpes. Corneal infections are almost always associated with significant conjunctival injection and edema.

Corneal cloudiness in one or both eyes is the most common presenting sign of *congenital glaucoma.* Congenital glaucoma is an uncommon ocular condition that is sometimes associated with other ocular or systemic disorders such as oculocerebrorenal syndrome or neurofibromatosis. It is due to the incomplete development of the normal channels that drain aqueous humor in the anterior chamber of the eye. Other common signs of congenital glaucoma include enlargement of the eye, light sensitivity, and poor visual acuity. Without early surgical intervention, blindness is the usual outcome.

Congenital ocular anomalies of the anterior segment of the eye may be characterized by a corneal opacity that is diffuse, focal, central, or peripheral. These anomalies usually occur in isolation, but have been described with a number of systemic syndromes including Axenfield-Rieger, congenital arthryogryposis, Warburg, and fetal alcohol.

Corneal cloudiness may occur with certain *metabolic disorders* such as mucopolysaccharidoses, mucolipidosis, and tyrosinemia. Typically, the newborn has a slight diffuse bilateral haze that progresses over months to years and results in marked visual impairment. Correction of the metabolic abnormality with bone marrow transplant may help to prevent progression of the corneal cloudiness in selected cases.

Birth trauma, usually with a forceps injury to one eye, can result in corneal clouding. Although the cloudiness generally improves within a few weeks after birth, the visual acuity may be permanently compromised. Finally, a rare cause for corneal clouding in infants is a hereditary *corneal dystrophy.* Both autosomal-dominant and autosomal-recessive inheritance patterns have been described.

Detection of corneal clouding in infants should prompt both a thorough ophthalmologic assessment and a systemic evaluation for congenital abnormalities and metabolic disorders. Prompt referral to an ophthalmologist is essential to determine the type of cornea pathology and to rule out other ocular abnormalities. The treatment of

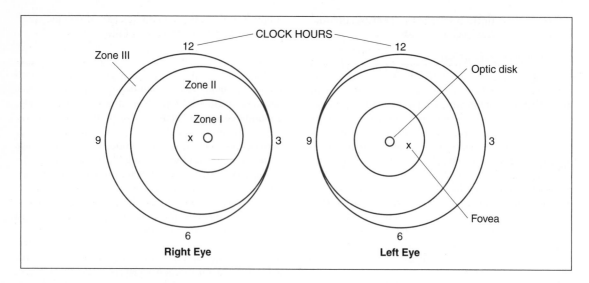

Location of disease

Described by a circle measured from the center of optic disk

> Zone I - Radius equal to twice the disc to fovea distance
>
> Zone II - Radius equal to disc to nasal ora serrata (peripheral edge of retina)
>
> Zone III - Circle encompasses all retina peripheral to Zone II

Stages of Acute ROP

> Stage 1 - Demarcation zone
>
> Stage 2 - Ridge
>
> Stage 3 - Ridge with extraretinal fibrovascular proliferation
>
> Stage 4 - Subtotal retinal detachment
>
> Stage 5 - Total retinal detachment (sub-classified according to shape)

Plus disease: Retinal vascular dilation and tortuosity in the posterior pole (often seen in severe disease)

Pre-threshold disease: Zone I disease with any stage; zone II disease with Stage 2 and plus disease, or Stage 3 without plus disease

Threshold disease: At least five contiguous or eight total clock hours of Stage 3 ROP involving zone I or II with plus disease

Figure 21–2. Description and classification of retinopathy of prematurity.

a cloudy cornea depends upon the cause. If glaucoma or a metabolic disorder is diagnosed, treatment of the underlying condition may improve the corneal opacification. If an underlying condition cannot be corrected, and the eye is otherwise relatively normal, then a corneal transplant may be indicated.

The Pediatric Red Eye

A pediatric red eye is the result of an inflammatory process involving the conjunctiva (Table 21–7). The inflammation may be caused by direct involvement with an infec-

tious, allergic, or toxic agent. In these cases, the clinical picture usually consists of an acute or subacute onset, moderate-to-severe ocular erythema and edema, and minimal pain. The conjunctiva may also become inflamed secondary to an intraocular, corneal, or ocular adnexal condition. The onset is often more insidious in these situations. The conjunctival injection is less severe and there may be significant pain, depending upon the etiology. Infectious causes of conjunctival inflammation are also discussed in Chap. 9, "Infectious Diseases."

The most common cause for a pediatric red eye is *viral conjunctivitis,* usually due to an adenovirus infection. Typ-

Table 21–5. Guidelines for the Evaluation of Infants at Risk for Retinopathy of Prematurity

One of the following criteria qualifies the patient for ROP screening
• Infants with a birth weight of ≤1500 g.
• Infants with an estimated gestational age at birth of ≤32 weeks.
• Infants who do not meet the first two criteria but are deemed at risk due to other medical conditions.
Method for determining the timing of the first ROP examination
• For infants born at ≤27 weeks gestation: The first eye examination is at 32 weeks postmenstrual age (gestation age at birth + chronological age).
• For infants born at >27 weeks gestation: The first eye examination is at five weeks chronological age.

ical findings include watery or mucoid discharge, conjunctival injection and edema involving both eyes asymmetrically or sequentially, preauricular lymphadenopathy, and upper respiratory infection. The condition is self-limiting and rarely requires treatment. Topical corticosteroids should be avoided. This condition is highly contagious for 7 to 10 days. Precautions, such as good hand washing and use of separate towels, should be undertaken to prevent spread of the infection.

Bacterial conjunctivitis is also common, particularly in the preschool-age group. The organisms most frequently implicated are *H. influenzae* and *Streptococcus Pneumo-*

Table 21–6. Cloudy Cornea in Infancy

Trauma
Corneal tear from forceps
Corneal perforation from aminocentesis
Congenital malformations
Anterior chamber cleavage syndromes
Peter anomaly
Sclerocornea
Congenital glaucoma
Corneal dystrophy
Posterior polymorphous dystrophy
Congenital hereditary endothelial dystrophy
Inborn errors of metabolism
Mucopolysaccharidoses types IH, IS
Mucolipidosis types I, III, IV
Tyrosinemia
Infectious/inflammatory
Rubella
Syphilis
Other bacteria
Herpes

niae. Bacterial conjunctivitis typically presents with a purulent discharge and no lymphadenopathy except in severe cases. On slit-lamp examination, the conjunctiva will have a papillary reaction in contrast to the follicular reaction found with viral infections. Cultures are usually not necessary except in severe cases or if improvement is not apparent within 48 to 72 h after instituting treatment. The condition is self-limiting, although it will resolve more rapidly with a broad-spectrum topical antibiotic such as polymyxinB/trimethaprim.

Acute infectious conjunctivitis due to *Chlamydia* has a more chronic onset than the previously mentioned bacterial infections, often resulting in moderate-to-severe ocular injection with lid swelling, mucopurulent discharge, and lymphadenopathy. One or both eyes may be involved. Conjunctival scrapings for cultures and immunofluorescent antibody testing will confirm the diagnosis in suspected cases. This condition is usually associated with a sexually active patient. With the possible exception of newborns, sexual abuse should be considered in all children with chlamydia conjunctivitis. A 14-day course of systemic erthryomycin is the treatment of choice for this infection.

Allergic conjunctivitis is characterized by an acute onset with more edema and less injection than is typically seen with an infectious conjunctivitis. The hallmark of an allergic conjunctivitis is itching. One or both eyes, often asymmetrically, are affected. Initial treatment consists of topical antihistamines, sometimes in conjunction with a mast-cell stabilizer. When allergic conjunctivitis is associated with other allergic symptoms (e.g., allergic rhinitis), a systemic antihistamine can be used. In severe cases, a short course of topical corticosteroids may be indicated.

A number of other ocular conditions can result in secondary inflammation of the conjunctiva and a red eye. *Corneal infection or injury* is almost always associated with ocular injection. In all red eyes, the cornea should be evaluated for focal opacities, abrasions, and foreign bodies. A common symptom in patients with acute corneal conditions, not usually found with an infectious conjunctivitis, is pain and photophobia . *Disorders of the ocular adnexa* are well-known causes for chronic ocular injection. Blepharitis (inflammation of the eyelid) can cause a toxic inflammatory response to the cornea or conjunctiva. Atopic dermatitis is frequently associated with ocular erythema. Chronic red eyes can also occur as a result of eyelid involvement with molluscum contagiosum.

Intraocular inflammatory conditions may manifest as a red eye. Uveitis (inflammation of the iris, ciliary body, or choroid) due to juvenile rheumatoid arthritis or sarcoidosis often presents with mild-to-moderate injection of the conjunctiva of one or both eyes. A red eye may also be the presenting sign of retinoblastoma. Finally, glaucoma is a rare cause for red eye in pediatric patients. Signs and symptoms that may be associated with intraocular causes of red

Table 21–7. The Pediatric Red Eye: Differential Diagnosis, Presentation, and Management

Disorder	Clinical Characteristics	Management
Blepharitis	Scaly lid debris, chronic mild conjunctival injection, hordeoli, chalazia	Lid hygiene, topical bacitracin or erythromycin ointment
Dacryostenosis	Epiphora, express purulent discharge with massage of the nasolacrimal sac	Massage, topical antibacterial, ophthalmology consult for nasolacrimal duct probing
Conjunctivitis[1]		
Toxic (i.e., UV light)	Acute onset, photophobia, watery discharge, history of exposure	Eliminate toxic agent, irrigation may be necessary, topical antibacterial, ocular lubricants
Allergic (i.e., hay fever)	Itching, watery or mucoid discharge, moderate conjunctival edema, minimal injection, history of antigen exposure	Cool compresses, topical antihistamines, systemic antihistamines
Viral		
Adenovirus	Watery discharge, preauricular lymphadenopathy, mild-to-severe injection	Cool compresses, topical antibacterial prn
Herpes	Watery discharge, history of herpes, lid lesions, corneal lesions	Tzank smear, Ag assays, culture, avoid corticosteroids, ophthalmology consult
Bacterial		
Acute (i.e., *Haemophilus influenzae*)	Mucopurulent discharge, moderate conjunctival injection and edema	Topical antibacterial
Hyperacute (i.e., gonoccocal)	Purulent discharge, marked conjunctival injection and edema, lid edema	Cultures, ophthalmology consult
Chronic	Present for more than 2 weeks	Ophthalmology consult
Chlamydial	Watery or mucoid discharge, moderate-to-severe edema and injection, more chronic course	Cultures, antigen or DNA assay, systemic erythromycin
Uveitis	Photophobia, irregular or miotic pupil, cloudy media	Ophthalmology consult
Keratitis	Pain, photophobia, corneal opacity or cloudy media, history of herpes, contact lens wear, or foreign body	Ophthalmology consult
Corneal abrasion	Pain, photophobia, tearing, history of trauma, corneal defect that stains with fluorescein	Topical antibacterial, pressure patch for large abrasions, daily examination until healed, ophthalmology consult if severe
Corneal or conjunctival foreign body (FB)	Pain, photophobia, tearing, presence of a foreign body	Rule out intraocular damage, remove FB with cotton applicator or irrigation, then treat as an abrasion, ophthalmology consult if severe
Ocular contusion	Eyelid edema, conjunctival hemorrhage, history of trauma	Rule out intraocular damage or orbital fracture, apply ice, head elevation, ophthalmology consult

[1] See also section on neonatal conjunctivitis.

eyes include decreased vision, photophobia, irregular or poorly responsive pupils, and an abnormal red reflex.

Leukocoria

Leukocoria, or a white pupil, is caused by ocular pathology at or behind the plane of the pupil, involving the lens, vitreous, retina, or optic nerve. Leukocoria is usually present for several months before it is recognized. Sometimes it is first noticed in a photograph. The abnormality is confirmed when obscuration of the red reflex is detected with the direct ophthalmoscope.

There are a number of ocular conditions that can present as leukocoria (Table 21–8). The most important of these is *retinoblastoma,* a malignancy of the retina. Retinoblastoma occurs in approximately 1 in 18,000 children and presents 90% of the time in the first 3 years of life, usually as leukocoria, strabismus, or red eye. Sixty percent of cases are sporadic, due to a somatic mutation in a single cell. The remaining 40% are germline mutations inherited in an autosomal-dominant fashion. In about 25% of the cases there is a family history of the disorder. Heritable retinoblastoma often involves both eyes with one or more tumors. Compared with the general population, patients with the heritable form of retinoblastoma have a much higher incidence of other malignancies during their lifetime. Approximately 3% of all retinoblastoma patients have a 13q14 chromosomal deletion.

A common cause for leukocoria is a *cataract* or an opacity of the crystalline lens. A cataract can present at any age and can affect one or both eyes. It may involve part of the lens or the entire lens. The location, size, and density of the lens opacity will determine if the cataract manifests as leukocoria. A pediatric cataract should raise other concerns besides the visual impairment. The possibility of an associated intraocular or systemic condition

Table 21–8. The Differential Diagnosis of Leukocoria

Cataract
Persistent hyperplasia of the primary vitreous
Retinopathy of prematurity
Vitreous hemorrhage
Uveitis (i.e., toxocariasis)
Retinal/optic nerve anomaly
Myelinated nerve fibers
Large optic nerve
Morning glory optic disc
Retinal or optic nerve coloboma
Retinal dysplasia
Persistent hyperplasia of the primary vitreous
Retinoblastoma
Retinal detachment

Table 21–9. Ocular and Systemic Conditions Associated with Pediatric Cataracts

Ocular Conditions
Microphthalmia
Persistent hyperplasia of the primary vitreous
Coloboma
Aniridia
Anterior segment dysgenesis
Systemic Conditions
Single gene disorder
Autosomal dominant
Autosomal recessive
X-linked recessive
Chromosomal anomalies
Trisomy 21
Trisomy 16–18
Trisomy 13
Prematurity
Intrauterine infections
Toxoplasmosis
Rubella
Cytomegalovirus
Herpes
Syphilis
Varicella
Metabolic disorders
Galactosemia
Lowe Syndrome
Neonatal hypoglycemia
Other syndromes
Hallerman Strief
Smith-Lemli-Opitz

should always be a consideration in the evaluation of a pediatric cataract (Table 21–9).

Retinopathy of prematurity, usually associated with a retinal detachment is another cause for leukocoria. Toxoplasmosis or other infections can present as leukocoria due to inflammatory lesions or scars of the retina or optic nerve. Retinal or optic nerve colobomas and other congenital anomalies may also present as leukocoria. Finally, trauma to the posterior segment of the eye such as a vitreous or retinal hemorrhage or retinal detachment may manifest as a leukocoria.

After the diagnosis of leukocoria is made, prompt referral to an ophthalmologist is crucial. Retinoblastoma tumors that present as leukocoria usually require removal of the affected eye, although newer treatments with adjunct chemotherapy and focal laser or cryotherapy have been employed. Cataracts, especially in young children, require prompt removal to prevent irreversible vision loss from amblyopia. If diagnosed early, a retinal detachment may be surgically repaired.

Learning Disorders

The visual system is often implicated as a cause or contributing factor to the development of dyslexia and other learning disorders. Normal reading and other academic achievements rely on vision. Word substitution, reversal of letters, and other apparent vision-related abnormalities are often manifestations of dyslexia. The link between abnormal ocular movements and reading difficulties is not well defined. Some vision "experts" promote treatments such as vision training or the use of color-tinted lenses as an effective approach for improving or curing learning disorders.

Despite this apparent association, the current scientific literature strongly suggests that learning disorders are not caused by visual system abnormalities but are due to perception and processing abnormalities in the brain. Slow reading speed and other ocular motor aberrations are thought to be a result of, rather than a cause for, learning disorders. Controlled studies have demonstrated no correlation between the treatment of any suspected visual system abnormality and an improvement in dyslexia.

Although visual system abnormalities are not the cause for learning disorders, there is a role for an ocular assessment of children with these problems. Ideally, all children with learning disorders should undergo a thorough ocular evaluation to rule out vision disorders that might contribute to difficulty with learning. This is particularly important if they demonstrate visual signs or symptoms such as holding reading material too closely near their eyes and complaining of poor visual acuity, double vision, or eye fatigue. Impaired sight from refractive errors or other more serious conditions may cause children to read more slowly, substitute words when they cannot see, and hold the reading material closer than normal. Although uncommon, convergence or accommodative disorders will make near visual tasks more difficult. Another important reason for the ocular examination is to reassure parents that the learning disorder is not due to a visual abnormality and does not require vision therapy. Once a vision problem is ruled out, optimal management should include an evaluation and treatment by a psychologist who has experience with learning disorders.

Ocular Trauma

Evaluation and management of ocular trauma in pediatric patients are especially challenging. Children are generally anxious and often in discomfort following eye trauma. The evaluation may also be difficult because of children's inability or unwillingness to provide an accurate history. Finally, with any pediatric eye injury, the possibility of child abuse should be considered.

The evaluation of children with a possible acute ocular or orbital injury requires a modification of the standard ocular examination. More patience is usually necessary. Decreasing the light intensity of the instruments often provides a better evaluation. If the extent of the injury cannot be determined due to a lack of cooperation, restraint or sedation and the use of an eyelid speculum may be required.

Every effort should be made to obtain the most accurate visual acuity possible. With few exceptions, normal vision is rarely found in the presence of a serious intraocular injury. Poor vision, in contrast, may be a result of poor cooperation or a minor injury that involves the visual axis such as a corneal abrasion. Ocular ductions should be assessed to rule out an orbital injury, especially if there is a history of blunt trauma and an orbital fracture is a consideration. An anterior segment evaluation will rule out an abrasion or laceration of the globe. Distortion of the pupil or an excessively deep anterior chamber suggests an occult posterior laceration. Assessment of the pupil reflexes and the red reflex, along with visual acuity, will help to rule out an injury to the posterior segment of the eye. If the injury is suspicious for a penetration or rupture of the globe, a metal eye shield should be applied and the patient referred to a specialist.

Conjunctival and corneal abrasions or foreign bodies are frequent occurrences in children. A slit-lamp examination is helpful in making the diagnosis. An evaluation of the cornea with a black light and fluorescein dye will usually confirm the diagnosis of an abrasion. Foreign bodies are often found on the cornea or under the upper eyelid. Eversion of the eyelid should always be performed. A foreign body can occasionally be removed with a cotton applicator. When necessary, a needle may be used to remove the foreign body under slit-lamp magnification. The treatment of an abrasion includes a topical antibiotic ointment with a daily examination to rule out infection until it has healed. Large abrasions may respond better with antibiotics and a firm eye patch changed daily.

Blunt injury to the orbital and globe is characterized by periorbital ecchymosis, lid swelling, and intraocular inflammation. Poor visual acuity, distortion of the pupil, or poor red reflex suggests a more serious injury such as a hyphema (blood in the anterior chamber), cataract, lens dislocation, rupture of the sclera, or a retinal detachment.

Trauma as a result of *child abuse* may cause any of the ocular injuries previously discussed. Approximately 40% of abused children will have ocular injuries with 95% of these occurring in children under 4 years of age. The most common ocular finding is retinal hemorrhages. These are usually bilateral and involve the posterior pole, although unilateral involvement has been described. When supported by the history and systemic findings, the presence of retinal hemorrhages in young children is highly suggested of child abuse.

In summary, the assessment and management of ocular trauma in children is challenging. Key findings that require immediate referral include hyphema, suspected penetrating ocular injury, scleral rupture, or suspected child abuse.

The Child with Suspected Vision Impairment

Suspected decrease in vision in one or both eyes in children is an important clinical presentation that includes a large differential diagnosis. Some of the more common causes for pediatric vision impairment include refractive errors, amblyopia, congenital ocular anomalies, and cerebral vision impairment. Because of its prominent role in many pediatric ocular disorders, amblyopia will be discussed in a separate section.

Pediatric patients with vision impairment typically present in one of two ways (Figure 21–3). The most common presentation is the preschool- or school-aged child with a mild bilateral or sometimes severe unilateral decrease in vision found during a vision screening or a routine physical examination. Occasionally, this is discovered by accident while covering one eye or when a parent compares their vision with their child's vision. Usually children have no symptoms, and there are no apparent signs. A frequent cause of mild-to-moderate vision impairment in older children is an uncorrected refractive error. The most common presentation is a decrease in vision for distant objects due to myopia or nearsightedness. In children less than 6 years of age, high refractive errors in one or both eyes may induce amblyopia, which will aggravate the visual impairment (see "Amblyopia" later). Other less common causes for vision impairment in older children include developmental cataracts, a progressive retinal dystrophy such as juvenile macular degeneration, and optic nerve conditions such as hereditary optic atrophy. Children with strabismus, afferent pupil defect, or visual acuity of less than 20/400 are more likely to have non-refractive, visual-impairing conditions.

The most important work-up in these cases is an assessment of vision, an evaluation of the visual axis to rule out any obstruction such as a cataract, and an assessment of the retina and optic nerve with the direct ophthalmoscope. A refractive error should be suspected if the visual acuity is better on a near optotype chart when compared with a chart placed at 20 ft (6.1 m) or if a pinhole device improves the vision. If the visual acuity cannot be measured, the presence of an afferent pupil defect or strabismus suggests the possibility of vision impairment.

A less common presentation for vision impairment is infants or very young children who are suspected of having little or no apparent vision in either eye. The parents usually note the children's inability to look directly at their face or to track objects. Nystagmus is another important finding in some cases of infantile vision impairment. Nystagmus is a rhythmic oscillation of the eyes. It is most often horizontal in direction, but can be vertical or rotary. Nystagmus associated with vision impairment in childhood usually has an onset between 2 and 3 months of age.

The possible causes for apparent vision impairment in infants and younger children can be divided into three groups. The first group includes children with neurological abnormalities that mimic vision impairment. Children with severe developmental delay or autism may demonstrate poor visual fixation behavior even with normal visual systems. Difficulty with ocular motor control due to cerebral palsy or congenital motor apraxia can result in slow fixation and following responses that mimic visual acuity impairment.

The second group includes children with vision impairment associated with nystagmus. Any disorder of the bilateral anterior visual pathways (cornea to the lateral geniculate body) that significantly affects the visual acuity in children less than 2 years of age almost always results in nystagmus. Some of the conditions included in this group are congenital cataracts, anterior segment anomalies of the eye, retinal degenerations or dystrophies such as congenital amaurosis of Leber (a dystrophy of the retinal photoreceptors), or anomalies of the optic nerve.

The third group consists of children with visual impairment without nystagmus. In this group the cause is almost always cortical visual impairment or delayed visual maturation. Cortical visual impairment is the result of an abnormality of the posterior visual pathways. Possible etiologies include hypoxia, hemorrhage, cerebral malformations, metabolic disorders, and infections. The visual acuity with cortical visual impairment often improves in the first few years of life; however, it never becomes normal.

Delayed visual maturation is a disorder of unknown etiology, possibly related to a delay in myelination of the visual pathways. The condition is often associated with other developmental deficits and visual disorders that make it difficult to diagnosis. Most children with delayed visual maturation demonstrate an improvement in vision responses between 4 and 10 months of age. If there are no other visual or systemic abnormalities, the visual prognosis is excellent.

The evaluation of infants and young children with suspected vision impairment differs from the examination of older children. Visual acuity is measured indirectly by children's ability to visually fixate on an object and follow its movement. Indirect signs of vision impairment such as strabismus, nystagmus, and abnormal pupil reflexes play a more important role. The red reflex test is crucial for determining the clarity of the visual axis.

All children with suspected visual impairment should be evaluated by an ophthalmologist. The cause for the vision impairment and any associated systemic condition must be determined. Many of the conditions can be improved or corrected with appropriate management.

Amblyopia

Amblyopia is a pathologic alteration of the visual system characterized by a reduction in visual acuity in one or both eyes with no clinically apparent organic abnormality that can completely account for the visual loss. It is

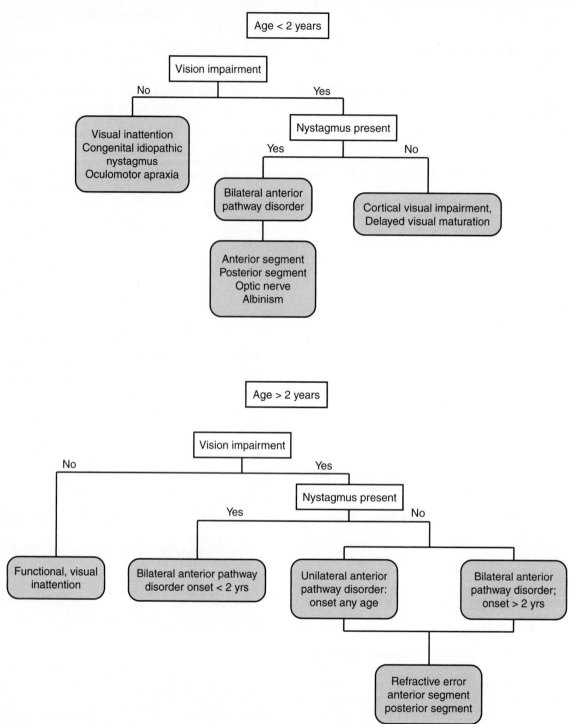

Figure 21–3. Evaluation of the child with suspected vision impairment.

due to a distortion of the normally clearly formed retinal image, an abnormal binocular interaction between the eyes with one eye competitively inhibiting the other eye, or a combination of both mechanisms. Amblyopia almost always has an onset before the age of 7 years. It is the most common cause of monocular vision impairment in the first 4 decades of life with a prevalence in the general population between 2 and 4%.

Amblyopia is most commonly classified according to the amblyopia-inducing condition with which it is associated. *Strabismus* (see "Strabismus" later) is the most common amblyopia-inducing condition. Approximately 40% of children with a manifest strabismus develop amblyopia. Esodeviations (inward eye deviations) are more frequently associated with amblyopia than are exodeviations (outward eye deviations), probably because most childhood exotropias are intermittent. *Refractive amblyopia* is due to a significant unilateral or bilateral refractive error. *Deprivational amblyopia* occurs from conditions that obstruct the visual axis, resulting in distortion of the visual image. The most common causes are cataracts and corneal opacities. In general, deprivational amblyopia results in more severe visual impairment than does amblyopia due to strabismus or refractive errors. *Organic amblyopia* refers to amblyopia superimposed upon an irreversible ocular abnormality that causes vision impairment. Retinal or optic nerve anomalies are the most common conditions accounting for this type of amblyopia. From a practical standpoint, it is important to note that many patients cannot be easily classified into one type of amblyopia since amblyopia-inducing conditions often coexist.

The treatment of amblyopia consists of techniques that provide the optimal visual image to the retina of the amblyopic eye and enhance the neural stimulus to the visual cortex. Surgical amelioration of visual axis impediments and correction of refractive errors are the most important methods for providing a clear retinal image. In most cases, the image to the visual cortex from the amblyopic eye is enhanced by limiting the stimulus to the nonamblyopic eye. This is achieved by patching the nonamblyopic eye or using an anticholinergic eye drop to impede accommodation. In general, the treatment of amblyopia is highly successful, but varies with the type of amblyopia, the age at onset of amblyopia, the age when treatment is initiated, and the consistency of the treatment. The older the child at the age of the onset of amblyopia and the shorter the time from the onset to the initiation of treatment, the better the prognosis.

Strabismus

Strabismus is a misalignment of one eye relative to the other eye in one or more positions of gaze. When strabismus is present in children, the most important concern is that it may be a sign of a more serious ocular or systemic disorder. Hurler, Gaucher, and fetal alcohol syndromes are a few of many systemic disorders known to be associated with strabismus. Any intracranial process affecting the third, fourth, or sixth cranial nerves almost always results in strabismus. Strabismus is also the second most common presenting sign of retinoblastoma.

Another concern when strabismus occurs is the possible loss of vision from amblyopia. Approximately 40% of children with strabismus will develop amblyopia. Early recognition and intervention can alleviate this problem in more than 90% of the cases. Those who receive treatment too late or are never treated will have permanent vision impairment.

Strabismus is commonly classified based on the characterics of the misalignment (i.e., direction of eye deviation) or the presumed etiology (i.e., sixth nerve palsy). Strabismus may be described as manifest or latent, and comitant or incomitant. A manifest strabismus is an ocular misalignment that occurs spontaneously and may be constant or intermittent. It is also known as a tropia. A latent strabismus, or a phoria, is an ocular misalignment that is apparent only when single binocular vision is disrupted, for example, with the alternate cover test. Strabismus is comitant if the misalignment is the same in all positions of gaze.

Esotropia is an inward or medial misalignment of one eye relative to the other. *Infantile esotropia,* also referred to as congenital esotropia, has an onset in the first 6 months of life. It is characterized by a large and constant misalignment. Other common findings include a limitation of abduction of one or both eyes, nystagmus, and incomitant vertical deviations. Glasses are usually not indicated for infantile esotropia. The recommended treatment is surgery. In general, the younger the age at surgical correction, the better the prognosis for long-term stability of the eye alignment and single binocular vision.

Acquired esotropia can be divided into accommodative and nonaccommodative types. Accommodative esotropia is associated with moderate or severe hyperopia (farsightedness). When children accommodate to overcome the hyperopia, the eyes converge. The typical onset is between 2 and 4 years of age, although accommodative esotropia has been diagnosed in infants. The degree of eye misalignment is generally less than that seen in infantile esotropia. It is often variable, depending upon how much accommodative effort children demonstrate at any given time. The treatment for accommodative esotropia is the correction of the hyperopia with glasses. The cause for acquired, nonaccommodative esotropia is unknown. Although rare, children with brainstem tumors or Arnold-Chiari malformation may have this type of misalignment. The condition can present at any age. The deviation is constant and small-to-moderate in degree. There is little or no farsightedness, and the esotropia does not respond to glasses. Strabismus surgery is usually necessary to correct the condition.

The most common cause for an incomitant esodeviation is a sixth nerve palsy or Duane syndrome. *Sixth nerve palsies* may be the result of central nervous system tumors, viral illness, trauma, or unknown causes. The typical manifestation of sixth nerve palsy is a limitation of abduction of the eye on the affected side. The evaluation includes a thorough history and physical examination and neuroimaging of the brainstem. *Duane syndrome* is a congenital strabismus condition due to abnormal ocular muscle innervation at the level of the brainstem. It is present at birth, although often not detected until children are older. The most common presentation is a small-to-moderate esodeviation of one eye with marked limitation of abduction and an abnormal turning of the head in the direction of the abduction deficit. Duane syndrome is commonly confused with sixth nerve palsy, although the two conditions are easily distinguished by an experienced examiner. Goldenhar syndrome and maternal thalidomide ingestion has been associated with Duane syndrome. In many cases of Duane syndrome, no treatment is necessary except to monitor for refractive errors and amblyopia. Surgery may be indicated when there is a significant ocular misalignment or abnormal head position.

Exotropia is an outward or lateral deviation of one eye relative to the other. Comitant childhood exodeviations usually appear as intermittent deviations with an onset between 2 and 5 years of age. Constant exodeviations are much less common in children. A constant exodeviation in infancy is frequently associated with a neurological disorder. Depending upon the characteristics of the misalignment, the treatment for exodeviations may include glasses, exercises, occlusion, or surgery.

Most *vertical strabismus* presents as an incomitant deviation due to a paresis or restriction of one or more extraocular muscles. The most common cause of vertical deviation is a paresis of the fourth cranial nerve. Acquired isolated fourth cranial nerve palsies are usually due to trauma. Patients often have an incomitant hypertropia that may improve by tilting the head, usually to the side opposite the palsied muscle. Management should include a thorough history and an evaluation of all the cranial nerves. Most symptomatic and stable fourth nerve palsies are best treated with strabismus surgery.

Blow-out fractures of the orbital floor can result in entrapment of the inferior rectus in the fracture site or, less commonly, an inferior rectus paresis. A history of blunt orbital trauma with a limitation of upgaze is a typical presentation of this condition. When a blow-out fracture is suspected, a thorough ocular examination is required because intraocular injuries are common. Surgical repair is usually required for large blow-out fractures or if patients have double vision.

Less frequent causes for a vertical misalignment of the eyes include Brown syndrome and monocular elevation deficiency. *Brown syndrome* is a congenital or sometimes acquired abnormality of the superior oblique tendon resulting in a restriction of elevation of the eye in adduction. *Monocular elevation deficiency* is a congenital oculomotor abnormality of unknown etiology characterized by a lack of supraduction of the one eye. Occasionally it is associated with a Marcus Gunn jaw winking reflex and ptosis. Surgery is usually recommended for both of these conditions if there is a significant ocular misalignment or abnormal head position.

REFERENCES

American Academy of Ophthalmology: *Amblyopia, Preferred Practice Pattern.* San Francisco, CA, American Academy of Ophthalmology, 1992.

American Academy of Ophthalmology: *Pediatric Eye Evaluations, Preferred Practice Pattern.* San Francisco, CA, American Academy of Ophthalmology, 1992.

American Academy of Pediatrics Policy Statement: *Learning Disabilities, Dyslexia, and Vision: A Subject Review* (RE 9825). 1998;102(5):1217.

American Academy of Pediatrics, American Association for Pediatric Ophthalmology and Strabismus, and American Academy of Ophthalmology Joint Policy Statement: *Screening Examination of Premature Infants for Retinopathy of Prematurity.* 1996.

American Academy of Pediatrics, Committee on Practice and Ambulatory Medicine and Section on Ophthalmology: Eye examination and vision screening in infants, children, and young adults. Pediatrics 1996;98:153.

Bateman JB: Microphthalmos. Intern Ophthalmol Clin 1984; 24(1):87.

Birch EE: Visual acuity testing in infants and young children. Ophthalmol Clin North Am 1989:369–389.

Cryotherapy for Retinopathy of Prematurity Cooperative Group: Multicenter trial of cryotherapy for retinopathy of prematurity: Snellen visual acuity and structural outcome at 5½ years after randomization. Archiv Ophthalmol 1996;114:417.

Gordon RA, Donzis PB: Refractive development of the human eye. Archiv Ophthalmol 1985;103:785.

Hoyt CS, Nickel BL, Billson FA: Ophthalmological examination of the infant. Surv Ophthalmol 1982;26:177.

Laga, et al: Prophylaxis of gonococcal and chlamydial ophthalmia neonatorum. New Engl J Med 1988;318:653.

Larsen JS: The sagittal growth of the eye. IV. Ultrasonic measurement of the axial length of the eye from birth to puberty. Acta Ophthalmologica 1971;49:873.

Levine AV: Ocular manifestations of child abuse. Ophthalmol Clin North Am 1990;3(2):249.

Ottar WL, Scott, WE, Holgado SI: Photoscreening for amblyogenic factors. J Pediatr Ophthalmol Strabis 1995;32:289.

Preslan MW, Novak A: Baltimore vision screening project. Ophthalmology 1996;103(1):105.

Smith BJ, O'Brien JM: The genetics of retinoblastoma and current diagnostic testing. J Pediatr Ophthalmol Strabis 1996;33:120.

Stoll C, Alembik Y, Dott B, Roth MP: Epidemiology of congenital eye malformations in 131,760 consecutive births. Ophthal Paediatr Genet 1992;12(3):179.

Orthopedic Problems in Children 22

John T. Smith, MD

INTRODUCTION

Orthopedic problems in children are common. Most problems present as an age-specific variation in normal development. These problems are usually straightforward but require a basic understanding of the growth and development of the musculoskeletal system to be managed properly. The ability to distinguish between age-specific variations of normal development and more serious problems provides optimal care for children and avoids unnecessary referrals and parental concern. This chapter will cover several common pediatric orthopedic problems that often present initially to the primary care provider. With the exception of sections on musculoskeletal trauma and sports medicine, conditions are grouped and presented in accordance with the typical age of their presentation.

ORTHOPEDIC PROBLEMS BY AGE

Orthopedic Problems in the First Year of Life

Many significant orthopedic deformities are apparent at birth. Severe malformations, limb deficiencies, and spina bifida are beyond the scope of this chapter. Deformities of the hips and feet are common and are discussed in the subsequent sections.

DEVELOPMENTAL DYSPLASIA OF THE HIP

Developmental dysplasia of the hip (DDH) represents a spectrum of hip problems ranging from mild positional instability of the newborn hip to frank dislocation of the femoral head from the acetabulum. About 1 in 100 children will have a dislocatable hip in the newborn nursery. The true incidence of hip dislocation in infants is about 1 in every 1000 births, implying that approximately 90% of positional instability resolves after the perinatal period. Several factors have been associated with the development of hip dysplasia (Table 22–1). Mechanical factors are suggested by the higher incidence of DDH observed in first-borns and in cases of breech presentation and oligohydramnios. Hormonal influences such as maternal estrogens and relaxins, genetic factors, and postnatal positioning may also contribute to the development of DDH in the perinatal period.

The diagnosis of DDH is made on physical examination and confirmed by ultrasound and radiographic stud-

ies. There are several clues to the early diagnosis of DDH in the nursery. Asymmetry of the skin folds of the thigh suggests a relative shortening of the leg because of the proximal dislocation of the femoral head out of the acetabulum. Similarly, the *Galiazzi test* (Figure 22–1) compares the level of the knees after the baby is carefully placed flat on the examination table with the hips and knees flexed. If one knee is higher than another, this may be indicative of a dislocated hip. In the *Ortolani maneuver* (Figure 22–2) reduction of a dislocated hip is detected by the sensation of a "clunk" when the hips are abducted with hips and knees flexed. The thighs should be able to abduct until they are flat against the examination table. The clunk represents the passive reduction of the femoral head back into the acetabulum. The Ortolani maneuver is usually combined with the *Barlow maneuver* (Figure 22–3), which attempts to dislocate an unstable hip from the acetabulum. Gentle but firm pressure directed posteriorly on the proximal medial thigh by the thumb while the hip is adducted elicits a clunk with subluxation or dislocation of the hip. With positional instability, the examiner can reproducibly move the hip in and out of the acetabulum with gentle pressure. It is important to note that the physical findings of DDH change with the age of the child. As an infant gets older, the dislocation may become fixed and the hip will no longer be reducible. After 3 to 4 months of age, the most reliable clinical finding in DDH is restricted abduction of the hip (Table 22–2).

Imaging studies are indicated when the diagnosis of DDH is suspected on physical examination. Prior to 3 months of age, hip ultrasound is the diagnostic study of choice. This is a dynamic test providing real-time information about acetabular development and the stability of the hip. The use of ultrasound requires an experienced radiologist for reliable interpretation. Because their femoral heads are made of cartilage, x-rays are of little diagnostic value in infants less that 3 months of age and have a 50% false-negative rate when used to rule out the diagnosis of DDH.

Once DDH is confirmed, treatment is dependent on the child's age at diagnosis. The goals of therapy are to obtain a concentric reduction of the hip into the acetabulum, maintain the reduction, and allow for normal growth stimulation of the acetabulum to correct associated acetabular dysplasia. Early diagnosis simplifies management and optimizes outcome. In infants less than 6 months of age, a

Table 22–1. Etiologic Factors Associated with Developmental Dysplasia of the Hip

Mechanical
Breech presentation
First-born
Oligohydramnios
Hormonal
Estrogens
Relaxin
Genetic
Environmental
Infant swaddling

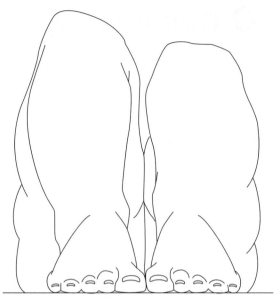

Figure 22–1. The Galiazzi test. (Reproduced with permission from Skinner SR: Orthopedic problems in childhood. In: Rudolph AM, et al (editors): *Rudolph's Pediatrics,* 20th ed. Appleton & Lange, 1996.)

dynamic splint called a Pavlic harness is used. This splint maintains, but does not rigidly fix, the hips in a flexed and abducted position. If reduction and/or stabilization cannot be achieved by using the Pavlic harness for a defined period (6 weeks or less), closed (nonoperative) reduction and spica casting are indicated. In children diagnosed between 6 months and 3 years of age, an attempt is made at closed reduction and spica casting, with or without a period of prereduction traction. If these efforts are unsuccessful, operative reduction is necessary.

FOOT PROBLEMS

Foot deformities are a source of considerable concern for parents and grandparents. Treatment myths abound but rarely have a scientific basis. Most problems are minor and have a favorable prognosis. However, some seemingly minor foot deformities may be the first sign of a more significant problem.

Evaluation of the foot begins with a thorough physical examination. When assessing a foot deformity, the ankle, hindfoot, and forefoot should be examined as sep-

arate entities. The position, alignment, and flexibility of each segment should be documented. By performing such a careful examination, the provider is generally able to identify and distinguish between the more common foot deformities. Radiographs may be necessary to establish the diagnosis. If so, these should always be obtained in a weight-bearing or simulated weight-bearing position. Several of the more common foot-deforming conditions identified during infancy are listed in Fig. 22–4 and described in the following sections.

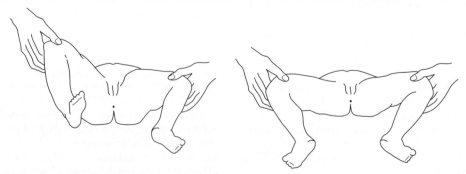

Figure 22–2. The Ortolani test. (See text for description.) (Reproduced with permission from Skinner SR: Orthopedic problems in childhood. In: Rudolph AM, et al (editors): *Rudolph's Pediatrics,* 20th ed. Appleton & Lange, 1996.)

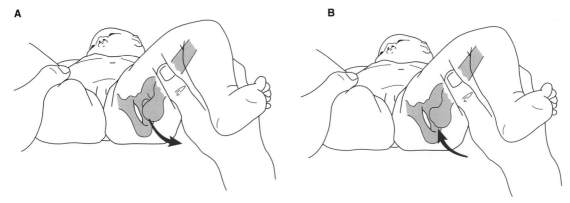

Figure 22–3. The Barlow maneuver. **A:** Gentle pressure by the thumb is first placed in the infant's groin in a posterior and lateral direction to dislocate the hip. **B:** The fingers then push the greater trochanter of the femur anteriorly and medially to return the femoral head to the acetabulum. (Reproduced with permission from Skinner SR: Orthopedic problems in childhood. I In: Rudolph AM, et al (editors): *Rudolph's Pediatrics*, 20th ed. Appleton & Lange, 1996.)

Clubfoot. The incidence of clubfeet in the general population is approximately 1.2 per 1000 live births. Increasingly, clubfeet are being diagnosed during prenatal ultrasound. A clubfoot is readily apparent at the time of birth and consists of three components, all of which must be present to make the diagnosis: extreme plantar flexion of the ankle (equinus), medial angulation of the hindfoot (varus), and adduction and supination of the forefoot (metatarsus adductus).

Clubfeet can generally be divided into three groups: Postural clubfeet result from intrauterine molding and correct rapidly after birth with stretching or serial casting. Congenital clubfeet are the most common form of this disorder and probably represent a true limb dysplasia. Congenital clubfeet rarely correct with casting and usually require surgical correction. Teratologic clubfeet are those associated with other problems, such as myelomeningocele or arthrogryposis, and also generally require surgery for correction.

Postural clubfeet may be treated with passive stretching exercises. For more severe deformities, therapy begins with the application of stretching casts, preferably in the newborn nursery. Serial casts are continued (changed at

1- to 2-week intervals) until either the foot is completely corrected or a plateau is reached. This plateau typically occurs at about 3 months of age. Clubfeet resistant to serial casting require surgery. This is best accomplished by a pediatric orthopedist when the child reaches the age of 4 to 6 months. The goals of surgical correction are to produce a flexible, plantagrade (fits flat on the floor) foot that functions normally and can utilize standard shoes.

Calcaneovalgus foot. A calcaneovalgus foot deformity is readily apparent at the time of birth. In this deformity, the dorsal surface of the foot is positioned up against the anterior surface of the tibia. This is felt to be the result of intrauterine molding. Although the initial appearance can be rather disturbing, the deformity is usually quite flexible and will generally respond to time and simple passive stretching exercises. Residual deformity is unusual.

Metatarsus adductus. Metatarsus adductus is a common disorder that results from intrauterine molding of the forefoot and is often noted shortly after birth. The forefoot is medially deviated causing the lateral border of the foot to be curved and giving the foot a kidney bean shape. Metatarsus adductus is often confused with a clubfoot but may be distinguished by the fact that the hindfoot is normal and there is no equinus at the ankle. Treatment consists of passive stretching exercises to counteract the curvature. Approximately 75% of cases of metatarsus adductus will correct spontaneously with stretching alone. If, however, the foot deformity is more rigid, serial casting may be necessary. A small percentage of children with metatarsus adductus will need surgical correction if the deformity has not corrected itself by 18 months of age.

Congenital vertical talus. Congenital vertical talus (CVT) is a rare deformity in which the talus is positioned

Table 22–2. Clinical Signs of Developmental Dysplasia of the Hip

	Age		
Test	**0–1 mo**	**1–3 mo**	**3–6 mo**
Ortolani (% +)	100	29	15
Limited abduction (% +)	7	67	86

Condition	Age at presentation	Appearance	Main feature	Treatment
Clubfeet	Birth	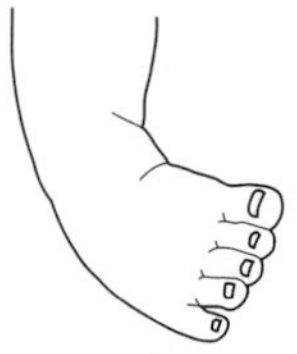	Fixed equinovarus	Serial casts; surgery in 80%
Calcaneovalgus feet	Birth	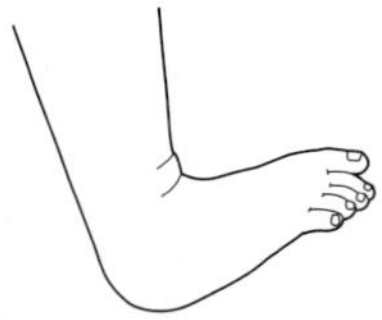	Dorsum of foot rests on shin	Reassurance, stretching
Metatarsus adductus	Birth	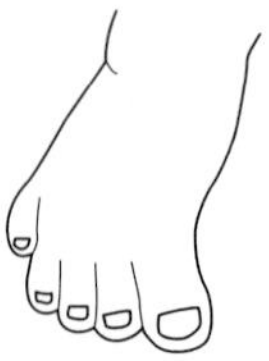	Forefoot adduction	Stretching, casting
Vertical talus	Birth	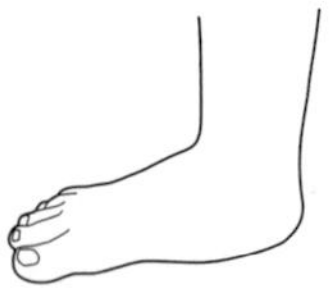	Rocker-bottom foot	Surgery

Figure 22–4. Common foot deformities in infancy.

in marked plantar flexion and the talonavicular joint is dislocated with the navicular positioned dorsally on the talus. The diagnosis is frequently delayed because CVT is often confused with a calcaneovalgus foot or a flexible flatfoot. It is distinguished by a rigid rocker-bottom deformity with equinus of the hindfoot, and dorsiflexion and abduction of the forefoot. The etiology of CVT is often neurologic in origin (e.g., spina bifida). A careful neurologic exam and often magnetic resonance imaging (MRI) of the spinal cord are indicated prior to initiating treatment. True CVT can only be corrected surgically: Stretching casts will improve the flexibility of the foot but are unable to restore the normal position of the talus in the ankle joint or reduce the talonavicular dislocation. Outcomes are optimal when treatment is completed prior to walking age.

CONGENITAL TORTICOLLIS

Congenital torticollis, or wryneck, is a unilateral contracture of the sternocleidomastoid muscle (SCM) that causes the infant's head to tilt toward the side with the shortened SCM with their chin pointed away. A smooth mass may also be palpated in the affected SCM, although this is often not apparent until 2 to 4 weeks of age. The precise etiology of congenital muscular torticollis is unknown, albeit intrauterine positioning and trauma to the SCM have both been implicated. There is a high association with developmental dysplasia of the hip (20%), and this should always be carefully investigated. Other causes of torticollis, or head tilt, though unusual in this age group, should also be considered, especially if the torticollis is severe, atypical, or associated with other physical findings. Radiographs of the neck will detect abnormalities of the cervical spine that can cause torticollis, but these abnormalities are rare.

Treatment for congenital torticollis begins with passive stretching. In 90% of patients, torticollis resolves with exercises aimed at stretching the SCM and strengthening the neck muscles. Although most congenital torticollis resolves without sequellae, plagiocephaly and facial asymmetry can result. Surgery may be necessary for those failing conservative treatment.

Orthopedic Problems in Toddlers

Variations in normal limb development as well as abnormalities become more apparent when the child is upright and walking. Common concerns at this time include torsional and angular deformities (intoeing and out-toeing; knock knees, and bowed legs) and flatfeet. These "deformities" usually represent variations of normal lower extremity development in children and have a favorable natural history. Toddlers are also prone to a variety of musculoskeletal injuries. Nursemaid's elbow is a particularly common injury in this age group and is discussed later. Pediatric fractures are covered in the subsequent section on musculoskeletal trauma.

Intoeing

Intoeing is defined as the turning in of the feet toward the midline during walking. A normal foot-progression angle (the position of the foot relative to the line of gait) ranges from 10° inward to 25° outward. The most common causes of intoeing in children are listed in Figure 22–5. Intoeing may result from factors at three anatomic locations: the femur, the tibia, and the foot. These can be easily differentiated by physical examination (Figure 22–6). An evaluation of intoeing should begin with observation of the child's gait. The child may then be placed in the prone position with hips extended, knees bent 90°, and the soles of the feet parallel to the examining table. In this position, internal and external rotation of the hips, the thigh foot axes, and the contour of the feet may be evaluated. Excessive internal rotation of the hip (normal 0 to 70°) is indicative of inward femoral torsion (anteversion of the femoral neck). An inturned thigh foot axis is characteristic of internal tibial torsion. With metatarsus adductus, the normally straight lateral border of the foot is curved and the line bisecting the heel intersects with the fourth or fifth toe (normally this occurs with the second).

Cause	Appearance	Age	Examination	Treatment
Metatarsus adductus	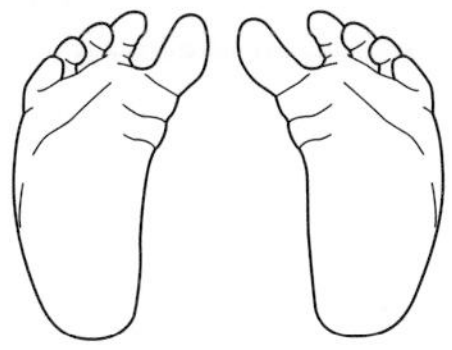	0–2 years	Curved lateral border of foot Heel bisector 4th–5th toe Flexibile versus rigid?	Flexible: stretch Rigid: cast
Inward tibial torsion	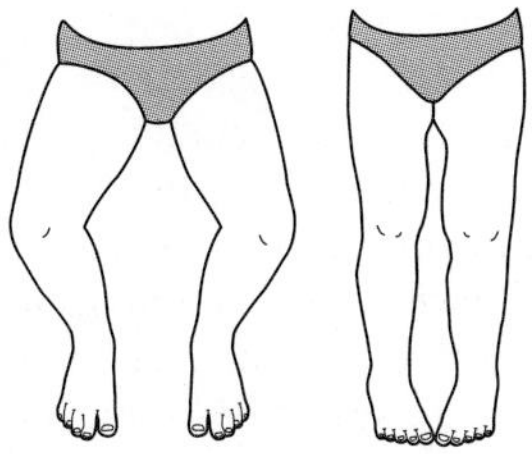	1–3 years	Inward thigh-foot angle Neutral transmalleolar axis	None
Inward femoral torsion	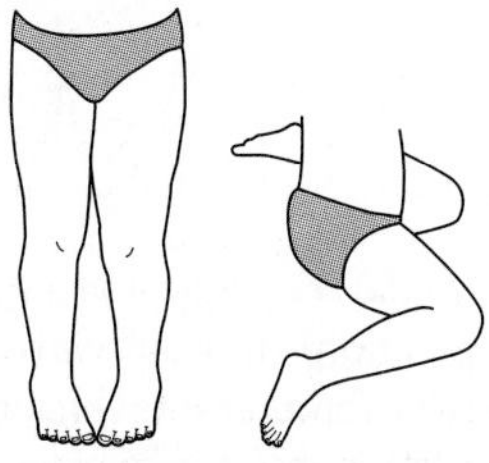	> 3 years	Increased inward hip rotation (prone)	None Surgery (rare)

Figure 22–5. Intoeing and its causes.

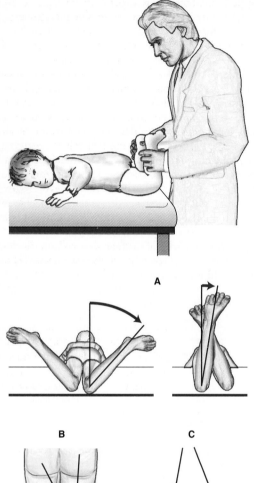

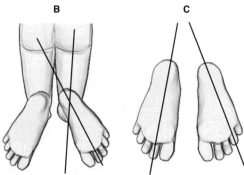

Metatarsus adductus is a common cause of intoeing in infants and young toddlers. The appearance of intoeing may be accentuated when this condition is associated with dynamic hallux varus of the first toe, also known as a searching or "monkey" toe. As previously discussed, most metatarsus adductus will correct spontaneously and is not associated with functional impairment (see "Orthopedic Problems of Infancy").

Internal tibial torsion is characterized by an excessive inward twisting of the tibiofibular unit and is the most common cause of intoeing in children younger than 3 years of age. It is thought to be a variation of normal limb development and may be exacerbated by intrauterine positioning. Internal tibial torsion corrects spontaneously with growth: Torsional bracing, despite its popularity, is rarely indicated and has never been proved efficacious.

Inward femoral torsion, or *excessive femoral anteversion,* is the most common cause of intoeing after 3 years of age. It is caused by increased anteversion of the femoral neck relative to the knee. The child may sit in a characteristic "reverse tailor" or "W" position (Figure 22–7). Although sitting and sleeping habits are often implicated, they are probably not etiologic. Inward femoral torsion generally corrects with growth by 10 years of age. Bracing has not been demonstrated to be of any benefit and is not indicated. About 1% of children require surgical correction for residual cosmetic or functional problems.

Figure 22–6. Examination of hip rotation, thigh-foot angle, and foot shape. **A:** Measurement of hip rotation: Thighs are rotated maintaining the pelvis level. Figure on left demonstrates internal rotation of hip. Figure on right demonstrates external rotation of hip. **B:** The thigh-foot angle is estimated by observing the foot and thigh from directly above. **C:** The lateral edge of the foot is normally straight with the heel bisector crossing the second toe. Metatarsus adductus is present in the foot on the right. (Modified and reproduced with permission from Staheli LT: Torsional deformity. Pediatr Clin North Am 1986;33:1373.)

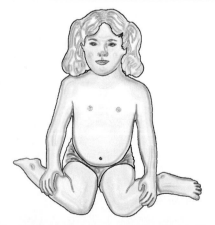

Figure 22–7. Typical sitting posture ("reverse tailor" or "W" position) of a girl with inward femoral torsion or excessive femoral anteversion. (Reproduced with permission from Staheli LT: Torsional deformity. Pediatr Clin NA 1986;33:1373.)

OUT-TOEING

Out-toeing is rarely a functional problem. Causes include outward rotation contracture of the hip (as commonly seen in infants), torsional variations in femoral and tibial development, and flexible flatfeet. Excess external hip rotation due to intrauterine positioning is a common cause of apparent out-toeing in infants and corrects spontaneously over time as ligaments loosen and mobility increases (Figure 22–8). Toddlers learning to walk often have a wide-based gait for stability, which looks like out-toeing. With initial efforts at weight bearing, flexible flatfeet have a tendency to pronate (weight is born on the inner border of the foot), which makes the foot turn outward. This improves as walking and strength develop. Out-toeing rarely requires treatment, and parents should be assured that spontaneous correction is the rule.

BOWLEGS (GENU VARUM)

Bowlegs and knock knees usually represent normal variations in limb development in children. At birth, the lower limbs are normally bowed. This becomes more apparent when the child begins to stand, but is often interpreted by parents as "getting worse." The range of normal physiologic bowing in toddlers is highly variable, but most show improvement by 2½ years of age. It is important to exclude pathologic causes of bowing such as rickets, Blount disease, and skeletal dysplasias. An orthopedic referral should be made if bowing is excessive or asym-

metrical, if findings are atypical for physiologic genu varum, and/or if the deformities persist beyond the normal age of resolution for physiologic bowing. In the absence of other referral criteria, an orthopedic consultation is indicated if bowing has not resolved by 3 years of age.

Blount disease, or tibia vara, is the most common cause of pathologic bowlegs in children and is characterized by a significant progressive bowing of the proximal tibia. Although the precise etiology is unknown, asymmetrical distribution of mechanical forces, exacerbated by such factors as early weight-bearing and obesity, may contribute to uneven growth of the medial tibial physis leading to the progressive bowing. In the infantile form (onset before 5 years), deformities are usually bilateral and associated with significant internal tibial torsion. Angulation occurs just below the knee and is generally more abrupt than the gentle curvature observed with physiologic genu vara. Radiographic studies assist in the diagnosis, although characteristic findings are not usually present before 2 years of age. Treatment of infantile tibia vara consists of bracing and, for more severe and/or progressive forms, surgical correction.

KNOCK KNEES (GENU VALGUM)

Between the ages of 3 and 5 years, most children develop some degree of genu valgum (knock knees) that corrects by 7 years of age. Genu valgum that is severe, asymmetrical, associated with other abnormalities, and/or has not

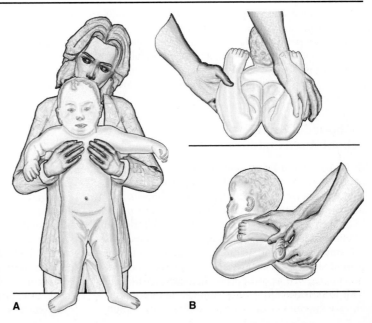

Figure 22–8. Excess external hip rotation due to intrauterine positioning. (Reproduced with permission from Staheli LT: Torsional deformity. Pediatr Clin North Am 1986;33:1373.)

A　　　　　　　**B**

resolved by age 7 years of age warrants referral to an orthopedist.

FLAT FEET (PES PLANUS)

Flatfeet occur when there is loss of the longitudinal arch of the foot. Most flatfeet are flexible and may be associated with generalized ligamentous laxity. This must be distinguished from a rigid flatfoot, which may be associated with neurologic disorders, congenital fusion of the tarsal bones, trauma, infection, tumors, and other problems.

Flexible flatfeet become especially apparent when children begin walking. With initial efforts at weight bearing, the feet tend to pronate so that the child stands on the inner borders of the feet. Parents will often say that it looks as if the child is "walking on their ankles." Time and growth will usually improve this appearance. Most children with flexible flatfeet can wear normal shoes and rarely have problems such as pain, excessive shoe wear, or functional difficulties. The use of arch supports, "orthopedic" shoes, and other treatment modalities to attempt to recreate a "normal" arch have no scientific basis. If a child has problems with excessive shoe wear and positioning problems, orthotics may be appropriate.

NURSEMAID'S ELBOW

Nursemaid's elbow is a common injury that is seen in the toddler age group. The usual mechanism of injury is forced hyperextension and supination of the forearm producing subluxation of the annular ligament around the radial neck at the elbow. This typically occurs when the child stumbles while holding onto an adult's hand or is playfully swung about by the hands. Children with subluxation of the annular ligament typically stop using their arm and avoid motion because of pain. Radiographs of the injury usually are normal. Nursemaid's elbow is easily reduced by rapidly taking the elbow through a full flexion, with pronation and supination of the wrist, and then into full extension. A palpable or audible "pop" may be felt, followed shortly by relief of pain, full range of motion, and return of normal function.

Orthopedic Problems in School-Aged Children

By 3 to 4 years of age, most children have developed an adult pattern of walking, and developmental variations related to growth have usually resolved. Orthopedic problems in this age group generally present with pain or limp. Such complaints in an otherwise active child demand careful evaluation, including a thorough history, physical examination, and selected laboratory and radiographic studies, as they may be indicative of a variety of systemic as well as orthopedic disorders. In the child with lower extremity pain or limp, it is important to observe the child's gait with both walking and running.

Joint range of motion and leg length measurements should also be obtained, paying particular attention to any asymmetric findings. Finally, it should be remembered that referred pain is common in children (e.g., a hip problem presenting as pain in the thigh or knee), and that the source of the problem may not always correspond to the location of pain. A more detailed approach to the child with musculoskeletal complaints is presented in Chap. 8, "Rheumatic Diseases." Common orthopedic conditions affecting school-aged children are discussed in the following sections.

LEGG-CALVÉ-PERTHES DISEASE

Legg-Calvé-Perthes (LCP) disease is an idiopathic process in which the capital femoral epiphysis becomes avascular, is resorbed, and then is revascularized. The etiology of LCP is uncertain, but hormonal, genetic, infectious, and traumatic factors may be involved. This disease is more common in boys, aged 4 to 10 years, who are short in stature and have delayed skeletal maturation.

Legg-Calvé-Perthes disease typically presents with a limp of insidious onset and associated pain in the groin and knee areas. Examination suggests an irritable hip with restricted range of movement, especially with abduction and inward rotation. This may be most apparent when hip rotation is assessed with the child in the prone position. These symptoms and findings are caused by an inflammatory synovitis of the hip associated with the resorption and revascularization of the healing femoral epiphysis. The diagnosis is confirmed with plain radiographs of the pelvis. Bone scans and MRI may be helpful for early diagnosis but are usually unnecessary.

Treatment takes advantage of the fact that, during the resorption and revascularization phase of LCP, the femoral head demonstrates "biologic plasticity" and responds to the forces placed on it. Therefore, the principle of treatment is to maintain containment of the femoral head in the acetabulum during the healing and remodeling process. This is achieved by either abduction bracing or surgery. Revascularization and healing of the femoral head usually takes 18 to 36 months. The prognosis is dependent on the age at onset, extent of femoral head involvement, and the stage of healing at the time treatment is initiated.

LEG LENGTH INEQUALITY

Leg length discrepancies may be caused by many different etiologies (Table 22–3). In infants, limb length is assessed in the supine position. Differences will be noted in the height of the knees when the hips are flexed (Galiazzi sign; see Figure 22–1) or when the legs are fully extended. In older children, limb length is best assessed in the standing position. Blocks used to visually level the pelvis provide very accurate measurements. Manual leg length measurements using a tape measure can be misleading. Flexion contractures around the hip or knees and abduction con-

Table 22–3. Causes of Limb-Length Inequality

Developmental dislocation of the hip

Abduction contracture of the hip

Congenital limb deficiencies
Proximal focal femoral deficiency
Congenital short femur
Tibial hypoplasia
Hemi-hypertrophy
Klippel-Trenaunay-Weber syndrome
Neurofibromatosis
Multiple hereditary osteochondromatosis

Acquired causes
Infection
Inflammatory conditions
Trauma

tractures around the hip can result in significant measurement inaccuracies. When suspected, limb length inequality can be confirmed by obtaining a standing radiograph of the lower extremities using a single long film. This provides both an estimate of the degree of difference in length as well as information regarding potential etiology.

The treatment and prognosis for limb length inequality depend on the etiology, severity, and the amount of growth potential that remains at the time of diagnosis. Treatment strategies are based on the projected limb length difference at skeletal maturity. Most adults will tolerate 2 cm of limb length difference without untoward effect. Minor differences can be treated with a shoe insert. When leg length differences are projected to exceed 2 cm at maturity, growth of the longer limb can be slowed to allow the shorter limb to catch up. Alternatively, the longer limb can be shortened at maturity. Extreme limb length differences (>5 cm) may require limb lengthening or prosthetic fitting.

Orthopedic Problems in Adolescents

A number of orthopedic conditions typically present during adolescence: Hormonal changes associated with puberty, rapid growth, and high physical demands all contribute to the appearance of these disorders at this time.

SLIPPED CAPITAL FEMORAL EPIPHYSIS

Slipped capital femoral epiphysis (SCFE) is a disorder in which the capital femoral epiphysis slips off the metaphysis through the growth plate (physis) producing deformity of the proximal femur. This disorder typically affects obese adolescents (girls age 10 to 12 years, boys age 12 to 14 years) during the adolescent growth spurt. The etiology is uncertain although mechanical and hormonal factors have been implicated.

Most children have an insidious onset of limping and pain that may suddenly increase in severity. The pain may localize to the knee, thigh, or groin, and the clinician can miss or delay this diagnosis if attention is focused only on the area presenting with pain. On examination, flexion of the hip reproduces symptoms and causes marked outward rotation of the hip. The diagnosis of SCFE is confirmed by obtaining anteroposterior and frog lateral radiographs of the pelvis. Early radiographic signs of SCFE, including widening and irregularity of the physis, a metaphyseal blanche, and/or varus position of the epiphysis relative to the metaphysis, may be subtle. As the slippage becomes more severe, the deformity becomes more obvious. In chronic SCFE, remodeling of the femoral neck becomes apparent.

Once recognized, SCFE requires immediate surgical treatment to prevent further slippage of the femoral epiphysis. Fusion of the capital femoral growth plate is accomplished through the percutaneous insertion of one or two cannulated screws. Early recognition and treatment are important to optimizing outcome.

OSTEOCHONDROSES

The osteochondroses are a group of growth-related conditions that typically occur in the adolescent age group. The etiology of these disorders remains uncertain. However, symptoms typically localize to areas where major ligaments insert into a growth plate (apophysis) under tension. Common locations include the knee (Osgood-Schlatter disease) and the heel (Sever disease). Symptoms vary with activity level and usually resolve by the end of the adolescent growth period.

Osgood-Schlatter disease is characterized by pain and swelling over the apophysis of the insertion of the patellar ligament at the tibial tubercle on the proximal tibia. It is most commonly seen in physically active boys, presenting with activity-related pain over the anterior knee and tibial tubercle. It is often bilateral. On examination there is obvious swelling over the tibial tubercle, which is painful to palpation. Radiographs show fragmentation of the tibial tubercle and soft-tissue swelling. Treatment consists of rest, activity restriction, and anti-inflammatory medications. The symptoms resolve at the completion of growth, however, some patients are left with a prominent tibial tubercle making kneeling painful as adults.

Sever disease presents as activity-related heel pain in adolescents. Palpation of the heel (calcaneal apophysis) is painful. Radiographs may demonstrate increased radiodensity and fragmentation of the calcaneal apophysis. Treatment is directed at controlling symptoms through the modification of activity and the use of proper shoes, heel lifts, and heel cups. Occasionally, casting, as a means of enforced rest, may be helpful. Sever disease resolves at the completion of growth with no significant long-term consequences.

BACK PROBLEMS

Scoliosis. Scoliosis is an asymmetry of the spine that causes both a lateral deviation (curvature in the frontal plane) and rotational abnormality (rib-cage asymmetry or rib hump on forward-bending test). It may occur at any point along the spine but is most often seen in the thoracolumbar region. Although scoliosis can be diagnosed at any age, idiopathic forms are usually detected in adolescence and late childhood during routine physical examinations and pre-sports participation screening programs. A previously insignificant curve may become more apparent during the adolescent growth spurt. Components of screening for scoliosis include observation of the exposed back in the standing position, the forward-bending test, and measurement of limb length in the standing position. The child must be undressed for optimal examination. Observation of the back allows identification of an obvious lateral curvature and signs of asymmetry in the levels of the shoulders, scapulae, and hips. The forward-bending test is performed by having the patient bend forward at the waist 90° with hands joined in the midline and allows the examiner to identify asymmetry of the ribs and spinous processes (Figure 22–9). Standing limb lengths should also be measured because discrepancies can cause a spinal curvature. Scoliosis that resolves in the sitting position may also indicate a leg length inequality. Radiographs should be obtained if a spinal curvature is detected. An upright posteroanterior view of the spine on a single film is the best initial study. Spinal curvature is

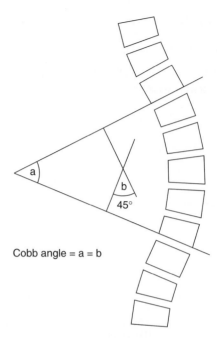

Figure 22–10. The Cobb method for measuring scoliosis.

then measured using the Cobb method (Figure 22–10). Special imaging studies such as MRI and bone scan are required only when a neurologic etiology is suspected or the curvature is painful.

Scoliosis is a physical finding, not a diagnosis. Its etiology is varied, and a specific cause must be sought before treatment is initiated (Table 22–4). A complete history, developmental assessment, and physical examination should be obtained. Idiopathic scoliosis is usually painless; a history of back pain should suggest another etiology. Because scoliosis can be the result of lesions and abnormalities in the spinal cord, a history of changes in bowel or bladder function, lower extremity spasticity, or other neuromuscular changes should be sought. Cutaneous abnormalities, such as dimpling or tufts of hair over the spine, may indicate underlying abnormalities of the spinal cord (spinal dysraphism). A careful neurologic examination may reveal weakness or altered reflexes, which may be indicative of a neuromuscular etiology.

Scoliosis is classified according to etiology, which greatly influences the treatment, natural history, and prognosis (see Table 22–4). *Idiopathic scoliosis* is the most common form of scoliosis in North America. It occurs primarily during the adolescent growth spurt and is much more common in females. Idiopathic scoliosis is a diagnosis of exclusion and other causes should be ruled out prior to initiating treatment. Most idiopathic curves are pain-

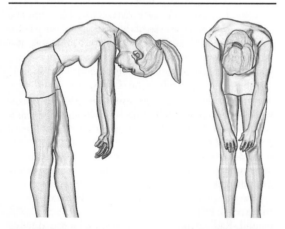

Figure 22–9. Forward-bending test: Examination of the spine for scoliosis is best carried out by observing for asymmetry and deformity as the patient bends forward. (Reproduced with permission from Rab GT: Pediatric orthopedic surgery. I In: Skinner HB (editor): *Current Diagnosis and Treatment in Orthopedics,* 2nd ed. New York, Lange Medical Books/McGraw-Hill, 2000.)

Table 22–4. Classification of Scoliosis

Idiopathic
 Infantile (0–3 years)
 Juvenile (4 years to puberty)
 Adolescent (puberty to epiphyseal closure)

Neuromuscular
 Cerebral palsy
 Myelomeningitis
 Spinal muscular atrophy
 Syringomyelia
 Friedreich ataxia
 Spinal cord tumor
 Spinal cord trauma

Myopathic
 Arthrogryposis
 Muscular dystrophy

Congenital
 Failures of formation (hemivertebrae)
 Failures of segmentation (unilateral unsegmented bar)
 Mixed

Mesenchymal
 Marfan syndrome
 Ehlers-Danlos syndrome

Other Causes
 Limb-length inequality
 Hysterical
 Metabolic
 Soft tissue contractures
 Osteochondrodystrophies

less and are associated with a normal neurologic exam. They are usually insidious in onset and have a typical curve pattern that usually involves the thoracolumbar region. Treatment decisions for idiopathic scoliosis are based on the risk for further curvature progression. The likelihood of progression increases with female sex, onset of curvature before menses, skeletal immaturity, and greater magnitude of curvature. An algorithm for the management of idiopathic scoliosis is given in Figure 22–11. Children with curvatures of <25° should be observed for further progression. Children with curvatures between 25 and 40° who are still growing warrant bracing. Most curvatures of >50°, regardless of skeletal maturity, will continue to progress slowly after growth is completed. These children therefore require surgery to prevent further progression and to restore structural balance to the spine

Congenital scoliosis is caused by the failure of formation or segmentation of the vertebrae during embryonic development. The resulting growth asymmetry, if severe, can cause curves of varying degrees which are often associated with a variety of other anomalies of the heart, kidneys, and other viscera. Anomalies of the spinal cord may also be present and must be investigated before any treatment is initiated. Management is guided by the expected growth imbalance of the spine over time based on the pattern of anomalies present. Treatment can involve either observation for small, nonprogressive curves or surgical stabilization for larger, progressive curves. Bracing is ineffective in controlling progression in congenital scoliosis.

A variety of neuromuscular problems are associated with scoliosis. This is especially true for children who are wheelchair-bound, have trunk weakness, and need support to sit. *Paralytic scoliosis* tends to be progressive and respond poorly to bracing. Treatment decisions must be individualized depending on the patient, the goals of treatment, the prognosis of the disease, and the impact of upright positioning on quality of life. Early surgical intervention facilitates maintenance of a sitting posture and minimizes potential risks associated with this patient population.

Kyphosis. Kyphosis is an exaggeration of the normal curvature of the thoracic spine in the saggital plane normal 20 to 50°). Two types of excessive kyphosis are seen in adolescents: *Scheuermann kyphosis* is a painful, progressive kyphosis that afflicts mainly teenage boys. Examination shows a sharp, well-demarcated kyphosis in the thoracic spine. Radiographs demonstrate a curvature of >50° with irregularity and anterior wedging of the involved vertebral endplates. Treatment is directed at pain control and prevention of progressive deformity. Bracing is often effective, however, surgical correction is indicated for curves exceeding 70° and those that continue to progress despite bracing. *Postural roundback* is an exaggerated kyphosis seen in adolescents due to poor posture. It can be differentiated from Scheuermann kyphosis by the flexible, gradual curvature and the absence of significant vertebral wedging or endplate irregularities on radiographs. Postural roundback resolves spontaneously and no treatment is necessary.

Back pain. In contrast to adults, back pain is unusual in children and should be thoroughly investigated. Potential etiologies are numerous ranging from simple muscular strain to serious local and systemic disorders. The reader is referred to Chap. 8, "Rheumatic Diseases," for a more detailed discussion of the assessment of the child with musculoskeletal complaints. A careful history and physical examination are mandatory, and spine radiographs should be obtained. For persistent symptoms, a bone scan and, in some instances, an MRI will be necessary in order to determine the etiology.

Spondylolysis is a defect in the lamina of the vertebrae in the pars interarticularis (usually in the lumbar spine) that is commonly seen in teenage gymnasts and football players and presents with activity-related lower back pain. It may occur as a congenital defect or be the result of repetitive trauma. Radiographic findings are subtle, but bone or computed tomography (CT) scans will usually detect the lesion. Initial treatment consists of activity modification.

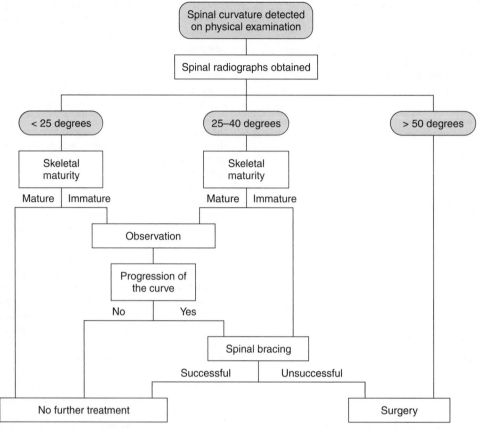

Figure 22–11. Algorithm for treatment of idiopathic scoliosis.

Bracing and surgical correction may be indicated for persistent symptoms. Spondylolysis also predisposes the teen to *spondylolisthesis,* a condition in which a superior vertebra slips forward on the adjacent inferior vertebra. Treatment with rest and analgesics may be effective initially. However, progressive spondylolisthesis usually requires surgical treatment.

KNEE PROBLEMS

A variety of conditions can cause chronic knee pain in the growing adolescent. Although most problems are self-limited and resolve at the completion of growth, each requires careful evaluation. Any knee pain associated with limping, swelling, or restriction of function should be evaluated radiographically. The clinician should bear in mind that the most common pitfall is to miss significant pathology of the hip that presents as referred pain to the knee. Acute knee injury is discussed in the section on sports medicine.

Peripatellar pain. Anterior peripatellar knee pain is common in children, especially adolescents. Overuse is a common etiology; patellar tendinitis, recurrent subluxation, and dislocation of the patella should also be considered. Radiographs, including patellar views, should be obtained but rarely confirm the diagnosis. Treatment is directed toward strengthening the quadriceps mechanism to restore proper patellar tracking and balance. Physical therapy often accelerates recovery.

Osgood-Schlatter disease. Osgood-Schlatter disease is a common cause of pain over the anterior knee and tibial tubercle in adolescent males and is discussed earlier (see section, "Osteochondroses").

Osteochondritis dissecans. Osteochondritis dissecans is a condition in which a small segment of subchondral bone becomes avascular. The etiology is uncertain, but trauma and endocrine problems have been suggested. Children often present with aching pain in the knee. The segment may become necrotic and then detached from the adjacent bone, producing catching or locking of the knee. Radiographs of the knee, especially a "tunnel or notch" view, are diagnostic. The lesion typically involves the lateral surface of the medial femoral condyle. In situ lesions are treated with rest and activity restriction, whereas detached fragments require surgical repair.

Popliteal cysts. Popliteal or Baker cysts frequently occur in the popliteal fossa under the medial head of the gastrocnemius muscle. They are an outpouching of the synovium of the capsule enclosing the knee joint. They are usually asymptomatic and their size frequently fluctuates. Spontaneous regression is to be expected. Indications for surgical excision include persistent pain, rapid change in size, uncertain diagnosis, and parental concern despite reassurance. The recurrence rate is 30% or greater after surgical excision.

MUSCULOSKELETAL TRAUMA

Musculoskeletal injuries in children account for 10 to 15% of all childhood injuries. The presence of open cartilaginous growth plates, greater elasticity of the bones, small size and blood volume, and the potential for growth disturbance are unique considerations in pediatric injuries and fractures. When evaluating a child with musculoskeletal injury, the possibility of nonaccidental trauma (NAT) should also always be kept in mind.

Fractures

PATHOPHYSIOLOGY: PEDIATRIC CONSIDERATIONS

Longitudinal growth of the axial skeleton occurs at the growth plate (physis) and is controlled by mechanical, local, and systemic factors. Physeal growth begins with the orderly multiplication of germinal cells on the epiphyseal side of the growth plate. These cells progress through a process of multiplication, hypertrophy, and vascular invasion, followed by ossification of physeal cartilage into metaphyseal bone. In this way the epiphysis "grows away" from the metaphysis resulting in limbs of symmetrical length and alignment.

Injuries involving the growth plate can interrupt this process and result in significant growth disturbance and angular deformity. The cartilaginous growth plate is vulnerable to injury because it is mechanically weaker than the surrounding bone and supporting ligaments. Fractures involving the growth plate may produce mechanical or vascular injury to the germinal cells of the physis. The Salter-Harris classification of growth-plate injuries correlates closely with the risk of subsequent growth disturbance (Figure 22–12). In type I injury, the fracture traverses the physis through the zone of hypertrophy and does not involve the germinal physeal fragment. Type II fractures involve the same zone of hypertrophy but also extend through a portion of the metaphysis. Type I and II injuries have a low incidence of subsequent growth disturbance and often can be managed with closed reduction and casting. Fractures of the distal femoral physis, however, are a major exception. Type III and IV injuries cross the germinal layer of the physis. Most of these injuries require surgical reduction and stabilization. Injury to this layer or an imperfect reduction can result in the formation of a bridge of bone across the physis, which functions as a tether to future growth. Angular deformity or limb-length inequality can result. Type V injury results from a crush injury to the germinal physeal cells; this diagnosis is made retrospectively. A common pitfall when treating pediatric injuries is to confuse a physeal separation with a "torn ligament," which is relatively rare in

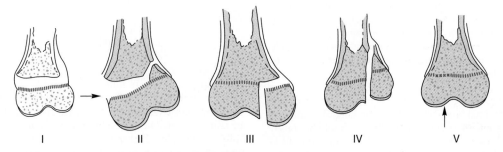

| I | II | III | IV | V |

Figure 22–12. The Salter-Harris classification of growth-plate injuries. Type I physeal fractures occur through the region of provisional calcification. The proliferating portion of the physis remains attached to the epiphysis and is not damaged. Type II fractures extend through a segment of the metaphysis. Again, the proliferative portions of the physis are intact. Type III fractures extend through a segment of the provisional calcification zone and then cross through the epiphysis to the articular surface. Type IV fractures extend obliquely from the metaphysis across the physis and into the epiphysis. They, too, are regular fractures. Type V fractures are crush injuries of all or a portion of the physis. The proliferative zones of the physis sustain irreversible damage. (Reproduced with permission from Salter RB, Harris WR: Injuries involving the epiphyseal plate. J Bone Joint Surg (Am) 1963;45:587.)

children. For example, an ankle injury in a skeletally immature patient is as likely to produce an injury to the distal fibular physis as is a simple ligamentous ankle sprain. A suspected physeal injury should be referred to an orthopedist.

Fractures in children, unlike their adult counterparts, have a considerable capacity to remodel with growth. This ability is dependent on the age of the child, the location of the fracture, the degree of deformity, and the proximity of the fracture to the growth plate. Growth and remodeling of long bone fractures will correct minor inaccuracies of alignment in many instances. Deformity in the plane of motion of a joint remodels readily. Angular deformity is slower to remodel, and rotational deformity has no capacity to correct with growth. The process of fracture healing also may produce stimulation of growth. Fracture healing begins with an inflammatory response facilitated by increased local blood flow. It is common to see 1 cm of "overgrowth" after healing of a femoral-shaft fracture. This must be accounted for at the time of treatment, or unequal limb lengths will result. Metaphyseal fractures of the medial aspect of the tibia can produce asymmetrical growth simulation, resulting in angular deformity (genu valgum). Most children's fractures heal rapidly with nonoperative care. Children tolerate prolonged immobilization physically and emotionally better than do adults.

EVALUATION

An algorithm for the management of a child with a fracture is presented in Fig. 22–13. The initial evaluation of a suspected fracture begins with a thorough physical examination. Deformity, point tenderness, pain on motion, neurocirculatory status, and skin integrity should be documented. History should be obtained as to the nature and circumstances of the injury. Any suspected fracture, regardless of how minor the trauma, must be assessed with radiographs in two planes. The joint above and below the suspected fracture should also be visualized. Comparison views of the opposite normal extremity may be helpful if the injury involves a growth plate. Splinting the extremity during the evaluation provides comfort and reassurance for the child.

Fractures seen in an urgent care setting often need splinting and transport to another facility for definitive care. Potential problems related to swelling, skin compromise, and neurovascular complications should be considered prior to transport. In general, fractures should be placed in a generously padded splint after the limb has been gently manipulated into a functional position. Any patient transported to another facility for definitive care should be given nothing by mouth until a decision can be made regarding the need for surgical reduction.

Children's fractures demand accurate description to facilitate communication between the primary care physician and the consulting physician. Fractures should be described by anatomic location, fracture pattern, align-

ment, and status of the surrounding soft tissues. Treatment of a given fracture must be individualized. The need for fracture reduction, splinting, and a plan for follow-up should be determined in conjunction with the consulting orthopedist.

COMMON FRACTURES IN CHILDREN

Forearm fractures. Forearm fractures are common in children and typically result from a fall on an outstretched arm. These fractures vary from a minimal buckle or torus fracture to an obviously displaced fracture of the radius and ulna that requires manipulation and reduction. These fractures may also involve the physis.

All suspected forearm fractures should be evaluated radiographically. When a fracture is present, a decision regarding reduction is made depending on the severity and degree of deformity. Torus fractures have little associated deformity and require only splinting or a below-elbow cast for protection; healing is rapid. Fractures with displacement, gross deformity, or angulation require manipulative reduction followed by splinting. A "sugar-tong" splint is preferred initially because it allows for swelling and provides sufficient ability to maintain fracture alignment. After swelling is reduced, a carefully molded cast is applied until radiographic union is achieved.

Elbow fractures. Elbow fractures are common in children and may be difficult to recognize. The ossification centers of the distal humeral epiphysis appear sequentially beginning at age 2 years and are all present by age 10. A large portion of the elbow is cartilaginous, making fractures difficult to visualize radiographically. Subtle physeal injuries are easily missed, resulting in adverse long-term outcomes. The normal development of the ossification centers of the elbow and their relation to each other are well established. An alteration in these normal relations or the presence of a joint effusion should lead to a strong suspicion that a fracture is present. Comparison views of the contralateral elbow, oblique views, and arthrography are often helpful adjuncts to making this diagnosis.

Treatment of elbow fractures in children must be individualized. Many of these fractures appear relatively benign radiographically yet are inherently unstable and require operative treatment. Good examples of this include supracondylar and lateral condylar fractures. The consequences of failure to recognize these injuries are angular deformity or non-union. Early referral and operative care, when appropriate, produce the best long-term outcome.

Femur fractures. Fractures of the femur are frequently the result of high-energy trauma and may be associated with major multisystem injury. In infants younger than 12 months, these injuries have a high association with nonaccidental trauma (NAT). These fractures are best treated by rapid stabilization to facilitate mobilization of the child to a center where both orthopedic and associated injuries can be managed concurrently. A variety of

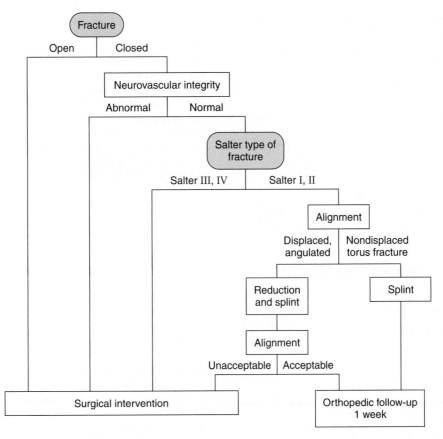

Figure 22–13. Algorithm for fracture care.

methods are used to treat these injuries, including immediate hip casting, prolonged skeletal traction, external fixation, and internal fixation. Treatment decisions are individualized on the basis of the age of the patient, associated injuries, and other factors.

Fractures of the femoral neck and proximal femur are surgical emergencies. They are often unstable and threaten the blood supply to the proximal femoral epiphysis. This problem can be minimized by early operative stabilization of the hip. Casting is successful in only a small percentage of stable fractures in this region.

Fractures of the distal femur often involve the distal femoral epiphysis. These injuries are easily mistaken for "knee sprains." Stress views of the distal femoral epiphysis readily distinguish these injuries. The distal femoral epiphysis tolerates injury poorly, with the incidence of subsequent growth disturbance as high as 30%. Most physeal injuries of the distal femur require anatomic reduction and pinning.

Tibia fractures. Fractures of the tibia are relatively common in children and can occur with seemingly minimal trauma. One common example is the so-called toddler's fracture, an oblique minimally displaced fracture of the tibial shaft without an associated fibular fracture. This injury usually results from a minor fall with a twisting component, followed by refusal to walk. The oblique nature of the fracture often makes it difficult to visualize on initial radiographs. Most of these injuries are stable, requiring only cast immobilization.

Fractures of the distal epiphysis of the tibia and fibula should be considered when evaluating any ankle injury. Until skeletal maturity, the yield strength of the physis is lower than that of the surrounding ligaments. Therefore, ankle sprains are easily confused with these fractures by physical examination but can be readily distinguished radiographically.

Compartment Syndrome

The development of compartment syndrome after an injury to an extremity can have serious consequences. Compartment syndrome develops when there is bleeding into a closed fascial space, producing progressive swelling and an increase in intracompartmental pressure. As the pressure increases, venous blood flow is impaired, followed by ischemia, which, if prolonged, will result in cell death of the surrounding muscle and nerves.

Compartment syndrome is characterized by the "five Ps": pain, pallor, paresthesia, pulselessness, and paralysis. The earliest sign of compartment syndrome is pain. A child with a splinted fracture should be comfortable with minimal analgesia. If not, compartment syndrome should be suspected. The remaining Ps are late findings. Compartment syndrome is confirmed by direct measurement of compartment pressures. If compartment syndrome is found, it is treated by immediate surgical fasciotomy. Without treatment, irreversible damage to the compartment structures occurs within 6 h after onset.

Child Abuse and Nonaccidental Trauma

Nonaccidental trauma (NAT), or battered child syndrome, must be recognized and reported by primary care physicians treating pediatric injuries. The diagnosis of NAT is rarely straightforward (see Chap. 10, "Injuries and Emergencies"). About 75% of abused children are younger than 3 years of age. The consequences of failure to diagnose NAT are significant, with a 35% risk of repeat injury and up to a 10% risk of death.

Child abuse covers a broad spectrum, from emotional neglect to physical injury. Several patterns of fracture strongly suggest the diagnosis of NAT and should prompt further investigation (Table 22–5). Fractures highly suggestive of NAT include multiple fractures in differing stages of radiographic healing, metaphyseal corner fractures, spinous process fractures, posterior rib fractures, complex skull fractures, and epiphyseal separations. Spiral fractures involving the femoral diaphysis in a child younger than 12 months should also prompt suspicion of NAT. Physical findings must always be correlated with the history of the injury. No single historical feature or behavior is consistently present in NAT. Abusive parents rarely offer accurate information. Stepparents or boyfriends are frequently implicated in documented cases. If the history is inconsistent with the physical findings, it is best to ensure the safety of the child and initiate further investigation into the circumstances of the injury.

PEDIATRIC SPORTS MEDICINE

Organized sports for children are increasing in the United States. The potential physical, psychological, and social benefits of participation in such programs are many. However, negative consequences can also occur. Both children and their parents are often driven by the many tangible rewards for exceptional performance. This has resulted in a major increase in injuries associated with organized sports. These can be divided into two groups and are addressed below. The reader is referred to Chap. 2, "Adolescence," for a discussion of relevant developmental issues and the adolescent pre-participation sports evaluation.

Overuse Syndromes

Overuse syndromes result from placing a highly repetitive stress on a given structure until injury occurs. This can produce several patterns of injury that are unique to the growing skeleton.

Shin Pain

Shin pain is a nonspecific symptom complex characterized by pain along the anterior aspect of the leg with activity. Persistent shin pain requires investigation to identify an underlying etiology. The differential diagnosis includes stress fractures, shin splints, periostitis, nerve entrapment, muscle strain, infection, tumors, and exercise-induced compartment syndrome.

Repetitive application of a load to a bone can produce a *stress fracture*. This usually presents with the gradual onset of activity-related pain. The tibia and metatarsals are the sites most common affected. Initial radiographs may be normal, whereas a bone scan will demonstrate early increased uptake. These findings must be interpreted carefully, because stress fractures can easily imitate infection, osteoid osteomas (an inflammatory lesion of bone), and malignant neoplasms. Treatment is directed at avoidance of the offending activity. Casting or bone grafting may be necessary if spontaneous healing fails.

Table 22–5. Fracture Patterns Suggesting Child Abuse

High specificity
  Metaphyseal lesions
  Posterior rib fractures
  Scapular fractures
  Spinous process fractures
  Sternal fractures

Moderate specificity
  Multiple fractures, bilateral
  Fractures of different ages
  Epiphyseal separations
  Vertebral body fractures
  Digital fractures
  Complex skull fractures

Common but low specificity
  Clavicular fractures
  Long bone fractures

Reproduced with permission from Kleinman PK (editor): *Diagnostic Imaging of Child Abuse.* Williams & Wilkins, 1987.

THROWING SYNDROMES

Most throwing syndromes result from repetitive valgus stress at the elbow. *Osteochondrosis of the capitellum*, or so-called *little league elbow,* is commonly seen in baseball pitchers and gymnasts. Patients complain of pain, grinding, and reduced range of motion of the elbow. Radiographs show fragmentation of the capitellum with or without a loose body. Treatment involves activity modification or avoidance, strengthening, and surgery if a loose body is present.

Other throwing syndromes seen less frequently include epiphysiolysis (slipping of the humeral epiphysis through the physis) of the proximal humerus, osteochondritis of the radial head, and stress injury or fracture to the medial epicondyle.

Sports Trauma

Ligamentous injuries and fractures of the ankle, knee, and shoulder often occur in association with participation in organized sports. Each injury requires careful evaluation to avoid confusing "simple" sprains with more complex physeal injuries or osteochondral fractures. Major swelling, hemarthrosis, or inability to bear weight should prompt x-ray evaluation.

ANKLE SPRAINS

Ankle sprains are a common sports injury. The usual mechanism is inversion of the ankle, producing varying degree of disruption to the lateral stabilizing ligaments or the anterior ankle capsule. Treatment is based on the severity of the injury and follows the basic principles of *r*est, *I*ce, *c*ompression, and *e*levation ("RICE"). For most sprains, rehabilitation exercises, taping, or a compressive ankle brace are adequate. More severe injuries may require casting or, rarely, surgical reconstruction of the ligaments. The reader is referred to the sports medicine section of Chap. 2, "Adolescence," for a more in depth discussion of the phases of rehabilitation for minor musculoskeletal sprains and strains.

ACUTE KNEE INJURIES

Acute knee injuries, especially those associated with hemarthrosis or inability to walk, require careful assessment. In the younger child, ligamentous injury is decidedly rare, with avulsions of bone at ligamentous insertions, osteochondral fractures, or physeal injury more common. In the adolescent, pure ligamentous disruption is similar to the adult pattern of injury. A clinical history of a forceful twisting injury to the knee, associated with a "pop," pain, and rapid onset of swelling, suggests a major injury. Examination of the knee after acute injury is often compromised by pain and swelling. Radiographs, includ-

ing standard, oblique, and stress views, are helpful. In some instances, examination under anesthesia may be necessary.

Treatment is age- and diagnosis-specific. Many problems, such as acute patellar dislocation, anterior cruciate ligament tears, and collateral ligament injuries, are initially managed with bracing and an aggressive rehabilitation program. In children, ligamentous reconstruction is delayed until skeletal maturity.

ACUTE SHOULDER DISLOCATION

Dislocation of the shoulder is rare in children but may occur in adolescence. The most common mechanism is that of forced abduction and external rotation of the shoulder producing an anterior dislocation. Immediate reduction under sedation is recommended. The incidence of chronic instability and recurrence is higher when the initial dislocation occurs before 20 years of age.

REFERENCES

American Academy of Pediatrics, Committee on Quality Improvement, Subcommittee on Developmental Dysplasia of the Hip: Clinical Practice Guideline: Early detection of developmental dysplasia of the hip. Pediatrics 2000;105:896.

Brooks WC, Gross RH: Genu varum in children: Diagnosis and treatment. J Am Acad Orthop Surg 1995;3:326.

Dietz FR: Intoeing–Fact, fiction, and opinion. Am Fam Physician 1994;50:1249.

Engle MG, Staheli LT: The natural history of the angle of gait, tibial torsion, knee angle, hip rotation, and development of the arch in normal children. Clin Orthop 1974;99:12.

Hensinger RN: Congenital dislocation of the hip. Treatment from infancy to walking age. Orthop Clin North Am 1987;18:597.

Huurman WW, Ginsburg GM: Musculoskeletal injury in children. Pediatr Clin North Am 1997;18:429.

Kling TF: Angular deformities of the lower limbs in children. Orthop Clin North Am 1987;18:513.

Marsh JS: Screening for scoliosis. Pediatr Rev 1993;14:297.

Rivara FP, Parish RA, Mueller BA: Extremity injuries in children: predictive value of clinical findings. Pediatrics 1986;78:803.

Robin NH: Congenital muscular torticollis. Pediatr Rev 1996;17:374.

Salenius P, Vankka E: The development of the tibiofemoral angle in children. J Bone Joint Surg [Am] 1975;57A:259.

Saperstein AL, Nicholas SJ: Pediatric and adolescent sports medicine. Pediatr Clin North Am 1996;43:1013.

Staheli LT: Torsional deformity. Pediatr Clin North Am 1986; 33:1373.

Staheli LT, et al: Lower extremity rotational problems in children: normal values to guide management. J Bone Joint Surg [Am] 1985;67A:39.

Wenger DR, et al: Corrective shoes and inserts as treatment for flexible flatfoot in infants and children. J Bone Joint Surg [Am] 71A:800, 1989.

Ethical Issues in Pediatrics

Bernard Lo, MD, & Ann Alpers, JD

Pediatricians and medical students commonly confront ethical issues in their clinical work. Some cases can present dramatic dilemmas, such as whether to discontinue mechanical ventilation on a 400 gm, 22 week infant with respiratory failure and intracerebral hemorrhage. More commonly, ethical issues are subtler, such as nagging doubts as to whether to tell a child a grave diagnosis or whether to tell parents that an adolescent has sought care for a sexually transmitted disease.

This chapter will suggest how to approach common ethical problems and analyze the reasons for and against conflicting courses of action. First, two fundamental questions will be addressed: What standards should be used in making decisions about the health care of children? Who should make medical decisions for children? Subsequently, life-sustaining interventions, the relationship of the pediatrician to parents and children, conflicts of interest, clinical research, and the role of the pediatrician and medical student will be discussed.

WHAT STANDARDS SHOULD BE USED IN MAKING DECISIONS?

Although the best interest of the child is the fundamental ethical guideline in pediatrics, other considerations may need to be taken into account.

The Best Interests of the Child

The expected benefits of a medical intervention should outweigh the possible harms. The "best interests" of the child are often vague and difficult to interpret. People may disagree over which factors comprise a child's best interests, which outcomes are desirable, and how to weigh the benefits and burdens of interventions. Promoting some of the child's interests may set back other interests of the child.

A child's best interests include both the duration and quality of life. For example, in deciding about chemotherapy for cancer, parents naturally consider not only the projected survival but also the likely side-effects of treatment and the expected level of functioning. But while quality-of-life judgments seem unavoidable, they may be ethically problematic. It is difficult to predict the future quality of life of a child. Healthy people tend to underestimate the quality of life of persons with chronic illness.

Quality of life should not be confounded with burdens to third parties or the costs to society. Despite these shortcomings, the concept of "best interests" is important because children deserve respect as individuals separate from their parents, with their own interests and rights.

The Preferences of the Child

To the extent that children have the capacity to make informed decisions about their medical care, their self-determination and their choices should be respected. When children are not capable of giving informed consent, their assent to interventions is still ethically important. It is disturbing to force interventions on children who are actively resisting them. Children's objections are not necessarily decisive; for instance, children who object to shots should still receive immunizations. But children's lack of assent should take on more weight as they are more capable of making informed decisions and as the medical indications for the intervention are less compelling.

Assessment of Futility

Some parents may insist on interventions that physicians regard as futile, in the strict sense that it has no pathophysiologic rationale, that it has already failed in the patient, or that cardiac arrest occurs despite maximal treatment. Physicians have no ethical obligation to provide such futile interventions, and parents are not entitled to demand such care.

In some cases, physicians use the term futile in a looser sense when they believe that the parents' goals for care are not worth pursuing, the likelihood of success is small, the child's quality of life is unacceptable, or the costs are prohibitive. In these circumstances, unilateral decisions by physicians to withhold interventions could be arbitrary and inconsistent. They are inappropriate unless authorized by society.

The Interests of Parents and Family Members

Parents and other family members have interests that must be considered. The time and expense of caring for a sick child may compromise the rearing of other children or jeopardize the family home or business. While parents and families should be expected to make some sacrifices, they cannot be expected to devote their entire lives to a sick child. Pediatricians should help provide parents with emotional and social support, so that they do not feel overwhelmed by the burdens of care.

Prevention of Harm to Others

Society has an interest in maintaining the public health and preventing the spread of infectious disease. For example, public health officials have the legal power to compel vaccination.

Just Allocation of Resources

Physicians should allocate limited health care resources in a fair manner. Pediatricians whose patients lack prenatal care and immunizations may be outraged when large amounts of money are spent on intensive care of neonates with a small likelihood of survival. The allocation of resources on a public policy level needs to be distinguished from rationing decisions at the bedside or in the office. Doctors can advocate for health insurance for all children and for more equitable allocation of resources. However, pediatricians should not limit beneficial care for one child to try to save money for other health care priorities, unless society or the parents have authorized them to do so. Attempts at bedside rationing are usually ineffective gestures because money saved on one patient cannot be redirected to more worthwhile social goals. In exceptional situations, however, providing scarce resources, such as a bed in the intensive care unit or extracorporeal membrane oxygenation, to one child would deny care to another child who would obtain much greater medical benefit. In such situations, it is appropriate to limit the care of the former child.

WHO SHOULD MAKE MEDICAL DECISIONS FOR CHILDREN?

Children generally cannot make informed decisions about their medical care or protect themselves from harm. Hence adults must make decisions for them and look after their welfare.

Presumption of Parental Decision-Making

Parents are presumed to be the appropriate decision-makers for children because in most cases love motivates them to act in the best interests of their children— United States culture prizes parental responsibility, the integrity of the family, and strong parent–child relationships. Society therefore grants parents considerable power and discretion to raise children according to their own values. The parents' view of what is best for their children usually should be respected. In most cases, parents give pediatricians permission to carry out recommended care. Parents are permitted to decline interventions when they believe the burdens outweigh the benefits.

EXCEPTIONS TO PARENTAL DECISION-MAKING

In some cases, the presumption of parental decision-making may be invalid. Some parents may be estranged from their children or unwilling to be involved in decisions about their care. Other parents lack the capacity to make informed decisions. For instance, they may be severely impaired by alcohol or substance abuse, developmental disability, or immaturity. Strictly speaking, parents should make decisions for children unless a court has appointed someone else as guardian. The courts, however, may be too slow in appointing guardians for medical decisions to be made in a timely manner. In practice, physicians often make informal arrangements for another relative to make decisions when parents are absent or incapable of making decisions.

In exceptional situations, the parents' assessment of their children's best interests may be overridden. For example, as discussed later, parents are not permitted to refuse highly effective life-saving therapy that has few side effects, such as antibiotics for bacterial meningitis in a previously healthy child.

EMERGENCIES

In emergencies, when a parent or guardian is not available, and delay in treatment would jeopardize the child's life or health, the physician should provide appropriate treatment without parental permission. The rationale is that it would violate the child's best interests to delay treatment until approval is obtained.

Adolescent Patients

As children mature, they develop the capacity to make informed decisions about their health care. By statute, adolescents over 18 years of age can give informed consent or refusal for medical care, without parental involvement. The law may also allow younger minors to make their own decisions about health care. Because statutes vary from state to state, pediatricians need to be familiar with the laws in their jurisdiction.

MATURE MINORS

Mature minors are those capable of giving informed consent. Ethically speaking, mature minors should be allowed to consent to or refuse medical treatment, just as would adults. Pediatricians need to assess an adolescent's capacity to give informed consent and to help him or her obtain appropriate support from parents or other adults. Physicians need to ask directly about the adolescent's understanding of the proposed intervention, the alternatives, the risks and benefits of each, and the likely consequences.

Generally, adolescents over 14 or 15 years of age can be shown to have such decision-making capacity, whereas younger children often have difficulty entertaining different alternatives, appreciating the consequences of decisions, and appraising their future realistically.

EMANCIPATED MINORS

Adolescents who are living apart from parents and managing their own finances, are married, have children, or have served in the armed forces are termed emancipated minors Most states regard them as de facto adults, capable of consenting to their own medical care. Some states require a judicial hearing and declaration of emancipation

TREATMENT OF SPECIFIED CONDITIONS

Most states allow minors to consent to treatment for sensitive conditions, such as sexually transmitted diseases, contraception, pregnancy, substance abuse, and psychiatric illness, without parental consent. Requiring parental permission would deter many adolescents from seeking treatment for important public health problems.

PARENTAL REQUESTS FOR TREATMENT

Parents may request that the physician test an adolescent for illicit drug use or pregnancy, without telling the child. While such requests are generally motivated by concern, surreptitious testing is unacceptable because it undermines the child's trust in the physician and compromises future care.

Institutional Ethics Committees

Interdisciplinary institutional ethics committees can provide a supportive forum to discuss difficult ethical issues, allow health care workers and parents to better understand each other's views, and suggest ways to resolve disagreements. These committees should serve an advisory role and do not relieve pediatricians of their responsibility for decisions.

The Courts

Courts have the power to intervene in health care decisions to protect the well-being of vulnerable children. Physicians may need to initiate legal proceedings to override parental decisions that severely violate the best interests of the child. This should be a last resort, because the adversarial legal process may polarize parents and health care workers, complicating subsequent care.

PEDIATRICIAN'S ROLE IN DECISION-MAKING

When ethical issues are complex, reasonable, well-meaning people may disagree. Pediatricians and medical students can play a key role in assuring that difficult decisions are made as wisely as possible.

Promote informed decision-making by parents and children. In addition to informing parents and older children of pertinent medical information, physicians help families deliberate by eliciting their concerns and questions, pointing out overlooked considerations, and recommending what they believe is best for the child. Whenever possible, one pediatrician should have primary, ongoing responsibility for care.

Act as the children's advocate. Pediatricians can remind everyone that the goal is to do what is best for the child. They need to try to persuade parents to accept highly effective interventions that have few side effects. In addition, physicians, together with social workers and nurses, can often mobilize emotional support and social resources.

Override parents only as a last resort. Pediatricians are understandably distressed when a child's care at home is suboptimal. They may consider asking the courts to remove the child from parental custody on the basis of neglect. Yet lifestyles that physicians may find objectionable, such as alcohol abuse or an untidy home, do not in themselves constitute neglect. While judicial intervention may be useful for limited interventions such as a single blood transfusion, it is usually impractical in chronic illness requiring ongoing care. Even if a child with asthma or diabetes is not receiving medications, disrupting the parent–child bond causes emotional distress for the child. Foster placement or institutionalization may be worse for the child than would be the attempts of well-meaning parents to cope with difficult circumstances. Generally, the best response is for pediatricians to try to mobilize more support and resources, so that the parents can provide better care.

DECISIONS ABOUT LIFE-SUSTAINING INTERVENTIONS

Dilemmas may occur when parents refuse life-sustaining interventions.

Refusal of Medical Interventions

Parents may refuse interventions that have limited effectiveness, impose significant side effects, are controversial, or require chronic treatment. In such situations, the parents' informed refusals should ordinarily be decisive. Pediatricians need to keep in mind the importance of parental discretion, family integrity, and ongoing care by parents.

Refusal of such life-sustaining interventions may be ethically appropriate even if the patient's life may be shortened.

EXTRAORDINARY AND ORDINARY CARE

The commonly used terms heroic, extraordinary, and ordinary, while intuitively plausible, are confusing and should be abandoned. Interventions such as mechanical ventilation are sometimes categorized as extraordinary because they are invasive, expensive, and highly technological. However, the crucial ethical issue is not whether a medical technology can be labeled as inherently heroic or ordinary, but how the benefits of the intervention compare to the burdens. Any medical intervention may be withheld if the burdens outweigh the benefits for a particular patient.

WITHHOLDING VERSUS WITHDRAWING INTERVENTIONS

Ethically and legally there is no difference between withdrawing interventions and withholding them, although there may be a great emotional difference. For example, many physicians or nurses are reluctant to stop mechanical ventilation in a child with severe cystic fibrosis, even though they would not have started it if they had known the child could not be weaned. This distinction, however, is not tenable. The reasons that justify not starting the intervention—refusal by parents or a mature child in the face of a poor prognosis—would also justify withdrawing the ventilator. Indeed the reasons to withdraw an intervention often are stronger because the prognosis is clearer after a trial of ventilatory support. Furthermore, if stopping the ventilator were not permitted, parents and pediatricians might forego at the onset a trial of intensive care, which would offer a chance that antibiotics would enable the child to survive.

"DO NOT RESUSCITATE" ORDERS

When a child is found to be in cardiopulmonary arrest, cardiopulmonary resuscitation (CPR) needs to be started immediately to have any prospect of success. Therefore, CPR is attempted unless a "do not resuscitate" (DNR) order has been written. Pediatricians caring for children with terminal or chronic illness need to raise the issue of DNR orders with parents or mature minors. The DNR orders would be appropriate if the parents or an informed, competent adolescent would refuse CPR or if the child would not survive the hospitalization even if CPR were administered.

The DNR orders should be written in the medical record, together with a progress note explaining the decision and plans for further care. "Slow" or shadow codes, in which CPR is perfunctorily administered in a manner known to be ineffective, are unethical because they deceive families into believing that maximal care is being provided. A DNR order means only that CPR will not be administered and does not preclude other interventions.

Everyone needs to understand that DNR does not mean withdrawal of all care or abandonment of the patient.

RELIEF OF DISTRESS

After a decision is made to withhold or withdraw life-sustaining interventions from children with terminal illness, pediatricians should provide adequate relief of distressful symptoms such as pain or shortness of breath. No predetermined ceiling on the dose of narcotics or sedatives should be set. If lower doses have not adequately controlled symptoms, the dosage should be increased to the level necessary to achieve this goal. In rare cases, the dose that provides adequate relief of distress may also depress respiration or even shorten life. In these circumstances, the appropriate goal of care is to relieve distress, not to try to prolong life.

THE DECISION-MAKING PROCESS

Decisions to withhold or withdraw interventions should be discussed with all health care workers caring for the patient, including house staff, students, nurses, and social workers. This allows them to understand the rationale for the decision; to voice their questions, concerns, and objections; and to make suggestions. This reasoning should also be clearly presented in the medical record.

Handicapped Infants

The federal "Baby Doe Regulations" apply to decisions to withhold medical treatment from disabled infants less than 1 year old. Their intent is to ensure interventions such as surgery for duodenal atresia or tracheal-esophageal fistula in infants with Down's syndrome.

The surgery would cure swallowing problems and allow the children to lead lives that they and their families generally find meaningful. Under the Baby Doe Regulations, treatment other than "appropriate nutrition, hydration, or medication" need not be provided in several situations: (1) when an infant is irreversibly comatose; (2) when treatment would merely prolong dying; (3) when treatment would not be effective in ameliorating or correcting all life-threatening conditions; (4) when treatment would be futile in terms of survival; or (5) when treatment would be virtually futile and would be inhumane under such circumstances. The implication is that medically appropriate nutrition, hydration, or medication must be provided in all cases. The pediatrician's reasonable medical judgment presumably determines what is medically appropriate. Physicians are not required to provide treatment that in their judgment is inappropriate. Decisions to withhold medically indicated treatment may not be based on "subjective opinions" about the child's future quality of life.

The Baby Doe Regulations have been sharply criticized. Many terms, such as *appropriate* and *futile*, are subject to conflicting interpretations. Parents are not mentioned in the decision-making process, despite their customary role as surrogates. Commentators point out that the regulations often are not literally followed, or strictly enforced.

Refusal of Effective Life-Saving Therapy with Few Side Effects

Parents sometimes refuse treatments that cure life-threatening conditions with few medical side effects. For example, Jehovah's Witnesses refuse blood transfusions for children who suffer acute trauma. Parents who are Christian Scientists often refuse antibiotics even for curable life-threatening infections such as bacterial meningitis. Physicians who are unable to persuade parents to accept such interventions should seek a court order to administer the treatment. As one court declared, while "parents may be free to become martyrs themselves, they are not free to make martyrs of their children."

RELATIONSHIP OF THE PEDIATRICIAN TO THE CHILD AND PARENTS

Physicians have ethical responsibilities concerning the disclosure of information, confidentiality, and truthtelling. These actions are important because they show respect for the child, lead to beneficial consequences, foster trust in the medical profession, and facilitate future care.

Disclosure of Information

In order for parents to make informed decisions, pediatricians must inform them of their children's prognosis, the alternatives for care, and the benefits, risks, and likely consequences of each alternative. Furthermore, to obtain assent from children, pediatricians need to inform children of their condition and the plan of care, in terms children can comprehend. Even when children cannot understand medical details, they still want to know what will be done to them.

Some parents do not want their children to know about a serious diagnoses, such as cancer. Pediatricians should elicit the parents' concerns and fears. Parents may believe that children will not be able to handle bad news or that peers will reject them. Physicians can explain how it can be beneficial for children to understand their diagnosis and the proposed therapy. Children may already suspect that something is seriously wrong and may cope better if they can discuss the situation with adults and receive support. Adherence to medical regimens may be enhanced if the children understand the rationale. Generally, physicians can persuade parents to disclose information to their children and help the family cope with the bad news.

Parental requests for secrecy are particularly difficult when adolescents are capable of making health care decisions. Pediatricians should ask adolescents whether they want to know what is wrong with them.

Physicians should never promise parents that their children will not learn the diagnosis. Other members of the health care team may disclose it. In addition, pediatricians should not deceive children who ask directly about their condition.

Confidentiality

Medical information should be kept confidential because the privacy of children and their parents deserves respect. Moreover, they would be less willing to seek care if sensitive information were disseminated inappropriately. However, confidentiality is not absolute, and it may be overridden when disclosure has been authorized by parents or adolescents, when the statutes or courts require it, and when it is necessary to protect the public health or prevent harm to identified third parties. Indeed, many adolescents expect confidentiality to be breached if serious harm can be averted. Whenever information is disclosed, physicians should disclose only information that is truly needed. For example, a school needs only to know that a child's absence was medically indicated, not the specific diagnosis.

CHILD ABUSE AND NEGLECT

Physicians and other health care workers are obligated by law to inform child protective services agencies about cases of suspected child abuse or neglect. Definitive proof of abuse and neglect is not required. The privacy of the parents is overridden in order to protect vulnerable children from the possibility of serious harm.

Intervention may enable parents to obtain enough assistance and support to prevent further abuse. In extreme cases, children may be removed from parental custody.

ADOLESCENTS' REQUESTS FOR CONFIDENTIALITY

Adolescents may wish to keep certain information confidential from their parents. For instance, they may not want parents to know that they are receiving care for psychiatric conditions, sexually transmitted diseases, pregnancy, or substance abuse. State laws generally protect confidentiality in such situations. Doctors should routinely offer adolescents an opportunity to talk privately, apart from their parents. Pediatricians usually should encourage adolescents to discuss medical decisions with their parents, who customarily can provide support and advice. Doctors can also help adolescents disclose information to their parents. In some situations, however, such disclosure may be counterproductive or even dangerous to adolescents, as when abuse has occurred.

Parental notification for abortion is particularly controversial. A number of states require minors who seek abortions to either have parental permission or to obtain a judicial waiver.

Truth-Telling

Some parents may ask physicians to misrepresent their children's diagnoses, for example, to excuse their child from school requirements or to obtain insurance coverage. Pediatricians understandably believe that children should receive needed care. Nonetheless, deception undermines trust in physicians. If physicians are willing to use deception to benefit patients, they might also deceive in other circumstances that could harm patients.

CONFLICTS OF INTEREST

As professionals, pediatricians and medical students should act for the best interests of their patients even if their own self-interest may be compromised. Conflicts of interest occur when advancing the interests of children would harm the self-interest of the physician or the interests of third parties, such as hospitals or insurers.

Financial Conflicts of Interest

Conflicts of interest may occur under any reimbursement system. Fee-for-service reimbursement and physician investment in health care facilities to which they refer patients create incentives for physicians to order services of little or no clinical utility. In contrast, prospective payment and capitated reimbursement offer physicians incentives to withhold expensive interventions that may benefit patients. Regardless of the reimbursement system, pediatricians should recommend tests and treatments that are likely to provide clinically meaningful benefit.

Medical Training and the Care of Children and Youth

Medical students and house officers need to assume clinical responsibility and to learn invasive procedures in order to benefit future patients. This need to learn may sometimes conflict with the needs of current patients. The attending pediatrician and trainee need to inform parents or children of the roles of members of the medical team and the identity of those performing procedures. Requests to exclude trainees from the case or from procedures should be honored whenever possible. Trainees should be adequately supervised and be willing to ask for help if they encounter difficulties during a procedure.

Responses to Mistakes

Many physicians and medical students feel uncomfortable calling attention to mistakes because their reputations and careers may suffer. Pediatricians may also be reluctant to tell parents or patients about mistakes, even those that clearly caused serious harm. They may fear that the family will worry needlessly, get angry, or sue. Yet there are cogent reasons to disclose mistakes. Families and patients often benefit from knowing what happened and what is being done to mitigate the mistake, particularly if changes in care are necessary. In teaching hospitals, discussing mistakes candidly in rounds and conferences enables others to learn from them.

Impaired or Incompetent Colleagues

Physicians and medical students may observe that a colleague is impaired, for example, because of alcohol abuse or depression. Physicians may be reluctant to report the problem to appropriate authorities, fearing that colleagues will regard them as snitches, or that the other physician will retaliate. Students and residents may be particularly reluctant to raise such issues because they fear their grades and recommendations will suffer. In such situations, the ethical ideal is clear: The well-being of patients should be paramount. Patients may be gravely harmed if an impaired or incompetent physician is allowed to continue to practice. Trainees can usually find ways to raise their concerns in a constructive manner; for example, by asking the chief resident to review the case.

RESEARCH ON CHILDREN

Traditionally, society has sought to protect children from the potential harms of clinical research. Because children cannot give their own consent, their participation in research has been limited. But clinical research is essential for improving pediatric care. The scientific basis for pediatric practice is compromised if therapies are not adequately tested in children. Increasingly, the public views research, not as exploitation of vulnerable children, but rather as access to promising new therapies for such grave conditions as HIV infection, cystic fibrosis, and cancer.

According to federal guidelines, several categories of pediatric research may be permitted: (1) research that presents no greater than minimal risk to children; (2) research that offers the prospect of direct benefit for participants, provided that the benefit: risk ratio is acceptable; and (3) research that is likely to yield vitally important knowledge about the subject's disorder or condition, provided that the risk is only slightly more than minimal. Parents or guardians must give their permission for their children to participate in the research. In addition, children must assent to the study if they are capable of doing so.

SUMMARY

In summary, when physicians respond to ethical dilemmas, it is not enough simply to be a good person or to follow one's personal beliefs. Pediatricians also need to formulate justifications for their plans, in order to persuade others of their approach. Ethical guidelines help assure that decisions in similar cases are consistent and fair. Yet guidelines cannot be applied by rote in difficult cases. Part of the art of clinical medicine is to act with discretion, compassion, and respect for the individual child and family.

REFERENCES

American Academy of Pediatrics Committee on Bioethics: informed consent, parental permission, and assent in pediatric practice. Pediatrics 1995;95:314.

Council of Ethical and Judicial Affairs of the American Medical Association: Mandatory parental consent to abortion. JAMA 1993; 269:82.

Fleischman AR, Nolan K, Dubler NN, et al: Caring for gravely ill children. Pediatrics 1994;94:433.

Holder AR: Minors' rights to consent to medical care. JAMA 1987; 257:3400.

Lo B: *Resolving Ethical Guidelines in Clinical Practice: A Guide for Clinicians,* 2d ed. Philadelphia, PA: Lippincott, 2000.

Society for Adolescent Medicine: Confidential health care for adolescents: position paper of the Society for Adolescent Medicine. J Adolesc Health 1997;21:408.

Traugott I, Alpers A: In their own hands: Adolescents' refusals of life-sustaining treatment. Arch Peds Adol Med 1997; 151:922.

Index

Page numbers followed by *i* or *t* indicate illustrations or tables.